PHTLS

Prehospital Trauma Life Support

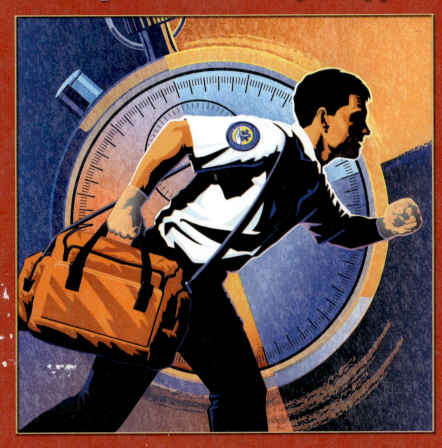

"The fate of the wounded rests in the hands of the one who applies the first dressing."

—Nicholas Senn, MD (1844–1908)
American Surgeon (Chicago, Illinois)
Founder, Association of Military Surgeons
of the United States

Seventh Edition

PHTLS

Prehospital Trauma Life Support

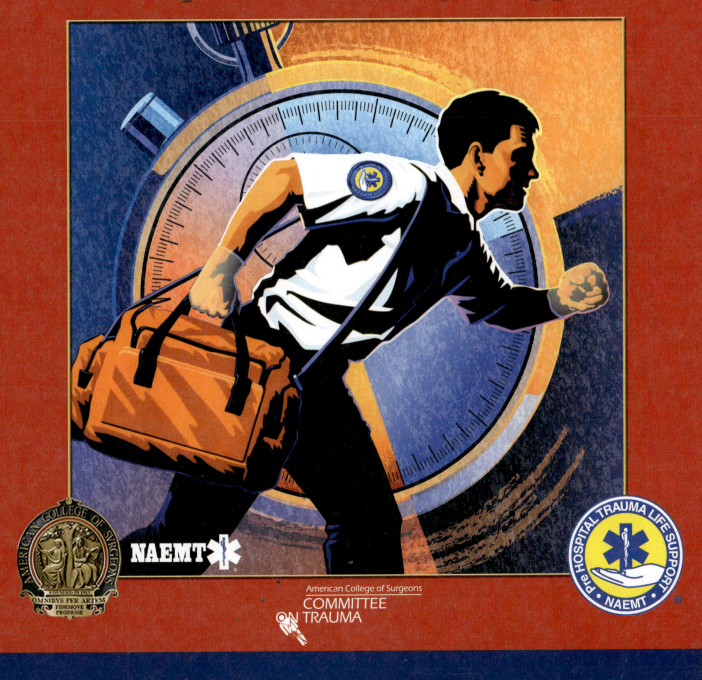

American College of Surgeons
COMMITTEE ON TRAUMA

ELSEVIER
MOSBY JEMS

Prehospital Trauma Life Support Committee of The National Association of Emergency Medical Technicians in Cooperation with The Committee on Trauma of The American College of Surgeons

MOSBY JEMS
ELSEVIER

3251 Riverport Lane
St. Louis, MO 63043

PHTLS PREHOSPITAL TRAUMA LIFE SUPPORT,   ISBN-13: 978-0-323-06502-3
SEVENTH EDITION   ISBN-10: 0-323-06502-3

Some material was previously published.

Notice

Knowledge and best practice in this field are constantly changing. As new research and experience broaden our knowledge, changes in practice, treatment, and drug therapy may become necessary or appropriate. Readers are advised to check the most current information provided (1) on procedures featured or (2) by the manufacturer of each product to be administered, to verify the recommended dose or formula, the method and duration of administration, and contraindications. It is the responsibility of the practitioner, relying on their own experience and knowledge of the patient, to make diagnoses, to determine dosages and the best treatment for each individual patient, and to take all appropriate safety precautions. To the fullest extent of the law, neither the Publisher nor the Editors assume any liability for any injury and/or damage to persons or property arising out of related to any use of the material contained in this book.

The Publisher

Previous editions copyrighted 1986, 1990 by Educational Direction, Inc., Akron, Ohio.
ISBN-13: 978-0-323-06502-3
ISBN-10: 0-323-06502-3

Publisher: Michael Ledbetter
Managing Editor: Laura Bayless
Publishing Services Manager: Catherine Jackson
Design Direction: Jessica Williams

Printed in Canada
Last digit is the print number: 9   8   7   6   5   4   3   2   1

CONTRIBUTORS

EDITORS

Jeffrey P. Salomone, MD, FACS, NREMT-P
Associate Medical Director, PHTLS
Associate Professor of Surgery
Emory University School of Medicine
Atlanta, Georgia

Peter T. Pons, MD, FACEP
Associate Medical Director, PHTLS
Emergency Medicine
Denver, Colorado

EDITOR-IN-CHIEF

Norman E. McSwain, Jr., MD, FACS, NREMT-P
Professor of Surgery
Medical Director, PHTLS
Tulane University Department of Surgery
New Orleans, Louisiana

ASSOCIATE EDITORS

Frank K. Butler, Jr., MD
CAPT MC USN (Ret)
Chairman
Committee on Tactical Combat Casualty Care
Defense Health Board

Will Chapleau, EMT-P, RN, TNS, CEN
Chairman, PHTLS Executive Council
Manager, ATLS Program
American College of Surgeons
Chicago, Illinois

Gregory Chapman, EMT-P, RRT
Vice Chairman, PHTLS Executive Council
Center for Prehospital Medicine
Department of Emergency Medicine
Carolinas Medical Center
Charlotte, North Carolina

Stephen D. Giebner, MD, MPH
CAPT, MC, USN (Ret)
Past Chairman
Developmental Editor
Committee on Tactical Combat Casualty Care
Defense Health Board

Jeffrey S. Guy, MD, MSc, MMHC, FACS, EMT-P
Associate Medical Director, PHTLS
Associate Professor of Surgery
Director, Regional Burn Center
Vanderbilt University School of Medicine
Nashville, Tennessee

EDITORS—MILITARY EDITION

Frank K. Butler, Jr., MD
CAPT MC USN (Ret)
Chairman
Committee on Tactical Combat Casualty Care
Defense Health Board

S. D. Giebner, MD, MPH
CAPT, MC, USN (Ret)
Past Chairman
Developmental Editor
Committee on Tactical Combat Casualty Care
Defense Health Board

CONTRIBUTORS

Brad L. Bennett, PhD, NREMT-P, FAWM
Captain, US Navy (Ret)
Adjunct Asst Professor, Military and Emergency
    Medicine Dept
Uniformed Services University of the Health Sciences
Bethesda, Maryland

Matthew Bitner, MD
Division of Emergency Medicine
Department of Surgery
Duke University, School of Medicine
Durham, North Carolina

Frank K. Butler, Jr., MD
CAPT MC USN (Ret)
Chairman
Committee on Tactical Combat Casualty Care
Defense Health Board

David W. Callaway, MD, MPA
Director, The Operational Medicine Institute
Instructor, Harvard Medical School
Beth Israel Deaconess Medical Center
Boston, Massachusetts

Howard Champion, MD, FRCS, FACS
Senior Advisory in Trauma
Professor of Surgery and Military and Emergency Medicine
Uniformed Services University of the Health Sciences
Washington, DC

Will Chapleau, EMT-P, RN, TNS, CEN
Chairman, PHTLS Executive Council
Manager, ATLS Program
American College of Surgeons
Chicago, Illinois

Gregory Chapman, EMT-P, RRT
Vice Chairman, PHTLS Executive Council
Center for Prehospital Medicine
Department of Emergency Medicine
Carolinas Medical Center
Charlotte, North Carolina

Jeffrey S. Guy, MD, MSc, MMHC, FACS, EMT-P
Associate Medical Director, PHTLS
Associate Professor of Surgery
Director, Regional Burn Center
Vanderbilt University School of Medicine
Nashville, Tennessee

Norman E. McSwain, Jr., MD, FACS, NREMT-P
Medical Director, PHTLS
Tulane University Department of Surgery
New Orleans, Louisiana

Peter T. Pons, MD, FACEP
Associate Medical Director, PHTLS
Emergency Medicine
Denver, Colorado

Jeffrey P. Salomone, MD, FACS, NREMT-P
Senior Associate Medical Director, PHTLS
Associate Professor of Surgery
Emory University School of Medicine
Atlanta, Georgia

Joseph A. Salomone, III, MD
Associate Professor of Emergency Medicine
University of Missouri, Kansas City
Kansas City, Missouri

INTERNATIONAL CONTRIBUTORS

Dr. Alberto Adduci, Italy

Shaikha M. Al-Alawi, Oman

Dhary Al Rasheed, Saudi Arabia

Dr. Saud Al Turki, Saudi Arabia

Stuart Alves, United Kingdom

Dr. Paul Barbevil, Uruguay

Dr. Jaime A. Cortés-Ojeda, Costa Rica

Kenneth D'Alessandro, Saudi Arabia

Jan Filippo, Netherlands

Dr. Subash Gautam, United Arab Emirates

Bernhard Gliwitzky, Germany

Steve Griesch, Luxemburg

Dr. Thorsten Hauer, Germany

Konstantin Karavasilis, Georgia

Fabrice Lamarche, Belgium

Dr. Salvijus Milasius, Lithuania

Dr. Ana Maria Montanez, Peru

Philip Nel, South Africa

Dr. Fernando Novo, Brazil

Dr. Gonzalo Ostria, Bolivia

Christoph Redelsteiner, Austria

John Richardsen, Norway

Dr. Osvaldo Rois, Argentina

Michal Soczynski, Poland

Dr. Javier Gonzales Uriarte, Spain

Lisbeth Wick, France

Patrick Wick, France

PUBLISHER ACKNOWLEDGMENTS

The publisher would also like to thank the following agencies for assisting us with the photos and videos created for this book:

Dixie Blatt and the staff at St. John's Mercy Medical Center

Creve Coeur Fire Protection District

Cabin John Park Volunteer Fire Department

Montgomery County Fire Rescue Service

Montgomery County Volunteer Fire Rescue Association

Annapolis Fire Department

Prince Georges County Fire Department

REVIEWERS

P. David Adelson, MD
Director, Children's Neuroscience Institute
Chief of Pediatric Neurosurgery
Phoenix Children's Hospital
Phoenix, Arizona

Kristen D. Borchelt, RN, NREMT-P
Cincinnati Children's Hospital
Cincinnati, Ohio

Timothy Scott Brisbin, RN, BSN, NREMT-P
Director
The Center for Prehospital Medicine, Department of
    Emergency Medicine
Carolinas Medical Center
Charlotte, North Carolina

Jeffrey S. Cain, MD
US Army Institute of Surgical Research
Fort Sam Houston, Texas

David W. Callaway, MD
Beth Israel Deaconess Medical Center
Boston, Massachusetts

Erik Carlsen, NREMT-P
Lead Instructor/Coordinator
EMS Education MAST Ambulance Inc./Kansas City
    Missouri Tactical Medic Team
Kansas City, Missouri

Greg Clarkes, EMT-P
Canadian College of EMS
Edmonton, Alberta, Canada

Jo Ann Cobble, Ed.D, Paramedic, RN
Dean, Division of Health Professions
Oklahoma City Community College
Oklahoma City, Oklahoma

Arthur Cooper, MD
Pediatric Surgeon
Metropolitan Hospital
New York, New York
Professor of Surgery
Columbia University College of Physicians & Surgeons

Phil Currance, EMT-P, RHSP
Deputy Commander Colorado-2 DMAT, National Medical
    Response Team – Central
National Disaster Medical System/St. Anthony
    Central Hospital
Denver, Colorado

Fidel O. Garcia, EMT-P
President
Professional EMS Education, LLC
Grand Junction, Colorado

Rudy Garrett, AS, NREMT-P, CCEMT-P
Flight Paramedic
Air Methods Kentucky
Somerset, Kentucky

J. Scott Hartley, NREMT-P, EMSI, PHTLS Affiliate Faculty
ALS Affiliates Inc.
Omaha, Nebraska

Gary Hoertz, Paramedic
EMS Division Chief
Kootenai Fire & Rescue
Post Falls, Idaho

Debra Houry, MD, MPH
Associate Professor
Vice Chair for Research, Department of Emergency Medicine
Director, Center for Injury Control
Emory University
Atlanta, Georgia

John M. Kirtley, BA, NREMT-P
EMS Program Coordinator
J. Sargeant Reynolds Community College
Richmond, Virginia

Glen Larson, CD, REMTP, RN, ASEMS, AS(n), BGS
EMT & Paramedic Instructor
Canadian College of EMS
Edmonton, Alberta, Canada

Douglas W. Lundy, MD
Orthopaedic Surgeon
Resurgens Orthopaedics
Marietta, Georgia

William T. McGovern, BS, EMT-P, EMS I, FSI
Quality Assurance Coordinator—Field Services/
    Assistant Fire Chief
Hunter's Ambulance Service/Yalesville Volunteer
    Fire Department
Meriden, Connecticut/Wallingford, Connecticut

Chad E. McIntyre, A.A.S, NREMT-P, FP-C
Shands Jacksonville Trauma & Flight Services
Jacksonville, Florida

Reylon Meeks, RN, PhDc
Clinical Nurse Specialist
Blank Children's Hospital
Des Moines, Iowa

Jeff J. Messerole, Paramedic
Clinical Instructor
Spencer Hospital
Spencer, Iowa

Gregory S. Neiman, BA, NREMT-P
BLS Training Specialist
Virginia Office of EMS
Richmond, Virginia

Dennis Parker, MA, EMT-P, I/C
EMS Program Coordinator
Tennessee Tech University
Cookeville, Tennessee

David Pecora, EMT-P, PA
Morgantown, West Virginia

Timothy Penic, NREMT-P CCP
Field Operations Supervisor
Medstar EMS
Fort Worth, Texas

Deborah L. Petty, BS, CICP, EMT-P I/C
Paramedic Training Officer
St. Charles County Ambulance District
St. Peters, Missouri

Jean-Cyrille Pitteloud, MD, DEAA
Hôpital du Valais
Sion, Switzerland

Larry Richmond, AS, NREMT-P, CCEMT-P
EMS Coordinator
Rapid City Indian Health Service Hospital
Rapid City, South Dakota

David Stamey, CCEMT-P
EMS Training Administrator
District of Columbia Fire & EMS Department
Washington, DC

Nerina Stepanovsky, PhD, RH, EMT-P
Emergency Medical Services Program
St. Petersburg College
St. Petersburg, Florida

Kevin M. Sullivan, MS, NREMT-P
Chief
Enfield EMS
Enfield, Conneticut

David M Tauber, NREMT-P, CCEMT-P, FP-C, I/C
Education Coordinator/Executive Director
New Haven Sponsor Hospital Program/Advanced Life
    Support Institute
New Haven, Connecticut/Conway, New Hampshire

Javier Uriarte, MD
Leioa, Bizkaia, Spain

Jason J. Zigmont, PhD, NREMT-P
Yale New Haven Health System
New Haven, Connecticut

NATIONAL ASSOCIATION OF EMTs BOARD OF DIRECTORS

Patrick F. Moore
President

Connie A. Meyer
President-Elect

Donald Walsh
Secretary

Richard Ellis, NREMT-P
Treasurer

Jerry Johnston
Immediate Past-President

DIRECTORS

Aimee Binning   KC Jones

Kenneth J. Bouvier   Chuck Kearns

Charlene Donahue   Don Lundy

Jennifer Frenette   Dennis Rowe

Paul Hinchey   James M. Slattery

Sue Jacobus

PHTLS EXECUTIVE COUNCIL

Will Chapleau, EMT-P, RN, TNS, CEN
Chairman, PHTLS Executive Council
Manager, ATLS Program
American College of Surgeons
Chicago, Illinois

Gregory Chapman, EMT-P, RRT
Vice Chairman, PHTLS Executive Council
Center for Prehospital Medicine
Department of Emergency Medicine
Carolinas Medical Center
Charlotte, North Carolina

Augie Bamonti, EMT-P
AFB Consulting
Chicago Heights Fire Department (Ret)
Chicago Heights, Illinois

Frank K. Butler, Jr., MD
CAPT MC USN (Ret)
Chairman
Committee on Tactical Combat Casualty Care
Defense Health Board

Corine Curd
PHTLS International Office Director
NAEMT Headquarters
Clinton, Mississippi

Jeffrey S. Guy, MD, MSc, MMHC, FACS, EMT-P
Associate Medical Director, PHTLS
Associate Professor of Surgery
Director, Regional Burn Center
Vanderbilt University School of Medicine
Nashville, Tennessee

Michael J. Hunter
Deputy Chief Worcester EMS
UMass Memorial Medical Center—University Campus
Worcester, Massachusetts

Craig H. Jacobus, EMT-P, BA/BS, DC
EMS Faculty Metro Community College
Fremont, Nebraska

Norman E. McSwain, Jr., MD, FACS, NREMT-P
Medical Director, PHTLS
Professor of Surgery
Tulane University School of Medicine
New Orleans, Louisiana

Steve Mercer, EMT-P, MEd
Paramedic Specialist
Ames, Iowa

Peter T. Pons, MD, FACEP
Associate Medical Director, PHTLS
Emergency Medicine
Denver, Colorado

Dennis Rowe, EMT-P
Director, Rural/Metro EMS
Lenoir City, Tennessee

PHTLS HONOR ROLL

PHTLS continues to prosper and promote high standards of trauma care all over the world. It would not be able to do this without the contributions of many dedicated and inspired individuals over the past three decades. Some of those mentioned below were instrumental in the development of our first textbook. Others were constantly "on the road" spreading the word. Still others "put out fires" and otherwise problem-solved to keep PHTLS growing. The PHTLS Executive Council, along with the editors and contributors of this, our seventh edition, would like to express our thanks to all of those listed below. PHTLS lives, breathes, and grows because of the efforts of those who volunteer their time to what they believe in.

Gregory H. Adkisson
Melissa Alexander
Jameel Ali
Augie Bamonti
J.M. Barnes
Morris L. Beard
Ann Bellows
Ernest Block
Chip Boehm
Don E. Boyle
Susan Brown
Susan Briggs
Jonathan Busko
Alexander Butman
H. Jeannie Butman
Christain E. Callsen, Jr.
Steve Carden
Edward A. Casker
Bud Caukin
Hank Christen
David Ciraulo
Victoria Cleary
Philip Coco
Frederick J. Cole
Keith Conover
Arthur Cooper
Jel Coward
Michael D'Auito
Alice "Twink" Dalton

Judith Demarest
Joseph P. Dineen
Leon Dontigney
Joan Drake-Olsen
Mark Elcock
Blaine L. Endersen
Betsy Ewing
Mary E. Fallat
Milton R. Fields, III
Scott B. Frame†
Sheryl G.A. Gabram
Bret Gilliam
Jack Grandey
Vincent A. Greco
Nita J. Ham
Larry Hatfield
Mark C. Hodges
Walter Idol
Alex Isakov
Len Jacobs
Craig Jacobus
Lou Jordan
Richard Judd
Jon A. King
Jon R. Krohmer
Peter LeTarte
Robert W. Letton, Jr.
Dawn Loehn
Mark Lockhart

Robert Loftus
Greg C. Lord
Fernando
    Magallenes-Negrete
Paul M. Maniscalco
Scott W. Martin
Don Mauger
William McConnell
Merry McSwain
John Mechtel
Claire Merrick
Bill Metcalf
George Moerkirk
Stephen Murphy
Lawrence D. Newell
Jeanne O'Brien
Dawn Orgeron
Eric Ossmann
James Paturas
Joseph Pearce
Thomas Petrich
Valerie J. Phillips
James Pierce
Brian Plaisier
Mark Reading
Brian Reiselbara
Lou Romig
Donald Scelza
John Sigafoos

Paul Silverston
David Skinner
Dale C. Smith
Richard Sobieray
Sheila Spaid
Michael Spain
Don Stamper
Kenneth G. Swan
Kenneth G. Swan, Jr.
David M. Tauber
Joseph J. Tepas III
Brian M. Tibbs
Josh Vayer
Richard Vomacka†
Robert K. Waddell, II
Michael Werdmann
Carl Werntz
Elizabeth Wertz
Keith Wesley
David E. Wesson
Roger D. White
Kenneth J. Wright
David Wuertz
Al Yellin
Steven Yevich
Doug York
Alida Zamboni

Again, thanks to all of you, and thanks to everyone around the world for making PHTLS work.
PHTLS Executive Council
Editors and Contributors of PHTLS

†Deceased.

ACKNOWLEDGMENTS

In 1624 John Donne wrote that "No man is an island, entire of itself." This describes in many ways the process of the publication of a book. Certainly, no editor is an island. Textbooks, such as the PHTLS book; courses, especially those that involve audiovisual material; and instructor manuals cannot be published by editors in isolation. As a matter of fact, much, if not most, of the work involved in publishing a textbook is done not by the editors and the authors whose names appear on the cover and on the inside of the book, but by the publisher's staff. The seventh edition of PHTLS is certainly no exception.

From the American College of Surgeons Committee on Trauma, Carol Williams, Executive Secretary of the Committee on Trauma; John Fildes, MD, FACS, the current Chairman of the Committee on Trauma; and Wayne Meredith, MD, FACS, the ACS Medical Director of Trauma, have provided outstanding support for this edition as well as for PHTLS.

Within Mosby, Linda Honeycutt led the effort to bring this edition out on time, Laura Bayless has been an outstanding editor, Megan Greiner at Graphic World Inc. has brought this project to fruition, and Joy Knobbe has worked hard on the public relations for this book.

The editors and authors whose wives, children, and significant others have tolerated the long hours in the preparation of the material are obviously the backbone of any publication.

Norman McSwain, MD, FACS, NREMT-P
Jeffrey Salomone, MD, FACS, NREMT-P
Peter T. Pons, MD, FACEP

FOREWORD

In Argentina, in Latin America, and around the world, trauma is a major cause of morbidity as a result of vehicle crashes, violence, and work-related accidents, among other causes.

A response to this issue began in Argentina in 1954 through the local chapter of the American College of Surgeons. It would take 35 more years for the first ATLS course to be conducted in 1989.

During the following years, trauma patient care became vital due to the growing number of victims and the poor training of people in prehospital care.

The thousands of people killed or permanently disabled in Argentina paid a heavy price, both socially and economically for the country. Thus, in 1996, the PHTLS program in Argentina was started by the international faculty of Norman McSwain, Will Chapleau, and Greg Chapman. Seventy instructors were trained, and Argentina was divided into eight regions comprising 23 provinces. Since its inception, the course was expanded throughout the country, becoming a golden milestone in the creation of integrated prehospital and hospital responses in the public and the private sphere.

From then until now, this course has trained physicians, nurses, firefighters, rescue groups, military personnel, and industrial brigades, from Argentina to neighboring Latin American countries. To date, the PHTLS program in our country has conducted International Conferences and Trauma Update Workshops for successive editions of this book.

With the support of the PHTLS international office, managed by Will Chapleau and Corine Curd, and with the generous collaboration of other Latin American coordinators from Mexico, Colombia, Brazil, Bolivia, as well as different faculty from the United States, we accomplish these activities. Also, the PHTLS Program in Argentina has contributed to and coordinated the implementation of the program in countries such as Bolivia, Uruguay, Chile, Peru, and now, Ecuador.

Personally, as an emergency doctor with more than 30 years of medical and scientific experience in academic societies related to the critically ill, I have to highlight the ongoing development of the program that, with its narrow sense based on scientific evidence, makes the PHTLS course universally adopted in over 40 countries in both the civilian and military worldwide.

It's been 15 years since the first course in our country. We have trained more than 7,500 students. Worldwide we have educated more than half a million providers. All this would not have been possible without the daily efforts of people like Norman McSwain, Will Chapleau, Jeff Salomone, and other greats, such as Scott Frame, who are no longer with us, and hundreds of managers and trainers in the other 50 countries that work day after day teaching and applying the concepts and skills of the program to their patients.

Today in Argentina, the initial management of trauma patient has a single protocol, "the PHTLS kind."

It is an honor shared by all of us who work on the scene, to feel part of this work philosophy and a sense of belonging. One takes great pride when a firefighter, a doctor, a soldier, or a brigade says "I'm PHTLS," and when we work among the victims of an accident, I feel that these 15 years of training have borne fruit and I understand "they are making a difference."

I will always remember a phrase from Norman McSwain in Argentina: "If one of us can once again save a victim, you can change the world." Thus, overcoming any geopolitical barrier, PHTLS is a bridge of knowledge over the world.

Oswaldo Rois, MD
President, Fundacion EMME
Director PHTLS Argentina

Prehospital care providers should accept the responsibility to provide patient care that is as close to absolutely perfect as possible. This cannot be achieved with insufficient knowledge of the subject. We must remember that the patient did not choose to be involved in a traumatic situation. The provider, on the other hand, has chosen to be there to take care of the patient. The prehospital care provider is obligated to give 100% of his or her effort during contact with every patient. The patient has had a bad day; the provider cannot also have a bad day. The prehospital care provider must be sharp and capable in the competition between the patient and death and disease.

The patient is the most important person at the scene of an emergency. There is no time to think about the order in which the patient assessment is performed or what treatments should take priority over others. There is no time to practice a skill before using it on a particular patient. There is no time to think about where equipment or supplies are housed within the jump kit. There is no time to think about where to transport the injured patient. All of this information and more must be stored in the mind and all supplies and equipment must be present in the jump kit when the provider arrives on the scene. Without the proper knowledge or equipment, the provider may neglect to do things that could potentially increase the patient's chance of survival. The responsibilities of a provider are too great to make such mistakes.

Those who deliver care in the prehospital setting are integral members of the trauma patient care team, as are the nurses or physicians in the emergency department, operating room, intensive care unit, ward, and rehabilitation unit. Prehospital care providers must be practiced in their skills so that they can move the patient quickly and efficiently out of the environment of the emergency and transport the patient quickly to the closest appropriate hospital.

WHY PHTLS?

Course Education Philosophy

Prehospital Trauma Life Support (PHTLS) focuses on principles, not preferences. By focusing on principles of good trauma care, PHTLS promotes critical thinking. The Executive Committee of the PHTLS Division of the National Association of Emergency Medical Technicians (NAEMT) believes that, given a good fund of knowledge, prehospital care providers are capable of making reasoned decisions regarding patient care. Rote memorization of mnemonics is discouraged.

Furthermore, there is no one "PHTLS way" of performing a specific skill. The principle of the skill is taught, and then one acceptable method of performing the skill that meets the principle is presented. The authors realize that no one method can apply to the myriad unique situations encountered in the prehospital setting.

Up-to-Date Information

Development of the PHTLS program began in 1981, immediately on the heels of the inception of the Advanced Trauma Life Support (ATLS) program for physicians. As the ATLS course is revised every 4 to 5 years, pertinent changes are incorporated into the next edition of PHTLS. This seventh edition of the PHTLS program has been revised based on the 2008 ATLS course as well as subsequent publications in the medical literature. Although following the ATLS principles, PHTLS is specifically designed for the unique requirements of caring for trauma patients in the prehospital setting. New chapters have been added, whereas others have been extensively revised. New chapters include information on the Art and Science of Medicine. Also included is a CD-ROM with video clips of skills and practice questions. Note throughout the book the symbol references indicating that more information can be found on the CD-ROM.

Scientific Base

The authors and editors have adopted an "evidence-based" approach that includes references from the medical literature supporting the key principles, and additional position papers published by the national organizations are cited when applicable. Many references have been added, allowing those providers with an inquisitive mind to read the scientific data supporting our recommendations.

Support for NAEMT

The NAEMT provides the administrative structure for the PHTLS program. No proceeds from the PHTLS program (surcharges or royalties from the text and audiovisuals) go to the editors or authors of this work or to the American College of Surgeons Committee on Trauma or any other physician-oriented organization. All profits from the PHTLS program are channelled back into NAEMT to provide funding for issues and programs that are of prime importance to EMS professionals, such as educational conferences and the lobbying of legislators on behalf of prehospital care providers.

PHTLS Is a World Leader

Because of the unprecedented success of the prior editions of PHTLS, the program has continued to grow by leaps and bounds. PHTLS courses continue to proliferate across the United States, and the US military has adopted it, teaching the program to US Armed Forces personnel at over 100 training sites worldwide. PHTLS has been exported to more than 50 nations, and many others are expressing interest in bringing PHTLS to their countries in efforts to improve prehospital trauma care levels.

Prehospital care providers have the responsibility to assimilate this knowledge and these skills in order to use them for the benefit of the patients for whom the providers are responsible. The editors and authors of this material and the Executive Committee of the PHTLS Division of the NAEMT hope that you will incorporate this information into your practice and daily rededicate yourself to the care of those persons who cannot care for themselves—the trauma patients.

Jeffrey P. Salomone, MD, FACS, NREMT-P
Peter T. Pons, MD, FACEP
Editors
Norman E. McSwain, Jr., MD, FACS, NREMT-P
Editor-in-Chief, PHTLS
Will Chapleau, EMT-P, RN, TNS, CEN
Gregory Chapman, EMT-P, RRT
Jeffrey S. Guy, MD, MSc, MMHC, FACS, EMT-P
Associate Editors

CONTENTS

DIVISION 1   Introduction

1   PHTLS: Past, Present, and Future, *1*
2   Injury Prevention, *15*

DIVISION 2   Assessment and Management

3   The Science and Art of Prehospital Care: Principles, Preferences, and Critical Thinking, *33*
4   Kinematics of Trauma, *43*
5   Scene Assessment, *87*
6   Patient Assessment and Management, *109*
7   Airway and Ventilation, *133*
8   Shock, *179*

DIVISION 3   Specific Injuries

9   Head Trauma, *217*
10   Spinal Trauma, *245*
11   Thoracic Trauma, *291*
12   Abdominal Trauma, *317*
13   Musculoskeletal Trauma, *333*
14   Burn Injuries, *355*
15   Pediatric Trauma, *377*
16   Geriatric Trauma, *403*

DIVISION 4   Summary

17   Golden Principles of Prehospital Trauma Care, *421*

DIVISION 5   Mass Casualties and Terrorism

18   Disaster Management, *431*
19   Explosions and Weapons of Mass Destruction, *447*

DIVISION 6   Special Considerations

20   Environmental Trauma I: Heat and Cold, *477*
21   Environmental Trauma II: Drowning, Lightning, Diving, and Altitude, *521*
22   Wilderness Trauma Care, *561*
23   Civilian Tactical Emergency Medical Support (TEMS), *579*
Glossary, *591*
Index, *605*

SPECIFIC SKILLS

DIVISION 2 Assessment and Management

7 Trauma Jaw Thrust, *158*
7 Alternate Jaw Thrust, *158*
7 Trauma Chin Lift (Two-Person), *159*
7 Oropharyngeal Airway (Tongue Jaw Lift Insertion Method), *160*
7 Oropharyngeal Airway (Tongue Blade Insertion Method), *161*
7 Nasopharyngeal Airway, *162*
7 Bag-Mask Ventilation (Two-Person), *164*
7 Combitube, *166*
7 King Airway, *168*
7 Laryngeal Mask Airway, *170*
7 Visualized Orotracheal Intubation of the Trauma Patient, *172*
7 Face-to-Face Orotracheal Intubation, *174*
7 Needle Cricothyrotomy and Percutaneus Transtracheal Ventilation, *176*
8 Intraosseous Vascular Access, *213*
8 Tourniquet Application: Israeli Trauma Bandage, *215*

DIVISION 3 Specific Injuries

10 Cervical Collar Sizing and Application, *267*
10 Log Roll/Supine, *269*
10 Log Roll/Prone or Semi-Prone, *271*
10 Standing Long Backboard Application (Three-Person), *273*
10 Standing Long Backboard Application (Two-Person), *275*
10 Sitting Immobilization (Vest Type), *277*
10 Rapid Extrication (Three-Person), *280*
10 Rapid Extrication (Two-Person), *283*
10 Infant Child Seat, *284*
10 Child Immobilization Device, *286*
10 Helmet Removal, *288*
11 Needle Decompression, *314*

ATLS

As happens so often in life, a personal experience brought about the changes in emergency care that resulted in the birth of the ATLS course (and eventually the PHTLS program). ATLS started in 1978, 2 years after a private plane crash in a rural area of Nebraska. The ATLS course was born out of that mangled mass of metal, the injured, and the dead.

The pilot, an orthopaedic surgeon, his wife, and family of four children were flying in their twin-engine airplane when it crashed. His wife was killed instantly. The children were critically injured. They waited for what seemed like an eternity for help to arrive, but it never did. After approximately 8 hours, he walked 5/8 of a mile along a dirt road to a highway and flagged down a car after two trucks didn't stop. They drove to the accident site and loaded the children in the car and drove to the closest hospital, a few miles south of the crash site.

When they approached the emergency room door of this rural hospital, they found it was locked and had to knock to get in. A little later the two general practitioners in this small farming community arrived. One of the doctors picked up one of the injured children by the shoulders and the knees and took him into the x-ray room. Later, he returned and announced there was no skull fracture. The cervical spine had not been considered. He then began suturing the laceration. Finally, the pilot called his physician partner and told him what had happened and that they would get to Lincoln as soon as they could.

The doctors and staff in this little hospital had little or no preparation for this type of situation. There was an obvious lack of training for triage and proper treatment.

Folks got tired of the criticism of the treatment received in the rural setting of the crash. The complaint was not about the care at any particular facility, but about the general lack of a delivery system to treat the acute trauma patient in the rural setting. They decided they wanted to educate rural physicians in a systematic way to treat trauma patients and chose to use a similar format to ACLS and call it ATLS.

A syllabus was created and organized into a logical approach to manage trauma. The "treat as you go" methodology was developed. The ABCs of trauma were developed to prioritize the order of assessment and treatment. The prototype was field tested in Auburn, Nebraska, in 1978 with the help of many. The course was presented to the University of Nebraska and, eventually, to the American College of Surgeons Committee on Trauma.

Since that first course in Auburn, Nebraska, three decades have passed and ATLS keeps spreading and growing. What was originally intended as a course for rural Nebraska became a course for the whole world in all types of trauma settings and served as the basis for PHTLS.

PHTLS

As Richard H. Carmona, MD, former United States Surgeon General, stated in his foreward to the sixth edition of this book, "It has been said that we stand on the shoulders of giants in many apparent successes, and PHTLS is no different. With great vision and passion, as well as challenges, a small group of leaders persevered and developed PHTLS over a quarter of a century ago."

Often referred to as "The Father of EMS," Joseph D. "Deke" Farrington, MD, FACS (1909–1982), penned the article "Death in a Ditch," which many believe signalled the turning point in modern EMS in the United States. In 1958, he convinced the Chicago Fire Department that firefighters should be trained to manage emergency patients. Working with Dr. Sam Banks, Deke started the Trauma Training Program in Chicago. Millions have been trained following the guidelines developed in this landmark program. Deke continued to work at every level of EMS from the field to education to legislation, ensuring that EMS would grow into the profession in which we 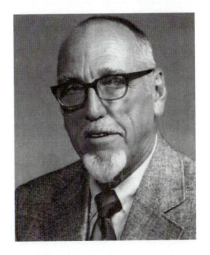 work today. The principles set forth by Deke's work form a part of the nucleus of PHTLS, and his are among the shoulders on which we all stand.

The first chairman of the ATLS ad hoc committee for the American College of Surgeons and Chairman of the Prehospital Care Subcommittee on Trauma for the American College of Surgeons, Dr. Norman E. McSwain, Jr., FACS, knew that what they had begun with ATLS would have a profound effect on the outcome of trauma patients. Moreover, he had a strong sense that an even greater effect could come from bringing this type of critical training to prehospital care providers.

Dr. McSwain, a founding member of the board of directors of the National Association of Emergency Medical Technicians (NAEMT), gained the support of the Association's president, Gary Labeau, and began to lay plans for a prehospital version of ATLS. President Labeau directed Dr. McSwain and Robert Nelson, NREMT-P, to determine the feasibility of an ATLS-type program for prehospital care providers.

As a professor of surgery at Tulane University School of Medicine in New Orleans, Louisiana, Dr. McSwain gained the university's support in putting together the draft curriculum of what was to become Prehospital Trauma Life Support (PHTLS). With this draft in place, a PHTLS committee was established in 1983. This committee continued to refine the curriculum, and later that same year, pilot courses were conducted in Lafayette and New Orleans, Louisiana, and at Marian Health Center in Sioux City, Iowa, Yale University School of Medicine in New Haven, Connecticut, and Norwalk Hospital in Norwalk, Connecticut.

Richard W. "Rick" Vomacka (1946–2001) was a part of the task force that developed the PHTLS course based on the Advanced Trauma Life Support program of the American College of Surgeons. PHTLS became his passion as the course came together, and he traveled around the country in the early 1980s conducting pilot courses and regional faculty workshops, and worked with Dr. McSwain and the other original task force members to fine-tune the program. Rick was the key to the close relationship that developed between PHTLS and the US military, and he also worked on the first international PHTLS course sites. Rick was a big part of PHTLS's beginnings and will always be remembered with gratitude for his hard work and dedication to the cause of improving care for trauma patients.

National dissemination began with three intensive workshops taught in Denver, Colorado, Bethesda, Maryland, and Orlando, Florida, between September 1984 and February 1985. The graduates of these early courses formed what would be the "Barnstormers," PHTLS national and regional faculty members who traveled the country training additional faculty members, spreading the word that PHTLS had arrived.

Alex Butman along with Rick Vomacka worked diligently, and frequently used money out of their own pockets, to bring the first two editions of the PHTLS program to fruition. Without their help and work, PHTLS would never have begun.

Early courses focused on advanced life support (ALS). In 1986, a course that encompassed basic life support (BLS) was developed. The course grew exponentially. Beginning with those first few enthusiastic faculty members, first dozens, then hundreds, and now thousands of providers annually participate in PHTLS courses all over the world.

As the course grew, the PHTLS committee became a division of the NAEMT. Course demand and the need to maintain course continuity and quality necessitated the building of networks of affiliate state, regional, and national faculty members. There are national coordinators for every country, and in each country, there are regional and state coordinators along with affiliate faculty members to make sure that information is disseminated and courses are consistent whether a provider participates in a program in Chicago Heights, Illinois, or Buenos Aires, Argentina.

Throughout the growth process, medical oversight has been provided through the American College of Surgeons Committee on Trauma. For nearly 20 years, the partnership between the American College of Surgeons and the NAEMT has ensured that course participants receive the opportunity to give trauma patients everywhere their best chance at survival.

More recently, Scott B. Frame, MD, FACS, FCCM (1952–2001), was the Associate Medical Director for the PHTLS program. His major emphasis was in the development of the audiovisuals for PHTLS and its promulgation internationally. At the time of his untimely death, he had assumed the responsibility of putting together the fifth edition of the PHTLS course. This included the revision not only of the textbook, but also of the instructor's manual and all of the associated teaching materials. He accepted the appointment to become Medical Director of the PHTLS course when the fifth edition was published. He published chapters and articles on EMS and trauma in major textbooks and scientific journals.

The PHTLS program grew tremendously under Scott's leadership and its continuation into the future is because of what Scott did and the part of his life that he lent to PHTLS and to his patients.

It is on the shoulders of these, and many more individuals too numerous to mention, that PHTLS stands and continues to grow.

PHTLS in the Military

Beginning in 1988, the US military aggressively set out to train its medics in PHTLS. Coordinated by DMRTI, the Defense Medical Readiness Training Institute at Fort Sam Houston in Texas, PHTLS is taught all over the United States, Europe, and Asia, and anywhere the flags of the US military fly. In 2001, the Army's 91WB program standardized the training of over 58,000 Army medics to include PHTLS. A military chapter was added in the fourth edition. After the fifth edition was initially published, a strong relationship was forged between the PHTLS organization and the newly established Committee on Tactical Combat Casualty Care. The initial fruit born of this relationship was an extensively revised military chapter in the fifth edition (revised), and a military version of the book was published in 2004. This collaboration has led to the creation of multiple military chapters for the sixth edition military PHTLS text. PHTLS has been taught numerous times "in theater" during the Afghanistan and Iraq wars and has contributed to the lowest mortality rate from any armed conflict in US history.

International PHTLS

The sound principles of prehospital trauma management emphasized in the PHTLS course have led prehospital care providers and physicians outside the United States to request the importation of the program to their various countries. ATLS faculty members presenting ATLS courses worldwide have assisted in this. This network provides medical direction and course continuity.

As PHTLS has moved across the United States and around the globe, we have been struck by the differences in our cultures and climates and also by the similarities of the people who devote their lives to caring for the sick and injured. All of us who have been blessed with the opportunity to teach overseas have experienced the fellowship with our international partners and know that we are all one people in pursuit of caring for those who need care the most.

The PHTLS family continues to grow with nearly a million students trained in 50 countries. Annually, we are running over 2,600 courses, with 34,000 students.

The nations in the ever-growing PHTLS family (as of the publication of this edition) include Argentina, Australia, Austria, Barbados, Belgium, Bolivia, Brazil, Canada, Chile, China and Hong Kong, Colombia, Costa Rica, Cyprus, Denmark, France, Georgia, Germany, Greece, Grenada, Ireland, Israel, Italy, Lithuania, Luxembourg, Mexico, Netherlands, New Zealand, Norway, Oman, Panama, Peru, Philippines, Poland, Portugal, Saudi Arabia, Scotland, Spain, Sweden, Switzerland, Trinidad and Tobago, United Arab Emirates, the United Kingdom, the United States, Uruguay, and Venezuela. Demonstration courses have been run in Bulgaria, Macedonia, and soon, Croatia, with hopes to establish faculty members there. Japan, Korea, South Africa, Ecuador, Paraguay, and Nigeria all hope to join the family in the near future.

Translations

Our growing international family has spawned translations of the text. The text is currently available in English, Spanish, Greek, Portuguese, French, Dutch, Georgian, Chinese, and Italian. Negotiations are ongoing to have the text published in a number of additional languages. Toward that end, there are subtitles in several languages on the CD-ROM that accompanies this book.

Vision for the Future

The vision for the future of PHTLS is family. The father of PHTLS, Dr. McSwain, remains the foundation for the growing family that provides vital training and contributes knowledge and experience to the world. The inaugural international PHTLS Trauma Symposium was held near Chicago, Illinois,

in the year 2000. In 2010, the first European PHTLS meeting was held. These programs bring the work of practitioners and researchers around the globe together to determine the standards of trauma care for the new millennium.

The support of the PHTLS family worldwide, all volunteering countless hours of their lives, allows the PHTLS leadership to keep PHTLS growing. This leadership consists of the following:

PHTLS Executive Council

International PHTLS Chairs

Will Chapleau, EMT-P, RN, TNS	1996-present
Elizabeth M. Wertz, RN, BSN, MPM	1992-1996
James L. Paturas	1991-1992
John Sinclair, EMT-P	1990-1991
David Wuertz, EMT-P	1988-1990
James L. Paturas	1985-1988
Richard Vomacka, REMT-P	1983-1985

Medical Director of PHTLS International

Norman E. McSwain, Jr., MD, FACS, NREMT-P	1983-present

Associate PHTLS Medical Directors

Jeffrey S. Guy, MD, FACS, EMT-P	2001-present
Peter T. Pons, MD, FACEP	2000-present
Jeffrey Salomone, MD, FACS, NREMT-P	1996-2010
Scott B. Frame, MC, FACS, FCCM	1994-2001

Executive Committee Members

Augie Bamonti, EMT-P
Gregory Chapman, EMT-P, RRT, Assoc. Chair, PHTLS
Frank K. Butler, MD
Michael J. Hunter, EMT-P
Craig Jacobus, EMT-P, DC
Steve Mercer, EMT-P, MEd
Dennis Rowe, EMT-P

As we continue to pursue the potential of the PHTLS course and the worldwide community of prehospital care providers, we must remember our commitment to the following:

- Rapid and accurate assessment
- Identification of shock and hypoxemia
- Initiation of the right interventions at the right time
- Timely transport to the right place

It is also fitting to reprise our mission statement, which was written in a marathon session at the NAEMT conference in 1997. The PHTLS mission continues to be to provide the highest quality prehospital trauma education to all who wish to avail themselves of this opportunity. The PHTLS mission also enhances the achievement of the NAEMT mission. The PHTLS program is committed to quality and performance improvement. As such, PHTLS is always attentive to changes in technology and methods of delivering prehospital trauma care that may be used to enhance the clinical and service quality of this program.

NAEMT was founded with the help of the National Registry of EMTs (NREMT) in 1975. Since its inception, the association has worked to promote professional status for prehospital care providers from the first responder to the administrator. Its educational programs began as a way of providing meaningful continuing education to providers at every level and have become the standard of prehospital continuing education all over the world.

NAEMT has reciprocal relationships with dozens of United States and international federal and private agencies that influence every aspect of prehospital care. The NAEMT's participation ensures that the voice of prehospital care is heard in determining the future of our practice.

National Association of Emergency Medical Technicians

The NAEMT represents the interests of prehospital care providers all over the world.

NAEMT MISSION

The mission of the National Association of Emergency Medical Technicians, Inc., is to be a professional representative organization that will receive and represent the views and opinions of prehospital care personnel and to influence the future advancement of EMS as an allied health profession. NAEMT will serve its professional membership through educational programs, liaison activity, development of national standards and reciprocity, and the development of programs to benefit prehospital care personnel.

With this mission clearly defined and passionately pursued, NAEMT will continue to provide leadership in this developing specialty of prehospital care into the future.

CHAPTER 1

PHTLS: Past, Present, and Future

CHAPTER OBJECTIVES

At the completion of this chapter, the reader will be able to do the following:

✓ Recognize the magnitude of the problem both in human and financial terms caused by traumatic injury.

✓ Understand the history and evolution of prehospital trauma care.

✓ Identify and recognize the components and importance of prehospital research and literature.

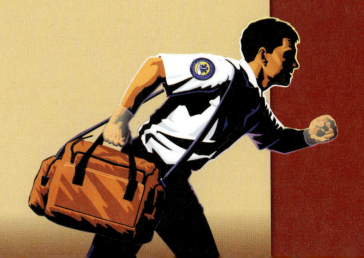

Introduction

Our patients did not choose us. We chose them. We could have chosen another profession, but we did not. We have accepted the responsibility for patient care in some of the worst situations: when we are tired or cold; when it is rainy and dark; when we cannot predict what conditions we will encounter. We must either accept this responsibility or surrender it. We must give to our patients the very best care that we can—not while we are daydreaming, not with unchecked equipment, not with incomplete supplies, and not with yesterday's knowledge. We cannot know what medical information is current, we cannot purport to be ready to care for our patients if we do not read and learn each day. The Pre-Hospital Trauma Life Support (PHTLS) course provides a part of that knowledge to the working EMT but, more important, it ultimately benefits the person who needs our all—the patient. At the end of each run, we should feel that the patient received nothing short of our very best.

Philosophy of PHTLS

PHTLS teaches knowledge that includes an understanding of anatomy and physiology, patient care skills and the limitations of time and blood loss, and the need to get the patient to the operating room as quickly as possible. This philosophy allows, nay requires, the provider to use critical thinking to make and carry out decisions that will enhance the survival of the trauma patient. PHTLS does not train providers to use protocols for patient care. Protocols are a robotic approach that does not allow better alternatives to be considered. Rather PHTLS provides and teaches understanding of medical care <u>and</u> critical thinking to achieve these goals. Each provider/patient contact involves a unique set of circumstances. If the provider understands the basis of medical care and the specific needs of this individual patient, then unique patient decisions can be made that provide the particular patient being treated with the greatest chance of survival.

It is the belief of the PHTLS educational process that providers are not medical technicians carrying out instructions sent down from "on high," but rather that they have a good fund of knowledge, are critical thinkers, and have appropriate care skills to make and carry out excellent patient care. PHTLS does not "tell" the provider what to do but supplies the provider with the appropriate knowledge and skills to use critical thinking to arrive that the best management of the specific trauma patient(s) at hand.

The opportunity for a prehospital care provider to help another person is greater in the management of trauma patients than in any other patient encounter. The number of trauma patients encountered is higher than most other patient populations, and the chance for survival of the trauma patient who receives excellent trauma care, both in the prehospital and the hospital setting, is probably greater than that of any other critically ill patient. The prehospital care provider can lengthen the life span and productive years of the trauma patient and benefit society by virtue of the care provided. The prehospital care provider, through effective management of the trauma patient, has a significant influence on society.

Understanding, learning, and practicing the principles of PHTLS is more beneficial to patients than any other educational program.[1] The following facts have led to the revised and expanded Chapter 2 on injury prevention in this edition of *Prehospital Trauma Life Support.*

The Problem

Trauma is the leading cause of death in persons between 1 and 44 years of age.[2] Approximately 80% of teenage deaths and 60% of childhood deaths are secondary to trauma. Trauma continues to be the seventh leading cause of death in elderly persons. Almost three times more Americans die of trauma *each year* than died in the entire Vietnam War and in the Iraq war through 2008.[3] Every 10 years, more Americans die of trauma than have died in all US military conflicts combined. Only in the fifth decade of life do cancer and heart disease compete with trauma as a leading cause of death. About 70 times as many Americans die yearly from blunt and penetrating trauma in the United States as died yearly in the Iraqi conflict through 2008.

Prehospital care providers can do little to increase the survival of a cancer patient. For the trauma patient, however, prehospital care providers can often make the difference between life and death; between temporary disablement and serious or permanent disability; or between a life of productivity and a life of destitution and welfare. In the United States, about 60 million injuries occur each year; 40 million will require emergency department care; 2.5 million will be hospitalized; and 9 million of these are disabling. About 8.7 million trauma patients will be temporarily disabled, and 300,000 will be permanently disabled.[4,5]

The cost for care of trauma patients is staggering. Billions of dollars are spent on the management of trauma patients, not including the dollars lost in wages, insurance administration costs, property damage, and employer costs. The National Safety Council estimates that the economic impact in 2007 from both fatal and non-fatal trauma is approximately $684 billion.[6] Lost productivity from disabled trauma patients is the equivalent of 5.1 million years at a cost of more than $65 billion annually. For patients who die, 5.3 million years of life are lost (34 years per person) at a cost of more than $50 billion. Comparatively, the costs per patient (measured in dollars and in years lost) for cancer and heart disease are much less, as illustrated in Figure 1-1. For example, proper protection of the fractured cervical spine by a prehospital care provider may make the difference between lifelong quadriplegia and a productive healthy life of unrestricted activity. Prehospital care providers encounter many more such examples almost every day.

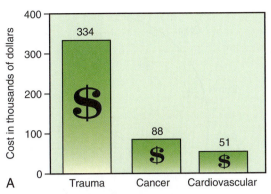

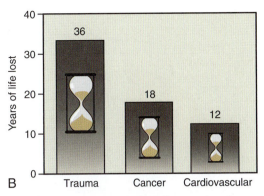

FIGURE 1-1 **A:** Comparative costs in thousands of dollars to US victims of trauma, cancer, and cardiovascular disease each year. **B:** Comparative number of years lost as a result of trauma, cancer, and cardiovascular disease.

The following data come from WHO Global Burden of Disease project, 2004:

Road traffic injuries are a huge public health and development problem—Road traffic crashes kill 1.3 million people a year or an average of 3242 people every day. Road traffic crashes injure or disable between 20 million and 50 million people a year. Road traffic crashes rank as the ninth leading cause of death and account for 2.2% of all deaths globally.

The majority of road traffic injuries affect people in low-income and middle-income countries, especially young males and vulnerable road users—90% of road traffic deaths occur in low-income and middle-income countries[7] (Figure 1-2).

The impact of preventable injuries is worldwide. Although the events that produce injuries and deaths may be of a differing etiologies from country to country, the consequences are not. Trauma is a worldwide problem. We who work in the trauma community have an obligation to our patients to prevent injuries, not just be able to treat them after they occur.

The often told story about EMS illustrates this point. On a long winding mountain road, there was one turn where cars would often slide off and land at the bottom, 100 feet below.

It was the decision of the community to station an ambulance at the bottom of the dangerous area to care for the patients that were involved. The better alternative would have been to place guard rails along the road on the curve to PREVENT the incident from occurring in the first place.

Trauma care is divided into three phases: pre-event, event, and postevent. The prehospital care provider has responsibilities in each phase.

Pre-event Phase

Trauma is no accident, even though it is often referred to as such. An *accident* is defined as either "an event occurring by chance or arising from unknown causes" or "an unfortunate occurrence resulting from carelessness, unawareness, ignorance." Most trauma deaths and injuries fit the second definition but not the first and are preventable. Traumatic incidents fall into two categories: *intentional* and *unintentional.*

The pre-event phase involves the circumstances leading up to an injury. Efforts in this phase are primarily focused on injury prevention. In working toward prevention of injuries, the public must be educated to increase the use of vehicle occupant restraint systems, promote methods to reduce the use of weapons in criminal activities, and promote nonviolent conflict resolution. In addition to caring for the trauma patient, all members

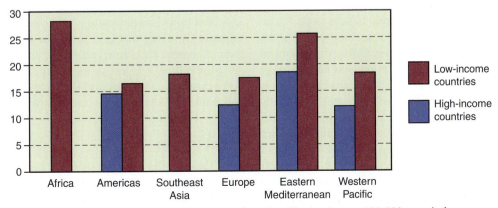

FIGURE 1-2 Worldwide distribution of road traffic deaths per 100,000 population.

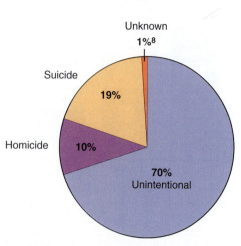

FIGURE 1-3   Unintentional trauma accounts for more deaths than all other causes of trauma death combined.
(Data from the National Center for Injury Prevention and Control: *Wisqars leading causes of death reports, 1999–2006.* Centers for Disease Control and Prevention.)

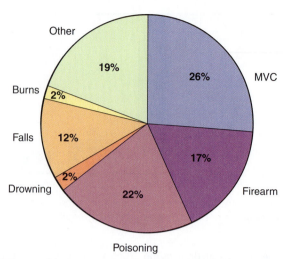

FIGURE 1-4   Motor vehicle trauma and firearms account for almost half of the deaths that result from traumatic injury.
(Data from the National Center for Injury Prevention and Control: *Wisqars leading causes of death reports, 1999–2006.* Centers for Disease Control and Prevention.)

of the health-care delivery team have a responsibility to reduce the number of victims. Currently, violence and unintentional trauma cause more deaths annually in the United States than all diseases combined. Violence accounts for more than one third of these deaths (Figure 1-3). Motor vehicles and firearms are involved in more than one half of all trauma deaths, most of which are preventable (Figure 1-4).

Motorcycle-helmet–usage laws are one example of legislation that has affected injury prevention. In 1966, the US Congress gave the Department of Transportation the authority to mandate that states pass legislation requiring the use of motorcycle helmets. The use of helmets subsequently increased to almost 100%, and the fatality rate from motorcycle crashes decreased dramatically. Congress rescinded this authority in 1975. More than half the states repealed or modified the existing legislation. As states reinstate or repeal these laws, mortality rates change. Recently, more states have repealed, rather than instituted, such laws, resulting in increased death rates in 2006 and 2007.[9] Motorcycle deaths are on the rise while deaths from automobiles are decreasing. The increase in motorcycle deaths was 11% in 2006.[10] The most likely cause for this dramatic increase in mortality is the decreased use of helmets while riding. Only 20 states have universal helmet laws. In states with such laws helmet usage is 74% whereas in states without such laws the usage rate is 42%.[11] The decreased number of states with such laws is the major factor from the drop in overall helmet usage from 71% in 2000 to 51% in 2006. As an example in one state (Florida), the change in the law in 2002 produced an increased death rate 24% greater than the increase in registrations would have predicted. In August 2008, US Secretary of Transportation, Mary Peters, reported a drop in highway fatalities in automobiles while at the same time there was an increase in

motorcycle fatalities. There has been major improvement in all aspects of vehicular safety except motorcycles.[12]

Another example of preventable trauma deaths involves drunk driving.[13] As a result of pressure to change state laws for the level of intoxication while driving and through the educational activities of such organizations as Mothers Against Drunk Drivers (MADD), the number of drunk drivers involved in fatal crashes has been consistently decreasing since 1989.

Another way to prevent trauma is through the use of child safety seats. Many trauma centers, law enforcement organizations, and emergency medical services (EMS) conduct programs to educate parents in the correct installation and use of child safety seats.

The other component of the pre-event phase is preparation by trauma care providers for the events that are not prevented. Preparation includes proper and complete education with updated information to the current medical care. It is just as important to update your knowledge with current medical practices and knowledge as it is to update your home computer or handheld device with the latest software. In addition, it is necessary to review the equipment on the response unit at the beginning of every shift and to review with your partner the individual responsibilities and expectations of who will carry out what duties. It is just as important to review the conduct of the care when you arrive on the scene as it is to decide who will drive and who will be in the back with the patient.

Event Phase

This phase is the moment of the actual trauma. Steps performed in the pre-event phase can influence the outcome of the event phase. This applies not only to our patients, but also to ourselves. Whether driving a personal vehicle or an emergency vehicle, prehospital care providers need to protect themselves and teach by example. It is important to always drive safely, follow traffic laws, not engage in distracting activities such as cell phone use or texting, and use the protective devices available, such as vehicle restraints, in the driving compartment and in the passenger or patient-care compartment.

Postevent Phase

Obviously, the worst possible outcome after a traumatic event is death of the patient. Donald Trunkey, MD, has described a trimodal categorization of trauma deaths.[14] The *first phase* of deaths occurs within the first few minutes and up to an hour after an incident. These deaths would likely occur even with prompt medical attention. The best way to combat these deaths is through injury prevention and safety strategies. The *second phase* of deaths occurs within the first few hours of an incident. These deaths can be prevented by good prehospital care and good hospital care. The *third phase* of deaths occurs several days to several weeks after the incident. These deaths are generally caused by multiple organ failure. Much more needs to be learned about managing and preventing multiple organ failure; however, early and aggressive management of shock in the prehospital setting can prevent some of these deaths (Figure 1-5).

R Adams Cowley, MD, founder of the Maryland Institute of Emergency Medical Services (MIEMS), one of the first trauma centers in the United States, described and defined what he called the "Golden Hour."[15] Based on his research, Cowley believed that patients who received definitive care soon after an injury had a much higher survival rate than those whose care was delayed. One reason for this improvement in survival is preservation of the body's ability to produce energy to maintain organ function. For the prehospital care provider, this translates into maintaining oxygenation and perfusion and providing rapid transportation to a facility that is prepared to continue the process of resuscitation using blood and plasma (Damage Control Resuscitation) and to not artificially elevate the blood pressure (<90 mmHg) using large volumes of crystalloid.

An average urban EMS system, in the United States, has a *response time* (from the time of notification that the incident occurred until arrival on the scene) of 6–8 minutes. A typical transport time to the receiving facility is another 8–10 minutes. Between 15 and 20 minutes of the magic "Golden Hour" are used just to arrive at the scene and transport the patient. If prehospital care at the scene is not efficient and well organized, an additional 30–40 minutes can be spent on the scene. With this time on the scene added to the transport time, the "Golden Hour" has already passed before the patient arrives at the hospital where the better resources of a well-prepared emergency department are available for the benefit of the patient. Research data are starting to support this concept.[16,17] One of these studies showed that critically injured patients had a significantly lower mortality rate (17.9% vs. 28.2%) when transported by a private vehicle rather than an ambulance.[16] This unexpected finding was most likely the result

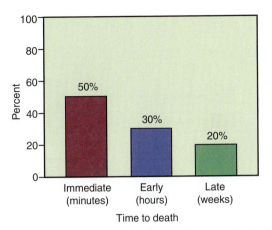

FIGURE 1-5 Immediate deaths can be prevented only by injury-prevention education because some patients' only chance for survival is for the incident not to have occurred. Early deaths can be prevented through timely, appropriate prehospital care to reduce mortality and morbidity. Late deaths can be prevented only through prompt transport to a hospital appropriately staffed for trauma care.

of prehospital care providers spending too much time on the scene. In the 1980s and 1990s, a trauma center documented that EMS scene times averaged 20–30 minutes for patients injured in motor vehicle crashes (MVCs) and for victims of penetrating trauma. This situation raises the questions that all prehospital providers need to ask: "Is what I am doing going to benefit the patient? Does that benefit outweigh the risk of delaying transport?" One of the most important responsibilities of a prehospital care provider is to spend as little time on the scene as possible. In the first precious minutes after arrival to a scene, a prehospital care provider rapidly assesses the patient, performs lifesaving maneuvers, and prepares the patient for transportation. In the 2000s, following the tenets of PHTLS prehospital, times have decreased and survival has increased.

A second responsibility is actually transporting the patient to an appropriate facility. The factor that is most critical to any patient's survival is the length of time that elapses between the incident and definitive care. For a cardiac arrest patient, definitive care is the restoration of a normal heart rhythm and adequate perfusion. Cardiopulmonary resuscitation (CPR) is merely a holding pattern. For a patient whose airway is compromised, definitive care is the management of the airway and restoration of adequate ventilation. The reestablishment of either ventilation or normal cardiac rhythm by defibrillation is usually easily achieved in the field. However, as critical care hospitals develop STEMI programs, the amount of time until balloon dilatation of the involved cardiac vessels is becoming more important.[18,19,20,21]

The management of trauma patients is different but time is just as critical, perhaps more so. Definitive care is usually hemorrhage control and restoration of adequate perfusion by replacement of fluids as near to whole blood as possible. Administration of packed red blood cells to plasma, in a ratio

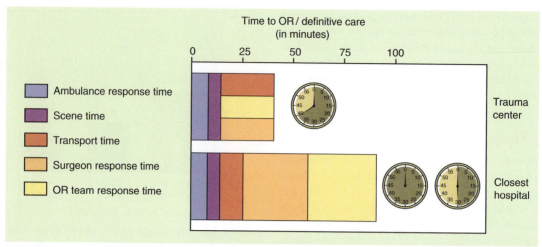

FIGURE 1-6   In locations in which trauma centers are available, bypassing hospitals not committed to the care of trauma patients can significantly improve patient care. In severely injured trauma patients, definitive patient care generally occurs in the operating room (OR). An extra 10 to 20 minutes spent en route to a hospital with an in-house surgeon and in-house OR staff will significantly reduce the time to definitive care in the OR. (*Blue,* EMS response time. *Purple,* on-scene time. *Red,* EMS transport time. *Orange,* surgical response from out of hospital. *Yellow,* OR team response from out of hospital.)

of 1:1 to replace lost blood, has produced impressive results by the military in Iraq and Afghanistan and now in the civilian community. These fluids are not available for use in the field and are another reason for rapid transport to the hospital. En route to the hospital balanced resuscitation (see Shock chapter) has proven to be important. Hemostasis (hemorrhage control) cannot always be achieved in the field or in the emergency department (ED); it must often be achieved in the operating room (OR). Therefore, in determining an appropriate facility to which a patient should be transported, it is important that the prehospital care provider consider the transport time to a given facility and the capabilities of that facility in the critical thinking process.

A trauma center that has a surgeon available either before or shortly after the arrival of the patient, a well-trained and trauma-experienced emergency medicine team, and an OR team immediately available can often have a trauma patient with life-threatening hemorrhage in the OR within 10–15 minutes of the patient's arrival and make the difference between life and death.

On the other hand, a hospital without such in-house surgical capabilities must await the arrival of the surgeon and the surgical team before transporting the patient from the ED to the OR. Additional time may then elapse before the hemorrhage can be controlled, resulting in an associated increase in mortality rate (Figure 1-6). There is a significant increase in survival if non-trauma centers are bypassed and all severely injured patients are taken to the trauma center.[22-29]

Experience, in addition to the initial training in surgery and trauma, is important. Studies have demonstrated that the more experienced surgeons in a busy trauma center had a better outcome than the less experienced trauma surgeons.[30,31]

History of Trauma Care in Emergency Medical Services

The stages and development of the management of the trauma patient can be divided roughly into four time periods as described by McSwain in the Scudder Oration of the American College of Surgeons in 1999.[32] This text, the PHTLS course, and care of the trauma patient are based on the principles developed and taught by the early pioneers of prehospital care. The list of these innovators is long; however, a few especially deserve recognition.

Ancient Period

All of the medical care that was accomplished in Egypt, Greece, and Rome, by the Israelites, and up to the time of Napoleon is classified as premodern EMS. There is much to be learned here, but most of the medical care was accomplished within some type of medical facility. Little was done by prehospital providers in the field.

Larrey Period

In the late 1700s, Baron Dominick Jean Larrey, Napoleon's chief military physician, recognized the need for prompt prehospital care. In 1797, he noted that "the remoteness of our ambulances deprive the wounded of the requisite attention. I was authorized to construct a carriage which I call flying ambulances."[33] He developed these horse-drawn "flying ambulances" for timely retrieval of warriors injured on the battlefield and introduced the premise that individuals working in these "flying ambulances" should be trained in medical care to provide on-scene and en route care for patients.

By the early 1800s, he had established the theory of prehospital care that we continue to use to this day:

- the "flying" ambulance
- proper training of medical personnel
- move into the field during battle for patient care and retrieval
- field control of hemorrhage
- transport to a nearby hospital
- provide care en route
- develop frontline hospitals

He also developed hospitals that were close to the front lines (much like the military of today) and stressed the rapid movement of patients from the field to medical care. Baron Larrey is now recognized as the **father of EMS in the modern era.**

Unfortunately, the type of care developed by Larrey was not used 60 years later at the beginning of the War Between the States by the Union Army in the United States. At the First Battle of Bull Run in August 1861, the wounded laid in the field—3000 for three days, 600 up to a week.[33,34] Jonathan Letterman was appointed Surgeon General and created a separate medical corps with better organized medical care. At the Second Battle of Bull Run a year later, there were 300 ambulances and attendants collected 10,000 wounded in 24 hours.[34]

In August 1864, the International Red Cross was created at the First Geneva Convention.[29] The convention recognized the neutrality of hospitals, of the sick and wounded, of all involved personnel, and of ambulances and guaranteed safe passage for ambulances and medical personnel to move the wounded. This was the first step in what we utilize today within the military as our Code of Conduct. This is an important component of the Tactical Combat Casualty Care Course, which is now an integral part of the PHTLS program.

Hospitals, Military, and Mortuaries

In 1865, the first private ambulance in the United States was created in Cincinnati, Ohio, at Cincinnati General Hospital.[34] Several EMS systems soon developed in the United States: Bellevue Hospital Ambulance[34] followed in New York in 1867; Grady Hospital Ambulance Service (the oldest continuously operating hospital-based ambulance) in Atlanta in the 1880s; Charity Hospital Ambulance Services created in 1885 by a surgeon, Dr. A. B. Miles in New Orleans; and many other facilities in the United States. These ambulance services were run basically by hospitals, by the military, or by mortuaries up until 1950.[32]

Some changes in medical care occurred during the various wars up until the end of World War II, but generally the system and the type of care rendered prior to arrival in the Battalion Aid station (Echelon II) or at the back door of the civilian hospital remained unchanged until the mid 1950s.

Many ambulances in the major cities with teaching hospitals were staffed by interns beginning their first year of training. The last ambulance service to require physicians on the ambulance runs was Charity Hospital in New Orleans in the 1960s. Despite the fact that physicians were present, most of the trauma care was primitive. The equipment and supplies were not changed from that used during the War Between the States.[32]

Farrington Era

The era of J.D. "Deke" Farrington, MD, began in 1950. Dr. Farrington, the **father of EMS in the United States**, stimulated the development of improved prehospital care with his landmark article, "Death in a Ditch."[35] In the late 1960s, Farrington and other early leaders, such as Oscar Hampton, MD, and Curtis Arts, MD, brought the United States into the modern era of EMS and prehospital care.[41] Dr. Farrington was actively involved in all aspects of ambulance care. His work as chairman of the committees that produced three of the initial documents establishing the basis of EMS—the essential equipment list for ambulances of the American College of Surgeons (ACS),[36] the KKK 1822 ambulance design specifications of the US Department of Transportation,[37] and the first emergency medical technician (EMT) basic training program—also propelled the idea and development of prehospital care. In addition to the efforts of Dr. Farrington, others actively helped promote the importance of prehospital care for the trauma victim. Robert Kennedy, MD, was the author of "Early Care of the Sick and Injured Patient."[38] Sam Banks, MD, with Dr. Farrington, taught the first prehospital training course to the Chicago Fire Department in 1957, which initiated proper care of the trauma patient.

A 1965 text edited and compiled by George J. Curry, MD, a leader of the ACS and its Committee on Trauma, stated: "Injuries sustained in accidents affect every part of the human body. They range from simple abrasions and contusions to multiple complex injuries involving many body tissues. This demands efficient and intelligent primary appraisal and care, on an individual basis, before transport. It is obvious that the services of trained ambulance attendants are essential. If we are to expect maximum efficiency from ambulance attendants, a special training program must be arranged."[38]

Although prehospital care was rudimentary when Curry wrote this passage, the words still hold true as prehospital care providers address the specific needs of the trauma patient in the field. The landmark white paper, "Accidental Death and Disability: the Neglected Disease of Modern Society," further accelerated the process in 1967.[39] The National Academy of Sciences/National Research Council issued this paper just one year after Curry's call.

Modern Era of Prehospital Care

The modern era of prehospital care began with the Dunlap and Associates report to the EMS Department of Transportation in 1968 defining the curriculum for EMT Ambulance Training. This training is now known as EMT-Basic.

The National Registry of EMTs was established in 1970 and developed the standards for testing and registration of trained EMS personal as advocated in the NSF/ACS white paper. Rocco Morando was the leader of the NREMT for many years and was associated with Drs. Farrington, Hampton, and Artz.

Curry's call for specialized training of ambulance attendants *for trauma* was initially answered by using the educational program developed by Drs. Farrington and Banks, by the publication of the "orange book" by the American Academy of Orthopedic Surgeons (first edited by Dr. Walter Hoyt), by the EMT training programs from NHTSA, and by the PHTLS training program during the past 25 years. The first training efforts were primitive but have progressed significantly in a relatively brief time.

The first textbook of this era was *Emergency Care and Transportation of the Sick and Injured.* This was the brain-child of Walter A. Hoyt Jr., MD, and was published in 1971 by the American Association of Orthopedic Surgeons.[32] This text is now in its 9th edition.

During this same period, the Glasgow Coma Scale was developed in Glasgow, Scotland, by Dr. Graham Teasdale and Dr. Bryan Jennett for research purposes. Dr. Howard Champion (the author of the Blast chapter in the military version of this textbook) brought it into the United States and incorporated it into the care of the trauma patient for assessment of the continued neurological status of the patient.[40] The Glasgow Coma Scale is a very sensitive indicator of improvement or deterioration of such patients.

In 1973, federal EMS legislation was created. Dr. David Boyd was in charge of this system. He divided the components of trauma care into 15 segments. One of these segments was education. This became the basis for the development of EMT-Basic, EMT-Intermediate, and EMT-Paramedic care throughout the United States. The curriculum was initially defined by the US Department of Transportation in the National Highway Traffic Safety Administration and became known as the National Standard Curriculum or the DOT curriculum. Dr. Nancy Caroline defined the standards and the curriculum for the first EMT-Paramedic program and wrote the initial textbook used in the training of EMT paramedics.

The Blue Star of Life was designed by the American Medical Association as the symbol of the "Medic Alert" indication that a patient had an important medical condition the EMS should note. It was given to the National Registry of EMTs (NREMT) by the AMA as the logo of that registration and testing organization. Because the American Red Cross would not allow the "Red Cross" logo to be used on ambulances as an emergency symbol, Lew Schwartz (chief of NHTSA's EMS branch) asked Dr. Farrington, who at the time was the chairman of the NREMT board, to allow NHTSA to use the emblem for ambulances. Permission was granted by Dr. Farrington and Rocco Morando (executive director of NREMT). It has since become an international symbol of Emergency Medical Services.[32] The National Association of EMTs was developed in 1975 by Jeffrey Harris with the financial support of NREMT.

The accomplishments of these great physicians, EMS providers, and organizations stand out; however, there are many more, too numerous to mention, who contributed to the development of EMS. To all of them, we owe a great debt of gratitude.

The modern era of EMS in the United States can essentially be divided into four periods[32]:

- Grab and run
  - No care—either in the field or en route, with rapid transportation to the hospital, frequently without anyone in the patient-care compartment—was the system prior to the 1950s.
- Field management and care
  - This period began with the publication of the national standard curriculum in 1969 continued until approximately 1975.
- Stay and play
  - From 1975 until mid-1980s, the trauma patient and the cardiac patient were treated exactly alike; that is, attempts to stabilize the patient in the field, often for prolonged amounts of time, were provided.
- No delay trauma care

In the mid-1980s it became apparent that the trauma patient was different from the cardiac patient. Trauma surgeons such as Frank Lewis, MD, and Donald Trunkey, MD, realized that, unlike the cardiac patient for whom all or most of the tools needed for re-establishment of cardiac output—CPR, external defibrillation, and supportive medications—were available to the properly trained EMT in the field, for the trauma patient, the most important tools—surgical control of internal hemorrhage and replacement of blood—were not available in the field. The importance of moving the patient rapidly to the correct hospital became apparent to both the field providers and the medical directors. This includes a facility with a well-trained trauma team comprised of emergency physicians, surgeons, trained nurses, O.R. staff, blood bank, registration and quality assurance processes, and all of the steps necessary for the management of the trauma patient. All of these resources are awaiting the arrival of the patient with the surgical team standing by to take the patient directly into the operating room. Over time, these standards have been modified to include such concepts as permissive hypotension (Dr. Ken Mattox) and Red Blood Cell: plasma transfusion (1:1) (Dr. John Holcomb). However, the bottom line of rapid availability of a well-equipped OR has not changed.

Rapid treatment of the trauma patient depends on a prehospital care system that offers easy access to the system. This access is aided by a single emergency phone number (e.g.,

9-1-1 in the United States, other numbers in other countries), a good communication system to dispatch the emergency medical unit, and well-prepared and well-trained prehospital care providers. Many people have been taught that early access and early CPR save the lives of those experiencing cardiac arrest. Trauma can be approached the same way. The principles just listed are the basis for good patient care; to these basic principles has been added the importance of internal hemorrhage control, which cannot be accomplished outside of the trauma center and operating room. Thus, rapid assessment, proper packaging, and rapid delivery of the patient to a facility with OR resources immediately available has become the additional principle that was not understood until the mid-1980s.

Reading the EMS Literature

A major goal of PHTLS has been to ensure that the practice recommendations presented in this text accurately represent the best medical evidence available at the time of publication in support of these recommendations. To that end, PHTLS began this process with the 6th edition and it is expanded in the 7th edition. We continue to add, as References and Suggested Readings, those manuscripts, sources, and resources that are fundamental components of each chapter and recommendation. (See Suggested Readings at the end of this chapter for further information on evaluating the EMS literature.) Every practitioner and health care provider should obtain, read, and critically evaluate the publications and sources that make up the basis for all the components of daily practice.

To accomplish this, an understanding of exactly what constitutes the medical literature and of how to interpret the various sources of information is essential. In many cases the first place that is accessed for information about a particular topic is a medical textbook. As our level of interest and sophistication grows, a search is undertaken to find the specific references that are referred to in those book chapters or to find what, if any, primary research studies have been performed and published. Then, after reviewing and analyzing the various sources, a decision can be made about the quality and strength of the evidence that will guide our decision making and patient care interventions.

Types of Evidence

There are a number of different systems for rating the quality and strength of medical evidence. Regardless of the exact rating system used, several common assessments can be found among them. The highest-quality source that leads to the strongest recommendation about the treatment under study is the randomized, double-blind controlled study. Studies of this type are usually referred to as *Class I evidence*. This type of study is considered to be the best type of study because: all patients entered into the study are *randomized* (meaning each patient has an equal chance of assignment to whatever type of treatment is being studied); the researchers as well as the patients do not know which type of treatment the subject is receiving *(double blinding)*; and investigators are controlling as many other aspects of the study as possible. These factors minimize the chances of any bias entering into the study or affecting the results or interpretation of the results.

Class II evidence generally includes the other types of studies that can be found in the medical literature, including nonrandomized non-blinded studies, retrospective case-control series, and cohort studies.

Finally, *Class III evidence* consists of case studies, case reports, consensus documents, textbook material, and medical opinion. Class III evidence is the weakest source of evidence, although often the easiest to obtain.

Unfortunately, if the literature related to prehospital care is critically reviewed, the majority qualifies as Class III evidence. There has been remarkably little research that would qualify as Class I. Much of the practice of medicine that has been applied to the prehospital setting has been adopted from and adapted to the out-of-hospital environment from the in-hospital delivery of emergency care. The result is that most of the prehospital care provided today is based on Class III evidence. However, more and more Class I and II studies related to prehospital care are being conducted. Unfortunately, Class I studies are limited in the United States by rigid informed-consent regulations. Specifically, with few exceptions, the medical practice of prehospital care is based on "expert" opinion usually found in textbook chapters, the credentials and qualifications of the individual offering that opinion, and the forcefulness and "volume" of the delivery of that opinion.

Recently, consensus seems to be building to utilize a system for grading the quality of evidence and the strength of a resulting clinical practice recommendation known as The Grades of Recommendation, Assessment, Development and Evaluation (GRADE). This system appraises the quality of evidence available and the benefits versus the risks of the intervention, and then develops a judgment about the strength of a particular treatment recommendation or intervention. Evidence is rated into one of four categories: high, moderate, low, very low quality. Based upon the quality of the evidence and the benefit/risk evaluation, the resulting recommendation is categorized as strong or weak.[1,42,43]

Steps in Evaluation

Every medical practitioner should read the medical literature and critically evaluate every study published that might alter treatment decisions in order to distinguish useful information and therapy from that which is useless or potentially even harmful. How, then, does one go about reading and critically evaluating the medical literature?

FIGURE 1-7 **Suggested Journals for Review**

Academic Emergency Medicine
American Journal of Emergency Medicine
Annals of Emergency Medicine
Journal of Emergency Medicine
Journal of Trauma
Prehospital Emergency Care

FIGURE 1-8 **Performing a Computerized Literature Search**

Medline can be accessed through the National Library of Medicine Web site at the following Web site address: www.ncbi.nlm.nih.gov/pubmed.

To perform a journal search for articles and studies, it is necessary to enter search terms into Medline that will be used as key words to find appropriate articles. The more specific that you can be with the terms, the more likely you are to find articles that will meet your needs. However, being too specific can occasionally exclude articles that might also apply. Therefore, a good strategy to follow is to first conduct a search using very specific terms and then do a follow-up search with more generic terms. For example, if you are interested in finding articles about cricothyroidotomy in the prehospital setting, the initial search you perform might be done using the terms "Cricothyroidotomy" and "Prehospital." The next search might be performed using the terms "Airway management" and "Emergency Medical Services," recognizing that "airway management" may yield articles that include not only cricothyroidotomy but other forms of airway management as well.

The first step in this process is to develop a list of journals that will form the foundation of a regular literature review. This list should comprise not only those journals with the desired specialty in their name, but also those publications that address related specialties or topics and have a high likelihood of also publishing applicable studies (Figure 1-7).

An alternative to reviewing multiple journals is to perform a computerized literature search if there is a particular topic of interest. The use of computerized search engines such as Medline or Ovid allows the computer to search a massive database of multiple medical journals and automatically develop a list of suggested studies and publications (Figure 1-8).

The next step is to review the title of every article in the table of contents of each of the selected journals to narrow down the article choices to those that clearly relate to the topic of interest. It would be impossible to read each of the selected journals from cover to cover, nor is it necessary. By reviewing the table of contents, articles that are of no interest can be immediately dismissed.

Once the selection has been narrowed, there are still a number of preliminary actions to take before reading the text of the article. Look at the authors listed on the articles to see if any are already known for their work in this area. Next, read the summary or abstract of the article to see if this overview of the article fulfils the expectations generated when the title was first reviewed. Then, review the site where the study was conducted to assess the similarities, differences, and applicability to the setting in which the results of the study may be subsequently applied. It must be stressed that reading the abstract alone is not enough. It serves only as the "teaser" to determine whether the full article should be reviewed. Medical practice should never be changed based on the abstract.

Once these initial points have been evaluated, the full text of the article is now read and critically assessed. In doing so, several specific issues are important to determine. The first issue is to *evaluate the study and the randomization of the patients* entered into the study. Every patient included should have had the same probability of receiving one or the other treatments or interventions being compared in the study, and that probability should be known beforehand. The method for assigning patients to their treatment should be described and should be similar to the flip of a coin.

Next, the *patient population* entered into the study is assessed to determine the similarities or differences with the target population for which the study conclusions will be implemented. To do so, adequate information must be provided in the text describing the clinical and sociodemographic makeup of the study population. Ideally, studies that will be used to alter the care provided in the prehospital setting should have been performed in the prehospital setting. As Dan Spaite, MD, stated "Strong evidence for efficacy of an intervention does not mean that it will be effective when applied in the field."[44]

The next issue for consideration is the *outcome measure* selected by the authors. All outcomes that are clinically relevant should be considered and reported in the study. For example, cardiac arrest studies may describe such endpoints or outcomes as cardiac rhythm conversion, return of spontaneous circulation, survival to hospital admission, or survival to discharge from the hospital.

Analysis of the *results* section also requires critical review. Just as it is important to evaluate the study population and entry criteria, it is equally important to see if all patients entered into the study at the beginning are accounted for at the end of the study. Specifically, the authors should describe any criteria used to exclude patients from the study analysis. Simple addition by the reader of the various treatment groups or subgroups will quickly confirm if all patients were accounted for. The authors should also describe occurrences that might introduce bias into the results. For example, the authors should report mishaps such as control patients accidentally receiving the treatment or study patients receiving other diagnostics or interventions.

In addition, the clinical, as well as the statistical, significance of the results are important to consider. Although the *statistical* analyses may be difficult to understand, a basic comprehension of statistical test selection and utilization will validate the statistical tests performed. Equal to and perhaps more important than the statistical significance of a result is the *clinical* significance of the reported result. For example, in evaluating the effect of a new antihypertensive medication, the statistical analysis may show that the new drug causes a statistically significant decrease in blood pressure of 4 mm Hg. Clinically, however, the reported decrease is insignificant. Thus, the health care provider must assess not only the statistical significance of the result but also the clinical significance.

If all the prior issues have been answered satisfactorily, the last issue relates to the *implementation* of the study results and conclusion in the reader's health care system. To determine the practicality of applying the therapy, the authors needed to describe the treatment in sufficient detail, the intervention or therapy must be available for use, and it must be clinically sensible in the planned setting.

Some differences exist in the evaluation of consensus statements, overviews, and textbook chapters. Ideally, the statement or overview should address a specific, focused question. The authors should describe the criteria used to select the articles included as references, and the reader will determine the appropriateness of these criteria. This in turn will help determine the likelihood that important studies were included and not missed. In addition, the reference list should be reviewed for known studies that should have been included.

A high-quality overview or consensus statement will include a discussion of the process by which the *validity* of the included studies was appraised. The validity assessment should be reproducible regardless of who actually performed the appraisal. Also, multiple studies with similar results help support the conclusions and ultimate decision about whether or not to change current practice.

Similar to the review of individual studies, the review and assessment of consensus statements, overviews, and textbook chapters include a determination of whether all clinically relevant outcomes were considered and discussed and whether the results can be applied to the reader's patient-care setting. This also includes an analysis of the benefits versus the potential risks and harm.

The final step in evaluation is to determine when a publication should cause a *change in daily medical practice*. Ideally, any change in medical practice will result from a study of the highest quality, specifically a randomized, controlled, double-blind study. The conclusion of that study will be based on results that have been critically evaluated, have both statistical and clinical significance, and have been reviewed and judged to be valid. The study should be the best information currently available on the issue. In addition, the change in practice must be feasible for the system planning to make the change, and the benefit of making the change must outweigh the risks.

All the medical practice in the out-of-hospital setting should be based on high-quality, Class I evidence that supports practice. As noted, however, most of the EMS literature qualifies as Class III evidence.

SUMMARY

Trauma is the leading cause of death in patients under the age of 44 years. An organized, systematic approach to the care of these patients can improve patient survival. This organized approach begins initially with efforts to prevent injury from occurring. When injury does occur, the organized and systematic response of the entire health care delivery team, beginning in the prehospital setting, will help decrease the morbidity and mortality of traumatic injury.

References

1. Guyatt G, Baumann M, Adrizzoo-Harris D, et al: Grading strength of recommendations and quality of evidence in clinical guidelines: Report from an American College of Chest Physicians task force. *Chest* 129:174, 2006.
2. American College of Surgeons Committee on Trauma: *Advanced Trauma Life Support (ATLS) Manual,* ed 8, 2008, American College of Surgeons, Chicago, IL.
3. US Casualties in Iraq. http://www.globalsecurity.org/military/ops/iraq_casualties.htm. Accessed February 9, 2010.
4. US Department of Transportation, National Highway Traffic Safety Administration: Not-in-Traffic Surveillance 2007—Highlights. In NHTSA's National Center for Statistics and Analysis: *Traffic Safety Facts,* HS 811 085, Washington, DC, 2009.
5. Townsend CM Jr, Beauchamp RD, Evers BM, Mattox KL (eds.): *Sabiston Textbook of Surgery,* ed 18, Philadelphia, 2008, Saunders.
6. National Safety Commission: *Highlights from Injury Facts, 2009 Edition.* http://www.nsc.org/news_resources/injury_and_death_statistics/Pages/HighlightsFromInjuryFacts.aspx. Accessed November 6, 2009.
7. World Health Organization: *Global Burden of Disease,* Switzerland, 2004 Update, WHO Press.
8. National Center for Injury Prevention and Control: *Wisqars leading causes of death reports, 1999–2006.* Centers for Disease Control and Prevention. http://webappa.cdc.gov/sasweb/ncipc/leadcaus10.html. Accessed November 6, 2009.
9. US Department of Transportation, National Highway Traffic Safety Administration: Motorcycles. In NHTSA's National Center

for Statistics and Analysis: *Traffic Safety Facts*, HS 810 990, Washington, DC, 2007.

10. Cars Blog: *Motorcycle Death Rates Doubled; Supersport Bikes the Most Dangerous.* September 18, 2007. http://blogs.consumerreports.org/cars/2007/09/motorcycle-deat.html. Accessed January 25, 2010.

11. Krisberg K: Motorcycle safety, helmets an issue as U S deaths increase: More Than 5,000 US Deaths in 2007. *The Nations Health* 38(9):1–20, November 1, 2008.

12. US Secretary of Transportation Mary Peters Announces Historic Drop in Highway Fatalities and Rate. August 14, 2008. www.dot.gov/affairs/dot11308.

13. Mothers Against Drunk Driving: Profile, Irving, TX, 2009, Center for Consumer Freedom. www.activistcash.com/organization_overview.cfm/oid/17. Accessed January 25, 2010.

14. Trunkey DD: Trauma. *Sci Am* 249(2):28, August 1983.

15. R Adams Cowley Shock Trauma Center: Tribute to R. Adams Cowley, MD. Accessed March 27, 2008. www.umm.edu/shocktrauma/history.htm.

16. Demetriades D, Chan L, Cornwell EE, et al: Paramedic vs. private transportation of trauma patients: Effect on outcome. *Arch Surg* 131(2):133–138, February 1996.

17. Cornwell EE, Belzberg H, Hennigan K, et al: Emergency medical services (EMS) vs. non-EMS transport of critically injured patients: A prospective evaluation. *Arch Surg* 135(3):315–319, March 2000.

18. Smith S, Hildebrandt D: Effect of workday vs. after-hours on door to balloon time with paramedic out-of-hospital catheterization laboratory activation for STEMI. *Acad Emerg Med* 14(5 Supp. 1): S126–127, May 2007.

19. Tantisiriwat W, Jiar W, Ngamkasem H, et al: Clinical outcomes of fast track managed care system for acute ST elevation myocardial infarction (STEMI) Patients: Chonburi Hospital Experience. *J Med Assoc Thai* 91(6):822–827, June 2008.

20. So DY, Ha AC, Turek MA, et al: Comparison of mortality patterns in patients with ST-elevation myocardial infarction arriving by emergency medical services vs. self-transport (From the Prospective Ottawa Hospital STEMI Registry). *Am J Cardiol* 97(4):458–461, February 15, 2006.

21. Bjorklund E, Stenestrand U, Lindback J, et al: Prehospital diagnosis and start of treatment reduces time delay and mortality in real-life patients with STEMI. *J Electrocardiol* 38(4 Supp.):186, October 2005.

22. Trauma Victims' Survival May Depend on Which Trauma Center Treats Them. October 2005. http://news.bio-medicine.org/medicine-news-3/Trauma-victims-survival-may-depend-on-which-trauma-center-treats-them-8343-1/. Accessed January 25, 2010.

23. Peleg K, Aharonson-Daniel L, Stein M, et al: Increased survival among severe trauma patients: The impact of a national trauma system. *Arch Surg* 139(11):1231–1236, November 2004.

24. Edwards W: Emergency medical systems significantly increase patient survival rates, Part 2. *Can Doct* 48(12):20–24, December 1982.

25. Haas B, Jurkovich GJ, Wang J, et al: Survival advantage in trauma centers: Expeditious intervention or experience? *J Am Coll* 208(1):28–36, January 2009.

26. Scheetz LJ: Differences in survival, length of stay, and discharge disposition of older trauma patients admitted to trauma centers and nontrauma center hospitals. *J Nurs Scholarsh* 37(4):361–366, 2005.

27. Norwood S, Fernandez L, England J: The early effects of implementing American College of Surgeons level II criteria on transfer and survival rates at a rurally based community hospital. *J Trauma* 39(2):240–244; discussion 244–245, August 1995.

28. Kane G, Wheeler NC, Cook S, et al: Impact of the Los Angeles county trauma system on the survival of seriously injured patients, *J Trauma* 32(5):576–583, May 1992.

29. Hedges JR, Adams AL, Gunnels MD: ATLS practices and survival at rural level III trauma hospitals, 1995–1999. *Prehosp Emerg Care* 6(3):299–305, July–September 2002.

30. Konvolinka CW, Copes WS, Sacco WJ: Institution and per-surgeon volume vs. survival outcome in Pennsylvania's trauma centers. *Am J Surg* 170(4):333–340, October 1995.

31. Margulies DR, Cryer HG, McArthur DL, et al: Patient volume per surgeon does not predict survival in adult level I trauma centers. *J Trauma* 50(4):597–601; discussion 601–603, April 2001.

32. McSwain NE: Prehospital care from Napoleon to Mars: The surgeon's role. *J Am Coll Surg* 200(44):487–504, April 2005.

33. Larrey, D. J.: *Mémoires de chirurgie militaire, et campagnes.* (Memoirs of Military Surgery and Campaigns of the French Armies) Paris, J. Smith and F. Buisson, 1812–1817. English translation with notes by R. W. Hall of volumes 1–3 in 2 volumes, Baltimore, 1814. English translation of volume 4 by J. C. Mercer, Philadelphia, 1832.

34. Rockwood CA, Mann CM, Farrington JD, et al: History of emergency medical services in the United States. *J Trauma* 16(4):299–308, April 1976.

35. Farrington JD: Death in a ditch. *Bull Am Coll Surg* 52(3):121–132, May–June 1967.

36. Federal Specifications for Ambulance, KKK-A-1822D. United States General Services Administration, Specifications Section, November 1994.

37. Iowa Department of Transportation: EMS History. Emergency Medical Services. December 2004. Accessed February 10, 2010.

38. Kennedy R: *Early Care of the Sick and Injured Patient*, Chicago, 1964, American College of Surgeons.

39. Committee on Trauma and Committee on Shock, Division of Medical Sciences: *Accidental Death and Disability: The Neglected Disease of Modern Society*, Washington, DC, 1966, National Academy of Sciences/National Research Council.

40. Champion H. Personal verbal communication, 1999.

41. Ali J, Adam RU, Gana TJ, et al: Effect of the Prehospital Trauma Life Support program (PHTLS) on prehospital trauma care. *J Trauma* 42(5):786–790, May 1997.

42. Atkins D, Best D, Briss PA, et al: Grading quality of evidence and strength of recommendations (GRADE). *BMJ* 328:1490, 2004.

43. Guyatt GH, Oxman AD, Vist G, et al: Rating quality of evidence and strength of recommendations GRADE: An emerging consensus on rating quality of evidence and strength of recommendations. *BMJ* 336:924, 2008.

44. Spaite D: Prehospital Evidence-Based Guidelines (presentation). From *Evidence to EMS Practice: Building the National Model,* a Consensus-Building Conference sponsored by The National Highway Traffic Safety Administration, the Federal Interagency Committee on EMS and The National EMS Advisory Council. September 2008.

Suggested Reading

Callaham M: Quantifying the scanty science of prehospital emergency care, *Ann Emerg Med* 30:785, 1997.

Cone DC, Lewis RJ: Should this study change my practice? *Acad Emerg Med* 10:417, 2003.

Haynes RB, McKibbon KA, Fitzgerald D, et al: How to keep up with the medical literature: II. Deciding which journals to read regularly. *Ann Intern Med* 105:309, 1986.

Keim SM, Spaite DW, Maio RF, et al: Establishing the scope and methodological approach to out-of-hospital outcomes and effectiveness research, *Acad Emerg Med* 11:1067, 2004.

Lewis RJ, Bessen HA: Statistical concepts and methods for the reader of clinical studies in emergency medicine, *J Emerg Med* 9:221, 1991.

MacAvley D: Critical appraisal of medical literature: an aid to rational decision making, *Fam Pract* 12:98, 1995.

Reed JF III, Salen P, Bagher P: Methodological and statistical techniques: What do residents really need to know about statistics? *J Med Syst* 27:233, 2003.

Sackett DL: How to read clinical journals: V. To distinguish useful from useless or even harmful therapy. *Can Med Assoc J* 124:1156, 1981.

CHAPTER 2

Injury Prevention

CHAPTER OBJECTIVES

At the completion of this chapter, the reader will be able to do the following:

✓ Describe the concept of energy as a cause of injury.

✓ Build a Haddon Matrix for a type of injury of interest.

✓ Relate the importance of accurate, attentive scene observations and documentation of data by emergency medical services (EMS) providers to the success of injury prevention initiatives.

✓ Assist in the development, implementation, and evaluation of injury prevention programs in his or her community or EMS organization.

✓ Describe and advocate for the role of EMS in injury prevention, to include:

  ✓ Individual
  ✓ Family
  ✓ Community
  ✓ Professional
  ✓ Organizational
  ✓ Coalitions of organizations

✓ Identify strategies that prehospital care providers can implement that will reduce the risk of injury.

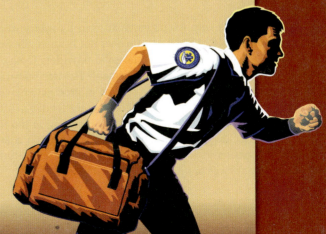

SCENARIO

Jose and Gwen are putting their rig back in service after a car crash that ended with three fatalities, including an infant and a child. "Jose, I just can't stop thinking about how this would have had a very different ending if this woman had put her babies in infant and child seats. She might have survived herself if she had used her seat belt and shoulder harness."

"I'm with you, Gwen. Someone needs to do something about compliance with seat belt and child seat laws around here."

"Do you think it's just ignorance of the dangers, or is it an economic issue, Jose?"

"Well, I suppose buying the seats might be an economic issue, but the unrestrained driver made a conscious decision not to use seat belts. There must be a way to get the message out."

Is prevention a realistic approach in preventing injury and death in car crashes and other causes of traumatic injury?

Is there evidence that compliance with seat belt and safety seats has an impact in preventing injury and death?

What can we as providers do to prevent these types of deaths and injuries?

A major impetus in the development of modern emergency medical services (EMS) systems was the publication of the 1966 white paper by the National Academy of Sciences/National Research Council (NAS/NRC), *Accidental Death and Disability: the Neglected Disease of Modern Society.* The paper spotlighted shortcomings in injury management in the United States and helped launch a formal system of on-scene care and rapid transport for patients injured as a result of "accidents." This educational initiative was instrumental in the creation of a more efficient system to deliver prehospital care to sick and injured patients.[1]

Death and disability from injury in the United States have fallen since the publication of the white paper.[2] Despite this progress, however, injury remains a major public health problem. More than 179,000 Americans die from injuries annually, and millions more are adversely affected to some degree.[3] However, injury is a global problem as well. Over 5 million people worldwide died from injuries in 2002, accounting for 9% of deaths worldwide. Injuries remain a leading cause of death for all age groups.[4] For some age groups, particularly children, teenagers, and young adults, injury is *the* leading cause of death.

The desire to care for patients stricken by injury draws many into the field of EMS. The Prehospital Trauma Life Support (PHTLS) course teaches prehospital providers to be efficient and effective in injury management. The need for well-trained prehospital providers to care for injured patients will always exist. However, the *most* efficient and effective method to combat injury is to prevent it from happening in the first place. Health care providers at all levels play an active role in injury prevention to achieve the best results for not only the community at large but for themselves as well.

Even in 1966, the authors of the NAS/NRC white paper recognized the importance of injury prevention when they wrote:

> The long-term solution to the injury problem is prevention ... Prevention of accidents involves training in the home, in the school, and at work, augmented by frequent pleas for safety in the news media; first aid courses and public meetings; and inspection and surveillance by regulatory agencies.[1]

Prehospital personnel can easily play an active role in most, if not all, of the current recommendations for injury prevention.

Prevention of some diseases, such as rabies, has been so effective that the occurrence of a single case makes front-page news. Public health officials recognize that prevention results in the greatest reward toward the amelioration of disease. Emergency medical technician (EMT) curricula have long included formal instruction in scene safety and personal protective equipment as a means of self-injury prevention for the EMT. To spur EMS systems to take a more active role in community prevention strategies, the *EMS Agenda for the Future*, developed by and for the EMS community, lists prevention as one of 14 attributes to develop further in order to "improve community health and result in more appropriate use of acute health resources."[5] To this end, the US Department of Transportation (DOT) paramedic curriculum and now the National EMS Core Content include community injury-prevention training.

EMS systems are transforming themselves from a solely reactionary discipline to a broader, more effective discipline that includes more emphasis on prevention. This chapter introduces key concepts of injury prevention to the prehospital care provider.

Scope of the Problem

Death from injuries is a major health problem worldwide, resulting in more than 14,000 deaths *daily* (Figure 2-1). In most countries, regardless of their level of development, injuries appear among the five leading causes of death.[4] Although causes of injury deaths vary little between countries, wide variability does exist between which causes have the greatest impact on specific age groups. Because of economic, social, and developmental issues, the cause of injury-

---

FIGURE 2-1   Worldwide Injury-Related Statistics, 2004

INJURY OVERALL

- The top eight injury-related causes of mortality in order were:
  1. Road traffic injuries
  2. Self-inflicted violence
  3. Interpersonal violence
  4. Drowning
  5. Poisoning
  6. War
  7. Falls
  8. Fires
- An estimated 5 million people die worldwide from injuries.
- Injuries accounted for 9% of the world's deaths and 16% of all disabilities.
- For persons aged 5–44, six of the top 10 leading causes of death are injury-related.
- The burden of disease related to injuries, particularly road traffic injuries, is expected to rise dramatically by the year 2020.
- Twice as many men die from injury as women; fire-related deaths are the notable exception.
- Males in Africa have the highest injury-related mortality rates.
- More than 90% of all injury-related deaths occur in low income and middle income countries.
- Injury accounts for 12% of the total *years of potential life lost* either from premature death or from disability.

ROAD TRAFFIC INJURY

- An estimated 1.2 million people died as a result of road traffic injuries, and 50 million more were injured or disabled.
- Road traffic injury is the leading cause of death for children and youth aged 10–24.
- Road traffic mortality for males is almost three times higher than for females.
- Southeast Asia accounts for the highest percentage of road traffic injury deaths.

FIRE-RELATED BURNS

- 300,000 fire-related burns occurred.
- Females in Southeast Asia have the highest fire-related burn mortality rates.
- Children under age 5 years and elderly persons have the highest fire-related mortality rates.
- Southeast Asia alone accounts for just over one half of fire-related burn deaths.

DROWNING

- 450,000 persons drowned in 2000.
- 97% of drowning deaths occurred in low- and middle-income countries.
- Among the various age groups, children under age 5 years have the highest drowning mortality rates, accounting for more than 50%.
- Males in Africa and the western Pacific have the highest drowning mortality rates.

FALLS

- 283,000 people died as a result of falls in 2000.
- A quarter of all fatal falls occurred in high-income countries.
- In all regions of the world, adults over age 70, particularly women, have the highest fall mortality rate.
- Europe and the western Pacific combined account for almost 60% of the total number of fall-related deaths.

POISONING

- An estimated 315,000 people died from poisoning worldwide.
- More than 94% of fatal poisonings occurred in low- and middle-income countries.
- The overall poisoning rate among males in Europe is approximately three times higher than the rate in either gender in any other world region.
- The European region accounts for more than one third of all poisoning deaths worldwide.

INTERPERSONAL VIOLENCE

- An estimated 520,000 people died worldwide as a result of interpersonal violence.
- 95% of homicides occurred in low- and middle-income countries.
- The highest interpersonal violence rates are found in the Americas among males age 15 to 29 years.
- Among females, Africa has the highest mortality rate from interpersonal violence.

SUICIDE

- 815,000 people worldwide committed suicide.
- 86% of all suicides occurred in low- and middle-income countries.
- Women in China have a suicide rate that is approximately twice that of women in other parts of the world.
- More than 50% of suicides occur in persons age 15 to 44 years.

All figures compiled from World Health Organization data.

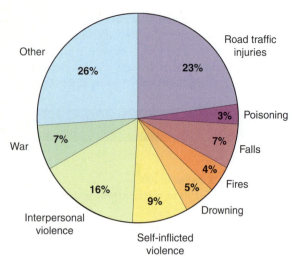

FIGURE 2-2 Distribution of global injury mortality by cause, 2000.
(From World Health Organization: *The Injury Chart Book,* Geneva, 2002, WHO.)

related death varies from country to country and even region to region within the same country.

For example, in low-income and middle-income countries of the western Pacific, the leading injury-related causes of death are road traffic injuries, drowning, and suicide, whereas in Africa the leading causes are road traffic injuries, war, and interpersonal violence. In high-income countries of the Americas, the leading cause of death among people between 15 and 29 years of age is road traffic injuries. In low-income and middle-income countries of the Americas, the leading cause is interpersonal violence for the same age group.[4] Figure 2-2 demonstrates that injury plays a leading role in the global burden of disease.

In the United States, injuries are the fifth leading cause of death, accounting for more than 179,000 deaths annually[3]

(Figure 2-3). Injury is an especially serious problem for the youth of America as well as of most industrialized nations of the world. In the United States, injury kills more children and young adults than all diseases combined (over 32,000 in 2006).[3]

Unfortunately, deaths from injury are only the tip of the iceberg. The "injury triangle" provides a more complete picture of the *public health impact* of injury (Figure 2-4). In the United States in 2006, in addition to the 167,000 people who died from injury, another 1.9 million were hospitalized because of nonfatal injuries. Injury also resulted in more than 31 million emergency-department visits.[3]

The impact can be further realized by examining the number of *years of potential life lost* (YPLL) as a result of injury. YPLL is calculated by subtracting age-at-death from a fixed age of the group under examination, usually 65 or 70 years or the life expectancy of the group. Injury unnecessarily kills or disables people of all ages, but it disproportionately affects children, youth, and young adults, especially in industrialized nations. Because injury is the leading killer of Americans between 1 and 44 years of age, it is responsible for more YPLL than any other cause. In 2006, injury stole an estimated 3.68 million years from its victims compared with 1.8 million years for cancer, even though cancer claims more lives than injury.[3]

A third measure of injury severity can be demonstrated financially. The *economics of injury* are felt far beyond the patient and the immediate family. The cost of injury is spread across a wide spectrum. All members of society feel the effect because the costs of injury are borne by federal and other agencies, private insurance programs that pass the expense on to other subscribers, and employers as well as the patient. As a result, everyone pays when an individual is seriously injured. Cost estimates for injury run as high as $325 billion annually, which includes the direct cost of medical care and indirect costs such as lost earnings.[6] Data from the World Health Organization (WHO) indicate that prevention activities are a good investment:

FIGURE 2-3 Ranking of Causes of Injury-Related Deaths by Age Groups, 2006

	Age Groups										All Ages (number of deaths)
	<1	1–4	5–9	10–14	15–24	25–34	35–44	45–54	55–64	65+	
Unintentional Injury (number of deaths)	5th (1,147)	Leading (1,610)	Leading (1,044)	Leading (1,214)	Leading (16,229)	Leading (14,954)	Leading (17,534)	3rd (19,675)	4th (11,446)	9th (36,689)	5th (121,599)
Intentional Injury Suicide	*	*	19th	4th	3rd	2nd	4th	5th	8th	18th	11th (33,300)
Homicide	14th	4th	4th	3rd	2nd	3rd	6th	13th	17th	*	15th (18,573)

*Data not applicable or available
Extracted from: National Vital Statistics System, National Center for Health Statistics, CDC, Office of Statistics and Programming, National Center for Injury Prevention and Control, CDC: Ranking of Causes of Injury-Related Deaths by Age Groups, 2006.

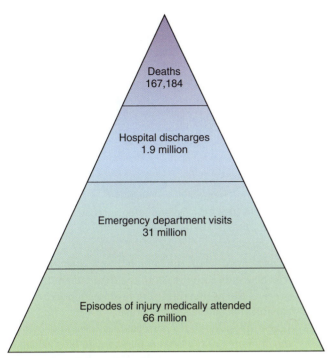

FIGURE 2-4   Injury triangle.
(Data from the US Department of Health and Human Services, Centers for Disease Control and Prevention, National Center for Health Statistics. *Injury in the United States 2007 Chartbook.*)

- Every US dollar invested in motorcycle helmets results in a $32 savings of medical costs.
- Seatbelts decrease the risk of ejection and suffering serious or fatal injury by 40–65%.

The toll of injury in terms of morbidity, mortality, and economic stress is excessive:

Injuries have always been a threat to the public's well-being, but until the mid-twentieth century, infectious diseases overshadowed the terrible contribution injury made to human morbidity and mortality. Public health's success in other areas has left injury as a major public health concern, one that has been termed "the neglected epidemic."[6]

Society is calling on all segments of the medical community to increase its prevention activities. With more than 600,000 prehospital providers in the United States alone, EMS systems can make a tremendous contribution to community-based injury-prevention efforts.

Injury in EMS

Obtaining a clear picture of the impact of injury on the EMS provider is difficult because no single, national data-gathering process deals with the industry. Even determining how many providers are in the United States is only an estimate of 600,000 to 832,000. However, several studies and publications have sought to answer this question.

EMS personnel are undoubtedly exposed to a wide variety of situations that can result in worker injury. They go where people are hurt and sick. Sometimes those scenes are unsecured, despite the best efforts of EMS personnel and law enforcement, because these scenes involve people in emotional and physical crisis. Even the very nature of the work presents opportunities for injury. Just driving to the scene can be hazardous. Lifting, exposure to environmental hazards and infectious diseases, and the stress of the job also present opportunities for injury.

For the years 1992 through 1997, an estimated 12.7 fatalities occurred per 100,000 workers per year in EMS.[7,8] This compares with a national average fatality rate of 5.0 per 100,000 for all workers over the same period. More than 58% of those EMS fatalities involved ambulance crashes; 9% involved assault or homicide. As with fatalities, estimating nonfatal injury can be difficult as well. However, one serious, disabling injury requiring hospitalization per 31,616 dispatches has been documented among urban providers.[9]

These numbers reveal a disturbing truth. "The most dangerous times for EMS personnel are when they are inside their truck when it is moving or when they are working at a crash scene near other moving vehicles."[10] It is critical that EMS personnel know and understand the concepts of injury and injury prevention so that the risks inherent in EMS can be identified and corrected. From almost the first day of EMT education, students are taught that no one is more important at the scene than the EMT, so his or her safety must come first. Seat belt use in the ambulance is the first step of safety.

Concepts of Injury

Definition of Injury

A discussion of injury prevention should begin with a definition of the term *injury*. The wide variability of the causes of injury initially represented a major hurdle in its study and prevention. For example, what does a fractured hip caused by an elderly person's fall have in common with a self-inflicted gunshot wound to the head of a young adult? All possible causes of injury—from vehicle crash, to stabbing, to suicide, to drowning—have one factor in common: energy transfer. *Injury* is now commonly defined as a harmful event that arises from the release of specific forms of physical energy or barriers to normal flow of energy.[11]

Typically, energy exists in five physical forms: mechanical, chemical, thermal, radiation, or electrical.

- *Mechanical energy* is the energy that an object contains when it is in motion. For example, mechanical energy, the most common cause of injury, is transferred from a vehicle when an unrestrained driver collides with the windshield during a vehicle crash.

- *Chemical energy* is the energy that results from the interaction of a chemical with exposed human tissue. For instance, chemical energy occurs when a curious child drinks ammonia found in an unlocked cabinet in the kitchen.
- *Thermal energy* is the energy associated with increased temperature and heat. For example, thermal energy causes injury when a cook sprays lighter fluid on actively burning charcoal in an outdoor grill, which then flashes in his face.
- *Radiation energy* is any electromagnetic wave that travels in rays (such as x-rays) and has no physical mass to it. Radiation energy produces sunburn to the teenager searching for a golden tan for the summer.
- *Electrical energy* results from the movement of electrons between two points. It is associated with direct injury as well as thermal injury and, for example, damages the skin, nerves, and blood vessels of a prehospital care provider who fails to do a proper scene assessment before touching a vehicle that hit a power pole.

The body requires basic elements, such as oxygen and heat, to produce the internal energy needed to function properly. If conditions arise that prevent the body from using these necessary elements, injury can result. Suffocation and hypothermia are physical injuries that result from an interruption of the body's normal energy flow.

Any form of physical energy in sufficient quantity can cause tissue damage. The body can tolerate energy transfer within certain limits; however, an injury results if this threshold is breached. A bullet fired from a pistol at point-blank range easily passes through skin and soft tissue, causing massive injury. If the intended victim is far enough away, theoretically, the potential victim can simply stick out a hand, and the bullet would hit his palm and fall harmlessly to the ground. As the energy dissipates in the air on its flight, the bullet does not have enough energy on impact to exceed the body's tolerance level. Such a situation rarely happens.

Energy Out of Control

People harness and use all five forms of energy in many productive endeavors every day. In these situations, energy is under control and is not allowed to affect the body adversely. A person's ability to maintain control of energy depends on two factors: task performance and task demand.[12] As long as a person's ability to perform a task exceeds the demands of a task, energy is released in a controlled, usable manner.

In the following three situations, however, demand may exceed performance, leading to an uncontrolled release of energy:

1. *When the difficulty of the task suddenly exceeds the individual's performance ability.* For example, a prehospital care provider may operate an ambulance safely during normal driving conditions but

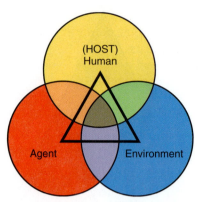

FIGURE 2-5   Epidemiological triad.

loses control when the vehicle hits a sheet of black ice. The sudden increase in the demands of the task exceeds the prehospital care provider's performance capabilities and leads to a crash.

2. *When the individual's performance level falls below the demands of the task.* A person who falls asleep at the wheel of a vehicle while driving down a country road experiences a sudden drop in performance with no change in task demand leading to a crash.

3. *When both factors change simultaneously.* Talking on a cellular phone while driving may reduce a driver's concentration on the road. If an animal darts in front of the vehicle, task demand suddenly rises. Under normal circumstances, the driver may be able to handle the increased demands of the task. A drop in concentration at the very moment when additional skill is required may lead to a crash.

Thus, injury may result when there is a release of energy in an uncontrolled manner in proximity to victims.

Injury as a Disease

The disease process has been studied for years. It is now understood that three factors must be present and interact simultaneously for an illness to occur: (1) an agent that causes the illness; (2) a host in which the agent can reside; and (3) a suitable environment in which the agent and host can come together. Once public health professionals recognized this "epidemiological triad," they discovered how to combat the disease (Figure 2-5). Eradication of certain diseases has been possible by vaccinating the host, destroying the agent with antibiotics, reducing environmental transmission through improved sanitation, or a combination of all three.

Only since the late 1940s has significant exploration of the *injury process* occurred. Pioneers in the study of injury demonstrated that despite the obviously different results, illness and injury behave similarly. Both require the presence of the three elements of the epidemiological triad, and therefore, both are treated as a disease:

1. For an injury to occur, a host (i.e., the human) must exist. As with illness, *susceptibility* of the host does not remain constant from individual to individual; it varies as a result of internal and external factors. *Internal* factors include intelligence, gender, and reaction time. *External* factors include intoxication, anger, and social beliefs. Susceptibility also varies over time within the same person.

2. As described previously, the agent of injury is *energy*. Velocity, shape, material, and time of exposure to the object that releases the energy all play a role in whether the host's tolerance level is overwhelmed.

3. The host and agent must come together in an environment that allows the two to interact. Typically, the environment is divided into physical and social components. *Physical* environmental factors can be seen and touched. *Social* environmental factors include attitudes, beliefs, and judgments. For example, teenagers are more likely to participate in risk-taking behavior (the physical component) because they have more of a sense of invincibility (the social component) than other age groups.

The characteristics of the host, agent, and environment change with time and circumstance:

To illustrate, think of the components of the Epidemiological Triad as constantly turning wheels. Inside each wheel are pie-shaped sections, one for each possible circumstantial variable—good and bad. The three wheels turn at different rates, so different characteristics interact (meet) at different times and in different combinations. Some combinations predict that no injury will occur; some predict disaster.[13]

In the case of injury, the host might be a curious, mobile 2-year-old child; the agent of injury might be a swimming pool filled with water with a beach ball floating just beyond the edge; the environment might be a pool gate left open while the babysitter runs inside to answer the telephone. With the host, agent, and environment all coming together at the same time, an unintentional injury—in this case, drowning—can occur.

Haddon Matrix

Dr. William J. Haddon, Jr., is considered the father of the science of injury prevention. Working within the concept of the epidemiological triad, in the mid-1960s, he recognized that an injury can be broken down into the following three temporal phases:

1. *Pre-event:* Before the injury.
2. *Event:* The point when harmful energy is released.
3. *Postevent:* The aftermath of the injury.

By examining the three factors of the epidemiological triad during each temporal phase, Haddon created a nine-cell "phase-factor" matrix (Figure 2-6). This grid has become known as the *Haddon Matrix*. It provides a means to depict graphically the events or actions that increase or decrease the odds that an injury will occur. It can also be used to identify prevention strategies. The Haddon Matrix demonstrates that *multiple* factors can lead to an injury, and therefore, multiple opportunities exist to prevent or reduce its severity. The matrix played a major role in dispelling the myth that injury is the result of a single cause, bad luck, or fate.

Figure 2-6 depicts a Haddon Matrix for an ambulance crash. The components in each cell of the matrix are different depending on the injury being examined. The *pre-event phase* includes factors that can contribute to the likelihood of a crash; however, energy is still under control. This phase may last from a few seconds to several years. The *event phase* depicts the factors that influence the severity of the injury. During this time, uncontrolled energy is released and injury occurs if energy transfer exceeds the body's tolerance. The event phase is typically very brief; it may last only a fraction of a second but rarely lasts more than a few minutes. Factors in the *postevent phase* affect the outcome once an injury has occurred. Depending on the type of event, it may last from a few seconds to the remaining life span of the host. (See also Chapter 1.)

Public Health programs have adopted the terminology of Primary, Secondary, and Tertiary Prevention. Primary prevention is aimed at avoiding the injury before it occurs. Secondary prevention refers to those actions taken to prevent the progression of an injury—for example, avoiding the occurrence of hypoxia or hypotension after a traumatic brain injury. Tertiary prevention is directed at minimizing death and disability of an injury (or disease) after it has occurred.

Swiss Cheese Model

British psychologist James Reason proposed another way of thinking about how accidents occur.[14] He likened the process to Swiss cheese. In every situation, a hazard exists that has the potential to cause injury or allow an error to occur. There are usually a series of safeguards or barriers to prevent this from happening. He suggested that each of these barriers or safeguards is like a piece of Swiss cheese. The holes in the cheese are flaws or failures that increase the potential for a hazard or error to cause injury. These flaws may be the result of deficiencies in the organization, administration or oversight of the system (latent conditions), or they may occur as a result of acts of omission or commission (active failures). Reason argued that every hazard has a trajectory, meaning that a series of failures generally must occur in order for there to be subsequent harm and that the trajectory must be such that it intersects with holes or failures that have aligned to allow all of the safeguards to fail and injury to occur (Figure 2-7).[16]

FIGURE 2-6   Haddon Matrix for an Ambulance Crash

| Time phases | Epidemiological Triad | | |
	Host	Agent	Environment
Pre-event	Driver's visual acuity Experience and judgment Amount of time in the ambulance per shift Level of fatigue Proper nutrition Stress level Adherence to company and community driving laws Quality of driver education courses	Maintenance of brakes, tires, etc. Defective equipment Ambulance's high center of gravity Speed Ease of control	Visibility hazards Road curvature and gradient Surface coefficient of friction Narrow road shoulder Traffic signals Speed limits
Event	Safety belt use Physical conditioning Injury threshold Ejection	Speed capability Ambulance size Automatic restraints Hardness and sharpness of contact surfaces Hardness and sharpness of loose items (e.g., clipboards, flashlights) Steering column Practice of safe driving habits: speed, use of lights/siren, passing, intersections, backing Practice of good partner habits en route: watching road, clearing intersections Park safely	Lack of guardrails Median barriers Distance between roadway and immovable objects Speed limits Other traffic Attitudes about safety belt use Maintain an escape route Make no assumptions about an environment being safe (e.g., "nice part of town," high-income home) Weather
Postevent	Age Physical condition Type or extent of injury	Fuel system integrity Entrapment	Emergency communication capability Distance to and quality of responding EMS Training of EMS personnel Availability of extrication equipment Trauma care system of the community Rehabilitation programs in the community

Classification of Injury

A common method to subclassify injuries is based on *intent*. Injury may result from either intentional or unintentional causes. Although this is a logical way to view injuries, it underscores the difficulty of injury prevention efforts.

Intentional injury is typically associated with an act of interpersonal or self-directed violence. Problems such as homicide, suicide, spousal abuse, and war fall into this category. Previously, prevention of intentional injury was thought to be the sole responsibility of the criminal justice and mental health systems. Although these agencies are integral to reducing violent deaths, intentional injuries can best be prevented through a broad, multidisciplinary approach, which includes the medical profession.

In the past, *unintentional injuries* were called "accidents." The authors of the NAS/NRC white paper appropriately referred to "accidental" death and disability; this was the vocabulary of the time.[1] Because it has since been understood that very specific

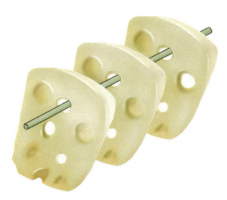

FIGURE 2-7   The Swiss cheese model.

factors must come together for an injury to occur, health care providers now realize that the term *accidental* does not describe unintentional injury resulting from events such as vehicle crashes, drownings, falls, and electrocutions. EMS systems have embraced this concept by using the term *motor vehicle crashes* (MVCs) rather than "motor vehicle accidents" (MVAs). However, public perception has changed much more slowly. News reporters still describe persons injured in "automobile accidents" or "accidental shootings." The term *accident* suggests that a person was injured as a result of fate, divine intervention, or bad luck. It implies that the injury was random and, therefore, unavoidable. As long as this misperception exists, implementation of corrective measures will be impeded.

Prevention as the Solution

Preventing injury is even more important than treating injury. When injury is prevented, it spares the patient and family from suffering and economic hardship. The National Center for Injury Prevention and Control (NCIPC) of the Centers for Disease Control and Prevention (CDC) estimates the following:

- $1 spent on smoke detectors saves $69.
- $1 spent on bicycle helmets saves $29.
- $1 spent on child-safety seats saves $32.
- $1 spent on center and edge lines on roads saves $3 in medical costs alone.
- $1 spent on counselling by pediatricians to prevent injuries saves $10.
- $1 spent on poison-control-center services saves $7 in medical expenses.[3]

In addition:

- A CDC-funded evaluation study of a regional trauma care system in Portland, Oregon, found a 35% decrease in the risk of dying for severely injured patients who were treated in the system.[15]
- A smoke detector distribution program in Oklahoma reduced burn-related injuries by 80%.[17]

Because of the variability among the host, agent, and environment at any given time, health care providers cannot always predict or prevent every individual injury. However, it is possible to identify high-risk populations (which include EMS providers), high-risk products, and high-risk environments. Prevention efforts focused on high-risk groups or settings influence as wide a range of society as possible. Health care providers can pursue prevention in multiple ways. Some strategies have proven successful across the United States and around the world. However, other strategies work in one region but not in another. Before implementing an injury prevention strategy, efforts must focus on determining if it will work. Although it is not necessary to "reinvent the wheel," health care providers may need to modify a prevention strategy to improve its chances of success. Methods for doing this are examined in the following section.

Concepts of Injury Prevention

Goal

The goal of injury prevention programs is to bring about a change in knowledge, attitude, and behavior on the part of a previously identified segment of society. Simply providing information to potential victims is not enough to prevent injury. A program must be implemented in a manner that will influence society's attitude and—most importantly—change behavior. The hope is that any change in behavior will be long term. This task is monumental but not insurmountable.

Opportunities for Intervention

Prevention strategies can be arranged according to their effect on the injury event. They coincide with the temporal phases of the Haddon Matrix. Pre-event interventions, known as *primary interventions,* strive to prevent the injury from occurring. Actions intended to keep intoxicated drivers off the road, lowering speed limits, and installing traffic lights are designed to prevent crashes from occurring. Event-phase interventions are intended to reduce injury severity by softening the blow of injuries that occur. Wearing safety belts, installing cushioned dashboards and airbags in vehicles, and enforcing child-safety-seat laws are means to reduce the severity of injury sustained in crashes. Postevent interventions provide a means to improve the likelihood of survival for those who are injured. Encouraging physical fitness, designing fuel systems for vehicles that do not explode on impact, and implementing high-quality EMS systems are intended to reduce the recovery time for persons who are injured.

FIGURE 2-8   Basic Strategies for Injury Countermeasures*

Strategy	Possible countermeasures
Prevent initial creation of the hazard	Do not produce firecrackers, three-wheeled all-terrain vehicles, or various poisons Eliminate spearing in high school football
Reduce amount of energy contained in the hazard	Limit the horsepower of motor vehicle engines Package toxic drugs in smaller, safer amounts **Obey or reduce speed limits** Mandate improved public transportation to reduce the number of privately-owned vehicles on the road **Reduce temperature on home hot water heaters** Limit the muzzle velocity of guns Limit the amount of gunpowder in firecrackers
Prevent release of a hazard that already exists	**Store firearms in locked containers or use gun locks** Close pools and beaches when no lifeguard is on duty **Use of non-slip surfaces in bathtubs and showers** **Childproof containers for all hazardous household drugs and chemicals** **Limit cell phone use in vehicles or use of hands-free models** Require safety shields on rotating farm machinery Improve vehicle handling
Modify rate or spatial distribution of the hazard	**Use of seat belts and child safety seats** Provide antilock brakes Use short cleats on football shoes so feet rotate rather than transmit sudden force to the knees Require vehicle air bags Provide hydraulic bumpers on vehicles Provide safety nets to protect workers from falls **Use of flame-retardant pajamas**
Separate in time or space the hazard from that which is to be protected	Provide pedestrian overpasses at high-volume crossings Keep roadsides clear of poles and trees Do not have play areas near unguarded bodies of water Install bike paths Spray pesticides at a time when people are not present Install sidewalks Route trucks carrying hazardous material along low-density roads **Use of smoke detectors in the home**
Separate the hazard from that which is to be protected by a material barrier	Install fencing around all sides of swimming pools **Use of protective eyewear for sports and occupational hazards** Build highway medians Build protective shields around hazardous machinery Install guardrails between sidewalks and roads Install reinforced panels in vehicle doors **Require health care workers to place used needles directly into a sharps container** **Use of helmets for motorcyclists, bicyclists, and high-risk sporting activites**
Modify basic nature of the hazard	Provide air bags in motor vehicles Provide collapsible steering columns Provide breakaway poles Make crib slats too narrow to strangle a baby Adopt breakaway baseball bases **Remove throw rugs in homes of the elderly**
Make what is to protected more resistant to the hazard	**Encourage calcium intake to reduce osteoporosis** Encourage musculoskeletal conditioning in athletes Prohibit alcohol sales and consumption near recreational water areas Treat medical conditions such as epilepsy to prevent episodes that can result in burns, drownings, and falls Check earthquake-resistant building codes in susceptible areas

FIGURE 2-8, cont'd

Strategy	Possible countermeasures
Begin to counter the damage already done by the hazard	**Provide emergency medical care** Employ systems to route injured persons to appropriately trained prehospital care providers **Develop school protocols for responding to injury emergencies** **Provide first-aid training to residents** Install automatic sprinkler systems
Stabilize, repair, and rehabilitate the object of the damage	Develop rehabilitation plans at an early stage of injury treatment Make use of occupational rehabilitation for paraplegic patients

*The examples listed are for illustrative purposes only and are not necessarily the official recommendations of PHTLS, the National Association of EMTs, or the American College of Surgeons Committee on Trauma.
BOLD = opportunities for EMS personnel to provide education and leadership

Prehospital systems have traditionally limited their community involvement to the postevent phase. Countless lives have been saved as a result. However, because of the limitations inherent in waiting until injury has occurred, the best results have not been achieved. EMS systems must look at entering the injury cycle earlier. Using the Haddon Matrix, EMS systems can identify opportunities to collaborate with other public health and public safety organizations to prevent injuries from occurring or to soften their blow.

Potential Strategies

No single strategy provides the best approach to injury prevention. The most effective option or options depends on the type of injury under study. However, Haddon developed a list of 10 generic strategies designed to break the chain of injury-producing events at numerous points (Figure 2-8). These strategies represent ways that the release of uncontrolled energy can be prevented or at least reduced to amounts the body can better tolerate. Figure 2-8 also presents countermeasures that can be taken in the pre-event, event, and postevent phases and that are directed toward the host, agent, or environment. This list is not complete and merely serves as a starting point to help determine the most effective options for the particular problem under study.

Most injury prevention strategies are either active or passive. *Passive strategies* require little or no action on the part of the individual; sprinkler systems and vehicle air bags are examples. *Active strategies* require the cooperation of the person being protected; examples include manual seat belts and choosing to wear a motorcycle or bicycle helmet. Passive measures are generally more effective because people do not need to consciously do anything to take advantage of the protection. Nonetheless, passive strategies are usually more difficult to implement because they can be expensive or require legislative or regulatory action. Sometimes a combination of active and passive strategies is the best option.

Strategy Implementation

Three common approaches to implementing an injury prevention strategy have become known as the "Three Es of Injury Prevention": *E*ducation, *E*nforcement, and *E*ngineering.

Education

Educational strategies are meant to impart information. To be effective, the target audience must embrace the new-found knowledge with enough enthusiasm to alter behavior in the manner prescribed by the program. Because the audience is required to do something, education is an active countermeasure. The target audience may be individuals who engage in high-risk activities, policymakers who have the authority to enact further prevention legislation or regulation, or prehospital care providers learning to become active participants in injury prevention. The NAS/NRC white paper is an example of an education initiative.

Education once was the primary means of implementing prevention programs because society believed that most injuries were simply the result of human error. Although this is true to a certain extent, many failed to recognize the role that energy and the environment play in causing injury. Education is still often used, however, and is probably the easiest of the three strategies to implement.

Experience has demonstrated that educational strategies have not met with overwhelming success for several reasons. The target audience may never hear the message. If the message is heard, some may reject it outright or not embrace it enough to alter behavior. Those who embrace it may do so sporadically or with declining enthusiasm over time.[19] However, education still can be particularly useful in reducing injury in the following four areas:

1. *Teaching young children basic safety behaviors and skills that stay with them later in life.* Examples include what to do when a smoke detector sounds an alarm, calling 9-1-1 for help in an emergency, or fastening seat belts.

2. *Teaching about certain types and causes of injury for certain age groups.* Education may be the only strategy available for these groups.

3. *Altering the public's perception of risk and acceptable risk to change social norms and attitudes.* This was used regarding drinking and driving and occurs now regarding wearing a helmet when riding a bicycle, scooter, skateboard, or rollerblades.

4. *Promoting policy change and educating consumers to demand safer products.*[7]

As a singular approach to injury prevention, educational programs have had disappointing results. Like many drugs, education needs to be "redosed" after a period of time in order to have a continued effect. However, when coupled with other forms of implementation strategies, education can be a valuable tool. Education often serves as a starting point to pave the way for enforcement and engineering strategies.

Enforcement

Enforcement seeks to tap the persuasive power of law to compel adherence to simple but effective prevention strategies. Certain government entities have the power to enact statutes, regulations, and laws in an effort to promote public health, safety, and general welfare even when such actions restrict individual autonomy to a limited degree. Generally, courts tend to uphold injury prevention laws that pose a minimal burden on individuals if they are fairly enforced and the public health benefit is substantial.

Statutory commands can either *require* or *prohibit,* and they can be directed at individual behavior (people), products (things), or environmental conditions (places), as follows:

- Legal requirements that apply to people are mandatory seat-belt, child-restraint, and helmet-use laws.
- Prohibitions that apply to people are drunk-driving laws, speed limits, and making assault a crime.
- Legal requirements that apply to products include design and performance standards, such as the federal Motor Vehicle Safety Standards.
- Prohibitions that apply to products include restrictions on dangerous animals and flammable fabrics.
- Legal requirements that apply to places include the installation of breakaway signposts along highways and fencing around swimming pools.
- Prohibitions that apply to places include the outlawing of rigid structures along highways and firearms in airport terminals.
- Legal requirements that apply to specific target groups and locations include the federal requirements that public safety and emergency responders wear high-visibility clothing at high-traffic crash sites.[6]

Enforcement is also an *active* countermeasure because people must obey the law to benefit from it. Enforcement typically has wide application because laws apply to all members of society within a given jurisdiction. The effectiveness of enforcement initiatives depends on the willingness of society to obey and the feasibility and visibility of their enforcement. The target audiences may be less likely to comply if they believe that the directive infringes on personal freedom, if they have little chance of getting caught, or if they will not face consequences of violating the law.

Because society as a whole tends to obey laws or at least stay within narrow limits around them, enforcement is often more effective than education. Enforcement in tandem with education appears to produce better results than either initiative alone.

Motorcycle-helmet laws provide an interesting case study in the role of enforcement in injury prevention. In states in which helmet laws have been repealed for motorcyclists, the rate of serious injuries and fatalities has increased.[18,19,20]

Engineering

Often the most effective means of injury prevention are those in which destructive energy release is permanently separated from the host. Passive countermeasures accomplish this goal with little or no effort on the part of the individual. Engineering strategies strive to build injury prevention into products or environments so that the host does not have to act differently to be protected. Engineering strategies help the people who actually need them, and they do so every time. Measures such as automatic sprinkler systems in buildings, flotation hulls in boats, and backup alarms on ambulances have all proven to save lives with little or no effort on the part of the host.

Engineering seems to be the perfect answer to injury prevention. It is passive, effective, and usually the least disruptive of the "Three Es." Unfortunately, it is often the most expensive to implement. Designing safety into a product usually makes it more expensive and may require legislative or regulatory initiation. The price may be more than the manufacturer is willing to absorb or the customer is willing to pay. Society dictates how much safety it wants built into a product and how much it is willing to support the endeavor financially.

Education initiatives should precede enforcement and engineering strategies. Ultimately, the most effective countermeasures may be those that incorporate all three implementation strategies.

Public Health Approach

Much has been learned about injury and injury prevention. Unfortunately, a wide discrepancy exists between what is known about injury and what is being done about it.[8] EMS systems are critical to help close that gap. Injury is a complex problem in all societies of the world. Unfortunately, a single person or single agency will usually have little impact. A public health approach has achieved success in dealing with other diseases and is making progress with injury prevention as well. EMS agencies that have joined forces with other public and private organizations have been able to accomplish as much or more than they could on their own. Partnerships bring together a community's expertise to tackle a complex and perplexing issue.

A public health approach creates a community-based coalition to combat a community-based disease through a four-step process, as follows:

1. Surveillance
2. Risk factor identification
3. Intervention evaluation
4. Implementation

The coalition is comprised of experts from such diverse fields as epidemiology, the medical community, schools of public health, public health agencies, community advocacy programs, economics, sociology, and criminal justice. EMS systems have an important place in a public health approach to injury prevention. Participating in a coalition to improve playground safety may not have the immediate effect of providing care at the scene of a horrific vehicle crash, but the results will be much more widespread.

Surveillance

Surveillance is the process of collecting data within a community. Collection of population-based data aids in the discovery of an injury's true magnitude and effect on the community. A community can be a neighborhood, city, county, state, or even the ambulance service itself. Support for the program, proper allocation of resources, and even knowing whom to include on the interdisciplinary team depend on understanding the scope of the problem.

Sources of information available within a community include the following:

- Mortality data
- Hospital admission and discharge statistics
- Medical records
- Trauma registries
- Police reports
- EMS run sheets
- Insurance reports
- Unique surveillance data collected solely for the study at hand

Risk Factor Identification

After a problem is identified and researched, it is necessary to know who is at risk to direct a prevention strategy at the correct population. "Shotgun" approaches to injury prevention are less successful than targeted ones. Identification of causes and risk factors determines who is injured; what types of injuries are sustained; and where, when, and why those injuries occur.[22] Sometimes a risk factor is obvious, such as the presence of alcohol in fatal vehicle crashes. At other times, research is required to discover the true risk factors involved in injury events. EMS systems can serve as the "eyes and ears" of public health at the scene of injuries to identify risk factors that no one else may be able to uncover. Risk factors can then be charted on a Haddon Matrix as they are properly identified.

Intervention Evaluation

As risk factors become clear, intervention strategies begin to emerge. Haddon's list of 10 injury prevention strategies serves as a starting point (see Figure 2-8). Even though communities have different characteristics, with modification, an injury prevention initiative from one community may work in another. Once a potential intervention has been selected, a pilot program using one or more of the "Three Es" may give indications of the success of full-scale implementation.

Implementation

The final step in the public health approach is implementation and evaluation of the intervention. Detailed implementation procedures are prepared so others interested in implementation of similar programs will have a guide to follow. Collection of evaluation data measures the effectiveness of a program. Answering the following three questions may help determine the success of a program:

1. Have attitudes, skills, or judgment changed?
2. Has behavior changed?
3. Does behavioral change lead to a favorable outcome?[11]

The public health approach provides a proven means to combat a disease such as injury. Through a multidisciplinary, community-based effort, it is possible to identify the "who, what, where, when, and why" of an injury problem and develop a plan of action. EMS systems need to play a much more substantial role in helping to close the gap between what is known about injury and what is being done about it. This approach can be thought of as a continuous loop. Continued surveillance occurs after implementation of an injury control strategy. This data is then used to modify or change the strategy. Successes in injury prevention can be broadened to wider populations at risk.

Evolving Role of EMS in Injury Prevention

Traditionally, the role of the prehospital care provider in health care focuses almost exclusively on postevent, one-on-one treatment of the individual. Little emphasis is placed on understanding the causes of the injuries or what a prehospital care provider could do to prevent them. As a result, patients may return to the same environment only to be injured again. In addition, information that could aid in the development of a community-wide prevention program to keep others from becoming injured in the first place may not be documented and, therefore, may remain unavailable to other sectors of public health.

The public health approach to injury is more proactive. It works to determine how to alter the host, agent, and environment to prevent injuries. Through coalitions that conduct surveillance and implement interventions, public health works to develop community-wide prevention programs. The *Emergency Medical Services Agenda for the Future* envisions closer ties between EMS systems and public health that would make both sectors of health care more effective.[5]

Prehospital care providers can take a more active role in development of community-wide injury prevention programs. EMS systems enjoy a unique position in the community. With more than 600,000 providers in the United States alone, basic and advanced prehospital care providers are widely distributed at the community level. Prehospital care providers enjoy a credible reputation in the community, making them high-profile role models. In addition, they are readily welcomed into homes and businesses. All phases of the public health approach to injury prevention benefit from an EMS presence.

One-on-One Interventions

EMS systems do not have to give up their one-on-one approach to patient care to conduct valuable injury prevention interventions. The one-on-one approach makes EMS systems uniquely able to conduct injury prevention initiatives. Prehospital care providers can bring injury prevention messages directly to high-risk individuals. One indicator of a successful educational program is that the information is received with enough enthusiasm to change behavior. Prehospital care providers can use their role-model status to deliver important prevention messages. Implicitly, people look up to role models, listen to what they have to say, and emulate what they do.

On-scene prevention counselling takes advantage of a "teachable moment." A teachable moment is the time when the patient who does not require critical medical interventions or the family members may be in a state that makes them more receptive to what a role model says. The prehospital care provider may think of the on-scene time as wasted when it becomes apparent that little or no medical interventions are necessary. However, this may be the best time to deliver primary prevention.[23]

Not every call allows for injury prevention counselling. Serious and life-threatening calls require concentration on acute care. However, as many as 95% of ambulance calls are nonlife-threatening. A significant proportion of EMS calls require minor, if any, treatment. One-on-one prevention counselling may be appropriate during these noncritical calls.

Patient interactions are typically short encounters, especially those that require little or no treatment. However, they provide enough time to discuss and demonstrate to patients and family members practices that may prevent an injury in the future. Prehospital care providers are in a unique position in that they are the only health care worker who enters the patient's environment, thereby viewing situations that may predispose to injury. A role model who discusses the importance of replacing a burned-out light bulb and removing a slippery throw rug in a dimly lit hallway may prevent a fall by an elderly resident. Prehospital care providers have an attentive audience during the ride to a hospital. Prevention is a more valuable topic to discuss than the weather or the local sports team. Teachable moments take 1 to 2 minutes to complete and do not interfere with treatment or transport.

Educational programs have been developed to train prehospital care providers to administer on-scene injury prevention counselling.[24] These types of programs must be further developed and evaluated to discover which are the most valuable and, therefore, worthy of inclusion in the primary education of a prehospital care provider.

Community-Wide Interventions

The public health approach to injury prevention is community-based and involves a multidisciplinary team. EMS personnel have the expertise to be valuable members of that team. Community-wide prevention strategies depend on data to address properly the "who, what, when, where, and why" of an injury problem. Multiple sources of information, as described previously, provide the needed data. Prehospital care providers, perhaps more than any other team member, have the opportunity to examine patient interaction with the environment at the time of the injury. This may allow identification of a high-risk individual, high-risk attitude, or high-risk behavior that is not present by the time the patient arrives at the emergency department.

The prehospital care provider can use documentation acquired en route to a medical facility in the following two ways:

1. Data can be used immediately by emergency personnel who receive the patient. Emergency physicians and nurses are also being called on to improve and increase their role in injury prevention. Their "teachable moment" can reinforce and supplement the prehospital care provider's on-scene counselling if they know what has already been discussed or demonstrated.
2. Others in public health can use injury data provided by prehospital care providers retrospectively to help develop a comprehensive, community-wide injury prevention program.

Prehospital care providers usually do not practice documentation to help support a community-wide prevention program. Knowing what to acquire and when to document information beneficial to the development of community-wide prevention programs requires opening a dialogue with other members of the public health team. Leaders in the EMS system need to build a coalition with others in public health to develop documentation policies that promote complete documentation of injuries.

EMS can be the spearhead for workable, effective injury prevention programs that make a profound impact in a community. Programs have been created out of the desire of a small group of EMS professionals to prevent childhood fatalities.[25,26] Services in Louisiana, Florida, Washington, Oregon, and Hawaii have been recognized for their efforts in designing, coordinating, and conducting injury prevention programs through the Nicholas Rosecrans Award for best practices in injury prevention in EMS.[27,28]

While opportunities exist for prehospital care providers to educate patients, one study by David Jaslow and colleagues suggests that only a minority do utilize the teachable moment. They found that only 33% routinely educate their patients on how to modify injury risk behaviors, and only 19% routinely provide instruction about proper use of protective devices.[28]

Injury Prevention for EMS Providers

"Who's the most important person at an incident scene?" EMT students are always asked this question early in their training to make them think about their own safety. Invariably, one or two students will say "the patient," which is what the instructor wanted to hear. This provides a teachable moment for the instructor to begin the course-long directive to reinforce the point that self-injury prevention is the most valuable service an EMT can provide.

Hostile environments resulting from terrorist activities or hazardous materials spills unfortunately make the news too often. However, the everyday activities of prehospital providers provide sufficient opportunity to end an EMT's career or life because of injury. The Bureau of Labor Statistics paints an accurate picture of the "normal" dangers in EMS:

EMTs and paramedics work both indoors and outdoors, in all types of weather. They are required to do considerable kneeling, bending, and heavy lifting. These workers risk noise-induced hearing loss from sirens and back injuries from lifting patients. In addition, EMTs and paramedics may be exposed to diseases such as hepatitis-B and AIDS, as well as violence from drug overdose victims or mentally unstable patients. The work is not only physically strenuous but also stressful, involving life-or-death situations and suffering patients.[29]

Providers can become complacent to the everyday dangers of the job. *Complacency* is a feeling of security or safety in the unacknowledged face of potential danger. Compounding the situation is the idealism and invincibility of youth typical to some EMS personnel.[30] Management is needed to create a culture of injury prevention by instituting prevention policy, maintaining adherence to procedure, and rewarding positive performance. It is necessary that the providers themselves be equally committed to the principles of injury prevention. Failure to do so by either management or providers can have potentially devastating effects.

Other factors to consider are the experience of personnel and fatigue. It's important to ensure that drivers are adequately prepared and trained to operate vehicles safely and that personnel are monitored to ensure they have adequate sleep to ensure safe operations. In a study that looked at common factors in EMS personnel involved in ambulance crashes, the odds were greater that the drivers involved in emergency vehicle crashes would be younger EMS professionals and those professionals reporting sleep problems.[31]

In a prehospital service, employees are not only the most valuable asset but also the most expensive. The service, community, and, most importantly, the EMT benefit when the employee remains uninjured. An in-house injury prevention program is worthwhile on its own merits. When conducted through a public health approach, however, it provides valuable experience for involvement in community injury-prevention initiatives as well. The community (e.g., the ambulance service) is small, there is 100% access to it, and surveillance is easier because the ambulance service has access to many of the data sources it may need. Identification of risk factors is simplified because the target audience consists of fellow employees. Gaining evaluation information should be almost immediate. Outcome data collection should be readily available as well.

J.M. Kinnane and colleagues mention in-house prevention programs that utilize education, enforcement, and engineering implementation strategies.[23] The wide variability of the programs demonstrates the dangers involved in EMS systems and the need for prevention initiatives. It also demonstrates the variability among EMS communities. Even though all EMS services are similar, individual services (communities) have different risk factors and different prevention priorities.

As described previously, education programs enhance wellness, prevent back injury, and increase awareness of the potential for violent patients. Enforcement programs introduce mandatory fitness programs and establish protocols to deal with violent patients. Engineering initiatives address increasing seat-belt use in the back of the ambulance by evaluating the position of equipment and location of the seat and reduced back injury through pre-employment screening and physical strengthening.

A small-scale, in-house injury prevention program may reap rewards beyond the most important outcome of improved employee health. Small successes lay the groundwork for participation in larger, more complicated endeavors. They provide a valuable on-the-job learning tool about injury prevention for all employees. In addition, in-house prevention programs provide an introduction of the EMS service to other public health agencies in the community that assist in in-house program implementation and evaluation.

SCENARIO SOLUTION

Jose and Gwen approached their supervisor about educating the public about the dangers of unrestrained driving and the importance of securing infants and children appropriately in vehicles. The supervisor contacted the local trauma center and was able to get them involved in community training and infant- and child-seat inspections. They became actively involved in educating the community and inspecting vehicles to ensure infants and children were properly restrained. After working in these programs throughout the year, they were able to see an increase in the number of restrained drivers, infants, and children in the vehicle crashes they responded to.

SUMMARY

- Trauma is the most neglected current epidemic—the health care industry has failed to measurably decrease the incidence of injuries.
- EMS providers are in a unique position to influence injury morbidity and mortality rates through prevention efforts. Many opportunities exist for EMS personnel to provide public education and leadership.

- The advancement of EMS systems in injury prevention depends on the adoption of this new role by each individual prehospital care provider.
- Armed with commitment to the effort and skill and knowledge of injury presentation, prehospital care providers may help prevent death and disability in their community.

References

1. National Academy of Sciences/National Research Council. *Accidental death and disability: the neglected disease of modern society,* Washington, DC, 1966, NAS/NRC.
2. National Center for Health Statistics. *Health, United States, 2000, with Adolescent Health Chartbook,* Hyattsville, MD, 2000, NCHS.
3. National Center for Injury Prevention and Control, Center for Disease Control and Prevention. http://www.cdc.gov/injury/wisqars/index.html. Accessed August 2009.
4. Peden M, McGee K, Sharma G. *The Injury Chart Book: A Graphical Overview of the Global Burden of Injuries,* Geneva, 2002, World Health Organization.
5. National Highway Traffic Safety Administration, US Department of Health and Human Services, Health Resources and Services Administration, Maternal and Child Health Bureau. *Emergency Medical Services Agenda for the Future,* Washington, DC, 1999, NHTSA.
6. Christoffel T, Gallagher SS. *Injury Prevention and Public Health: Practical Knowledge, Skills, and Strategies,* Gaithersburg, MD, 1999, Aspen.
7. Maguire BJ, Huntington KL, Smith GS, Levick NR. Occupational fatalities in emergency medical services: a hidden crisis. *Ann Emerg Med* 40:6, 2002.
8. Centers for Disease Control and Prevention (CDC): Ambulance crash-related injuries among Emergency Medical Services workers—United States, 1991–2002. *MMWR Morb Mortal Wkly Rep*28;52(8):154–156, 2003.
9. Tortella BJ, Lavery RF: Disabling job injuries among EMS providers. *Prehosp Disaster Med* 9, 1994.
10. Garrison HG: Keeping rescuers safe. *Ann Emerg Med* 40:6, 2002.
11. Martinez R: Injury control: a primer for physicians. *Ann Emerg Med* 19:1, 1990.
12. Waller JA: *Injury control: A Guide to the Causes and Prevention of Trauma,* Lexington, MA, 1985, Lexington Books.
13. PIER: *Public Information, Education, and Relations for EMS Injury Prevention Modules,* DOT HS 809 520, Washington, DC, 2002, US Department of Transportation, National Highway Traffic Safety Administration.
14. Reason J: Human Error: Models and Management. *BMJ* 320:768–770, 2000.
15. Mullins RJ, Veum-Stone J, Helfand M, et al: Outcome of hospitalized injured patients after institution of a trauma system in an urban area. *JAMA* 271(24):1919-1924, 1994.
16. Haddix AC, Mallonee S, Waxweiler R, et al: Cost effectiveness analysis of a smoke alarm giveaway program in Oklahoma City, Oklahoma. *Inj Prevention* 7:276-281, 2001.
17. Kellerman AL, Hutson HR: Injury Control. In Schwartz GR: *Principles and Practice of Emergency Medicine*, Philadelphia, 1992, Lea & Febiger.
18. Mertz KJ, Weiss HB: Changes in motorcycle-related head injury deaths, hospitalizations, and hospital charges following repeal of

Pennsylvania's mandatory motorcycle helmet law. *Am J Public Health.* 98(8):1464-1467. Epub June 12, 2008.

19. Bledsoe GH, Li G: Trends in Arkansas motorcycle trauma after helmet law repeal. *South Med J* 98(4):436–440, 2005.

20. Chenier TC, Evans L: Motorcyclist fatalities and the repeal of mandatory helmet wearing laws. *Accid Anal Prev* 19(2):133–139, 1987.

21. Kellerman AL, Todd KH: Injury control. In Tintinelli JE, Kelen GD, Stapczynski JS, editors: *Emergency Medicine: A Comprehensive Study Guide*, New York, 1999, McGraw-Hill.

22. Todd KH: *Accident's Aren't: Proposal for Evaluation of an Injury Prevention Curriculum for EMS Providers: a grant proposal to the National Association of State EMS Directors,* Atlanta, 1998, Department of Emergency Medicine, Emory University School of Medicine.

23. Kinnane JM, Garrison HG, Coben JH, et al: Injury Prevention: Is there a role for out-of-hospital emergency medical services? *Acad Emerg Med* 4:306, 1997.

24. EPIC Medics: http://www.epicmedics.ord. Accessed July 2004.

25. Hawkins ER, Brice JH, Overby BA: Welcome to the world: Findings from an emergency medical services pediatric injury prevention program. *Pediatr Emerg Care* 23(11):790–795, 2007.

26. Griffiths K: Best practices in injury prevention. *J Emerg Med Serv* 27:8, 2002.

27. Krimston J, Griffiths K: Best practices in injury prevention. *J Emerg Med Serv* 28:9, 2003.

28. Jaslow D, Ufberg J, Marsh R: Primary injury prevention in an urban EMS system. *J Emerg Med* 25(2):167–170, 2003.

29. US Department of Labor: Emergency Medical Technicians and Paramedics. In US Department of Labor, Bureau of Labor Statistics: *Occupational Outlook Handbook, 2004–2005 Edition,* http://stats.bls.gov/oco/ocos101.htm. Accessed July 2004.

30. Federal Emergency Management Agency, US Fire Administration: EMS safety: Techniques and applications. International Association of Fire Fighters, FEMA contract EMW-91-C-3592.

31. Studnek JR, Fernandez AR: Characteristics of emergency medical technicians involved in ambulance crashes. *Prehosp Disaster Med* 23(5):432–437, 2008.javascript:PopUpMenu2_Set(Menu19189612);

Suggested Reading

American College of Surgeons Committee on Trauma: *Advanced Trauma Life Support for Doctors, Student Course Manual*, ed 7, Chicago, 2004, ACS.

CHAPTER 3

The Science and Art of Prehospital Care: Principles, Preferences, and Critical Thinking

CHAPTER OBJECTIVES

At the completion of this chapter, the reader will be able to do the following:

✓ Describe the difference between principles and preferences.

✓ Discuss how principles and preferences relate to decision making in the field.

✓ Given a trauma scenario, discuss the principles of trauma care and choice of preference for the specific situation, conditions, knowledge and skill level, and available equipment.

✓ Given a trauma scenario, use critical-thinking skills to determine the preferred method for accomplishing the principles of emergency trauma care.

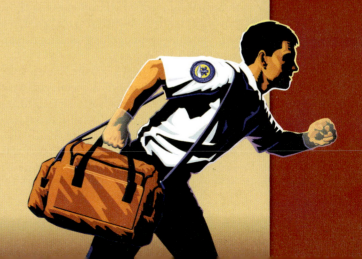

SCENARIO

You and your partner arrive to the scene of a single-car crash into a tree on a rural road in a wooded area. The weather is clear and dark (time 0200 hours). The transport time by ground to the trauma center is 35 minutes. A medical helicopter can be dispatched by prehospital providers on the scene with approval of medical control. Startup time for the helicopter is 5 minutes, and travel time is 15 minutes; a non-trauma center hospital is 15 minutes away and has a helistop.

The patient is breathing with difficulty at a rate of 30 breaths per minute, his heart rate is 110, blood pressure is 90 mm Hg by palpation, and his GCS is 11 (E3V3M5). He is in his mid 20s, he was not wearing a seat belt, and his position is against the dash away from the driver-side airbag. He has a deformed right leg at mid-thigh and an open left ankle fracture with significant hemorrhage. There is approximately 1 liter of blood on the floorboard near the ankle.

You and your partner have been working together for 2 years. Both of you are NREMT-P certified. The last update training for endotracheal use was 1 year ago. You last placed an ET tube 2 months ago; your partner placed one a month ago. You are not authorized to use paralytic drugs for ET insertion, but you can use sedation if necessary. You were just trained on hemorrhage control using tourniquets and hemostatic agents.

You have complete EMT-P equipment that you checked at the beginning of the shift. Your equipment includes ET tubes, laryngoscopes, tourniquets and other equipment and supplies as indicated by the ACS/ACEP equipment list. You have all the appropriate drugs including hemostatic agents.

What judgment decisions do you have to make based on science (Principles), and how do you make them—the art of medicine (Preferences)?

Introduction

It has been understood and accepted for many years that medicine is not an exact science and that there is much art in the practice of medicine. This includes all aspects of medicine and all practitioners from allied health personnel to nurses to physicians. In recent decades, technology has advanced at a rapid rate as electronics have developed and as research has allowed us to better understand patient care. The practice of medicine has become more and more a science and less and less an art. However, the art remains, and medicine is still a long way from the precise science of math or physics.

At the founding of Tulane Medical School in 1834, students were matriculated into the first medical school class in January of 1835 and graduated in June of 1836. Not much knowledge was available to be imparted, and this short curriculum was not unusual for medical education at the time. Many students simply apprenticed themselves to a practicing physician for several months or a couple of years and then went out on their own.

Medicine has changed a great deal since the famous 1891 painting of Sir Luke Fildes that shows the concern and frustration of a physician sitting at the bedside of a sick child. At that time, there were no antibiotics, a minimal understanding of not only childhood illness, but all disease and illness, only rudimentary surgery was available, and medication was mostly herbal remedies. We have moved a long way toward the science side of medicine.

It was not until the 1950s that there was thought to be any benefit to training those who encountered the patient prior to arrival to the emergency room, which was literally a "room," usually at the back of the hospital and often locked until someone came to open it. The fund of knowledge provided to the prehospital provider has significantly advanced in the years since. With this growth comes the major responsibility that each prehospital provider assures that he or she is up-to-date with the latest knowledge and that skills are finely honed. Knowledge is gained from reading and continuing medical education (CME) classes, and skills improve with experience and critique, like those of a surgeon or an airplane pilot. Just as a pilot does not solo after one flight, the emergency medical technician (EMT) does not mature from using a skill once or in one situation.

The science of prehospital care and the understanding to make fully correct decisions when treating a patient includes a working knowledge of: 1) anatomy—the organs, bones, muscles, arteries, nerves, and veins (perhaps not all of the names but certainly where they are in the patient); 2) physiology—including how the body produces and maintains heat, Starling's Law of the heart (increasing preload increases stroke volume), and the Ficke principle; and 3) pharmacology and the physiologic actions produced by the various drugs and their interaction with each other inside the body.

A major improvement in the science of medicine has been in technical components and the diagnostic equipment available. The ability to diagnose and treat a patient has been dramatically improved with the imaging techniques of CT scans, ultrasound and MRI; with sophisticated clinical laboratories that can measure almost any electrolyte, hormone, or substance produced metabolically; with the sophistication of complex medications produced by the pharmaceutical industry; with the technical advances in surgery, medicine, and invasive radiology; with the EMS communication improvements and logistic equipment such as GPS to improve access to the patient; and with the advanced care that can be provided by physicians and EMS personnel working together as part of the same medical-care team. The science of medicine has become much more advanced.

Yet, with all of these advances, it is the art of medicine that continues to rely on health care providers to use their knowledge and critical-thinking skills to make appropriate judgments and decisions to identify the correct diagnostic device, the proper medication, or the most efficient EMS procedures that will most benefit the patient. For prehospital providers, this is the determination of which patient is potentially seriously injured; which patient needs rapid transportation to which hospital; how much should be done on the scene versus during transport; what techniques should be used to accomplish needed interventions; and what equipment is the best to use in a particular situation. This is all the art of medicine, or *preference*. Which technique, procedure, or device does the EMS provider have in their armamentarium that, in his or her hands, will suit the needs of the patient in the situation that exists at the time? Which is the preferred method?

Principles and Preferences

The science of medicine provides the *principles* of medical care. Simply stated, principles are those things that must be present, accomplished, or assured by the health care provider in order to optimize patient survival and outcome. How these principles are implemented by the individual provider to most efficiently manage the patient at the time of patient contact depends on *preferences,* based on the situation that exists at the specific time, the clinical condition of the patient, individual training and skills, and the equipment available. This is how the **Science** of medicine **and** the **Art** of medicine come together for the good of patient care.

The importance of and difference between *principle* and *preference* can be illustrated by using airway management as an example. The *principle* is that air, containing oxygen, must be moved through an open airway into the lungs to provide oxygenation of the red cells as they course through the lungs and on to the tissue cells. This principle is true for all patients. The *preference* is in how airway management is carried out in a particular patient. In some cases,

---

FIGURE 3-1   Principles versus Preferences

Principle—what is necessary for patient improvement or survival

Preference—how the principle is achieved in the time needed and by the provider available

The preference used to accomplish the principle depends upon four factors:

- *Situation* that exists
- *Condition* of the patient
- *Fund of knowledge* of the provider
- *Equipment* available

---

patients will manage this on their own; in others, the prehospital provider will have to decide what devices are to be used, whether or not assisted ventilation is required, etc. In other words, what is the best way to assure that the air passages are open to get oxygen into the lungs and, secondarily, to get carbon dioxide out. The art is how the prehospital provider makes this determination and carries it out to achieve the principle.

The preferences of how to accomplish the principles depend upon four factors (Figure 3-1).

The philosophy of the PHTLS program is that each situation and patient is different. PHTLS teaches the importance of having a strong understanding of the subject matter and the skills necessary to accomplish needed interventions. The judgments and decisions made on the scene should be individualized to the needs of this specific patient being managed at this specific time and in this specific situation. Protocols are not the final answer. Protocols are inflexible to the variability of the event. The provider must know the scene, the situation, the abilities of the providers involved, and the equipment available. Understanding what can and should be accomplished for a particular patient is based on this information. By understanding the principles involved and using **critical-thinking** skills, appropriate decisions can be made. Preferences describe the way that an individual prehospital provider can best accomplish the principle. The principle will not be done the same way in every situation or for every condition of every patient. Not all providers have skill in every available technique. The tools to carry out these techniques are not necessarily available at the site of all emergencies. Just because one instructor, lecturer, or physician director prefers one technique does not mean that it is the best technique for every provider in every situation. The important point is to achieve the principle. How this is done and how the care is provided to the patient depend on the four factors listed in Figure 3-1 and described in more detail in the following section.

Situation

The situation involves all of the factors at a scene that can affect what care is provided to a patient. These include, but are certainly not limited to, the following: hazards on the scene, number of patients involved, location of the patient, position of the vehicle, contamination or hazardous materials concerns, fire (or chance of fire), weather, scene control and security by law enforcement, time/distance to medical care (including qualifications of the closest hospital and the trauma center if different), number of EMS providers and other possible helpers on the scene, bystanders, transportation available on the scene, other transportation available at a distance (i.e., helicopters, additional ambulances), and many more factors. For the military provider, the scene situation will include whether or not combat is presently going on, the location of the enemy, the combat situation, and what protection is available for sheltering the wounded. All of these conditions may be constantly changing in both the civilian and military setting. These factors and many others will change the way that you, as a prehospital provider, can respond to the needs of the patient.

In the opening scenario in this chapter, the situation was as follows: a single-car crash into a tree on a rural road in a wooded area. The weather is clear and dark (time 0200 hours). The transport time by ground to the trauma center is 35 minutes. A medical helicopter can be dispatched by prehospital providers on the scene with approval of medical control. Startup time for the helicopter is 5 minutes and travel time is 15 minutes, a nontrauma center hospital is 15 minutes away and has a helistop.

Some examples of how the situation affects a procedure such as spinal immobilization include:

Situation 1:
- Automobile crash
- Bull's-eye fracture of the windscreen
- Warm, sunny day
- No traffic on the road

Management:
- Patient is examined in the car
- Cervical collar applied
- Secured to the short backboard
- Rotated onto the long back board
- Removed from the car
- Placed on the stretcher
- Physical assessment completed
- Patient transported to the hospital

Situation 2:
- Same as above except gasoline is dripping from the gas tank
- Concern for fire

Management:
- Rapid extraction techniques used
- Patient moved significant distance from the vehicle
- Physical assessment completed
- Patient transported to the hospital

Situation 3:
- House fully involved in flames
- Patient unable to move

Management:
- No assessment
- Patient dragged from the fire
- Placed on backboard
- Moved quickly to a distance from the fire
- Patient assessment completed
- Transported quickly to the hospital depending on the patient's condition

Situation 4:
- Combat situation with nearby perpetrator or enemy combatants actively shooting (police or military action)
- Officer (or soldier) with GSW to the knee and significant bleeding

Management:
- Assessment from a distance (binoculars)
- Presence of other wounds
- Ability to still fire his weapon
- Tell him to apply tourniquet on upper leg
- Tell him to pull himself to a protected position
- Rescue when conditions permit

Condition of the Patient

This component of the decision-making process concerns the medical condition of the patient. The major question that will affect decision making is "How sick is the patient?" Some examples of issues that will help this determination include the cause of the medical condition, the age of the patient, physiologic factors that affect energy production (blood pressure, pulse, ventilatory rate, skin temperature, etc.), the etiology of the trauma, the patient's medical condition prior to the event, medication that the patient is using, illicit drug use, alcohol use, and many others.

Again, in the opening scenario, the condition was: The patient is breathing with difficulty at a rate of 30 breaths per minute, his heart rate is 110, blood pressure is 90 mm Hg by palpation, and his GCS is 11 (E3V3M5); he is in his mid 20s, was not wearing a seat belt, and his position is against the dash away from the driver-side airbag; he has a deformed right leg at mid-thigh and an open left ankle fracture with significant hemorrhage. There is approximately 1 liter of blood on the floorboard near the ankle.

Fund of Knowledge of the Provider

The **fund of knowledge** of the provider comes from several sources including initial training, recent CME courses, experience in the field, experience with this specific condition, and skill with the available potential procedures that the patient might require.

For example, consider airway control. The level of the provider has a significant impact of the available choice of preference. The authorized airway interventions depend on the level of the provider at the scene. In addition, skill with a particular intervention and comfort with performing it depend a great deal on the frequency with which it has been performed. As the provider, you might consider: When was the last time that you had to actively manage an airway? What device did you use? When is the last time that you did an intubation? How comfortable are you with the laryngoscope? How many times have you done a cricothyrotomy on a live patient or even an animal training model? Without the appropriate skills and experience, the patient would likely be better off and the operator would be more comfortable by choosing an oral airway plus bag mask device rather than a more advanced intervention such as endotracheal intubation or a surgical airway as the *preference* for management.

Back to the opening scenario: You and your partner have been working together for 2 years. Both of you are NREMT-P certified. The last update training for endotracheal use was 1 year ago. You last placed an ET tube 2 months ago; your partner placed one a month ago. You are not authorized to use paralytic drugs for ET insertion, but you can use sedation if necessary. You were just trained on hemorrhage control using tourniquets and hemostatic agents.

Equipment Available

The experience of any operator with the most sophisticated equipment in the world does no good if that sophisticated equipment is not available. The prehospital provider must use the equipment or supplies that are available. As an example, blood may be the best resuscitation fluid for trauma victims. However, this is not available in the field; therefore, the resuscitation fluid at hand (crystalloid) is the best available choice, depending on the situation. Another consideration is whether hypotensive resuscitation (permissive hypotension) would be a better choice given the nature of the patient's injuries. This particular issue is discussed in more detail in the chapter about shock.

Finally, the opening scenario once again: there is complete EMT-P equipment that was checked at the beginning of the shift. It includes ET tubes, laryngoscopes, tourniquets, and other equipment and supplies as indicated by the ACS/ACEP equipment list. You have all the appropriate drugs including hemostatic agents.

The foundation of PHTLS is to teach the prehospital provider to make appropriate decisions for patient care based on knowledge, not based on protocol. The goal of patient care is to achieve the principle. How this is achieved and the decision made by the prehospital provider to manage the patient is the preference based on the situation, patient condition, fund of knowledge and skill, and equipment available at the time—the four components outlined above.

Referring back to the airway management example and the choice of devices will help to understand these concepts. When a nonbreathing patient is encountered, the **principle** is that the airway must be opened and oxygen delivered to the lungs. The **preference** chosen depends on those four factors described above; a bystander on the street with only CPR training may perform mouth-to-mask ventilation; the EMT-B may choose an oral airway and bag-mask ventilation; the EMT-P may choose to place an endotracheal tube or may decide that it is more advantageous to use the bag-mask with rapid transportation; the corpsman in combat may chose a cricothyroidotomy or nothing at all if the enemy fire is too intense; and the physician in the ED may chose paralytic drugs or fiber optic-guided ET tube placement. None of the choices are wrong at a specific point in time for a given patient (situation, patient condition, fund of knowledge, experience/skill, equipment available) and, in the same way, none are correct all of the time for the same reasons.

This concept of principle and preference for the care of the trauma patient has its most dramatic application in the combat situation in the military. For this reason, the Tactical Combat Casualty Care Committee (TCCC) wrote the military component of the PHTLS program. Although this critical difference in situation leading to alterations in preference for patient care is most apparent in the military, similar considerations exist in the civilian setting for tactical-situation responders and those providers who work in hazardous environments such as fire scenes. For example, in the middle of a house that is fully involved in fire, a medic coming upon a patient who is down cannot stop to check the basic principles of patient assessment, such as airway and cardiac output. The first step is to get the victim outside and away from the immediate danger of the fire and then to check for airway and pulse.

For the military medic potentially involved in combat, the four step process for casualty management developed by the TCCC is: management in the middle of a fire fight (Care Under Fire); management after the shooting is over but danger still exists (Tactical Field Care); moving the patient out of the hazardous situation (casualty evacuation or CASEVAC); and finally, moving from a lower level hospital (Echelon II in the military) to a higher level hospital (Echelon III or above) or medical evacuation (MEDEVAC). While the principles of patient care are not changed, the preferences of patient care may be dramatically different due to one or more of the factors outlined above. For other discussion, details, and clarification, refer to the military version of PHTLS. These situational differences are described in more detail in the chapter about situation assessment.

Critical Thinking

In order to successfully accomplish the principle needed for a particular patient and to choose the best preference to implement the principle, critical-thinking skills are as important

FIGURE 3-2   Steps in Critical Thinking

ASSESSMENT

What is going on? What needs to be done? What are the resources to achieve the goal? Analysis will involve: the scene survey, identification of any hazards to either the patient or to the provider, condition of the patient, rapidity required for resolution, location of the care (in the field, during transport, and after arrival to the hospital), number of patients on the scene, number of transport vehicles required, need for more rapid transportation (aeromedical), and destination of the patient for the appropriate care.

ANALYSIS

Each of the above described conditions needs to be individually and rapidly analyzed, cross-referenced with the provider's fund of knowledge and the resources available, and steps defined to provide the best care.

CONSTRUCTION OF A PLAN

The plan to achieve the best outcome for the patient is developed and critically reviewed. Is any step false? Are the planned steps all achievable? Are the resources available that will allow the plan to move forward? Will they, more likely than not, lead to a successful outcome?

ACTION

The plan is enacted and started in motion. This is done decisively and with strength of command so that there is no question or hesitation on the part of any of the individuals involved as to

what needs to be accomplished, who is in command, and who is making the decisions. If the decisions are incorrect, incomplete, or causing difficulties or complications, the person in command must make appropriate changes. The input for change can come from observations of the commander or from other sources available.

REASSESSMENT

Is the process moving correctly? Has the situation on scene changed? What is the patient's condition? How has the treatment plan changed the patient's condition? Does anything in the action plan need to be changed?

CHANGES ALONG THE WAY

Any changes that are identified by the commander are assessed and analyzed as above and alterations made as appropriate so as to continue the best possible care to the patient. Decision making and reassessing the patient must be done without the worry of, "If I change, is that a sign of weakness or poor decision making initially?" Such change based on patient need is not weakness, but rather strength. Once a decision is made, as the process continues and the situation and patient respond, the provider reassesses and makes appropriate changes as required to provide the best possible care to the patient.

---

as—and may be even more important than—the manual skills that will be used to perform an intervention. Critical thinking in medicine is a process in which the medical care provider assesses the situation, the patient, and all of the resources that are available. This information is then rapidly analyzed and integrated to provide the best care possible to the patient. This requires that the provider develop a plan of action, initiate this plan, reassess the plan as the process of caring for the patient moves forward, and make adjustments in the plan as the patient's condition changes until that phase of care is completed (Figure 3-2). Critical thinking is a learned skill that improves with use and experience, just as all skills do.[1] If students are to function successfully as health care providers, then they must be equipped with the lifelong learning and critical-thinking skills necessary to acquire and process information in a rapidly and an ever-changing world.[2]

For the prehospital provider, this process begins with the initial information provided at the time of dispatch and continues until the hand off in the hospital to the next component in the chain of patient care. This critical-thinking process first

requires that the prehospital care provider assess and reassess the situation in which the patient is encountered. Then, the patient's condition must be assessed and frequently reassessed during the time on the scene and while en route to the best/appropriate facility. Critical thinking is also involved in the selection of best/appropriate facility for the patient, the resources available, and the transportation time to the various facilities in the vicinity. All of these critical decisions are based upon the situation, the patient condition, the fund of knowledge of the prehospital provider, and the equipment available.

By using, analyzing and integrating all of this information, the field care provider will develop an initial plan for caring for the injured trauma victim and move that plan forward. For each step along the way, the provider must reassess exactly how the patient has responded to this process. Prehospital providers must either continue the treatment plan or take steps to change the process as additional information becomes available. All of this depends on the critical-thinking skills used by providers to carry out their responsibilities. Critical thinking is based on accepting nothing at face value and always asking the question "Why?" as taught by Socrates and on the theory of falsifiability taught by Popper.[3]

The critical-thinking process cannot be dogmatic or gullible but must be open-minded with skepticism.[4] The provider must question the scientific accuracy of all approaches. This is the reason that the patient care provider must have a strong, well-grounded fund of knowledge that can be used to make appropriate decisions. However, this cannot be taken too far. Aristotle suggested that one should not require more certainty than the subject allows.[5]

In other words, critical thinking involves how to best provide the principles of patient care needed by the patient based on the current circumstances that the provider has noted. This uses the basis of appropriate medical care advocated by PHTLS: "Judgment based on knowledge." Robert Carroll described critical thinking as based on concepts and principles, not hard-and-fast rules or step-by-step procedures.[4] The emphasis throughout PHTLS education is that protocols involving robotic recall are not beneficial for patient management. Guidelines for patient care must be flexible. Critical thinking requires that flexibility. Protocols should simply serve as guidelines to assist the provider in aligning the thought process. They are not the definitive, be-all-end-all steps that cannot be violated by thoughtful, insightful analysis of the situation and application of appropriate steps to assure the best possible patient care in each unique situation.

In addition, all medical providers have biases that can affect the critical-thinking process and decision making about the patient. These biases must be recognized and not allowed to intrude during the patient care process. These biases usually arise from previous experiences that resulted in either a significant positive or negative impact. By becoming aware of and controlling biases, all conditions are taken into consideration and action is based on the admonition of "assume the worst possible injury is present and prove that it is not there" as well as "do no further harm." The patient's management plan is designed regardless of the attitudes of the provider regarding the "apparent" conditions that might have lead to the current circumstances. For example, the initial impression that a driver is intoxicated may be correct but other conditions may exist as well. Because a victim is found to be intoxicated does not mean he or she is not injured too. Because the victim is intoxicated with impaired mental facilities does not mean that some of that impairment might not be due to brain injury or decreased cerebral perfusion because of shock.

Frequently the answers to these sorts of questions cannot be obtained until the patient arrives at the hospital (or maybe even several days thereafter); therefore, the critical thinking and response of the prehospital provider must be based on a worst-case scenario. Judgments must be made on the best information available. The critical thinker is constantly looking for "other information" as it becomes available and acting on it, another sign of a good critical thinker. The critical thinking process must continue throughout the assessment of the patient, of the situation, and of the conditions. The brain

of the critical thinker is always looking for new information, making and revising judgments, and planning two to three steps beyond the current activity.

EMS is a field of quick action and reliance on the innate ability of the provider to respond decisively to varying presentations and varying diseases. These quick actions require the skill of critical thinking and the ability to decide, based on the current knowledge, which steps provide the best chance for patient survival—preference not rigidity.

Critical thinking at the site of an emergency must be swift, thorough, flexible, and objective. The EMS provider at the site of an emergency may have only seconds to assess the situation, the condition of the patient(s), and the resources in order to make decisions and commence patient care. This encompasses the processes of discernment, analysis, evaluation, judgment, re-evaluation, and making new decisions until the patient finally arrives at the hospital. The critical-care thinking process of an administrator may, on the other hand, allow for several days, weeks, or even months to work through the decision-making process. In EMS, a strong fund of knowledge possessed by the provider and the ability to communicate these judgments with strength and conviction to all involved in the response to the patient are the foundation for critical thinking.

As taught in the assessment chapter, information is gathered using all of the provider's senses—vision, smell, touch, hearing—and simultaneously fed into the "computer" inside the brain. The provider then analyzes the data obtained based on the predetermined priorities of the primary survey (airway, ventilation and circulation), resuscitation, and rapid transportation to the appropriate medical facility to select the appropriate management steps for the individual needs of that particular patient. Typically, the process of evaluating a trauma patient begins with the ABCDE priorities. However, if the patient is in shock because of severe ongoing external hemorrhage, then a pressure dressing (and tourniquet if that fails) over the site of severe hemorrhage is the appropriate initial step. Critical thinking is the recognition that following the standard ABCDE priority may lead to a patient who has an airway but who has now exsanguinated; so, instead of attention to the airway, control of the bleeding was the appropriate first step. Critical thinking is the process of recognizing that if direct pressure and the pressure dressing are not working, something more needs to be done, and application of a tourniquet is the next best step to stop the hemorrhage. How the brain of the provider functionally arrived at this decision is *critical thinking*. It is based on the assessment of the situation, the condition of the patient, the fund of knowledge of the prehospital provider, the skills of the provider, and the equipment available. "Critical thinking is a pervasive skill that involves scrutinizing, differentiating, and appraising information and reflecting on the information gained in order to make judgments and inform clinical decisions."[6]

The art and science of medicine, the knowledge of principles, and the appropriate application of preferences will lead to the anticipated outcome of the very best care possible for the patient in the circumstances in which the care is provided. There are essentially four steps in the process of caring for patients with acute injuries: (1) the prehospital phase; (2) the initial (resuscitative) phase in the hospital; (3) the stabilization and definitive care phase; and (4) the long-term resolution and rehabilitation to return the patient to a functional status. All of these phases use the same principles of patient care in each step. All of the providers throughout the phases of the patient's care must use critical thinking. Critical-thinking steps continue from the time of the injury until the time that the patient goes home. Each critical-thinking step along the way varies according to the resources that are available to provide this care and the condition of the patient during each individual step. Therefore, understanding the principles of management, the options available, the reassessment as the situation and the conditions change, and the modification of the management plan throughout the patient's entire care requires use of the critical-thinking process.

EMS personnel are directly involved in the initial (prehospital) phase of care but must use critical thinking and be aware of the entire process in order to produce seamless patient care as the patient moves through the system. The field care provider must think beyond the current situation to the definitive care needs and the patient's ultimate outcome. The goal is to manage the patient's injuries so that they heal and that the patient can be discharged from the hospital in the best possible condition.

SUMMARY

- Principles or science
  - What the patient must have in order to optimize outcome and survival
- Preferences or art
  - Methods of achieving the principle
  - Considerations for choosing the method
    - Situation that currently exists
    - Condition of the patient
    - Knowledge and experience
    - Equipment available
- Critical thinking
  - The assessment of all concerns and components of the traumatic event at hand

- Critical thinking—continued
  - Use all senses to achieve assessment
  - Review the need for additional information, equipment, and personnel
  - Identification of hospitals in the vicinity and their capabilities
  - Develop a plan of action and management
  - Reassessment of the situation, patient, response to the action plan
  - Midcourse correction(s) as necessary
  - Goal is successful management
  - Critical thinking is NOT following protocols
  - Critical thinking IS swift, flexible, objective

SCENARIO SOLUTION

The answer to the question of patient management requires critical thinking and must be based on addressing the four components of patient management: situation, condition, knowledge and experience, and the equipment that you have available:

Questions about the situation that you will have to analyze include:

1. How long will it take to extricate the patient from the vehicle?
2. Do you have adequate resources on the scene for such things as lighting, extrication and rescue, personnel, etc.?

Questions about the patient condition that you will have to analyze include:

1. Does the patient require airway intervention?
2. What has to be done to control the hemorrhage?
3. Does pressure control the hemorrhage?
4. If you place a tourniquet and go to the nontrauma center, how long will it stay on prior to definitive control in this facility?
5. Does the patient have an urgent need for immediate replacement of oxygen-carrying fluid (blood)?
6. If yes, will the patient get that blood faster in the farther trauma center or the closer nontrauma center?

Questions about knowledge and experience that you will have to analyze include:

1. How will the airway be managed given the personnel available on scene?

2. If available, should the patient undergo endotracheal intubation, or should ventilation be assisted with a bag-mask device?
3. Who is the most experienced person available to manage the airway and when was the last time he or she had to do so?

Questions about resources and equipment that you will have to analyze include:

1. If you load the patient immediately in your ambulance, how long will it take to get to the trauma center?
2. If you call for a helicopter, how long will it take to get the patient to the trauma center?
3. Should you rendezvous with the helicopter at the nontrauma center helistop?
4. Should you take the patient to the nontrauma center first?

Critical thinking is very important. Decisions must be made based on the knowledge of the entire incident as it is before you. The answers are yours. The situation is unique. The responsibility is yours. The patient may live or die based on what you do.

References

1. Hendricson WD, Andrieu SC, Chadwick DG, et al: As educational strategies associated with development of problem-solving, critical thinking, and self-directed learning. *J Dent Educ* 70(9):925–936, 2006.
2. Cotter AJ: Developing critical-thinking skills. *EMS Mag* 36(7):86, 2007.
3. Wang SY, Tsai JC, Chiang HC, et al: Socrates, problem-based learning and critical thinking—a philosophic point of view. *Kaohsiung J Med Sci* 24(3 Suppl):S6–13, 2008.
4. Carroll, RT: *Becoming a Critical Thinker: A Guide for the New Millenium,* ed 2, 2005, Pearson Custom Publishing, Boston, MA.
5. Aristotle: *Nichomachean Ethics,* (Book I, part 3). Translation by W.D. Ross, The Internet Classics Archive, 1994–2000, http://classics.mit.edu//Aristotle/nicomachaen.html.
6. Banning M: Measures that can be used to instill critical-thinking skills in nurse prescribers. *Nurse Educ Pract* 6(2):98–105, 2006.

CHAPTER 4

Kinematics of Trauma

CHAPTER OBJECTIVES

At the completion of this chapter, the reader will be able to do the following:

✓ Define energy in the context of production of injury.

✓ Describe the association between the laws of motion, energy, and the kinematics of trauma.

✓ Describe the relationship of injury and energy exchange to speed.

✓ Discuss energy exchange and the production of cavitation.

✓ Given the description of a motor vehicle crash, use kinematics to predict the likely injury pattern for an unrestrained occupant.

✓ Associate the principles of energy exchange with the pathophysiology of injury to the head, spine, thorax, abdomen, and extremities resulting from that exchange.

✓ Describe the specific injuries and their causes as related to interior and exterior vehicle damage.

✓ Describe the function of restraint systems for vehicle occupants.

✓ Relate the laws of motion and energy to mechanisms other than motor vehicle crashes (e.g., blasts, falls).

✓ Describe the five phases of blast injury and the injuries produced in each phase.

✓ Describe the differences in the production of injury with low-medium-, and high-energy weapons.

✓ Discuss the relationship of the frontal surface of an impacting object to energy exchange and injury production.

✓ Integrate principles of the kinematics of trauma into patient assessment.

SCENARIO

You and your partner are dispatched to a two-car collision. The day is warm and sunny. The scene is secured by law enforcement when you arrive.

On arrival, you confirm that there are only two cars involved. The first car is in the ditch on the right side of the road and has impacted a tree at the passenger-side door. There are bullet holes in the left-front door. At least three holes are visible to you. There are two occupants in the vehicle.

The other car veered off the left side of the road and hit a utility pole, centered between the two headlights. There are two people in that car. It is an old vehicle without air bags. There is a bent steering wheel, and, there is a bull's-eye fracture of the windshield on the driver's side. As you look into the car on the passenger side, you find an indentation in the lower part of the passenger-side dash. None of the passengers in either vehicle are wearing a safety belt. You are dealing with four injured patients—two in each car—and all have remained in the cars.

You are the senior EMT-paramedic on the scene. It is your responsibility to assess the patients and assign priority for transportation. Take the patients one at a time and describe them based on the kinematics.

How would you describe each patient based upon the kinematics?

What injuries do you expect to find?

Unexpected traumatic injuries are responsible for more than 169,000 deaths in the United States each year.[1] Vehicle collisions accounted for more than 37,000 deaths and more than 4 million injured persons in 2008.[2] This problem is not limited to the United States; other countries have an equal frequency of vehicular trauma, although the vehicles may be different. Penetrating trauma from guns is very high in the United States. In 2006, there were almost 31,000 deaths from firearms. Of these, over 13,000 were homicides.[1] In 2008, there were over 78,000 nonfatal firearm injuries reported.[3] Blast injuries are a major cause of injuries in many countries, whereas penetrating injuries from knives are prominent in others. Successful management of trauma patients depends on identification of injuries or potential injuries and the use of good assessment skills. It is frequently difficult to determine the exact injury produced, but understanding the potential for injury and the potential for significant blood loss will allow the critical-thinking process of the provider to recognize this likelihood and make appropriate triage, management, and transportation decisions.

The management of any patient begins (after initial resuscitation) with the history of the patient's injury. In trauma, the history is the story of the impact and the energy exchange that resulted from this impact.[4] An understanding of the energy exchange process will lead to the suspicion of 95% of the potential injuries.

When the provider, at any level of care, does not understand the principles of kinematics or the mechanisms involved, injuries may be missed. An understanding of these principles will increase the level of suspicion based on the pattern of injuries likely associated with the survey of the scene on arrival. This information and the suspected injuries can be used to properly assess the patient on the scene and can be transmitted to the physicians and nurses in the emergency department (ED). At the scene and en route, these suspected injuries can be managed to provide the most appropriate patient care and "do no further harm."

Injuries that are not obvious but are still severe can be fatal if they are not managed at the scene and en route to the trauma center or appropriate hospital. Knowing where to look and how to assess for injuries is as important as knowing what to do after finding injuries. A complete, accurate history of a traumatic incident and proper interpretation of this data will provide such information. Most of a patient's injuries can be predicted by a proper survey of the scene, even before examining the patient.

This chapter discusses the general principles and mechanical principles involved in the kinematics of trauma, and the sections on the regional effects of blunt and penetrating trauma address local injury pathophysiology. The general principles are the laws of physics that govern energy exchange and the general effects of the energy exchange. Mechanical principles address the interaction of the human body with the components of the crash for blunt trauma (e.g., motor vehicles, three- and two-wheeled vehicles, and falls), penetrating trauma, and blasts. A crash is the energy exchange that occurs when an object with energy, usually something solid, impacts the human body. It is not only the collision of a motor vehicle, but also the crash of a falling body onto the pavement, the impact of a bullet on the external and internal tissues of the body, and the overpressure and debris of a blast. All of these involve energy exchange, all result in injury, all involve potentially life-threatening conditions, and all require the correct management by a knowledgeable and insightful prehospital care provider.

General Principles

A traumatic event is divided into three phases: precrash, crash, and postcrash. Again, the term *crash* does not necessarily mean a vehicular crash. The crash of a vehicle into a pedestrian, a missile (bullet) into the abdomen, and a construction worker striking the asphalt after a fall are all examples of a crash. In each case, energy is exchanged between a moving object and the tissue of the human body or between the moving human body and a stationary object.

The *precrash phase* includes all of the events that preceded the incident. Conditions that are present before the incident, but important in the management of the patient's injuries, are assessed as part of the precrash history. These include such things as a patient's acute or pre-existing medical conditions (and medications to treat those conditions), ingestion of recreational substances (illegal and prescription drugs, alcohol, etc.), and a patient's state of mind. Typically, young trauma patients do not have chronic illnesses. With older patients, however, medical conditions that are present before the trauma event can cause serious complications in the prehospital assessment and management of the patient and can significantly influence the outcome. For example, the elderly driver of a vehicle that has struck a utility pole may have chest pain indicative of a myocardial infarction (heart attack). Did the driver hit the utility pole and have a heart attack, or did he have a heart attack and then strike the utility pole? Does the patient take medication (e.g., beta blocker) that will prevent elevation of the pulse in shock? Most of these conditions not only directly influence the assessment and management strategies discussed in Chapters 4 and 5, but are important in overall patient care as well, even if they do not necessarily influence the kinematics of the crash.

The *crash phase* begins at the time of impact between one moving object and a second object. The second object can be moving or stationary and can be either an object or a person. Three impacts occur in most vehicular crashes: (1) the impact of the two objects; (2) the impact of the occupants into the vehicle; and (3) the impact of the vital organs inside the occupants. For example, when a vehicle strikes a tree, the first impact is the collision of the vehicle with the tree. The second impact is the occupant of the vehicle striking the steering wheel or windshield. If the patient is restrained, an impact occurs between the occupant and the seat belt. The third impact is between the patient's internal organs and his or her chest wall, abdominal wall, or skull. (In a fall, only the second and third impacts are involved.)

The direction in which the energy exchange occurs, the amount of energy that is exchanged, and the effect that these forces have on the patient are all important considerations as assessment begins.

During the *postcrash phase* the information gathered about the crash and precrash phases is used to assess and manage a patient. This phase begins as soon as the energy from the crash is absorbed. The onset of the complications from life-threatening trauma can be slow or fast (or these complications can be prevented or significantly reduced), depending in part on the care provided at the scene and en route to the hospital. In the postcrash phase, the understanding of the kinematics of trauma, the index of suspicion regarding injuries, and strong assessment skills all become crucial to the patient outcome.

Simply stated, the **precrash** phase is the prevention phase. The **crash** phase is that portion of the traumatic event that involves the exchange of energy or the kinematics (mechanics of energy). Lastly, the **postcrash** is the patient care phase.

To understand the effects of the forces that produce bodily injury, the prehospital care provider needs first to understand two components—energy exchange and human anatomy. For example, in a motor vehicle crash (MVC), what does the scene look like? Who hit what and at what speed? How long was the stopping time? Were the victims using appropriate restraint devices such as seat belts? Did the air bag deploy? Were the children restrained properly in child seats, or were they unrestrained and thrown about the vehicle? Were occupants thrown from the vehicle? Did they strike objects? If so, how many objects and what was the nature of those objects? These and many other questions must be answered if the prehospital care provider is to understand the exchange of forces that took place and translate this information into a prediction of injuries and appropriate patient care.

The process of surveying the scene to determine what forces and motion were involved and what injuries might have resulted from those forces is called *kinematics*. Because kinematics is based on fundamental principles of physics, an understanding of the pertinent laws of physics is necessary.

Energy

The initial component in obtaining a history is to evaluate the events that occurred at the time of the crash (Figure 4-1), to estimate the energy that was exchanged with the human body, and to make a gross approximation of the specific conditions that resulted.

Laws of Energy and Motion

Newton's first law of motion states that a body at rest will remain at rest and a body in motion will remain in motion unless acted on by an outside force. The skier in Figure 4-2

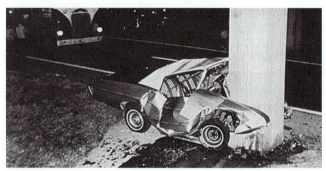

FIGURE 4-1 Evaluating the scene of an incident is critical. Such information as direction of impact, passenger-compartment intrusion, and amount of energy exchange provides insight into the possible injuries of the occupants. Although an older-model vehicle, this photograph shows the concept of mechanism of injury.

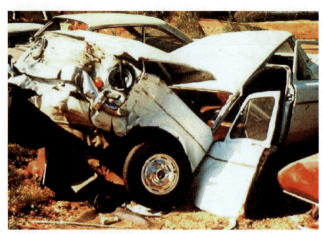

FIGURE 4-3 Vehicle stops suddenly against a dirt embankment.

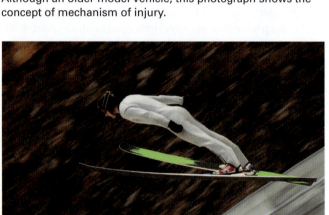

FIGURE 4-2 A skier was stationary until the energy from gravity moved him down the slope. Once in motion, although he leaves the ground, the momentum will keep him in motion until he hits something or returns to the ground, and the transfer of energy (friction or a collision) causes him to come to a stop.

was stationary until the energy from gravity moved him down the slope. Once in motion, although he leaves the ground, he will remain in motion until he hits something or returns to the ground and comes to a stop.

As previously mentioned, in any collision, when the body of the potential patient is in motion, there are three collisions: 1) the vehicle hitting an object, moving or stationary; 2) the potential patient hitting the inside of the vehicle, crashing into an object, or being struck by energy in an explosion; and 3) the internal organs interacting with the walls of a compartment of the body or being torn loose from their supporting structures. An example is a person sitting

in the front seat of a vehicle. When the vehicle hits a tree and stops, the unrestrained person continues in motion—at the same rate of speed—until he or she hits the steering column, dashboard, and windshield. The impact with these objects stops the forward motion of the torso or head, but the internal organs of the person remain in motion until the organs hit the inside of the chest wall, abdominal wall, or skull, halting the forward motion.

The *law of conservation of energy* combined with *Newton's second law of motion* describes that energy cannot be created or destroyed but can be changed in form. The motion of the vehicle is a form of energy. To start the vehicle, gasoline explodes within the cylinder of the engine. This moves the pistons. The motion of the pistons is transferred by a set of gears to the wheels, which grasp the road as they turn and impart motion to the vehicle. To stop the vehicle, the energy of its motion must be changed to another form, such as heating up the brakes or crashing into an object and bending the frame. When a driver brakes, the energy of motion is converted into the heat of friction (thermal energy) by the brake pads on the brake drums/disk and by the tires on the roadway. The vehicle decelerates.

Just as the mechanical energy of a vehicle that crashes into a wall is dissipated by the bending of the frame or other parts of the vehicle (Figure 4-3), the energy of motion of the organs and the structures inside of the body must be dissipated as these organs stop their forward motion. The same concepts apply to the human body when it is stationary and comes into contact and interacts with an object in motion such as a knife, a bullet, or a baseball bat.

Kinetic energy is a function of an object's mass and velocity. Although they are not exactly the same, a victim's weight is used to represent his or her mass. Likewise, speed is used to represent velocity (which really is speed and direction). The relationship between weight and speed as it affects kinetic energy is as follows:

Kinetic energy = One-half the mass times the velocity squared

$$KE = \frac{1}{2}mv^2$$

Thus, the kinetic energy involved when a 150-lb (68-kg) person travels at 30 mph (48 km/hr) is calculated as follows:

$$KE = \frac{150}{2} \times 30^2$$

$$KE = 67{,}500 \text{ units}$$

For the purpose of this discussion, no specific physical unit of measure (e.g., foot-pounds, joules) is used. The units are used merely to illustrate how this formula affects the change in the amount of energy. As just shown, a 150-lb (68-kg) person travelling at 30 mph (48 km/hr) would have 67,500 units of energy that has to be converted to another form when he or she stops. This change takes the form of damage to the vehicle and injury to the person in it unless the energy dissipation can take some less harmful form, such as on a seat belt or into an air bag.

Which factor in the formula, however, has the greatest effect on the amount of kinetic energy produced: mass or velocity? Consider adding 10 lbs to the 150-lb person travelling at 30 mph (48 km/hr) in the prior example now making the mass equal to 160 lbs (72 kg):

$$KE = \frac{160}{2} \times 30^2$$

$$KE = 72{,}000 \text{ units}$$

As the mass has increased, so has the amount of kinetic energy.

Finally, returning to this same example of a 150-lb (68-kg) person, instead of increasing the mass by 10, if the speed is increased by 10 mph (16 km/hr), the kinetic energy is as follows:

$$KE = \frac{150}{2} \times 40^2$$

$$KE = 120{,}000 \text{ units}$$

These calculations demonstrate that increasing the velocity (speed) increases the kinetic energy much more than increasing the mass. Much more energy exchange will occur (and, therefore, produce greater injury to either the occupant or the vehicle or both) in a high-speed crash than in a crash at a slower speed. The velocity is exponential and the mass is linear; this is critical even when there is a great mass disparity between two objects.

Mass × acceleration = force = mass × deceleration

Force (energy) is required to put a structure into motion. This force (energy) is required to create a specific speed. The speed imparted is dependent on the weight (mass) of the structure. Once this energy is passed on to the structure and it is placed in motion, the motion will remain until the energy is given up (Newton's first law of motion). This loss of energy will place other components in motion (tissue particles) or be lost as heat (dissipated into the brake disks on the wheels). An example of this process is the gun and the patient. In the chamber of a gun is a cartridge that contains gunpowder. If this gunpowder is ignited, it burns rapidly creating energy that pushes the bullet out of the barrel at a great speed. This speed is equivalent to the weight of the bullet and the amount of energy produced by the burning of the gunpowder or force. To slow down (Newton's first law of motion), the bullet must give up its energy into the structure that it hits. This will produce an explosion in the tissue that is equal to the explosion that occurred in the chamber of the gun when the initial speed was given to the bullet. The same phenomenon occurs in the moving automobile, the patient falling from a building, or the explosion of an improvised explosive device (IED).

Another important factor in a crash is the *stopping distance*. The shorter the stopping distance and the quicker the rate of that stop, the more energy transferred to the patient and the more damage or injury that is done to the patient. A vehicle that stops against a brick wall or one that stops when the brakes are applied dissipates the same amount of energy, just in a different manner. The rate of energy exchange (into the vehicle body or into the brake disks) is different and occurs over a different distance and time. In the first instance, the energy is absorbed in a very short distance and amount of time by the bending of the frame of the vehicle. In the latter case, the energy is absorbed over a longer distance and period of time by the heat of the brakes. The forward motion of the occupant of the vehicle (energy) is absorbed in the first instance by damage to the soft tissue and bones of the occupant. In the latter case, the energy is dissipated, along with the energy of the vehicle, into the brakes.

This inverse relationship between stopping distance and injury also applies to falls. A person has a better chance of surviving a fall if he or she lands on a compressible surface, such as deep, powder snow. The same fall terminating on a hard surface, such as concrete, can produce more severe injuries. The compressible material (i.e., the snow) increases the stopping distance and absorbs at least some of the energy rather than allowing all of the energy to be absorbed by the body. The result is decreased injury and damage to the body. This principle also applies to other types of crashes. In addition, an unrestrained driver will be more severely injured than a restrained driver. The restraint system, rather than the body, will absorb a significant portion of the energy transfer.

Therefore, once an object is in motion and has energy in the form of motion, in order for it to come to a complete rest, the object must lose all of its energy by converting the energy to another form or transferring it to another

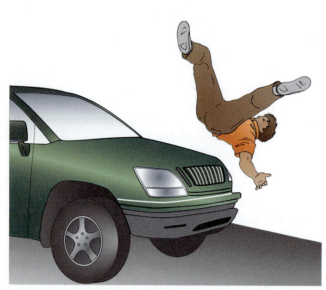

FIGURE 4-4   The energy exchange from a moving vehicle to a pedestrian crushes tissue and imparts speed and energy to the pedestrian to knock the victim away from the point of impact. Injury to the patient can occur at the point of impact as the pedestrian is hit by the vehicle and as the pedestrian is thrown to the ground or into another vehicle.

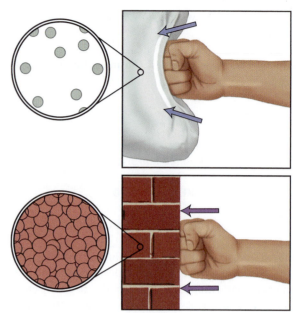

FIGURE 4-5   The fist absorbs more energy colliding with the dense brick wall than with the less dense feather pillow, which dissipates the force.

object. For example, if a vehicle strikes a pedestrian, the pedestrian is knocked away from the vehicle (Figure 4-4). Although the vehicle is somewhat slowed by the impact, the greater force of the vehicle imparts much more acceleration to the lighter-weight pedestrian than it loses in speed because of the mass difference between the two. The softer body parts of the pedestrian versus the harder body parts of the vehicle also means more damage to the pedestrian than to the vehicle.

Energy Exchange between a Solid Object and the Human Body

When the human body collides with a solid object, or vice versa, the number of body tissue particles that are impacted by the solid object determines the amount of energy exchange that takes place. This transfer of energy produces the amount of damage (injury) that occurs to the patient. The number of tissue particles affected is determined by (1) the density (particles per volume) of the tissue and (2) the size of the contact area of the impact.

Density

The denser a tissue is (measured in particles per volume), the greater the number of particles that will be hit by a moving object and, therefore, the greater the rate and the total amount

of energy exchanged. Driving a fist into a feather pillow and driving a fist at the same speed into a brick wall will produce different effects on the hand. The fist absorbs more energy colliding with the dense brick wall than with the less dense feather pillow (Figure 4-5).

Simplistically, the body has three different types of tissue densities: *air density* (much of the lung and some portions of the intestine), *water density* (muscle and most solid organs; e.g., liver, spleen), and *solid density* (bone). Therefore, the amount of energy exchange (with resultant injury) will depend on which type of organ is impacted.

Contact Area

Wind exerts pressure on a hand when it is extended out of the window of a moving vehicle. When the palm of the hand is horizontal and parallel to the direction of the flow through the wind, some backward pressure is exerted on the front of the hand (fingers) as the particles of air strike the hand. Rotating the hand 90 degrees to a vertical position places a larger surface area into the wind; thus, more air particles make contact with the hand, increasing the amount of force on it.

For trauma events, the energy imparted and the resulting damage can be modified by any change in the size of the impact surface area. Examples of this effect on the human body include the front of an automobile, a baseball bat, rifle

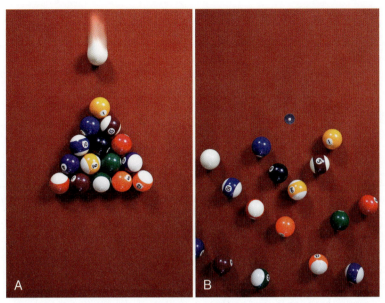

FIGURE 4-6   **A.** The energy of a cue ball is transferred to each of the other balls. **B.** The energy exchange pushes the balls apart to create a cavity.

bullet or shotgun. The automobile's front surface contacts a large portion of the victim. A baseball bat contacts a smaller area and a bullet contacts a very small area. The amount of energy exchange that would produce damage to the patient depends then on the energy of the object and the density of the tissue in the pathway of the energy exchange.

If all of the impact energy is in a small area and this force exceeds the resistance of the skin, the object is forced though the skin. This is the definition of **penetrating trauma.** If the force is spread out over a larger area and the skin it not penetrated, then it fits the definition of **blunt trauma.** In either instance, a cavity in the patient is created by the force of the impacting object. Even with something like a bullet, the impact surface area can be different based on such factors as bullet size, its motion (tumble) within the body, deformation ("mushroom"), and fragmentation.

Cavitation

The basic mechanics of energy exchange are relatively simple. The impact on the tissue particles accelerates those tissue particles away from the point of impact. These tissues then become moving objects themselves and crash into other tissue particles, producing a "falling domino" effect. A common game that provides a visual effect of cavitation is pool.

The cue ball is driven down the length of a pool table by the force of the muscles in the arm. The cue ball crashes into the racked balls at the other end of the table. The energy from the arm into the cue ball is thus transferred onto each of the racked balls (Figure 4-6). The cue ball gives up its energy to the other balls. The other balls began to move while the cue ball, which has lost its energy, slows or even stops. The other balls take on this energy as motion and move away from the impact point. A cavity has been created where the rack of balls once was. The same kind of energy exchange occurs when a bowling ball rolls down the alley, hitting the set of pins at the other end. The result of this energy exchange is a cavity. This sort of energy exchange occurs in both blunt and penetrating trauma.

Similarly, when a solid object strikes the human body or when the human body is in motion and strikes a stationary object, the tissue particles of the human body are knocked out of their normal position, creating a hole or cavity. Thus, this process is called *cavitation.*

Two types of cavities are created:

1. A temporary cavity is caused by the stretching of the tissues that occurs at the time of impact. Because of the elastic properties of the body's tissues, some or all of the contents of the temporary cavity return to their previous position. The size, shape, and portions of the cavity that become part of the permanent damage depend on the tissue type, the elasticity of the tissue, and how much rebound of tissue occurs. This extent of this cavity is usually not visible when the prehospital or hospital provider examines the patient, even seconds after the impact.

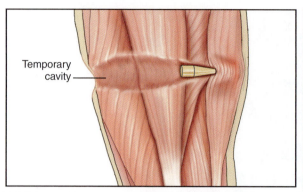
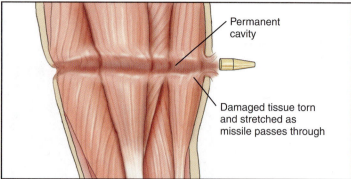

Temporary cavity

Permanent cavity

Damaged tissue torn and stretched as missile passes through

FIGURE 4-7   Damage to tissue is greater than the permanent cavity that remains from a missile injury. The faster or heavier the missile, the larger the temporary cavity and the greater the zone of tissue damage.

2. A permanent cavity is left after the temporary cavity collapses and is the visible part of the tissue destruction. In addition, there is a crush cavity that is produced by the direct impact of the object on the tissue. Both of these can be seen when the patient is examined[5] (Figure 4-7).

The amount of the temporary cavity that remains as a permanent cavity is related to the elasticity (stretch ability) of the tissue involved. For example, forcefully swinging a baseball bat

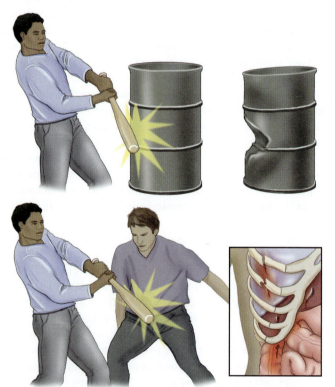

FIGURE 4-8   A. Swinging a baseball bat into a steel drum leaves a dent, or cavity, in its side. **B.** Swinging a baseball bat into a person usually leaves no visible cavity as the elasticity of the trunk returns the body back to its normal shape.

into a steel drum leaves a dent, or cavity, in its side. Swinging the same baseball bat with the same force into a mass of foam rubber of similar size and shape will leave no dent once the bat is removed (Figure 4-8). The difference is *elasticity*—the foam rubber is more elastic than the steel drum. The human body is more like the foam rubber than the steel drum. If a person punches a fist into another person's abdomen, he or she would feel the fist go in. However, when the person pulls the fist away, a dent is not left. Similarly, a baseball bat swung into the chest will leave no obvious cavity in the thoracic wall, but it would cause damage, both from direct contact and the cavity created by the energy exchange. The history of the incident and its interpretation will provide the information needed to determine the potential size of the temporary cavity at the time of impact. The organs or the structures involved predict injuries.

When the trigger of a loaded gun is pulled, the firing pin strikes the cap and produces an explosion in the cartridge. The energy created by this explosion is exchanged onto the bullet, which speeds from the muzzle of the weapon. The bullet now has energy, or force (acceleration × mass = force). Once such force is imparted, the bullet cannot slow down until acted on by an outside force (Newton's first law of motion). In order for the bullet to stop inside the human body, an explosion must occur within the tissues that is equivalent to the explosion in the weapon (acceleration × mass = force = mass × deceleration) (Figure 4-9). This explosion is the result of energy exchange accelerating the tissue particles out of their normal position, creating a cavity.

Blunt and Penetrating Trauma

Trauma is generally classified as either blunt or penetrating. However, the energy exchange and the injury produced are similar in both types of trauma. Cavitation occurs in both; only the type and direction are different. The only real difference is penetration of the skin. If an object's entire energy is concentrated on one small area of skin, the skin likely will tear, and the object will enter the body and create a more concentrated energy exchange along the pathway. This

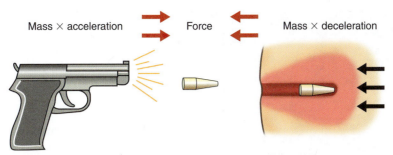

Mass × acceleration   Force   Mass × deceleration

FIGURE 4-9 As a bullet travels through tissue, its kinetic energy is transferred to the tissue that it comes in contact with, accelerating it away from the bullet.

can result in greater destructive power to one area. A larger object whose energy is dispersed over a much larger area of skin may not penetrate the skin. The damage will be distributed over a larger area of the body, and the injury pattern will be less localized. An example is difference in the impact of a large truck into a pedestrian versus a gunshot impact (Figure 4-10).

The cavitation in blunt trauma is frequently only a temporary cavity and is directed away from the point of impact. Pene-

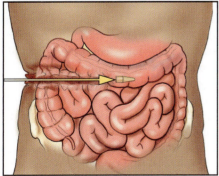

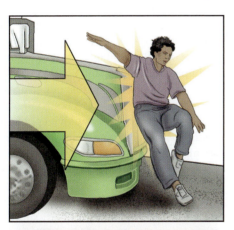

FIGURE 4-10 The force from a collision of a vehicle with a person is generally distributed over a large area, whereas the force of the collision between a bullet and person is localized to a very small area and results in penetration of the body and underlying structures.

trating trauma creates both a permanent and a temporary cavity. The temporary cavity that is created will spread away from the pathway of this missile in both frontal and lateral directions.

Blunt Trauma

Mechanical Principles

This section is divided into two major parts. The mechanical and structural effects on the vehicle of a crash are discussed first, and then the internal effects on the organs and body structures are addressed. Both are important and must be understood to properly assess the trauma patient and the potential injuries that exist after the crash.

The on-scene observations of the probable circumstances that led to a crash resulting in blunt trauma provide clues as to the severity of the injuries and the potential organs involved. The factors to assess are: (1) direction of the impact; (2) external damage to the vehicle (type and severity); and (3) internal damage (e.g., occupant-compartment intrusion, steering wheel/column bending, windshield bull's-eye fractures, mirror damage, dashboard knee impacts).

In blunt trauma, two forces are involved in the impact: shear and compression, both of which may result in cavitation. *Shear* is the result of one organ or structure (or part of an organ or structure) changing speed faster than another organ or structure (or part of an organ or structure). This difference in acceleration (or deceleration) causes the parts to separate and tear. *Compression* is the result of an organ or structure (or part of an organ or structure) being directly squeezed between other organs or structures. Injury can result from any type of impact, such as MVCs (vehicle or motorcycle), pedestrian collisions with vehicles, falls, sports injuries, or blast injuries. All of these mechanisms are discussed separately, followed by the results of this energy exchange on the specific anatomy in each of the body regions.

As discussed previously in this chapter, three collisions occur in blunt trauma. The first is the collision of the vehicle

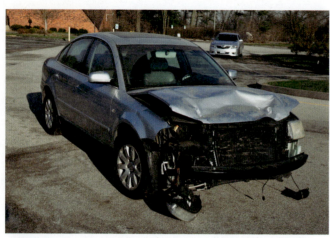

FIGURE 4-11 As a vehicle impacts a utility pole, the front of the car stops but the rear portion of the vehicle continues traveling forward, causing deformation of the vehicle.

into another object. The second is the collision that occurs when the potential patient strikes the inside of the vehicular passenger compartment, strikes the ground at the end of a fall, or is stuck by the force created in an explosion. The third is when the structures within the various regions of the body (head, chest, abdomen, etc.) strike the wall of that region or are torn (shear force) from their attachment within this compartment. The first of these will be discussed as it relates to vehicle crashes, falls, and explosions. The latter two will be discussed in the specific regions involved.

Motor Vehicle Crashes

Many forms of blunt trauma occur, but MVCs (including motorcycle crashes) are the most common. In 2008, 86% of fatalities were vehicle occupants. The remaining 14% were pedestrians, cyclists, and other nonoccupants, as reported by the U.S. National Highway Traffic Safety Administration (NHTSA).[6]

MVCs can be divided into the following five types:

1. Frontal impact
2. Rear impact
3. Lateral impact
4. Rotational impact
5. Rollover[7]

Although each pattern has variations, accurate identification of the five patterns will provide insight into other, similar types of crashes.

One method to estimate the potential for injury to the occupant is to look at the vehicle and determine which of the five types of collisions occurred, the energy exchange involved, and the direction of the impact. The occupant receives the same type of force as the vehicle from the same direction as the vehicle. The amount of force exchanged with the occupant, however, may be somewhat reduced by absorption of energy by the vehicle.

Frontal Impact

In Figure 4-11, for example, the vehicle has hit a utility pole in the center of the car. The impact point stopped its forward motion, but the rest of the car continued forward until the energy was absorbed by the bending of the car. The same type of motion occurs to the driver resulting in injury. The stable steering column is impacted by the chest, perhaps in the center of the sternum. Just as the car continued in forward motion, significantly deforming the front of the vehicle, so too will the driver's chest. As the sternum stops forward motion against the dash, the posterior thoracic wall continues until the energy is absorbed by the bending and possible fracture of the ribs. This process will also crush the heart and the lungs, which are trapped between the sternum and the vertebral column and the posterior thoracic wall.

The amount of damage to the vehicle indicates the approximate speed of the vehicle at the time of impact. The greater the intrusion into the body of the vehicle, the greater is the speed at the time of impact. The greater the vehicle speed, the greater the energy exchange and the more likely the occupants are to be injured.

Although the vehicle suddenly ceases to move forward in a frontal impact, the occupant continues to move and will follow one of two possible paths: either up-and-over or down-and-under.

The use of a seat belt and the deployment of an air bag or restraint system will absorb some or most of the energy, thus reducing the injury to the victim. For clarity and simplicity of discussion, the occupant is these examples will be assumed to be without restraint.

Up-and-Over Path. In this sequence, the body's forward motion carries it up and over the steering wheel (Figure 14-12). The head is usually the lead body portion striking the windshield, windshield frame, or roof. The head then stops its forward motion. The torso continues in motion until its energy/force is absorbed along the spine. The cervical spine is the least protected segment of the spine. The chest or abdomen then collides with the steering column, depending on the position of the torso. Impact of the chest into the steering column produces thoracic cage, cardiac, lung, and aortic injuries (see Regional Effects of Blunt Trauma). Impact of the abdomen into the steering column can compress and crush the solid organs, produce overpressure injuries (especially to the diaphragm), and rupture of the hollow organs. The kidneys, spleen, and liver are also subject to shear injury as the abdomen strikes the steering wheel and abruptly stops.

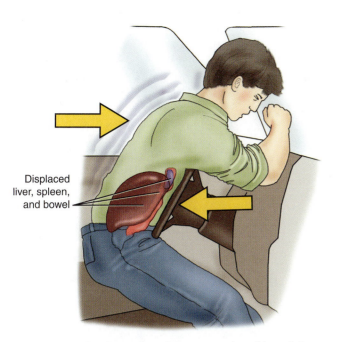

FIGURE 4-12   Configuration of the seat and position of the occupant can direct the initial force on the upper torso, with the head as the lead point.

Displaced liver, spleen, and bowel

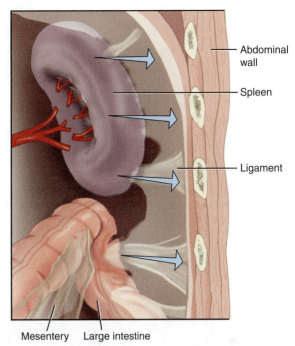

Abdominal wall

Spleen

Ligament

Mesentery   Large intestine

FIGURE 4-13   Organs can tear away from their point of attachment to the abdominal wall. The spleen, kidney, and small intestine are particularly susceptible to these types of shear forces.

An organ may be torn from its normal anatomic restraints and supporting tissues (Figure 4-13). For example, the continued forward motion of the kidneys after the vertebral column has stopped moving produces shear along the attachment of the organs at their blood supply. The aorta and vena cava are tethered tightly to the posterior abdominal wall and vertebral column. The continued forward motion of the kidneys can stretch the renal vessels to the point of rupture. A similar action may tear the aorta in the chest as the unattached arch becomes the tightly adhered descending aorta (Figure 4-14).

Down-and-Under Path. In a down-and-under path, the occupant moves forward, downward, and out of the seat into the dashboard (Figure 4-15). The importance of understanding kinematics is illustrated by the injuries produced to the lower extremity in this pathway. Because many of the injuries are difficult to identify, an understanding of the mechanism of injury is very important.

The foot, if planted on the floor panel or on the brake pedal with a straight knee, can twist as the continued torso motion angulates and fractures the ankle joint. More often, however, the knees are already bent, and the force is not directed to the ankle. Therefore, the knees strike the dashboard.

The knee has two possible impact points against the dashboard, the tibia and the femur (Figure 4-16A). If the tibia hits the dashboard and stops first, the femur remains in motion and overrides it. A dislocated knee, with torn ligaments, tendons, and other supporting structures, can result. Because the popliteal artery lies close to the knee joint, dislocation of the joint is frequently associated with injury to the vessel. The artery can be completely disrupted or the lining alone (intima) may be damaged (Figure 4-16B). In either case, a blood clot may form in the injured vessel, resulting in significantly decreased blood flow to the leg tissues below the knee. Early recognition of the knee injury and the potential for vascular injury will alert the physicians to the need for assessment of the vessel in this area.

Early identification and treatment of such a popliteal artery injury significantly decreases the complications of distal limb ischemia. Perfusion to this tissue needs to be re-established within about 6 hours. Delays could occur because the prehospital care provider failed to consider the kinematics of the injury or overlooked important clues during assessment of the patient.

Although most of these patients have evidence of injury to the knee, an imprint on the dashboard where the knee impacted is a key indicator that significant energy was

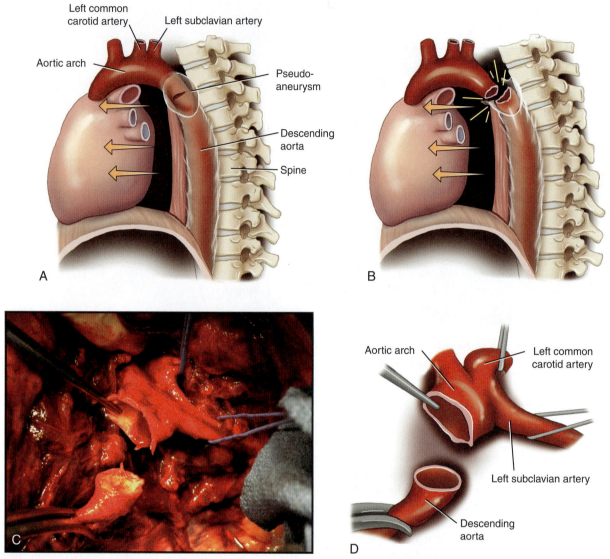

FIGURE 4-14 **A.** The descending aorta is a fixed structure that moves with the thoracic spine. The arch, aorta, and heart are freely movable. Acceleration of the torso in a lateral-impact collision or rapid deceleration of the torso in a frontal-impact collision produces a different rate of motion between the arch-heart complex and the descending aorta. This motion may result in a tear of the inner lining of the aorta that is contained within the outermost layer, producing a pseudo-aneurysm. **B.** Tears at the junction of the arch and descending aorta may also result in a complete rupture, leading to immediate exsanguination in the chest. **C** and **D.** Operative photograph and drawing of a traumatic aortic tear.
(**A** from McSwain NE Jr, Paturas JL: The Basic EMT: Comprehensive Prehospital Patient Care, ed 2, St. Louis, 2001, Mosby.)

focused on this joint and adjacent structures (Figure 4-17). Further investigation is needed in the hospital to better eliminate the possible injuries.

When the femur is the point of impact, the energy is absorbed on the bone shaft, which can then break (Figure 4-18). The continued forward motion of the pelvis onto the femur that remains intact can override the femoral head, resulting in a posterior dislocation of the acetabular joint (Figure 4-19).

After the knees and legs stop their forward motion, the upper body will bend forward into the steering column or dashboard. The unrestrained victim may then sustain many of the same injuries described previously for the up-and-over pathway.

Recognizing these potential injuries and relaying the information to the ED physicians can result in long-term benefits to the patient.

Rear Impact

Rear-impact collisions occur when a slower-moving or stationary vehicle is struck from behind by a vehicle moving at a faster rate of speed. For ease of understanding, the more rapidly moving vehicle is called the "bullet vehicle" and the slower-moving or stopped object is called the "target vehicle." In such collisions, the energy of the bullet vehicle at the moment of impact is converted to acceleration of the target

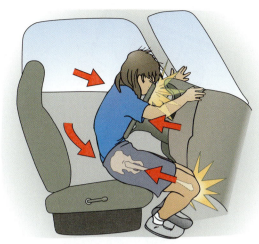

FIGURE 4-15   The occupant and the vehicle travel forward together. The vehicle stops, and the unrestrained occupant continues forward until something stops that motion.

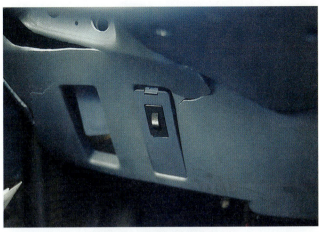

FIGURE 4-17   The impact point of the knee on the dashboard indicates both a down-and-under pathway and a significant absorption of energy along the lower extremity.

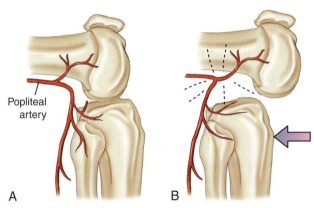

FIGURE 4-16   **A.** The knee has two possible impact points in a motor vehicle crash: the femur and the tibia. **B.** The popliteal artery lies close to the joint, tightly tied to the femur above and tibia below. Separation of these two bones stretches, kinks, and tears the artery.

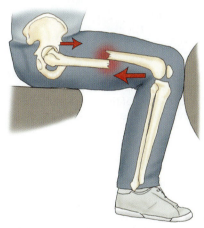

FIGURE 4-18   When the femur is the point of impact, the energy is absorbed on the bone shaft, which can then break.

vehicle and damage results to both vehicles. The greater the difference in the momentum of the two vehicles, the greater the force of the initial impact and the more energy is available to create damage and acceleration.

During a rear-impact collision, the target vehicle in front is accelerated forward. Everything that is attached to the frame will also move forward at the same rate of speed. This includes the seats in which the occupants are riding. The unattached objects in the vehicle, including the occupants, will begin forward motion only after something in contact with the frame begins to transmit the energy of the frame motion to these objects or occupants. As an example, the torso is accelerated by the back of the seat after some of the energy has been absorbed by the springs in the seats. If the headrest is improperly positioned behind and below the occiput of the head, the head will

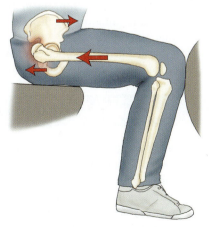

FIGURE 4-19   The continued forward motion of the pelvis onto the femur can override the femur's head, resulting in a posterior dislocation of the acetabular joint.

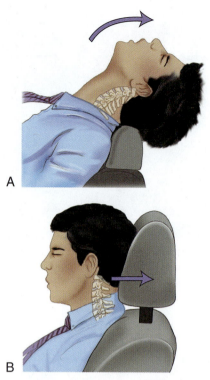

FIGURE 4-20 **A.** A rear-impact collision forces the torso forward. If the headrest is improperly positioned, the head is hyperextended over the top of the headrest. **B.** If the headrest is up, the head moves with the torso, and neck injury is prevented.

begin its forward motion after the torso, resulting in hyperextension of the neck. Shear and stretching of the ligaments and other support structures, especially in the anterior part of the neck, can result in injury (Figure 4-20A).

If the headrest is properly positioned, the head moves at approximately the same time as the torso without hyperextension (Figures 4-20B, 4-21). If the target vehicle is allowed to move forward without interference until it slows to a stop, the occupant will probably not suffer significant injury because most of the body's motion is supported by the seat, similar to an astronaut launching into orbit.

However, if the vehicle strikes another vehicle or object or if the driver slams on the brakes and stops suddenly, the

---

FIGURE 4-21 **Head Rests**

If it can be proved that the victim's headrest was not properly positioned when the neck injury occurred, some courts consider reducing the liability of the party at fault in the crash on the grounds that the victim's negligence contributed to the injuries *(contributory negligence)*. Similar measures have been considered in cases of failure to use occupant restraints. Elderly patients have a high frequency of injury.[35]

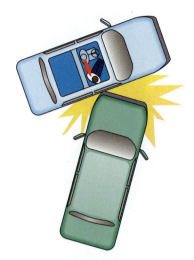

FIGURE 4-22 Lateral impact of the vehicle pushes the entire vehicle into the unrestrained passenger. A restrained passenger moves laterally with the vehicle.

occupants will continue forward, following the characteristic pattern of a frontal-impact collision. The collision then involves two impacts—rear and frontal. The double impact increases the likelihood of injury.

Lateral Impact

Lateral-impact mechanisms come into play when the vehicle is involved in an intersection ("T-bone") collision or when the vehicle veers off the road and impacts sideways a utility pole, tree, or other obstacle on the roadside. If the collision is at an intersection, the target vehicle is accelerated from the impact in the direction away from the force created by the bullet vehicle. The side of the vehicle or the door that is struck is thrust against the side of the occupant. The occupants may then be injured as they are accelerated laterally (Figure 4-22) or as the passenger compartment is bent inward by the door's projection (Figure 4-23). Injury caused by the

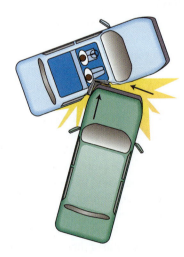

FIGURE 4-23 Intrusion of the side panels into the passenger compartment provides another source of injury.

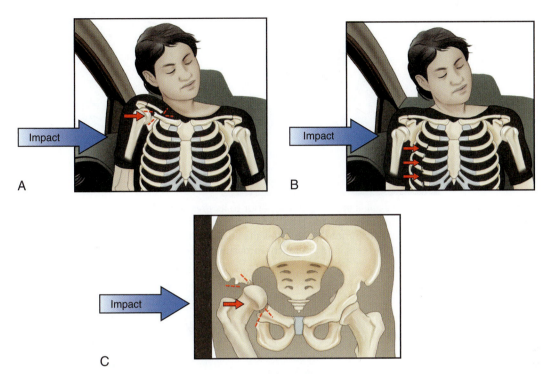

FIGURE 4-24 **A.** Compression of the shoulder against the clavicle produces midshaft fractures of this bone. **B.** Compression against the lateral chest and abdominal wall can fracture ribs and injure the underlying spleen, liver, and kidney. **C.** Lateral impact on the femur pushes the head through the acetabulum or fractures the pelvis.

vehicle's movement is less severe if the occupant is restrained and moves with the initial motion of the vehicle.[9]

Five body regions can sustain injury in a lateral impact:

1. *Clavicle.* The clavicle can be compressed and fractured if the force is against the shoulder (Figure 4-24).
2. *Chest.* Compression of the thoracic wall inward can result in fractured ribs, pulmonary contusion, or compression injury of the solid organs beneath the rib cage, as well as overpressure injuries (e.g., pneumothorax) (Figure 4-24B). Shear injuries of the aorta can result from the lateral acceleration (25% of aortic shear injuries occur in lateral-impact collisions). [10, 11, 12]
3. *Abdomen and pelvis.* The intrusion compresses and fractures the pelvis and pushes the head of the femur through the acetabulum (Figure 4-24C). Occupants on the driver's side are vulnerable to spleen injuries because the spleen is on the left side of the body, whereas those on the passenger side are more likely to receive an injury to the liver.
4. *Neck.* The torso can move out from under the head in lateral collisions as well as in rear impacts. The attachment point of the head is posterior and inferior to the center of gravity of the head. Therefore, the motion of the head in relationship to the neck is lateral flexion and rotation. The contralateral side of the spine will be opened (distraction) and the ipsilateral side compressed. This

can fracture the vertebrae or more likely produce jumped facets and possible dislocation as well as spinal cord injury (Figure 4-25).
5. *Head.* The head can impact the frame of the door.

Near-side impacts produce more injuries than far-side impacts.

Rotational Impact

Rotational-impact collisions occur when one corner of a vehicle strikes an immovable object, the corner of another vehicle, or a vehicle moving slower or in the opposite direction of the first vehicle. Following Newton's first law of motion, this corner of the vehicle will stop while the rest of the vehicle continues its forward motion until all its energy is completely transformed.

Rotational-impact collisions result in injuries that are a combination of those seen in frontal impacts and lateral collisions. The victim continues to move forward and then is hit by the side of the vehicle (as in a lateral collision) as the vehicle rotates around the point of impact (Figure 4-26). *More severe injuries are seen in the victim closest to the point of impact.*

Rollover

During a rollover, a vehicle may undergo several impacts at many different angles, as may the unrestrained occupant's body and internal organs (Figure 4-27). Injury and damage

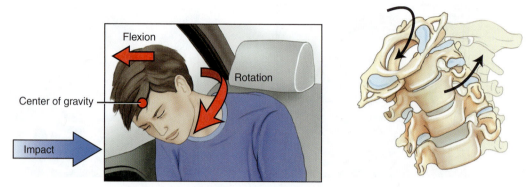

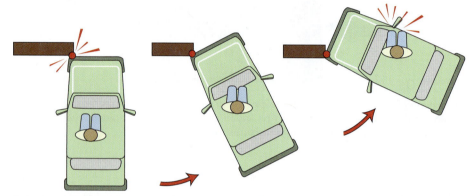

FIGURE 4-25   The center of gravity of the skull is anterior and superior to its pivot point between the skull and cervical spine. During a lateral impact, when the torso is rapidly accelerated out from under the head, the head turns toward the point of impact, in both lateral and anterior-posterior angles. Such motion separates the vertebral bodies from the side of opposite impact and rotates them apart. Jumped facets, ligaments, tears, and lateral compression fractures result.

FIGURE 4-26   The victim in a rotational-impact crash first moves forward and then laterally as the vehicle pivots around the impact point.

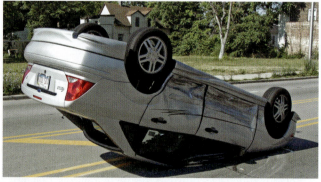

FIGURE 4-27   During a rollover, the unrestrained occupant can be wholly or partially ejected out of the vehicle or can bounce around inside the vehicle. This action produces multiple and somewhat unpredictable injuries that are usually severe.

can occur with each of these impacts. In rollover collisions, a restrained occupant often sustains shearing-type injuries because of the significant forces created by a rolling vehicle. The forces are similar to the forces of a spinning carnival ride. Although the occupants are held securely by restraints, the

internal organs still move and can tear at the connecting tissue areas. More serious injuries result from being unrestrained. In many cases, the occupants are ejected from the vehicle as it rolls and are either crushed as the vehicle rolls over them or sustain injuries from the impact with the ground. If the occupants are ejected onto the roadway, they can be struck by oncoming traffic. The NHTSA reports that in crashes involving fatalities in the year 2008, 77% of occupants who were totally ejected from a vehicle were killed.[13]

Vehicle Incompatibility

The type of vehicles involved in the crash plays a significant role in the potential for injury and death to the occupants. For example, in a lateral impact between two cars that lack air bags, the occupants of the car struck on its lateral aspect are 5.6 times more likely to die than the occupants in the vehicle striking that car. This can be largely explained by the relative lack of protection on the side of a car compared with the large amount of deformation that can occur to the front end of a vehicle before there is intrusion into the passenger compartment. However, when the vehicle that is struck in a lateral collision (by a car) is a sport utility vehicle (SUV),

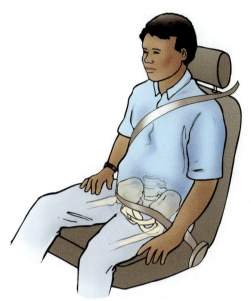

FIGURE 4-28   A properly positioned seat belt is located below the anterior-superior iliac spine on each side, above the femur, and is tight enough to remain in this position. The bowl-shaped pelvis protects the soft intra-abdominal organs.

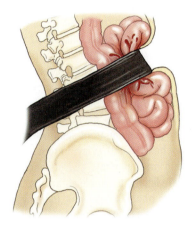

FIGURE 4-29   A seat belt that is incorrectly positioned above the brim of the pelvis allows the abdominal organs to be trapped between the moving posterior wall and the belt. Injuries to the pancreas and other retroperitoneal organs result, as well as blowout ruptures of the small intestine and colon.

van, or pickup truck rather than a car, the risk of death to occupants is almost the same for all vehicles involved. Thus, SUVs, vans, and pickup trucks provide additional protection to their occupants because the passenger compartment sits higher off the ground than that of a car, and the occupants sustain less of a direct blow in a lateral impact.

More serious injuries and a greatly increased risk of death to vehicle occupants have been documented when a car is struck on its lateral aspect by a van, SUV, or pickup. In a lateral-impact collision between a van and a car, the occupants of the car struck broadside are 13 times more likely to die than those in the van. If the striking vehicle is a pickup truck or SUV, the occupants of the car struck broadside are 25 to 30 times more likely to die than those in the pickup truck or SUV. This tremendous disparity results from the higher center of gravity and increased mass of the van, SUV, or pickup truck. Knowledge of vehicle types in which occupants were located in a crash may lead the prehospital care provider to have a higher index of suspicion for serious injury.

Occupant Protective and Restraining Systems

Seat Belts. In the injury patterns described previously, the victims were assumed to be unrestrained. The NHTSA reported that, in 2008, only 17% of occupants were unrestrained compared with 67% in a 1999 NHTSA report.[14] Ejection from vehicles accounted for approximately 25% of the 44,000 vehicular deaths in 2002. About 77% of passenger vehicle occupants who were totally ejected were killed[13]; 1 in 13 ejection victims sustained a spine fracture. After ejection from a vehicle, the body is subjected to a second impact as the body

strikes the ground (or another object) outside the vehicle. This second impact can result in injuries that are even more severe than the initial impact. The risk of death for ejected victims is six times greater than for those who are not ejected. Clearly, seat belts save lives.[7]

The NHTSA reports that 49 states and the District of Columbia have safety-belt legislation. From 2004 through 2008, more than 75,000 lives were saved by the use of these restraining devices.[15] The NHTSA estimates that over 255,000 lives have been saved in the United States alone since 1975. Also, the NHTSA reports that over 13,000 lives were saved by seat belts in the United States in 2008 and that if all occupants wore restraints, the total lives saved would have been more than 17,000.

What occurs when the victims are restrained? If a seat belt is positioned properly, the pressure of the impact is absorbed by the pelvis and the chest, resulting in few, if any, serious injuries (Figure 4-28). The proper use of restraints transfers the force of the impact from the patient's body to the restraint belts and restraint system. With restraints, the chance of receiving life-threatening injuries is greatly reduced.[7,15,16]

Seat belts must be worn properly to be effective. An improperly worn belt may not protect against injury in the event of a crash, and it may even cause injury. When lap belts are worn loosely or are strapped above the pelvis, compression injuries of the soft abdominal organs can occur. Injuries of the soft intra-abdominal organs (spleen, liver, and pancreas) result from compression between the seat belt and the posterior abdominal wall (Figure 4-29). Increased intra-abdominal pressure can cause diaphragmatic rupture and herniation of abdominal organs. Lap belts should also not be worn alone

Front-seat passenger air bags have been shown to be dangerous to children and small adults, especially when children are placed in incorrect positions in the front seat or in incorrectly installed child seats. Children 12 years of age and younger should always be in the proper restraint device for their size and should be in the back seat. At least one study has demonstrated that almost 99% of the parents checked did not know how to properly install child restraining systems.[3]

Drivers should always be at least 10 inches (25 cm) from the air bag cover, and front-seat passengers should be at least 18 inches (45 cm) away. In most cases, when the proper seating arrangements and distances are used, air bag injuries are limited to simple abrasions.

Air bags are now also available in many vehicles in the sides and tops of the doors.

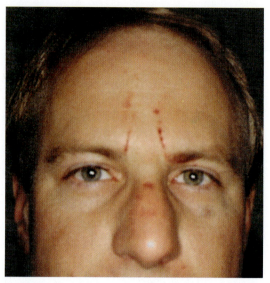

FIGURE 4-32   Expansion of the air bag into eyeglasses produces abrasions.
(From McSwain NE Jr, Paturas JL: The Basic EMT: Comprehensive Prehospital Patient Care, ed 2, St Louis, 2001, Mosby.)

As mandatory laws on seat belt use are passed and enforced, the overall severity of injuries decreases, and the number of fatal crashes is significantly reduced.

Air Bags. Air bags (in addition to seat belts) provide supplemental protection to the occupant of a vehicle. Originally, front-seat driver and passenger air bag systems were designed to cushion the forward motion of only the front-seat occupants. The air bags absorb energy slowly by increasing the body's stopping distance. They are extremely effective in the first collision of frontal and near-frontal impacts (the 65% to 70% of crashes that occur within 30 degrees of the headlights). However, air bags deflate immediately after the impact and, therefore, are not effective in multiple-impact or rear-impact collisions. An air bag deploys and deflates within 0.5 second. As the vehicle veers into the path of an oncoming vehicle or off the road into a tree after the initial impact, no air bag protection is left. Side air bags do add to the protection of occupants.

When air bags deploy, they can produce minor but noticeable injuries that the prehospital care provider needs to manage (Figure 4-30). These include abrasions of the arms, chest, and face (Figure 4-31); foreign bodies to the face and eyes; and injuries caused by the occupant's eyeglasses (Figure 4-32). Air bags that do not deploy can still be dangerous to both the patient and the prehospital care provider. Air bags can be deactivated by an extrication specialist trained to do so properly and safely. Such deactivation should *not* delay patient care or extrication of the critical patient.

Air bags pose a significant hazard to infants and children if the child is either unrestrained or placed in a rear-facing child seat in the front-passenger compartment. Of the over 290 deaths from air-bag deployments, almost 70% were passengers in the front seat, and 90% of those were infants or children.

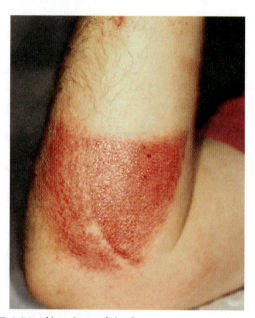

FIGURE 4-31   Abrasions of the forearm are secondary to rapid expansion of the air bag when the hands are tight against the steering wheel.
(From McSwain NE Jr, Paturas JL: The Basic EMT: Comprehensive Prehospital Patient Care, ed 2, St Louis, 2001, Mosby.)

but in combination with a shoulder restraint. Anterior compression fractures of the lumbar spine can occur as the upper and lower parts of the torso pivot over the lap belt and the restrained twelfth thoracic (T12), first lumbar (L1), and second lumbar (L2) vertebrae. Many occupants of vehicles still place the diagonal strap under the arm and not over the shoulder, risking serious injury.

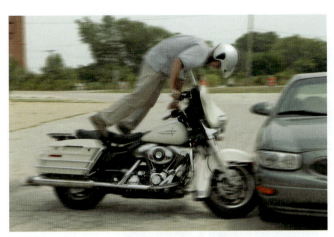

FIGURE 4-33   The position of a motorcycle driver is above the pivot point of the front wheel as the motorcycle impacts an object head-on.

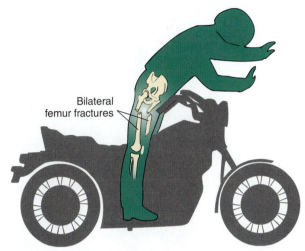

FIGURE 4-34   The body travels forward and over the motorcycle, impacting the thighs and the femurs into the handlebars. The driver can also be ejected.

Motorcycle Crashes

Motorcycle crashes account for a significant number of the motor vehicle deaths each year. While the laws of physics for motorcycle crashes are the same, the mechanism of injury varies from automobile and truck crashes. This variance occurs in each of the following types of impacts: head-on, angular, and ejection. An additional factor that leads to increased death, disability, and injury is the lack of structural framework around the biker that is present in other motor vehicles.

Head-on Impact

A head-on collision into a solid object stops the forward motion of a motorcycle (Figure 4-33). Because the motorcycle's center of gravity is above and behind the front axle, which is the pivot point in such a collision, the motorcycle will tip forward, and the rider will crash into the handlebars. The rider may receive injuries to the head, chest, abdomen, or pelvis, depending on which part of the anatomy strikes the handlebars. If the rider's feet remain on the pegs of the motorcycle and the thighs hit the handlebars, the forward motion will be absorbed by the midshaft of the femur, usually resulting in bilateral femoral fractures (Figure 4-34). "Open-book" pelvic fractures are a common result of the interaction between the biker's pelvis and the handle bars.

Angular Impact

In an angular-impact collision, the motorcycle hits an object at an angle. The motorcycle will then collapse on the rider or cause the rider to be crushed between the motorcycle and the object that was struck. Injuries to the upper or lower extremities can occur, resulting in fractures and extensive soft tissue injury (Figure 4-35). Injuries can also occur to organs of the abdominal cavity as a result of energy exchange.

Ejection Impact

Because of the lack of restraint, the rider is susceptible to ejection. The rider will continue in flight until the head, arms, chest, abdomen, or legs strike another object, such as a motor vehicle, a telephone pole, or the road. Injury will occur at the point of impact and will radiate to the rest of the body as the energy is absorbed.[7]

Injury Prevention

Many riders do not use proper protection. Protection for motorcyclists includes boots, leather clothing, and helmets. Of the three, the *helmet* affords the best protection. It is built similar to the skull: strong and supportive externally and energy-absorbent internally. The helmet's structure absorbs much of the impact, thereby decreasing injury to the face, skull, and brain. Failure to use helmets has been shown to increase head injuries by more than 300%. The helmet provides only minimal protection for the neck but does not cause neck injuries. Mandatory helmet laws work. For example, Louisiana had a 60% reduction in head injuries in the first 6 years after passing a helmet law. Most states that have passed mandatory helmet legislation have found an associated reduction in motorcycle incidents.

"Laying the bike down" is a protective maneuver used by bikers to separate them from the motorcycle in an impending crash (Figure 4-36). The rider turns the motorcycle sideways and drags the inside leg on the ground. This action slows the rider more than the motorcycle so that the motorcycle will move out from under the rider. The rider will then slide along on the pavement but will not be trapped between the motorcycle and any object it hits. These riders usually receive abrasions ("road rash") and minor fractures but generally avoid the severe injuries associated with the other types of impact, unless they directly strike another object (Figure 4-37).

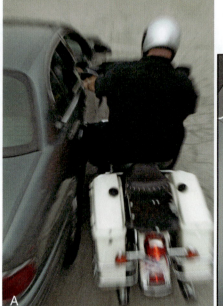
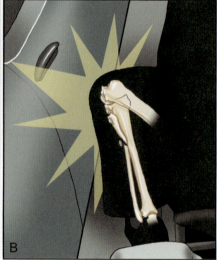

FIGURE 4-35   **A.** If the motorcycle does not hit an object head-on, it collapses like a pair of scissors. **B.** This collapse traps the rider's lower extremity between the object that was impacted and the motorcycle.

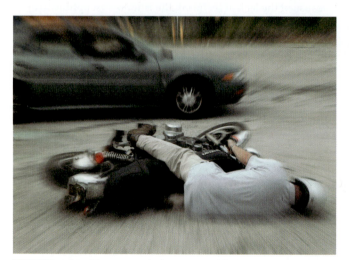

FIGURE 4-36   To prevent being trapped between two pieces of steel (motorcycle and vehicle), the rider "lays the bike down" to dissipate the injury. This often causes abrasions ("road rash") as the rider's speed is slowed on the asphalt.

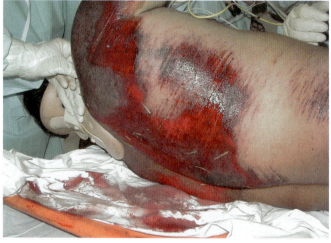

FIGURE 4-37   Road burns after a motorcycle crash without protective clothing.

Pedestrian Injuries

Pedestrian collisions with MVCs have three separate phases, each with its own injury pattern, as follows:

1. The initial impact is to the legs and sometimes the hips (Figure 4-38A).
2. The torso rolls onto the hood of the vehicle (and may strike the windshield) (Figure 4-38B).
3. The victim falls off the vehicle and onto the ground, usually headfirst, with possible cervical spine trauma (Figure 4-38C).

The injuries produced in pedestrian crashes vary according to the height of the victim and the height of the vehicle (Figure 4-39). The impact points on a child and an adult standing in front of a car present different anatomical structures to the vehicles. Because they are shorter, children are initially struck higher on the body than adults (Figure 4-40A). The first impact generally occurs when the bumper strikes the child's legs (above the knees) or pelvis, damaging the femur or pelvic girdle. The second impact occurs almost instantly afterward as the front of the vehicle's hood continues forward and strikes the child's thorax. Then, the head and face strike

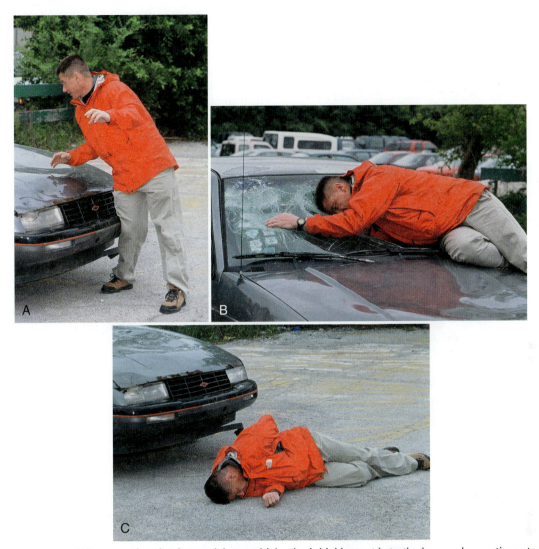

FIGURE 4-38   **A.** *Phase 1.* When a pedestrian is struck by a vehicle, the initial impact is to the legs and sometimes to the hips. **B.** *Phase 2.* The torso of the pedestrian rolls onto the hood of the vehicle. **C.** *Phase 3.* The pedestrian falls off the vehicle and hits the ground.

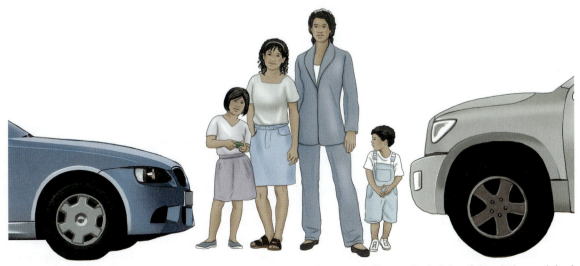

FIGURE 4-39   The injuries resulting from vehicle-pedestrian crashes vary according to the height of the victim and the height of the vehicle.

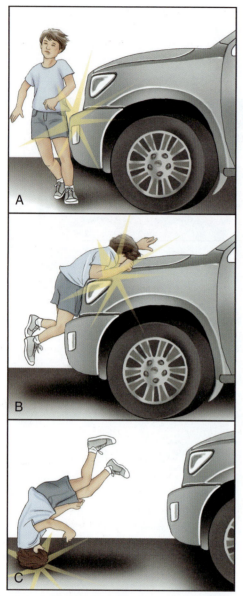

FIGURE 4-40   **A.** The initial impact on a child occurs when the vehicle strikes the child's upper leg or pelvis. **B.** The second impact occurs when the child's head and face strike the front or top of the vehicle's hood. **C.** A child may not be thrown clear of a vehicle but may be trapped and dragged by the vehicle.

later, as will the planted foot. The energy exchange moving the torso but not the feet will fracture the pelvis and shear the femur, producing severe angulation at the point of impact and possible spine injury as well.

To complicate these injuries further, a child will likely turn toward the car out of curiosity, exposing the anterior body and face to injuries, whereas an adult will attempt to escape and will be hit in the back or the side.

Adults are usually struck first by the vehicle's bumper in the lower legs, fracturing the tibia and fibula. The collision continues into the pelvis and chest as the victim is impacted. As the victim is impacted by the front of the vehicle's hood, depending on the height of the hood, the abdomen and thorax are struck by the top of the hood and the windshield. This substantial second strike can result in fractures of the upper femur, pelvis, ribs, and spine, producing intra-abdominal or intrathoracic crush and shear. If the victim's head strikes the hood or if the victim continues to move up the hood so that the head strikes the windshield, injury to the face, head, and cervical and thoracic spine can occur. If the vehicle has a large frontal area (trucks and SUVs), the entire potential patient is hit simultaneously.

The third impact occurs as the victim is thrown off the vehicle and strikes the pavement. The victim can receive a significant blow on one side of the body, injuring the hip, shoulder, and head. Head injury often occurs when the victim strikes either the vehicle or the pavement. Similarly, because all three impacts produce sudden, violent movement of the torso, neck, and head, an unstable spine fracture may result. After falling, the victim may be struck by a second vehicle travelling next to or behind the first.

As with an adult, any child struck by a vehicle can receive some type of head injury. Because of the sudden, violent forces acting on the head, neck, and torso, cervical spine injuries are high on the suspicion list.

Knowing the specific sequence of multiple impacts in pedestrian versus motor vehicle crashes and understanding the multiple underlying injuries that they can produce are keys to making an initial assessment and determining the appropriate management of a patient.

Falls

Victims of falls can also sustain injury from multiple impacts. An estimation of the height of the fall, the surface on which the victim landed, and the part of the body struck first are important factors to determine since these are indications of the energy involved and, thus, the energy exchange that occurred. Victims who fall from greater heights have a higher incidence of injury because their velocity increases as they fall. Falls from greater than three times the height of the victim are frequently severe. The type of surface on which the victim lands and its degree of *compressibility* (ability to be deformed by the transfer of energy) also have an effect on stopping distance.

The pattern of injury in falls occurring feet first is called the *Don Juan syndrome.* Only in the movies can the character Don Juan jump from a high balcony, land on his feet, and

the front or top of the vehicle's hood (Figure 4-40B). Because of the child's smaller size and weight, the child may not be thrown clear of the vehicle, as usually occurs with an adult. Instead, the child may be dragged by the vehicle while partially under the vehicle's front end (Figure 4-40C). If the child falls to the side, the lower limbs may also be run over by a front wheel. If the child falls backward, ending up completely under the vehicle, almost any injury can occur (e.g., being dragged, struck by projections, or run over by a wheel).

If the foot is planted on the ground at the time of impact, the child will receive energy exchange at the upper leg, hip, and abdomen. This will force the hips and abdomen away from the impact. The upper part of the torso will come along

walk painlessly away. In real life, bilateral fractures of the calcaneus (heel bone), compression or shear fractures of the ankles, and distal tibial or fibular fractures are often associated with this syndrome. After the feet land and stop moving, the legs are the next body part to absorb energy. Tibial plateau fractures of the knee, long-bone fractures, and hip fractures can result. The body is compressed by the weight of the head and torso, which are still moving, and can cause compression fractures of the spinal column in the thoracic and lumbar areas. Hyperflexion occurs at each concave bend of the S-shaped spine, producing compression injuries on the concave side and distraction injuries occur on the convex side. This victim is often described as breaking his or her "S."

If a victim falls forward onto the outstretched hands, the result can be bilateral compression and flexion (Colles') fractures of the wrists. If the victim did not land on the feet, the prehospital care provider will assess the part of the body that struck first, evaluate the pathway of energy displacement, and determine the injury pattern.

If the falling victim lands on the head with the body almost inline, as often occurs in shallow-water diving injuries, the entire weight and force of the moving torso, pelvis, and legs compress the head and cervical spine. A fracture of the cervical spine is a frequent result, as with the up-and-over pathway of the frontal-impact collision.

Sports Injuries

Severe injury can occur during many sports or recreational activities, such as skiing, diving, baseball, and football. These injuries can be caused by sudden deceleration forces or by excessive compression, twisting, hyperextension, or hyperflexion. In recent years, various sports activities have become available to a wide spectrum of occasional, recreational participants who often lack the necessary training and conditioning or the proper protective equipment. Recreational sports and activities include participants of all ages. Sports such as downhill skiing, waterskiing, bicycling, and skateboarding are all potentially high-velocity activities. Other sports, such as trailbiking, all-terrain vehicle (ATV) riding, and snowmobiling, can produce velocity deceleration, collisions, and impacts similar to motorcycle crashes or MVCs.

The potential injuries of a victim who is in a high-speed collision and then ejected from a skateboard, snowmobile, or bicycle are similar to those sustained when a person is ejected from an automobile at the same speed because the amount of energy is the same. The specific mechanisms of MVCs and motorcycle crashes were described earlier.

The potential mechanisms associated with each sport are too numerous to list in detail. However, the general principles are the same as for MVCs. While assessing the mechanism of injury, the prehospital care provider considers the following questions to assist in the identification of injuries:

- What forces acted on the victim, and how?
- What are the apparent injuries?

- To what object or part of the body was the energy transmitted?
- What other injuries are likely to have been produced by this energy transfer?
- Was protective gear being worn?
- Was there sudden compression, deceleration, or acceleration?
- What injury-producing movements occurred (e.g., hyperflexion, hyperextension, compression, excessive lateral bending)?

When the mechanism of injury involves a high-speed collision between two participants, as in a crash between two skiers, reconstruction of the exact sequence of events from eyewitness accounts is often difficult. In such crashes, the injuries sustained by one skier are often guidelines for examination of the other. In general, which part of one victim struck what part of the other victim and what injury resulted from the energy transfer are important. For example, if one victim sustains an impact fracture of the hip, a part of the other skier's body must have been struck with substantial force and, therefore, must have sustained a similar high-impact injury. If the second skier's head struck the first skier's hip, the prehospital care provider will suspect potentially serious head injury and an unstable spine for the second skier.

Broken or damaged equipment is also an important indicator of injury and must be included in the evaluation of the mechanism of injury. A broken sports helmet is evidence of the magnitude of the force with which it struck. Because skis are made of highly durable material, a broken ski indicates that extreme localized force came to bear, even when the mechanism of injury may appear unimpressive. A snowmobile with a severely dented front end indicates the force with which it struck a tree. The presence of a broken stick after an ice hockey skirmish raises the question of whose body broke it, how, and, specifically, what part of the victim's body was struck by the stick or fell on it.

Victims of significant crashes who complain of no apparent injuries must be assessed as if severe injuries exist. The steps are as follows:

1. Evaluate the patient for life-threatening injury.
2. Evaluate the patient for mechanism of injury. (What happened and exactly how did it happen?)
3. Determine how the forces that produced injury in one victim may have affected any other person.
4. Determine whether any protective gear was worn (it may have already been removed).
5. Assess damage to the protective equipment. (What are the implications of this damage relative to the patient's body?)
6. Assess the patient for possible associated injuries.

High-speed falls, collisions, and falls from heights without serious injury are common in many contact sports. The ability of athletes to experience incredible collisions and falls and sustain only minor injury—largely as a result of

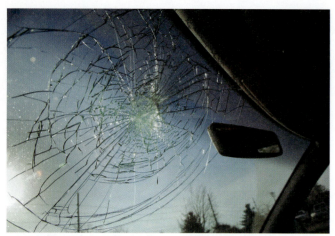

FIGURE 4-41   A bull's-eye fracture of the windshield is a major indication of skull impact and energy exchange to both the skull and the cervical spine.

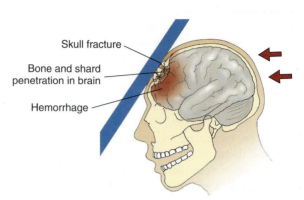

FIGURE 4-42   As the skull impacts a movable object, pieces of bone are fractured and are pushed into the brain substance.

impact-absorbing equipment—may be confusing. The potential for injury in sports participants may be overlooked. The principles of kinematics and careful consideration of the exact sequence and mechanism of injury will provide insight into sports collisions in which greater forces than usual came to bear. Kinematics is an essential tool in identifying possible underlying injuries and determining which patients require further evaluation and treatment at a medical facility.

Regional Effects of Blunt Trauma

The body can be divided into several regions: head, neck, thorax, abdomen, pelvis, and extremities. Each body region is subdivided into (1) the external part of the body, usually composed of skin, bone, soft tissue, vessels, and nerves, and (2) the internal part of the body, usually vital internal organs. The injuries produced as a result of shear, cavitation, and compression forces are used to provide an overview in each component and region for potential injuries.

Head

The only external indication that compression and shear injuries have occurred to the patient's head may be a soft tissue injury to the scalp, a contusion of the scalp, or a bull's-eye fracture of the windshield (Figure 4-41).

Compression. When the body is travelling forward with the head leading the way, as in a frontal vehicular crash or a head-first fall, the head is the first structure to receive the impact and the energy exchange. The continued momentum of the torso then compresses the head. The initial energy exchange occurs on the scalp and the skull. The skull can be compressed and fractured, pushing the broken, bony segments of the skull into the brain (Figure 4-42).

Shear. After the skull stops its forward motion, the brain continues to move forward, compressing against the intact or frac-

tured skull with resultant concussion, contusions, or lacerations. The brain is soft and compressible; therefore, its length is shortened. The posterior part of the brain can continue forward, pulling away from the skull, which has already stopped moving. As the brain separates from the skull, stretching or breaking (shearing) of brain tissue itself or any blood vessels in the area occurs (Figure 4-43). Hemorrhage into the epidural, subdural, or subarachnoid space can then result, as well as diffuse axonal injury of the brain. If the brain separates from the spinal cord, it will most likely occur at the brain stem.

Neck

Compression. The dome of the skull is fairly strong and can absorb the impact of a collision; however, the cervical spine is much more flexible. The continued pressure from the momentum of the torso toward the stationary skull produces angulation or compression (Figure 4-44). Hyperextension or hyperflexion of the neck often results in fracture or dislocation of one or more vertebra and injury to the spinal cord. The result can be jumped (dislocated) facets, potential fractures, spinal cord compression or unstable neck fractures (Figure 4-45). Direct inline compression crushes the bony vertebral bodies. Both angulation and inline compression can result in an unstable spine.

Shear. The skull's center of gravity is anterior and cephalad to the point at which the skull attaches to the bony spine. Therefore, a lateral impact on the torso when the neck is unrestrained will produce lateral flexion and rotation of the neck (see Figure 4-25). Extreme flexion or hyperextension may also cause stretching injuries to the soft tissues of the neck.

Thorax

Compression. If the impact of a collision is centered on the anterior part of the chest, the sternum will receive the ini-

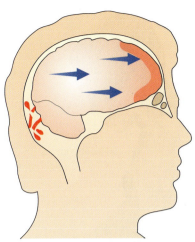

FIGURE 4-43 As the skull stops its forward motion, the brain continues to move forward. The part of the brain nearest the impact is compressed, bruised, and perhaps even lacerated. The portion farthest from the impact is separated from the skull, with tearing and lacerations of the vessels involved.

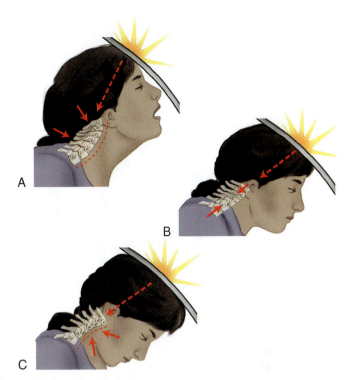

FIGURE 4-45 The spine can be compressed directly along its own axis or angled in hyperextension or hyperflexion.

tial energy exchange. When the sternum stops moving, the posterior thoracic wall (muscles and thoracic spine) and the organs in the thoracic cavity continue to move forward until the organs strike and are compressed against the sternum.

The continued forward motion of the posterior thorax bends the ribs. If the tensile strength of the ribs is exceeded, fractured ribs and a flail chest can develop (Figure 4-46). This is similar to what happens when a vehicle stops suddenly against a dirt embankment (see Figure 4-3). The frame of the vehicle bends, which absorbs some of the energy. The rear of the vehicle continues to move forward until the bending of the frame absorbs all the energy. In the same way, the posterior thoracic wall continues to move until the ribs absorb all the energy.

Compression of the chest wall is common with frontal and lateral impacts and produces an interesting phenomenon called the *paper bag effect*, which may result in a pneumothorax. A

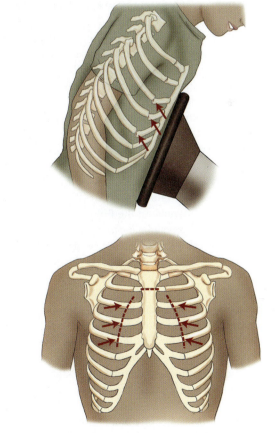

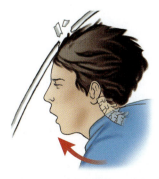

FIGURE 4-44 The skull frequently stops its forward motion, but the torso does not. As the brain compresses within the skull, the torso continues its forward motion until its energy is absorbed. The weakest point of this forward motion is the cervical spine.

FIGURE 4-46 Ribs forced into the thoracic cavity by external compression, usually fracture in multiple places, producing the clinical condition known as *flail chest.*

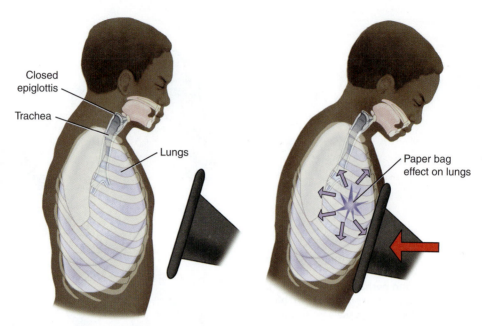

FIGURE 4-47 Compression of the lung against a closed glottis, by impact on either the anterior or the lateral chest wall, produces an effect similar to compressing a paper bag when the opening is closed tightly by the hands. The paper bag ruptures, as does the lung.

victim instinctively takes a deep breath and holds it just before impact. This closes the glottis, effectively sealing off the lungs. With a significant energy exchange on impact and compression of the chest wall, the lungs may then burst, like a paper bag full of air that is popped (Figure 4-47). The lungs can also become compressed and contused, compromising ventilation.

Compression injuries of the internal structures of the thorax may also include cardiac contusion, which occurs as the heart is compressed between the sternum and the spine and can result in significant dysrhythmias. Perhaps a more frequent injury is compression of the lungs leading to pulmonary contusion. Although the clinical consequences may develop over time, immediate loss of the ability of the patient to properly ventilate may occur. Pulmonary contusion can have consequences in the field for the prehospital provider and for the physicians during resuscitation after arrival in the hospital. In situations in which long transportation times are required, this condition can play a role en route.

Shear. The heart, ascending aorta, and aortic arch are relatively unrestrained within the thorax. The descending aorta, however, is tightly adhered to the posterior thoracic wall and the vertebral column. The resultant motion of the aorta is similar to holding the flexible tubes of a stethoscope just below where the rigid tubes from the earpiece end and swinging the acoustic head of the stethoscope from side to side. As the skeletal frame stops abruptly in a collision, the heart and the initial segment of the aorta continue their forward motion. The shear forces produced can tear the aorta at the junction of

the portion that moves freely with the tightly bound portion (see Figure 4-14).

An aortic tear may result in an immediate, complete transection of the aorta followed by rapid exsanguination. Some aortic tears are only partial, and one or more layers of tissue remain intact. However, the remaining layers are under great pressure, and a traumatic aneurysm often develops, similar to the bubble that can form on a weak part of a tire. The aneurysm can eventually rupture within minutes, hours, or days after the original injury. Approximately 80% of these patients die on the scene at the time of the initial impact. Of the remaining 20%, one-third will die within 6 hours, one-third will die within 24 hours, and one-third will live 3 days or longer. It is important that the prehospital care provider recognizes the potential for such injuries and relays this information to the hospital personnel.

Abdomen

Compression. Internal organs pressed by the vertebral column into the steering wheel or dashboard during a frontal collision may rupture. The effect of this sudden increase in pressure is similar to the effect of placing the internal organ on an anvil and striking it with a hammer. Solid organs frequently injured in this manner include the pancreas, spleen, liver, and kidneys.

Injury may also result from overpressure within the abdomen. The *diaphragm* is a ¼-inch thick (5mm) muscle located across the top of the abdomen that separates the abdominal cavity from the thoracic cavity. Its contraction causes the pleural cavity to expand for ventilation. The anterior abdomi-

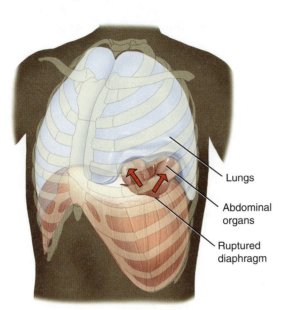

FIGURE 4-48 With increased pressure inside the abdomen, the diaphragm can rupture.

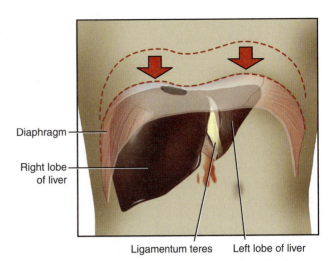

FIGURE 4-49 The liver is not supported by any fixed structure. Its major support is from the diaphragm, which moves freely. As the body travels in the down-and-under pathway, so does the liver. When the torso stops but the liver does not, the liver continues downward onto the ligamentum teres, tearing the liver. This is much like pushing a cheese-cutting wire into a block of cheese.

nal wall comprises two layers of fascia and one very strong muscle. Laterally, there are three muscle layers with associated fascia, and the lumbar spine and its associated muscles provide strength to the posterior abdominal wall. The diaphragm is the weakest of all the walls and structures surrounding the abdominal cavity. It may be torn or ruptured as the intra-abdominal pressure increases (Figure 4-48). This injury has four common consequences, as follows:

1. The "bellows" effect that is usually created by the diaphragm is lost and ventilation is affected.
2. The abdominal organs can enter the thoracic cavity and reduce the space available for lung expansion.
3. The displaced organs can become ischemic from compression of their blood supply.
4. If intra-abdominal hemorrhage is present, the blood can also cause a hemothorax.

Another injury caused by increased abdominal pressure is from sudden retrograde blood flow up the aorta and against the aortic valve. This force against the valve can rupture it. This injury is rare but does exist. It occurs when a collision with the steering wheel or involvement in another type of incident (e.g., ditch or tunnel cave-in) has produced a rapid increase in intra-abdominal pressure. This rapid pressure increase results in a sudden increase of aortic blood pressure. Blood is pushed back (retrograde) against the aortic valve with enough pressure to cause rupture of the valve cusps.

Shear. Injury to the abdominal organs occurs at their points of attachment to the mesentery. During a collision, the for-

ward motion of the body stops, but the organs continue to move forward, causing tears at the points of attachment of organs to the abdominal wall. If the organ is attached by a pedicle (a stalk of tissue), the tear can occur where the pedicle attaches to the organ, where it attaches to the abdominal wall, or anywhere along the length of the pedicle (see Figure 4-13). Organs that can shear this way are the kidneys, small intestine, large intestine, and spleen.

Another type of injury that often occurs during deceleration is laceration of the liver caused by its impact with the ligamentum teres. The liver is suspended from the diaphragm but is only minimally attached to the posterior abdomen near the lumbar vertebrae. The ligamentum teres attaches to the anterior abdominal wall at the umbilicus and to the left lobe of the liver in the midline of the body. (The liver is not a midline structure; it lies more on the right than on the left.) A down-and-under pathway in a frontal impact or a feet-first fall causes the liver to bring the diaphragm with it as it descends into the ligamentum teres (Figure 4-49). The ligamentum teres will fracture or transect the liver, analogous to a cheese slicer cutting cheese.

Pelvic fractures are the result of damage to the external abdomen and may cause injury to the bladder or lacerations of the blood vessels in the pelvic cavity. Approximately 10% of patients with pelvic fractures also have a genitourinary injury.

Pelvic fractures resulting from compression from the side, usually due to a lateral impact collision, have two components. One is the compression of the proximal femur into the pelvis which pushes the head of the femur through the acetabulum itself. This frequently produces radiating fractures that involve the entire joint. Further compression of the femur and/or of the lateral walls of the pelvis produce compression fractures of the pelvic bones or the ring of the pelvis. Since a ring generally cannot be fractured in only one place, this usually means two fractures to the ring, although some of the fractures may involve the acetabulum.

Shear fractures usually involve the ilium and the sacral area. This shearing force tears the joint open. Since the joints in a ring, such as the pelvis, must be generally fractured in two places, this frequently produces a fracture somewhere else along the pelvic ring.

The other type of compression fracture occurs anteriorly when the compression force is directly over the symphysis pubis. This will either break the symphysis by pushing in on both sides or break one side and push it back towards the sacra-iliac joint. This opens the joint producing the so-called "open-book."

For more detailed information about pelvic fractures, Andrew Burgess and his co-authors have discussed these mechanisms of injury.[17]

Penetrating Trauma

Physics of Penetrating Trauma

The principles of physics discussed earlier are equally important when dealing with penetrating injuries. Again, the kinetic energy that a striking object transfers to body tissue is represented by the following formula:

$$KE = \frac{1}{2}mv^2$$

Energy cannot be created or destroyed, but it can be changed in form. This principle is important in understanding penetrating trauma. For example, although a lead bullet is in the brass cartridge casing that is filled with explosive powder, the bullet has no force. However, when the primer explodes, the powder burns, producing rapidly expanding gases that are transformed into force. The bullet then moves out of the gun and toward its target.

According to Newton's first law of motion, after this force has acted on the missile, the bullet will remain at that speed and force until it is acted on by an outside force. When the bullet hits something, such as a human body, it strikes the individual tissue cells. The energy (speed and mass) of the bullet's motion is exchanged for the energy that crushes these cells and moves them away (cavitation) from the path of the bullet:

Mass × acceleration = force = mass × deceleration

Factors That Affect the Size of the Frontal Area

The larger the frontal area of the moving missile, the greater is the number of particles that will be hit—therefore, the greater

FIGURE 4-50 Expanding Bullets

A munitions factory in Dum Dum, India, manufactured a bullet that expanded when it hit the skin. Ballistic experts recognized this design as one that would cause more damage than is necessary in war; therefore, these bullets were prohibited in military conflicts. The Petersburg Declaration of 1868 and the Hague Convention of 1899 affirmed this principle, denouncing these "dum-dum" projectiles and other expanding missiles, such as silver tips, hollow-points, scored-lead cartridges or jackets, and partially jacketed bullets, and outlawing their use in war.

the energy exchange that occurs and the larger the cavity that is created. The size of the frontal surface area of a projectile is influenced by three factors: profile, tumble, and fragmentation. Energy exchange or potential energy exchange can be analyzed based on these factors.

Profile. *Profile* describes an object's initial size and whether that size changes at the time of impact. The profile, or frontal area, of an ice pick is much smaller than that of a baseball bat, which in turn is much smaller than that of a truck. A hollow-point bullet flattens and spreads on impact (Figure 4-50). This change enlarges the frontal area so that it hits more tissue particles and produces greater energy exchange. As a result, a larger cavity forms and more injury occurs.

In general, a bullet should remain very aerodynamic as it travels through the air en route to the target. Low resistance while passing through the air (hitting as few air particles as possible) is a good thing. This will allow it to maintain most of its speed. To achieve this, the frontal area is kept small in a conical shape. A lot of drag (resistance to travel) is a bad thing. A good bullet design would have very little drag while passing through the air but much more drag when passing through the body's tissues. If that missile strikes the skin and becomes deformed, covering a larger area and creating much more drag, then a much greater energy exchange will occur. Therefore, the ideal bullet is designed to keep its shape while in the air and only deform on impact.

Tumble. *Tumble* describes whether the object turns over and over and assumes a different angle inside the body than the angle it assumed as it entered the body, thus creating more drag inside the body than in the air. A wedge-shaped bullet's center of gravity is located nearer to the base than to the nose of the bullet. When the nose of the bullet strikes something, it slows rapidly. Momentum continues to carry the base of the bullet forward, with the center of gravity seeking to become the leading point of the bullet. A slightly asymmetrical shape causes an end-over-end motion, or tumble. As the bullet tumbles, the normally horizontal sides of the

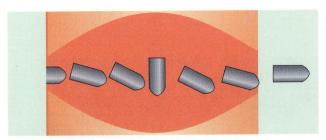

FIGURE 4-51   Tumble motion of a missile maximizes its damage at 90 degrees.

bullet become its leading edges, thus striking far more particles than when bullet was in the air (Figure 4-51). More energy exchange is produced, and therefore, greater tissue damage occurs.

Fragmentation. *Fragmentation* describes whether the object breaks up to produce multiple parts or rubble and, therefore, more drag and more energy exchange. There are two types of fragmentation rounds: 1) fragmentation on leaving the weapon (e.g., shotgun pellets) (Figure 4-52); and 2) fragmentation after entering the body. This can be active or passive fragmentation. Active fragmentation involves a bullet that has an explosive inside it that detonates inside the skin. Bullets with soft noses or vertical cuts in the nose and safety slugs that contain many small fragments to increase body damage by breaking apart on impact are examples of passive fragmentation. The resulting mass of fragments creates a larger frontal area than a single solid bullet, and energy is dispersed rapidly into the tissue. If the missile shatters, it will spread out over a wider area, with two results: (1) more tissue particles will be struck by the larger frontal projection; and (2) the injuries will be distributed over a larger portion of the body because more organs will be struck (Figure 4-53). The multiple pieces of shot from a shotgun blast produce similar results. Shotgun wounds are an excellent example of the fragmentation injury pattern.

Damage and Energy Levels

The damage caused in a penetrating injury can be estimated by classifying penetrating objects into three categories according to their energy capacity: low-, medium-, and high-energy weapons.

Low-Energy Weapons

Low-energy weapons include hand-driven weapons such as a knife or an ice pick. These missiles produce damage only with their sharp points or cutting edges. Because these are low-velocity injuries, they are usually associated with less secondary trauma (i.e., less cavitation will occur). Injury in these victims can be predicted by tracing the path of the weapon into the body. If the weapon has been removed, the prehospital care provider should try to identify the type of weapon used.

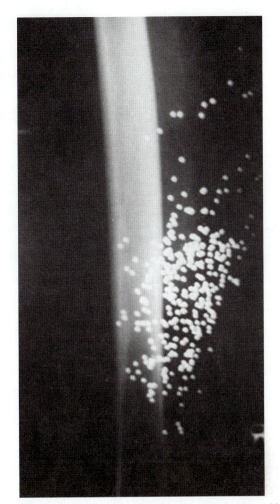

FIGURE 4-52   Maximum fragmentation damage is caused by a shotgun.

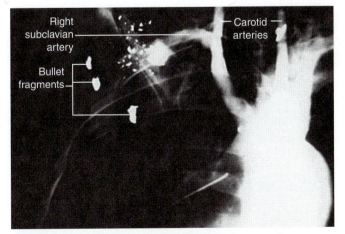

FIGURE 4-53   When the missile breaks up into smaller particles, this fragmentation increases its frontal area and increases the energy distribution.
(From McSwain NE Jr: Pulmonary chest trauma. In Moylan JA, editor: *Principles of Trauma,* New York, 1992, Gower.)

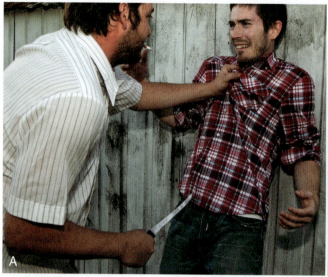
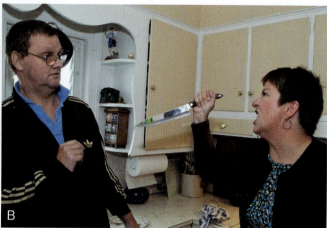

FIGURE 4-54 The gender of an attacker often determines the trajectory of the wound in stabbing incidents. Male attackers tend to stab upwards whereas female attackers tend to stab downwards.

The gender of the attacker is an important factor in determining the trajectory of a knife. Men tend to thrust with the blade on the thumb side of the hand and with an upward or inward motion, whereas women tend to hold the blade on the little finger side and stab downward (Figure 4-54).

An attacker may stab a victim and then move the knife around inside the body. A simple appearing entrance wound may produce a false sense of security. The entrance wound may be small, but the damage inside may be extensive. The potential scope of the movement of the inserted blade is an area of possible damage (Figure 4-55).

Evaluation of the patient for associated injury is important. For example, the diaphragm can reach as high as the nipple line on deep expiration. A stab wound to the lower chest can injure intra-abdominal as well as intrathoracic structures, and a wound of the upper abdomen may also involve the lower chest.

Penetrating trauma can result from impaled objects such as fence posts and street signs in vehicle crashes and falls, ski poles in snow sports, and handlebar injuries in bicycling.

Medium-Energy and High-Energy Weapons

Firearms fall into two groups: medium energy and high energy. Medium-energy weapons include handguns and some rifles whose muzzle velocity is 1000 ft/sec. The temporary cavity created by this weapon is three to five times the caliber of the bullet. High energy weapons have muzzle velocity in excess of 2000 ft/sec and significantly greater muzzle energy. They create a temporary cavity 25 times or greater than the caliber of the bullet. It is obvious that as the amount of gunpowder in the cartridge increases and the size of the bullet increases, the speed and mass of the bullet and, therefore, its kinetic energy increase (Figure 4-56A–B). The mass of the bullet is an important, but smaller, component **(KE = $\frac{1}{2}$ mv^2)**. However, the bullet mass is not to be discounted. In the War Between the States, the Kentucky Long rifle 0.55 caliber Minie Ball had almost the same muzzle energy as the modern M16. The mass of the missile becomes more important when considering the damage produced by a 12-gauge shotgun at close range or an Improvised Explosive Device (IED). Additional information is available in the blast chapter of the military edition of PHTLS.

In general, medium-energy and high-energy weapons damage not only the tissue directly in the path of the missile, but also the tissue involved in the temporary cavity on each side of the missile's path. The variables of missile profile, tumble, and fragmentation influence the rapidity of the

FIGURE 4-55 Damage produced by a knife depends on the movement of the blade inside the victim.

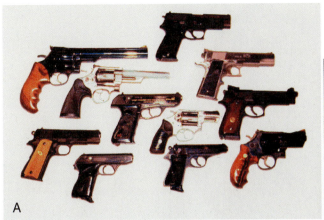
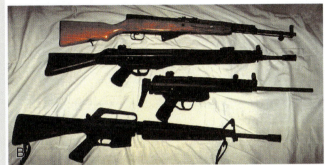

FIGURE 4-56 **A.** Medium-energy weapons are usually guns that have short barrels and contain cartridges with less power. **B.** High-energy weapons.
(From McSwain NE Jr, Paturas JL: The Basic EMT: Comprehensive Prehospital Patient Care, ed 2, St Louis, 2001, Mosby.)

energy exchange and, therefore, the extent and direction of the injury. The force of the tissue particles moved out of the direct path of the missile compresses and stretches the surrounding tissue (Figure 4-57).

High-energy weapons discharge high-energy missiles (Figure 4-58A–B). Tissue damage is much more extensive with a high-energy penetrating object than with one of medium energy. The vacuum created in the cavity created by this high-speed missile can pull clothing, bacteria, and other debris from the surface into the wound.

A consideration in predicting the damage from a gunshot wound is the range or *distance* from which the gun (either medium- or high-energy) is fired. Air resistance slows the bullet; therefore, increasing the distance will decrease the energy at the time of impact and will result in less injury. Most shootings are done at close range with handguns, so the probability of serious injury is related to both the anatomy involved and the energy of the weapon rather than loss of kinetic energy.

High-Energy Weapons

Cavitation. Fackler and Malinowski described the unusual injury pattern of an AK-47. Because of its eccentricity, the bullet tumbles and travels almost at a right angle to the area of entrance. During this tumble action, the rotation carries it over and over so that there are two or sometimes even three (depending on how long the bullet stays in the body) cavitations.[18] The very high energy exchange produces the cavitation and a significant amount of damage.

The size of the permanent cavity is associated with the elasticity in the tissue struck by the missile. For example, if the same bullet going the same speed penetrates both muscle and the liver, the results are very different. Muscle has much more elasticity and will expand and return to a relatively small, permanent cavity. On the other hand, the liver has

very little elasticity, so it develops fracture lines and a much larger, permanent cavity than the same energy exchange in muscle.[19,20]

Fragmentation. The combination of a high-energy weapon with fragmentation can produce significant damage. If the high-energy missile fragments on impact (which many do not), the initial entrance site may be very large and may have significant soft tissue injury. On the other hand, if the bullet only fragments when it hits a hard structure in the body (such as bone), this large cavitation occurs at this impact point and the bony fragments themselves become part of the damage-producing component. Significant destruction to the bone and nearby organs and vessels may result.[18]

Emil Theodor Kocher, a surgeon living at the latter part of the 19th century, was extremely active in the understanding of ballistics and the damage produced by the weapons. He was a strong advocate of not using the "dum-dum" bullet (produced

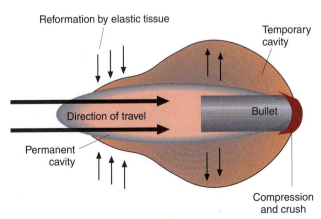

FIGURE 4-57 A bullet crushes tissues directly in its path. A cavity is created in the wake of the bullet. The crushed part is permanent. The temporary expansion can also produce injury.

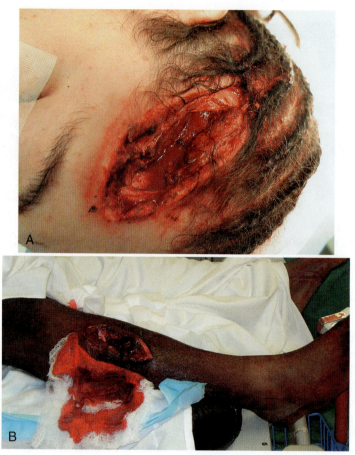

FIGURE 4-58 **A.** Graze wound to the scalp created by a projectile from a high-velocity weapon. The skull was not fractured. **B.** High-velocity gunshot wound to the leg demonstrating the large, permanent cavity.

by the arsenal in Dum Dum, India).[21] The St. Petersburg Declaration of 1868 outlawed explosive projectiles less than 400 grams in weight. This was followed by the Hague Convention of 1899, which outlawed the use of dum-dum bullets in war.

Anatomy

Entrance and Exit Wounds

Tissue damage will occur at the site of missile entry into the body, along the path of the penetrating object, and on exit from the body. Knowledge of the victim's position, the attacker's position, and the weapon used is helpful in determining the path of injury. If the entrance wound and the exit wound can be related, the anatomical structures that would likely be in this pathway can be approximated.

Evaluating wound sites provides valuable information to direct the management of the patient and to relay to the receiving facility. Do two holes in the victim's abdomen indicate that a single missile entered and exited or that two missiles entered and are both still inside the patient? Did the missile cross the midline (usually causing more severe injury) or remain on the same side? In what direction did the mis-

sile travel? What internal organs are likely to have been in its path?

Entrance and exit wounds usually, but not always, produce identifiable injury patterns to soft tissue. Evaluation of the apparent trajectory of a penetrating object is very helpful to the clinician. This information should be given to the physicians in the hospital. On the other hand, prehospital providers (and most physicians) do not have the experience or the expertise of a forensic pathologist; therefore, the assessment of which wound is an entrance and which is an exit is fraught with uncertainty. Such information is solely for patient care to try to gauge the trajectory of the missile and not for legal purposes to determine specifics about the incident. These two issues should not be confused. The provider must have as much information as possible to determine the potential injuries sustained by the patient and to best decide how the patient is to be managed. The legal issues related to the specifics of entrance and exit wounds are best left to others. An entrance wound from a gunshot lies against the underlying tissue, but an exit wound has no support. The former is typically a round or oval wound depending on the entry path, and the latter is

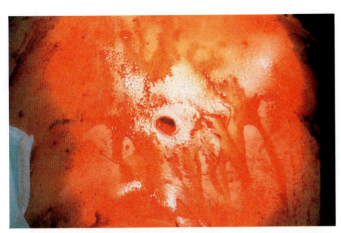

FIGURE 4-59 Entrance wound is round or oval in shape, and exit wound is stellate or linear.

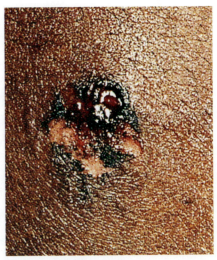

FIGURE 4-61 Hot gases coming from the end of a muzzle held in proximity to the skin produce partial-thickness and full-thickness burns on the skin.

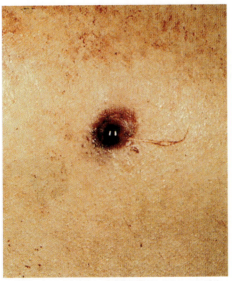

FIGURE 4-60 The abraded edge indicates that the bullet traveled from top right to bottom left.

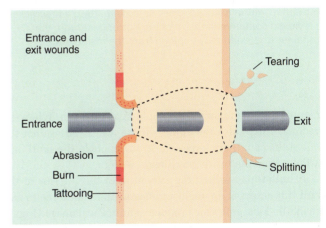

FIGURE 4-62 Spin and compression of the bullet on entrance produce round or oval holes. On exit, the wound is pressed open.

usually a *stellate* (starburst) wound (Figure 4-59). Because the missile is spinning as it enters the skin, it leaves a small area of abrasion (1 to 2 mm in size) that is pink (Figure 4-60). Abrasion is not present on the exit side. If the muzzle was placed directly against the skin at the time of discharge, the expanding gases will enter the tissue and produce crepitus on examination (Figure 4-61). If the muzzle is within 2 to 3 inches (5 to 7 cm), the hot gases that exit will burn the skin; at 2 to 6 inches (5 to 15 cm) the smoke will adhere to the skin; and inside 10 inches (25 cm) the burning cordite particles will tattoo the skin with small (1 to 2 mm) burned areas (Figure 4-62).

Regional Effects of Penetrating Trauma

This section discusses the injuries sustained by various parts of the body during penetrating trauma.

Head

After a missile penetrates the skull, its energy is distributed within a closed space. Particles accelerating away from the missile are forced against the unyielding skull, which cannot expand as can skin, muscle or even the abdomen. Thus, the brain tissue is compressed against the inside of the skull, producing more injury than would otherwise occur if it could expand freely. It is similar to putting a firecracker in

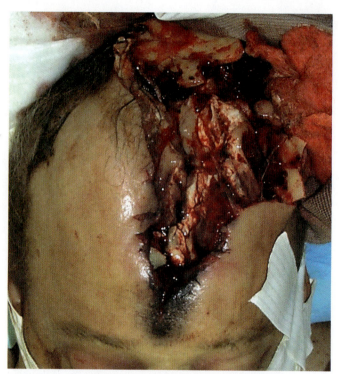

FIGURE 4-63   After a missile penetrates the skull, its energy is distributed within a closed space. It is like putting a firecracker in a closed container. If the forces are strong enough, the container (the skull) may explode from the inside out.

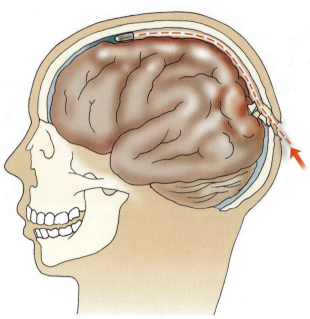

FIGURE 4-64   The bullet may follow the curvature of the skull. (From McSwain NE Jr, Paturas JL: The Basic EMT: Comprehensive Prehospital Patient Care, ed 2, St Louis, 2001, Mosby).

an apple and then placing the apple in a metal can. When the firecracker explodes the apple will be destroyed against the wall of the can. If the forces are strong enough, the skull may explode from the inside out (Figure 4-63).

A bullet may follow the curvature of the interior of the skull if it enters at an angle and has insufficient force to exit the skull. This path can produce significant damage (Figure 4-64). Because of this characteristic, small caliber, medium-velocity weapons, such as the 0.22-caliber or 0.25-caliber pistol, have been called the "assassin's weapon." They go in and exchange all of their energy into the brain.

Thorax

Three major groups of structures are inside the thoracic cavity: the pulmonary system, vascular system, and gastrointestinal tract. This does not include the bone and muscle of the chest wall and spine. One or more of the anatomic structures of these systems may be injured by a penetrating object.

Pulmonary System. Lung tissue is less dense than blood, solid organs, or bone; therefore, a penetrating object will hit fewer particles, exchange less energy and do less damage to lung tissue. Damage to the lungs can be clinically significant (Figure 4-65), but fewer than 15% of patients will require surgical exploration. [22]

Vascular System. Smaller vessels that are not attached to the chest wall may be pushed aside without significant damage. However, larger vessels, such as the aorta and vena cava, are less mobile because they are tethered to the spine or the heart. They cannot move aside easily and are more susceptible to damage.

The myocardium (almost totally muscle) stretches as the bullet passes through and then contracts, leaving a smaller defect. The thickness of the muscle may control a low-energy penetration, such as by a knife, or even a small, medium-energy 0.22-caliber bullet. This closure can prevent immediate exsanguination and allow time to transport the victim to an appropriate facility.

Gastrointestinal Tract. The *esophagus,* the part of the gastrointestinal tract that traverses the thoracic cavity, can be penetrated and can leak its contents into the thoracic cavity. The signs and symptoms of such an injury may be delayed for several hours or several days.

Abdomen

The abdomen contains structures of three types: air-filled, solid, and bony. Penetration by a low-energy missile may not cause significant damage; only 30% of knife wounds penetrating the abdominal cavity require surgical explora-

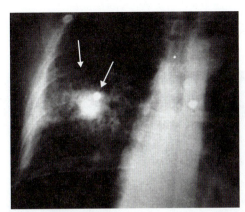

FIGURE 4-65 Lung damaged produced by the cavity at a distance from the point of impact.

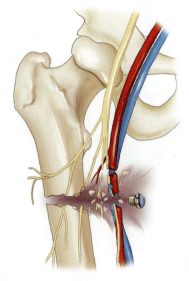

FIGURE 4-66 Bone fragments become secondary missiles themselves, producing damage by the same mechanism as the original penetrating object.

tion to repair damage. A medium-energy injury (e.g., handgun wound) is more damaging; 85% to 95% require surgical repair. However, in injuries caused by medium-energy missiles, the damage to solid and vascular structures frequently does not produce immediate exsanguination. This enables prehospital care providers to transport the patient to an appropriate facility in time for effective surgical intervention.

Extremities

Penetrating injuries to the extremities can include damage to bones, muscles, nerves, or vessels. When bones are hit, bony fragments become secondary missiles, lacerating surrounding tissue (Figure 4-66). Muscles often expand away from the path of the missile, causing hemorrhage. The missile may penetrate blood vessels, or a near-miss may damage the lining of a blood vessel, causing clotting and obstruction of the vessel within minutes or hours.

Shotgun Wounds

Although shotguns are not high-velocity weapons, they are high-energy weapons and, at close range, they can be more lethal than some of the highest-energy rifles. Handguns and rifles predominantly use *rifling* (grooves) on the inside of the barrel to spin a single missile in a flight pattern toward the target. In contrast, most shotguns possess a smooth, cylindrical tube barrel that directs a load of missiles in the direction of the target. Devices known as *chokes* and *diverters* can be attached to the end of a shotgun barrel to shape and form the column of missiles into specific patterns (e.g., cylindrical or rectangular). Regardless, when a shotgun is fired, a large number of missiles are ejected in a *spread,* or *spray,* pattern. The

barrels may be shortened ("sawed off") to prematurely widen the trajectory of the missiles.

Although shotguns may use various types of ammunition, the structure of most shotgun shells is similar. A typical shotgun shell contains gunpowder, wadding, and projectiles. When discharged, all these individual components are propelled from the muzzle and can inflict injury on the victim. Certain types of gunpowder can *stipple* ("tattoo") the skin in close-range injuries. Wadding, which is usually lubricated paper, fibers, or plastic used to separate the shot (missiles) from the charge of gunpowder, can provide another source of infection in the wound if not removed. The missiles can vary in size, weight, and composition. A wide variety of missiles are available, from compressed metal powders to *birdshot* (small metal pellets), *buckshot* (larger metal pellets), *slugs* (a single metal missile), and more recently, plastic and rubber alternatives. The average shell is loaded with 1 to 1½ ounces of shot. Fillers that are placed with the shot (polyethylene or polypropylene granules) can become embedded in the superficial layers of the skin.

An average birdshot shell may contain 200 to 2000 pellets, whereas a buckshot shell may contain only 6 to 20 pellets (Figure 4-67). It is important to note that as the size of the buckshot pellets increases, they approach the wounding characteristics of 0.22-caliber missiles in regard to effective range and energy transfer characteristics. Larger or "magnum" shells are also available. These shells may contain more shot and a larger charge of gunpowder or only the larger powder charge to boost the muzzle velocity of the shot.

The type of ammunition used is important in gauging injuries, but the *range* (distance) at which the patient was shot provides the most important variable when evaluating the shotgun-injury victim. Shotguns eject a large number of

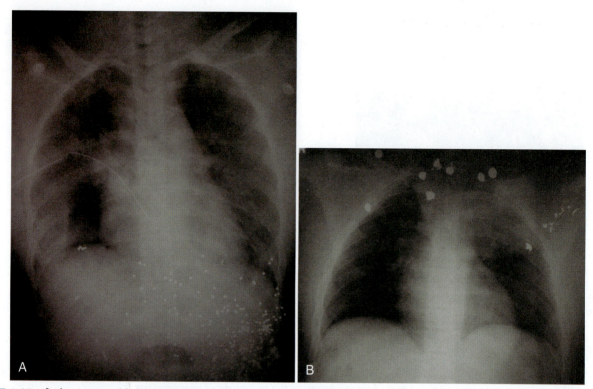

FIGURE 4-67 **A.** An average birdshot shell may contain 200 to 2000 pellets. **B.** A buckshot shell may contain only 6 to 20 pellets.

missiles, most of which are spherical. These projectiles are especially susceptible to the effects of air resistance, thereby quickly slowing once they exit the muzzle (Figure 4-68). The effect of air resistance on the projectiles decreases the effective range of the weapon and changes the basic characteristics of the wounds that it generates. Consequently, shotgun wounds have been classified into four major categories: contact, close-range, intermediate-range, and long-range wounds (Figure 4-69).

Contact wounds occur when the muzzle is touching the victim at the time the weapon is discharged. This typically results in circular entrance wounds, which may or may not have soot or an imprint of the muzzle (see Figure 4-61). Searing or burning of the wound edges is common, secondary to the high temperatures and the expansion of hot gases as the

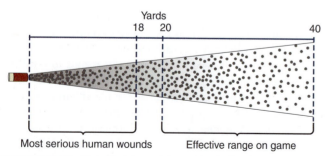

FIGURE 4-68 The diameter of the spread of a shot column expands as range increases.
(From DeMuth WE: The mechanism of gunshot wounds. *J Trauma* 11:219, 1971.)

missiles exit the muzzle. Some contact wounds may be more stellate (star-shaped) in appearance, caused by the superheated gases from the barrel escaping from the tissue. Contact wounds usually result in widespread tissue damage and are associated with high mortality. The length of a standard shotgun barrel makes it difficult to commit suicide with this weapon, since it is difficult to reach and pull the trigger. Such attempts usually result in a split face without the shot reaching the brain.

Close-range wounds (less than 6 feet), although still typically characterized by circular entrance wounds, will likely have more evidence of soot, gunpowder, or filler stippling around the wound margins than contact wounds. Additionally, abrasions and markings from the impact of the wadding that coincide with the wounds from the missiles may be found. Close-range wounds also create significant damage in the patient; missiles fired from this range still retain sufficient energy to penetrate deep structures and exhibit a slightly wider spread pattern. This increases the extent of injury as missiles travel through soft tissue.

Intermediate-range wounds are characterized by the appearance of satellite pellet holes emerging from the border around a central entrance wound. This pattern is a result of individual pellets spreading from the main column of shot and generally occurs at a range of 6 to 18 feet. These injuries are a mixture of deep, penetrating wounds and superficial wounds and abrasions. Because of the deep, penetrating components of this injury, however, victims may still have a relatively high mortality rate.

FIGURE 4-69 **Patterns of Shotgun Injury**

Type	Wound Appearance	Injury	Mortality
Contact		Widespread tissue damage	85%–90%
Close		Penetrates beyond deep fascia	15%–20%
Intermediate		Penetrates SQ tissue and deep fascia	0–5%
Long Range		Superficial skin penetration	0%

(Modified from: Sherman RT, Parrish RA: Management of shotgun injuries: a review of 152 cases. *J Trauma* 18:236, 1978.)

Long-range wounds are rarely lethal. These wounds are typically characterized by the classic spread of scattered pellet wounds and result from a range of greater than 18 feet. However, even at these slower velocities, the pellets can cause significant damage to certain sensitive tissues (e.g., eyes). In addition, larger buckshot pellets can retain sufficient velocity to inflict damage to deep structures, even at long range. The prehospital care provider also needs to consider the cumulative effects of many small missile wounds and their locations, focusing on sensitive tissues. *Adequate exposure* is essential when examining all patients involved in trauma, and shotgun injuries are no exception.

These varying characteristics need to be taken into account when evaluating injury patterns in patients with shotgun injuries. For example, a single, circular, shotgun wound could represent a contact or close-range injury with birdshot or buckshot in which the missiles have retained a tight column or grouping. Conversely, this may also represent an intermediate-range to long-range injury with a slug or solitary missile. Only detailed examination of the wound will allow differentiation of these injuries that will likely involve significant damage to internal structures despite strikingly different missile characteristics.

Contact and close-range wounds to the chest may result in a large, visually impressive wound resulting in an open pneumothorax, and bowel may eviscerate from such wounds to the abdomen. On occasion, a single pellet from an intermediate-range wound may penetrate deep enough to perforate the bowel, leading eventually to peritonitis, or may damage a major artery, resulting in vascular compromise to an extremity. Alternatively, a patient who exhibits multiple small wounds in a spread pattern may have dozens of entrance wounds. However, none of the missiles may have retained enough energy to penetrate through fascia, let alone produce significant damage to internal structures.

Although immediate patient care must always remain the priority, any information (shell type, suspected range of the patient from the weapon, number of shots fired) that prehospital care providers can gather from the scene and relay to the receiving facility can assist with appropriate diagnostic evaluation and treatment of the shotgun-injured patient. Furthermore, recognition of various wound types can aid providers in maintaining a high index of suspicion for internal injury regardless of the initial impression of the injury.

Blast Injuries

Injury from Explosions

Explosive devices are the most frequently used weapons in combat and by terrorists. Explosive devices cause human injury by multiple mechanisms, some of which are exceedingly complex. The greatest challenges for clinicians at all levels of care in the aftermath of an explosion are the large numbers of casualties and multiple, penetrating injuries (Figure 4-70).[23]

Physics of Blast

Explosions are physical, chemical, or nuclear reactions that result in the almost instantaneous release of large amounts of energy in the form of heat and rapidly expanding, highly compressed gas, capable of projecting fragments at extremely high velocities. The energy associated with an explosion can take multiple forms: kinetic and heat energy in the "blast wave"; kinetic energy of fragments formed by the breakup of the weapon casing and surrounding debris; and electromagnetic energy.

Blast waves can travel at greater than 16,400 feet (5000 meters)/second and are composed of static and dynamic components. The static component ("blast overpressure") surrounds

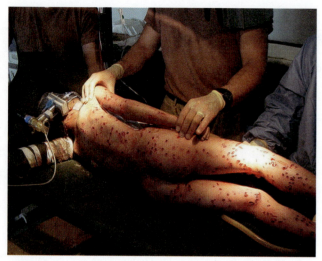

FIGURE 4-70   Patient with multiple fragment wounds from a bomb blast.

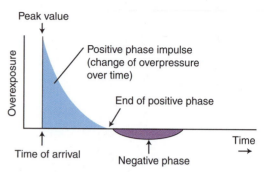

FIGURE 4-71   Pressure-time history of a blast wave. This graph shows the sudden massive increase in pressure (blast overpressure) following the decrease in pressure and negative pressure phase.
(From Bowen TE and Bellamy RF, editors, *Emergency War Surgery,* Washington, DC, 1988, United States Government Printing Office.)

objects in the flow field of the explosion, loading them on all sides with a discontinuous rise in pressure called the "shock front" or "shock wave" up to a "peak overpressure" value. Following the shock front, the overpressure drops down to ambient pressure, and then a partial vacuum is often formed as a result of air being sucked back (Figure 4-71). The dynamic component ("dynamic pressure") is directional and is experienced as a blast "wind." The primary significance of the blast wind is that it propels fragments at speeds in excess of several thousand meters per second (faster than standard ballistic weapons such as bullets and shells).[24] Whereas the effective range of both the static and dynamic pressure is measured in tens of feet, the fragments accelerated by the dynamic pressure will quickly outpace the blast wave to become the dominant cause of injury out to ranges of thousands of feet.

Interaction of Blast Waves with the Body

Blast waves interact with the body and other structures by transmitting energy from the blast wave into the structure. This energy causes the structure to deform in a manner dependent on the strength and the natural period of oscillation of the structure being affected. Changing density interfaces within a structure cause complex re-formations, convergences, and couplings of the transmitted blast waves. This occurs particularly with large density interfaces such as solid tissue to air or liquid (e.g., lung, heart, liver, and bowel).

Explosion-Related Injuries

Injuries from explosions are generally classified as primary, secondary, tertiary, quaternary, and quinary after the injury taxonomy described in Department of Defense Directive 6025.21E[24] (Figure 4-72). Detonation of an explosive device sets off a chain

of interactions in the objects and people in its path.[23] If an individual is close enough, the initial blast wave increases pressure in the body, causing stress and shear, particularly in gas-filled organs such as the ears, lungs, and (rarely) bowels (Figure 4-73). These primary blast injuries are more prevalent when the explosion occurs in an enclosed space because the blast wave bounces off surfaces, thus enhancing the destructive potential of the pressure waves.[25] Immediate death from pulmonary barotrauma (blast lung) occurs more often in enclosed-space than in open-air bombings.[26,27,28] Most (95%) explosion injuries in Iraq and Afghanistan occur in open-space explosions.[29] The most common form of primary blast injury is tympanic membrane rupture.[30,31] Tympanic membrane rupture, which may occur at pressures as low as 5 psi,[32,33] is often the only significant overpressure injury experienced. The next major injury occurs at less than 40 psi, a threshold known to be associated with pulmonary injuries including pneumothorax, air embolism, interstitial and subcutaneous emphysema, and pneuomediastinum.[34] Data from burned soldiers from Operation Iraqi Freedom (OIF) confirm that tympanic membrane rupture is not predictive of lung injury.

The shock front of the blast wave quickly dissipates and is followed by the blast wind, which propels fragments to create multiple penetrating injuries. Although these are termed secondary injuries, they are usually the predominant wounding agent.[23] The blast wind also propels large objects into people or people onto hard surfaces (whole or partial body translocation), creating blunt (tertiary blast) injuries; this category of injury also includes crush injuries caused by structural collapse.[34] Heat, flames, gas, and smoke generated during explosions cause quaternary injuries that include burns, inhalation injury, and asphyxiation.[25] Quinary injuries are produced when bacteria, chemicals, or radioactive materials are added to the explosive device and released upon detonation.

FIGURE 4-72   **Blast Injury Categories**

Category	Definition	Typical Injuries
Primary	▪ Produced by contact of blast shockwave with body ▪ Stress and shear waves occur in tissues ▪ Waves reinforced/reflected at tissue density interfaces ▪ Gas-filled organs (lungs, ears, etc.) at particular risk	▪ Tympanic membrane rupture ▪ Blast lung ▪ Eye injuries ▪ Concussion ▪ Tympanic membrane rupture
Secondary	▪ Ballistic wounds produced by: ▪ Primary fragments (pieces of exploding weapon) ▪ Secondary fragments (environmental fragments, e.g., glass) ▪ Threat of fragment injury extends further than that from blast wave	▪ Penetrating injuries ▪ Traumatic amputations ▪ Lacerations
Tertiary	▪ Blast wave propels individuals onto surfaces/objects or objects onto individuals, causing whole body translocation ▪ Crush injuries caused by structural damage and building collapse	▪ Blunt injuries ▪ Crush syndrome ▪ Compartment syndrome
Quaternary	▪ Other explosion-related injuries, illnesses, or diseases	▪ Burns ▪ Toxic gas and other inhalation injury ▪ Injury from environmental contamination
Quinary	▪ Injuries resulting from specific additives such as bacteria and radiation ("dirty bombs")	

(From: *NAEMT: PHTLS Prehospital Trauma Life Support:* Military edition, ed 7, St Louis, 2011, Mosby.)

Injury from Fragments

Conventional explosive weapons are designed to maximize damage caused by fragments. With initial velocities of many thousands of feet per second, the distance that fragments may be thrown for a 50-lb (23-kg) bomb will be well over 1000 feet (0.3 km), whereas the lethal radius of the blast overpressure is approximately 50 feet (15 meters). The developers of both military and terrorist weapons, therefore, design weapons to maximize fragmentation injury so as to significantly increase the damage radius of a free-field explosive.

Very few explosive devices cause injury solely by blast overpressure, and serious primary blast injury is relatively rare compared to the predominant numbers of secondary and tertiary injuries. Thus, few patients have injuries dominated by primary blast effects. The entire array of explosion-related injuries is often referred to en masse as "blast injuries," leading to major confusion as to what constitutes a blast injury. Because energy from the blast wave dissipates rapidly, most explosive devices are constructed to cause damage primarily from fragments. These may be primary fragments generated through the breakup of the casing surrounding the explosive or secondary fragments created from debris in the surrounding environment. Regardless of whether the fragments are created from shattered munitions casing, flying debris, or embedded objects that terrorists often pack into homemade bombs, they

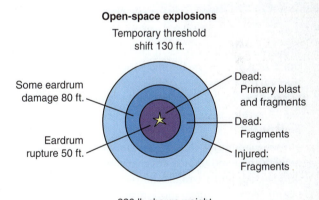

Open-space explosions

FIGURE 4-73   Morbidity and mortality as a function of distance from open-space detonation of a 220-lb (100-kg) explosive.

exponentially increase the range and lethality of explosives and are the primary cause of explosion-related injury.

Multi-Etiology Injury

In addition to the direct effects of an explosion, health care providers must be mindful of the other causes of injury from attacks with explosions. For instance, an IED that targets a vehicle may result in minimal initial damage to the vehicle occupants. However, the vehicle itself may be displaced vertically or vectored off course resulting in occupant blunt trauma from collision, from flipping upside down as part of the vertical displacement process, or from rollover, for instance, down an embankment or culvert. In these circumstances, occupants sustain injury based on the mechanisms previously described for blunt trauma. In the military setting, a vehicle's occupants may be afforded some protection from blunt injury by virtue of their body armor. Furthermore, the occupants of a vehicle disabled following an IED attack may be attacked with gunfire as they exit the vehicle and are subject to ambush, thus potentially becoming victims of penetrating injury.

Using Kinematics in Assessment

The assessment of a trauma patient must involve knowledge of kinematics. For example, a driver who hits the steering wheel (blunt trauma) will have a large cavity in the anterior chest at the time of impact; however, the chest rapidly returns to, or near to, its original shape as the driver rebounds from the steering wheel. If two prehospital care providers examine the patient separately—one who understands kinematics and another who does not—the one without knowledge of kinematics will be concerned only with the bruise visible on the patient's chest. The prehospital care provider who understands kinematics will recognize that a large cavity was present at the time of impact, that the ribs had to bend in for the cavity to form, and that the heart, lungs, and great vessels were compressed by the formation of the cavity. Therefore, the knowledgeable provider will suspect injury to the heart, lungs, great vessels, and chest wall. The other prehospital care provider will not even be aware of these possibilities.

The knowledgeable prehospital care provider suspecting serious intrathoracic injuries will assess for these potential injuries, manage the patient, and initiate transport more aggressively, rather than react to what otherwise appears to be only a minor, closed, soft-tissue injury. Early identification, adequate understanding, and appropriate treatment of underlying injury will significantly influence whether a patient lives or dies.

SUMMARY

- Integrating the principles of the kinematics of trauma into the assessment of the trauma patient is key to discovering the potential for severe or life-threatening injuries.
- Up to 95% of the injuries can be anticipated by understanding the energy exchange that occurs with the human body at the time of a collision. Knowledge of kinematics allows for injuries that are not immediately apparent to be identified and treated appropriately. Left unsuspected, undetected, and therefore untreated, these injuries contribute significantly to morbidity and mortality resulting from trauma.
- Energy cannot be created or destroyed, only changed in form. The kinetic energy of an object, expressed as a function of both velocity (speed) and mass (weight), is transferred to another object on contact.
- Damage to the object or body tissue impacted is not only a function of the amount of kinetic energy applied to it, but also a function of the tissue's ability to tolerate the forces applied to it.

Blunt trauma
- The direction of the impact determines the pattern of and potential for injury: frontal, lateral, rear, rotational, rollover, or angular.
- Ejection from a car reduces the protection on impact.

- Energy-absorbing protective devices are very important. These include seat belts, air bags, drop-down engines, and energy-absorbing auto parts, such as bumpers, collapsible steering wheels, dashboards, and helmets. On arrival, the damage to the vehicles and the direction of the impact will indicate which victims are most likely to have been more severely injured.
- Pedestrian injures vary according to the height of the victim and which part of the patient had direct contact with the vehicle.

Falls
- Distance travelled before impact affects the severity of the injury sustained.
- Energy-absorbing capability of the target at the end of the fall (concrete versus soft snow) affects the severity of the injury.
- Victim body parts that hit the target and progression of the energy exchange through the victim's body are important.

Penetrating trauma
- The energy varies depending on the primary injuring agent:
- Low energy—handheld cutting devices

- Medium energy—most handguns
- High energy—high-powered rifles, assault weapons, etc.
- The distance of the victim to the perpetrator and the objects that the bullet might have struck will affect the amount of energy at the time of impact with the body and, therefore, the available energy to be dissipated into the patient to produce damage to the body parts.
- Organs in proximity of the pathway of the penetrating object determine the potential life-threatening conditions.
- The pathway of the penetrating trauma is determined by the wound of entrance and the wound of exit.

Blasts

- There are 5 types of injury in a blast:
  - Primary—over-and-under pressure
  - Secondary—projectiles (the most common source of injury from blasts)
  - Tertiary—propulsion of the body into another object
  - Quaternary—heat and flames
  - Quinary—Radiation, chemicals, bacteria.

SCENARIO SOLUTION

Patient #1: Driver of the vehicle with side impact. Two bullets traversed the door of the car. The patient has two left-side bullet wounds, one below the ribs and one above the ribs. The patient's blood pressure was low; therefore, the likely injuries in the chest include pneumothorax, hemothorax, penetration of the heart, and possibly major vessels. Below the ribs, penetration into the abdominal cavity could involve any of the abdominal organs with associated hemorrhage.

Patient #2: Passenger side with side impact of car. Because of the energy exchanged between the door and the occupant, you should suspect injury in all four side impact areas—the shoulder (clavicle), chest wall and the thoracic cavity, the abdominal cavity, and the pelvis. The potential injuries in these areas include: 1) fractured clavicle; 2) fractured ribs (potential flail chest); 3) pulmonary contusions; 4) sheering related to the aorta; 5) pneumothorax; 6) abdomen (fractured liver or spleen); 7) deceleration injury to the kidney; 8) fractured pelvis; and 9) rotational injury of the cervical spine.

Patient #3: Driver of the vehicle. With the bent steering wheel, you suspect an up-and-over pathway at the time of the collision into the pole, with frontal chest impact into the steering wheel and head impact into the windshield. Potential injuries include: 1) myocardial contusion; 2) pneumothorax; 3) flail chest; 4) pulmonary contusion; 5) overpressure injury in the abdomen; 6) fractured liver and spleen; 7) cervical spine facture; and 8) brain injury.

Patient #4: You suspect down-and-under pathway: 1) fracture of the lower extremities (ankle, shaft of the femur, hip dislocation; 2) facial injuries; and 3) cervical spine injury.

One other additional important assessment to consider: How did the bullet holes get in the first car? Did you search the occupants for weapons?

References

1. http://webappa.cdc.gov/sasweb/ncipc/mortrate10_sy.html. Accessed December 4, 2009.
2. http://www-fars.nhtsa.dot.gov/Main/index.aspx, http://webappa.cdc.gov/sasweb/ncipc/nfirates.html. Accessed December 4, 2009.
3. http://webappa.cdc.gov/sasweb/ncipc/nfirates2001.html. Accessed December 4, 2009.
4. Rogers CD, Pagliarello G, McLellan BA, et al: Mechanism of injury influences the pattern of injuries sustained by patients involved in vehicular trauma. *Can J Surg* 34(3):283–286, June 1991.
5. Hollerman JJ, Fackler ML, Coldwell DM, et al: Gunshot wounds: 1. Bullets, ballistics, and mechanisms of injury. *AJR J Roentgenol* 155(4):685–690, October 1990.
6. http://www-fars.nhtsa.dot.gov/Main/index.aspx. Accessed December 4, 2009.
7. Simon BJ, Legere P, Emhoff T, et al: Vehicular trauma triage by mechanism: Avoidance of the unproductive evaluation. *J Trauma* 37(4):645–649, October 1994.
8. Hernandez IA, Fyfe KR, Heo G, et al: Kinematics of head movement in simulated low velocity rear-end impacts. *Clin Biomech* 20(10):1011–1018, December 2005.
9. Kumaresan S, Sances A, Carlin F, et al: Biomechanics of side-impact injuries: Evaluation of seat belt restraint system, occupant kinematics, and injury potential. *Conf Proc IEEE Eng Med Biol Soc* 1:87–90, 2006.

10. Siegel JH, Yang KH, Smith JA, et al: Computer simulation and validation of the Archimedes Lever hypothesis as a mechanism for aortic isthmus disruption in a case of lateral impact motor vehicle crash: A Crash Injury Research Engineering Network (CIREN) study. *J Trauma* 60(5):1072–1082, May 2006.

11. Horton TG, Cohn SM, Heid MP, et al: Identification of trauma patients at risk of thoracic aortic tear by mechanism of injury. *J Trauma* 48(6):1008–1013; discussion 1013–1014, June 2000.

12. Dyer DS, Moore EE, Ilke DN, et al: Thoracic aortic injury: How predictive is mechanism and is chest computed tomography a reliable screening tool? A prospective study of 1,561 patients. *J Trauma* 48(4):673–682; discussion 682–683, April 2000.

13. http://www-nrd.nhtsa.dot.gov/Pubs/811160.PDF. Accessed December 4, 2009.

14. http://www-nrd.nhtsa.dot.gov/Pubs/811106.PDF. Accessed December 4, 2009.

15. http://www-nrd.nhtsa.dot.gov/Pubs/811153.PDF. December 5, 2009.

16. Siegel AW: Automobile collisions, kinematics, and related injury patterns. *Calif Med* 116(2):16–22, February 1972.

17. Burgess AR, Eastridge BJ, Young JW, et al: Pelvic ring disruptions: Effective classification system and treatment protocols. *J Trauma* 30(7):848–856, 1990.

18. Fackler ML, Malinowski JA. Internal deformation of the AK-74: A possible cause for its erratic path in tissue. *J Trauma* 28(Suppl 1) S72–75, January 1988.

19. Fackler ML, Surinchak JS, Malinowski JA, et al: Wounding potential of the Russian AK-74 assault rifle. *J Trauma* 24(3):263–266, March 1984.

20. Fackler ML, Surinchak JS, Malinowski JA, et al: Bullet fragmentation: A major cause of tissue disruption, *J Trauma* 24(1):35–39, January 1984.

21. Fackler ML, Dougherty PJ: Theodor Kocher and the Scientific Foundation of Wound Ballistics. *Surg Gynecol Obstet* 172(2):153–160, February 1991.

22. American College of Surgeons (ACS) Committee on Trauma: *Advanced trauma life support course,* Chicago, 2002, ACS.

23. Wade CE, Ritenour AE, Eastridge BJ, et al: Explosion injuries treated at combat support hospitals in the Global War on Terrorism. In Elsayed N, Atkins J, editors: *Explosion and Blast-Related Injuries.* Burlington, MA, 2008, Elsevier.

24. Champion HR, Baskin T, Holcomb JB: Injuries from explosives. In: McSwain NE, et al, editors: *National Association of Emergency Medical Technicians: PHTLS Basic and Advanced Prehospital Trauma Life Support: Military Edition,* ed. 2, St. Louis, 2006, Mosby.

25. Department of Defense Directive: Medical Research for Prevention, Mitigation, and Treatment of Blast Injuries. Number 6025:21E, 2006. http://www.dtic.mil/whs/directives/corres/html/602521.htm. Accessed April 15, 2008.

26. Gutierrez de Ceballos JP, Turégano-Fuentes F, Perez-Diaz D, et al: The terrorist bomb explosions in Madrid, Spain—An analysis of the logistics, injuries sustained, and clinical management of casualties treated at the closest hospital. *Crit Care Med* 9:104–111, 2005.

27. Gutierrez de Ceballos JP, Turégano Fuentes F, Perez Diaz D, et al: Casualties treated at the closest hospital in the Madrid, March 11, terrorist bombings. Crit Care Med 33(1 Suppl):S107–112, 2005.

28. Avidan V, Hersch M, Armon Y, et al: Blast lung injury: Clinical manifestations, treatment, and outcome. *Am J Surg* 190:927–931, 2005.

29. Ritenour AE, Blackbourne LH, Kelly JF, et al: Primary blast injury in the global war on terrorism: 2003–2006. Unpublished data.

30. Leibovici D, Gofrit ON, Stein M, et al: Blast injuries: Bus versus open-air bombings—a comparative study of injuries in survivors of open-air versus confined-space explosions. *J Trauma* 41:1030–1035, 1996.

31. Ritenour AE, Wickley A, Ritenour JS, et al: Tympanic membrane perforation and hearing loss from blast overpressure in Operation Enduring Freedom and Operation Iraqi Freedom wounded. *J Trauma* 64:S174–178, 2008.

32. Zalewski T: Experimentelle Untersuchungen uber die Resistenzfahigkeit des Trommelfells. *Z Ohrenheilkd* 52:109, 1906.

33. Helling ER: Otologic blast injuries due to the Kenya embassy bombing. *Mil Med* 169:872–876, 2004.

34. Nixon RG, Stewart C: When things go boom: Blast injuries. *Fire Engineering,* May 1, 2004. http://www.fireengineering.com/articles/article_display.html?id=204602. Accessed April 15, 2008.

35. Lomoschitz FM, Blackmore CC, Mirza SK, et al: Cervical spine injuries in patients 65 years old and older: Epidemiologic analysis regarding the effects of age and injury mechanism on distribution, type, and stability of injuries. *AJR Am J Roentgenol* 178(3):573–577, March 2002.

36. Dalal SA, Burgess AR, Siegel JH, et al: Pelvic fracture in multiple trauma: classification by mechanism is key to pattern of organ injury, resuscitative requirements, and outcome. *J Trauma* 29(7):981–1000; discussion 1000–1002, July, 1989.

Suggested Reading

Alderman B, Anderson A: Possible effect of air bag inflation on a standing child. In *Proceedings of 18th American Association of Automotive Medicine,* September 1974.

American College of Surgeons (ACS) Committee on Trauma: *Advanced trauma life support course,* Chicago, 2002, ACS.

Anderson PA, Henley MB, Rivara P, et al: Flexion distraction and chance injuries to the thoracolumbar spine. *J Orthop Trauma* 5(2):153, 1991.

Anderson PA, Rivara FP, Maier RV, et al: The epidemiology of seatbelt-associated injuries. *J Trauma* 31(1):60, 1991.

Bartlett CS: Gunshot wound ballistics. *Clin Orthop* 408:28, 2003.

DePalma RG, Burris DG, Champion HR, et al: Current concepts: Blast injuries. *N Engl J Med* 352:1335, 2005.

Di Maio VJM: Gunshot wounds: practical aspects of firearms, ballistics and forensic techniques, Boca Raton, Fla, 1999, CRC Press.

Fackler ML, Surinchak JS, Malinowski JA, et al: Bullet fragmentation: A major cause of tissue disruption. *J Trauma* 24:35, 1984.

Fackler ML, Surinchak JS, Malinowski JA, et al: Wounding potential of the Russian AK-47 assault rifle. *J Trauma* 24:263, 1984.

Garrett JW, Braunstein PW: The seat belt syndrome. *J Trauma* 2:220, 1962.

Huelke DF, Mackay GM, Morris A: Vertebral column injuries and lap-shoulder belts. *J Trauma* 38:547, 1995.

Huelke DF, Moore JL, Ostrom M: Air bag injuries and occupant protection. *J Trauma* 33(6):894, 1992.

Joksch H, Massie D, Pichler R: *Vehicle aggessivity: Fleet characterization using traffic collision data,* Washington, DC, 1998, NHTSA/Department of Transportation.

McSwain NE Jr: Kinematics. In Mattox KL, Feliciano DV, Moore EE, editors: *Trauma,* ed 4, New York, 1999, McGraw-Hill.

McSwain NE Jr, Brent CR: Trauma rounds: Lipstick sign. *Emerg Med* 21:46, 1898.

National Safety Council (NSC): *Accident facts 1994*, Chicago, 1994, NSC.

Ordog GJ, Wasserberger JN, Balasubramaniam S: Shotgun wound ballistics. *J Trauma* 28:624, 1988.

Oreskovich MR, Howard JD, Compass MK, et al: Geriatric trauma: Injury patterns and outcome. *J Trauma* 24:565, 1984.

Rutledge R, Thomason M, Oller D, et al: The spectrum of abdominal injuries associated with the use of seat belts. *J Trauma* 31(6):820, 1991.

States JD, Annechiarico RP, Good RG, et al: A time comparison study of the New York State Safety Belt Use Law utilizing hospital admission and police accident report information. *Accid Anal Prev* 22(6):509, 1990.

Swierzewski MJ, Feliciano DV, Lillis RP, et al: Deaths from motor vehicle crashes: Patterns of injury in restrained and unrestrained victims. *J Trauma* 37(3):404, 1994.

Sykes LN, Champion HR, Fouty WJ: Dum-dums, hollowpoints, and devastators: Techniques designed to increase wounding potential of bullets. *J Trauma* 28:618, 1988.

CHAPTER 5

Scene Assessment

CHAPTER OBJECTIVES

At the completion of this chapter, the reader will be able to do the following:

- ✓ Identify potential threats to the safety of the patient, bystanders, and emergency personnel that are common to all emergency scenes.

- ✓ Identify potential threats that are unique to a given scenario, such as a motor vehicle crash (MVC).

- ✓ Integrate analysis of scene safety, scene situation, and kinematics into assessment of the trauma patient to make patient care decisions.

- ✓ Describe appropriate steps to take to mitigate potential threats to safety.

- ✓ Given a mass-casualty incident (MCI) scenario (hazardous material incident, weapon of mass destruction), integrate the use of a triage system into the management of the scene and make triage decisions based on assessment findings.

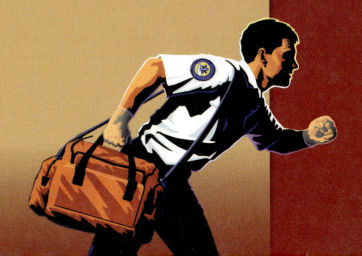

SCENARIO

You are dispatched to the scene of a tanker-truck crash. As you begin to respond, you notice that it has just begun to snow. Dispatch provides the additional information that the driver of the truck is reported to be unconscious and bleeding from a large scalp laceration. In addition, a witness states that liquid from the vehicle is leaking onto the street. As you arrive on the scene, what considerations are important before you contact the patient?

What are your concerns about the scene?

The prehospital care provider has the following three priorities upon arrival to a scene:

1. The first priority for everyone involved at a trauma incident is assessment of the scene. *Scene assessment* involves establishing that the scene is safe and carefully considering the exact nature of the situation. As well as ensuring patient and EMT safety, the determination needs to be made as to what alteration in patient care is indicated by the current conditions. Assessment of scene safety and the situation is initiated while en route to the scene based on information from the dispatcher. It continues as the emergency medical services (EMS) unit arrives on the scene, and as the providers approach the patient. The issues identified in this evaluation must be addressed before beginning assessment of individual patients. In some situations, such as combat or tactical situations, this becomes even more critical and can alter the methods of how the principles of patient care are accomplished.

2. After performing the scene assessment, attention is turned to evaluating individual patients (Chapter 6 discusses this in detail). Scene assessment includes an initial abbreviated form of triage so that the most severely injured patients are assessed first. The emphasis in order of priority is (a) conditions that may result in the loss of life, (b) conditions that may result in the loss of limb, and (c) all other conditions that do not threaten life or limb.

3. If the scene involves more than one patient, the situation is classified as either a multiple-patient incident or a mass-casualty incident (MCI). In an MCI, the priority shifts from focusing all resources on the most injured patient to saving the maximum number of patients; that is, providing the greatest good to the greatest number. Triage is discussed in the final section of this chapter.

cess by providing the initial information about the incident and the patient, based on bystander reports or information provided by other public safety or prehospital care units first on the scene. The on-scene information-gathering process begins immediately upon arrival at the incident. Before making contact with the patient, the prehospital care provider can evaluate the scene by (1) obtaining a general impression of the situation for scene safety, (2) looking at the cause and results of the incident, and (3) observing family members and bystanders. A majority of patient injuries can be predicted based on an understanding of the kinematics and the effects on the patients. Taking the time to prepare mentally for a call and practicing basic communication between partners may be the difference between a well-managed scene and a hostile confrontation (or a physical assault). Good observation, perception, and communication skills are the best tools. The scene's appearance creates an impression that influences the entire assessment; therefore, correct evaluation of the scene is crucial. A wealth of information is gathered by simply looking, watching, listening, and cataloguing as much information as possible, including the mechanisms of injury, the present situation, and the overall degree of safety. Just as the patient's condition can improve or deteriorate, so can the condition of the scene. Evaluating the scene initially then failing to reassess how the scene may be changing can result in serious consequences to the care providers and the patient.

Scene assessment includes the following two major components:

1. *Safety.* The primary consideration when approaching any scene is the safety of the medical and rescue personnel. Rescue attempts should not be done by those untrained in the techniques required. When medical personnel become victims, they will no longer be able to assist other injured people and will add to the number of patients and decrease the number of care providers. Patient care needs to wait until the scene is secured.

   Scene safety involves not only rescuer safety but also patient safety. In general, patients in a hazardous situation should be moved to a safe area before assessment and treatment begin. Threatening conditions to patient or rescuer safety include fire, downed electrical lines, explo-

Scene Assessment

Patient assessment starts long before the prehospital care provider arrives at the patient's side. Dispatch begins the pro-

sives, hazardous materials (including blood or body fluid, traffic, floodwater, and weapons such as guns, knives), and environmental conditions. Also, an assailant may still be on the scene and may intervene to harm the patient, rescuers, or others.

The preferences employed for patient care can be drastically altered by the conditions on the scene. For example, an industrial explosion or chemical spill can produce dangerous conditions for the prehospital care provider that take precedent and alter the methods by which patient care is provided. (For more information on principle versus preference, see Chapter 3.)

2. *Situation.* Assessment of the situation follows the safety assessment. Many issues must be assessed based upon the individual situation:

- What really happened at the scene?
- Why was help summoned?
- What was the mechanism of injury (kinematics), and what forces and energies led to the victims' injuries? (See Chapter 4.)
- How many people are involved, and what are their ages?
- Are additional EMS units needed for treatment or transport?
- Is mutual aid needed? Are any other personnel or resources needed (e.g., law enforcement, fire department, power company)?
- Is special extrication or rescue equipment needed?
- Is helicopter transport necessary?
- Is a physician needed to assist with triage or on-scene medical care issues?
- Could a medical problem be the instigating factor that led to the trauma (e.g., a vehicle crash that resulted from the driver's heart attack)?

Issues related to both safety and situation have significant overlap; many safety topics are also specific to certain situations, and certain situations pose serious safety hazards. These issues are discussed in further detail in the following sections.

Safety Issues

Traffic Safety

The majority of EMS responders who are killed or injured each year are involved in motor vehicle–related incidents (Figure 5-1).[1] Although most of these are related to direct ambulance collisions during the response phase, a subset of these fatalities and injuries occurs while working on the scene of a motor vehicle crash (MVC). In the United States, MVCs resulted in more than 1.9 million EMS responses in 2003. Many factors can result in prehospital care providers being injured or killed on the scene of an MVC (Figure 5-2). Some factors, such as

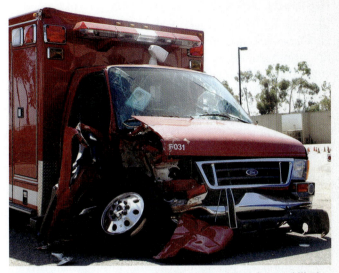

FIGURE 5-1 The majority of EMS responders who are killed or injured each year are involved in motor vehicle–related incidents.

weather conditions (e.g., snow, ice, rain, fog) and road design (e.g., limited-access or rural roads), cannot be changed; however, the responder can be aware that these conditions exist and can act appropriately to mitigate these situations.[2]

Weather/Light Conditions

Many prehospital care responses to MVCs take place in adverse weather conditions and at night. These weather conditions vary by geographic location and time of the year. Providers in many areas need to deal with ice and snow during the winter months, whereas those in coastal and mountainous areas often confront fog. Rainstorms are common in most geographic areas, and sandstorms affect other regions. Incoming traffic may not see or be able to stop in time to avoid emergency vehicles or personnel parked on the scene.

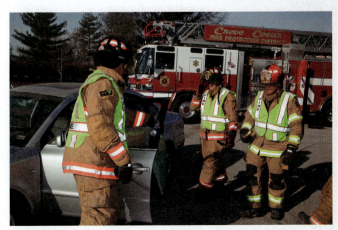

FIGURE 5-2 A significant number of prehospital care providers who are injured or killed are working at the scene of a motor vehicle crash.

Highway Design

High-speed, limited-access highways have made moving large amounts of traffic efficient, but when a crash occurs, the resulting traffic backup and "rubber necking" by drivers create dangerous situations for responders. Law enforcement is usually reluctant to shut down a limited-access highway and strives to keep the flow of traffic moving. Although this may appear to produce further danger to responders, it may prevent additional rear-end collisions caused by the backup of vehicles.

Rural roads present other problems. Although the volume of traffic is much less than on urban roadways, the winding, narrow, and hilly nature of these roads creates short sight distances for drivers as they approach the scene of an MVC. Rural roads may not be as well maintained as those in urban areas, resulting in slippery conditions long after a storm has passed and catching unsuspecting drivers off guard. Isolated areas of snow, ice, or fog that caused the original MVC may still be present, may hinder EMS arrival, and may result in suboptimal conditions for oncoming drivers.

Mitigation Strategies

It would be safest to respond to MVCs only during daylight hours on clear days; unfortunately, prehospital care providers need to respond at all times of day and in any weather condition. However, steps can be taken to reduce the risks of becoming a victim while working at an MVC. The best way is to not be there, particularly on limited-access highways. The number of people on the scene at any given time should be the number needed to accomplish the tasks at hand; for example, having three ambulances and a supervisor's vehicle at a scene that has only one patient dramatically increases the risk of a provider being hit by a passing vehicle. *Although many dispatch protocols require multiple-ambulance response to limited-access highways, all but the initial ambulance should be staged at an on-ramp nearby unless immediately needed.*

The location of equipment on the ambulance also plays a role in safety. Equipment should be placed so that it can be gathered without stepping into the traffic flow. The passenger's side of the ambulance is usually toward the guardrails, and placing the equipment most often used at MVCs in these compartments will keep responders out of the traffic flow.

Reflective Clothing

In most cases of prehospital care responders hit by oncoming vehicles, the drivers stated that they did not see the responder in the road. Both the National Fire Protection Association and the Occupational Safety and Health Administration (OSHA) have standards for reflective warning garments used on highways. OSHA has three levels of protection for workers on highways, with the highest level (level 3) to be used at night

on a high-speed roadway. The Federal Highway Administration has mandated that all workers, including public safety and first responders, wear American National Standards Institute (ANSI) Class 2 or Class 3 reflective vests when responding to an incident on a highway funded by federal aid. Common sense dictates that prehospital care providers should wear reflective clothing at all motor vehicle crashes as a safety measure. The ANSI standards can be met either by affixing reflective material to the outer jacket or by wearing an approved reflective vest.

Vehicle Positioning and Warning Devices

Vehicle positioning at the scene of an MVC is of the utmost importance. The incident commander or the safety officer should ensure that the responding vehicles are placed in the best positions to protect prehospital care providers. It is important for the first arriving emergency vehicles to "take the lane" of the accident (Figure 5-3). Although placement of the ambulance behind the scene will not facilitate the loading of the patient, it will protect the responders and patient from oncoming traffic. As additional emergency vehicles arrive, they should generally be placed on the same side of the road as the incident. These vehicles should be placed farther away from the incident to give increased warning time to oncoming drivers.

Headlights, especially high beams, should be turned off so as not to blind oncoming drivers, except if the beams are in use to illuminate the scene. The number of warning lights at the scene should be evaluated; too many lights will only serve to confuse oncoming drivers. Many departments use warning signs stating "accident ahead" to give ample warning time for drivers. Flares may be arranged to warn and direct traffic flow; however, care should be used in dry conditions so as not to start grass fires. Reflective cones serve as good devices to direct traffic flow away from the lane taken up by the emergency (Figure 5-4).

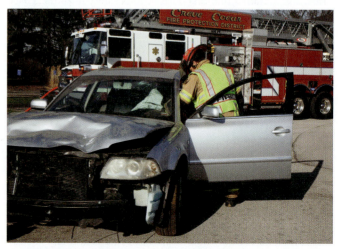

FIGURE 5-3 Correct positioning of emergency vehicle.

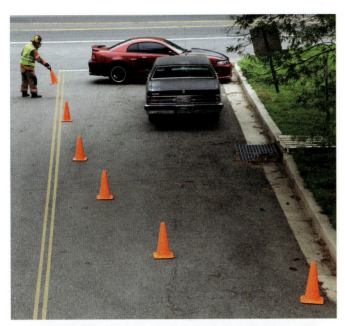

FIGURE 5-4   Placement of traffic delineation devices.

If traffic needs to be directed, this should be done by law enforcement or those with special training in traffic control. Confusing or contradicting instructions given to drivers only create additional safety risks. The best situations are created when traffic is not impeded and normal flow can be maintained around the emergency. Construction sites provide an example of traffic flow around obstructions. Traffic issues at crash scenes can be handled in much the same way; prehospital care providers can observe construction sites to gain insight into how traffic flow may work better at an MVC.

Violence

Each call has the potential to take the EMS provider into an emotionally charged environment. Some EMS agencies have a policy that requires the presence of law enforcement before providers enter a scene of violence or potential violence. Even a scene that appears benign has the potential to deteriorate into violence; therefore, providers must always be alert to subtle clues suggesting a change in situation. The patient, family, or bystanders on the scene may not be able to perceive the situation rationally. These individuals may think that the response time was too long, may be oversensitive to words or actions, and may misunderstand the "usual" approach to patient assessment. Maintaining a confident and professional manner while demonstrating respect and concern is important to gain the patient's trust and achieve control of the scene.

It is important that EMS personnel train themselves to "observe" the scene and not just "look" at it. Learn to notice numbers and locations of individuals when arriving on the scene, movement of bystanders into or out of the scene, indicators of stress or tension, unexpected or unusual reactions to EMS presence, or other "gut" feelings that may be developing. Watch the hands; look for unusual bulges in waistbands, clothing that is "out of season" such as wearing an overcoat in warm weather, or oversized clothing that could easily hide a weapon.

If a developing threat is perceived, immediately begin preparing to leave the scene. An assessment or a procedure may need to be finished in the ambulance. The safety of the prehospital care providers takes priority. Consider the following situation: You and your partner are in the living room of your patient's home. While your partner is checking the patient's blood pressure, an apparently intoxicated individual enters the room from the back of the house. He looks angry, and you notice what appears to be the butt of a gun sticking out of the waistband of his pants. Your partner does not see or hear this person enter the room because he is focused on the patient. The suspicious person begins to question your presence and is extremely agitated about your uniform and your badge. His hands repeatedly move toward, then away from, his waist. He begins to pace and mumble. How can you and your partner prepare for this sort of situation?

Managing the Violent Scene

Prior to the beginning of the day's EMS calls, the partners need to discuss and agree on methods to handle the violent or disruptive patient. Attempting to develop a process when the event in ongoing is not the correct approach. Partners can use a hands-on/hands-off approach, as well as predetermined code words and hand signals, for emergencies.

- The role of the *hands-on* prehospital care provider is to take charge of the patient assessment, giving necessary attention to the patient. The *hands-off* provider stands back (until needed) to observe the scene, interact with family or bystanders, collect necessary information, and create better access and egress. In essence, the hands-off provider is monitoring the scene and "covering" his partner's back.
- A predetermined *code word* and *hand signals* allow partners to communicate a threat without alerting others of their concerns. In many situations, *tension* and *anxiety* are immediately reduced when an attentive prehospital care provider begins interacting with and assessing the patient.

If both providers have all of their attention focused on the patient, the scene can quickly become threatening, and early clues (as well as opportunities to retreat) may be missed.

There are various methods for dealing with a scene that has become dangerous such as:

1. **Don't be there.** When responding to a known violent scene, stage at a safe location until the scene has been

rendered safe by law enforcement and clearance to respond has been given.

2. **Retreat.** If threats are presented when approaching the scene, tactfully retreat to the vehicle and leave the scene. Stage at a safe location and notify appropriate personnel.

3. **Diffuse.** If a scene becomes threatening during patient care, use verbal diffusion skills to reduce tension and aggression (while preparing to leave the scene).

4. **Defend.** *As a last resort,* the prehospital care provider may find it necessary to defend him- or herself. It is important that such efforts are to "disengage and get away." Do not attempt to chase or subdue an aggressive party. Ensure that law enforcement personnel have been notified and are en route. Again, the safety of the providers is the priority.

Blood-borne Pathogens

Before the recognition of acquired immunodeficiency syndrome (AIDS) in the early 1980s, health care workers (HCWs) showed little concern over exposure to blood and body fluids. Despite knowledge that blood was known to transmit certain hepatitis viruses, prehospital care providers and others involved in emergency medical care often viewed contact with a patient's blood as an annoyance rather than an occupational hazard. Because of the high mortality rate associated with contracting AIDS and the recognition that human immunodeficiency virus (HIV)—the causative agent of AIDS—could be transmitted in blood, HCWs became much more concerned about the patient as a vector of disease. Federal agencies, such as the Centers for Disease Control and Prevention (CDC) and OSHA, developed guidelines and mandates for HCWs to minimize exposure to blood-borne illness, including HIV and hepatitis. The primary infections transmitted through blood include both hepatitis B (HBV) and hepatitis C (HCV) viruses and HIV. Although this issue became a concern because of HIV, it is important to note that infection by hepatitis is much easier to contract than infection with HIV and requires much less inoculum than HIV. It also carries a high mortality rate and is without specific treatment.

Epidemiologic data demonstrate that HCWs are much more likely to contract blood-borne illness from their patients than their patients are to contract disease from health professionals. Exposures to blood are typically characterized as either percutaneous or mucocutaneous. *Percutaneous exposures* occur when an individual sustains a puncture wound from a contaminated sharp object, such as a needle or scalpel, with the risk of transmission directly related to both the contaminating agent and the volume of infected blood introduced by the injury. *Mucocutaneous exposures* typically are less likely to result in transmission and include exposure of blood to non-intact skin, such as a soft tissue wound (e.g., abrasion, superficial laceration) or a skin condition (e.g., acne), or to mucous membranes (e.g., conjunctiva of eye).

FIGURE 5-5 Hepatitis

The clinical manifestations of viral hepatitis are right upper-quadrant pain, fatigue, loss of appetite, nausea, vomiting, and alteration in liver function. Jaundice, a yellowish coloration of the skin, results from an increased level of bilirubin in the bloodstream. Although most individuals with hepatitis recover without serious problems, a small percentage of patients develop *acute fulminant hepatic failure* and may die. A significant number of those who recover will develop a carrier state in which their blood can transmit the virus.

As in HBV, infection with HCV can range from a mild, asymptomatic course to liver failure and death. The incubation period for HCV is somewhat shorter than for HBV, typically 6 to 9 weeks. Chronic infections with HCV are much more common than with HBV, and about 80% to 85% of those who contract HCV will develop persistently abnormal liver function, predisposing them to *hepatocellular carcinoma*. Hepatitis C is primarily transmitted through blood, whereas hepatitis B can be transmitted through blood or sexual contact. About two-thirds of intravenous drug abusers have been infected with HCV. Before routine testing of donated blood for presence of HBV and HCV, blood transfusion was the primary reason patients contracted hepatitis.

Viral Hepatitis

Hepatitis can be transmitted to HCWs through needle sticks and mucocutaneous exposures on non-intact skin.

Although a number of hepatitis viruses have been identified, HBV and HCV are of most concern to HCWs experiencing a blood exposure. Viral hepatitis causes acute inflammation of the liver (Figure 5-5). The incubation period, from exposure to manifestation of symptoms, is generally 60 to 90 days. Up to 30% of those infected with HBV may have an asymptomatic course.

A vaccine derived from the hepatitis B surface antigen (HBsAg) can immunize individuals against HBV.[3] Before the development of this vaccine, more than 10,000 HCWs became infected with HBV annually, and several hundred would die each year from either severe hepatitis or complications of chronic HBV infection. OSHA now requires employers to offer HBV vaccine to those workers in high-risk environments. All prehospital care providers should be immunized against HBV. Almost all those who complete the series of three vaccines will develop antibody (Ab) to HBsAg, and immunity can be determined by testing blood for the presence of HBsAb. If a HCW is exposed to blood from a patient who is potentially infected with HBV before the HCW has developed immunity (i.e., before completing the vaccine series), passive protection from HBV can be conferred to the HCW with the administration of hepatitis B immune globulin (HBIG).

FIGURE 5-6   Human Immunodeficiency Virus

Two serotypes of HIV have been identified. *HIV-1* accounts for virtually all AIDS in the United States and equatorial Africa, and *HIV-2* is found almost exclusively in Western Africa. Although early victims of HIV were male homosexuals, intravenous drug users, or hemophiliacs, HIV disease is now found in many teenage and adult heterosexual populations, with the fastest-growing numbers in minority communities. The screening test for HIV is very sensitive, and false-positive tests occasionally occur. All positive screening tests should be confirmed with a more specific technique (e.g., Western blot electrophoresis).

After infection with HIV, when patients develop one of the opportunistic infections or cancers, they transition from being *HIV positive* to having AIDS. In the last decade, significant advances have been made in the treatment of HIV disease, primarily in developing new drugs to combat its effects. This has resulted in many individuals with HIV infection able to lead fairly normal lives because the progression of the disease is slowed dramatically.

Although HCWs typically are more concerned about contracting HIV because of its uniformly fatal prognosis, they are at greater risk of contracting HBV or HCV.

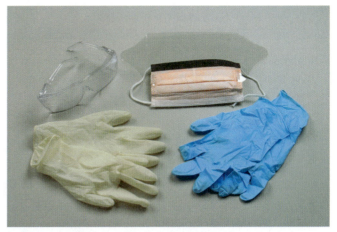

FIGURE 5-7   At a minimum, personal protective equipment for prehospital care providers should consist of gloves, mask, and eye protection.
(From Chapleau W: *Emergency First Responder,* St Louis, 2004, Mosby.)

At present, no immune globulin or vaccine is available to protect HCWs from exposure to HCV, emphasizing the need for using Standard Precautions.

Human Immunodeficiency Virus

After infection, HIV targets the immune system of its new host. Over time, the number of certain types of white blood cells falls dramatically, leaving the individual prone to developing unusual infections or cancers (Figure 5-6).

Only about 0.3% (about 1 in 300) of needle-stick exposures to HIV-positive blood lead to infection, compared to infection rates of 23% to 62% (1 in 4 to 1 in 2) with exposure to HBV-infected needles. Infection with HCV falls between these two rates (1.8%; 1 in 50). The probable explanation for the varying rates of infection is the relative concentration of virus particles found in infected blood. In general, HBV-positive blood contains 100 million to 1 billion virus particles/mL, whereas HCV-positive and HIV-positive blood contains 1 million and 100 to 10,000 particles/mL, respectively. The risk of infection appears higher with exposure to a larger quantity of blood, exposure to blood from a patient with a more advanced stage of disease, a deep percutaneous injury, or an injury from a hollow-bore, blood-filled needle. HIV is primarily transmitted through infected blood or semen, but vaginal secretions and pericardial, peritoneal, pleural, amniotic, and cerebrospinal fluids are all considered potentially infected. Unless obvious blood is present, tears, urine, sweat, feces, and saliva are generally considered noninfectious.

Standard Precautions

Because clinical examination cannot reliably identify all patients who pose a potential threat to HCWs, Standard Precautions were developed to prevent HCWs from coming into direct contact with a patient's blood or body fluid (e.g., saliva, vomit). OSHA has developed regulations that mandate employers and their employees to follow Standard Precautions in the workplace. Standard Precautions consist of both physical barriers to blood and body fluid and exposure as well as safe-handling practices for needles and other "sharps." Because trauma patients often have external hemorrhage and because blood is an extremely high-risk body fluid, protective devices should be worn while caring for patients.

Physical Barriers

Gloves. Gloves should be worn when touching non-intact skin, mucous membranes, or areas contaminated by gross blood or other body fluids. Because perforations may readily occur in gloves while caring for a patient, gloves should be examined regularly for defects and changed immediately if a problem is noted (Figure 5-7).

Masks and Face Shields. Masks serve to protect the HCW's oral and nasal mucous membranes from exposure to infectious agents, especially in situations in which airborne pathogens are known or suspected. Masks and face shields should be changed immediately if they become wet or soiled.

Eye Protection. Eye protection must be worn in circumstances in which droplets of infected fluid may be splattered, such as while providing airway management to a patient with blood

---

FIGURE 5-8 Preventing Sharps Injury

Prehospital care providers are at significant risk for injury from needles and other sharps. Strategies for reducing sharps injuries include the following:

- Use safety devices, such as shielded or retracting needles and scalpels and automatically retracting lancets.
- Use "needleless" systems that allow injection of medication at ports without needles.
- Refrain from recapping needles and other sharps.
- Immediately dispose of contaminated needles into rigid sharps containers rather than setting them down or handing them to someone else for disposal.
- Use prefilled medication syringes rather than drawing medication from an ampule.
- Provide a written exposure control plan and ensure that all employees are aware of the plan.
- Maintain a sharps injury log.

---

in the oropharynx. Standard eyeglasses are not considered adequate because they lack side shields.

Gowns. Disposable gowns with impervious plastic liners offer the best protection, but they may be extremely uncomfortable and impractical in the prehospital environment. Gowns or clothing should be changed immediately if significant soilage occurs.

Resuscitation Equipment. HCWs should have access to bag-mask devices or mouthpieces to protect them from direct contact with a patient's saliva, blood, and vomit.

Hand Washing

Hand washing is a fundamental principle of infection control. Hands should be washed with soap and running water if gross contamination with blood or body fluid occurs. Alcohol-based hand antiseptics are useful toward preventing transmission of many infectious agents but are not appropriate for situations in which obvious soiling has occurred; however, they can provide some cleansing and protective effect in situations in which running water and soap are not available. After removal of gloves, hands should be cleansed with either soap and water or an alcohol-based antiseptic.

Preventing Sharps Injury

As noted earlier, percutaneous exposure to a patient's blood or body fluid constitutes a significant manner in which viral infections could be transmitted to HCWs. Many percutaneous exposures are caused by injuries from needle sticks with contaminated needles or other sharps. Eliminate unnecessary needles and sharps, never recap a used needle, and implement safety devices when possible (Figure 5-8).

Management of Occupational Exposure

In the United States, OSHA mandates that every organization providing health care have a control plan for managing occupational exposures of its employees to blood and body fluids. Each exposure should be thoroughly documented, including the type of injury and estimation of the volume of inoculate. If a HCW has a mucocutaneous or percutaneous exposure to blood or sustains an injury from a contaminated sharp, efforts are taken to prevent bacterial infection, including tetanus, and HBV and HIV infection. No prophylactic therapy to prevent HCV infection is currently approved or available. Figure 5-9 describes a typical blood and body-fluid exposure protocol.

Hazardous Materials

Understanding the prehospital care provider's risk of exposure to hazardous materials is not as simple as recognizing environments that have obvious potential for hazardous material exposure. Hazardous materials are widespread in the modern world; vehicles, buildings, and even homes have hazardous-material potential. For this reason, all prehospital care providers require training to a minimum awareness level.

There are four levels of hazardous materials training:

- *Awareness:* This is the first of four levels of training available to responders and is designed to provide a basic level of knowledge.
- *Operations:* These responders are trained to set up perimeters and safety zones, limiting the spread of the event. Whereas awareness represents the minimum level of training, the operations level would be helpful for all responders, as well as providing the training to help control the event.
- *Technician:* Technicians are trained to work within the hazardous area and stop the release of hazardous materials.
- *Specialist:* This advanced level allows the responder to provide command and support skills to a hazardous materials ("hazmat," HazMat) event.

Prehospital care providers accept that scene safety is the first part of the approach to every patient and every scene. An important part of determining the safety of the scene is to evaluate for the potential of hazmat exposure. Assessment of potential hazards should begin with dispatch. The information given by dispatch may establish a high index of suspicion. Additional information can be requested while en route if prehospital care providers have any concerns or questions that could be relayed to the scene.

Once a scene has been determined to have hazmat involvement, the focus must shift to securing the scene and summoning help to safely isolate the involved area and remove and decontaminate the patients. The general simple rule is, "If the scene is not safe, make it safe." If the provider cannot make

---

FIGURE 5-9   Sample Exposure Protocol

After a percutaneous or mucocutaneous exposure to blood or other potentially infected body fluids, taking the appropriate actions and instituting appropriate postexposure prophylaxis (PEP) can help minimize the potential for acquiring viral hepatitis or HIV infection. Appropriate steps include:

1. Prevention of bacterial infection.
   - Cleanse exposed skin thoroughly with germicidal soap and water; exposed mucous membranes (mouth, eyes) should be irrigated with copious amounts of water.
   - Administer tetanus toxoid booster, if not received in previous 5 years.
2. Baseline laboratory studies are performed on both the exposed health care worker (HCW) and the source patient, if known.
   - *HCW:* Hepatitis B surface antibody (HBsAb), hepatitis C virus (HCV), and human immunodeficiency virus (HIV) tests.
   - *Source patient:* Hepatitis B and C serology and HIV test.
3. Prevention of hepatitis B virus (HBV) infection.
   - If the HCW has not been immunized against hepatitis B, the first dose of HBV vaccine is administered along with hepatitis B immune globulin (HBIG).
   - If the HCW has begun but not yet completed the HBV vaccine series, or if the HCW has completed all HBV immunizations, HBIG is given if the HBsAb test fails to show the presence of protective antibodies and the source patient's tests demonstrate active infection with HBV. HBIG may be administered up to 7 days after an exposure and still be effective.
4. Prevention of HIV infection.
   - PEP depends upon the route of exposure (percutaneous versus mucocutaneous) and the likelihood and severity of HIV infection in the source patient. If the source patient is known to be negative, PEP is not indicated regardless of exposure route. In the past, when recommended, PEP has generally involved a two-drug regimen. With the development of numerous anti-retroviral medications, the number of drug regimen combinations has increased. In addition, three-drug treatment is also warranted in specific cases involving high risk of transmission. Therefore, it is recommended that an exposed prehospital provider be evaluated by an expert to determine the most appropriate PEP regimen, given the circumstances of the particular exposure.

---

the scene safe, help should be summoned. The *Emergency Response Guidebook* (ERG), produced by the US Department of Transportation, can be used to identify potential hazards (Figure 5-10). The book uses a simple system that allows identification of a material by its name or placard number. The text then refers the reader to a guide page that provides basic information about safe distances for rescuers, life and fire hazards, and the patient's likely complaints. Binoculars should be used to read labels; if labels can be read without the use of viewing devices, the provider is too close and likely to be exposed.

At a hazmat scene, security must be ensured: "nobody in, nobody out." The staging area should be established upwind and upgrade at a safe distance from the hazard. Entry into and exit from the scene should be denied until the arrival of hazmat specialists. In most cases, patient care will begin when the decontaminated patient is delivered to the prehospital care provider.

It is important for the prehospital care provider to understand the command system and structure of the work zones in a hazmat operation. Hazmat control operations are set up in zones:

- HOT—The "hot" zone is the area of highest contamination, and only specially trained and protected workers may enter this area. If patients are in this area, the hazmat team will bring them out.

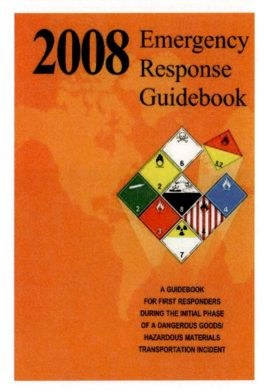

FIGURE 5-10 The *Emergency Response Guidebook* produced by the US Department of Transportation provides critical information at the scene of a potential hazardous material ("hazmat") incident.

■ WARM—A contamination reduction corridor runs through the next zone, called the "warm" zone, in which the patients will be decontaminated by the hazmat team. From here, they will move into the "cold" zone.

■ COLD—The cold zone is an area that is free from contamination. Patient care activities generally occur outside the cold zone. The command post, treatment, and triage areas will be outside the cold zone. (See Weapons of Mass Destruction for further hazmat considerations.)

Situation Issues

Crime Scenes

Unfortunately, a sizable percentage of trauma patients encountered by many prehospital care providers, especially in urban settings, are intentionally injured. In addition to shootings and stabbings, patients may be victims of other types of violent crimes, including assaults with fists or blunt objects and attempted strangulation. In other cases, victims may have been intentionally struck by a vehicle or pushed from a structure, resulting in a significant fall. Even an MVC can be considered a crime scene if one of the drivers is thought to be under the influence of alcohol or other intoxicants, driving recklessly, or speeding (Figure 5-11).

When managing these types of patients, prehospital care personnel interact with law enforcement personnel. Although both EMS and law enforcement share the goal of preserving life, prehospital care providers and law enforcement personnel occasionally find that their duties at a crime scene come into conflict. EMS personnel focus on the need to assess a victim for signs of life and viability, whereas law enforcement personnel are concerned with preserving evidence at a crime scene or bringing a perpetrator to justice.

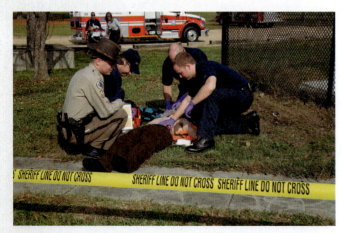

FIGURE 5-11 Prehospital care providers often have to manage patients at the scene of a crime and need to collaborate with law enforcement to preserve evidence.

With awareness of the general approach taken by law enforcement personnel at a crime scene, prehospital care providers not only may aid their patient, but also may better cooperate with law enforcement personnel, leading to the arrest of their patient's assailant.

At the scene of a major crime (homicide, suspicious death, rape, traffic death), most law enforcement agencies will collect and process evidence. Officers will typically perform the following duties:

■ Initially canvass the scene to identify all evidence, including weapons and shell casings.

■ Photograph the scene.

■ Sketch the scene.

■ Create a log of everyone who has entered the scene.

■ Conduct a more thorough search of the entire scene, looking for all potential evidence.

■ Look for and collect trace evidence, ranging from fingerprints to items that may contain DNA evidence (e.g., cigarette butts, strands of hair, fibers).

Police investigators believe that everyone who enters a crime scene brings some type of evidence to the scene and unknowingly removes some evidence from the scene. To solve the crime, a detective's goal is to identify the evidence deposited and removed by the perpetrator. To accomplish this, the investigators have to account for any evidence left or removed by other law enforcement officers, EMS personnel, and citizens who may have entered the scene. Careless behavior by prehospital care personnel at a crime scene may disrupt, destroy, or contaminate vital evidence, hampering a criminal investigation.

On occasion, prehospital care providers arrive at a potential crime scene before any law enforcement officers. If the victim is obviously dead, providers should carefully back out of the location without touching any items and await the arrival of officers. Although they would prefer that a crime scene not be disturbed, investigators realize that in some circumstances, prehospital care providers need to turn a body or move objects at a crime scene to access a victim and determine viability. If providers needed to transport a patient or move a body or other objects in the area before the arrival of law enforcement, investigators will typically ascertain the following:

■ When were the alterations made to the scene?

■ What was the purpose of the movement?

■ Who made the alterations?

■ At what time was the person's death identified by EMS personnel?

If prehospital care providers entered a crime scene before law enforcement personnel, investigators may want to interview and formally take a statement from the providers regarding their actions or observations. Prehospital care providers should never be alarmed or concerned about such a request. The purpose of the interview is not to critique the actions of the providers but to learn information that may prove helpful to the investigator in solving the case. Investigators may also request to take fingerprints of the prehospital care personnel if items in the crime scene were touched or handled by the crew without gloves.

Proper handling of a patient's clothing may preserve valuable evidence. If a patient's clothing needs to be removed, law enforcement officers and medical examiners prefer that prehospital care providers refrain from cutting through bullet or knife holes in the clothing. If the clothing is cut, investigators may ask what alterations were made to the clothing, who made the alterations, and the reason for alterations. Any clothing that is removed should be placed in a paper (not plastic) bag and turned over to investigators.

One final important issue involving victims of violent crimes is the value of any statements made by the patient while under the care of prehospital care providers. Some patients, realizing the critical nature of their injuries, may tell providers who inflicted their injuries. This information should be documented and passed on to investigators. If possible, prehospital care personnel should inform officers of the critical nature of a patient's injuries so that a sworn officer can be present if the patient is capable of providing any information regarding the perpetrator: a "dying declaration."

Weapons of Mass Destruction

The response to a scene involving hazardous materials, as discussed earlier, includes safety and other concerns similar to the response to the scene involving a weapon of mass destruction (WMD).

Every scene that involves multiple victims or that was reported to have resulted from an explosion should trigger two questions: (1) Was a WMD was involved, and (2) Could there be a secondary device intended to harm responders? In particular, when many victims complain of similar symptoms or present with similar findings, a WMD should be considered. (See the chapter on WMD for greater detail.)

The prehospital care provider needs to approach such scenes with extreme caution and resist the urge to rush in to care for the sickest victim. This natural response of providers only serves to increase the victim count. Instead, the provider should approach the scene from an upwind position and take a moment to stop, look, and listen for clues that will alert the team to the possible presence of a WMD. Obvious spills of wet or dry material, visible vapors, and smoke should be avoided until the nature of the material has been ascertained. Enclosed or confined spaces should never be entered without appropriate personal protective equipment (PPE).

Once a WMD has been included as a possible cause, the prehospital care provider needs to take all appropriate steps for self-protection. These steps include the use of PPE appropriate to the function of the individual provider. Information

that this may be a WMD incident should be relayed back to dispatch to alert incoming responders from all services. Staging areas for additional equipment, responders, and helicopters should be established upwind and at a safe distance from the site.

The scene should be secured and zones indicating hot, warm, and cold areas designated. Sites for decontamination should also be determined. Once the nature of the agent has been determined (chemical, biologic, or radiologic), specific requests for antidote or antibiotics can be made.

Scene Control Zones

To limit the spread of a hazardous material or WMD, the National Institute of Occupational Safety and Health (NIOSH) and the Environmental Protection Agency (EPA) have developed and advocated the use of control zones. The objective of this concept is to perform specific activities in specific zones. Adherence to such principles reduces the likelihood of spread of contamination and injury to rescue personnel and bystanders.

The zones are three concentric circles (Figure 5-12). The innermost zone, the *hot zone,* is the region immediately adjacent to the hazmat or WMD incident. The task of rescuers in this region is to evacuate the contaminated, injured patient, with no provision of patient care. In order to do so, generally the highest level of PPE must be utilized. The next zone, the *warm zone,* is where decontamination of victims, personnel, and equipment occurs. In this zone, the only patient care administered is primary assessment and spinal immobilization. The outermost zone, the *cold zone,* is where equipment and personnel are staged. Once the patient is evacuated to the cold zone, providers can deliver definitive patient care. Figure 5-13 lists safe evacuation distances for bomb threats.

If a patient is delivered to the hospital or aid station from a hazmat or WMD scene, it is most prudent to re-evaluate if that patient has been decontaminated and to mimic the concepts of these zones (see Figure 5-12).

Decontamination

Whether the incident involves a hazmat situation or a WMD, decontamination of an exposed individual often may be required. *Decontamination* is the reduction or removal of hazardous chemical, biologic, or radiologic agents. The provider's highest priority in the care of an exposed patient, as in any emergency, is personal and scene safety. If there is any question of a continued exposure hazard, assurance of personal safety is the first priority. Failure to do so will only produce an additional victim (the provider) and deprive those already injured of the provider's skills. Decontamination of the patient is the next priority. This will minimize the exposure risk to the provider during assessment and treatment of the patient and will prevent contamination of equipment,

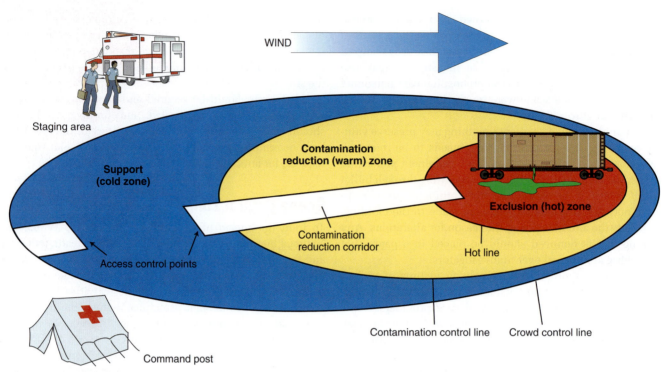

FIGURE 5-12 The scene of a WMD or hazmat incident is generally divided into hot, warm, and cold zones.
(From Chapleau W: *Emergency First Responder,* St Louis, 2004, Mosby.)

FIGURE 5-13   Bomb Threats: Safe Evacuation Distances

Threat Description		Explosives Capacity (TNT Capacity) (pounds)	Building Evacuation Distance (feet)	Outdoor Evacuation Distance (feet)
	Pipe bomb	5	70	850
	Briefcase/suitcase bomb	50	150	1,850
	Compact sedan	500	320	1,500
	Full-size sedan	1,000	400	1,750
	Passenger/cargo van	4,000	650	2,750
	Small moving van, delivery truck	10,000	860	3,750
	Moving van, small tank truck	30,000	1,240	6,500
	Semitrailer	60,000	1,570	7,000

(Modified from Messier *DM:* Explosive Prospects: terrorist bombings present multifaceted response challenge. *Homeland Response* 2(1), 2004.)

thereby avoiding the risk of exposure of other individuals from contaminated equipment and vehicles.

OSHA provides regulatory guidelines for PPE used by prehospital care providers during the emergency care of victims in a potentially hazardous environment. Individuals providing medical care in environments of an unknown hazard must have a minimum of appropriate training and be supplied and trained with level B protection. Level B protection consists of splash-protective, chemical-resistant clothing and self-contained breathing sources. Training in advance of the need to use this level of PPE is required.

If the patient is conscious and able to assist, it is best to enlist their cooperation to have them perform as much of the decontamination as possible to reduce the likelihood of cross-contamination to providers. Carefully remove the patient's clothes and jewelry and place these in plastic bags. Transfer the removed clothing carefully so as not to spread any particulate matter or splash any liquid onto noncontaminated personnel or surfaces. Brush any particulate matter off the patient, then irrigate copiously with water. Washing with water will dilute the concentration of the potentially hazardous material and remove any remaining agent. A common axiom is, "The solution to pollution is dilution." Successful decontamination requires large amounts of water. A common mistake made by the inexperienced prehospital care provider is to irrigate the patient with water only until the irrigant begins to spill onto the floor, which usually occurs after 1 or 2 liters of irrigation. This practice has two problems: the area of body contamination is increased, and the offending agent is not diluted sufficiently to render the agent harmless. Failure to provide for adequate runoff and drainage of lavage fluid may cause injury to previously unexposed areas of the body as the contaminated lavage accumulates. Neutralizing agents for chemical burns are typically avoided. In the neutralizing process, the agents often give off heat in an exothermic reaction. Therefore, a well-meaning provider may create a thermal burn in addition to the chemical burn. Most commercially available decontamination solutions are made for the purpose of decontaminating equipment, not people.

Secondary Devices

Within months after the bombing at the 1996 Atlanta Summer Olympics, the metropolitan Atlanta area experienced two additional bombings. These bombings, at an abortion clinic and a nightclub, had secondary bombs planted and represented the first time in 17 years in the United States that secondary bombs had been planted, presumably to kill or injure rescuers responding to the scene of the first blast. Unfortunately, the secondary device at the abortion clinic was not detected prior to its detonation and there were six casualties. Secondary devices have been used with regularity by terrorists in many countries. All prehospital care personnel need to be mindful of the potential presence of a secondary device. After these incidents, the Georgia Emergency Management

Agency developed the following guidelines for rescuers and prehospital care personnel responding to the scene of a bombing at which a secondary bomb might be planted:

1. *Refrain from use of electronic devices.* Sound waves from cell phones and radios may cause a secondary device to detonate, especially if used close to the bomb. Equipment used by the news media may also trigger a detonation.
2. *Ensure sufficient boundaries for the scene.* The potential zone of danger (hot zone) should extend 1000 feet in all directions (including vertically) from the original blast site. As more powerful bombs are created, shrapnel may travel further. The initial bomb blast may damage infrastructure, including gas lines and power lines, which may jeopardize the safety of rescuers. Access to and exit from the hot zone should be carefully controlled.
3. *Provide rapid evacuation of victims from the scene and hot zone.* Because the scene of a bomb blast is considered unsafe, triage of victims should not occur in the hot zone. An EMS command post (or triage area) should be established 2000 to 4000 feet from the scene of the initial bombing. Rescuers can rapidly evacuate victims from the bombing site with minimal interventions until victims and rescuers are out of the hot zone.
4. *Collaborate with law enforcement personnel on preserving and recovering evidence.* Bombing sites constitute a crime scene, and rescuers should disrupt the scene only as necessary to evacuate victims. Any potential evidence that is inadvertently removed from the scene with a victim should be documented and turned over to law enforcement personnel to ensure proper chain of custody. Prehospital care personnel can document exactly where they were in the scene and which items they touched.

Command Structure

An EMT ambulance responding to a call will usually have one person in charge (the incident commander) and another person assisting in a rudimentary incident command structure. As an incident grows larger and more responders from various public safety and other agencies respond to the scene, the need for a formal system and structure to oversee and control the response becomes increasingly important.

Incident Command

The *incident command system* (ICS) has developed over the years as an outgrowth of planning systems used by firefighting services for multiple-service responses to major fire situations. The program gained acceptance particularly from the experience of wildland firefighters battling expansive fire fronts, with deployment of dozens of diverse agencies. The collective wisdom of their efforts resulted in FIRESCOPE, or Firefighting Resources of California Organized for Potential Emergencies. In addition, the Phoenix Fire Department developed the Fire Ground Command System (FGC). Although many similarities existed between these two approaches, there were also differences, and attempts were made to combine the two systems into one comprehensive command structure.

In 1987, the National Fire Protection Association (NFPA) published NFPA Standard 1561, the Standard on Fire Department Incident Command Management System. NFPA 1561 was later revised as the *Standard on Emergency Services Incident Management.* This version can be implemented and adjusted to any type or size of event by any agency managing an incident. In the 1990s, the National Fire Incident Management System (IMS) was created, which further refined the single-incident management approach.

Dealing with any incident, large or small, is enhanced by the precise command structure afforded by the ICS. At the core of ICS are the establishment of centralized command at the scene and the subsequent buildup of divisional responsibilities. The first arriving unit establishes the command center, and communications are established through command for the buildup of the response. The five key elements of the incident command system are as follows:

1. *Command* provides overall control of the event and the communications that will coordinate the movement of resources in and patients out of the incident scene.
2. *Operations* include divisions to handle the tactical needs of the event. Fire suppression, EMS, and rescue are examples of operational divisions.
3. *Planning* is a continuous process of evaluating immediate and potential needs of the incident and planning the response. Throughout the event, this element will be used to evaluate the effectiveness of operations and to make suggested alterations in the response and tactical approach.
4. *Logistics* handles the task of acquiring resources and moving them where needed; these include personnel, shelter, vehicles, and equipment.
5. *Finance* tracks the money. Response personnel from all involved agencies as well as contractors, personnel, and vendors brought into service in the incident will be tracked so that the cost of the event can be determined and these groups can be paid for goods, supplies, equipment, and services.

Unified Command

An expansion of the ICS is the *unified command system.* This expansion takes into account the needs of coordinating agencies from across jurisdictional boundaries. The technical aspects of bringing resources to bear from multiple communities, counties, and states are covered by this additional coordinating structure.

National Incident Management System

On February 28, 2003, President George W. Bush directed the secretary of Homeland Security through Presidential Directive HSPD-5 to produce a National Incident Management System (NIMS). This would establish a consistent, nationwide approach for federal, state, and local governments to work effectively together to prepare for, respond to, and recover from domestic incidents regardless of cause, size, or complexity. The Department of Homeland Security authorized NIMS on March 1, 2004, after collaborating with detailed working groups consisting of state and local government officials and representatives of the National Association of Emergency Medical Technicians (NAEMT), Fraternal Order of Police (FOP), International Association of Fire Chiefs (IAFC), and International Association of Emergency Managers (IAEM), as well as a wide range of other public safety organizations.

NIMS focuses on the following incident management characteristics:

- Common terminology
- Modular organization
- Management by objectives
- Reliance on an incident action plan
- Manageable span of control
- Predesignated "incident mobilization center" locations and facilities
- Comprehensive resource management
- Integrated communications
- Establishment of transfer of command
- Chain of command and unity of command
- Unified command
- Accountability of resources and personnel
- Deployment
- Information and intelligence management

The key elements of NIMS are as follows:

1. ICS
2. Communications and information management
3. Preparedness
4. Joint information systems (consistent public information)
5. National Incident Management Integration Center (NIC)

Command

Command comprises the *incident commander* (IC) and command staff. Command staff positions are made as appropriate to the size and nature of the event and may include public information officer (PIO), safety officer (SO), and liaison officer. Other positions can be created as deemed necessary by the IC.

As described earlier, unified command is an enhancement to incident command in situations involving multiple jurisdictions. In a single-command situation, the IC is solely responsible for the incident management. In a unified command structure, individuals representing various jurisdictions jointly determine objectives, plans, and priorities. The unified command system seeks to solve problems involving differences in communications and operational standards (Figure 5-14).

One element not included in ICS that is added with unified command and NIMS is *intelligence.* Based on the size of the event, intelligence and information gathering related to national security may also include risk-management assessment, medical intelligence, weather information, structural design of buildings, and information on toxic containment. Although these functions are typically handled in the planning section, the IC may separate information gathering from planning in certain situations.

In NIMS the IC can assign intelligence and information as follows:

- Within the command staff
- As a unit of the planning section
- As a branch of operations
- As a separate general staff function

Incident Action Plans

Incident action plans (IAPs) include overall incident objectives and strategies established by the IC or unified command. The planning section develops and documents the IAP. The IAP also addresses the tactical objectives and support activities for the operational period, which is generally 12 to 24 hours. The planning section also provides an ongoing critique, or "lessons learned" process, to ensure the response meets the needs of the event.

In very large incidents, multiple ICS organizations may be established. Area command may be established to manage multiple ICS organizations. Area command does not have operational responsibilities but will perform the following duties:

1. Set overall incident-related priorities for the agency
2. Allocate critical resources according to established priorities
3. Ensure that incidents are managed properly
4. Ensure effective communications
5. Ensure that incident management objectives are met and do not conflict with each other or with agency policies
6. Identify critical resource needs and report to the Emergency Operations Center(s)
7. Ensure that short-term emergency recovery is coordinated to assist in the transition to full-recovery operations
8. Provide for personnel accountability and safe operating environments

Detailed information and training programs about the Incident Command System and the National Incident Management System can found on the Federal Emergency Management Agency's Web site (Figure 5-15).

Patient Assessment and Triage

Once all the preceding issues have been addressed, the actual process of assessing and treating patients can begin. The greatest challenge occurs when the prehospital care provider is faced with multiple victims.

Mass-casualty incidents (MCIs) occur in many sizes. Most rescuers have responded to incidents with more than one victim, but large-scale events with hundreds or thousands of victims are rarely encountered.

Triage is a French word meaning "to sort." Triage is a process that will be used to assign priority for treatment and transport. In the prehospital environment, triage is used in two different contexts:

1. **Sufficient resources are available to manage all patients.** In this triage situation, the most severely injured patients are treated and transported first, and those with lesser injuries are treated and transported later.
2. **The number of patients exceeds the immediate capacity of on-scene resources.** The objective in such triage is to ensure survival of the largest possible number of injured patients. Patients are sorted into categories for patient care. In an MCI, patient care must be rationed because the number of patients exceeds the available resources. Relatively few prehospital care providers ever experience an MCI with 50 to 100 or more simultaneously injured persons, but many will be involved in MCIs with 10 to 20 patients, and most prehospital veterans have managed an incident with 2 to 10 patients.

Incidents that involve sufficient rescuers and medical resources allow for treatment and transport of the most severely injured patients first. In a large-scale MCI, limited resources will require that patient treatment and transport be prioritized to salvage the victims with the greatest chance of survival. These victims are prioritized for treatment and transport (Figure 5-16).

The goal of patient management at the MCI scene is to do the most good for the most patients with the resources available. It is the responsibility of the prehospital care provider to make decisions about who is to be managed first. The usual rules about saving lives are different in MCIs. The decision is always to save the most lives; however, when the available resources are not sufficient for the needs of all the injured patients present, these resources should be used for the patients who have the best chance of surviving. In a choice between a patient with

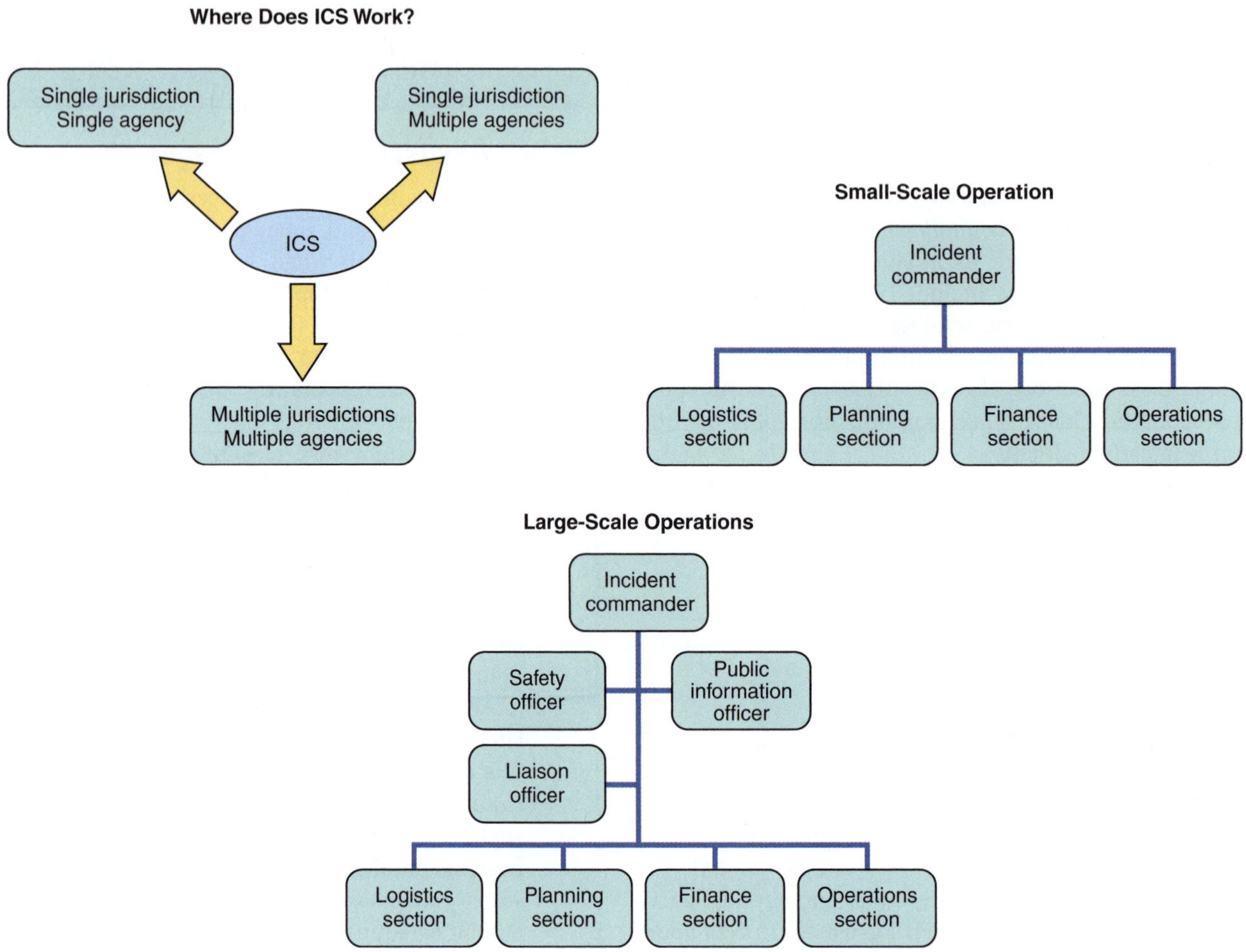

Where Does ICS Work?

Small-Scale Operation

Large-Scale Operations

FIGURE 5-14 The incident command structure is flexible and can be expanded or decreased based on the number of patients and the complexity of the event. The operational functions of each of the sections under incident command are the branches. The Medical Services Branch is the operational component that is responsible for coordinating and providing medical services needed to meet the tactical objectives of the incident. This includes marshalling equipment and personnel, triage, communications with medical facilities, and transport.

a catastrophic injury such as severe brain trauma and a patient with acute intra-abdominal hemorrhage, the proper course of action in an MCI is to manage first the salvageable patient—the victim with the abdominal hemorrhage. Treating the patient with severe head trauma first will probably result in the loss of both patients; the head trauma patient may die because he or she may not be salvageable, and the abdominal hemorrhage patient may die because time, equipment, and personnel spent managing the unsalvageable patient kept this salvageable patient from receiving the simple care needed to survive until definitive surgical care was available.

In a triage MCI situation, the catastrophically injured patient may need to be considered "lower priority," with treatment delayed until more help and equipment become available. These are difficult decisions and circumstances, but a prehospital care provider must respond quickly and properly. A medical care team should not make efforts to resuscitate a traumatic cardiac arrest patient with little or no chance of survival while three other patients die because of airway compromise or external hemorrhage. The "sorting scheme" most often used divides patients into five categories based on need of care and chance of survival:

1. *Immediate*—Patients whose injuries are critical, but who will require only minimal time or equipment to manage and who have a good prognosis for survival. An example is the patient with a compromised airway or massive external hemorrhage.

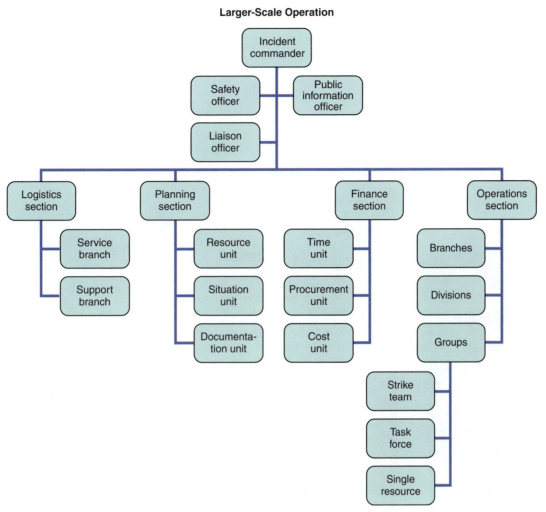

FIGURE 5-14, cont'd

FIGURE 5-15   **Incident Command Training Resources**

Federal Emergency Management Agency (FEMA): Incident command system (ICS) training:

■ ICS-100.a, Introduction to ICS (http://training.fema.gov/EMIWeb/IS/IS100A.asp)
■ ICS-200.a, Basic ICS (http://training.fema.gov/EMIWeb/IS/IS200A.asp)
■ ICS-700.a, NIMS an Introduction (http://training.fema.gov/EMIWeb/IS/is700a.asp)
■ ICS-800.b, National Response Framework, an Introduction (http://training.fema.gov/EMIWeb/IS/IS800b.asp)

National Incident Management System (NIMS) and FEMA training:

■ Contact your state Emergency Management Agency or Emergency Management Institute and National Fire Academy, Emmitsburg, Md. A variety of online correspondence and onsite courses are available. (http://training.fema.gov/IS/crslist.asp)

For more information on NIMS, contact the NIMS Integrations Center: www.dhs.gov.

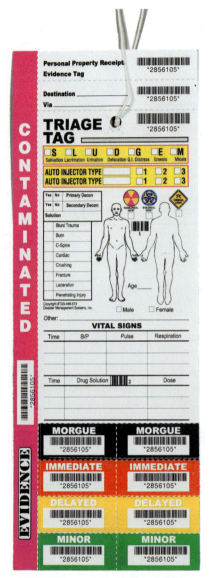

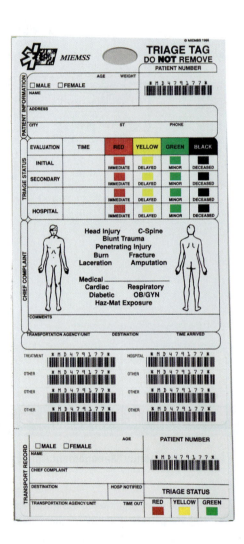

FIGURE 5-16 Examples of triage tags.

2. *Delayed*—Patients whose injuries are debilitating, but who do not require immediate management to salvage life or limb. An example is the patient with a long-bone fracture.
3. *Minor*—Patients, often called the "walking wounded," who have minor injuries that can wait for treatment or who may even assist in the interim by comforting other patients or helping as litter bearers.
4. *Expectant*—Patients whose injuries are so severe that they have only a minimal chance of survival. An example is the patient with a 90% full-thickness burn and thermal pulmonary injury.

5. *Dead*—Patients who are unresponsive, pulseless, and breathless. In a disaster, resources rarely allow for attempted resuscitation of cardiac arrest patients.

Figures 5-17 through 5-19 describe a commonly used triage scheme known as START, which uses only four categories: Immediate, Delayed, Minor, and Dead. (For more information, please see the Disaster Chapter.)
Figures 5-20 and 5-21 describe the recently published SALT triage system.[4]

FIGURE 5-17   START Triage

In 1983, medical personnel from Hoag Memorial Hospital and firefighter-paramedics from the Newport Beach Fire Department created a triage process for first responders, *Simple Triage and Rapid Treatment* (START) (see Figure 5-18). This triage process was designed to identify critically injured patients easily and quickly. START does not establish a medical diagnosis, but instead provides a rapid and simple sorting process. START uses three simple assessments to identify those victims most at risk to die from their injuries. Typically, the process takes 30 to 60 seconds per victim. START requires no tools, specialized medical equipment, or special knowledge.

HOW DOES START WORK?
The first step is to direct anyone who can walk to a designated safe area. If the victims can walk and follow commands, their condition is categorized as "minor," and they will be further triaged and tagged when more rescuers arrive. This now leads to a smaller group of presumably more seriously injured victims remaining for rescuers to triage. The mnemonic "30-2-can-do" is used as the START triage prompt (see Figure 5-19). The "30" refers to the patient's respiratory rate, the "2" refers to capillary refill, and the "can-do" refers to the ability of the patient to follow commands. Any victim with respirations fewer than 30 per minute, capillary refill of less than 2 seconds, and the ability to follow verbal commands and to walk is categorized as a "minor" patient. When victims meet these criteria but cannot walk, they are categorized as "delayed." Victims who are unconscious or have rapid breathing, or who have delayed capillary refill or absent radial pulse are categorized as "immediate." While at the victim's side, two basic lifesaving measures can be performed: opening the airway and controlling external hemorrhage. For those victims who are not breathing, the rescuer should open the airway, and if breathing resumes, the victim is categorized as "immediate." No cardiopulmonary resuscitation (CPR) should be attempted. If the victim does not resume breathing, the victim is categorized as "dead." Bystanders or the "walking wounded" can be directed by the rescuer to help maintain the airway and hemorrhage control.

Retriage is also needed if lack of transportation prolongs the time the victims remain at the scene. Using START criteria, significantly injured victims may be categorized as "delayed." The longer they remain without treatment, the greater the chance their condition will deteriorate. Therefore, repeat evaluation and triage are appropriate over time.

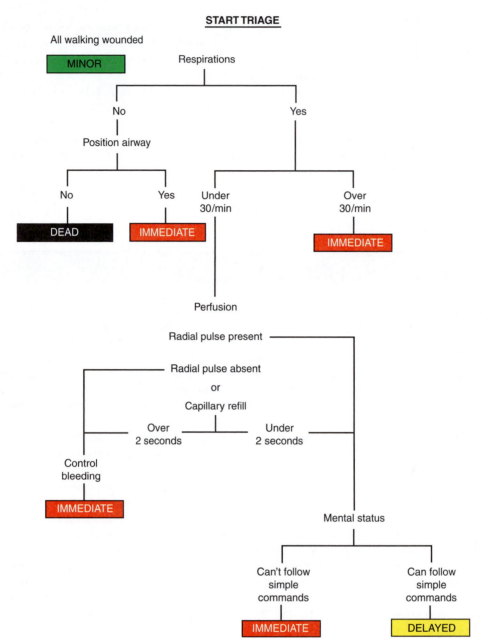

FIGURE 5-18 START triage algorithm.

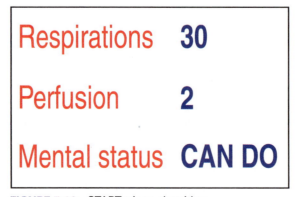

FIGURE 5-19 START triage algorithm.
(Courtesy of Newport Beach Fire Department, Newport Beach, Cal.)

FIGURE 5-20 SALT Triage

This system begins by using a global sorting process: asking patients to walk or wave (follow commands). Those patients who do not respond are then assessed for life threats and subsequently categorized into immediate, delayed, minimal, or dead (see Figure 5-21).

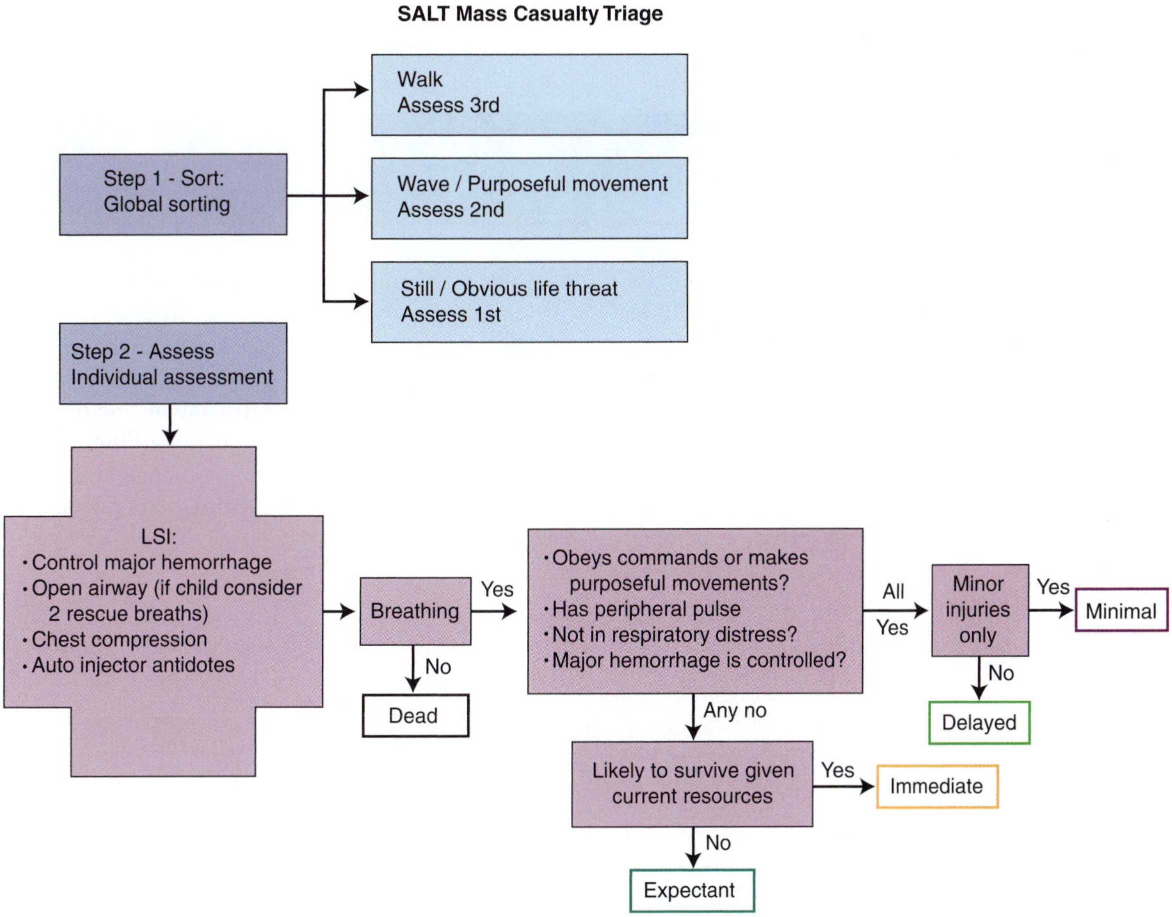

SALT Mass Casualty Triage

Step 1 - Sort:
Global sorting

- Walk
  Assess 3rd
- Wave / Purposeful movement
  Assess 2nd
- Still / Obvious life threat
  Assess 1st

Step 2 - Assess
Individual assessment

LSI:
- Control major hemorrhage
- Open airway (if child consider 2 rescue breaths)
- Chest compression
- Auto injector antidotes

Breathing → No → Dead

Breathing → Yes →
- Obeys commands or makes purposeful movements?
- Has peripheral pulse
- Not in respiratory distress?
- Major hemorrhage is controlled?

All Yes → Minor injuries only → Yes → Minimal

Minor injuries only → No → Delayed

Any no → Likely to survive given current resources → Yes → Immediate

Likely to survive given current resources → No → Expectant

FIGURE 5-21 SALT triage algorithm.

SCENARIO SOLUTION

Assessment of the scene reveals many potential hazards, the most apparent being the environmental conditions. Snow not only obscures vision, but also makes the roadway slippery and increases stopping distances. Lying on the ground in the cold and snow may predispose the patient to hypothermia. Providing emergency medical care along roadsides ranks as one of the most dangerous situations encountered by prehospital care providers. If this incident occurred at night, the darkness adds to the risk and makes it imperative that personnel wear reflective clothing. Law enforcement personnel are essential for traffic control along the scene. Fuel spills, chemical cargo, and other vehicle fluids may create a hazardous material situation. Fire department personnel can isolate or neutralize the fluids while monitoring the scene for fires that may erupt. In addition, a bloody patient exposes prehospital care personnel to the risks of blood-borne infections, and the caregivers should wear physical barriers, including gloves, masks, and eye protection.

SUMMARY

■ As a part of assessing the scene for provider safety in each and every patient contact, it is important to assess for hazards of all types. Hazards include traffic issues, environmental concerns, violence, blood-borne pathogens, and hazardous materials.

■ Assessing the scene will assure that provider personnel and equipment are not compromised and unavailable for others and ensure that other health care professionals are protected from hazards that are not isolated or removed.

■ Sometimes hazards will be ruled out quickly, but if they are not looked for, they won't be seen, and this is what can cause harm.

■ Certain situations such as crime scene or intentional acts including the use of weapons of mass destruction will affect how the provider deals with the scene and the patients at that scene.

■ Incidents will be managed using an Incident Command System structure, and EMS is one of the components in that structure. Providers must know and understand the ICS system and their role within that system.

References

1. Maguire BJ, Hunting KL, Smith GS, et al. Occupational fatalities in emergency medical services. *Ann Emerg Med* 40(6):625, 2002.
2. Schaeffer J. Prevent run downs: best practices for roadside incident management, 2002. http://www.jems.com/jems/news02/0903a.html. Accessed September 2002.
3. Poland GA, Jacobson RM. Prevention of hepatitis B with the hepatitis B vaccine. *N Engl J Med* 351:2832, 2004.
4. Lerner EB, Schwartz RB, Coule PL, et al. Mass casualty triage: An evaluation of the data and development of a proposed national guideline. *Disaster Med Public Health Prep* 2:S25-S34, 2008.

Suggested Reading

Centers for Disease Control and Prevention: See website for information on Standard Precautions and postexposure prophylaxis, www.cdc.gov.

Rinnert KJ: A review of infection control practices, risk reduction, and legislative regulations for blood-borne disease: Applications for emergency medical services. *Prehosp Emerg Care* 2(1):70, 1998.

Rinnert KJ, O'Connor RE, Delbridge T: Risk reduction for exposure to blood-borne pathogens in EMS: National Association of EMS Physicians. *Prehosp Emerg Care* 2(1):62, 1998.

CHAPTER 6

Patient Assessment and Management

CHAPTER OBJECTIVES

At the completion of this chapter, the reader will be able to do the following:

- ✓ Provide an illustration of the significance of patient assessment in the context of overall management of the trauma patient.

- ✓ Systematize the discrete steps involved in assessing and managing the trauma patient into an organized and rational process.

- ✓ Given a scenario, adapt the 15-second global survey and primary survey to the particulars of the situation.

- ✓ Employ a process of critical questioning in order to associate the physical examination and scene findings with their likely causes and consequences.

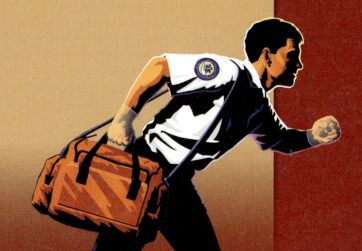

SCENARIO

You are awakened at 0400 on a Saturday to respond to the scene of a person who fell from a third-floor balcony. As you go to the ambulance, you notice the temperature is 50°F (10°C). According to dispatch, bystanders report that the patient lost consciousness but now is awake. On arrival, you detect no threats to safety in your scene assessment. Bystanders state that he was partying in the apartment above and had been drinking some alcohol. They report that he seemed to land feet first onto the ground below and confirm that they witnessed the patient's loss of consciousness for a period of "several minutes." Approaching the patient, a young adult male, you kneel at his head, observing that he is conscious. You position your hands to provide cervical spine stabilization. In response to your questioning, you discover that the patient's chief complaint is foot and back pain. Your questioning serves the dual purpose of obtaining the patient's complaint and assessing his ventilatory effort. Detecting no shortness of breath, you proceed with further questioning as your partner obtains the patient's vital signs. The patient answers your questions appropriately to establish that he is oriented to person, place, and event.

Based on kinematics as they relate to this incident, what potential injuries do you anticipate finding during your assessment? What are your next priorities? How will you proceed with this patient?

Assessment is the cornerstone of excellent patient care. For the trauma patient, as for other critically ill patients, assessment is the foundation on which all management and transportation decisions are based. The first goal in assessment is to determine a patient's current condition. In doing so, an overall impression of a patient's status is developed and baseline values for the status of the patient's respiratory, circulatory, and neurologic systems established. Life-threatening conditions are rapidly assessed and urgent intervention and resuscitation initiated. Any other conditions that require attention are identified and addressed before a patient is moved. If time allows, a secondary survey for nonlife-or-limb-threatening injuries is conducted. Often this occurs during transportation of the patient.

All of these steps are performed quickly and efficiently with a goal of minimizing time spent on the scene. Critical patients should not remain in the field for care other than that needed to stabilize them for transport, unless they are trapped or other complications exist that prevent early transportation. By applying the principles learned in this course, on-scene delay can be minimized and patients moved rapidly to an appropriate medical facility. Successful assessment and intervention require a strong knowledge base of trauma physiology and a well-developed plan of management that is carried out quickly and effectively.

The trauma management literature frequently mentions the need to transport the trauma patient to definitive surgical care within an absolute minimum amount of time after the onset of the injury. This is because a critical trauma patient who does not respond to initial therapy is most likely bleeding internally. This blood loss will continue until the hemorrhage is controlled. Except for the most basic external bleeding, this hemorrhage control can be accomplished only in the operating room (OR).

The primary concerns for assessment and management of the trauma patient, in order of importance, are: (1) airway, (2) ventilation, (3) oxygenation, (4) hemorrhage control, (5) perfusion, and (6) neurologic function. This sequence protects the ability of the body to oxygenate and the ability of the red blood cells (RBCs) to deliver oxygen to the tissues. Hemorrhage control, which is only temporary in the field, but permanent in the OR, depends on rapid transportation by the prehospital care providers and the presence of a trauma team that is immediately available on arrival at the medical facility.

R Adams Cowley, MD, developed the concept of the "Golden Hour" of trauma. He believed that the time between injury occurrence and definitive care was critical. During this period, when bleeding is uncontrolled and inadequate tissue oxygenation is occurring because of decreased perfusion, damage occurs throughout the body. If bleeding is not controlled and tissue oxygenation is not restored within 1 hour of the injury, the patient's chances of survival plummet.

The Golden Hour is now referred to as the "Golden Period" because this critical time period is not necessarily 1 hour. Some patients have less than an hour in which to receive care whereas others have more time. A prehospital care provider is responsible for recognizing the urgency of a given situation and transporting a patient as quickly as possible to a facility in which definitive care can be accomplished. To deliver the trauma patient to definitive care, the

FIGURE 6-1 Assessment Terminology

PHTLS	National EMS Education Standards
Scene assessment	Scene size-up
Primary survey	Primary assessment
Secondary survey	Secondary assessment
Monitoring and reassessment	Reassessment

seriousness of the patient's life-threatening injuries must be quickly identified; only essential, lifesaving care at the scene provided; and rapid transportation to an appropriate medical facility undertaken. In many urban prehospital systems, the average time between injury and arrival to the scene is 8 to 9 minutes. Usually another 8 to 9 minutes are spent transporting the patient. If the providers spend only 10 minutes on the scene, 30 minutes of the Golden Period will have passed by the time a patient arrives at the receiving facility. Every additional minute spent on the scene is additional time that the patient is bleeding, and valuable time is ticking away from the Golden Period. To address this critical trauma management issue, quick, efficient evaluation and management of the patient is the ultimate objective. Scene time should not exceed 10 minutes; the shorter the scene time, the better. The longer the patient is kept on scene, the greater the potential for blood loss and death. These time parameters change as delayed extrication, delayed transport, and other unexpected circumstances arise.

This chapter covers the essentials of patient assessment and initial management in the field and is based on the approach taught to physicians in the Advanced Trauma Life Support (ATLS) program.[1] The principles described are identical to those learned in initial basic- or advanced-provider training programs, although different terminology may occasionally be used. For example, the phrase "primary survey" is used in the ATLS and Prehospital Trauma Life Support (PHTLS) programs to describe the patient assessment activity known as "primary assessment" in the National EMS Education Standards. What the PHTLS course refers to as the "secondary survey" is essentially the same activity that the basic provider learns as the "secondary assessment" of the trauma patient. For the most part, the activities performed in each phase are exactly the same; the various courses simply use different terminology (Figure 6-1).

Establishing Priorities

There are three priorities on arrival to a scene:

1. The first priority for everyone involved at a trauma incident is assessment of the scene. Chapter 5 discusses this in detail.

2. Recognition of the existence of multiple-patient incidents and mass-casualty incidents (MCIs). In an MCI, the priority shifts from focusing all resources on the most injured patient to saving the maximum number of patients (providing the greatest good to the greatest number). Chapter 5 also discusses triage.

3. Once a brief scene assessment has been performed, attention can be turned to evaluating individual patients. The assessment and management process begins by focusing on the patient or patients who have been identified as most critical, as resources allow. Emphasis is placed on the following, in this order: (a) conditions that may result in the loss of life; (b) conditions that may result in the loss of limb; and (c) all other conditions that do not threaten life or limb. Depending on the severity of the injury, the number of injured patients, and the proximity to the receiving facility, conditions that do not threaten life or limb may never be addressed.

Most of this chapter focuses on the *critical thinking* skills required to conduct a proper assessment, interpret the findings, and set priorities for proper patient care.

Primary Survey (Initial Assessment)

In the critical multisystem trauma patient, the priority for care is the rapid identification and management of life-threatening conditions (Figure 6-2). More than 90% of trauma patients have simple injuries that involve only one system (e.g., an isolated limb fracture). For these single-system trauma patients, there is time to be thorough in both the primary and the secondary survey. For the critically injured patient, the provider may never conduct more than a primary survey. The emphasis is on rapid

FIGURE 6-2 Multisystem versus Single-System Trauma Patient

- A *multisystem trauma patient* has injuries involving more than one body system, including the pulmonary, circulatory, neurologic, gastrointestinal, musculoskeletal, and integumentary systems. An example would be a patient involved in a motor vehicle crash who has a traumatic brain injury, pulmonary contusions, a splenic injury with shock, and a femur fracture.
- A *single-system trauma patient* has injury to only one body system. An example would be a patient with a simple ankle fracture and no evidence of blood loss or shock.

evaluation, initiation of resuscitation, and transportation to an appropriate medical facility. This does not eliminate the need for prehospital management; it means that it needs to be *done faster, done more efficiently, and done en route to the receiving facility.*

Quick establishment of priorities and the initial evaluation of life-threatening injuries must be routine. Therefore, the components of the primary and secondary surveys need to be memorized and the logical progression of priority-based assessment and treatment understood. A prehospital care provider must think about the pathophysiology of a patient's injuries and conditions; the provider cannot waste time trying to remember which priorities are the most important.

The most common basis of life-threatening injuries is lack of adequate tissue oxygenation, which leads to anaerobic (without oxygen) metabolism (energy production). Decreased energy production that occurs with anaerobic metabolism is termed *shock*. Three components are necessary for normal metabolism: (1) oxygenation of RBCs in the lungs; (2) delivery of RBCs to the cells throughout the body; and (3) off-loading of oxygen to these cells. The activities involved in the primary survey are aimed at identifying and correcting problems with the first two components.

General Impression

The primary survey begins with a simultaneous, or *global,* overview of the status of a patient's respiratory, circulatory, and neurologic systems to identify obvious, significant external problems with oxygenation, circulation, hemorrhage, or gross deformities. When initially approaching a patient, the prehospital care provider observes whether the patient appears to be moving air effectively, is awake or unresponsive, is holding him- or herself up, and is moving spontaneously. Once at the patient's side, a reasonable starting point is to ask the patient, "What happened to you?" If the patient answers with a coherent explanation in complete sentences, the prehospital care provider can conclude that the patient has a patent airway, sufficient respiratory function to support speech, adequate cerebral perfusion, and reasonable neurologic functioning; that is, there are probably no immediate threats to this patient's life.

If a patient is unable to provide such an answer, a detailed primary survey to identify life-threatening problems is begun. While asking follow-up questions (e.g., "Where do you hurt?"), airway patency is further assessed and respiratory function observed. A quick check of the radial pulse allows the prehospital care provider to evaluate the presence, quality, and rate (very fast, very slow, or generally normal) of circulatory activity. The provider can simultaneously feel the temperature and moistness of the skin while noting skin color and capillary refill. The patient's level of consciousness and mentation are determined by the appropriateness of the verbal responses. Then, a rapid scan of the patient from head to foot, looking for signs of hemorrhage while gathering all the preliminary data

for the primary survey, is performed. By doing these things, a quick, overall look at the patient has been accomplished, making the first few seconds with the patient a global survey of overall condition and an evaluation of life-threatening possibilities. The information obtained will help determine priorities, categorize the severity of the patient's injuries and conditions, and identify which injury or condition needs to be managed first. Within 15 to 30 seconds, a general impression of the patient's overall condition has been obtained.

The general impression establishes whether the patient is presently or imminently in a critical condition and rapidly evaluates the patient's overall systemic condition. The global overview and general impression often provide all of the information necessary to determine whether additional resources, such as advanced life support (ALS), are required. If helicopter transportation to a trauma facility is appropriate, this is often when the decision to request the helicopter is made. Delay in deciding that additional resources are necessary will only extend on-scene time. Early decision making will ultimately shorten scene time. Once a general impression of the patient's condition is obtained, the primary survey is performed unless a complication requires more care or evaluation.

The primary survey must proceed rapidly. The following discussion addresses the specific components of the primary survey and the order of priority for optimal patient management.

The following are the five steps involved in the primary survey, in order of priority:

A—Airway management and cervical spine stabilization
B—Breathing (ventilation)
C—Circulation and bleeding
D—Disability
E—Expose/environment

Step A—Airway Management and Cervical Spine Stabilization

Airway

The patient's airway is quickly checked to ensure that it is *patent* (open and clear) and that no danger of obstruction exists. If the airway is compromised, it will have to be opened, initially using manual methods (trauma chin lift or trauma jaw thrust), and cleared of blood, body substances, and foreign bodies, if necessary (Figure 6-3). Eventually, as equipment and time become available, airway management can advance to mechanical means (oral airway, nasal airway, supraglottic airways, or endotracheal intubation) or to transtracheal methods (percutaneous transtracheal ventilation) (see Chapter 7).

Cervical Spine Stabilization

As learned in the initial training program, every trauma patient with a significant mechanism of injury is suspected

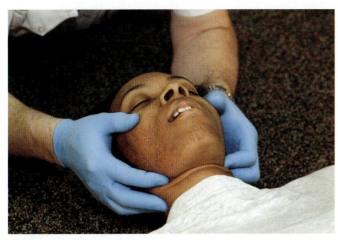

FIGURE 6-3 If the airway appears compromised, it must be opened while continuing to protect the spine.

of spinal injury until spinal injury is conclusively ruled out. (See Chapter 10 for a complete list of indications for spinal immobilization.) Therefore, when establishing an open airway, the possibility of cervical spine injury must always be considered. Excessive movement could either produce or aggravate neurologic damage because bony compression of the spinal cord may occur in the presence of a fractured spine. The solution is to ensure that the patient's neck is manually maintained in the neutral position during the opening of the airway and the administration of necessary ventilation. This does not mean that the necessary airway maintenance procedures just described cannot or should not be applied. Instead, it means that the procedures will be performed while protecting the patient's spine from unnecessary movement. After initiating precautions for cervical injury, the patient's entire spine must be immobilized. Therefore, the patient's entire body must be in-line and secured.

Step B—Breathing (Ventilation)

The first step is to effectively deliver oxygen to a patient's lungs to help maintain the aerobic metabolic process. Hypoxia can result from inadequate ventilation of the lungs and leads to lack of oxygenation of the patient's tissues. Once the patient's airway is open, the quality and quantity of the patient's breathing (ventilation) can be evaluated as follows:

1. Check to see if the patient is breathing.
2. If the patient is not breathing (apneic), immediately begin assisting ventilations with a bag-mask device with supplemental oxygen before continuing the assessment.
3. Ensure that the patient's airway is patent, continue assisted ventilation and prepare to insert an oral, nasal,

Although commonly referred to as the "respiratory rate," a more correct term is *ventilatory rate*. *Ventilation* refers to the process of inhalation and exhalation, whereas *respiration* best describes the physiologic process of gas exchange between the arteries and the alveoli. This text uses the term *ventilatory rate* rather than *respiratory rate*.

or supraglottic airway, intubate, or provide other means of mechanical airway protection.
4. If the patient is breathing, estimate the adequacy of the ventilatory rate and depth to determine whether the patient is moving enough air, and assess oxygenation. Ensure that the inspired oxygen concentration is 85% or greater.
5. Quickly observe the patient's chest rise, and if the patient is conscious, listen to the patient talk to assess whether he or she can speak a full sentence without difficulty.

The ventilatory rate can be divided into the following five levels:

1. *Apneic.* The patient is not breathing.
2. *Slow.* A very slow ventilatory rate may indicate ischemia (decreased supply of oxygen) of the brain. If the ventilatory rate has dropped below 12 breaths/minute (*bradypnea*), it is necessary to either assist or completely take over the patient's breathing with a bag-mask device. Assisted or total ventilatory support with the bag-mask device should include supplemental oxygen that achieves an oxygen concentration of 85% or greater, or a fraction of inspired oxygen (FiO_2) of 0.85 or greater (Figure 6-4).

FIGURE 6-4 **Airway Management Based on Spontaneous Ventilation Rate**

Ventilatory Rate (breaths/minute)	Management
Slow (<12)	Assisted or total ventilation with ≥ 85% oxygen (FiO_2 ≥ 0.85)
Normal (12–20)	Observation; consider supplemental oxygen
Too fast (20–30)	Administration of ≥ 85% oxygen (FiO_2 ≥ 0.85)
Abnormally fast (>30)	Assisted ventilation (FiO_2 ≥ 0.85)

FiO₂, Fraction of inspired oxygen concentration.

3. *Normal.* If the ventilatory rate is between 12 and 20 breaths/minute (*eupnea*, a normal rate for an adult), the prehospital care provider watches the patient closely. Although the patient may appear stable, supplemental oxygen should be considered.

4. *Fast.* If the ventilatory rate is between 20 and 30 breaths/minute *(tachypnea)*, the patient must be watched closely to see whether the patient is improving or deteriorating. The drive for increasing the ventilatory rate is increased accumulation of carbon dioxide (CO_2) in the blood or a decreased level of blood oxygen (O_2). When a patient displays an abnormal ventilatory rate, the reason why must be investigated. A rapid rate indicates that not enough oxygen is reaching the body tissue. This lack of oxygen initiates anaerobic metabolism (see Chapter 7) and, ultimately, an increase in CO_2. The body's detection system recognizes an increased level of CO_2 and tells the ventilatory system to speed up to exhale this excess. Therefore, an increased ventilatory rate may indicate that the patient needs better perfusion or oxygenation, or both. Administration of supplemental oxygen to achieve an oxygen concentration of 85% or greater ($FiO_2 \geq 0.85$) is indicated for this patient, at least until the patient's overall status is determined. Concern must remain about the patient's ability to maintain adequate ventilation and remains alert for any deterioration in overall condition.

5. *Abnormally fast.* A ventilatory rate greater than 30 breaths/minute *(severe tachypnea)* indicates hypoxia, anaerobic metabolism, or both, with a resultant acidosis. Ventilation with supplemental oxygen must be assisted immediately with a BVM device that achieves an inspired oxygen concentration of 85% or greater ($FiO_2 \geq 0.85$). A search for the cause of the rapid ventilatory rate should begin at once to ascertain if the etiology is an oxygenation problem or an RBC delivery problem. Once the cause is identified, the intervention must occur immediately to correct the problem.

In the patient with abnormal ventilation, the chest must be exposed, observed, and palpated rapidly. Then, auscultation of the lungs will identify abnormal, diminished, or absent breath sounds. Injuries that may impede ventilation include tension pneumothorax, spinal cord injuries, and traumatic brain injuries. These injuries should be identified during the primary survey and require that ventilatory support be initiated at once.

When assessing the trauma patient's ventilatory status, the ventilatory *depth* as well as the *rate* is assessed. A patient can be breathing at a normal ventilatory rate of 16 breaths/minute but have a greatly decreased ventilatory depth. Conversely, a patient can have a normal ventilatory depth but an increased or decreased ventilatory rate. The ventilatory depth and rate combine to produce the *total minute ventilation* of the patient (see Chapter 7).

Step C—Circulation (Hemorrhage and Perfusion)

Assessing for circulatory-system compromise or failure is the next step in caring for the trauma patient. Oxygenation of the RBCs without delivery to the tissue cells is of no benefit to the patient. In the primary survey of a trauma patient, external hemorrhage must be identified and controlled. The provider can then obtain an adequate overall estimate of the patient's cardiac output and perfusion status.

Hemorrhage Control

External hemorrhage is identified and controlled in the primary survey. Hemorrhage control is included in the assessment of circulation because if gross bleeding is not controlled as soon as possible, the potential for the patient's death increases dramatically. The three types of external hemorrhage are:

1. *Capillary bleeding* is caused by abrasions that have scraped open the tiny capillaries just below the skin's surface. Usually capillary bleeding will have slowed or even stopped before the arrival of prehospital care.

2. *Venous bleeding* is from deeper areas within the tissue and is usually controlled with a small amount of direct pressure. Venous bleeding is usually not life threatening unless the injury is severe or blood loss is not controlled.

3. *Arterial bleeding* is caused by an injury that has lacerated an artery. This is the most important and most difficult type of blood loss to control. It is characterized by spurting blood that is bright red in color. Even a small, deep, arterial puncture wound can produce life-threatening arterial blood loss.

Hemorrhage control is a priority because every red blood cell counts. Rapid control of blood loss is one of the most important goals in the care of a trauma patient. The primary survey cannot advance unless hemorrhage is controlled.

In cases of external hemorrhage, application of direct pressure will control most major hemorrhage until the prehospital care provider can transport the patient to a hospital in which an operating room (OR) and adequate equipment are available. Hemorrhage control is initiated during the primary survey and maintained throughout transport. The provider may require assistance to accomplish both ventilation and bleeding control.

Hemorrhage can be controlled in the following ways:

1. *Direct pressure.* Direct pressure is exactly what the name implies—applying pressure to the site of bleeding. This is accomplished by placing a dressing (e.g., 4 x 4 inch gauze) or abdominal pads directly over the site and applying pressure. The application and maintenance of direct pressure will require all of one provider's attention, preventing the provider from participating in other aspects of patient care.

However, if assistance is limited, a pressure dressing can be fashioned out of gauze pads and an elastic bandage. If bleeding is not controlled, it will not matter how much oxygen or fluid the patient receives; perfusion will not improve in the face of ongoing hemorrhage.

2. *Tourniquets.* Tourniquets have often been described as the technique of "last resort." Military experience in Afghanistan and Iraq, plus the routine and safe use of tourniquets by surgeons, has led to reconsideration of this approach.[2,3,4] The use of "elevation" and pressure on "pressure points" is no longer recommended because of insufficient data supporting their effectiveness.[5,6] Tourniquets are very effective in controlling severe hemorrhage and should be used if direct pressure or a pressure dressing fails to control hemorrhage from an extremity.

If internal hemorrhage is suspected, the thorax and abdomen are exposed to quickly inspect and palpate for signs of injury. The pelvis is also palpated because a pelvic fracture is a major source of intra-abdominal bleeding. Pelvic fractures are managed with rapid transport, use of a pneumatic antishock garment (PASG) if available and the pelvis is felt to be unstable, and rapid, warm intravenous (IV) fluid replacement.

Many causes of hemorrhage are not easy to control outside the hospital. The prehospital treatment is rapid delivery of the patient to a facility equipped and staffed for rapid control of hemorrhage in the OR (e.g., trauma center, if available).

Perfusion

The patient's overall circulatory status can be determined by checking the pulse; skin color, temperature, and moisture; and capillary refilling time.

Pulse. The pulse is evaluated for presence, quality, and regularity. The presence of a palpable peripheral pulse also provides an estimate of blood pressure. A quick check of the pulse reveals whether the patient has tachycardia, bradycardia, or an irregular rhythm. It can also reveal information about the systolic blood pressure. If a radial pulse is not palpable in an uninjured extremity, the patient has likely entered the *decompensated phase* of shock, a late sign of the patient's critical condition. In the primary survey, determination of an exact pulse rate is not necessary. Instead, a gross estimate is rapidly obtained, and assessment moves on to other gross evaluations. The actual pulse rate is obtained later in the process. If the patient lacks a palpable carotid or femoral pulse, he or she is in cardiopulmonary arrest (see later discussion).

Skin

Color. Adequate perfusion produces a pinkish hue to the skin. Skin becomes pale when blood is shunted away from an area. Pale coloration is associated with poor perfusion. Bluish col-

oration indicates incomplete oxygenation. The bluish color is caused by lack of blood or oxygen to that region of the body. Skin pigmentation can often make this determination difficult. Examination of the color of nail beds and mucous membranes serves to overcome this challenge because these changes in color usually first appear in the lips, gums, or fingertips.

Temperature. As with overall skin evaluation, skin temperature is influenced by environmental conditions. Cool skin indicates decreased perfusion, regardless of the cause. The prehospital care provider usually assesses skin temperature by touching the patient with the back of the hand; therefore, an accurate determination can be difficult with gloves donned. Normal skin temperature is warm to touch, neither cool nor hot. Normally the blood vessels are not dilated and do not bring the heat of the body to the surface of the skin.

Moisture. Dry skin indicates good perfusion. Moist skin is associated with shock and decreased perfusion. This decrease in perfusion is caused by blood being shunted to the core organs of the body as a result of vasoconstriction of peripheral vessels.

Capillary Refilling Time. The capillary refilling time is checked by pressing over the nail beds. This removes the blood from the visible capillary bed. The rate of return of blood to the nail beds (refilling time) is a tool for estimating blood flow through this most distal part of the circulation. A capillary refilling time of greater than 2 seconds indicates that the capillary beds are not receiving adequate perfusion. However, capillary refilling time by itself is a poor indicator of shock because it is influenced by so many other factors. For example, peripheral vascular disease (arteriosclerosis), cold temperatures, the use of pharmacologic vasodilators or constrictors, or the presence of neurogenic shock can skew the result. Refilling becomes a less useful check of cardiovascular function in these cases. Capillary refilling time has a place in the evaluation of circulatory adequacy, but it should always be used in conjunction with other physical examination findings, just as the prehospital care provider uses other indicators (e.g., blood pressure).

Step D—Disability

Having evaluated and corrected, to the extent possible, the factors involved in delivering oxygen to the lungs and circulating it throughout the body, the next step in the primary survey is assessment of cerebral function, which is an indirect measurement of cerebral oxygenation. The goal is to determine the patient's level of consciousness (LOC) and ascertain the potential for hypoxia.

The prehospital care provider can infer that a confused, belligerent, combative, or uncooperative patient is hypoxic until proved otherwise. Most patients want help when their lives are medically threatened. If a patient refuses help, the

Eye Opening	Points
Spontaneous eye opening	4
Eye opening on command	3
Eye opening to painful stimulus	2
No eye opening	1
Best Verbal Response	
Answers appropriately (oriented)	5
Gives confused answers	4
Inappropriate response	3
Makes unintelligible noises	2
Makes no verbal response	1
Best Motor Response	
Follows command	6
Localizes painful stimuli	5
Withdrawal to pain	4
Responds with abnormal flexion to painful stimuli (decorticate)	3
Responds with abnormal extension to pain (decerebrate)	2
Gives no motor response	1
Total	

FIGURE 6-5 Glasgow Coma Scale (GCS).

reason must be questioned. Does the patient feel threatened by the presence of a prehospital care provider on the scene? If so, further attempts to establish rapport will often help to gain the patient's trust. If nothing in the situation seems to be threatening, the source of the behavior should be considered physiologic and reversible conditions identified and treated. During the assessment, the history can help determine whether the patient lost consciousness at any time since the injury occurred, what toxic substances might be involved, and whether the patient has any pre-existing conditions that may produce a decreased LOC or aberrant behavior.

A decreased LOC alerts a prehospital care provider to the following four possibilities:

1. Decreased cerebral oxygenation (caused by hypoxia/hypoperfusion)
2. Central nervous system (CNS) injury
3. Drug or alcohol overdose
4. Metabolic derangement (diabetes, seizure, cardiac arrest)

The Glasgow Coma Scale (GCS) score is a tool used for determining LOC.[7] It is a quick, simple method for determining cerebral function and is predictive of patient outcome, especially the best motor response. It also provides a baseline of cerebral function for serial neurologic evaluations. The GCS score is divided into three sections: (1) *eye* opening, (2) best *verbal* response, and (3) best *motor* response (EVM). The patient is assigned a score according to the *best*

response to each component of the EVM (Figure 6-5). For example, if a patient's right eye is so severely swollen that the patient cannot open it, but the left eye opens spontaneously, the patient receives a "4" for the best eye movement. If a patient lacks spontaneous eye opening, the provider should use a verbal command ("Open your eyes"). If the patient does not respond to a verbal stimulus, a painful stimulus, such as nail bed pressure with a pen or squeezing of the axillary tissue, can be applied.

The patient's verbal response is determined by using a question such as, "What happened to you?" If fully oriented, the patient will supply a coherent answer. Otherwise, the patient's verbal response is scored as confused, inappropriate, unintelligible, or absent. If a patient is intubated, the GCS score contains only the eye and motor scales, and a "T" is added to note the inability to assess the verbal response (e.g., "8T").

The third component of the GCS is the motor score. A simple, unambiguous command, such as "Hold up two fingers," or "Show me a hitchhiker's sign," is given to the patient. If the patient complies with the command, the highest score of "6" is given. A patient who squeezes or grasps the finger of a provider may simply be demonstrating a grasping reflex and not purposefully following a command. If the patient fails to follow a command, a painful stimulus, as noted previously, should be used, and the patient's *best* motor response should be scored. A patient who attempts to push away a painful stimulus is considered to be "localizing." Other possible responses to pain include withdrawal from the stimulus, abnormal flexion (*decorticate posturing*) or extension (*decerebrate posturing*) of the upper extremities, or absence of motor function. Recent evidence suggests that the motor component of the GCS alone is essentially as good in evaluating a patient as the entire score.[8]

The maximum GCS score is 15, indicating a patient with no disability, whereas the lowest score of 3 is generally an ominous sign. A score of less than 8 indicates a major injury, 9 to 12 a moderate injury, and 13 to 15 a minor injury. A GCS score of 8 is an indication for considering active airway management of the patient. The prehospital care provider can easily calculate and relate the individual components of the score and will include them in the verbal report to the receiving facility as well as in the patient care record.

If a patient is not awake, oriented, or able to follow commands, the prehospital care provider can assess the pupils quickly. Are the pupils equal and round, reactive to light (PEARRL)? Are the pupils equal to each other? Is each pupil round and of normal appearance, and does it appropriately react to light by constricting, or is it unresponsive and dilated? A GCS score of less than 14 in combination with an abnormal pupil examination can indicate the presence of a life-threatening traumatic brain injury (see Chapter 9).

The acronym AVPU is often used to describe the patient's LOC. In this system, *A* stands for *alert, V* for responds to *verbal* stimulus, *P* for responds to *painful* stimulus, and *U* for *unre-*

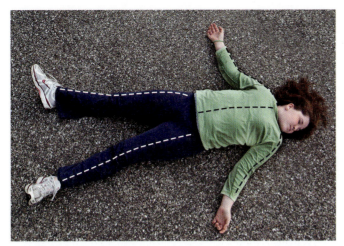

FIGURE 6-6 Clothing can be quickly removed by cutting, as indicated by the dotted lines.

sponsive. This approach, although very simple, fails to provide information as to specifically *how* the patient responds to verbal or painful stimuli. In other words, if the patient responds to verbal questioning, is the patient oriented, confused, or mumbling incomprehensibly? Likewise, when the patient responds to painful stimulus, does the patient localize, withdraw, or demonstrate decorticate or decerebrate posturing? Because of its lack of precision, the use of AVPU has fallen into disfavor. Although the GCS is more complicated to remember than AVPU, repeated practice will make this crucial assessment second nature.

Step E—Expose/Environment

An early step in the assessment process is to remove a patient's clothes because exposure of the trauma patient is critical to finding all injuries (Figure 6-6). The saying, "The one part of the body that is not exposed will be the most severely injured part," may not always be true, but it is true often enough to warrant a total body examination. Also, blood can collect in and be absorbed by clothing and, thereby, go unnoticed. After seeing the patient's entire body, the prehospital care provider can then cover the patient again to conserve body heat. Although it is important to expose a trauma patient's body to complete an effective assessment, *hypothermia* is a serious problem in the management of a trauma patient. Only what is necessary should be exposed to the outside environment. Once the patient has been moved inside the warm emergency medical services (EMS) unit, the complete examination can be accomplished and the patient covered again as quickly as possible.

The amount of the patient's clothing that should be removed during an assessment varies depending on the conditions or injuries found. A general rule is to remove as much clothing as necessary to determine the presence or absence of a condition or injury. The prehospital care provider need not be afraid to remove clothing if it is the only way to com-

plete the assessment and treatment properly. On occasion, patients can sustain multiple mechanisms of injury, such as experiencing a motor vehicle crash after being shot. Potentially life-threatening injuries may be missed if the patient is inadequately examined. Injuries cannot be treated if they are not first identified. Special care should be taken when cutting and removing clothing from a victim of a crime so as not to inadvertently destroy evidence (Figure 6-7).

Resuscitation

Resuscitation describes treatment steps taken to correct life-threatening problems as identified in the primary survey. PHTLS assessment is based on a "treat as you go" philosophy, in which treatment is initiated as each threat to life is identified or at the earliest possible moment (Figure 6-8).

Limited Scene Intervention

Airway problems are managed as the top priority. If the airway is open but the patient is not breathing, ventilatory support is initiated. Ventilatory support includes administration of high concentrations of oxygen ($\geq 85\%$; $FiO_2 \geq 0.85$) as early as possible. If the patient is exhibiting signs of ventilatory distress and lowered levels of air exchange, ventilatory assistance is needed by way of a bag-mask device. Cardiac arrest is identified during the assessment of circulation and chest compressions begun, if appropriate. Exsanguinating hemorrhage is also controlled during this step. In a patient

---

FIGURE 6-8   Simultaneous Evaluation

In discussing the process of patient assessment, management, and decision making, the information must be presented in a sequential format (i.e., step A followed by step B followed by step C, etc.). Although presentation of information in this manner makes explanation easier and perhaps makes the concepts easier for a student to understand, it is not how the real world functions. In reality, these steps are accomplished virtually simultaneously. The prehospital care provider's brain is similar to a computer that can receive input from several sources at once (cerebral multitasking). The brain can assess data received simultaneously and is capable of prioritizing the information from all input sources, sorting it in such a way that orderly decision making follows.

The brain can gather most data in about 15 seconds. Simultaneous processing of these data and appropriate prioritization of the information by the prehospital care provider can identify the component that the provider must manage first. Although the ABCDE approach described in this chapter may not necessarily be the order in which the prehospital care provider collects or receives the information, it does serve to establish priorities for management.

The primary survey addresses life-threatening conditions. The secondary survey of the patient identifies possible limb-threatening injuries as well as other, less significant problems.

FIGURE 6-9   Critical Trauma Patient

Limit scene time to 10 minutes or less when any of the following life-threatening conditions are present:

1. Inadequate or threatened airway
2. Impaired ventilation, as demonstrated by the following:
   - Abnormally fast or slow ventilatory rate
   - Hypoxia ($Spo_2 < 95\%$ even with supplemental oxygen)
   - Dyspnea
   - Open pneumothorax or flail chest
   - Suspected pneumothorax
3. Significant external hemorrhage or suspected internal hemorrhage
4. Abnormal neurologic status
   - GCS score ≤ 13
   - Seizure activity
   - Sensory or motor deficit
5. Penetrating trauma to the head, neck, or torso, or proximal to elbow and knee in the extremities
6. Amputation or near-amputation proximal to the fingers or toes
7. Any trauma in the presence of the following:
   - History of serious medical conditions (e.g., coronary artery disease, chronic obstructive pulmonary disease, bleeding disorder)
   - Age >55 years
   - Hypothermia
   - Burns
   - Pregnancy

---

with adequate airway and breathing, hypoxia and shock (anaerobic metabolism), if present, can be rapidly corrected.

Transport

If life-threatening conditions are identified during the primary survey, the patient should be rapidly "packaged" after initiating limited field intervention. Transport of critically injured trauma patients to the closest appropriate facility should be initiated as soon as possible (Figure 6-9). Unless complicating circumstances exist, scene time should be limited to 10 minutes or less for these patients. Limited scene time and initiation of rapid transport to the closest appropriate facility—preferably a trauma center—are fundamental aspects of prehospital trauma resuscitation.

Fluid Therapy

Another important step in resuscitation is the restoration of the cardiovascular system to an adequate perfusing volume as quickly as possible. Because blood is usually not available

in the prehospital setting, *lactated Ringer's* is the preferred solution for trauma resuscitation. In addition to sodium and chloride, lactated Ringer's solution contains small amounts of potassium, calcium, and lactate and is an effective volume expander. Crystalloid solutions, such as lactated Ringer's, however, do not replace the oxygen-carrying capacity of the lost RBCs or the lost platelets that are necessary for clotting and bleeding control. Therefore, rapid transportation of a severely injured patient to an appropriate facility is an absolute necessity.

En route to the receiving facility, two large-bore (14- or 16-gauge) IV catheters may be placed in the patient's forearm or antecubital veins, if possible. In general, central IV lines (subclavian, internal jugular, or femoral) are not appropriate for the field management of trauma patients. The rate of fluid administration depends on the clinical scenario, primarily whether or not the patient's hemorrhage has been controlled when the IV fluid is initiated, or if the patient has evidence of CNS injury. Chapter 8 provides guidelines for fluid resuscitation.

Starting an IV line at the scene only prolongs on-scene time and delays transport. As addressed previously, the definitive treatment for the trauma patient can only be accomplished in the hospital. For example, a patient with an injury to the spleen who is losing 50 ml of blood per minute will continue to bleed at that rate for each additional minute that delays arrival in the OR. Initiating IV lines on the scene instead of early transportation will not only increase blood loss, but also may decrease the patient's chance of survival. Exceptions exist, such as entrapment, when a patient simply cannot be moved immediately. Also, aggressive and continual volume replacement is not a substitute for manual hemorrhage control whenever possible.

Basic Provider Level

At the basic provider level, the key steps in resuscitating a critically injured trauma patient include (1) immediate control of major external hemorrhage, (2) rapid packaging of the patient for transportation, and (3) quickly initiated, rapid but safe transport of the patient to the closest appropriate facility. If transport time is prolonged, it may be appropriate to call for aid from a nearby ALS service that can intercept the basic unit en route. Helicopter evacuation to a trauma center is another option. Both the ALS service and the flight service will allow advanced airway management, ventilatory management, and earlier fluid replacement.

Secondary Survey (Detailed History and Physical Examination)

The secondary survey is a head-to-toe evaluation of a patient. The secondary survey is performed only after the primary survey is completed, all life-threatening injuries have been identified and treated, and resuscitation initiated (Figure 6-10). The objective of the secondary survey is to identify injuries or problems that were not identified during the primary survey. Because a well-performed primary survey will identify all life-threatening conditions, the secondary survey, by definition, deals with less serious problems. Therefore, a critical trauma patient is transported as soon as possible after conclusion of the primary survey and not held in the field for either IV initiation or a secondary survey.

The secondary survey uses a "look, listen, and feel" approach to evaluate the skin and everything it contains. Rather than looking at the entire body at one time, returning to listen to all areas, and finally returning to palpate all areas, the prehospital care provider "searches" the body. The provider identifies injuries and correlates physical findings region by region, beginning at the head and proceeding through the neck, chest, and abdomen to the extremities, concluding with a detailed neurologic examination. The fol-

lowing phrases capture the essence of the entire assessment process:

See, don't just look.
Hear, don't just listen.
Feel, don't just touch.

The definition of the word *see* is "to perceive with the eye" or "to discover," whereas *look* is defined as "to exercise the power of vision." *Listen* is defined as "to monitor without participation," and *hear* is defined as "to listen with attention." While examining the patient, all available information is used to formulate a patient care plan. The provider not only provides the patient with transport, but also does everything possible to ensure survival of the patient.

See

- Examine all of the skin of each region.
- Be attentive for external hemorrhage or signs of internal hemorrhage, such as distension of the abdomen, marked tenseness of an extremity, or an expanding hematoma.
- Make note of soft tissue injuries, including abrasions, burns, contusions, hematomas, lacerations, and puncture wounds.
- Make note of any masses or swelling or deformation of bones.
- Make note of abnormal indentations on the skin and the skin's color.
- Make note of anything that does not "look right."

Hear

- Make note of any unusual sounds when the patient inhales or exhales.
- Make note of any abnormal sounds when auscultating the chest.
- Verify whether the breath sounds are equal in both lung fields.
- Auscultate over the carotid arteries and other vessels.
- Make note of any unusual sounds (bruits) over the vessels that would indicate vascular damage.

Feel

- Carefully move each bone in the region. Note whether this produces crepitus, pain, or unusual movement.
- Firmly palpate all parts of the region. Note whether anything moves that should not, whether anything feels "squishy," if the patient complains of tenderness, where pulses are felt, whether pulsations are felt that should not be present, and whether all pulses are present.

Vital Signs

The quality of the pulse and ventilatory rates and the other components of the primary survey are continually re-evaluated because significant changes can occur rapidly. Quantitative vital signs are measured and motor and sensory

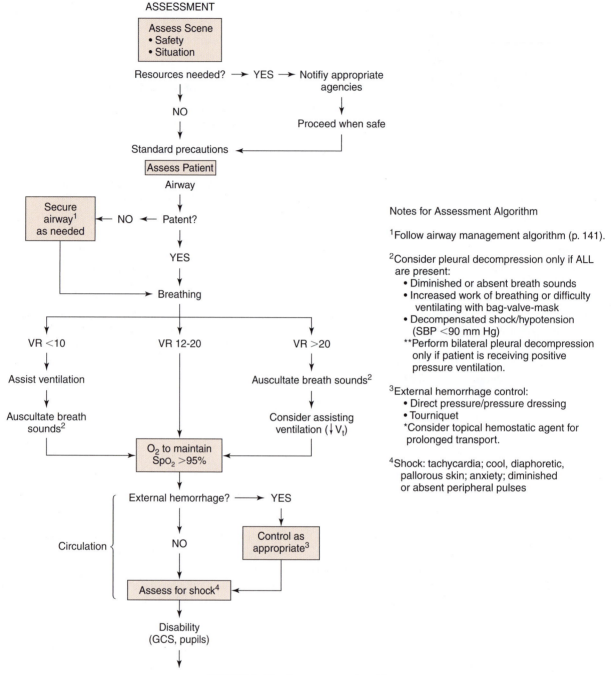

ASSESSMENT

Assess Scene
• Safety
• Situation

Resources needed? → YES → Notifiy appropriate agencies

NO

Proceed when safe

Standard precautions

Assess Patient

Airway

Secure airway[1] as needed ← NO ← Patent?

YES

Breathing

VR <10 | VR 12-20 | VR >20

Assist ventilation

Auscultate breath sounds[2]

Auscultate breath sounds[2]

Consider assisting ventilation ($\downarrow V_t$)

O_2 to maintain SpO_2 >95%

External hemorrhage? → YES

NO

Control as appropriate[3]

Circulation

Assess for shock[4]

Disability (GCS, pupils)

Notes for Assessment Algorithm

[1]Follow airway management algorithm (p. 141).

[2]Consider pleural decompression only if ALL are present:
• Diminished or absent breath sounds
• Increased work of breathing or difficulty ventilating with bag-valve-mask
• Decompensated shock/hypotension (SBP <90 mm Hg)
**Perform bilateral pleural decompression only if patient is receiving positive pressure ventilation.

[3]External hemorrhage control:
• Direct pressure/pressure dressing
• Tourniquet
*Consider topical hemostatic agent for prolonged transport.

[4]Shock: tachycardia; cool, diaphoretic, pallorous skin; anxiety; diminished or absent peripheral pulses

FIGURE 6-10 Assessment algorithm.

status evaluated in all four extremities as soon as possible, although this is normally not accomplished until the conclusion of the primary survey. Depending on the situation, a second provider may obtain vital signs while the first provider completes the primary survey, to avoid further delay. However, exact "numbers" for pulse rate, ventilatory rate, and blood pressure are not critical in the initial management of the patient with severe multisystem trauma. There-

fore, the measurement of the exact numbers can be delayed until completion of the essential steps of resuscitation and stabilization.

A set of complete vital signs includes blood pressure, pulse rate and quality, ventilatory rate (including breath sounds), and skin color and temperature. A complete set of vital signs are evaluated and recorded every 3 to 5 minutes, as often as possible, or at the time of any change in condition

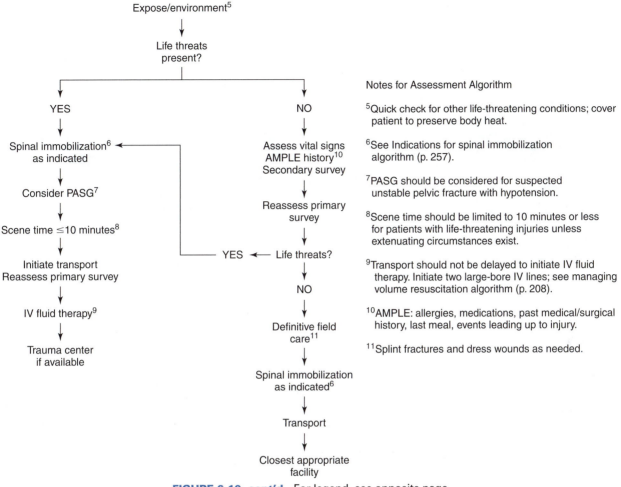

FIGURE 6-10, cont'd   For legend, see opposite page

or a medical problem. Even if an automated, noninvasive blood pressure device is available, the initial blood pressure should be taken manually. Automatic blood pressure devices may be inaccurate when the patient is significantly hypotensive.

SAMPLE History

A quick history is obtained on the patient. This information should be documented on the patient care report and passed on to the medical personnel at the receiving facility. The mnemonic SAMPLE serves as a reminder for the key components:

- *Symptoms:* What does the patient complain of? Pain? Trouble breathing? Numbness? Tingling?
- *Allergies:* Primarily to medications.
- *Medications:* Prescription and nonprescription drugs that the patient takes regularly.
- *Past medical and surgical history:* Significant medical problems for which the patient receives ongoing medical care; includes prior surgeries.

- *Last meal:* Many trauma patients will require surgery, and recent food intake increases the risk of aspiration during induction of anesthesia.
- *Events:* Leading up to the injury.

Head

Visual examination of the head and face will reveal contusions, abrasions, lacerations, bone asymmetry, hemorrhage, bony defects of the face and supportive skull, and abnormalities of the eye, eyelid, external ear, mouth, and mandible. The following are included during a head examination:

- Search thoroughly through the patient's hair for any soft tissue injuries.
- Check pupil size for reactivity to light, equality, accommodation, roundness, and irregular shape.
- Carefully palpate the bones of the face and skull to identify crepitus, deviation, depression, or abnormal mobility. (This is extremely important in the nonradiographic evaluation for head injury.) Figure 6-11 reviews the boney anatomy of the skull.

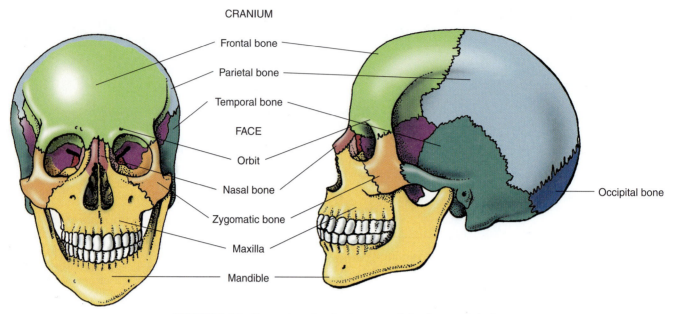

CRANIUM

Frontal bone

Parietal bone

Temporal bone

FACE

Orbit

Nasal bone

Zygomatic bone

Maxilla

Mandible

Occipital bone

FIGURE 6-11 Normal anatomic structure of the face and skull.

Neck

Visual examination of the neck for contusions, abrasions, lacerations, and deformities will alert the prehospital care provider to the possibility of underlying injuries. Palpation may reveal subcutaneous emphysema of a laryngeal, tracheal, or pulmonary origin. Crepitus of the larynx, hoarseness, and subcutaneous emphysema constitute a triad classically indicative of laryngeal fracture. Lack of tenderness of the cervical spine may help rule out cervical spine fractures (when combined with strict criteria), whereas tenderness may frequently indicate the presence of a fracture, dislocation, or ligamentous injury. Such palpation is performed carefully, ensuring that the cervical spine remains in a neutral, in-line position.

Figure 6-12 reviews the normal anatomic structure of the neck.

Chest

Because the thorax is strong, resilient, and elastic, it can absorb a significant amount of trauma. Close visual examination of the chest for deformities, areas of paradoxical movement, contusions, and abrasions is necessary to identify underlying injuries. Other signs for which the prehospital care provider should watch closely include splinting and guarding, unequal bilateral chest excursion, and intercostal, suprasternal, or supraclavicular bulging or retraction.

For example, a contusion over the sternum may be the only indication of a cardiac injury. A stab wound near the sternum may indicate cardiac tamponade. A line traced from the fourth intercostal space anteriorly to the sixth intercostal space laterally and to the eighth intercostal space posteriorly

defines the upward excursion of the diaphragm at full expiration (Figure 6-13). A penetrating injury that occurs below this line or with a path that may have taken it below this line should be considered to have traversed both the thoracic and abdominal cavities.

Except for the eyes and hands, the stethoscope is the most important instrument a prehospital care provider can use for chest examination. A patient will most often be in a supine position so that only the anterior and lateral chest is available for auscultation. It is important to recognize normal and decreased breath sounds with a patient in this position. A small area of rib fractures may indicate a severe underlying pulmonary contusion. Any type of compression injury to the chest can result in a pneumothorax (Figure 6-14). Diminished or absent breath sounds indicate a possible pneumothorax, tension pneumothorax, or hemothorax. Crackles heard posteriorly (when the patient is logrolled) or laterally may indicate pulmonary contusion. Cardiac tamponade is characterized by distant heart sounds; however, these may be difficult to ascertain given the commotion at the scene or road noise during transport. The thorax is palpated for the presence of subcutaneous emphysema.

Abdomen

The abdominal examination begins, as with the other parts of the body, by visual evaluation. Abrasions and ecchymosis indicate the possibility of underlying injury. The abdomen should be examined carefully, near the umbilicus, for a telltale transverse contusion, which suggests that an incorrectly worn seat belt has caused underlying injury. Almost 50% of patients with

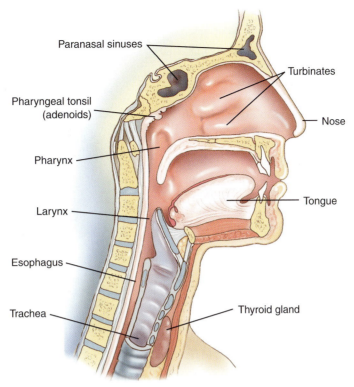

FIGURE 6-12 Normal anatomy of the neck.

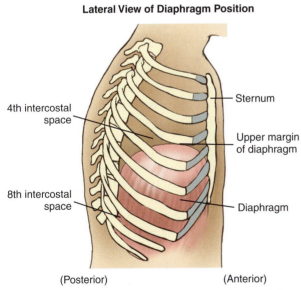

FIGURE 6-13 Lateral view of diaphragm position at full expiration.

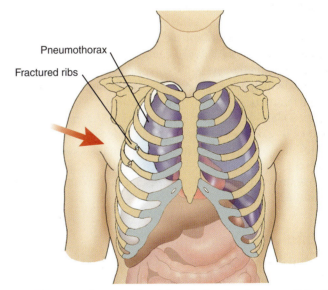

FIGURE 6-14 Compression injury to the chest can result in rib fracture and subsequent pneumothorax.

this sign will have an intestinal injury. Lumbar spine fractures may also be associated with the "seat belt sign."

Examination of the abdomen also includes palpation of each quadrant to evaluate tenderness, abdominal muscle guarding, and masses. When palpating, the prehospital care provider notes whether the abdomen is soft and whether rigidity or guarding is present. There is no need to continue palpating after discovering abdominal tenderness or pain. Additional information will not alter prehospital management, and the only outcomes of a continued abdominal examination are further discomfort to the patient and delayed transportation to the receiving facility. Similarly, auscultation of the abdomen adds virtually nothing to the assessment of a trauma patient.

Pelvis

The pelvis is evaluated by observation and palpation. The pelvis is first visually examined for abrasions, contusions, lacerations, open fractures, and signs of distension. Pelvic fractures can produce massive internal hemorrhage, resulting in rapid deterioration of a patient's condition.

The pelvis is palpated only once for instability as part of the secondary survey. Because palpation can aggravate hemorrhage, this examination step should only be performed once and not repeated. Palpation is accomplished by first gently applying anterior-to-posterior pressure with the heels of the hands on the symphysis pubis and then medial pressure to the iliac crests bilaterally, evaluating for pain and abnormal movement. Any evidence of instability raises the likelihood of internal hemorrhage.

Back

The back of the torso should be examined for evidence of injury. This is best accomplished when logrolling the patient for placement onto the long backboard. Breath sounds can be auscultated over the posterior thorax, and the spine should be palpated for tenderness and deformity.

Extremities

The examination of the extremities begins at the clavicle in the upper extremity and the pelvis in the lower extremity and then proceeds toward the most distal portion of each extremity. Each individual bone and joint is evaluated by visual examination for deformity, hematoma, or ecchymosis and by palpation to determine the presence of crepitus, pain, tenderness, or unusual movements. Any suspected fracture should be immobilized until radiographic confirmation of its presence or absence is possible. Circulation and motor and sensory nerve function at the distal end of each extremity are also checked. If an extremity is immobilized, pulses, movement, and sensation should be rechecked after splinting.

Neurologic Examination

As with the other regional examinations described, the neurologic examination in the secondary survey is conducted in much greater detail than in the primary survey. Calculation of the GCS score, evaluation of motor and sensory function, and observation of pupillary response are all included. When examining a patient's pupils, equality of response in addition to equality of size are evaluated. A small but significant portion of the population has pupils of differing sizes as a normal condition *(anisocoria)*. Even in these patients, however, the pupils should react to light in a similar manner. Pupils that react at differing speeds to the introduction of light are considered to be unequal. Unequal pupils in an unconscious trauma patient may indicate increased intracra-

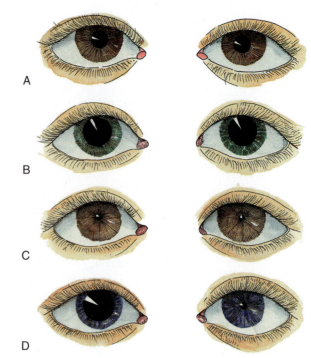

FIGURE 6-15   **A.** Normal pupils. **B.** Pupil dilation. **C.** Pupil constriction. **D.** Unequal pupils.

nial pressure or pressure on the third cranial nerve, caused by either cerebral edema or a rapidly expanding intracranial hematoma (Figure 6-15). Direct eye injury can also cause unequal pupils.

A gross examination of sensory capability and response will determine the presence or absence of weakness or loss of sensation in the extremities and will identify areas that require further examination. The entire length of the spine, and thus the entire patient, need to be immobilized. Use of a long backboard, cervical collar, head pads, and straps is required. Immobilizing only the head and neck is inadequate to accomplish the necessary stabilization. If the body is not immobilized, a shift in the patient's body resulting from lifting or ambulance movement will cause the body to move but not the head which has been restrained, potentially causing further injury to the spinal cord. Protection of the entire spinal cord is required at all times.

Definitive Care in the Field

Included in assessment and management are the skills of packaging, transportation, and communication. Definitive care is the end phase of patient care. The following are examples of definitive care:

- For a patient with cardiac arrest, definitive care is defibrillation with resultant normal rhythm; cardiopulmonary resuscitation (CPR) is just a holding pattern until defibrillation can be accomplished.

- For a patient in a diabetic hypoglycemic coma, definitive care is IV glucose and a return to normal blood glucose levels.
- For a patient with an obstructed airway, definitive care is relief of the obstruction, which may be accomplished by the jaw thrust and assisted ventilation.
- For the patient with severe bleeding, definitive care is hemorrhage control and resuscitation from shock.

In general, definitive care for many of the injuries sustained by the trauma patient can only be provided in the OR. Anything that delays the administration of that definitive care will lessen the patient's chance for survival. The care given to the trauma patient in the field is similar to CPR for the cardiac arrest patient. It keeps the patient alive until something definitive can be done. For the trauma patient, the care given in the field is frequently only temporizing—buying the additional minutes needed to reach the OR.

Packaging

As discussed previously, spinal injury must be suspected in all trauma patients. Therefore, when indicated, stabilization of the spine should be an integral component of packaging the trauma patient. If time is available, the following are accomplished:

- Careful stabilization of extremity fractures using specific splints.

- If the patient is in critical condition, immobilization of all fractures as the patient is stabilized on a long backboard ("trauma" board).
- Bandaging of wounds as necessary and appropriate.

Transport

Transportation should begin as soon as the patient is loaded and stabilized. As discussed previously, delay at the scene to start an IV line or to complete the secondary survey only extends the period before the receiving facility can administer blood and control hemorrhage. Continued evaluation and further resuscitation occur en route to the receiving facility. *For some critically injured trauma patients, initiation of transport is the single most important aspect of definitive care in the field.*

A patient whose condition is not critical can receive attention for individual injuries before transportation, but even this patient should be transported rapidly before a hidden condition becomes critical.

Revised Trauma Score

The Trauma Score (TS), originally developed by surgeon Howard Champion and colleagues, is a good predictor of survival of blunt trauma patients. The Revised Trauma Score (RTS), published in 1989, eliminated two components of the older TS and is equally useful in predicting survival after serious injury.[9] The RTS is composed of scores for the GCS, systolic blood pressure, and ventilatory rate (Figure 6-16). Each of these three components is assigned a value from 4 (best) to 0 (worst). The combined score indicates the patient's condition.

		Score	Start of Transport	End of Transport
A. Ventilatory rate	10-29/min	4		
	>29/min	3		
	6-9/min	2		
	1-5/min	1		
	0	0		
B. Systolic blood pressure	>89 mm Hg	4		
	76-89 mm Hg	3		
	50-75 mm Hg	2		
	1-49 mm Hg	1		
	No pulse	0		
C. Glasgow coma scale score	13-15 =	4		
	9-12 =	3		
	6-8 =	2		
	4-5 =	1		
	3 =	0		
Trauma score total = A + B + C				

FIGURE 6-16 Revised Trauma Score (RTS). A trauma score can be numerically calculated en route to the hospital. Such information is extremely helpful in preparing to manage a patient.
(Modified from Champion HR, Sacco WJ, Copes WS, et al: A revision of the trauma score. *J Trauma* 29(5):624, 1989.)

The lowest possible combined score, 0, is obviously the most critical; the highest, 12, is the least critical. The combined score is valuable to analyze the care given to a patient, but it is not necessarily a prehospital triage tool. In many prehospital systems, the score is calculated and recorded at the receiving facility based on information provided in the radio report, but prehospital care providers are neither required nor expected to compute it before arrival.

Field Triage Scheme

The Triage Decision Scheme, originally published by the American College of Surgeons (ACS) Committee on Trauma, is more useful than the RTS in making prehospital patient triage decisions (Figure 6-17).[10] In some systems, the Triage Decision Scheme is used in the process of determining the most appropriate receiving facility for a trauma patient. As with any schematic tool, however, it should be used as a guideline and not as a replacement for good judgment. The Triage Decision Scheme divides triage into three prioritized steps that will assist in the decision as to when it is best to transport a patient to a trauma center, if available: (1) physiologic criteria, (2) anatomic criteria, and (3) mechanism of injury (kinematics). Following this scheme results in *overtriage* (not all patients taken to the trauma center will actually need a trauma center level of care), but this outcome is better than *undertriage* (patients needing a trauma center level of care are taken to nontrauma centers). Medical directors or local medical control boards should establish local protocols to familiarize prehospital field personnel with trauma centers. The field triage decision scheme on page 127 was revised by an expert panel representing emergency medical services, emergency medicine, trauma surgery, and public health.[11] The panel was convened by the Centers for Disease Control and Prevention (CDC) with support from the National Highway Traffic Safety Administration (NHTSA). Its contents are the recommendations of the expert panel and do not necessarily represent the official views of CDC and NHTSA.

Duration of Transport

The prehospital care provider should choose a receiving facility according to the severity of the patient's injury. In simple terms, the patient should be transported to the closest appropriate facility (i.e., the closest facility most capable of managing the patient's problems). If the patient's injuries are severe or indicate the possibility of continuing hemorrhage, the provider can take the patient to a facility that will provide definitive care as quickly as possible (i.e., a trauma center, if available).

For example, if an ambulance responds to a call in 8 minutes and the prehospital team spends 6 minutes on the scene to package and load the patient into the transporting unit, 14 minutes of the Golden Period have passed.

The closest hospital is 5 minutes away, and the trauma center is 14 minutes away. On arrival at the trauma center, the surgeon is in the emergency department (ED) with the emergency physician and the entire trauma team. The OR is staffed and ready. After 10 minutes in the ED for resuscitation, necessary radiographs, and blood work, the patient is taken to the OR. The total time since the incident is now 38 minutes. In comparison, the closest hospital has an available emergency physician, but the surgeon and OR team are out of the hospital. The patient's 10 minutes in the ED for resuscitation could stretch to 45 minutes by the time the surgeon arrives and examines the patient. Another 30 minutes could elapse while waiting for the OR team to arrive once the surgeon has examined the patient and decided to operate. The total time is 94 minutes, or 2½ times longer than the first scenario. The 9 minutes saved by the shorter ambulance ride actually cost 57 minutes, during which time operative management could have been started and hemorrhage control achieved.

In a rural community, the transport time to an awaiting trauma team may be 45 to 60 minutes or even longer. In this situation, the closest hospital with an on-call trauma team is the appropriate receiving facility.

Method of Transport

Another aspect of the transportation decision is the transportation method. Some systems offer an alternative option of air transportation. Air medical services may offer a higher level of care than ground units. Air transportation may also be quicker and smoother than ground transportation in some circumstances. As previously mentioned, if air transportation is available in a community and is appropriate for the specific situation, the earlier in the assessment process that the decision is made to call for air transport, the greater the likely benefit to the patient.

Monitoring and Reassessment (Ongoing Assessment)

After the primary survey and initial care are complete, the patient must continuously be monitored, the vital signs reassessed, and the primary survey repeated several times while en route to the receiving facility or at the scene if transport is delayed. Continuous reassessment of the components of the primary survey will help ensure that unrecognized compromise of vital functions does not occur. Particular attention must be paid to any significant change in a patient's condition and management re-evaluated if the patient's condition changes. Furthermore, the continued monitoring of a patient

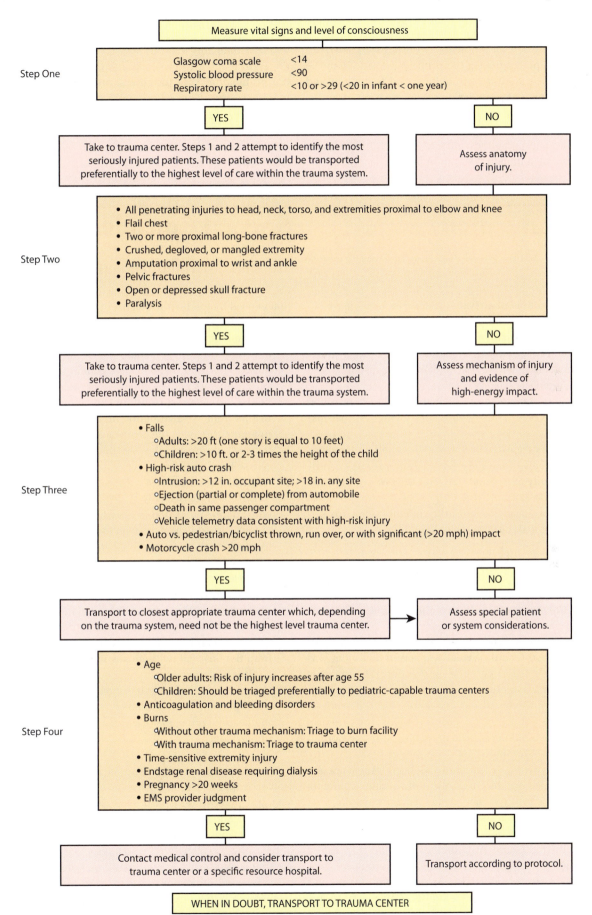

FIGURE 6-17   Deciding where to transport a patient is critical, with consideration of the type and location of available facilities. Situations that will most likely require an in-house trauma team are detailed in the Triage Decision Scheme.

helps reveal conditions or problems that may have been overlooked or not apparent during the primary survey. Often the patient's condition will be not obvious, and looking at and listening to the patient provides much information. How the information is gathered is not as important as ensuring that *all* the information is gathered. Reassessment should be conducted as quickly and thoroughly as possible. Monitoring during a prolonged transport situation is described later.

Communication

Communication with medical direction and the receiving facility should be undertaken as soon as possible. The information transmitted about a patient's condition, management, and the expected time of arrival will give the receiving facility time to prepare for the patient. Transmission of information about the mechanism of injury, the characteristics of the scene, the number of patients, and other pertinent facts allows the receiving facility staff to best coordinate its resources and meet each patient's needs.

Equally important is the written *prehospital care report* (PCR). A good PCR is valuable for the following two reasons:

1. It gives the receiving facility staff a thorough understanding of the events that occurred and of the patient's condition should any questions arise after the prehospital care providers have left.
2. It helps ensure quality control throughout the prehospital system by making case review possible.

For these reasons, it is important that the prehospital care provider fill out the PCR accurately and completely and provide it to the receiving facility. The report should stay with the patient; the report is of little use if it does not arrive until hours or days after the patient arrives.

The PCR often becomes a part of the patient's medical record. It is a legal record of what was found and what was done and can be used as part of a legal action. The report is considered to be a complete record of the injuries found and the actions taken. A good adage to remember is, "If it is not on the report, it was not done." All that the prehospital care provider knows, sees, and does to the patient should be recorded in the report. Another important reason for providing a copy of the PCR to the receiving facility is that most trauma centers maintain a "trauma registry," a database of all trauma patients admitted to their facility. The prehospital information is an important aspect of this database and may aid in valuable research.

The prehospital care provider also verbally transfers responsibility for a patient ("sign off," "report off," or "transfer over") to the physician or nurse who takes over the patient's care at the receiving facility. This verbal report is typically more detailed than the radio report and less detailed than the written record, providing an overview of the significant history of the incident, the action taken by the prehospital care providers, and the patient's response to this action. The report must highlight any significant changes in the patient's condition that have taken place since transmitting the radio report. Transfer of important prehospital information further emphasizes the team concept of patient care.

Special Considerations

Traumatic Cardiopulmonary Arrest

Cardiopulmonary arrest resulting from trauma differs from that caused by medical problems in three significant ways:

1. Most medical cardiac arrests are the result of either a respiratory problem, such as a foreign body airway obstruction, or a cardiac dysrhythmia that prehospital care providers may be able to treat definitively in the field. Cardiac arrest resulting from injury most often results from exsanguination or, less often, a problem incompatible with life, such as a devastating brain or spinal cord injury, and the patient cannot be appropriately resuscitated in the field.
2. Medical arrests are best managed with attempts at stabilization at the scene (e.g., removal of airway foreign body, defibrillation). In contrast, traumatic cardiopulmonary arrest is best managed with immediate transport to a facility that offers immediate blood and emergent surgery.
3. Because of the differences in etiology and management, patients with traumatic cardiopulmonary arrest in the prehospital setting have an extremely low likelihood of survival. Less than 4% of trauma patients who require CPR in the prehospital setting survive to be discharged from the hospital, with most studies documenting that victims of penetrating trauma have a slightly increased chance of survival over those of blunt trauma. Of the small percentage of patients who are discharged from the hospital alive, many sustain significant neurologic impairment.

In addition to the extremely low survival rate, resuscitation attempts in patients who are extremely unlikely to survive put prehospital care providers at risk from exposure to blood and body fluids as well as injuries sustained in motor vehicle crashes during transport. Such unsuccessful attempts at resuscitation may divert resources away from patients who are viable and have a greater likelihood of survival. For these reasons, good judgment needs to be exercised regarding the decision to initiate resuscitation attempts for victims of traumatic cardiopulmonary arrest.

The National Association of EMS Physicians collaborated with the ACS Committee on Trauma to develop guidelines for withholding or terminating CPR in the prehospital setting. Victims of drowning, lightning strike, or hypothermia and patients in whom the mechanism of injury does not correlate with the clinical situation (suggesting a nontraumatic cause) deserve special consideration before a decision is made to withhold or terminate resuscitation. A patient found in cardiopulmonary arrest at the scene of a traumatic event may have experienced the arrest because of a medical problem (e.g., myocardial infarction), especially if the patient is elderly and evidence of injury is minimal.

Withholding Cardiopulmonary Resuscitation

If, during the primary survey, patients are found to meet the following criteria, CPR may be withheld and the patient declared dead:

- For victims of blunt trauma, resuscitation efforts may be withheld if the patient is pulseless and apneic on arrival of prehospital care providers.
- For victims of penetrating trauma, resuscitation efforts may be withheld if there are no signs of life (no pupillary reflexes, no spontaneous movement, no organized cardiac rhythm on ECG >40 beats/minute).
- Resuscitation efforts are not indicated when the patient has sustained an obviously fatal injury (e.g., decapitation) or when evidence exists of dependent lividity, rigor mortis, and decomposition.[12]

Basic Life Support

Guidelines for managing cardiopulmonary arrest have recently been revised and published by the American Heart Association.[13] After opening the airway with a jaw thrust, ventilatory effort is assessed. If the patient is apneic, the prehospital care provider delivers two rescue breaths. These breaths are delivered slowly to prevent gastric inflation. Any obvious, exsanguinating hemorrhage should be controlled. The carotid pulse is then assessed for up to 10 seconds. If no pulse is present, chest compressions are initiated. Cycles of compressions and ventilations are given, with a brief pause in compressions to deliver the two breaths. Once an advanced airway is in place, compressions are delivered at 100 per minute without pausing for ventilations; ventilations are administered at a rate of 8 to 10 per minute. The individual delivering chest compressions is changed every 2 minutes to prevent fatigue. If an automatic external defibrillator (AED) is available, the patient's cardiac rhythm is assessed and defibrillation performed if ventricular fibrillation is present.

Advanced Life Support

The airway is secured while simultaneously ensuring in-line stabilization of the cervical spine. Breath sounds should be auscultated and the possible presence of a tension pneumothorax ruled out. A tension pneumothorax may be present when a decrease in breath sounds is noted, with inadequate chest excursion during ventilation. If any doubt exists that the patient may have a tension pneumothorax, chest decompression is performed. Bilateral chest decompression should be performed only if the patient is receiving positive pressure ventilation.

Large-bore venous access is obtained, and isotonic crystalloid solution is delivered through a wide-open line if hypovolemic shock is a possible cause of the cardiac arrest. Electrocardiogram (ECG) monitoring is performed and cardiac rhythm assessed. The following dysrhythmias may be noted:

- *Pulseless electrical activity* (PEA). A patient found in PEA should be assessed for the presence of hypovolemia, hypothermia, tension pneumothorax, and cardiac tamponade. Fluids, warming, and chest decompression should be performed if indicated. Epinephrine and atropine may be administered.
- *Bradyasystole.* A patient found in this rhythm should be assessed for severe hypoxia and hypovolemia. The location of the airway should be confirmed and volume resuscitation initiated. Epinephrine and atropine may be administered.
- *Ventricular fibrillation/pulseless ventricular tachycardia.* The primary therapy for these dysrhythmias is defibrillation. If the available defibrillator is biphasic, a shock of 120 to 200 joules is delivered. If a monophasic defibrillator is present, a shock of 360 joules is used. Epinephrine, antidysrhythmics (amiodarone or lidocaine), and magnesium may be used in the management of this rhythm.

Terminating Cardiopulmonary Resuscitation

Termination of CPR and ALS measures may be considered in the prehospital setting in the following circumstances: 1) trauma patients with an EMS-witnessed cardiopulmonary arrest and 15 minutes of unsuccessful resuscitation and CPR; and 2) patients with traumatic cardiopulmonary arrest who would require transport longer than 15 minutes to reach an ED or trauma center.[12]

Pain Management

Pain management *(analgesia)* is often used in the prehospital setting for pain caused by angina or myocardial infarction. Traditionally, pain management has had a limited role in the management of trauma patients, primarily because of the concern that side effects (decreased ventilatory drive and vasodilatation) of narcotics may aggravate pre-existing hypoxia and hypotension. This concern has resulted in pain relief being denied to some patients with appropriate indications, such as an isolated limb injury or spinal fracture. The prehospital care provider may consider pain management in such patients, particularly if prolonged transport occurs, provided that signs of ventilatory impairment or shock are not present.

Chapter 13 devotes a section to pain management as it relates to isolated extremity injuries and fractures. Morphine sulfate is typically the agent of choice and should be titrated intravenously in 1 mg to 2 mg increments until some degree of pain relief is obtained or a change in the patient's vital signs occurs. Pulse oximetry and serial vital signs must be monitored if any narcotics are administered to a trauma patient. Sedation with an agent such as a benzodiazepine should be reserved for exceptional circumstances, such as a combative intubated patient, because the combination of a narcotic and benzodiazepine may result in respiratory arrest. Prehospital personnel can collaborate with their medical control to develop appropriate protocols.

Abuse

A prehospital care provider is often the first person on the scene, allowing the provider to observe a potentially abusive situation. The provider inside a house can observe and relay the details at the scene to the receiving facility so that the appropriate social services in the area can be alerted. The prehospital care provider is usually the first, and sometimes the only, medically trained person to be in a position to observe, suspect, and relay information about this silent danger.

Anyone at any age can be a potential abuser or victim of abuse. A pregnant woman, infant, toddler, child, adolescent, young adult, middle-age adult, and older adult are all at risk for abuse. Several different types of abuse exist, including physical, psychological (emotional), and financial. Abuse may occur by *commission,* in which a purposeful act results in an injury (physical abuse or sexual abuse), or by *omission* (e.g., neglectful care of a dependent). This section does not discuss types of abuse and only introduces the general characteristics and heightens a prehospital care provider's awareness and suspicion of abuse.

General characteristics of a potential abuser include dishonesty, the "story" not correlating with the injuries, a negative attitude, and abrasiveness with prehospital personnel. General characteristics of the abused patient include quietness, not wanting to elaborate on details of the incident, constant eye contact or lack of eye contact with someone at the scene, and minimization of personal injuries. Abuse, abusers, and the abused can take many different forms, and prehospital care providers need to keep suspicion high if the scene and the story do not correlate. The provider is required to relay suspicions and any information to the proper authorities.

Prolonged Transport

Although most urban or suburban EMS transports take 30 minutes or less, many prehospital care providers in rural and frontier settings routinely manage patients for much lon-

ger periods of time during transport. Additionally, providers are called on to manage patients during transfer from one medical facility to another, either by ground or air. These transfers may take up to several hours.

Special preparations need to be taken when prehospital care providers are involved in the prolonged transport of a trauma patient. The issues that must be considered before undertaking such a transport can be divided into those dealing with the patient, the prehospital crew, and equipment.

Patient Issues

Of preeminent importance is providing a safe, warm, and secure environment in which the patient is transported. The gurney should be appropriately secured to the ambulance, and the patient secured to the gurney. As emphasized throughout this text, hypothermia is a potentially deadly complication in a trauma patient, and the patient compartment must be sufficiently warm. The patient should be secured in a position that allows maximum access to the patient, especially the injured areas. Before transport, the security of any airway devices placed must be assured, and adjuncts (e.g., monitors, oxygen tanks) should be secured so that they do not become projectiles in the event that the ambulance has to swerve in an evasive action or is involved in a motor vehicle crash. Adjuncts should not rest on the patient because pressure ulcers might be created during a prolonged transport. During transport, all IV lines and catheters must be securely fastened to prevent loss of the access.

The patient should receive serial assessments of the primary survey and vital signs at routine intervals. Pulse oximetry and ECG are monitored continuously for virtually all patients, as well as end tidal CO_2, if available, in an intubated patient. The prehospital care providers accompanying the patient should be trained at a level appropriate to the anticipated needs of the patient. Critically injured patients should generally be managed by providers with advanced training. If the patient is anticipated to require blood transfusion during transport, an individual should be in attendance whose scope of practice allows this procedure; in the United States, this generally requires a registered nurse.

Two management plans should be devised. The first, a medical plan, is developed to manage either anticipated or unexpected problems with the patient during transport. Necessary equipment, medications, and supplies should be readily available. The second plan involves identifying the most expeditious route to the receiving hospital. Weather conditions, road conditions (e.g., construction), and traffic concerns should be identified and anticipated. Additionally, the providers should be knowledgeable about the medical facilities along the transport route in case a problem arises that cannot be managed en route to the primary destination.

Crew

The safety of the EMS crew is as important as that of the patient. The prehospital crew needs to have appropriate safety devices, such as seat belts, and they should be secured during transport unless an issue involving patient care prevents this. The crew members use Standard Precautions and ensure that sufficient gloves and other personal protective equipment (PPE) are available for the trip.

Equipment

Equipment issues during prolonged transport involve the ambulance, supplies and medications, monitors, and communications. The ambulance must be in good working order, including an adequate amount of fuel and a spare tire. The crew must make sure that sufficient supplies and medications are available and accessible for the transport, including gauze and pads for reinforcing dressings, IV fluids, oxygen, and pain medications. Drug supplies are based on anticipated patient needs and include sedatives, paralytic agents, analgesics and antibiotics. A good rule of thumb is to provision the ambulance with about 50% more supplies and medications than the anticipated need in case a significant delay is encountered. Patient care equipment must be in good working order, including monitors (with functioning alarms), oxygen regulators, and suction devices. Also, success of a prolonged transport may depend on functional communications, including the ability to communicate with other crew members, medical control, and the destination facility.

The management of specific injuries during prolonged transport is discussed in the subsequent corresponding chapters of this text.

SUMMARY

- Chances of survival for a patient with traumatic injuries depend on the immediate identification and mitigation of conditions that interfere with tissue perfusion.
- The identification of these conditions requires a systematic, prioritized, logical process of collecting information and acting on it. This process is referred to as *patient assessment*.
- Patient assessment begins with scene assessment and includes the formation of a general impression of the patient, a primary survey, and when the patient's condition and availability of additional EMS personnel permit, a secondary survey.
- The information obtained through this process is analyzed and used as the basis for patient care and transport decisions.
- In the care of the trauma patient, a missed problem is a missed opportunity to aid potentially in an individual's survival.
- After the simultaneous determination of scene safety and general impression of the situation, the focus is on the priorities of patient assessment—on the patency of the patient's airway, the ventilatory status, and the circulatory status. This primary survey follows the ABCDE format for evaluation of the patient's airway, breathing, circulation, disability (initial neurologic examination), and exposure (removing the patient's clothing to discover additional significant injuries). Although the sequential nature of language limits the ability to describe the simultaneity of these actions, the primary survey of the patient is a process of actions that occur essentially at the same time.
- Immediate threats to the patient's life are quickly corrected in a "find and fix" manner. Once the provider manages the patient's airway and breathing and controls exsanguinating hemorrhage, he or she packages the patient and begins transportation without additional treatment at the scene. The limitations of field management of trauma require the safe, expedient delivery of the patient to definitive care.

SCENARIO SOLUTION

You have been on the scene for 1 minute, yet you have obtained much important information to guide further assessment and treatment of the patient. In the first 15 seconds of patient contact, you have developed a general impression of the patient, determining that resuscitation is not necessary. With a few simple actions you have evaluated the A, B, C, and D of the initial assessment. The patient spoke to you without difficulty, indicating that his airway is open and he is breathing with no signs of distress. At the same time, with an awareness of the mechanism of injury, you have stabilized the cervical spine. You have noted no obvious bleeding, your partner has assessed the radial pulse, and you have observed the patient's skin color, temperature, and moisture. These findings indicate no immediate threats to the patient's circulatory status. Additionally, you have simultaneously found no initial evidence of disability because the patient is awake, alert, and answers questions appropriately. This information, along with information about the fall, will help you determine the need for additional resources, the type of transportation indicated, and to what type of facility you should deliver the patient.

Now that you have completed these steps and no immediate lifesaving intervention is necessary, you will proceed with step E of the primary survey early in the evaluation process and then obtain vital signs. You will expose the patient to look for additional injuries and bleeding that may have been concealed by clothing, then cover the patient to protect him from the environment. During this process, you will perform a more detailed examination, noting less serious injuries. The next steps you will take are packaging the patient, including splinting the entire spine and extremity injuries and bandaging wounds if time allows; initiating transportation; and communicating with medical direction and the receiving facility. During the trip to the hospital, you will continue to re-evaluate and monitor the patient. Your knowledge of kinematics and the patient's witnessed loss of consciousness will generate a high index of suspicion for traumatic brain injury, lower extremity injuries, and injuries to the spine. In an advanced life support (ALS) system, intravenous (IV) access will be established en route to the receiving facility.

References

1. Advanced Trauma Life Support (ATLS) Subcommittee, Committee on Trauma: Initial assessment and management. In *Advanced Trauma Life Support Course for Doctors, Student Course Manual,* ed 7, Chicago, 2004, ACS.

2. Kragh JF, Littrel ML, Jones JA, et al: Battle casualty survival with emergency tourniquet use to stop limb bleeding. *J Emerg Med* 2009, epub (in press).

3. Beekley AC, Sebesta JA, Blackbourne LH, et al: Pehospital tourniquet use in Operation Iraqi Freedom: Effect on hemorrhage control and outcomes. *J Trauma* 64:S28-S37, 2008.

4. Doyle GS, Taillac PP: Tourniquets: A review of current use with proposals for expanded prehospital use. *Prehosp Emerg Care* 12:241–256, 2008.

5. First Aid Science Advisory Board: First aid. *Circulation* 112(III):115, 2005.

6. Swan KG Jr, Wright DS, Barbagiovanni SS, et al: Tourniquets revisited. *J Trauma* 66:672–675, 2009.

7. Teasdale G, Jennett B: Assessment of coma and impaired consciousness: A practical scale. *Lancet* 2:81, 1974.

8. Healey C, Osler TM, Rogers FB, et al: Improving the Glasgow Coma Scale score: Motor score alone is a better predictor. *J Trauma* 54:671, 2003.

9. Champion HR, Sacco WJ, Copes WS, et al: A revision of the Trauma Score. *J Trauma* 29(5):623, 1989.

10. Committee on Trauma: *Resources for optimal care of the injured patient: 1999,* Chicago, 1998, American College of Surgeons.

11. Centers for Disease Control and Prevention: Guidelines for field triage of injured patients: Recommendations of the national expert panel on field triage. MMWR 58: 1–35, 2009.

12. Hopson LR, Hirsh E, Delgado J, et al: Guidelines for withholding or termination of resuscitation in prehospital traumatic cardio-pulmonary arrest. *Prehosp Emerg Care* 7:141, 2003.

13. American Heart Association: 2005 guidelines for cardio-pulmonary resuscitation and emergency cardiovascular care. *Circulation* 112(IV):1, 2005.

Suggested Reading

American Heart Association: Cardiac arrest associated with trauma. *Circulation* 112(IV):146, 2005.

CHAPTER 7

Airway and Ventilation

CHAPTER OBJECTIVES

At the completion of this chapter, the reader will be able to do the following:

- ✓ Integrate the principles of ventilation and gas exchange with the pathophysiology of trauma to identify patients with inadequate perfusion.

- ✓ Relate the concepts of minute volume and oxygenation to the pathophysiology of trauma.

- ✓ Explain the mechanisms by which supplemental oxygen and ventilatory support are beneficial to the trauma patient.

- ✓ Given a scenario that involves a trauma patient, select the most effective means of providing a patent airway to suit the needs of the patient.

- ✓ Given a scenario that involves a patient who requires ventilatory support, select the most effective means available to suit the needs of the trauma patient.

- ✓ Given situations that involve various trauma patients, formulate a plan for airway management and ventilation.

- ✓ Given current research, understand the risks versus benefits when discussing new invasive procedures.

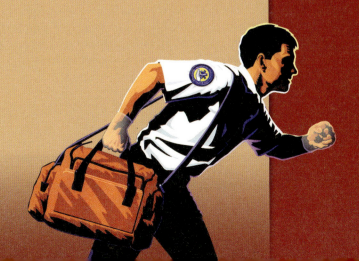

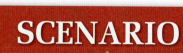

SCENARIO

You and your partner are dispatched to a pedestrian who has been hit by a motor vehicle. You find that your patient has been thrown about 30 feet from the point of impact. The car has damage to the grill and a spider web mark on the windshield. The driver of the car is out of the vehicle standing by his car. The pedestrian is being attended to by a police officer who is maintaining an open airway of the patient. The patient looks to be in his 30s, weighing around 280 lbs (125kg). The police officer has inserted an oropharyngeal airway (OPA) and is administering oxygen by facemask. The officer reports that since her arrival the patient has been unconscious. You note bleeding from the scalp and an angulated right femur. You are within 8 minutes of the local trauma center by ground.

What indicators of airway compromise are evident in this patient? What other information, if any, would you seek from witnesses or the first responders? Describe the sequence of actions you would take to manage this patient before and during transport.

Airway management plays a prominent role in the management of trauma patients. Its importance is recognized now even more than in years past. The failure to maintain oxygenation and ventilation causes secondary brain injury, compounding the primary brain injury produced by the initial trauma. Ensuring patency of the airway and maintaining the patient's oxygenation and supporting ventilation, when necessary, are critical steps in minimizing the overall brain injury and improving the likelihood of good outcome.

Cerebral oxygenation and oxygen delivery to other parts of the body provided by adequate airway management and ventilation remain the most important components of prehospital patient care. Because techniques and adjunct devices are changing and will continue to change, keeping abreast of these changes is important.

The respiratory system serves two primary functions:

1. The system provides oxygen to the red blood cells,which carry the oxygen to all of the cells in the body.
2. The system removes carbon dioxide (CO_2) from the body.

Inability of the respiratory system to provide oxygen to the cells or inability of the cells to use the oxygen supplied results in *anaerobic metabolism* and can quickly lead to death. Failure to eliminate CO_2 can lead to coma and acidosis.

Anatomy

The respiratory system is comprised of the upper airway and the lower airway, including the lungs (Figure 7-1). Each part of the system plays an important role in ensuring gas exchange—the process by which oxygen enters the bloodstream and CO_2 is removed.

Upper Airway

The upper airway consists of the nasal cavity and the oral cavity (Figure 7-2). Air entering the nasal cavity is warmed, humidified, and filtered to remove impurities. Beyond these cavities is the area known as the *pharynx,* which runs from the back of the soft palate to the upper end of the esophagus. The pharynx is composed of muscle lined with mucous membranes. The pharynx is divided into three discrete sections: the *nasopharynx* (upper portion), the *oropharynx* (middle portion), and the *hypopharynx* (lower or distal end of the pharynx). Below the pharynx are the *esophagus,* which leads to the stomach, and the *trachea,* at which point the lower airway begins. Above the trachea is the *larynx* (Figure 7-3), which contains the vocal cords, and the muscles that make them work, housed in a strong cartilaginous box. The vocal cords are folds of tissue that meet in the midline. The false cords, or *vestibular folds,* direct the airflow through the vocal cords. Supporting the cords posteriorly is the arytenoid cartilage. Directly above the larynx is a leaf-shaped structure called the *epiglottis.* Acting as a gate or flapper valve, the epiglottis directs air into the trachea and solids and liquids into the esophagus.

Lower Airway

The lower airway consists of the trachea, its branches, and the lungs. On inspiration, air travels through the upper airway and into the lower airway before reaching the alveoli, where the actual gas exchange occurs. The trachea divides into the

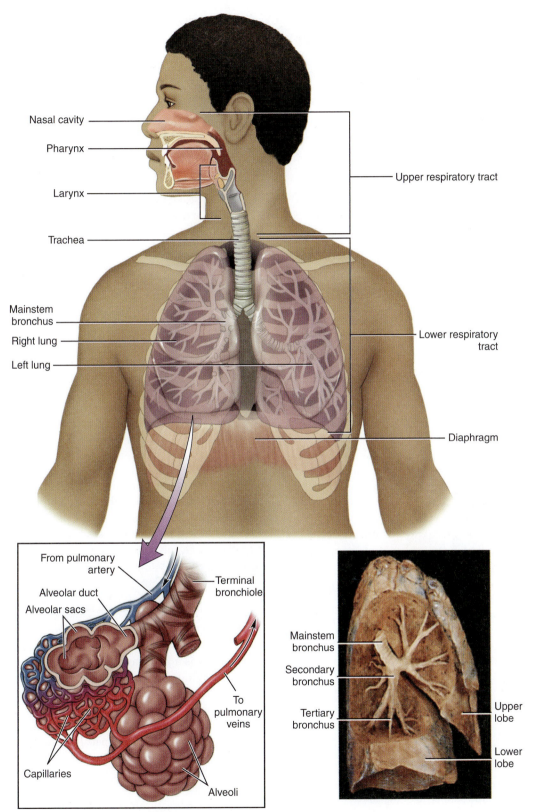

Nasal cavity

Pharynx

Larynx

Trachea

Mainstem bronchus

Right lung

Left lung

Upper respiratory tract

Lower respiratory tract

Diaphragm

From pulmonary artery

Alveolar duct

Alveolar sacs

Terminal bronchiole

To pulmonary veins

Capillaries

Alveoli

Mainstem bronchus

Secondary bronchus

Tertiary bronchus

Upper lobe

Lower lobe

FIGURE 7-1   Organs of the respiratory system: upper respiratory tract and lower respiratory tract. (Modified from Herlihy B, Maebius WK: *The Human Body in Health and Disease,* Philadelphia, 2000, Saunders.)

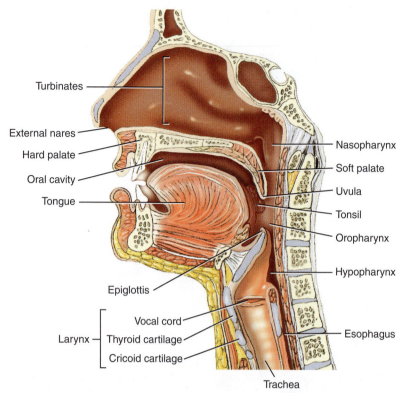

FIGURE 7-2 Sagittal section through the nasal cavity and pharynx viewed from the medial side.

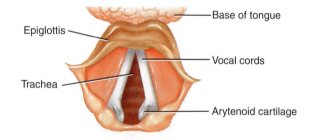

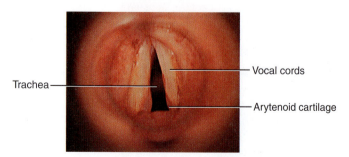

FIGURE 7-3 Vocal cords viewed from above, showing their relationship to the paired cartilages of the larynx and the epiglottis.
(Custom Medical Stock photo, modified from Thibodeau GA: *Structure and Function,* ed 9, St Louis, 1992, Mosby.)

right and left *main stem bronchi.* Each of the main stem bronchi subdivides into several primary bronchi and then into bronchioles. *Bronchioles* (very small bronchial tubes) terminate at the *alveoli,* which are tiny air sacs surrounded by capillaries. The alveoli are the site of gas exchange where the respiratory and circulatory systems meet.

Physiology

The airway is a pathway that leads atmospheric air through the nose, mouth, pharynx, trachea, and bronchi to the alveoli. With each breath, the average adult takes in approximately 500 ml of air. The airway system holds up to 150 ml of air that never actually reaches the alveoli to participate in the critical gas-exchange process. The space in which this air is held is known as *dead space.* The air inside this dead space is not available to the body to be used for oxygenation because it never reaches the alveoli.

With each breath, air is drawn into the lungs. When atmospheric air reaches the alveoli, oxygen moves from the alveoli, across the alveolar-capillary membrane, and into the red blood cells (RBCs). The circulatory system then delivers the oxygen-carrying RBCs to the body tissues, where oxygen is used as fuel for metabolism.

As oxygen is transferred from inside the alveoli to the RBCs, CO_2 is exchanged in the opposite direction, from the plasma to the alveoli. Carbon dioxide, which is carried in the plasma, not in the RBCs, moves from the bloodstream, across the alveolar-capillary membrane, and into the alveoli, where it is eliminated during exhalation (Figure 7-4). On completion of this exchange, the oxygenated RBCs and plasma with a low CO_2 level return to the left side of the heart to be pumped to all the cells in the body.

Once at the cell, the oxygenated RBCs deliver their oxygen, which the cells then use for aerobic metabolism. Carbon dioxide, a by-product of aerobic metabolism, is released into the blood plasma. Deoxygenated blood returns to the right side of the heart. The blood is pumped to the lungs, where it is again supplied with oxygen, and the CO_2 is eliminated by diffusion.

The alveoli must be constantly replenished with a fresh supply of air that contains an adequate amount of oxygen. This replenishment of air, known as *ventilation,* is essential for the elimination of CO_2. Ventilation is measurable. The size of each breath, called the *tidal volume,* multiplied by the ventilatory rate for 1 minute equals the *minute volume:*

Minute volume =
Tidal volume × Ventilatory rate per minute

During normal resting ventilation, about 500 ml of air is taken into the lungs. As mentioned previously, part of this volume, 150 ml, remains in the airway system as dead space and does not participate in gas exchange. If the tidal volume is 500 ml and the ventilatory rate is 14 breaths/minute, the minute volume can be calculated as follows:

Minute volume = 500 ml × 14 breaths/minute
Minute volume = 7000 ml/minute, or 7 liters/minute

Therefore, at rest, about 7 liters of air must move in and out of the lungs each minute to maintain adequate CO_2 elimination and oxygenation. If the minute volume falls below normal, the patient has inadequate ventilation, a condition called *hypoventilation.* Hypoventilation leads to a build-up of CO_2 in the body. Hypoventilation is common when head or chest trauma causes an altered breathing pattern or an inability to move the chest wall adequately. For example, a patient with rib fractures who is breathing quickly and shallowly because of the pain of the injury may have a tidal volume of 100 ml and a ventilatory rate of 40 breaths/minute. This patient's minute volume can be calculated as follows:

Minute volume = 100 ml × 40 breaths/minute
Minute volume = 4000 ml/minute, or 4 liters/minute

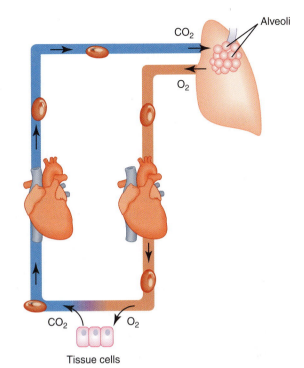

FIGURE 7-4 Oxygen (O_2) moves into the red blood cells from the alveoli. The O_2 is transferred to the tissue cell on the hemoglobin molecule. After leaving the hemoglobin molecule, the O_2 travels into the tissue cell. Carbon dioxide *(CO_2)* travels in the reverse direction, but not on the hemoglobin molecule. It travels in the plasma as CO_2.

If 7 liters/minute is necessary for adequate gas exchange in a nontraumatized person at rest, 4 liters/minute is much less than the body requires to eliminate CO_2 effectively, indicating hypoventilation. Furthermore, 150 ml of air is necessary to overcome dead space. If tidal volume is 100 ml, oxygenated air will never reach the alveoli. If left untreated, this hypoventilation will quickly lead to severe distress and, ultimately, death.

In the previous example, the patient is hypoventilating even though the ventilatory rate is 40 breaths/minute. Evaluating a patient's ability to exchange air involves assessing both ventilatory rate and depth. A common mistake is assuming that any patient with a fast ventilatory rate is hyperventilating. A much better measure of ventilatory status is the amount of CO_2 eliminated, which can be determined using CO_2 monitors. The effect of CO_2 elimination on metabolism is discussed with the Fick principle and aerobic and anaerobic metabolism in Chapter 8.

Assessment of ventilatory function always includes an evaluation of how well a patient is taking in, diffusing, and delivering oxygen. Without proper intake and processing of oxygen, anaerobic metabolism will begin. In addition, effective ventilation must also be assured. A patient may accomplish ventilation completely, partially, or not at all. Aggressive assessment and management of these inadequacies in both oxygenation and ventilation are paramount to a successful outcome.

Oxygenation and Ventilation of the Trauma Patient

The oxygenation process within the human body involves the following three phases:

1. *External respiration* is the transfer of oxygen (O_2) molecules from the atmosphere to the blood. All alveolar oxygen exists as free gas; therefore, each O_2 molecule exerts pressure. Increasing the percentage of oxygen in the inspired atmosphere will increase alveolar O_2 tension. Air contains 21% oxygen with most of the remainder made up of nitrogen. When supplemental oxygen is provided, the percent of oxygen in each inspiration increases, causing an increase in the amount of oxygen in each alveolus.

2. *Oxygen delivery* is the result of O_2 transfer from the atmosphere to the RBCs during ventilation and the transportation of these RBCs to the tissues via the cardiovascular system. This process primarily involves cardiac output, hemoglobin concentration, and oxyhemoglobin saturation. The volume of oxygen consumed by the body in 1 minute is known as *oxygen consumption.* One could describe the RBCs as the body's "oxygen tankers." These tankers move along the vascular system "highways" to "off-load" their O_2 supply at the body's distribution points, the capillary beds.

3. *Internal (cellular) respiration* is the movement, or diffusion, of oxygen from the RBCs into the tissue cells. Metabolism normally occurs through glycolysis and the Krebs cycle to produce energy. Because the actual exchange of oxygen between the RBCs and the tissues occurs in the thin-walled capillaries, any factor that interrupts a supply of oxygen will disrupt this cycle. Supplemental oxygen can help overcome some of these factors. The tissues cannot consume adequate oxygen if adequate amounts are not available.

Adequate oxygenation depends on all three of these phases. Although the ability to assess tissue oxygenation in prehospital situations is improving rapidly, appropriate ventilatory support for all trauma patients begins by providing supplemental oxygen to help ensure that hypoxia is corrected or averted entirely.

Pathophysiology

Trauma can affect the respiratory system's ability to adequately provide oxygen and eliminate carbon dioxide in the following ways:

1. Hypoventilation can result from loss of ventilatory drive, usually because of decreased neurologic function, most often after a traumatic brain injury.
2. Hypoventilation can result from obstruction of airflow through the upper and lower airways.
3. Hypoventilation can be caused by decreased expansion of the lungs.
4. *Hypoxemia* (decreased oxygen level in the blood) can result from decreased diffusion of oxygen across the alveolar-capillary membrane.
5. *Hypoxia* (deficient tissue oxygenation) can be caused by decreased blood flow to the alveoli.
6. Hypoxia can result from the inability of the air to reach the capillaries, usually because the alveoli are filled with fluid or debris.
7. Hypoxia can be caused at the end cellular level by decreased blood flow to the tissue cells.

The first three ways involve hypoventilation as a result of the reduction of minute volume. If left untreated, hypoventilation results in CO_2 build-up, acidosis, and eventually death. Management involves improving the patient's ventilatory rate and depth by correcting existing airway problems and assisting ventilation as appropriate.

The following sections discuss the first two causes of inadequate ventilation: decreased neurologic function and mechanical obstruction. The third cause, a reduction in minute volume as a result of decreased pulmonary expansion, is discussed in Chapter 10. The last four causes are discussed in Chapter 8.

Decreased Neurologic Function

Decreased minute volume can be caused by two clinical conditions related to decreased neurologic function: flaccidity of the tongue and a decreased level of consciousness (LOC).

Flaccidity of the tongue associated with a reduced LOC allows the tongue to fall into a dependent position (toward the lowest area of the body). If a patient is supine, the base of the tongue will fall backward and occlude the hypopharynx (Figure 7-5). This complication commonly presents as snoring with respirations. To prevent the tongue from occluding the hypopharynx or correct the problem when it occurs, maintaining an open airway must be assured in any supine patient with a diminished LOC, regardless of whether signs of ventilatory compromise exist. Such patients may also require periodic suctioning because secretions, saliva, blood, or vomitus may accumulate in the oropharynx. A decreased LOC will also affect ventilatory drive and may reduce the rate of ventilation, the volume of ventilation, or both. This reduction in minute volume may be temporary or permanent.

Mechanical Obstruction

Another cause of decreased minute volume is mechanical airway obstruction. The source of these obstructions may be neurologically influenced or purely mechanical in nature. Neurologic insults that alter the LOC may disrupt the "controls" that normally hold the tongue in an anatomically neutral (nonobstructing) position. If these "controls" are compromised, the tongue falls rearward, occluding the hypopharynx (see Figure 7-5).

Foreign bodies in the airway may be objects that were in the patient's mouth at the time of the injury, such as false teeth, chewing gum, tobacco, real teeth, and bone. Outside materi-

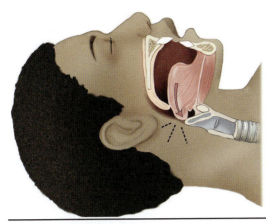

FIGURE 7-5   In an unconscious patient the tongue has lost its muscle tone and falls back into the hypopharnyx, occluding the airway and preventing passage of oxygen into the trachea and lungs.

als, such as glass from a broken windshield or any object that is near the patient's mouth on injury, may also threaten airway patency. Upper and lower airway obstructions may also be caused by bone or cartilage collapse from a fractured larynx or trachea, by mucous membrane avulsed from the hypopharynx or tongue, or by facial damage in which blood and fragments of bone and tissue create an obstruction.

Management of mechanical airway obstructions can be extremely challenging. Foreign bodies in the oral cavity may become lodged and create occlusions in the hypopharynx or the larynx. Crush injuries to the larynx and edema of the vocal cords may be present. Patients with facial injuries present with two of the most common foreign body obstructions: blood and vomit. Treatment of these problems is aimed at immediate recognition of the obstruction and the steps taken to ensure airway patency.

Assessment of the Airway and Ventilation

The ability to assess the airway is required in order to effectively manage it. Certainly we do many aspects of assessing the airway without even thinking about them. A patient who is alert and talking to us as we walk through the door has an open and patent airway. But when the patients' level of conciseness is decreased, it is essential to thoroughly assess the airway prior to moving to other injuries. When examining the airway during the primary survey, the following need to be assessed.

Positioning of the Airway and Patient

As you make visual contact with the patient, you observe the positioning of the patient. Patients in a supine position are at risk for airway obstruction from the tongue falling back into the airway. Most trauma patients will be placed in the supine position on a backboard for spinal immobilization. Any patient exhibiting signs of decreased level of consciousness will need constant re-examination for airway obstruction and the placement of an adjunctive device to assure an open airway. Patients who present with an open airway while lying on their side may obstruct their airways when placed supine on a backboard. Patients with massive facial trauma and active bleeding may need to be maintained in the position that they are found if they are maintaining their own airway. Placing these patients supine on a backboard may cause obstruction to the airway and possible aspiration of blood. In these cases, if the patient is maintaining their own airway, the best course of action may be to let them continue.

Any Sounds Emanating from the Upper Airway

Noise coming from the upper airway is never a good sign. These noises can often be heard as you approach the patient. These noises are usually a result of a partial airway obstruction caused by either the tongue or blood or foreign bodies in the upper airway. Stridorous breath sounds point to a partially obstructed upper airway. This obstruction may be an anatomical obstruction like the tongue that has fallen back into the airway or an edematous epiglottis or airway. It may also be caused by foreign bodies. An edematous, or swollen, airway is an emergent situation that demands quick action to prevent total airway obstruction. Steps must be taken immediately to alleviate the obstructions and maintain an open airway.

Examine the Airway for Obstructions

Look in the mouth for any obvious foreign matter or any gross anatomical malformations. Remove foreign bodies found.

Look for Chest Rise

Limited chest rise may be a sign of an obstructed airway. The use of accessory muscles and the appearance of increased work of breathing should lead to a high index of suspicion of airway compromise.

Management

Airway Control

Ensuring a patent airway is the first priority of trauma management and resuscitation, and no action is more crucial in airway management than appropriate assessment of the airway (Figure 7-6). Regardless of how the airway is managed, a cervical spine injury must be considered. The use of any of these methods of airway control requires simultaneous manual stabilization of the cervical spine in a neutral position until the patient has been completely immobilized (see Chapter 9).

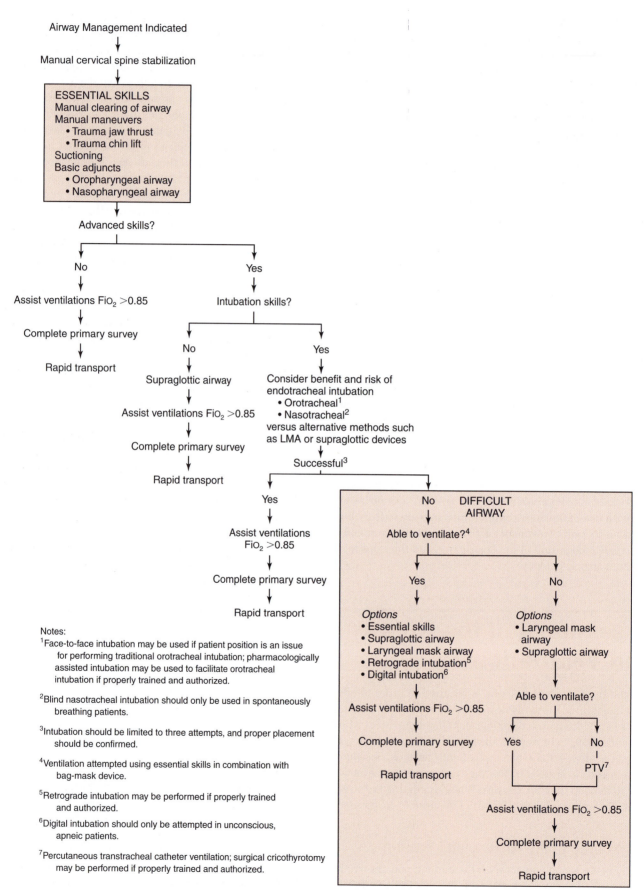

Airway Management Indicated

↓

Manual cervical spine stabilization

↓

ESSENTIAL SKILLS
Manual clearing of airway
Manual maneuvers
• Trauma jaw thrust
• Trauma chin lift
Suctioning
Basic adjuncts
• Oropharyngeal airway
• Nasopharyngeal airway

↓

Advanced skills?

No → Assist ventilations FiO_2 >0.85 → Complete primary survey → Rapid transport

Yes → Intubation skills?

    No → Supraglottic airway → Assist ventilations FiO_2 >0.85 → Complete primary survey → Rapid transport

    Yes → Consider benefit and risk of endotracheal intubation
• Orotracheal[1]
• Nasotracheal[2]
versus alternative methods such as LMA or supraglottic devices

↓

Successful[3]

Yes → Assist ventilations FiO_2 >0.85 → Complete primary survey → Rapid transport

No — DIFFICULT AIRWAY

Able to ventilate?[4]

Yes →
Options
• Essential skills
• Supraglottic airway
• Laryngeal mask airway
• Retrograde intubation[5]
• Digital intubation[6]

Assist ventilations FiO_2 >0.85 → Complete primary survey → Rapid transport

No →
Options
• Laryngeal mask airway
• Supraglottic airway

↓

Able to ventilate?

Yes / **No** → PTV[7]

Assist ventilations FiO_2 >0.85 → Complete primary survey → Rapid transport

Notes:

[1]Face-to-face intubation may be used if patient position is an issue for performing traditional orotracheal intubation; pharmacologically assisted intubation may be used to facilitate orotracheal intubation if properly trained and authorized.

[2]Blind nasotracheal intubation should only be used in spontaneously breathing patients.

[3]Intubation should be limited to three attempts, and proper placement should be confirmed.

[4]Ventilation attempted using essential skills in combination with bag-mask device.

[5]Retrograde intubation may be performed if properly trained and authorized.

[6]Digital intubation should only be attempted in unconscious, apneic patients.

[7]Percutaneous transtracheal catheter ventilation; surgical cricothyrotomy may be performed if properly trained and authorized.

FIGURE 7-6 Airway management algorithm.

Essential Skills

Management of the airway in trauma patients takes precedence over all other procedures because without an adequate airway, a positive outcome cannot be achieved. Management of the airway can be challenging, but in most patients, basic-level procedures may be sufficient initially.[1] Even prehospital care providers who have been trained in more advanced airway techniques need to maintain their ability to perform these essential, basic skills, because these methods provide an acceptable alternative when more advanced techniques fail. Providers with advanced skills always weigh the risk versus the benefit of performing these highly invasive procedures. Furthermore, maintenance of advanced skill proficiency, quality assurance, and close oversight by the medical director are necessary.

Manual Clearing of the Airway. The first step in airway management is a quick visual inspection of the oropharyngeal cavity. Foreign material (e.g., pieces of food) or broken teeth and blood may be found in the mouth of a trauma patient. These are swept out of the mouth using a gloved finger or, in the case of blood or vomitus, may be suctioned away. In addition, positioning of the patient on the side, when not contraindicated by possible spinal trauma, will allow for gravity assisted clearing of secretions, blood and vomitus.

Manual Maneuvers. In unresponsive patients, the tongue becomes flaccid, falling back and blocking the hypopharynx (see Figure 7-5). The tongue is the most common cause of airway obstruction. Manual methods to clear this type of obstruction can easily be accomplished because the tongue is attached to the mandible (jaw) and moves forward with it. Any maneuver that moves the mandible forward will pull the tongue out of the hypopharynx:

■ *Trauma jaw thrust.* In patients with suspected head, neck, or facial trauma, the cervical spine is maintained in a neutral in-line position. The trauma jaw thrust maneuver allows the prehospital care provider to open the airway

with little or no movement of the head and cervical spine (Figure 7-7). The mandible is thrust forward by placing the thumbs on each zygoma (cheekbone), placing the index and long fingers on the mandible, and at the same angle, pushing the mandible forward.

■ *Trauma chin lift.* The trauma chin lift maneuver is used to relieve a variety of anatomic airway obstructions in patients who are breathing spontaneously (Figure 7-8). The chin and lower incisors are grasped and then lifted to pull the mandible forward. The prehospital care provider wears gloves to avoid body fluid contamination.

Both these techniques result in movement of the lower mandible anteriorly (upward) and slightly caudal (toward the feet), pulling the tongue forward, away from the posterior airway, and opening the mouth. The trauma jaw thrust pushes the mandible forward, whereas the trauma chin lift pulls the mandible. The trauma jaw thrust and the trauma chin lift are modifications of the conventional jaw thrust and chin lift. The modifications provide protection to the patient's cervical spine while opening the airway by displacing the tongue from the posterior pharynx.

Suctioning. A trauma patient may not be capable of effectively clearing the build-up of secretions, vomitus, blood, or foreign objects from the trachea. Providing suction is an important part of maintaining a patent airway.

The most significant complication of suctioning is that suctioning for prolonged periods will produce hypoxemia, which may manifest as a cardiac abnormality (e.g., tachycardia). Preoxygenation of the trauma patient by providing supplemental oxygen will help prevent hypoxemia. In addition, during an extended period of suctioning, cardiac dysrhythmias may occur from arterial hypoxemia, and lead to myocardial hypoxemia or vagal stimulation secondary to tracheal irritation. True vagal stimulation may lead to profound bradycardia and hypotension.

The trauma patient not yet intubated may require aggressive suctioning of the upper airway. Much larger amounts

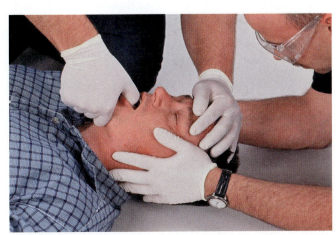

FIGURE 7-7 Trauma jaw thrust. The thumb is placed on each zygoma with the index and long fingers at the angle of the mandible. The mandible is lifted superiorly.

FIGURE 7-8 Trauma chin lift. The chin lift performs a function similar to that of the trauma jaw thrust. It moves the mandible forward by moving the tongue.

of blood and vomit may be in the airway on the arrival of emergency medical services (EMS) than a suction unit can quickly clear. If so, the patient may be rolled onto his or her side while maintaining cervical spine stabilization; gravity will then assist in clearing the airway. A rigid suction device is preferred to clear the oropharynx. Although hypoxia can result from prolonged suctioning, a totally obstructed airway will provide no air exchange. Aggressive suctioning and patient positioning are done until the airway is at least partially clear. At that point, hyperoxygenation followed by repeated suctioning can be performed. Hyperoxygenation, like preoxygenation, may be accomplished with either a nonrebreather mask on a high flow of oxygen or with a bag-mask running at 15 liters per minute. The goal when hyperoxygenating is to maintain an SPO$_2$ at or above 95% at sea level.

When suctioning intubated patients through the *endotracheal tube* (ET), the suction catheter should be made of soft material to limit trauma to the tracheal mucosa and to minimize frictional resistance. It needs to be long enough to pass the tip of the artificial airway (20–22 inches/50–55 cm) and should have smooth ends to prevent mucosal trauma. The soft catheter will probably not be effective in suctioning copious amounts of foreign material or fluid from the pharynx of a trauma patient, in which case the device of choice will be one with a tonsil-tip or Yankauer design. Under no circumstances should a tonsil-tip or Yankauer rigid suction device be placed in the end of the endotracheal tube.

When suctioning an intubated patient, aseptic procedures are vital. This technique includes the following steps:

1. Preoxygenate the trauma patient with 100% oxygen (Fio$_2$ of 1.0).
2. Prepare equipment while maintaining sterility.
3. Insert the catheter without suction. Suctioning is then initiated and continued for up to 15 to 30 seconds while withdrawing the catheter.
4. Re-oxygenate the patient, and ventilate for at least five assisted ventilations.
5. Repeat as necessary, allowing time for re-oxygenation to take place between procedures.

Selection of Adjunctive Device

If any problems are found with the airway during the primary survey, the provider needs to take immediate action to establish and maintain a patent airway. Once a basic airway has been established using manual maneuvers such as a trauma jaw thrust, it is necessary to use an adjunctive device to maintain the airway in an open position. The particular device should be selected based on the provider's level of training and proficiency with that particular device. This should then be included in a risk benefit analysis for the use of various types of devices and techniques that may be needed for this particular patient. The choice of the airway adjunct should be patient driven, "what is the best airway for this particular patient in this particular situation." During original training as well as during ongoing continuing education, providers at various levels are exposed to various adjunctive devices to help maintain an open airway. The amount of training directly relates to the difficulty in placement of the device. At the emergency medical responder level, providers are trained to place oral and nasal pharyngeal airways. At the other end of the spectrum, advanced providers have been trained to use advanced airway devices with some protocols allowing surgical airway procedures.

With skills such as intubation, the more times a skill is performed, the better the chance for a successful outcome. A new paramedic who only has performed intubations in the operating room has less of a chance of intubating a difficult patient compared to a 10-year veteran with over a hundred intubations during his or her career. The more steps there are in a procedure, the more difficult they are to learn. These also lend themselves to a greater probability of failure. As a skill increases in difficulty, so do the educational requirements, both in initial training and ongoing skills maintenance (Figures 7-9, 7-10). Generally the more difficult a procedure is to perform, the greater the penalty to the patient for failure. With airway procedures, this is particularly true. Careful evaluation of the airway prior to selecting the airway adjunct for any particular patient is essential to the best possible patient outcome.

Basic Adjuncts. When manual airway maneuvers are unsuccessful or when continued maintenance of an open airway is necessary, the use of an artificial airway is the next step.

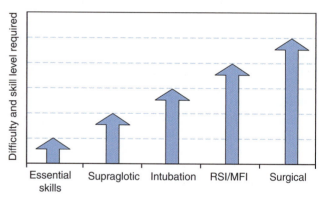

FIGURE 7-9   Airway skills.

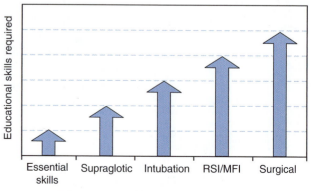

FIGURE 7-10   Educational skills required.

Oropharyngeal Airway. The most frequently used artificial airway is the oropharyngeal airway (OPA) (Figure 7-11). The OPA is inserted in either a direct or an inverted manner.

Indications

- Patient who is unable to maintain his or her airway
- To prevent an intubated patient from biting an ET tube

Contraindications

- Patient who is conscious or semiconscious

Complications

- Because it stimulates the gag reflex, use of the OPA may lead to gagging, vomiting, and laryngospasm in patients who are conscious.

Nasopharyngeal Airway. The nasopharyngeal airway (NPA) is a soft, rubberlike device that is inserted through one of the nares and then along the curvature of the posterior wall of the nasopharynx and oropharynx (Figure 7-12).

Indications

- Patient who is unable to maintain his or her airway

Contraindications

- No need for an airway adjunct

Complications

- Bleeding caused by insertion may be a complication

Supraglottic Airways. Supraglottic airways offer a functional alternative airway to endotracheal intubation (Figure 7-13 and Figure 7-14). Many jurisdictions allow the use of these devices because minimal training is required to achieve and retain competency. These types of devices are inserted without direct visualization of the vocal cords. These devices are also a useful backup airway when endotracheal intubation attempts are unsuccessful, even when rapid-sequence intubation has been attempted, or when, after careful evaluation of the airway, the provider feels that the chance for successful placement is higher than for endotracheal intubation. The primary advantage of supraglottic airways is that they may be inserted independent of the patient's position, which may be especially important in trauma patients with access and extrication difficulties or a high suspicion of cervical injury. Some manufacturers have developed supraglottic airways in pediatric sizes. Providers should assure proper

> **FIGURE 7-13   Common Supraglottic Airways**
>
> - King LT airway
> - Combi-Tube
> - Laryngeal mask airway (LMA)
> - Intubating LMA

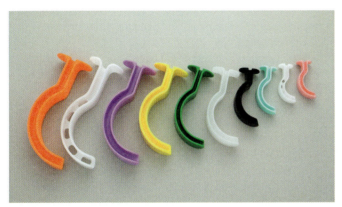

FIGURE 7-11   Oropharyngeal airways.
(From McSwain NE Jr, Paturas JL: *The Basic EMT: Comprehensive Prehospital Patient Care,* ed 2, St Louis, 2001, Mosby.)

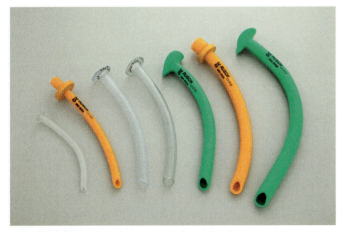

FIGURE 7-12   Nasopharyngeal airways.
(From McSwain NE Jr, Paturas JL: *The Basic EMT: Comprehensive Prehospital Patient Care,* ed 2, St Louis, 2001, Mosby.)

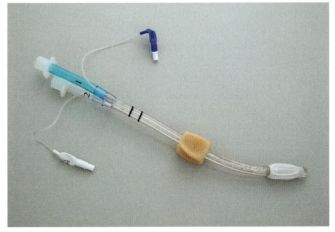

FIGURE 7-14   Supraglottic airways.

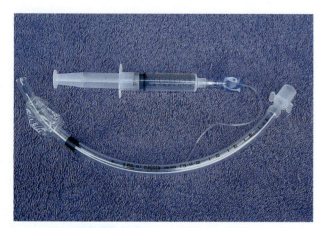

FIGURE 7-15   Endotracheal tube.

sizing according to the manufacturers' specifications if using these types of airways on pediatric patients.

Indications

- *Basic providers.* If the provider is trained and authorized, a supraglottic airway is the primary airway device for an unconscious trauma patient who lacks a gag reflex and is apneic or ventilating at a rate of less than 10 breaths/minute.
- *Advanced providers.* A supraglottic airway is the alternative airway device when the provider is unable to perform endotracheal intubation and cannot easily ventilate the patient with a bag-mask device and an OPA or NPA.

Contraindications

- Intact gag reflex
- Nonfasting (recent meal)
- Known esophageal disease
- Recent ingestion of caustic substances

Complications

- Gagging and vomiting, if gag reflex is intact
- Aspiration
- Damage to the esophagus
- Hypoxia if ventilated using the incorrect lumen

Endotracheal Intubation

Endotracheal intubation traditionally has been the preferred method for achieving maximum control of the airway in trauma patients who are either apneic or who require assisted ventilation (Figures 7-15 and 7-16). Recent studies, however, have shown that in an urban environment, critically injured trauma patients with endotracheal intubation had no better outcome than those transported with a bag-mask and OPA.[1] The decision to perform endotracheal intubation or use an alternative device should be

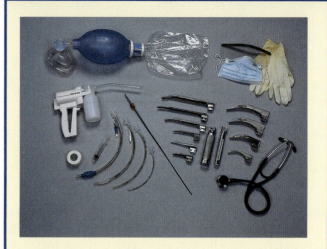

FIGURE 7-16   Equipment for Endotracheal Intubation

As with any advanced life support skill, prehospital care providers need to have the proper equipment. The standard components of an intubation kit should include the following:

- Laryngoscope with adult- and pediatric-sized straight and curved blades
- Extra batteries and spare light bulbs
- Suction equipment including ridged and flexible catheters
- Adult- and pediatric-sized endotracheal tubes
- Stylet
- Gum Elastic Bougie
- 10-ml syringe
- Water-soluble lubricant
- Magill forceps
- End-tidal detection device (ETDD) for end-tidal carbon dioxide detection
- Wave form capnography
- Tube-securing device

made after assessment of the airway has determined the difficulty of the intubation. The risk of hypoxia from prolonged intubation attempts of a patient that has a difficult airway needs to be weighed against the need to insert the endotracheal tube.

Prediction of potentially difficult endotracheal intubation. It is imperative that prior to performing endotracheal intubation an assessment of the difficulty of the intubation be done. There are many factors that can result in a difficult intubation of the trauma patient (Figure 7-17). Some of these are directly related to the trauma that they have sustained, oth-

FIGURE 7-17 Factors That Contribute to Difficult Intubation

- Receding chin
- Short neck
- Large tongue
- Small mouth opening
- Cervical immobilization or stiff neck
- Facial trauma
- Bleeding into the airway
- Active vomiting
- Access to the patient

ers are due to anatomical anomalies of their face and upper airway.

A mnemonic LEMON has been developed to assist in the assessment of the relative difficulty that will be involved in a particular intubation (Figures 7-18). Although not all components of the LEMON mnemonic may be applied to the trauma patient in the field, an understanding of the components can help the provider prepare for the difficult intubation. Alternative procedures or devices may be selected if the difficulty of the procedure is deemed high. Transport time may also be a factor when deciding the appropriate modality; an example may be a patient that is being maintained effectively with an OPA and bag-mask with a short transport time to the trauma center. The provider may elect not to intubate but rather transport while maintaining the airway using BLS techniques. Providers need to assess the risks versus the benefits when making the decision to perform advanced level airway procedures.

Despite this, endotracheal intubation still remains the preferred method of airway control because it does the following:

- Isolates the airway
- Allows for ventilation with 100% oxygen (Fio_2 of 1.0)
- Eliminates the need to maintain an adequate mask-to-face seal
- Significantly decreases the risk of aspiration (vomitus, foreign material, blood)
- Facilitates deep tracheal suctioning
- Prevents gastric insufflation
- Provides an additional (although limited) route for medication administration

Indications
- Patient who is unable to protect his or her airway
- Patient with significant oxygenation problem, requiring administration of high concentrations of oxygen

- Patient with significant ventilatory impairment requiring assisted ventilation

Contraindications
- Lack of training in technique
- Lack of proper indications
- Proximity to receiving facility (relative contraindication)
- High probability of failed airway

Complications
- Hypoxemia from prolonged intubation attempts
- Vagal stimulation causing bradycardia
- Trauma to the airway with resultant hemorrhage and edema
- Right main stem bronchus intubation
- Esophageal intubation
- Vomiting leading to aspiration
- Loose or broken teeth
- Injury to the vocal cords
- Conversion of a cervical spine injury without neurologic deficit to one with neurologic deficit

Research studies have shown that practice increases the likelihood of success when intubating. Although no correlation was found between success rate and length of time as a paramedic, there was a correlation between the number of patients intubated by the paramedic and the success rate. Experience with the procedure increases the likelihood of successful performance.[2]

As with all procedures, the prehospital care provider, along with the system medical director, makes a risk/benefit judgment when using any advanced procedures. Performing procedures simply because "the protocols allow it" is inappropriate. Think of the possible benefits and the possible risks, and form a plan based on the best interest of the patient in a given situation. Situations differ drastically based on transport time, location (urban vs. rural), and provider level of comfort in performing a given procedure.

Methods of Endotracheal Intubation. Several alternative methods are available for performing endotracheal intubation. The method of choice depends on such factors as the patient's needs, the level of urgency (orotracheal vs. nasotracheal), patient positioning (face-to-face), or training and scope of practice (pharmacologically assisted intubation). Regardless of the method selected, the patient's head and neck should be stabilized in a neutral position during the procedure and until spinal immobilization is completed. In general, if intubation is not successful after three attempts, consider a backup technique.

Orotracheal Intubation. Orotracheal intubation involves placing an ET tube into the trachea through the mouth. The nontrauma patient is often placed in a "sniffing" position to

FIGURE 7-18   LEMON Assessment for Difficult Intubation.

L = Look Externally: Look for characteristics that are known to cause difficult intubation or ventilation.

E = Evaluate the 3–3–2 Rule (see below): To allow for alignment of the pharyngeal, laryngeal, and oral axes, and therefore simple intubation, the following relationships should be observed:

■ The distance between the patient's incisor teeth should be at least 3 finger breadths (3)

■ The distance between the hyoid bone and the chin should be at least 3 finger breadths (3)

■ The distance between the thyroid notch and floor of the mouth should be at least 2 finger breadths (2)

M = Mallampati (see below): The hypopharynx should be visualized adequately. This has been done traditionally by assessing the Mallampati classification.

■ When possible, the patient is asked to sit upright, open the mouth fully, and protrude the tongue as far as possible. The examiner then looks into the mouth with a light to assess the degree of hypopharynx visible. In supine patients, the Mallampati score can be estimated by asking the patient to open the mouth fully and protrude the tongue; a laryngoscopy light is then shone into the hypopharynx from above.

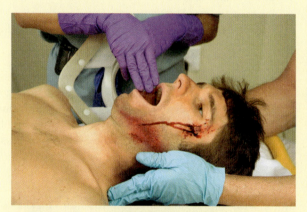

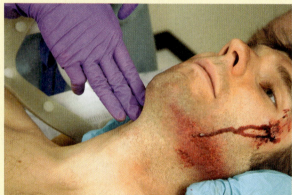

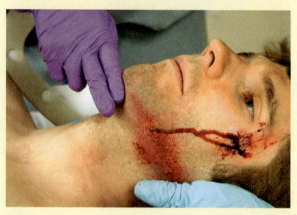

The 3–3–2 Rule. To allow for alignment of the pharyngeal, laryngeal, and oral axes and, therefore, simple intubation, the following relationships should be observed: **A.** The distance between the patient's incisor teeth should be at least 3 finger breadths, **B.** The distance between the hyoid bone and the chin should be at least 3 finger breadths, and **C.** The distance between the thyroid notch and floor of the mouth should be at least 2 finger breadths.

Modified with permission from: Reed, MJ, Dunn MJG, McKeown DW. Can an airway assessment score predict difficulty at intubation in the emergency department? *Emerg Med J* 2005;22:99–102. (In American College of Surgeons: *Advanced Trauma Life Support for Doctors,* Chicago, 2008, American College of Surgeons.)

facilitate intubation. Because this position hyperextends the cervical spine at C1-C2 (the second most common site for cervical spine fractures in the trauma patient) and hyperflexes it at C5-C6 (the most common site for cervical spine fractures in the trauma patient), it should not be used for trauma patients (Figure 7-19).

Nasotracheal Intubation. In conscious trauma patients or in those with an intact gag reflex, endotracheal intubation may be difficult to accomplish. If spontaneous ventilations are present, blind nasotracheal intubation (BNTI) may be attempted if the benefit outweighs the risk. Although nasotracheal intubation is often more difficult to perform than

FIGURE 7-18, cont'd

O = Obstruction: Any condition that can cause obstruction of the airway will make laryngoscopy and ventilation difficult. Such conditions include epiglottitis, peritonsillar abscess, and trauma.

N = Neck Mobility: This is a vital requirement for successful intubation. It can be assessed easily by asking the patient to place his or her chin onto the chest and then extending the neck so that he or she is looking toward the ceiling. Patients in a hard collar neck immobilizer obviously have no neck movement and are, therefore, more difficult to intubate.

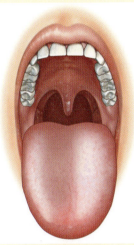 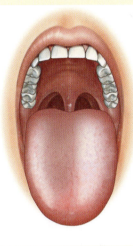 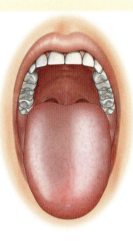 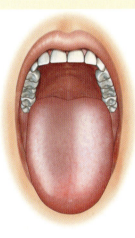

| Class I: soft palate, uvula, fauces, pillars visible | Class II: soft palate, uvula, fauces visible | Class III: soft palate, base of uvula visible | Class IV: hard palate only visible |

Mallampati Classifications. Used to visualize the hypopharynx. **Class I:** soft palate, uvula, fauces, pillars visible. **Class II:** soft palate, uvula, fauces visible. **Class III:** soft palate, base of uvula visible. **Class IV:** hard palate only visible. (From NAEMT: ATLS)

direct visualization and oral intubation, a 90% success rate has been reported in traumatized patients. During BNTI, the patient must be breathing to ensure that the ET tube is passed through the vocal cords. Many texts suggest that BNTI is contraindicated in the presence of midface trauma or fractures, but an exhaustive literature search reveals no documentation of an ET tube entering the cranial vault. Apnea is a contraindication specific to BNTI. In addition, no stylet is used when BNTI is performed.

Face-to-Face Intubation. Face-to-face intubation is indicated when standard trauma intubation techniques cannot be used

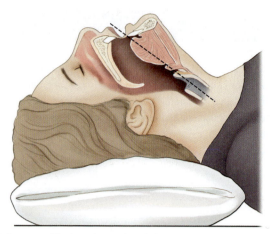

FIGURE 7-19 Placing the patient's head in the "sniffing" position provides ideal visualization of the larynx through the mouth. However, such positioning hyperextends the patient's neck at C1 and C2 and hyperflexes it at C5 and C6. These are the two most common points of fracture of the cervical spine.

because of the inability of the rescuer to assume the standard position at the head of the trauma patient. These situations include but are not limited to the following:

- Vehicle entrapment
- Pinning of the patient in rubble

Pharmacologically-Assisted Intubation. Intubation using pharmacologic agents may occasionally be required to facilitate ET tube placement in injured patients. In skilled hands, this technique can facilitate effective airway control when other methods fail or are otherwise not acceptable. To maximize the effectiveness of this procedure and ensure patient safety, personnel using drugs to assist with intubation need to be familiar with applicable local protocols, medications, and indications for use of the technique. The use of drugs to assist with intubation, particularly rapid-sequence intubation, does have risks. Pharmacologically-assisted intubation is a procedure of necessity, not convenience. Intubation using drugs falls into the following two categories:

1. *Intubation using sedatives or narcotics.* Medications such as diazepam, midazolam, fentanyl, or morphine are used alone or in combination, with the goal being to relax the patient enough to permit intubation but not to abolish protective reflexes or breathing. The effectiveness of a single pharmacologic agent, such as midazolam, has been well documented.[3]
2. *Rapid-sequence intubation (RSI) using paralytic agents* (Figure 7-20). The patient is chemically paralyzed after first being sedated. This provides complete muscle paralysis but removes all protective reflexes and causes apnea. Studies of this method of airway management have demonstrated successful performance of the technique

in the field, with intubation success rates reported in the mid-90% range. However, few studies have critically evaluated whether or not patient outcome is affected.[4] One center reported its experience with RSI in the field and documented that patients with traumatic brain injury who underwent RSI had a poorer outcome than those who did not require RSI.[5] Subsequent analysis has shown that unrecognized hyperventilation leading to hypocarbia and unrecognized hypoxia were major contributors to the poor outcome.[6]

Also, pharmacologically-assisted intubation of any type requires time to accomplish. For every trauma patient for whom this intubation is contemplated, the benefits of securing an airway are weighed against the additional time spent on the scene to perform the procedure.

Indications

- A patient who requires a secure airway and is difficult to intubate because of uncooperative behavior (as induced by hypoxia, traumatic brain injury, hypotension, or intoxication)

Relative Contraindications

- Availability of an alternative airway (e.g., dual lumen)
- Severe facial trauma that would impair or preclude successful intubation
- Neck deformity or swelling that complicates or precludes placement of a surgical airway
- Known allergies to indicated medications
- Medical problems that would preclude use of indicated medications
- Inability to intubate

Complications

- Inability to insert the ET tube in a sedated or paralyzed patient no longer able to protect his or her airway or breathe spontaneously; patients who are medicated and then cannot be intubated require prolonged bag-mask ventilation until the medication wears off
- Development of hypoxia or hypercarbia during prolonged intubation attempts
- Aspiration
- Hypotension—virtually all the drugs have the side effect of decreasing blood pressure

Patients who are mildly or moderately hypovolemic but compensating may have a profound drop in blood pressure associated with the intravenous administration of many of these drugs. Exercise caution whenever the use of medications for intubation is considered (Figure 7-21).

Verification of Endotracheal-Tube Placement. Once intubation has been performed, take specific measures to ensure that the tube has been properly placed in the trachea. An improperly

FIGURE 7-20   Sample Protocol for Rapid-Sequence Intubation (RSI)

1. Ensure availability of required equipment.
   a. Oxygen supply
   b. Bag-mask of appropriate size and type
   c. Nonrebreathing mask
   d. Laryngoscope with blades
   e. Endotracheal (ET) tubes
   f. Gum Elastic Bougie
   g. Surgical and alternative airway equipment
   h. RSI medications
   i. Materials or devices to secure ET tube after placement
   j. Suction equipment
2. Ensure that at least one (but preferably two) patent intravenous (IV) line is present.
3. Preoxygenate the patient using a nonrebreathing mask or bag-mask with 100% oxygen. Preoxygenation for 3 to 4 minutes is preferred.
4. Apply cardiac and pulse oximetry monitors.
5. If the patient is conscious, strongly consider the use of sedative agents.
6. Consider the administration of sedative agents and lidocaine in the presence of potential or confirmed traumatic brain injury (TBI).
7. After administration of paralytic agents, use the Sellick maneuver (cricoid pressure) to decrease the potential for aspiration.
8. Confirm tube placement immediately after intubation. Continuous cardiac and pulse oximeter monitoring is required during and after RSI. Reconfirm tube placement periodically throughout transport and each time the patient is moved.
9. Use repeat doses of sedation and paralytic agents as needed.

PROCEDURE

1. Assemble the required equipment.
2. Ensure the patency of the IV lines.
3. Preoxygenate the patient with 100% oxygen for approximately 3 to 4 minutes if possible.
4. Place the patient on cardiac and pulse oximeter monitors.
5. Administer a sedative, such as midazolam, if appropriate.
6. In the presence of confirmed or potential TBI, administer lidocaine (1.5 mg/kg) 2 to 3 minutes before administration of a paralytic agent.
7. For pediatric patients, administer atropine (0.01–0.02 mg/kg) 1 to 3 minutes before paralytic administration to minimize the vagal response to intubation.
8. Administer a short-acting paralytic agent intravenously, such as succinylcholine. Paralysis and relaxation should occur within 30 seconds. Using the Sellick maneuver may also be helpful.
   a. Adult: 1 to 2 mg/kg
   b. Pediatric: 1 to 2 mg/kg
9. Insert an ET tube. If initial attempts are unsuccessful, precede repeat attempts with preoxygenation.
10. Confirm ET tube placement.
11. If repeated attempts to achieve endotracheal intubation fail, consider placement of an alternative or surgical airway.
12. Use doses of a long-acting paralytic agent, such as vecuronium, to continue paralysis.
    a. Initial dose: 0.1 mg/kg IV push
    b. Subsequent doses: 0.01 mg/kg every 30 to 45 minutes
13. Repeat doses of sedation may also be needed.

Note: Requirements vary with individual patients.

positioned ET tube, if unrecognized for only a brief period, may result in profound hypoxia, with resultant brain injury (hypoxic encephalopathy) and even death. Therefore, it is important that proper placement be confirmed. Techniques to verify intubation include the use of both clinical assessments and adjunct devices.[7] Clinical assessments include the following:

- Direct visualization of the ET tube passing through the vocal cords
- Presence of bilateral breath sounds (auscultate laterally below the axilla) *and* absence of air sounds over the epigastrium
- Visualization of the chest rising and falling during ventilation
- Fogging (water vapor condensation) in the ET tube on expiration

Unfortunately, none of these techniques is 100% reliable *by itself* for verifying proper tube placement. Therefore, prudent practice involves assessing and documenting *all* these clinical signs, if possible. On rare occasions, because of difficult anatomy, visualization of the ET tube passing through the vocal cords may not possible. In a moving vehicle (ground or aeromedical), engine noise may make auscultation of breath sounds almost impossible. Obesity and chronic obstructive pulmonary disease (COPD) may interfere with the ability to see chest movement during ventilation.

Monitoring devices include the following:

- End-tidal CO_2 monitoring (capnography)
- Esophageal detector device
- Colorimetric CO_2 detector
- Pulse oximetry

FIGURE 7-21   Common Drugs Used for Pharmacologically Assisted Intubation

Drug	Dose (Adult)	Dose (Pediatric)	Indications	Complications/ Side Effects
PRETREATMENT				
Oxygen	High flow; Assist ventilation as needed to achieve oxygen saturation of 100% if possible	High flow; Assist ventilation as needed to achieve oxygen saturation of 100% if possible intubation	All patients undergoing pharmacologically assisted	
Lidocaine	1–1.5 mg/kg	1.5 mg/kg IV	Brain injury	Seizure
Atropine		0.01–0.02 mg/kg IV **(min. dose: 0.1 mg)**	Pediatric intubation, prevention of bradycardia and excess secretions	Tachycardia
INDUCTION OF SEDATION				
Midazolam (Versed)	0.1–0.15 mg/kg up to 0.3 mg/kg IV	0.1–0.15 mg/kg up to 0.3 mg/kg IV	Sedation	Respiratory depression/ apnea, hypotension
Fentanyl (Sublimaze)	2–3 mcg/kg IV	1–3 mcg/kg IV	Sedation	Respiratory depression/ apnea, hypotension, bradycardia
Etomidate	0.2–0.3 mg/kg IV	Not approved for patients under 10 years of age	Sedation, induced anesthesia	Apnea, hypotension, vomiting
CHEMICAL PARALYSIS				
Succinylcholine	1–2 mg/kg	1–2 mg/kg	Muscle relaxation and paralysis (short duration)	Hyperkalemia, muscle fasciculations
Vecuronium (Norcuron)	0.1 mg/kg	0.1 mg/kg	Muscle relaxation and paralysis (intermediate duration)	Hypotension
Pancuronium (Pavulon)	0.04–0.1 mg/kg	0.04–0.1 mg/kg	Muscle relaxation and paralysis (long duration	Tachycardia, hypertension, salivation

As with the clinical assessments, none of these adjuncts is 100% accurate in all patients. In a patient with a perfusing rhythm, end-tidal CO_2 monitoring (capnography) serves as the "gold standard" for determining ET tube placement. This technique should be used in the prehospital setting whenever available. Patients in cardiopulmonary arrest do not exhale CO_2, and therefore, neither colorimetric detectors nor capnography may be useful in patients who lack a perfusing cardiac rhythm.

Because none of these techniques is universally reliable, all the clinical assessments noted previously should be performed, unless impractical, followed by use of at least one of the monitoring devices. If any of the techniques used to verify proper placement suggests that the ET tube may not be properly positioned, the tube should be immediately removed and reinserted, with placement verified again. All the techniques used to verify tube placement should be noted on the patient care report.

Securing an Endotracheal Tube. Once endotracheal intubation has been performed, the tube must be manually held in place and proper tube placement verified; the depth of tube insertion at the central incisors (front teeth) should be noted. Next, the ET tube is secured in place. The most common method used is to tape the tube to the patient's face. Unfortunately, blood and secretions often prevent the tape from adhering satisfactorily, allowing movement and potential dislodging of the ET tube. Several commercially available products may serve to secure the ET tube adequately. Ideally, if sufficient personnel are present, someone should be assigned the task of manually holding the tube in proper position to ensure that it does not move.

Continuous pulse oximetry should be considered *necessary* for all patients who require endotracheal intubation. Any decline in the pulse oximetry reading (SpO_2) or development of cyanosis requires reverification of ET tube placement. Additionally, an ET tube may also become dislodged during any movement of the patient. Reverify tube position after every move of a patient, such as logrolling to a long backboard or carrying the patient down a staircase.

Back-up Techniques

If endotracheal intubation has been unsuccessful after three attempts, consideration of airway management using the essential skills described previously and ventilating with a bag-mask device is appropriate. *If the receiving facility is reasonably close, these techniques may be the most prudent option for airway management when faced with a brief transport time.* If the nearest appropriate facility is more distant, one of the following backup techniques may be considered.

Digital Intubation. Digital, or *tactile,* intubation was a precursor to the current use of laryngoscopes for endotracheal intubation. Essentially, the intubator's fingers act in similar fashion to a laryngoscope blade by manipulating the epiglottis and acting as a guide for placement of the ET tube.

Indications
- Patients in whom endotracheal intubation failed but for whom ventilations can be assisted with a bag-mask device
- When laryngoscope is unavailable or fails
- When the airway is obscured or blocked because of large volumes of blood or vomitus
- Entrapment with inability to perform face-to-face intubation

Contraindications
- Any patient who is not comatose and may bite the intubator's fingers (dental clamp or bite stick may be used to hold the patient's mouth open)

Complications
- Esophageal intubation
- Lacerations or crush injuries to the prehospital care provider's fingers
- Hypoxia or hypercarbia during the procedure
- Damage to the vocal cords

Laryngeal Mask Airway. The laryngeal mask airway (LMA) is another alternative for unconscious or seriously obtunded

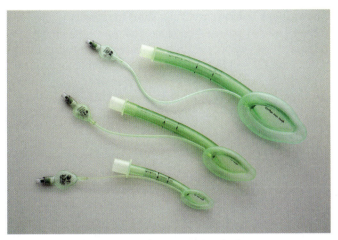

FIGURE 7-22   Laryngeal mask airway.

adult and pediatric patients. The device consists of an inflatable silicone ring attached diagonally to a silicone tube (Figure 7-22). When inserted, the ring creates a low-pressure seal between the LMA and the glottic opening, without direct insertion of the device into the larynx.

Advantages of the LMA include the following:

1. The device is designed for blind insertion. Direct visualization of the trachea and vocal cords is unnecessary.
2. With proper cleaning and storage, the LMA can be reused multiple times.
3. Disposable LMAs are now available.
4. The LMA is available in a range of sizes to accommodate both pediatric and adult patient groups.

Prehospital use of the LMA thus far has been more prevalent in Europe than in North America. A recent development is the introduction of an "intubating LMA." This device is inserted similar to the original LMA, but a flexible ET tube is then passed though the LMA, intubating the trachea. This secures the airway without the need to visualize the vocal cords.

Indications
- When unable to perform endotracheal intubation and the patient cannot be ventilated using a bag-mask device

Contraindications
- When endotracheal intubation can be performed
- Insufficient training

Complications
- Aspiration, because LMA does not completely prevent regurgitation and protect the trachea
- Laryngospasm

Percutaneous Transtracheal Ventilation. In rare cases, a trauma patient's airway obstruction cannot be relieved by the methods previously discussed. In these patients, a needle tracheostomy may be performed using a percutaneously placed catheter. It has been shown that adequate oxygenation can be achieved using percutaneous transtracheal ventilation (PTV), with acceptable levels of CO_2 maintained for 30 minutes.[8]

Advantages of PTV include the following:

1. Ease of access (landmarks usually easily recognized)
2. Ease of insertion
3. Minimal equipment required
4. No incision necessary
5. Minimal training required

Indications

- When all other alternative methods of airway management fail or are impractical and the patient cannot be ventilated with a bag-mask device

Contraindications

- Insufficient training
- Lack of proper equipment
- Ability to secure airway by another technique (as described previously) or ability to ventilate with a bag-mask device

Complications

- Hypercarbia from prolonged use (CO_2 elimination not as effective as with other methods of ventilation)[8]
- Damage to surrounding structures, including the larynx, thyroid gland, carotid arteries, jugular veins, and esophagus

Surgical Cricothyrotomy. Surgical cricothyrotomy involves the creation of a surgical opening in the *cricothyroid membrane,* which lies between the larynx (thyroid cartilage) and the cricoid cartilage. In most patients, the skin is very thin in this location, making it amenable to immediate access to the airway.[9] Consider this a technique of "last resort" in prehospital airway management.

The use of this surgical airway in the prehospital arena is controversial. Proficient endotracheal intubation skills should minimize the need even to consider its use. *Surgical cricothyrotomy should never be the initial airway control method.* Insufficient data exist at this time to support a recommendation that surgical cricothyrotomy be established as a national standard for routine use in prehospital airway management. Local protocols should govern the implementation of surgical cricothyrotomy.

Indications

- Massive midface trauma precluding the use of a bag-mask device

- Inability to control the airway using less invasive maneuvers
- Ongoing tracheobronchial hemorrhage

Contraindications

- Any patient who can be safely intubated, either orally or nasally
- Patients with laryngotracheal injuries
- Children under 10 years of age
- Patients with acute laryngeal disease of traumatic or infectious origin
- Insufficient training

Complications

- Prolonged procedure time
- Hemorrhage
- Aspiration
- Misplacement or false passage of the ET tube
- Injury to neck structures or vessels
- Perforation of the esophagus

Continuous Quality Improvement (CQI)

With the literature questioning the effectiveness of prehospital intubation of the trauma patient, it is important that the EMS service medical director or his or her designee individually review all out-of-hospital intubations or invasive airway techniques. This is even more imperative if medications have been used to facilitate the intubation attempt. Specific points include the following:

- Adherence to protocol and procedures
- Number of attempts
- Confirmation of tube placement and the procedures used for verification
- Outcome and complications
- Proper indications for the use of induction agents if used
- Proper documentation of drug dosage routes and monitoring of the patient during and after intubation

An effective CQI program for airway management must not be seen as a "punishment" but rather as an educational opportunity by the providers, management, and the medical director. Since most CQI programs are self-reporting, any results that are used to discipline a particular provider may result in misreporting. CQI should be tied directly to the continuing education program within an organization. After identifying a problem in performance, an educational component should be developed that addresses those issues. Follow up evaluations should take place to determine if the educational component has been effective.

Ventilatory Devices

All trauma patients receive appropriate ventilatory support with supplemental oxygen to ensure that hypoxia is corrected or averted entirely. In deciding which method or equipment to use, prehospital care providers should consider the following devices and their respective oxygen concentrations (Figure 7-23).

Pocket Masks

Regardless of which mask is chosen to support ventilation of the trauma patient, the ideal mask has the following characteristics:

1. Is a good fit.
2. Is equipped with a one-way valve.
3. Is made of a transparent material.
4. Has a supplemental oxygen port.
5. Is available in infant, pediatric, and adult sizes.

Mouth-to-mask ventilation satisfactorily delivers adequate tidal volumes by ensuring a tight face seal even when performed by those who do not use this skill often.

Bag-Mask

The bag-mask consists of a self-inflating bag and a nonrebreathing device; it can be used with basic (OPA, NPA) or advanced (endotracheal, nasotracheal) airway devices. Most bag-mask devices currently on the market have a volume of 1600 ml and can deliver an O_2 concentration of 90% to 100%. Some models also have a built-in colorimetric CO_2 detector. However, a *single* provider attempting to ventilate with a bag-mask may create poor tidal volumes secondary to the inability to create a tight face seal and to squeeze the bag adequately. Ongoing practice of this skill is necessary to ensure that the technique is effective and that the trauma patient receives adequate ventilatory support.

Manually Triggered (Oxygen-Powered) Devices

Manually triggered devices can deliver O_2 concentrations of 100%. Because these devices do not permit the provider to feel the compliance of the chest during the ventilation process, care is taken not to overinflate the lungs. Maintaining a tight face seal with the device is easy because the trigger mechanism requires only one hand to operate. Complications may include gastric distension, over inflation of the lungs, barotrauma, and lung rupture. These devices should not be used in the field except in unusual circumstances.

Positive-Pressure Ventilators

Positive-pressure volume ventilators during prolonged transport have long been used in the aeromedical environment. However, more ground units are now adopting the use of mechanical ventilation as a means of controlling rate, depth, and minute volume in trauma patients. Importantly, only volume ventilators with appropriate alarms and pressure control/relief should be used. These ventilators do not need to be as sophisticated as those used in the hospital and only have a few simple modes of ventilation as follows.

FIGURE 7-23 Ventilatory Devices and Oxygen Concentration

Device	Liter Flow (L/min)	Oxygen Concentration*
WITHOUT SUPPLEMENTAL OXYGEN		
Mouth-to-mouth	N/A	16%
Mouth-to-mask	N/A	16%
Bag-mask	N/A	21%
WITH SUPPLEMENTAL OXYGEN		
Nasal cannula	1–6	24%–45%
Mouth-to-mask	10	50%
Simple face mask	8–10	40%–60%
Bag-mask without reservoir	8–10	40%–60%
Bag-mask with reservoir	10–15	90%–100%
Nonrebreather mask with reservoir	10–15	90%–100%
Demand valve	N/A	90%–100%
Ventilator	N/A	21%–100%

*Percentages indicated are approximate.
N/A, Not applicable.

Assist Control (A/C). A/C ventilation is probably the most widely used mode of ventilation in prehospital transport from the scene to the emergency department. The A/C setting delivers ventilations at a preset rate and tidal volume. If patients initiate a breath on their own, an additional ventilation of the full tidal volume is delivered, which may lead to breath-stacking and overinflation of the lungs.

Intermittent Mandatory Ventilation (IMV). IMV delivers a set rate and tidal volume to patients. If patients initiate their own breath, only the amount that they actually pull on their own will be delivered.

Positive End-Expiratory Pressure (PEEP). PEEP provides an elevated level of pressure at the end of expiration, thus keeping the alveolar sacs and small airways open and filled with air for a longer time. This intervention provides greater oxygenation. However, by increasing the end-expiratory pressure and, therefore, the overall intrathoracic pressure, PEEP may decrease blood return to the heart. In hemodynamically unstable patients, PEEP may further decrease blood pressure. PEEP should also be avoided in patients with traumatic brain injuries. The increase in thoracic pressure can cause an elevation in intracranial pressure.

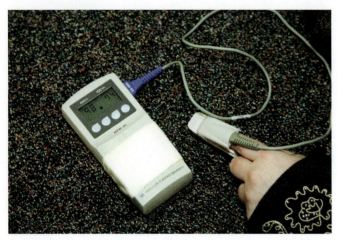

FIGURE 7-24   Pulse oximeter.

Initial settings for mechanical ventilations

Rate. The rate is set initially at between 10 and 12 breaths per minute on nonbreathing adult patients. In the hospital, the rate is increased or decreased depending upon the levels of CO_2 in arterial blood ($PaCO_2$). It should be noted that in the multisystem trauma patient, the end-tidal CO_2 reading may not correlate with the actual $PaCO_2$ readings. Due to this, the increasing or decreasing of rate based strictly upon $ETCO_2$ should be done with caution. The $ETCO_2$ should be used in combination with other readings and vital signs to determine the best course of action for the patient. $ETCO_2$ that has been correlated to an arterial blood gas can, however, be used as a trend of actual $PaCO_2$. This may be seen in interfaculty transports of these patients.

Tidal Volume (vt). The tidal volume should be set using 5–7 ml/kg of the patient's ideal body weight. This should be used as a guide and may need to be adjusted in the trauma patient.

PEEP

Positive End Expiratory Pressure should be set initially at 5 cm H_2O. This will maintain what is known as physiological PEEP. This is the amount of PEEP that is normally present in the airway prior to intubation. Once intubated, this positive pressure is taken away. Although increased levels of PEEP may be needed as the traumatic insult worsens, this rarely ever takes place in the first couple of hours following the traumatic event. The prehospital care provider may encounter patients requiring high levels of PEEP during a transfer of a patient from one hospital to another. The hospital staff prior to the transfer will have established these levels of PEEP. Care must be taken if PEEP is increased, as there can be adverse complications:

■ Decreased blood pressure secondary to decreased thoracic return

■ Increased intracranial pressure
■ Increased intrathoracic pressure leading to pneumothorax or tension pneumothorax

Oxygen Concentration. The oxygen concentration should be set to maintain a saturation of 95% or greater at sea level in the trauma patient.

High-Pressure Alarm/Pop-Off. The high-pressure alarm and pressure relief pop-off should be set at no more than 10 cm H_2O above the pressure needed to normally ventilate the patient (peak inspiratory pressure). Care should be taken when setting the alarm above 40 cm H_2O. Levels above this have been shown to produce barotrauma and a higher possibility of a pneumothorax. Should more than 40 cm H_2O be required to deliver the desired tidal volume, reassessment of the airway and preset tidal volume should be done. Decreasing the tidal volume and increasing the rate to maintain the same alveolar minute ventilation may be the prudent action in this case. As with any alarm, should the high-pressure alarm continue to activate for more than a few breaths, the patient should be removed from the ventilator and manually ventilated with a bag-mask while the ventilator circuit and endotracheal tube are evaluated. The patient should also be re-evaluated for an increase in compliance. This increase in compliance or resistance may be caused by many factors. The most common, early in the care of the trauma patient, is either tension pneumothorax or an increasing level of consciousness causing "bucking" on the tube. The tension pneumothorax should be treated with chest decompression as indicated. An increasing level of conciseness should be treated with the administration of a sedative agent if available. Other potential problems include displacement or obstruction of the tube. In no case should the provider simply just continue to increase the upper pressure limit and alarm.

Low Pressure Alarm. The low-pressure alarm alerts the provider if the connection between the patient and the ventilator is disconnected or is losing significant volume though a leak in the ventilator circuit. In most transport ventilators, this alarm is preset and cannot be adjusted.

Evaluation
Pulse Oximetry

Over the past few years, use of pulse oximetry has increased in the prehospital environment. Appropriate use of pulse oximetry devices allows early detection of pulmonary compromise or cardiovascular deterioration before physical signs are evident. Pulse oximeters are particularly useful in prehospital applications because of their high reliability, portability, ease of application, and applicability across all age ranges and races (Figure 7-24).

Pulse oximeters provide measurements of arterial oxyhemoglobin saturation (SpO_2) and pulse rate. SpO_2 is determined by measuring the absorption ratio of red and infrared light passed through tissue. A small microprocessor correlates changes in light absorption caused by the pulsation of blood through vascular beds to determine arterial saturation and pulse rate. Normal SpO_2 is between 93% and 95% at sea level. When SpO_2 falls below 90%, severe compromise of oxygen delivery to the tissues is most likely present. At higher altitudes, the acceptable levels of SpO2 are at 90%. Sound clinical judgment should be used to determine what acceptable levels are given higher altitudes.

To ensure accurate pulse oximetry readings, the following general guidelines should be followed:

1. Use the appropriate size and type of sensor.
2. Ensure proper alignment of sensor light.
3. Ensure that sources and photodetectors are clean, dry, and in good repair.
4. Avoid sensor placement on grossly edematous sites.

Common problems that can produce inaccurate SpO_2 measurement include the following:

- Excessive motion
- Moisture in SpO_2 sensors
- Improper sensor application and placement
- Poor patient perfusion or vasoconstriction from hypothermia
- Anemia
- Carbon monoxide poisoning

In a critical trauma patient, pulse oximetry may be less than accurate because of poor capillary perfusion status. Therefore, pulse oximetry is only a valuable addition to the prehospital care provider's "toolbox" when combined with a thorough knowledge of trauma pathophysiology and strong assessment and intervention skills.

Capnography

Capnography, or end-tidal carbon dioxide ($ETCO_2$) monitoring, has been used in critical care units for many years. Recent advances in technology have allowed smaller, more durable units to be produced for prehospital use (Figure 7-25). Capnography measures the partial pressure of carbon dioxide (PCO_2, or $ETCO_2$) in a sample of gas. If this sample is taken at the end of exhalation, it correlates closely to arterial PCO_2 ($PaCO_2$).

Most critical care units within the hospital setting use the *mainstream technique*. This technique places a sensor directly into the "mainstream" of the exhaled gas. In the patient being ventilated with a bag-mask, the sensor is placed between the bag-mask and the ET tube. In the critical patient, the $PaCO_2$ is generally 2 to 5 mm Hg higher than the $ETCO_2$. (A normal $ETCO_2$ reading in a critical trauma patient is 30 to 40 mm Hg.) Although these readings may not totally reflect the patient's $PaCO_2$, maintaining readings between normal levels will usually be beneficial to the patient.

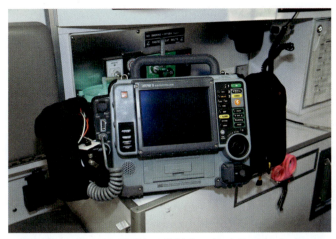

FIGURE 7-25 Handheld end-tidal carbon dioxide detector.

Although capnography correlates closely with $PaCO_2$, certain conditions will cause variations in accuracy. These conditions are often seen in the prehospital environment and include severe hypotension, high intrathoracic pressure, and any increase in dead space ventilation, as with pulmonary embolism. Therefore, following trends in $ETCO_2$ levels may be more important than focusing on specific readings. Continuous capnography provides another tool in the prehospital management of a trauma patient and is correlated with all other information about a patient. Initial transport decisions are based on physical and environmental conditions. For example, it would be inappropriate to take time to place the patient on monitors if the patient is losing blood. Instead, capnography should be used to monitor ET tube placement and continuously monitor patient status during transport. A sudden drop in expired CO_2 may result either from dislodgement of the ET tube or decreased perfusion and should prompt a re-evaluation of patient status and ET tube position.[10]

Prolonged Transport

Airway management of a patient prior to and during a prolonged transport requires complex decision making on the part of the prehospital care provider. Intervention to control and secure the airway, especially with advanced techniques, depends on numerous factors, including the patient's injuries, the clinical skills of the prehospital care provider, the equipment available, and the distance and transport time to definitive care. Risks and benefits of all the airway options available should be considered prior to making a final airway decision. Both a longer distance of transport and a longer transport time lower the threshold for securing the airway with endotracheal intubation. For transports of 15 to 20 minutes, essential skills, including an oral airway and bag-mask ventilation, may be sufficient. Use of air medical transport also lowers the threshold to perform endotracheal intubation, as a cramped, noisy environment makes ongoing airway assessment and management difficult.

Any patient requiring airway management or ventilatory support requires ongoing patient monitoring. Continuous pulse oximetry should be performed on all trauma patients during transport, and capnography should be strongly considered for all intubated patients. Loss of end-tidal CO_2 ($ETCO_2$) indicates that the ventilator circuit has become disconnected or, more importantly, the endotracheal tube has been dislodged, or the patient's perfusion has decreased significantly. All of these possible causes require immediate action. Serial vital signs should also be recorded on patients requiring airway or ventilation interventions. Confirmation of endotracheal intubation, as described above, should be performed each time the patient is moved or repositioned. It is also a good idea to frequently confirm the security of any airway device.

Any patient who requires increasing FiO_2 or PEEP in order to maintain oxygenation needs to be carefully re-evaluated. Possible etiologies include the development of a pneumothorax or worsening of pulmonary contusions. Any known or suspected pneumothorax must be monitored closely for the development of a tension pneumothorax, and pleural decompression should be performed if hemodynamic compromise occurs. Burn patients should receive supplemental oxygen to maintain SpO_2 $\geq 95\%$, whereas those with known or suspected carbon monoxide poisoning should receive 100% oxygen. Remember that positive pressure ventilation can convert a simple pneumothorax to a tension pneumothorax. If the patient has had an open pneumothorax sealed, the dressing should be opened to release any pressure that may have accumulated. Prior to embarking on a prolonged transport of a patient, potential oxygen needs should be calculated, and sufficient amounts of oxygen should be available for the transport. A good rule of thumb is to bring 50% more oxygen than anticipated.

Intermittent sedation may be required for an agitated intubated patient. Sedation may also decrease the work of breathing and any "fighting the ventilator" when mechanical ventilation is being used. Small doses of benzodiazepines should be titrated intravenously. The use of neuromuscular blocking agents may also be considered if the patient is significantly combative, the airway is secured with an endotracheal tube, *and* prehospital care personnel are properly trained and credentialed.

SUMMARY

The trauma patient is susceptible to various injuries that may impair ventilation and gas exchange. Trauma to the chest, airway obstruction, central nervous system injury, and hemorrhage can all result in inadequate tissue perfusion. Proper care for the trauma patient requires that the provider understands or has the ability to:

- Integrate the principles of ventilation and gas exchange with the pathophysiology of trauma to identify patients with inadequate perfusion.
- Relate the concepts of minute volume and oxygenation to the pathophysiology of trauma.
- Explain the mechanisms by which supplemental oxygen and ventilatory support are beneficial to the trauma patient.
- Given situations that involve various trauma patients, formulate a plan for airway management and ventilation.

- Given current research, understand the risks versus benefits when discussing new, invasive procedures.
- Determine by examination of the patient the relative difficulty of endotracheal intubation.
- Given a scenario, can develop a plan for airway management on a given patient in a given location.

Managing the airway is not without risks. When applying certain skills and modalities, the risk has to be weighed against the potential benefit for that particular patient. What may be the best choice for one patient in a certain situation may not be for another with a similar presentation. Sound critical-thinking skills need to be in place to make the best judgments for the trauma patient.

SCENARIO SOLUTION

Physical evidence at the scene suggests that the driver has likely been subjected to kinetic forces capable of creating life-threatening injuries. The position of the patient suggests that multiple impacts have occurred.

The patient exhibits several signs of airway compromise and ventilatory insufficiency. His ventilations are sonorous and irregular, he has an altered level of consciousness, and he requires frequent suctioning. Bleeding from the nares and ears and the early presence of "raccoon eyes" strongly suggest the presence of a basilar skull fracture. The primary survey indicates a rapidly deteriorating patient who requires aggressive airway care and rapid transport.

First responder personnel are already administering oxygen with ventilatory assistance using a bag-mask without difficulty. Continue ventilatory support and cervical spine stabilization while assessing the difficulty for endotracheal intubation. Be careful to ensure that the airway remains clear and that manual ventilations are effective.

After assessing the patient's airway for the difficulty of an intubation attempt, you determine that it will be a difficult intubation. You decide that, due to the 4-minute transport time, the anticipated high difficulty intubating the patient, and the ease in which bag-mask ventilations are being administered, you will manage the patient's airway and breathing with a bag-mask and OPA. You establish intravenous access while the patient is en route to a trauma receiving facility. You take care to maintain the effectiveness of immobilization efforts and frequently reassess the patient's condition. To ensure proper activation of the receiving facility's trauma response, you notify the trauma center during transport. On arrival at the trauma center, you concisely convey all pertinent information regarding the incident, the patient, and medical interventions to the receiving physician or other appropriate trauma team member. ■

References

1. Stockinger ZT, McSwain NE Jr. Prehospital endotracheal intubation for trauma does not improve survival over bag-mask ventilation. *J Trauma* 56(3):531, 2004.
2. Garza AG, Gratton MC, Coontz D, et al. Effect of paramedic experience on orotracheal intubation success rates. *J Emerg Med* 25(3):251, 2003.
3. Dickinson ET, Cohen JE, Mechem CC. The effectiveness of midazolam as a single pharmacologic agent to facilitate endotracheal intubation by paramedics. *Prehosp Emerg Care* 3(3):191, 1999.
4. Wang HE, Davis DP, O'Connor RE, et al. Drug-assisted intubation in the prehospital setting. *Prehosp Emerg Care* 10(2):261, 2006.
5. Davis DP, Hoyt DB, Ochs M, et al. The effect of paramedic rapid sequence intubation on an outcome in patients with severe trauma brain injury. *J Trauma* 54:444, 2003.
6. Davis DP, Dunford JV, Poste JC, et al. The impact of hypoxia and hyperventilation on outcome after paramedic rapid sequence intubation of severely head-injured patient. *J Trauma* 57:1, 2004.
7. O'Connor RE, Swor RA. Verification of endotracheal tube placement following intubation. *Prehosp Emerg Care* 3:248, 1999.
8. Frame SB, Simon JM, Kerstein MD, et al. Percutaneous transtracheal catheter ventilation (PTCV) in complete airway obstruction: a canine model. *J Trauma* 29:774, 1989.
9. American College of Surgeons Committee on Trauma. Airway management and ventilation. In *Advanced trauma life support for doctors, student course manual*, ed 7, Chicago, 2004, ACS.
10. Silvestri S, Ralis GA, Krauss B, et al: The effectiveness of out-of-hospital use of continuous end-tidal carbon dioxide monitoring on the rate of unrecognized misplaced intubations within a regional emergency medical services system. *Ann Emerg Med* 45:497, 2005.

Suggested Reading

American College of Surgeons Committee on Trauma: *Advanced trauma life support for doctors, student course manual,* ed 7, Chicago, 2004, ACS.

Brainard C: Whose tube is it? *JEMS* 31:62, 2006.

Dunford JV, David DP, Ochs M, et al: The incidence of transient hypoxia and heart rate reactivity during paramedic rapid sequence intubation. *Ann Emerg Med* 42:721, 2003.

Soubani AO: Noninvasive monitoring of oxygen and carbon dioxide. *Am J Emerg Med* 19:141, 2001.

Walls RM, Murphy MF (editors): *Manual of Emergency Airway Management,* ed 3, Philadelphia, 2008, Lippincott Williams Wilkins Publishers/Wolters Kluwer Health.

Weitzel N, Kendal J, Pons P: Blind nasotracheal intubation for patients with penetrating neck trauma. *J Trauma* 56(5):1097, 2004.

SPECIFIC SKILLS

Airway Management and Ventilation Skills

Trauma Jaw Thrust

Principle: To open the airway without moving the cervical spine.

In both the trauma jaw thrust and the trauma chin lift, manual neutral in-line stabilization of the head and neck is maintained while the mandible is moved anteriorly (forward). This maneuver moves the tongue forward, away from the hypopharynx, and holds the mouth slightly open.

From a position above the patient's head, the prehospital care provider positions his or her hands on either side of the patient's head, fingers pointing caudad (toward the patient's feet).

Depending on the size of the provider's hands, the fingers are spread across the face and around the angle of the patient's mandible.

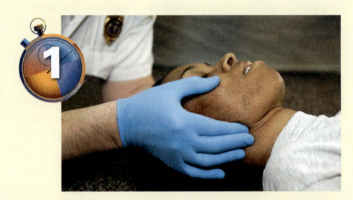

Gentle, equal pressure is applied with these digits to move the patient's mandible anteriorly (forward) and slightly downward (toward the patient's feet).

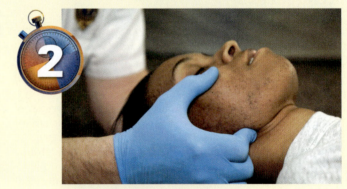

Alternate Trauma Jaw Thrust

Principle: To open the airway without moving the cervical spine.

The trauma jaw thrust can also be performed while positioned beside the patient, facing toward the patient's head. The provider's fingers point cephalad (toward the top of the patient's head). Depending on the size of the provider's hands, the fingers are spread across the face and around the angle of the patient's mandible. Gentle, equal pressure is applied with these digits to move the patient's mandible anteriorly (forward) and slightly downward (toward the patient's feet).

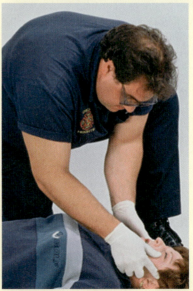

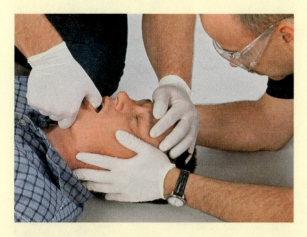

Trauma Chin Lift 💿

Principle: To open the airway without moving the cervical spine.

From a position above the patient's head, the patient's head and neck are moved into a neutral in-line position, and manual stabilization is maintained. The prehospital care provider positions himself or herself at the patient's side between the patient's shoulders and hips, facing the patient's head. With the hand closest to the patient's feet, the provider grasps the patient's teeth or the lower mandible between his or her thumb and first two fingers beneath the patient's chin. The provider now pulls the patient's chin anteriorly and slightly caudad, elevating the mandible and opening the mouth.

Oropharyngeal Airway

Principle: An adjunct used to maintain an open airway mechanically in a patient without a gag reflex.

The oropharyngeal airway (OPA) is designed to hold the patient's tongue anteriorly out of the pharynx. The OPA is available in various sizes. Proper sizing to the patient is required to ensure a patent airway. *Placement of an OPA in the hypopharynx is contraindicated in patients who have an intact gag reflex.*

Two methods for insertion of the OPA are effective: the tongue jaw lift insertion method and the tongue blade insertion method. Regardless of which method is used, the first provider stabilizes the patient's head and neck in a neutral in-line position while the second provider measures and inserts the OPA.

SPECIFIC SKILLS

Tongue Jaw Lift Insertion Method

The first provider brings the patient's head and neck into a neutral in-line position and maintains stabilization while opening the patient's airway with a trauma jaw thrust maneuver. The second provider selects and measures for a properly sized OPA. The distance from the corner of the patient's mouth to the earlobe is a good estimate for proper size.

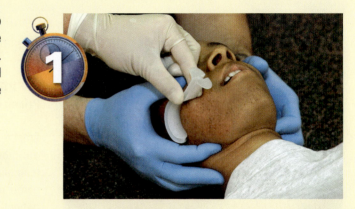

The patient's airway is opened with the chin lift maneuver. The OPA is turned so that the distal tip is pointing toward the top of the patient's head (flanged end pointing toward patient's head) and tilted toward the mouth opening.

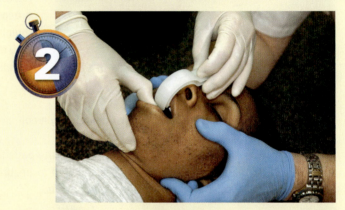

The OPA is inserted into the patient's mouth and rotated to fit the contours of the patient's anatomy.

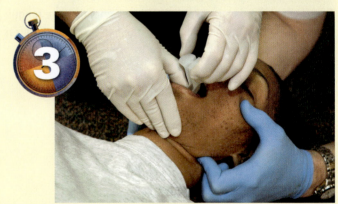

The OPA is rotated until its inside curve is resting against the tongue and holding it out of the posterior pharynx. The flanges of the OPA should be resting against the outside surface of the patient's teeth.

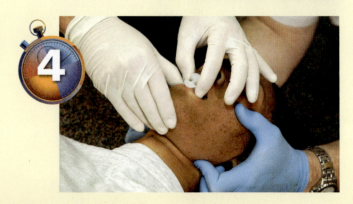

Tongue Blade Insertion Method

The tongue blade insertion method is probably a safer method than the tongue jaw lift because it eliminates the accidental tearing or puncturing of gloves or skin by sharp, pointed, or broken teeth. This method also eliminates the possibility of being bitten if the patient's level of consciousness (LOC) is not as deep as previously assessed or if any seizure activity occurs.

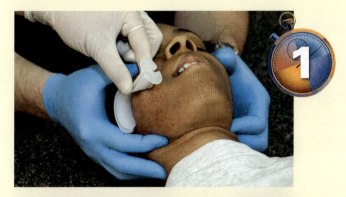

The first provider brings the patient's head and neck into a neutral in-line position and maintains stabilization while opening the patient's airway with the trauma jaw thrust maneuver. The second provider selects and measures for a properly sized OPA.

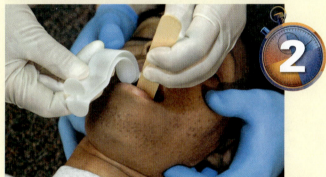

The second provider pulls the patient's mouth open by the chin and places a tongue blade into the patient's mouth to move the tongue forward in place and keep the airway open.

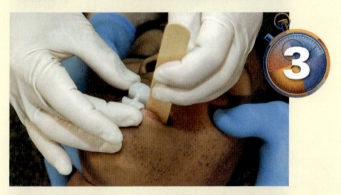

The device is inserted with the flanged end pointing toward the patient's feet and the distal tip pointing into the patient's mouth, following the curvature of the airway.

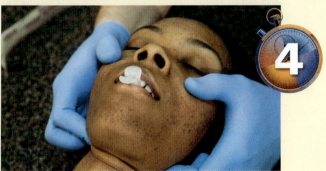

The OPA is advanced until the flanged end of the OPA rests against the outside surface of the patient's teeth.

SPECIFIC SKILLS

Nasopharyngeal Airway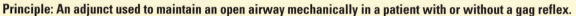

Principle: An adjunct used to maintain an open airway mechanically in a patient with or without a gag reflex.

The nasopharyngeal airway (NPA) is a simple airway adjunct that provides an effective way to maintain a patent airway in patients who may still have an intact gag reflex. Most patients will tolerate the NPA if properly sized. NPAs are available in a range of diameters (internal diameters of 5–9 mm), and the length varies appropriately with the size of the diameter. NPAs are usually made of a flexible, rubberlike material. Rigid NPAs are not recommended for field use.

The first provider brings the patient's head and neck into a neutral in-line position and maintains stabilization while opening the patient's airway with the trauma jaw thrust maneuver. A second provider examines the patient's nostrils with a light and selects the one that is the largest and least deviated or obstructed (usually the right nostril). The second provider selects the appropriately sized NPA for the patient's nostril, a size slightly smaller in diameter than the size of the nostril opening (frequently the diameter of the patient's little finger).

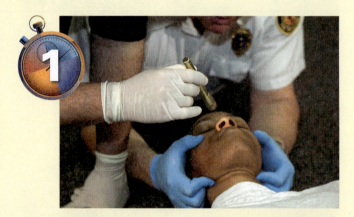

The length of the NPA is also important. The NPA needs to be long enough to supply an air passage between the patient's tongue and the posterior pharynx. The distance from the patient's nose to the earlobe is a good estimate for proper size.

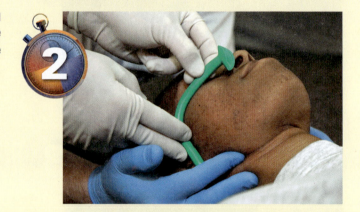

The distal tip (nonflanged end) of the NPA is lubricated liberally with a water-soluble jelly.

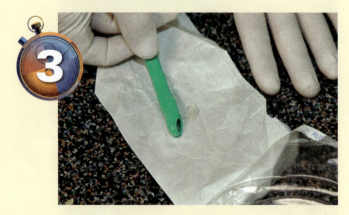

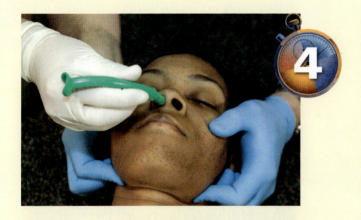

The NPA is slowly inserted into the nostril of choice. Insertion should be in an anterior-to-posterior direction along the floor of the nasal cavity, not in a superior-to-inferior direction. If resistance is met at the posterior end of the nostril, a gentle back-and-forth rotation of the NPA between the fingers will usually aid in passing beyond the turbinate bones of the nasal cavity without damage. Should the NPA continue to meet with resistance, the NPA should not be forced past the obstruction but rather should be withdrawn, and the distal tip should be relubricated and inserted into the other nostril.

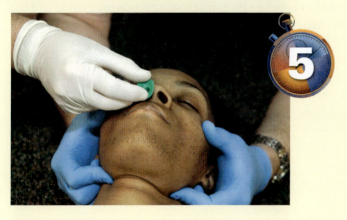

The second provider continues insertion until the flange end of the NPA is next to the anterior nares or until the patient gags. If the patient gags, the NPA is withdrawn slightly.

SPECIFIC SKILLS

Bag-Mask Ventilation

Principle: The preferred method of providing assisted ventilation.

Ventilation using a bag-mask system has an advantage over other ventilatory support systems because it gives a prehospital care provider feedback by the feel of the bag (compliance). Positive feedback ensures the operator of successful ventilations; changes in the feedback indicate a loss of mask seal, the presence of a pathologic airway, or a thoracic problem interfering with the delivery of successful ventilations. This "feel" and the control it provides also make the bag-mask suitable for assisting ventilations. The bag-mask's portability and readiness for immediate use make it useful for immediate delivery of ventilations on identification of the need.

Without supplemental oxygen, however, a bag-mask provides an oxygen concentration of only 21%, or a fraction of inspired oxygen (FiO_2) of 0.21; as soon as time allows, an oxygen reservoir and high-concentration supplemental oxygen should be connected to the bag-mask. When oxygen is connected without a reservoir, the FiO_2 is limited to 0.50 or less; with a reservoir, the FiO_2 is 0.85 or greater.

If the patient being ventilated is unconscious without a gag reflex, a properly sized oropharyngeal airway should be inserted before attempting to ventilate with the bag-mask. If the patient has an intact gag reflex, a properly sized nasopharyngeal airway should be inserted before attempting to assist ventilations.

Various bag-mask devices are available, including disposable single-patient-use models that are relatively inexpensive. Different brands have varying bag, valve, and reservoir designs. All the parts used should be of the same model and brand because these parts are usually not safely interchangeable.

Bag-mask units are available in adult, pediatric, and neonatal sizes. Although an adult bag can be used with the properly sized pediatric mask in an emergency, use of the correct bag size is recommended as a safe practice. Adequate ventilations of an adult patient are achieved when a minimum of 800 ml/breath is delivered (1000–1200 ml/breath preferred).

When ventilating with any positive-pressure device, inflation should stop once the chest has risen maximally. When using the bag-mask, the chest should be visualized for maximum inflation and the bag felt to recognize any marked increased resistance in the bag when lung expansion is at its maximum. Adequate time for exhalation is needed (1:3 ratio between time for inhalation and time for exhalation). If enough time is not allowed, "stepped or stacked breaths" occur, providing a greater volume of inspiration than expiration. Stepped breaths produce poor air exchange and result in hyperinflation, increased pressure, opening of the esophagus, and gastric distension.

Two-Provider Method

Two or more prehospital care providers performing ventilations with a bag-mask device is easier than with only one provider. The first provider can focus attention on maintaining an adequate mask seal, while the second provides good delivery volume by using both hands to squeeze (deflate) the bag.

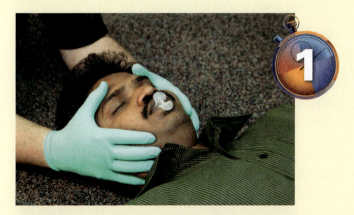

The first provider kneels above the patient's head and maintains manual stabilization of the patient's head and neck in a neutral in-line position.

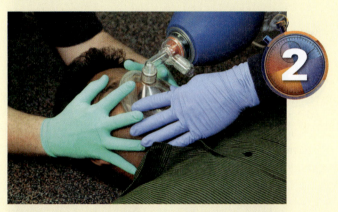

The facemask is placed over the patient's nose and mouth, and the mask is held in place with the thumbs on the lateral portion of the mask while pulling the mandible up into the mask. The other fingers provide the manual stabilization and maintain a patent airway.

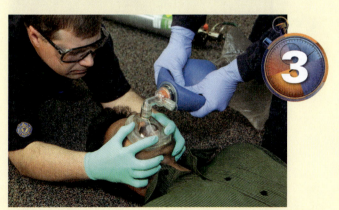

The second provider kneels at the side of the patient and squeezes the bag with both hands to inflate the lungs.

SPECIFIC SKILLS

Supraglottic Airway

Note: The Combitube and the King Airways are used in the following illustrations for demonstration purposes only. Other brands of supraglottic airways may be used as per local preference.

Combitube

Principle: A mechanical device used for opening and maintaining an airway when unable to intubate.

The supraglottic airway provides prehospital care providers with a functional alternative airway. These combination airways are an acceptable prehospital field device and typically do not require extensive training to achieve competency. The airway's greatest advantage is that it can be inserted independent of the patient's position ("blindly" inserted), which may be especially important in trauma patients with high suspicion of cervical injury. The indications for placement of a supraglottic airway are the same as for the placement of any airway: the necessity of obtaining a patent airway in a patient. Each manufacturer of the supraglottic airway will identify age and size requirements pertinent to their airway. The provider should always follow the manufacturer's recommendations for size selection, contraindications, and specific insertion procedures.

As with any other invasive airway, the patient is preoxygenated with a high concentration of oxygen using a simple airway adjunct or manual airway procedure before insertion of a supraglottic airway.

As with any other piece of medical equipment, the dual lumen should be inspected and each part tested before insertion. The distal end of the airway should be lubricated with a water-soluble lubricant.

The provider stops ventilations and removes all other airway adjuncts. If the patient is supine, the tongue and lower jaw are lifted upward with one hand (chin lift).

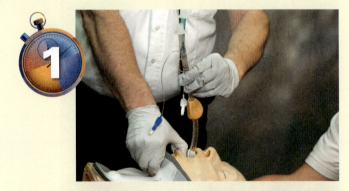

The end of the tube is inserted (tearing the cuff when inserting the airway past broken teeth or dental appliances should be avoided).

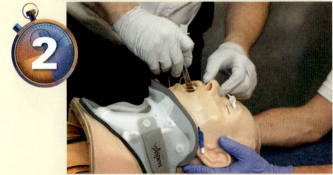

The Combitube is inserted until the marker rings line up with the patient's teeth.

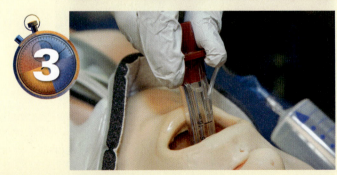

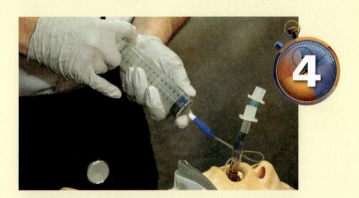

Using the large syringe, the pharyngeal cuff is inflated with 100 ml of air and the syringe removed. The device should seat itself in the posterior pharynx just behind the hard palate.

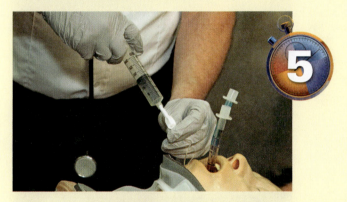

Using the small syringe, the distal cuff is inflated with 15 ml of air and the syringe removed. Typically the balloon will be placed (inflated) in the patient's esophagus. The provider begins ventilation through the esophageal tube (generally marked with a #1).

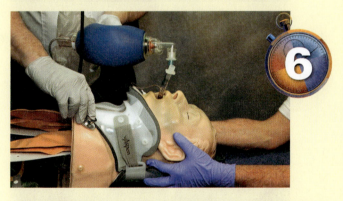

If auscultation of breath sounds is positive and gastric insufflation is negative, the provider continues ventilation through the esophageal tube.

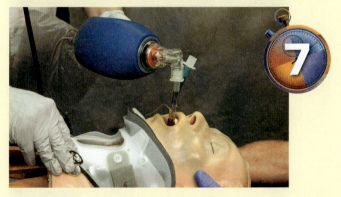

If auscultation of breath sounds is negative and gastric insufflation is positive, the provider immediately ventilates with the shortened tracheal tube (generally marked with a #2), after which reauscultation of breath sounds and gastric sounds is done to affirm proper tube placement. The provider continues to ventilate the patient and initiate immediate transport to an appropriate facility.

All esophageal airways require the patient to have no gag reflex. If the patient regains consciousness and begins to gag or vomit, these devices are removed immediately. Extubation of esophageal airways almost always causes vomiting or regurgitation. Consequently, suction equipment must be readily available when the device is removed. Observe Standard Precautions.

SPECIFIC SKILLS

King Airway
Principle: The King LT single lumen airway is a blindly inserted device used to provide ventilation of the traumatized patient.

It may be used in patients over 4 feet in height and in whom the risk of aspiration is considered to be low. The King LT is a single lumen tube with both a distal and oral (proximal) cuff. Unlike dual lumen airways, there is only one ventilatory tube and one cuff-inflation port. This simplifies the insertion procedure of this device. It should be noted that the KING LT does not provide protection from aspiration. In fact, the manufacturer lists lack of fasting as a contraindication to its use as well as "situations where gastric contents may be present (that) include, but are not limited to…multiple or massive injury, acute abdominal or thoracic injury…." Therefore, significant care must be taken to avoid aspiration when the King airway is used in these situations.

Choose the correct KING LT size, based on patient height. Test cuff-inflation system by injecting the maximum recommended volume of air into the cuff.

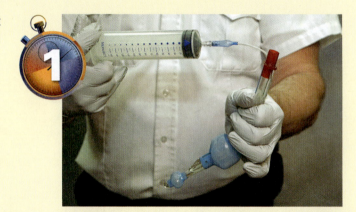

Apply a water-based lubricant to the beveled distal tip and posterior aspect of the tube. Pre-oxygenate. Hold the KING LT with dominant hand. With the non-dominant hand, hold the mouth open and apply chin lift while maintaining cervical spine stabilization.

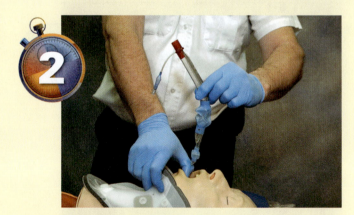

Introduce tip into mouth and advance behind the base of tongue. Rotate the tube back to the midline as the tip reaches the posterior wall of the pharynx.

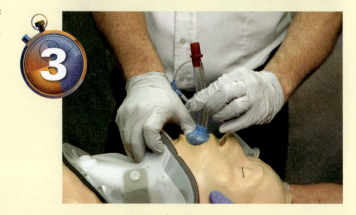

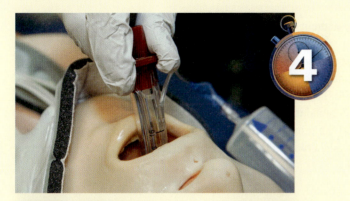

Advance KING LT until base of connector is aligned with teeth.

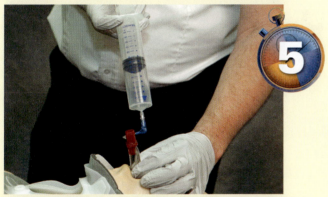

Inflate the cuffs. Typical inflation volumes are as follows:
Size 3 45–60ml
Size 4 60–80ml
Size 5 70–90ml

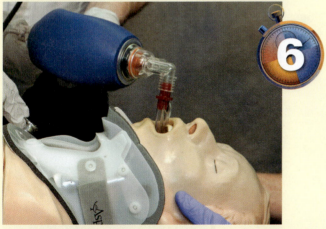

Attach a bag-mask to the KING LT. While gently ventilating the patient to assess ventilation, simultaneously withdraw the airway until ventilation is easy and free flowing (large tidal volume with minimal airway pressure). Reference marks are provided at the proximal end of the KING LT which, when aligned with the upper teeth, give an indication of the depth of insertion.

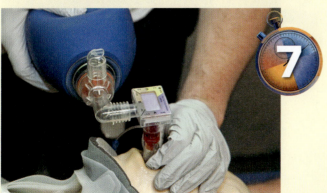

Confirm proper position by auscultation, chest movement and verification of CO_2 by capnography.

Readjust cuff inflation to 60 cm H_2O (or to just seal volume).

Secure KING LT to patient using tape or other accepted means. A bite block can also be used, if desired.

*Adapted from King LT manufacturer's instructions.

SPECIFIC SKILLS

Laryngeal Mask Airway 💿

Principle: A mechanical device used to maintain an open airway without direct visualization of the airway.

The LMA is an airway device that can be inserted by the prehospital provider without the need for direct visualization of the vocal cords. This blind insertion technique has advantages over endotracheal intubation as initial training requirements are less and skill retention is easier to accomplish. The disadvantage to the LMA is that although it forms a seal around the glottic opening, this seal is not as occlusive as that of an endotracheal tube cuff. Aspiration remains a potential problem. Another potential problem is that in order to insert an LMA, it is necessary for the provider to insert the provider's fingers into the mouth of the patient. This limits the usefulness of the LMA to fully unconscious patients. As with any airway in the trauma patient, cervical stabilization must be maintained for the duration of the procedure.

Deflate the cuff of the mask and apply a water-soluble lubricant to the posterior surface. Hold the LMA in the dominant hand, between the thumb and the other fingers, at the junction of the cuff and the tube.

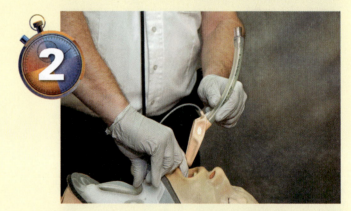

Grasp the mandible with the other hand and open the mouth. Insert the LMA into the mouth and press the tip of the cuff upward against the hard palate and flatten the cuff against it.

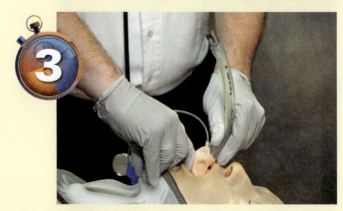

Guide (do not use force) the LMA into the mouth and advance it into the pharynx.

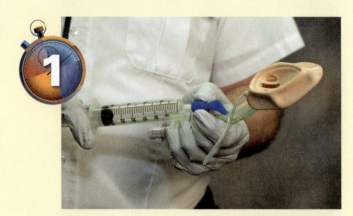

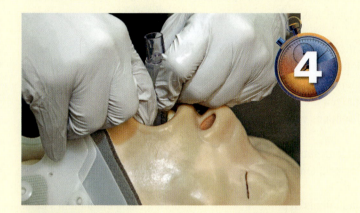

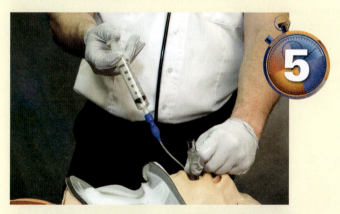

Continue to advance the LMA into the hypopharynx until a definite resistance is felt. Hold the end of the airway tube in place while removing your fingers from the patient's mouth.

Inflate the cuff with enough air to maintain a seal. Never over-inflate the cuff as this can cause damage to the airway structures.

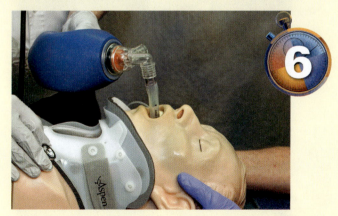

Attach a bag-mask device to the tube and confirm breath sounds with bagging.

SPECIFIC SKILLS

Visualized Orotracheal Intubation of the Trauma Patient

Principle: To secure a definitive airway without manipulating the cervical spine.

Visualized orotracheal intubation of the trauma patient is done with the patient's head and neck stabilized in a neutral in-line position. Orotracheal intubation while maintaining manual in-line stabilization requires additional training and practice beyond that for intubation of nontrauma patients. As with all skills, training requires observation, critique, and certification initially and at least twice a year by the medical director or designee.

In hypoxic trauma patients who are not in cardiac arrest, intubation should not be the initial airway maneuver. The provider should perform intubation only after he or she has preoxygenated the patient with a high concentration of oxygen using a simple airway adjunct or manual maneuver. Contact with the deep pharynx when intubating a severely hypoxic patient without preoxygenation can easily produce vagal stimulation, resulting in a dangerous bradycardia.

The provider should not interrupt ventilation for more than 20 seconds when intubating the patient. Ventilation should never be interrupted for more than 30 seconds for any reason.

Visualized orotracheal intubation is extremely difficult in conscious patients or patients with an intact gag reflex. The provider should consider use of topical anesthesia or paralytic agents after additional training, protocol development, and approval by the EMS medical director.

For the novice provider, the use of a straight laryngoscope blade tends to produce less rotary force (pulling the patient's head toward a "sniffing" position) than that produced by the use of a curved blade. However, because the success rate of intubation is often related to the provider's comfort with a given design, the style of blade selection for the laryngoscope remains a matter of individual preference.

Note: The cervical collar will limit forward motion of the mandible and complete opening of the mouth. Therefore, after adequate spinal immobilization is ensured, the cervical collar is removed, manual stabilization of the cervical spine is held, and intubation is attempted. Once intubation is accomplished the collar is reapplied.

Before attempting intubation, the providers should assemble and test all required equipment and follow Standard Precautions. The first provider kneels at the patient's head and ventilates the patient with a bag-mask and high-concentration oxygen. The second provider, kneeling at the patient's side, provides manual stabilization of the patient's head and neck.

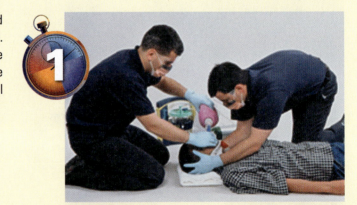

After preoxygenation, the first provider stops ventilations and grasps the laryngoscope in the left hand and the endotracheal (ET) tube (with syringe attached to pilot valve) in the right hand. If a stylet is used, this should have been inserted when the equipment was inspected and tested. The distal end of the stylet should be inserted just short of the ET tube's distal opening.

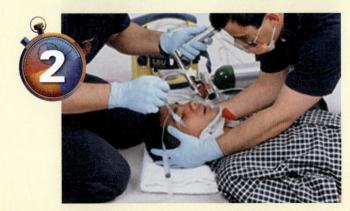

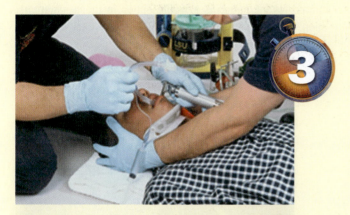

The laryngoscope blade is inserted into the right side of the patient's airway to the correct depth, sweeping toward the center of the airway while observing the desired landmarks.

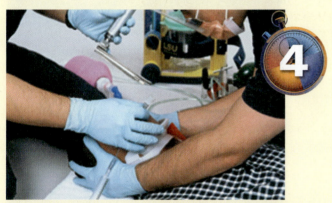

After identification of desired landmarks, the ET tube is inserted between the patient's vocal cords to the desired depth. The laryngoscope is then removed while holding the ET tube in place; the depth marking on the side of the ET tube is noted. If a malleable stylet has been used, it should be removed at this time.

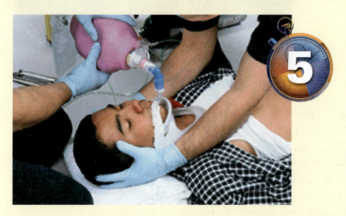

The pilot valve is inflated with enough air to complete the seal between the patient's trachea and the cuff of the ET tube (usually 8–10 ml of air), and the syringe is removed from the pilot valve. The first provider attaches the bag-valve system with a reservoir attached to the proximal end of the ET tube, and ventilation is resumed while observing the rise of the patient's chest with each delivered breath. Manual stabilization of the patient's head and neck is maintained throughout the process. Bilateral breath sounds and absence of air sounds over the epigastrium and other indications of proper ET tube placement (as described in the earlier section entitled **Verification of Endotracheal-Tube Placement page 148)** including wave form capnography are checked. Once tube placement is confirmed, the ET tube is secured in place. Although the use of tape or other commercially available devices is adequate in controlled situations in which the patient is not moved, *the best way to guard against displacement of the ET tube in the prehospital situation is to physically hold onto the tube at all times.*

SPECIFIC SKILLS

Face-to-Face Orotracheal Intubation

Principle: An alternative method of securing a definitive airway when patient positioning limits use of traditional methods.

Situations may arise in the prehospital setting in which the provider cannot take a position above the patient's head to initiate endotracheal intubation in a traditional manner. The face-to-face method for intubation is a viable option in these situations. The basic concepts of intubation still apply with face-to-face intubation: preoxygenate the patient with a bag-mask and high-concentration oxygen before attempting intubation, maintain manual stabilization of the patient's head and neck throughout the intubation, and do not interrupt ventilation for longer than 20 to 30 seconds at a time.

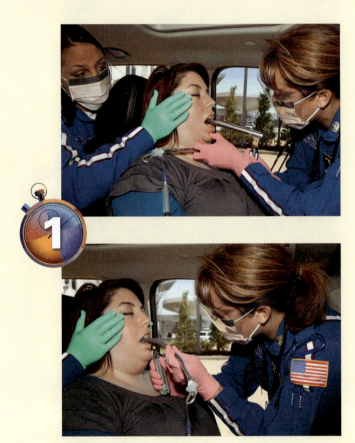

While manual stabilization of the patient's head and neck in a neutral in-line position is held, the prehospital care provider positions himself or herself in front of the patient, "face to face." The laryngoscope is held in the right hand with the blade on the patient's tongue. The blade moves the tongue down and out rather than up and out. The patient's airway is opened with the left hand, and the laryngoscope is placed into the patient's airway. After the laryngoscope blade is placed in the patient's airway, the desired landmarks are found. Looking into the airway from a position above the open airway provides the best view.

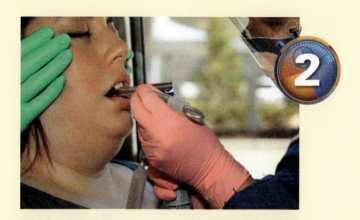

2 After identification of desired landmarks, the ET tube is passed between the patient's vocal cords to the desired depth with the left hand. The cuff is inflated with air to form the seal, and the syringe is removed. A bag-valve device is attached, and placement of the ET tube is confirmed.

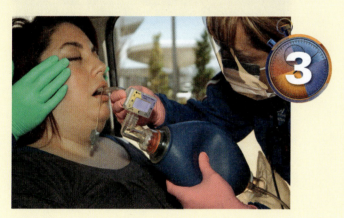

3 After confirmation of ET tube placement, the patient is ventilated while the provider holds onto the ET tube and maintains manual stabilization of the patient's head and neck. The ET tube should then be secured into place.

An alternative method for face-to-face intubation is to hold the laryngoscope in the left hand and place the ET tube with the right hand. This method may block the visualization of the lower airway as the ET tube is placed.

SPECIFIC SKILLS

Needle Cricothyrotomy and Percutaneous Transtracheal Ventilation

Principle: A method of providing oxygenation to a patient who cannot be intubated or ventilated with a bag-mask.

All parts except the needle, tank, and regulator should be modified as needed, preassembled, and packaged for ready availability in the field. This will ensure successful assembly. When this technique is needed, time will be of the essence. The equipment should be ready to use, requiring only connection to the regulator and needle. The prehospital care provider can use a commercially available product that contains all of the necessary equipment. If this is not available, the following equipment is required:

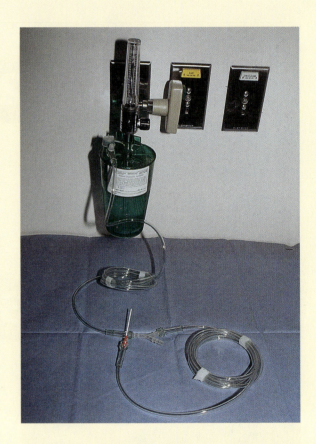

- Syringe: 10 to 30 ml
- To allow for inflation and deflation of the lung while there is constant flow from the oxygen source, some type of bypass is necessary. The following are two examples:
  1. A hole approximately 40% of the circumference of the oxygen delivery tube, cut in the side, that can be occluded by the thumb
  2. A plastic "T" or "Y" connector of a size compatible with the oxygen tubing used and connected to the oxygen source with a length of standard universal oxygen tubing
- A short piece of tubing that will fasten over the lower end of the "T" or "Y" and snugly fit into the hub of the needle (This leaves one opening of the "T" or "Y" connector free with nothing attached to it.)
- An oxygen tank with a regulator that has a 50 psi delivery pressure at its supplemental oxygen nipple
- Strips of $\frac{1}{2}$-inch adhesive tape

The patient should be in the supine position while manual in-line stabilization is maintained.

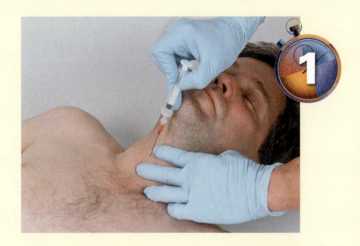

The larynx and trachea are stabilized with the fingers of one hand. The needle, attached to the syringe, is placed midline over the cricothyroid membrane or directly into the trachea at a slightly downward angle. As the needle is inserted into the trachea, the plunger of the syringe is withdrawn to create a negative pressure. Once the needle enters into the trachea, air will be sucked into the syringe, confirming that the tip of the needle is properly located. The needle is advanced an additional centimeter, and then the syringe is removed from the needle. The inner needle is removed, leaving the catheter in place. The provider quickly forms a loop with adhesive tape around the needle or the hub of the catheter and places the ends of tape on the patient's neck to secure the airway. The provider should use caution when securing the catheter to prevent kinking it.

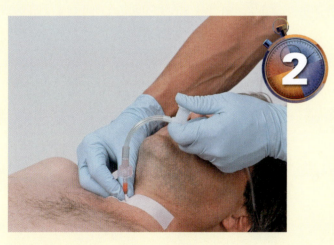

The oxygen delivery tube with a vent is connected to the hub of the needle while the hand that initially stabilized the trachea is moved to hold the needle in place. Ventilation is begun by occluding the opening of the tubing assembly with the thumb for 1 second. The patient's chest may or may not rise to indicate that inhalation is occurring. To stop the flow of oxygen into the lungs, the thumb is removed from the opening.

Note: The passive process of exhalation takes three to four times as long as inhalation with a normal airway. In this process, exhalation will require a longer time period because of the smaller opening.

The patient is oxygenated by alternately closing the hole to provide the positive flow of oxygen for inhalation and opening the same hole to stop the oxygen flow and allow deflation. The proper time sequence for these maneuvers is 1 second of occlusion of the opening for inhalation and 4 seconds of leaving the hole open for passive deflation. This process is continued until a more definitive airway is established.

After percutaneous transtracheal ventilation (PTV) of 45 to 60 minutes, this technique can provide a high $Paco_2$ level because of carbon dioxide retention as a result of the restricted expirations. Therefore, the patient should have a more definitive airway established as soon as possible.

Warning: *Patients being ventilated using PTV may remain hypoxic and unstable. Prehospital care providers should initiate transportation to a suitable facility without delay because the patient is in urgent need of a more definitive surgical transtracheal procedure (cricothyroidotomy) for adequate ventilation and oxygenation.*

CHAPTER 8

Shock

CHAPTER OBJECTIVES

At the completion of this chapter, the reader will be able to do the following:

✓ Define shock.

✓ Explain how preload, afterload, and contractility affect cardiac output.

✓ Classify shock on an etiologic basis.

✓ Explain the pathophysiology of shock and its progression through phases.

✓ Relate shock to energy production, etiology, prevention, and treatment

✓ Describe the physical findings in shock.

✓ Clinically differentiate the different types of shock.

✓ Discuss the limitations of the field management of shock.

✓ Recognize the need for rapid transport and early definitive management in various forms of shock.

✓ Apply principles of management of shock in the trauma patient.

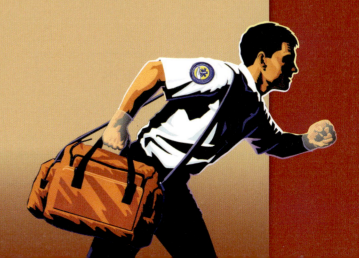

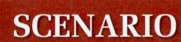

SCENARIO

You and you partner are dispatched to the scene of a multiple-victim shooting. The scene is in the middle of a dark street. Police are already present and state that the scene is secured. You find the first person with multiple bullet holes in his upper and lower back. He is breathing rapidly and you see air moving in and out of the holes in his chest. He is lying on top of a woman of similar age (late 20s). You roll him off her and note that he also has several wounds in his abdomen. One of the wounds in the anterior abdomen has a loop of bowel protruding. His pulse is weak and very fast. He has protected the female from the bullets with his body except for some bullet holes in her legs. You note that there is a large amount of blood running onto the pavement from one of the wounds of her legs at the knee.

What injuries do you expect in these patients? How would you manage them in the field? You are 15 minutes away from the nearest trauma center. How does this alter your management plans?

A lthough shock following trauma has been recognized for more than three centuries, its description by Samuel Gross in 1872 as a "rude unhinging of the machinery of life"[1] and by John Collins Warren as "a momentary pause in the act of death"[2] emphasizes its continuing central role in the causes of major morbidity and mortality in the trauma patient. Prompt diagnosis, resuscitation, and definitive management of shock resulting from trauma are all essential in determining patient outcome. The prehospital care provider faces significant challenges in accomplishing all these essential actions for shock. To improve survival from shock, a clear understanding of the definition, pathophysiology, and clinical features is essential.

In the prehospital setting, the therapeutic challenge posed by the patient in shock is compounded by the need to assess and manage such patients in a relatively primitive, and sometimes dangerous, environment in which sophisticated diagnostic and management tools are either unavailable or impractical to apply. This chapter defines and classifies shock and describes the pathophysiologic changes present in shock to help direct management strategies. It emphasizes the importance of energy production and the preservation of aerobic metabolism in the manufacture of energy, which is the key to life.

Definition of Shock

Although it has many definitions, shock is most often regarded as a state of generalized cellular hypoperfusion in which the delivery of oxygen at the cellular level is inadequate to meet metabolic needs. Based on this definition, shock can be classified in terms of the determinants of cellular perfusion and oxygenation. An understanding of the cellular changes arising from this state of hypoperfusion, as well as the endocrine, microvascular, cardiovascular, tissue, and end-organ effects, will also assist in directing treatment strategies.

Probably no better definition exists today to describe the devastating impact of this process on the patient than that of Samuel Gross. More recent definitions tend to be concerned with identifying the mechanism of shock and the effects on the patient's homeostasis. They are more specific and perhaps give a better picture of the particular pathophysiology dysfunctions that take place. It is a basic tenet of prehospital care that shock is not defined as low blood pressure, rapid pulse rates, or cool, clammy skin; these are merely systemic manifestations of the entire pathologic process called shock. The correct definition of shock is a lack of tissue perfusion (oxygenation) at the cellular level that leads to anaerobic metabolism and loss of energy production needed to support life.

If the EMT, or any provider, is to understand this abnormal condition and be able to develop a treatment plan to prevent or reverse shock, it is important that he or she knows and understands what is happening to the body at a cellular level. The normal physiologic responses the body uses to protect itself from the development of shock must be understood, recognized, and interpreted. Only then can a rational approach for managing the problems of the patient in shock be developed. The critical word is "understand."

Shock can kill a patient in the field, the emergency department, the operating room, or in the intensive care unit. Although actual death may be delayed for several hours to several days or even weeks, the most common cause of that death is the failure of early resuscitation. The lack of perfusion of cells by oxygenated blood results in anaerobic metabolism and decreased function for organ survival. Even when some cells are initially spared, death can occur later, because the remaining cells are unable to carry out the function of that organ indefinitely. This chapter explains this phenomenon and presents methods to prevent such an outcome.

Physiology

Metabolism: The Human Motor

The human body consists of over 100 million cells and each one of these cells requires oxygen to function and produce energy. The cells take in oxygen and metabolize it through a complicated physiologic process that produces energy. The metabolism of the cell requires energy, and cells must have fuel—glucose—to carry out this process. As in any combustion event, a by-product is also produced. In the body, oxygen and glucose are metabolized to produce energy, water (H_2O), and carbon dioxide (CO_2).

This is similar to the process that occurs in a motor vehicle engine when gasoline and air are mixed and burned to produce energy, and carbon monoxide (CO) is created as a by-product. The motor moves the car, the heater warms the driver, and the electricity generated is used for the lights to show the road, all because of the burning of gasoline to produce energy.

Aerobic metabolism describes the use of oxygen by cells. This form of metabolism is the body's principle combustion process. It produces energy using oxygen in a complicated process known as the Krebs cycle. Cells in the body do contain an alternate power source. **Anaerobic metabolism** occurs without the use of oxygen. It is the back-up power system in the body and uses stored body fat as its energy source.

As a comparison, alternate fuel sources are also available in automobiles; it is possible to drive a car powered only by its battery and electric starting motor if air and gasoline are not available. The automobile could move only as long as the energy stored in the battery lasted. This movement would be much slower and much less efficient than that powered by gasoline and air. However, it would work, in a fashion, although the battery would soon run down and there would be no more energy to move the car, even if air and gasoline again became available. In the body, the problems with using anaerobic metabolism to provide power are similar to the disadvantages of using a battery to run an automobile: it can only run for a short time, it does not produce as much energy, it produces by-products that are harmful to the body, and it may ultimately be irreversible.

The major by-product of anaerobic metabolism is excessive amounts of acid. In addition, energy production is reduced 15-fold. If anaerobic metabolism is not reversed quickly, cells cannot continue to function and will die. If a sufficient number of cells in any one organ die, the entire organ ceases to function. If a large number of cells in an organ die, but not enough cells to kill it, the organ's function will be significantly reduced and the remaining cells in that organ will have to work even harder than usual to keep the organ functioning. These overworked cells may or may not be able to support the function of the entire organ. Even with some cells remaining, the organ may still die. An example is a patient who has suffered a heart attack. Blood flow and oxygen are shut off to one portion of the myocardium (heart muscle), and some cells of the heart die, thus decreasing cardiac output and the oxygen supply to the rest of the heart. This, in turn, causes a further reduction in oxygenation of the remaining heart cells. If not enough other cells remain or if they are not strong enough to take over the entire function of the heart to meet the blood flow needs of the body, heart failure can result. Unless major improvement in cardiac output and oxygenation occur, the patient eventually will not survive.

Another example of this deadly process occurs in the kidneys. When the kidneys are injured or are deprived of adequate oxygenated blood, some of the kidney cells begin to die and kidney function decreases. Other cells may be compromised yet continue to function for a while before dying. If enough cells die, the decreased level of function in the kidneys results in inadequate elimination of toxic byproducts of metabolism, further exacerbating cell death. If this systemic deterioration continues, more and more organs die and, eventually, the entire organism (the human) dies. Depending on the organ initially involved, the progression from cell death to organism death can be rapid or delayed. It can take as long as 2 or 3 weeks before the damage caused by hypoxia or hypoperfusion in the first minutes posttrauma results in the patient's death. The effectiveness of the EMT's actions to reverse or prevent **hypoxia** (insufficient oxygen available to meet cell requirements) and **hypoperfusion** (inadequate blood passing to tissue cells) in the critical prehospital time period may not be immediately apparent. However, these resuscitation measures are unquestionably necessary if the patient is to ultimately survive. These initial actions are a critical component of the "golden hour" of trauma care referred to by R Adams Cowley, M.D.

The sensitivity of cells to the lack of oxygen and the usefulness of anaerobic metabolism varies from organ system to organ system. This sensitivity is called **ischemic** (lack of oxygen) sensitivity and it is greatest in the brain, heart, and lungs. It may take only 4 to 6 minutes of anaerobic metabolism before one or more of these vital organs are injured beyond repair. Skin and muscle tissue have a significantly longer ischemic sensitivity—as long as 4 to 6 hours. The abdominal organs generally fall between these two groups and are able to survive 45 to 90 minutes of anaerobic metabolism (Figure 8-1).

Long-term survival of the individual organs and the body as a whole requires delivery of important nutrients (oxygen and glucose) to the tissue cells. Other nutrients are also important, but because the resupply of these other materials is not a component of the prehospital EMS system, they are not discussed here. Although these factors are important, they are beyond the scope of the EMT's practice and resources. The most important supply item is oxygen.

FIGURE 8-1 Organ Tolerance to Ischemia

Organ	Warm Ischemia Time
Heart, brain, lungs	4–6 minutes
Kidneys, liver, gastrointestinal tract	45–90 minutes
Muscle, bone, skin	4–6 hours

(American College of Surgeons Committee on Trauma: *Advanced trauma life support for doctors, student course manual*, ed 7, Chicago, 2004, ACS.)

The Fick Principle

The Fick principle is a description of the components necessary for oxygenation of the body cells. Simply stated these three components are:

1. On-loading of oxygen to red blood cells (RBCs) in the lung
2. Delivery of RBCs to tissue cells
3. Off-loading of oxygen from RBCs to tissue cells

A crucial part of this entire process is that the patient must have enough red blood cells (RBCs) available to deliver adequate amounts of oxygen to tissue cells throughout the body, so that these cells can produce energy. Additionally, the patient's airway must be patent and adequate volume, and depth of respirations present. (See Chapter 7: Airway & Ventilation.)

The prehospital treatment of shock is directed at assuring that critical components of the Fick principle are maintained with the goal of preventing or reversing anaerobic metabolism, thus avoiding cellular death and, ultimately, patient death. These components should be the major emphasis of the prehospital care provider and are implemented in the management of the trauma patient by the following actions:

■ Maintaining an adequate airway and ventilation, thus providing adequate oxygen to the red blood cells
■ Judicious use of supplemental oxygen as part of ventilating the patient
■ Maintaining adequate circulation, thus perfusing tissue cells with oxygenated blood

The first component (oxygenation of the lungs and red blood cells) is covered in Chapter 7: Airway & Ventilation. The second component of the Fick principle involves perfusion, which is the delivery of blood to the tissue cells. A helpful analogy to use in describing perfusion is to think of the RBCs as transport vans, the lungs as oxygen warehouses, the blood vessels as roads and highways, and the body tissue cells as the oxygen's destination. An insufficient number of transport vans, obstructions along the roads and highways, and/or slow transport vans can all contribute to decreased oxygen delivery and the eventual starvation of the tissue cells.

The fluid component of the circulatory system—blood—contains not only RBCs but infection-fighting factors (white blood cells and antibodies), platelets and factors to support clotting in hemorrhage, protein for cellular rebuilding, nutrition in the form of glucose, and other substances necessary for metabolism and survival.

Classification of Shock

The prime determinants of cellular perfusion are: the heart (acting as the pump or the motor of the system); fluid volume (acting as the hydraulic fluid); the blood vessels (serving as the conduits or plumbing); and, finally, the cells of the body.

Based on these components of the perfusion system, shock may be classified into the following categories:

1. *Hypovolemic*—primarily hemorrhagic in the trauma patient, related to loss of circulating blood volume. This is the most common cause of shock in the trauma patient.
2. *Distributive* (or vasogenic)—related to abnormality in vascular tone arising from several different causes.
3. *Cardiogenic*—related to interference with the pump action of the heart.

By far the most common cause of shock in the trauma patient is hemorrhage, and the safest approach in managing the trauma patient in shock is to consider the cause of the shock as hemorrhagic until proven otherwise.

More detailed descriptions of these different types of shock follow after a discussion of the relevant anatomy and pathophysiology of shock.

Anatomy and Pathophysiology

Cardiovascular, Hemodynamic, and Endocrine Responses

Heart

The heart consists of two receiving chambers *(atria)* and two major pumping chambers *(ventricles)*. The function of the atria is to accumulate and store blood so that the ventricles can fill rapidly, minimizing delay in the pumping cycle. The right atrium receives blood from the veins of the body and pumps it to the right ventricle. With each contraction of the right ventricle (Figure 8-2), blood is pumped through the lungs for on-loading of oxygen to the red blood cells (RBC's) (Figure 8-3).

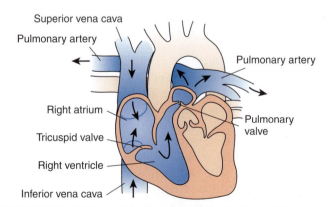

FIGURE 8-2 With each contraction of the right ventricle, blood is pumped through the lungs. Blood from the lungs enters the left side of the heart, and the left ventricle pumps it into the systemic vascular system.

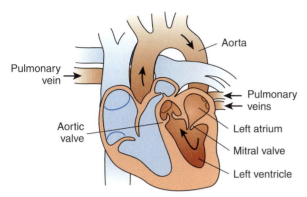

FIGURE 8-3 Blood returning from the lungs is pumped out of the heart and through the aorta to the rest of the body by left ventricular contraction.

The oxygenated blood from the lungs is returned to the left atrium and is pumped into the left ventricle. Then, the RBCs are pumped by the contractions of the ventricle throughout the arteries of the body to the tissue cells (Figure 8-4).

Although it is one organ, the heart actually has two subsystems. The right atrium, which receives blood from the body, and the right ventricle, which pumps blood to the lungs, are referred to as the "right heart." The left atrium, which receives oxygenated blood from the lungs, and the left ventricle, which pumps blood to the body, are referred to as the "left heart" (Figure 8.5). Preload (volume of blood entering into the heart) and afterload (pressure against which the blood has to push when it is squeezed out of the ventricle) of the right heart *(pulmonary)* and left heart *(systemic)* pumping systems are important concepts to understand.

Blood is forced through the circulatory system by the contraction of the left ventricle. This sudden pressure increase produces a pulse wave to push blood through the system. The peak of the pressure increase is the systolic blood pressure and represents the force of the pulse wave produced by ventricular contraction *(systole)*. The resting pressure in the vessels between ventricular contractions is the diastolic blood pressure and represents the force that remains in the blood vessels that continues to move blood through the vessels while the ventricle is refilling for the next pulse of blood

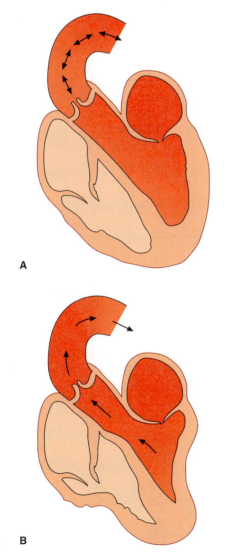

FIGURE 8-4 In a relaxed position (diastole), the ventricle fills with blood from the contractions of the atrium. During this time, blood is gradually flowing out of the major vessels as the pressure gradually decreases. During the contraction of the ventricle (systole), a large amount of blood flows into the vascular system, which raises the pressure. Cardiac action and blood flow is demonstrated in **A** and the pulse wave is seen in **B**.

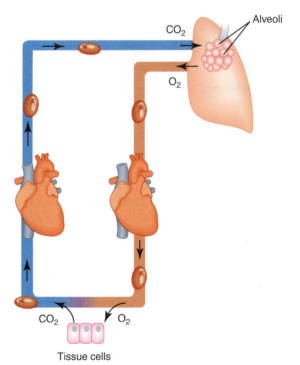

FIGURE 8-5 Although the heart seems to be one organ, it functions as if it were two organs. Unoxygenated blood is received into the "right heart" from the superior and inferior venae cavae and pumped through the pulmonary artery into the lungs. The blood is oxygenated in the lungs, flows back into the heart through the pulmonary vein, and is pumped out of the left ventricle.

(diastole). The difference between the systolic and diastolic pressures is called *pulse pressure.* This is the pressure of the blood as it is being pushed out into the circulation. It is the pressure felt against the finger tip as the pulse is checked.

Another term used in the discussion of shock management but often not emphasized in the prehospital setting is *mean arterial pressure* (MAP). This number gives a more realistic assessment of the overall pressure to produce blood flow than either the systolic or the diastolic pressures alone.

The MAP is the average pressure in the vascular system and is calculated as follows:

MAP = Diastolic pressure + ⅓ Pulse pressure

For example, the MAP of a patient with a blood pressure of 120/80 mm Hg is calculated as follows:

MAP = 80 + ([120 − 80]/3)
= 80 + (40/3)
= 80 + 13.3
= 93.3, rounded to 93

Many automatic, noninvasive blood pressure devices automatically calculate and report the MAP in addition to the systolic and diastolic pressures.

The volume of fluid pumped into the system with each contraction of the ventricle is called the *stroke volume,* and the volume of blood pumped into the system over 1 minute is called the *cardiac output.* The formula for cardiac output (CO) is as follows:

Cardiac output (CO) =
Heart rate (HR) × Stroke volume (SV)

Cardiac output is reported in liters per minute (LPM, or l/min). Cardiac output is not measured in the prehospital environment. However, understanding cardiac output and its relationship to stroke volume is important in understanding shock management. For the heart to work effectively, an adequate volume of blood must be present in the vena cava and pulmonary veins to fill the ventricles.

Starling's law of the heart is an important concept explaining how this relationship works. This pressure that fills the heart *(preload)* stretches the myocardial muscle fibers. The more the ventricles fill, the greater the strength of the contraction of the heart, until the point of overstretching. Significant hemorrhage or relative hypovolemia decreases cardiac preload so that a reduced volume of blood is present and the fibers are not stretched as much, resulting in a lower stroke volume. If the filling pressure of the heart is too great, the cardiac muscle fibers become overstretched and can fail to deliver a satisfactory stroke volume.

The resistance to blood flow that the left ventricle must overcome to pump blood out into the arterial system is called *afterload,* or systemic vascular resistance (SVR). As periph-

eral arterial vasoconstriction increases, the resistance to blood flow increases and the heart has to generate a greater force to pump blood into the arterial system. Conversely, widespread peripheral vasodilation decreases afterload.

The systemic circulation contains more capillaries and a greater length of blood vessels than the pulmonary circulation. Therefore, the left (or *left-sided*) heart system works at a higher pressure and bears a greater workload than the right (or *right-sided*) heart system. Anatomically, the muscle of the left ventricle is thicker and stronger than that of the right ventricle.

Blood Vessels

The blood vessels contain the blood and route it to the various areas and cells of the body. They are the "highways" of the physiologic process of circulation. The single, large exit tube from the heart, the *aorta,* cannot serve every individual cell in the body and, therefore, splits into multiple arteries of decreasing size, the smallest of which are the capillaries (Figure 8-6). A capillary may be only one cell wide; therefore, oxygen and nutrients carried by red blood cells (RBCs) and plasma are able to diffuse easily through the walls of the capillary into the tissue cell (Figure 8-7a). Each tissue cell has a membranous covering called the *cell membrane.* Interstitial fluid is located

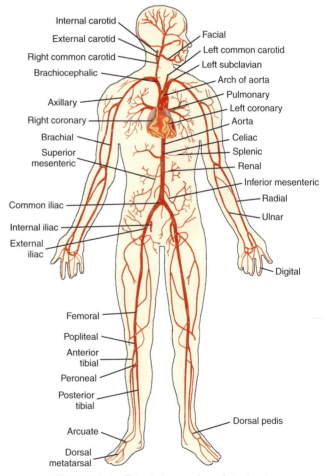

FIGURE 8-6   Principle arteries of the body.

between the cell membrane and the capillary wall. The amount of interstitial fluid varies tremendously. If little interstitial fluid is present, the cell membrane and the capillary wall are closer together and oxygen can easily diffuse between them (Figure 8-8). When there is extra fluid (edema) forced into this space (such as occurs in over resuscitation with crystalloid fluids), the cells move further away from the capillaries, making transfer of oxygen and nutrients less efficient (Figure 8-7b).

The size of the vascular "container" is controlled by smooth muscles in the walls of the arteries and arterioles and, to a lesser extent, by muscles in the walls of the venules and veins. These muscles respond to signals from the brain via the sympathetic nervous system, to the circulating hormones epinephrine and norepinephrine, and to other chemicals, such as nitric oxide (NO). Depending on whether they are being stimulated to contract or allowed to relax, these muscle fibers in the walls of the vessels result in either the constriction or dilation of the blood vessels, thus changing the size of the container component of the cardiovascular system and thus affecting the patient's blood pressure.

There are three fluid compartments: intravascular fluid (fluid that is inside the vessels), intracellular fluid (fluid that is inside the cells), and interstitial fluid (fluid that is between the cells and the vessels). Interstitial fluid in excess of normal amounts produces edema and causes the spongy, boggy feeling when the skin is compressed with a finger.

Blood

The fluid component of the circulatory system—the blood—contains not only RBCs but also infection-fighting factors (white blood cells [WBCs] and antibodies), platelets and clotting factors essential for blood clotting at times of vascular injury, protein for cellular rebuilding, nutrients such as glucose, and other substances necessary for metabolism and survival. The volume of fluid within the vascular system must

equal the capacity of the blood vessels if it is to adequately fill the container and maintain perfusion. Any variance in the volume of the vascular system container compared to the volume of blood in that container will affect the flow of blood either positively or negatively.

The human body is 60% water, which is the base of all body fluids. A person who weighs 154 pounds (70kg) contains approximately 40 liters of water. Body water is present in two components: intracellular and extracellular fluid. As noted above, each type of fluid has specific, important properties (Figure 8-9). *Intracellular fluid,* the fluid within the cells, accounts for approximately 45% of body weight. *Extracellular fluid,* the fluid outside the cells, can be further classified into two subtypes: interstitial fluid and intravascular

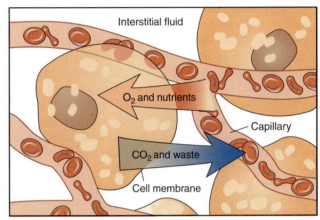

FIGURE 8-8   Oxygen and nutrients diffuse from the red blood cells through the capillary wall, the interstitial fluid, and the cell membrane into the cell. Acid production is a byproduct of cellular energy production during the Krebs cycle. By way of the buffer system of the body, this acid is converted into carbon dioxide and travels with the red blood cells and in the plasma to be eliminated from the circulatory system by the lungs.

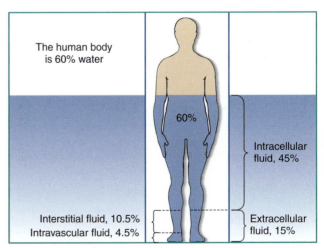

FIGURE 8-7   **A.** If the tissue cells are close to the capillary, oxygen can easily diffuse into them, and carbon dioxide can diffuse out. **B.** If tissue cells are separated from capillary walls by increased edema (interstitial fluid), it is much more difficult for the oxygen and carbon dioxide to diffuse.

FIGURE 8-9   Body water represents 60% of body weight. This water is divided into intracellular and extracellular fluid. The extracellular fluid is further divided into interstitial and intravascular fluid.

fluid. *Interstitial fluid,* which surrounds the tissue cells and also includes cerebrospinal fluid (found in the brain and spinal canal) and synovial fluid (found in the joints), accounts for approximately 10.5% of body weight. *Intravascular fluid,* which is found in the vessels and carries the formed components of blood as well as oxygen and other vital nutrients, accounts for approximately 4.5% of body weight.

A review of some key concepts is helpful in this discussion of how fluids operate in the body. Besides movement of fluid through the vascular system, there are two major types of fluid movement: (1) movement between the plasma and interstitial fluid (across capillaries); and (2) movement between the intracellular and interstitial fluid compartments (across cell membranes).

The movement of fluid across capillaries is determined by (1) the difference between the hydrostatic pressure within the capillary (which tends to push fluid out) and the hydrostatic pressure outside the capillary (which tends to push fluid in); (2) the difference in the oncotic pressure from protein concentration within the capillary (which keeps fluid in) and the oncotic pressure outside the capillary (which pulls fluid out); and (3) the "leakiness" or permeability of the capillary (Figure 8-10). Hydrostatic pressure, oncotic pressure, and capillary permeability are all affected by the shock state itself, as well as by the type and volume of fluid resuscitation, leading to alterations in circulating blood volume, hemodynamics, and tissue or pulmonary edema.

Movement of fluid between the intracellular and interstitial space occurs across cellular membranes, which is determined primarily by osmotic effects. *Osmosis* is the process by which solutes separated by a membrane to which the solutes are impermeable govern the movement of water across that semipermeable membrane based on the concentration of the solute. Water moves from the compartment of lower solute concentration to that of higher solute concentration to maintain osmotic equilibrium across the semipermeable membrane (Figure 8-11).

Nervous System

The *autonomic nervous system* directs and controls the involuntary functions of the body, such as respiration, digestion, and cardiovascular function. It is divided into two subsystems—the sympathetic and parasympathetic nervous systems. These systems oppose each other to keep vital body systems in balance.

The *sympathetic nervous system* produces the fight-or-flight response. This response simultaneously causes the heart to beat faster and stronger, increases the ventilatory rate, and constricts the blood vessels to nonessential organs (skin and gastrointestinal tract) while dilating vessels and improving blood flow to muscles. The goal of this response is to maintain sufficient amounts of oxygenated blood to critical tissues so that an individual can respond to an emergency situation while shunting blood away from nonessential areas. In contrast, the *parasympathetic system* slows the heart rate, decreases the ventilatory rate, and increases gastrointestinal activity.

In patients who are hemorrhaging after sustaining trauma, the body attempts to compensate for the blood loss. The cardiovascular system is regulated by the vasomotor center in the medulla. In response to a transient fall in blood pressure, stimuli travel to the brain via cranial nerves IX and X from stretch receptors in the carotid sinus and the aortic arch. This leads to increased sympathetic nervous system activity, with increased peripheral vascular resistance resulting from arteriolar constriction and increased cardiac output from an increased rate and force of cardiac contraction. Increased venous tone enhances circulatory blood volume. Blood is thus diverted from the extremities, bowel, and kidney to more vital areas—the heart and brain—in which vessels constrict very little under intense sympathetic stimulation. These responses result in cold, cyanotic extremities, decreased urine output, and decreased bowel perfusion.

A decrease in the left atrial filling pressure, a fall in blood pressure, and changes in plasma osmolality cause release of antidiuretic hormone (ADH) from the pituitary

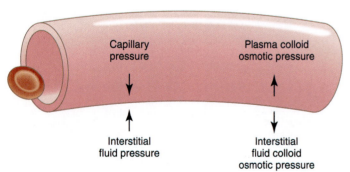

FIGURE 8-10 Forces governing fluid flux across capillaries.
(Source: From Guyton AC, Hall JE: *Textbook of medical physiology,* ed 10, Philadelphia, 2000, Saunders.)

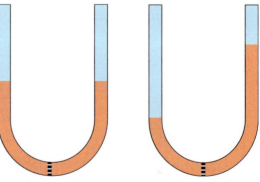

FIGURE 8-11 A U-tube, in which the two halves are separated by a semipermeable membrane, contains equal amounts of water and solid particles. If a solute that cannot diffuse through the semipermeable membrane is added to one side but not to the other, fluid will flow across to dilute the added particles. The pressure difference of the height of fluid in the U-tube is known as *osmotic pressure.*

gland and aldosterone from the adrenal glands, which enhances retention of sodium and water by the kidneys. This also helps to expand the intravascular volume; however, many hours are required for this mechanism to make a difference clinically.

Types of Shock

There are three types of shock:

- Hypovolemic shock
  - Vascular volume smaller than normal vascular size
    - Loss of fluid and electrolytes
      - Dehydration
    - Loss of blood and fluid
      - Hemorrhagic shock
- Distributive shock
  - Vascular space is larger than normal
    - Neurogenic "shock" (hypotension)
    - Psychogenic shock
    - Septic shock
    - Anaphylactic shock
- Cardiogenic shock
  - Pump failure

Hypovolemic Shock

Acute loss of blood volume, either from dehydration (loss of fluid and electrolytes) or hemorrhage (loss of plasma and RBCs), causes an imbalance in the relationship of fluid volume to the size of the container. The container retains its normal size, but the fluid volume is decreased. *Hypovolemic*

shock is the most common cause of shock encountered in the prehospital environment, and blood loss is by far the most common cause of shock in trauma patients and the most dangerous for the patient.

When blood is lost from the circulation, the heart is stimulated to increase cardiac output by increasing the strength and rate of contractions. This is caused by the release of *epinephrine* from the adrenal glands. The sympathetic nervous system releases *norepinephrine* to trigger constriction of the blood vessels to reduce the size of the container and bring it more into proportion with the volume of remaining fluid. Vasoconstriction results in closing of the peripheral capillaries, which reduces oxygen delivery, and forces the switch from aerobic to anaerobic metabolism at the cellular level.

These compensatory defense mechanisms work well up to a point. When the defense mechanisms can no longer compensate for the volume reduction, a patient's blood pressure will drop. A decrease in blood pressure marks the switch from compensated to decompensated shock—a sign of impending death. A patient who has signs of compensation such as tachycardia is already in shock, not "going into shock." Unless aggressive resuscitation occurs, the patient who enters decompensated shock has only one more stage of decline left—irreversible shock, leading to death.

Hemorrhagic Shock

Hemorrhagic shock (hypovolemic shock resulting from blood loss) can be categorized into four classes, depending on the severity of hemorrhage, as follows (Figure 8-12):

1. *Class I hemorrhage* represents a loss of up to 15% of blood volume in the adult (up to 750 ml). This stage has few clinical manifestations. Tachycardia is often mini-

FIGURE 8-12   Classification of Hemorrhagic Shock

	CLASS I	CLASS II	CLASS III	CLASS IV
Blood loss (mL)	Up to 750	750-1500	1500-2000	>2000
Blood loss (% blood volume)	Up to 15%	15%-30%	30%-40%	>40%
Pulse rate	<100	100-120	120-140	>140
Blood pressure	Normal	Normal	Decreased	Decreased
Pulse pressure (mm Hg)	Normal or increased	Decreased	Decreased	Decreased
Respiratory rate	14-20	20-30	30-40	>35
Urine output (mL/hr)	>30	20-30	5-15	Negligible
CNS/mental status	Slightly anxious	Mildly anxious	Anxious, confused	Confused, lethargic
Fluid replacement	Crystalloid	Crystalloid	Crystalloid and blood	Crystalloid and blood

(From American College of Surgeons Committee on Trauma: *Advanced trauma life support for doctors, student course manual,* ed 8, Chicago, 2008, ACS.)

mal, and no measurable changes in blood pressure, pulse pressure, or ventilatory rate occur. Most healthy patients sustaining this amount of hemorrhage require only maintenance fluid as long as no further blood loss occurs. The body's compensatory mechanisms restore the intravascular container/fluid volume ratio and assists in the maintenance of blood pressure.

2. *Class II hemorrhage* represents a loss of 15% to 30% of blood volume (750–1500 ml). Most adults are capable of compensating for this amount of blood loss by activation of the sympathetic nervous system which will maintain their blood pressure. Clinical findings include increased ventilatory rate, tachycardia, and a narrowed pulse pressure. The clinical clues to this phase are tachycardia, tachypnea, and normal systolic blood pressure. Because the blood pressure is normal, this is "compensated shock:" the patient is in shock but able to compensate for the time being. The patient often demonstrates anxiety or fright. Urine output drops slightly to between 20 and 30 ml/hour in an adult, although this is not usually measured in the field. On occasion, these patients may require blood transfusion; however, most will respond well to crystalloid infusion if hemorrhage is controlled at this point.

3. *Class III hemorrhage* represents a loss of 30% to 40% of blood volume (1500–2000 ml). When blood loss reaches this point, most patients are no longer able to compensate for the volume loss, and hypotension occurs. The classic findings of shock are obvious and include tachycardia (heart rate >120 beats/minute), tachypnea (ventilatory rate 30–40 breaths/minute), and severe anxiety or confusion. Urine output falls to 5 to 15 ml/hour. Many of these patients will require blood transfusion and surgical intervention for adequate resuscitation and control of hemorrhage.

4. *Class IV hemorrhage* represents a loss of more than 40% of blood volume (>2000 ml). This stage of severe shock is characterized by marked tachycardia (heart rate >140 beats/minute), tachypnea (ventilatory rate >35 breaths/minute), profound confusion or lethargy, and greatly decreased systolic blood pressure, typically in the range of 60 mm Hg. These patients truly have only minutes to live. Survival depends on immediate control of hemorrhage (surgery for internal hemorrhage) and aggressive resuscitation, including blood and plasma transfusions with minimal crystalloid.

The rapidity with which a patient develops shock depends on how fast blood is lost from the circulation. Bernoulli, a Swiss mathematician, developed the mathematical physics formula that calculates the rate of fluid loss from within a tube to the outside of the tube. The details are not required for the understanding of blood loss and the production of shock, but the basics of the principle are required. From a simplistic approach, the Bernoulli Principle says that the rate of fluid loss from a tube is directly proportional to the size of the hole in the wall of the tube and to the differential pressure of the intraluminal pressure versus the extraluminal pressure. These same principles apply to blood vessels.

Imagine the blood vessels as plumbing inside a home and the blood inside the vessels as water in the pipes. If the plumbing has a leak, the amount of water lost is directly related to the size of the hole and the difference in pressure inside and outside the pipe. For example, if the hole in the pipe is 1 inch (2.5cm) in diameter and the pressure inside the plumbing is 100 psi, more water will leak out than if the hole is 1 inch in diameter and the pressure inside the plumbing is 50 psi. Similarly, the blood flow from a wound in a vessel is proportional to the difference between the size of the hole in the vessel wall and the difference between intraluminal (inside the vessel) and extraluminal (outside the vessel) pressures.

The *definitive management for volume deficit* is to stop the fluid loss and replace the lost fluid. A dehydrated patient needs fluid replacement with water and salt, whereas a trauma patient who has lost blood needs to have the source of blood loss stopped and, if significant blood loss has occurred, blood replacement needs to be accomplished. Mild to moderate dehydration can be treated with an electrolyte solution that a conscious patient can drink. An unconscious or severely dehydrated patient should receive the replacement intravenously. Blood replacement is usually not available in the prehospital environment; therefore, trauma patients with hemorrhagic shock must have measures to control external blood loss instituted, receive minimal intravenous electrolyte solution, and receive rapid transportation to the hospital where blood, plasma, and clotting factors are available and emergent operative steps as necessary to control blood loss can be performed.

Shock research has demonstrated that for lost blood, the replacement ratio with electrolyte solution should be 3 liters of replacement for each liter of blood lost.[3] This is because only about ¼–⅓ of the volume of an isotonic crystalloid solution remains in the intravascular space 30–60 minutes after infusing it. The administration of a limited volume of electrolyte solution before blood replacement is the correct approach while en route to the hospital. The result of over-infusion of crystalloid is increased interstitial fluid (edema), resulting in reduced oxygen transfer to the remaining RBCs and into the tissue cells. The goal is NOT to raise the blood pressure to normal levels but to provide only enough fluid to maintain perfusion and continue to provide oxygenated RBCs to the heart, brain, and lungs. The best crystalloid solution for treating hemorrhagic shock is Ringer's Lactate solution (RL). Normal saline is another isotonic crystalloid solution that can be used for volume replacement, but its use may produce hyperchloremia (marked increase in the blood chloride level), leading to acidosis.

Newer research[4,5] has shown that with significant blood loss, the replacement fluid should ideally be as near to whole blood as possible. The first step is administration of packed RBCs and plasma at a ratio of 1:1 or 1:2. This is only available in the hospital in the civilian environment. Platelets, cryoprecipitate, and other clotting factors are added as needed. Plasma contains a large number of the clotting factors and other components needed to control blood loss from small vessels. There are 13 factors in the coagulation cascade. In patients with massive blood loss requiring large volumes of blood replacement, most of the factors have been lost. Plasma transfusion is a reliable source of most of these factors. If major blood loss has occurred, the control of hemorrhage from large vessels requires operative management or, in some cases, endovascular placements of coils or clotting sponges.

Distributive (Vasogenic) Shock

Distributive shock, or vasogenic shock, occurs when the vascular container enlarges without a proportional increase in fluid volume. Although the amount of intravascular fluid has not changed, relatively less fluid is available for the size of the container. As a result, the volume of fluid available for the heart to pump (preload) decreases and results in a decreasing cardiac output. In most situations, fluid has not been lost from the vascular system. This form of shock is not a cause of hypovolemia, in which fluid has been lost through hemorrhage, vomiting, or diarrhea. Instead, the problem is the size of the container which is now larger than the fluid available to fill it. For this reason, this condition is sometimes referred to as *relative hypovolemia.* Although some of the presenting signs and symptoms may closely mimic those of hypovolemic shock, the cause of the two conditions is different.

In distributive shock, resistance to blood flow is decreased because of the relatively larger size of the blood vessels. This reduced resistance causes a decrease in the diastolic blood pressure. When this reduced resistance is combined with the reduced preload and, therefore, a reduced cardiac output, the net result is a decrease in both systolic and diastolic blood pressures. Tissue oxygenation may remain adequate in the neurogenic form of shock and blood flow remains normal although the pressure is low (neurogenic hypotension). In addition, energy production remains adequate in neurogenic hypotension.

Distributive shock can result from loss of autonomic nervous system control of the smooth muscles that control the size of the blood vessels or release of chemicals that result in peripheral vasodilation. This loss of control can stem from spinal cord trauma, simple fainting, severe infections, or allergic reactions. Management of distributive shock is directed toward improving oxygenation of the blood and improving or maintaining blood flow to the brain and vital organs.

Neurogenic "Shock"

Neurogenic shock, or more appropriately neurogenic hypotension, occurs when a spinal cord injury interrupts the sympathetic nervous system pathway. This usually involves injury to the thoracolumbar area. Because of the loss of sympathetic control of the vascular system, which controls the smooth muscles in the walls of the blood vessels, the peripheral vessels dilate below the level of injury. The marked decrease in systemic vascular resistance and peripheral vasodilation that occurs as the container for the blood volume increases results in relative hypovolemia. The patient is not really hypovolemic, but the normal blood volume insufficiently fills an expanded container. This decrease in blood pressure does not alter perfusion or compromise energy production and, therefore, is *not* shock since energy production remains unaffected. However, since there is less resistance to blood flow, the systolic and diastolic pressures are lower.

Decompensated hypovolemic shock and neurogenic shock both produce a decreased systolic blood pressure. However, the other vital and clinical signs, as well as the treatment for each, are different (Figure 8-13). Decreased systolic and diastolic pressures and a narrow pulse pressure characterize hypovolemic shock. Neurogenic shock also displays decreased systolic and diastolic pressures, but the pulse pressure remains normal or is widened. Hypovolemia produces cold, clammy, pale, or cyanotic skin and delayed capillary refilling time. In neurogenic shock the patient has warm, dry skin, especially below the area of injury. The pulse in hypovolemic shock patients is weak, thready, and rapid. In neurogenic shock, because of unopposed parasympathetic activity on the heart, bradycardia is typically seen rather than tachycardia, but the pulse quality may be weak. Hypovolemia produces a decreased level of

FIGURE 8-13 Signs Associated with Types of Shock

Vital Sign	Hypovolemic	Neurogenic	Septic	Cardiogenic
Skin temperature	Cool, clammy	Warm, dry	Cool, clammy	Cool, clammy
Skin color	Pale, cyanotic	Pink	Pale, mottled	Pale, cyanotic
Blood pressure	Drops	Drops	Drops	Drops
Level of consciousness	Altered	Lucid	Altered	Altered
Capillary refilling time	Slowed	Normal	Slowed	Slowed

consciousness (LOC), or, at least, anxiety and, often, combativeness. In the absence of a traumatic brain injury, the patient with neurogenic shock is usually alert, oriented, and lucid when in the supine position (Figure 8-14).

Patients with neurogenic shock frequently may have associated injuries that produce significant hemorrhage. Therefore, a patient who has neurogenic shock and signs of hypovolemia, such as tachycardia, should be treated as if blood loss is present.

Psychogenic (Vasovagal) "Shock"

Psychogenic shock is typically mediated through the parasympathetic nervous system. Stimulation of the tenth cranial nerve (vagus nerve) produces bradycardia. The increased parasympathetic activity may also result in transient peripheral vasodilation and hypotension. If the bradycardia and vasodilation are severe enough, cardiac output falls dramatically, resulting in insufficient blood flow to the brain. Vasovagal syncope (fainting) occurs when the patient loses consciousness. Compared to neurogenic shock, the periods of bradycardia and vasodilation are generally very brief and limited to no more than a few minutes, whereas neurogenic shock may last up to several days. In psychogenic shock patients, normal blood pressure is quickly restored when the patient is placed in a horizontal position. Because it is self-limited, a vasovagal episode is unlikely to result in true "shock" and the body quickly recovers before significant systemic impairment of perfusion occurs.

Septic Shock

Septic shock, seen in patients with life-threatening infections, is another condition that exhibits vascular dilation. Cytokines, released in response to the infection, cause damage to the walls of the blood vessels, peripheral vasodilation, and leakage of fluid from the capillaries into the interstitial space. Thus, septic shock has characteristics of both distributive shock and hypovolemic shock. Preload is diminished because of the vasodilation and loss of fluid, and hypotension occurs when the heart can no longer compensate. Septic shock is virtually never encountered within minutes of an injury; however, the prehospital care provider may be called on to care for a trauma patient in septic shock during an interfacility transfer or if a patient sustains an injury to the gastrointestinal tract and did not promptly seek medical attention.

Anaphylactic Shock

Anaphylactic shock is a severe, life-threatening allergic reaction that involves numerous body organ systems. When an individual is exposed to an allergen for the first time, they become sensitized to it. If they are later re-exposed to that same allergen, a systemic response occurs. In addition to the more common symptoms of allergic reaction such as erythema of the skin, development of hives, and itching, more serious findings are noted, including respiratory distress, airway obstruction, and vasodilation leading to shock. Active airway management may be needed in some cases. Treatment involves administration of epinephrine, antihistamines, and steroids in the hospital.

Cardiogenic Shock

Cardiogenic shock, or failure of the heart's pumping activity, results from causes that can be categorized as either intrinsic (a result of direct damage to the heart itself) or extrinsic (related to a problem outside the heart).

Intrinsic Causes

Heart Muscle Damage. Any process that weakens the cardiac muscle will affect its output. The damage may result from an acute interruption of the heart's own blood supply (as in a myocardial infarction from coronary artery disease) or from a direct bruise to the heart muscle (as in a blunt cardiac injury). A recurring cycle will ensue: decreased oxygenation causes decreased contractibility, which results in decreased cardiac output and, therefore, decreased systemic perfusion. Decreased perfusion results in a continuing decrease in oxygenation and, thus, a continuation of the cycle. As with any muscle, the cardiac muscle does not work as efficiently when it becomes bruised or damaged.

Dysrhythmia. The development of a cardiac dysrhythmia can affect the efficiency of contractions, resulting in impaired systemic perfusion. Hypoxia may lead to myocardial ischemia and cause dysrhythmias, such as premature contractions and tachycardia. Because cardiac output is a result of the volume ejected with each contraction (stroke volume), any dysrhythmia that results in a slow rate of contractions (bradycardia) or shortens the left ventricle's filling time (tachycardia) can decrease stroke volume, and cardiac output. Blunt cardiac injury may also result in dysrhythmias, the most common of which is a mild, persistent tachycardia.

Valvular Disruption. A sudden, forceful compressing blow to the chest or abdomen (see Chapter 4) may damage the valves

---

FIGURE 8-14 Neurogenic Shock versus Spinal Shock

As discussed in this chapter, the term *neurogenic shock* refers to a disruption of the sympathetic nervous system, typically from injury to the spinal cord, which results in significant dilation of the peripheral arteries. If untreated, this may result in impaired perfusion to the body's tissues. This condition should not be confused with *spinal shock*, a term that refers to an injury to the spinal cord that results in temporary loss.

of the heart. Severe valvular injury results in acute regurgitation, in which a significant amount of blood leaks back into the chamber from which it was just pumped. These patients often rapidly develop CHF, manifested by pulmonary edema and cardiogenic shock. The presence of a new heart murmur is an important clue in making this diagnosis.

Extrinsic Causes

Cardiac Tamponade. Fluid in the pericardial sac will prevent the heart from refilling completely during the diastolic (relaxation) phase. In the case of trauma, blood leaks into the pericardial sac and the walls of the ventricle cannot fully expand. In addition, inadequate filling means the cardiac muscle is not stretched and results in diminished strength of the cardiac contraction. In the case of penetrating cardiac trauma, more blood may be squeezed out of the cardiac wound and enter the pericardial sac with each contraction, further compromising cardiac output. Severe shock and death may rapidly follow.

Tension Pneumothorax. When the thoracic cavity becomes filled with air that is under pressure, the lung collapses and is prevented from refilling with air from the outside and reduces blood flow into the lungs. If the volume of air and pressure inside the injured chest is great enough, the mediastinum is pushed away from the side of the injury. As the mediastinum shifts, compression and kinking of the superior and inferior venae cavae and the increased pulmonary vascular resistance drastically impede venous return to the heart, producing a significant drop in preload. Because of its impaired filling, the heart loses its efficiency as a pump, and shock rapidly ensues.

Complications of Shock

Several complications may result in patients with persistent or inadequately resuscitated shock, which is why early recognition and aggressive management of shock are essential. The quality of care delivered in the prehospital setting can alter a patient's hospital course and outcome. *Failure to recognize shock and initiate proper treatment in the prehospital setting may extend the patient's hospital length of stay or result in death.* The following complications of shock are not often seen in the prehospital setting, but they are a result of shock in the field and in the ED. In addition, they may be encountered when transferring patients between facilities. Knowing the outcome of the process of shock helps in the understanding of the severity of the condition, the importance of rapid hemorrhage control, and appropriate fluid replacement.

Acute Renal Failure

Impaired circulation to the kidneys, resulting from prolonged shock, can result in temporary or permanent renal failure. The cells that make up the renal tubules are most sensitive to ischemia and may die if their oxygen delivery is impaired for more than 45 to 60 minutes. This *acute tubular necrosis* (ATN) may cause the kidneys to fail. Because the kidneys are no longer functioning, excess fluid is not excreted, and volume overload may result. Also, the kidneys lose their ability to excrete metabolic acids and electrolytes, leading to a metabolic acidosis and hyperkalemia (increased blood potassium). These patients often require dialysis for several weeks or months. Most patients who develop ATN resulting from shock will eventually recover normal renal function, provided they survive.

Acute Respiratory Distress Syndrome

Acute respiratory distress syndrome (ARDS) is the result of damage to the lining of the capillaries in the lung and decreased energy production to maintain the metabolism of these cells. This leads to the leakage of fluid into the interstitial spaces and alveoli of the lungs, making it much more difficult for oxygen to diffuse across the alveolar walls and into the capillaries and bind with the RBCs. Although these patients do have pulmonary edema, it is not the result of impaired cardiac function, as in CHF (*cardiogenic* pulmonary edema). ARDS represents *noncardiogenic* pulmonary edema, and initial care is supportive and does not involve diuretic therapy. Many factors have been associated with the development of ARDS, including shock, fluid overload, aspiration, and severe infection. ARDS is associated with a mortality rate of about 40%, and the patients who survive may require mechanical ventilation for up to several months.

Hematologic Failure

The term *coagulopathy* refers to impairment in the normal blood-clotting capabilities. This may result from hypothermia (decreased body temperature), dilution of clotting factors from transfusion of fluids, or depletion of the clotting substances as they are used in an effort to control bleeding (*consumptive coagulopathy*). The normal blood-clotting cascade involves several enzymes and eventually results in the creation of fibrin molecules that serve as a matrix to trap platelets and form a plug in a vessel wall. These enzymes function best in a narrow temperature range (i.e., near-normal body temperature). As the core temperature of the body falls and energy production lessens, blood clotting decreases, leading to continued hemorrhage. The blood-clotting factors may also be used up as they form blood clots in an effort to slow and control hemorrhage. The decreased body temperature worsens the clotting problems, which exacerbates hemorrhage, which further reduces the body temperature. Thus, with inadequate resuscitation, this becomes an ever-worsening cycle. Several studies have reported fewer difficulties with coagulopathy since the increase in use of plasma for resuscitation.[4]

Hepatic Failure

Severe damage to the liver is a less common result of prolonged shock. Liver failure is manifested by persistent hypoglycemia (low blood sugar), a persistent lactic acidosis, and jaundice. Because the liver produces many of the clotting factors necessary for hemostasis, a coagulopathy may accompany liver failure.

Overwhelming Infection

There is increased risk of infection associated with severe shock. This is thought to be from several causes:

a) A marked decrease in the number of WBCs, predisposing the shock patient to infection is another manifestation of hematologic failure.
b) The ischemia and reduction in energy production in the cells of the wall of the bowel in the patient with shock may allow bacteria to leak out into the peritoneal cavity.
c) There is decreased function of the immune system in the face of ischemia and loss of energy production.

Multiple Organ Failure

Shock, if not successfully treated, can lead to dysfunction first in one organ, then followed by several organs simultaneously with sepsis as a common accompaniment, leading to the multiple organ dysfunction syndrome.

Failure of one major body system (e.g., lungs, kidneys, blood-clotting cascade, liver) is associated with a mortality rate of about 40%. As an organ system fails, the shock state worsens. By the time four organ systems fail, the mortality rate is essentially 100%.[6] Cardiovascular failure, in the form of cardiogenic and septic shock, can only occasionally be reversed.

Assessment

As was discussed earlier, shock is a condition resulting from decreased perfusion and diminished energy production, and heralds the potential onset of death. If not quickly treated, this lack of energy production can become irreversible. The loss of energy production when the body switches from aerobic to anaerobic metabolism results in a 15-fold decrease in ATP production and the energy needed to maintain aerobic metabolism in all the cells of the body. The body responds to this decrease in energy production by selectively decreasing perfusion in nonessential parts of the body and increasing cardiovascular function to compensate and better perfuse other, more critical, organs of the body.

When shock develops, the physiologic response results in clinical signs that indicate the body has responded and is attempting to compensate.

The body's response is identified by reduction of perfusion to nonvital organs such as the skin, which will feel cold and may look mottled, decreased pulse character in the extremities, cold cyanotic extremities with decreased capillary refill, and decreased mentation as a result of the decline in oxygenated blood perfusion to the brain. Acidosis from anaerobic metabolism produces rapid ventilations as the body attempts to blow off the carbon dioxide byproduct. Decreased energy production is identified by sluggish body responses, cold skin, and decreased core temperature. The patient may be shivering in an effort to maintain body heat.

The assessment for the presence of shock must include looking for the subtle early evidence of this state of hypoperfusion. In the prehospital setting, this requires the assessment of organs and systems that are immediately accessible. Signs of hypoperfusion manifest as malfunction of these accessible organs or systems. Such systems are the brain and central nervous system (CNS), heart and cardiovascular system, respiratory system, skin and extremities, and the kidneys. The signs of decreased perfusion and energy production and the body's response include the following:

- Decreased LOC, anxiety, disorientation, belligerence, bizarre behavior (brain and CNS)
- Tachycardia, decreased systolic and pulse pressure (heart and cardiovascular system)
- Rapid, shallow breathing (respiratory system)
- Cold, pale, clammy, diaphoretic or even cyanotic skin with decreased capillary refill time (skin and extremities)
- Decreased urine output (kidneys), identified only rarely in the prehospital setting in situations of prolonged or delayed transport when a urinary catheter is present

Because hemorrhage is the most common cause of shock in the trauma patient, all shock should be considered as hemorrhagic until proven otherwise. The first priority is to examine for external sources of hemorrhage and control them as quickly and completely as possible. This may involve such techniques as application of pressure dressing, tourniquets, or splinting of extremity fractures. If there is no evidence of external hemorrhage, internal hemorrhage should be suspected. Although definitive management of internal hemorrhage is not practical in the prehospital setting, identification of an internal source mandates rapid transport to the definitive care institution. Internal hemorrhage can occur in the chest, abdomen, pelvis, or retroperitoneum. Evidence of blunt or penetrating chest injury, with decreased breath sounds and dullness to percussion, would suggest a thoracic source. The abdomen, pelvis, and retroperitoneum can be a source of bleeding with evidence of blunt trauma (e.g., ecchymosis) or penetrating trauma, abdominal distension or tenderness, pelvic instability, leg-length inequality, pain in the pelvic area aggravated by movement, perineal ecchymosis, and blood at the urethral meatus. As a general rule, patients who meet National Trauma Triage Protocol (NTTP) criteria 1 or 2 (or both) need rapid transport to the nearest trauma center (Figure 8-15).

If the assessment does not suggest hemorrhage as the cause of the shock, nonhemorrhagic causes should be suspected. These include cardiac tamponade and tension pneumothorax (both evident by distended neck veins vs. collapsed neck veins in hemorrhagic shock) and neurogenic shock. Decreased breath sounds and hyper-resonance on the side of the chest injury, respiratory distress (tachypnea), and tracheal deviation (rarely seen in the field) suggest tension pneumothorax. Presence of these signs suggests the need for immediate needle decompression. Different sources of cardiogenic

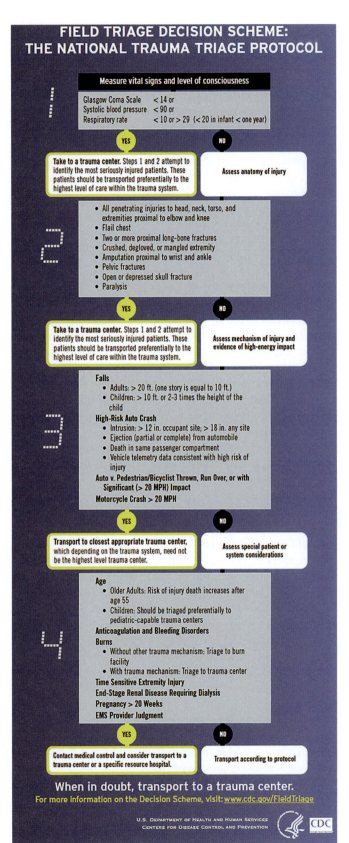

FIGURE 8-15 Field Triage Decision Scheme: The National Trauma Triage Protocol.
(From the US Department of Health and Human Services, Centers for Disease Control and Prevention.)

shock are suspected with blunt or penetrating chest trauma, muffled heart sounds suggesting cardiac tamponade (difficult to detect in the noisy prehospital environment), dysrhythmias, and neurogenic shock with signs of spinal trauma, bradycardia, and warm extremities. Most, if not all, of these features can be detected by the astute prehospital care provider who can determine the cause of the shock and the need for appropriate intervention when feasible in the field.

Areas of patient evaluation include status of the airway, ventilation, perfusion, skin color and temperature, capillary refilling time, and blood pressure. Each is presented separately here in the context of both the primary survey (initial assessment) and the secondary survey (focused history and physical examination). Simultaneous evaluation is an important part of patient assessment to gather and process information from different sources simultaneously. If all systems are functioning normally, no alarm is set off.

Primary Survey

Lord Kelvin said, "When you can measure what you are speaking about and express it in numbers, you know something about it, when you cannot express it in numbers, your knowledge is of a meager and unsatisfactory kind." Although this is often how we feel about vital signs, the first step in patient assessment is to get a general impression as quickly as possible of the patient's condition. It is only after that general impression that time can be taken to gather the numbers for a more specific assessment. The following signs identify the need for suspicion of life-threatening conditions:

- Mild anxiety, progressing to confusion or altered LOC
- Mild tachypnea, leading to rapid, labored ventilations
- Mild tachycardia, progressing to marked tachycardia
- Weakened radial pulse, progressing to an absent radial pulse
- Pale or cyanotic skin color
- Prolonged capillary-refilling time
- Loss of pulses in the extremities
- Hypothermia

Any compromise or failure of the airway, breathing, or circulatory system must be managed before proceeding. The following steps are described in an ordered series; however, all of these assessments are carried out more or less simultaneously.

Airway

Assessment should include evaluation of the airway to ensure its patency (see Chapter 7).

Breathing

As noted earlier, the anaerobic metabolism associated with decreased cellular oxygenation will produce an increase in lactic acid. The hydrogen ions (H^+) from the acidosis and hypoxia lead to stimulation of the respiratory center to increase the rate and depth of ventilation. Thus, tachypnea is frequently one of the earliest signs of shock. In the primary survey, time is not taken to measure a ventilatory rate. Instead, ventilations should be estimated to be slow, normal, fast, or very fast. A slow ventilatory rate, in conjunction with shock, generally indicates that a patient is in profound shock and may be moments away from cardiac arrest. Any fast ventilatory rate is a concern and should serve as an impetus to search for the cause of shock. A patient who tries to remove an oxygen mask, particularly when such action is associated with anxiety and belligerence, is displaying another sign of cerebral ischemia. This patient has "air hunger" and feels the need for more ventilation. The presence of a mask over the nose and mouth creates a psychological feeling of ventilatory restriction. This action should be a clue that the patient is not receiving enough oxygen and is hypoxic. Decreased oxygen saturation, as measured by the pulse oximeter, will confirm this suspicion. Any pulse oximeter reading below 95% (at sea level) is worrisome and should serve as a stimulus to identify the cause of hypoxia.

Circulation

There are two components in the assessment of circulation:

- Hemorrhage
- Perfusion with oxygenated blood
  - Total body
  - Regional

The data accumulated during the cardiac assessment help to make a quick initial determination of the patient's total blood volume and perfusion status and, secondarily, provide a similar assessment of specific regions of the body. For example, when checking the capillary-refill time, the pulse, skin color, and temperature of a lower extremity may show compromised perfusion while the same signs may be normal in the upper extremity. This does not mean the signs are inaccurate, only that one part is different from another. The immediate question that must be answered is "WHY?" It is important to check for these circulatory and perfusion findings in more than one part of the body and to remember that the assessment of the total body condition should not be based on a single part.

Hemorrhage. Assessment of circulation begins with a rapid scan for significant external hemorrhage. The patient may be lying on the major source of the hemorrhage, or it may be hidden by the patient's clothes. Efforts at restoring perfusion will be much less effective in the face of ongoing hemorrhage. The patient can lose a significant volume of blood from scalp lacerations because of the high concentration of blood vessels or from wounds that damage major blood vessels (subclavian, axillary, brachial, radial, ulnar, carotid, femoral, or popliteal). Examine the entire body to identify external hemorrhage sources.

Pulse. The next important assessment point for perfusion is the pulse. Initial evaluation of the pulse determines whether it is palpable at the artery being examined. In general, loss of a radial pulse indicates severe hypovolemia (or vascular damage to the arm), especially when a central pulse, such as the carotid or femoral artery, is weak, thready, and extremely fast, indicating the status of the total body circulatory system. If the pulse is palpable, its character and strength should be noted, as follows:

- Is the rate strong or weak and thready?
- Is the rate normal, too fast, or too slow?
- Is the rate regular or irregular?

Although many individuals involved in the management of trauma patients focus on blood pressure, precious time should not be spent during the primary survey to obtain a blood pressure. The exact level of the blood pressure is much less important in the primary survey than other signs. Significant information can be determined from the pulse rate and character. In one series of trauma patients, a radial pulse characterized by prehospital care providers as "weak" was associated with blood pressure that averaged 26mm Hg lower than a pulse thought to be "normal." More importantly, trauma patients with a weak radial pulse were 15 times more likely to die than those with a normal pulse.[9] Although generally obtained at the beginning of the secondary survey, blood pressure can be palpated or auscultated earlier in the assessment if sufficient assistance is present, or once the primary survey has been completed and life-threatening issues are being addressed during transport.

Level of Consciousness (LOC)

Mental status is part of the disability evaluation, but altered mental status can represent impaired cerebral perfusion. This represents an assessment of end-organ perfusion. An anxious, belligerent patient should be assumed to have cerebral ischemia and anaerobic metabolism until another cause is identified. Drug and alcohol overdose and cerebral contusion are conditions that cannot be treated rapidly, but cerebral ischemia can be treated. Therefore, all patients in whom cerebral ischemia might be present should be managed as if it is present.

Skin Color. Pink skin color generally indicates a well-oxygenated patient without anaerobic metabolism. Blue (cyanotic) or mottled skin indicates unoxygenated hemoglobin and a lack of adequate oxygenation to the periphery. Pale, mottled, or cyanotic skin has inadequate blood flow resulting from one of the following three causes:

1. Peripheral vasoconstriction (most often associated with hypovolemia)
2. Decreased supply of RBCs (acute anemia)
3. Interruption of blood supply to that portion of the body, such as might be found with a fracture or injury of a blood vessel supplying that part of the body

Pale skin may be a localized or generalized finding with different implications. Other findings, such as tachycardia, should be used to resolve these differences and to determine if the pale skin is a localized, regional, or systemic condition. Also, cyanosis may not develop in hypoxic patients who have lost a significant number of their RBCs from hemorrhage. In patients who have dark-pigmented skin, cyanosis may be noted in the lips, gums, and palms.

Skin Temperature. As the body shunts blood away from the skin to more important parts of the body, skin temperature decreases. Skin that is cool to the touch indicates decreased cutaneous perfusion and decreased energy production and, therefore, shock. Because a significant amount of heat can be lost during the assessment phase, steps should be taken to preserve the patient's body temperature.

A good sign of adequate resuscitation is a warm, dry, pink toe. The environmental conditions in which the determination is made can affect the results, as can an isolated injury that affects perfusion.

Capillary-Refilling Time. The ability of the cardiovascular system to refill the capillaries after the blood has been "removed" represents an important support system. Analyzing this support system's level of function by compressing the capillaries to remove all the blood and then measuring the refilling time provides insight into the perfusion of the capillary bed being assessed. Generally, the body shuts down circulation in the most distal parts first and restores this circulation last. Evaluation of the nail bed of the big toe or thumb provides the earliest indication that hypoperfusion is developing. Additionally, it provides a strong indication as to when resuscitation is complete. However, as with many other signs that a patient may exhibit, several conditions—both environmental and physiologic—can alter the results. A test of the capillary-refilling time is a measurement of the time required to reperfuse the skin and, therefore, an indirect measurement of the actual perfusion of that part of the body. It is not a diagnostic test of any specific disease process or injury.

Capillary-refilling time has been described as a poor test of shock. However, it is not a test of shock, but rather a test of perfusion of the capillary bed being analyzed. Used along with other tests and components of the assessment, it is a good indicator of perfusion and suggestive of shock.

Shock may be the cause for poor perfusion and delayed capillary refilling, but there are other causes, such as: arterial interruption from a fracture, a gunshot wound of the vessel, hypothermia, and even arteriosclerosis. Another cause of poor capillary refilling is decreased cardiac output resulting from hypovolemia (other than from hemorrhage).

Capillary-refilling time is a helpful diagnostic sign that can also be used to monitor the progress of resuscitation.

Disability

One regional system that can be readily evaluated in the field is brain function. At least five conditions can produce an altered LOC or change in behavior (combativeness or belligerence) in trauma patients:

1. Hypoxia
2. Shock with impaired cerebral perfusion
3. Traumatic brain injury
4. Intoxication with alcohol or drugs
5. Metabolic processes such as diabetes, seizures, and eclampsia

Of these five conditions, the easiest to treat—and the one that will kill the patient most quickly if not treated—is hypoxia. Any patient with an altered LOC should be treated as if decreased cerebral oxygenation is the cause. An altered LOC is usually one of the first visible signs of shock. Brain injury may be considered *primary* (caused by direct trauma to brain tissue) or *secondary* (caused by the effects of hypoxia, hypoperfusion, edema, loss of energy production, etc.). There is no effective treatment in the prehospital setting for the primary brain injury, but secondary brain injury can essentially be prevented or significantly reduced by maintaining oxygenation and perfusion.

The brain's ability to function decreases as perfusion and oxygenation drop and ischemia develops. This decreased function evolves through various stages as different areas of the brain become affected. Anxiety and belligerent behavior are usually the first signs, followed by a slowing of the thought processes and a decrease of the body's motor and sensory functions. The level of cerebral function is an important and measurable prehospital sign of shock. A belligerent, combative, anxious patient or one with a decreased LOC should be assumed to have a hypoxic, hypoperfused brain until another cause can be identified. Hypoperfusion and cerebral hypoxia frequently accompany brain injury and make the long-term result even worse. Even brief episodes of hypoxia and shock may worsen the original brain injury and result in poorer outcomes.

Body Exposure/Environment

The patient's body is exposed to assess for less obvious sites of external blood loss and for clues that may indicate internal hemorrhage. The possibility of hypothermia is also considered. This exposure is best done in the patient compartment of the ambulance in order to protect the patient from the environment and the prying eyes of the public.

Secondary Survey

In some cases, the patient's injuries may be too severe for an adequate secondary survey to be completed in the field. If time permits, the secondary survey can be done while en route to the hospital if no other issues need to be addressed.

Vital Signs

Measurement of an accurate set of vital signs is one of the first steps in the secondary survey or, after reassessing the primary survey, when a few minutes are available during transport.

Ventilatory Rate. A rate of 20 to 30 breaths/minute indicates a borderline abnormal rate and the need for supplemental oxygen. A rate greater than 30 breaths/minute indicates a late stage of shock and the need for assisted ventilation. The physiologic drive for the increased ventilatory rate is the acidosis caused by shock, but it is usually associated with a decreased tidal volume. Both of these ventilatory rates indicate the need to look for the potential sources of impaired perfusion.

Pulse. In the secondary survey, the pulse rate is determined more precisely. The normal pulse range for an adult is 60 to 100 beats/minute. With lower rates, except in extremely athletic individuals, an ischemic heart or a pathologic condition such as complete heart block should be considered. A pulse in the range of 100 to 120 beats/minute identifies a patient who has early shock, with an initial cardiac response of tachycardia. A pulse above 120 beats/minute is a definite sign of shock unless it is caused by pain or fear, and a pulse over 140 beats/minute is considered extremely critical and near-death.

Blood Pressure. Blood pressure is one of the least sensitive signs of shock. Blood pressure does not begin to drop until a patient is profoundly hypovolemic (from either true fluid loss or container-enlarged relative hypovolemia). Decreased blood pressure indicates that the patient can no longer compensate for the hypovolemia and hypoperfusion. In otherwise healthy patients, blood loss must exceed 30% of blood volume before the patient's compensatory mechanisms fail and systolic blood pressure drops below 90 mm Hg. For this reason, ventilatory rate, pulse rate and character, capillary-refilling time, and LOC are more sensitive indicators of hypovolemia than is blood pressure.

When the patient's pressure has begun to drop, an extremely critical situation exists, and rapid intervention is required. In the prehospital environment, a patient who is found to be hypotensive already has lost a significant volume of blood and ongoing blood loss is likely. The development of hypotension as a first sign of shock means that earlier signs may have been overlooked.

The severity of the situation and the appropriate type of intervention vary based on the cause of the condition. For example, low blood pressure associated with neurogenic shock is not nearly as critical as low blood pressure from hypovolemic shock. Figure 8-16 presents the signs used to assess compensated and decompensated hypovolemic shock.

One important pitfall to avoid involves equating systolic blood pressure with cardiac output and tissue perfusion. As emphasized in this chapter, significant blood loss is typically required before the patient becomes hypotensive (Class III hemorrhage). Thus, patients will have decreased cardiac output and impaired tissue oxygenation when they have lost 15% to 30% of their blood volume, despite having a normal systolic blood pressure. Ideally, shock will be recognized and treated in the earlier stages before decompensation occurs.

FIGURE 8-16 Shock Assessment in Compensated and Decompensated Hypovolemic Shock

Vital Sign	Compensated	Decompensated
Pulse	Increased; tachycardia	Greatly increased; marked tachycardia that can progress to bradycardia
Skin	White, cool, moist	White, cold, waxy
Blood pressure range	Normal	Decreased
Level of consciousness	Unaltered	Altered, ranging from disoriented to coma

Brain injuries do not cause hypotension until the brain begins to herniate through the incisura and foramen magnum. Therefore, a patient with a brain injury, who is hypotensive, should be assumed to have hypovolemia (usually blood loss) from other injuries and not from the brain injury. Young infants (less than 6 months of age) are the exception to this rule because they may bleed inside their head into hypovolemic shock as a result of open sutures and fontanelles.

Musculoskeletal Injuries

Significant internal hemorrhage can occur with fractures (Figure 8-17). Fractures of the femur and pelvis are of greatest concern. A single femoral fracture may be associated with up to 2 to 4 units (1000–2000 ml) of blood loss into a thigh. This injury alone could potentially result in the loss of 30% to 40% of an adult's blood volume, resulting in decompensated hypovolemic shock. Pelvic fractures, especially those resulting from significant falls or crushing mechanisms, can be associated with massive internal hemorrhage into the retroperitoneal space. A victim of blunt trauma can have multiple fractures and Class III or IV shock but no evidence of external blood loss, hemothoraces, intra-abdominal bleeding, or pelvic fracture. For example, an adult pedestrian struck by a vehicle and sustaining four rib fractures, a humerus fracture, a femur fracture, and bilateral tibia/fibula fractures may experience internal bleeding of 3000 to 5500 ml of blood. This potential blood loss is enough for the patient to die from shock if it is unrecognized and inappropriately treated.

Confounding Factors

Numerous factors can confound the assessment because they obscure the usual signs of shock in the trauma patient.

FIGURE 8-17 Approximate Internal Blood Loss Associated with Fractures

Type of Fracture	Internal Blood Loss (ml)
Rib	125
Radius or ulna	250–500
Humerus	500–750
Tibia or fibula	500–1000
Femur	1000–2000
Pelvis	1000–massive

Age

Patients at the extremes of life—the very young (neonates) and the elderly—have diminished capability to compensate for acute blood loss and other shock states. Thus, a relatively minor injury may produce decompensated shock in these individuals. On the other hand, children and young adults have a tremendous ability to compensate for blood loss and may appear relatively normal on a quick scan. A closer look may reveal subtle signs of shock, such as mild tachycardia and tachypnea, pale skin with delayed capillary-refilling time, and anxiety. Because of their powerful compensatory mechanisms, children found in decompensated shock represent dire emergencies. Elderly individuals may be more prone to certain complications of prolonged shock, such as acute renal failure.

Athletic Status

Well-conditioned athletes often have enhanced compensatory capabilities. Many have resting heart rates in the range of 40 to 50 beats/minute. Thus, a heart rate of 100 to 110 beats/minute or hypotension may be warning signs that indicate significant hemorrhage in a well-conditioned athlete.

Pregnancy

During pregnancy, a woman's blood volume may increase 45–50%. Heart rate and cardiac output during pregnancy are also increased. Because of this, a pregnant female may not demonstrate signs of shock until her blood loss exceeds 30% to 35% of her total blood volume. Also, well before the mother demonstrates signs of hypoperfusion, the fetus may be adversely affected because the placental circulation is more sensitive to the vasoconstrictive effects of catecholamine released in response to the shock state. During the third trimester, the gravid uterus may compress the inferior vena cava, greatly diminishing venous return to the heart and resulting in hypotension. Elevation of the patient's right side once she has been immobilized to a long backboard may alleviate this. Hypotension in a pregnant female that persists after performing this maneuver typically represents life-threatening blood loss.

Pre-existing Medical Conditions

Patients with serious pre-existing medical conditions, such as coronary artery disease and chronic obstructive pulmonary disease (COPD), are typically less able to compensate for hemorrhage and shock. These patients may experience angina as their heart rate increases in an effort to maintain their blood pressure. Patients with implanted fixed-rate pacemakers are typically unable to develop the compensatory tachycardia necessary to maintain blood pressure.

Medications

Numerous medications may interfere with the body's compensatory mechanisms. Beta-adrenergic blocking agents and calcium channel blockers used to treat hypertension may prevent an individual from developing a compensatory tachycardia to maintain blood pressure. Additionally, nonsteroidal anti-inflammatory drugs (NSAIDs), used in the treatment of arthritis and musculoskeletal pain, may impair platelet activity and blood clotting, and may result in increased hemorrhage.

Time between Injury and Treatment

In situations in which the emergency medical services (EMS) response time has been brief, patients may be encountered who have life-threatening internal hemorrhage but have not yet lost enough blood to manifest severe shock (Class III or IV hemorrhage). Even patients with penetrating wounds to their aorta, venae cavae, or iliac vessels may arrive at the receiving facility with a normal systolic blood pressure if the EMS response, scene, and transport times are brief. The assumption that patients are not bleeding internally just because they "look good" is frequently very wrong. The patient who "looks good" may well be because the patient's condition is compensated shock or because not enough time has elapsed for the signs of shock to manifest themselves. Patients should be thoroughly assessed for even the subtlest signs of shock, and internal hemorrhage should be assumed to be present until it is definitively ruled out. This is one reason why continued reassessment of trauma patients is essential.

Management

Steps in the management of shock are:

1) Insure oxygenation (adequate airway and ventilation)
2) Identify hemorrhage (control external bleeding)
3) Transport to definitive care
4) Fluids in route as appropriate

In addition to securing the airway and providing ventilation to maintain oxygenation, the prime goals of treatment of shock include identifying the source or cause, treating the cause as specifically as possible, and supporting the circulation. In the prehospital setting, external sources of bleeding should be identified and directly controlled immediately. Internal causes of shock usually cannot be definitively treated in the prehospital setting; therefore, the approach is to transport the patient rapidly to the definitive care setting while supporting the circulation in the best way possible. Resuscitation in the prehospital setting includes the following:

- Improve oxygenation of the RBCs in the lungs through:
  - Appropriate airway management; and
  - Providing ventilatory support with a bag- mask, and delivering a high concentration of supplemental oxygen (FiO$_2$ >0.85).
- Control both external hemorrhage and internal hemorrhage, to the extent possible in the prehospital setting. *Every red blood cell counts.*
- Improve circulation to deliver the oxygenated RBCs more efficiently to the systemic tissues, and improve oxygenation and energy production at the cellular level.
- Maintain body heat.
- Reach definitive care as soon as possible for hemorrhage control and replacement of lost RBCs, plasma, coagulation factors, and platelets.

Without appropriate measures, a patient will continue to deteriorate rapidly until he or she reaches the ultimate "stable" condition—death.

The following four questions need to be addressed when deciding what treatment to provide for a patient in shock:

1. What is the cause of the patient's shock?
2. What is the definitive care for the patient's shock?
3. Where can the patient best receive this definitive care?
4. What interim steps can be taken to support the patient and manage the condition while the patient is being transported to definitive care?

Although the first question may be difficult to answer accurately in the field, identification of the possible source of the shock assists in defining which facility is best suited to meet the patient's need and what measures may be necessary during transport to improve the patient's chances of survival.

Airway

The airway should be evaluated initially in all patients. Patients in need of immediate management of their airway include those with the following conditions, in order of importance:

1. Patients who are not breathing
2. Patients who have obvious airway compromise
3. Patients who have ventilatory rates greater than 20 breaths/minute
4. Patients who have noisy sounds of ventilation

Advanced techniques for securing the airway and maintaining ventilation may be required in the prehospital setting, as outlined in Chapter 7. The importance of essential airway skills, especially when transport times are brief, should not be underestimated.

Breathing

Once a patent airway is ensured, patients in shock or those at risk for developing shock (almost all trauma patients) should initially receive supplemental oxygen in a concentration as close to 100% (FiO$_2$ of 1.0) as possible. This level of oxygenation can be achieved only with a device that has a reservoir attached to the oxygen source. Nasal prongs, a nasal cannula, or a simple facemask do not meet this requirement. *Oxygen saturation (SpO$_2$) should be monitored by pulse oximetry in virtually all trauma patients and maintained above 95% (at sea level).*

A nonbreathing patient, or one who is breathing without an adequate depth and rate, needs ventilatory assistance using a bag-mask unit immediately. Hyperventilation during assisted ventilation produces a negative physiologic response, especially in the patient with hypovolemic shock. Ventilating too deeply and too quickly can make the patient alkalotic. This chemical response increases the affinity of hemoglobin for oxygen, resulting in decreased oxygen delivery to the tissue. In addition, hyperventilation may increase the intrathoracic pressure, leading to impaired venous return to the heart and hypotension. Data from animal experiments utilizing a hypovolemic shock model suggest normal or higher ventilatory rates in animals with even moderate hemorrhage impaired hemodynamic functioning, as exhibited by lower systolic blood pressure and cardiac output.[7,8] The increase in intrathoracic pressure could result from either large tidal volumes (10–12 ml/kg body weight) or from the creation of "auto-PEEP" (positive end-expiratory pressure) when ventilated too quickly (inadequate exhalation leads to air trapping in the lungs). For an adult patient, giving a reasonable tidal volume (350–500ml) at a rate of 10 ventilations/minute is probably sufficient. If available, end-tidal carbon dioxide (ETCO$_2$) monitoring may be used in conjunction with pulse oximetry to maintain the patient in a eucapneic state (normal blood CO$_2$ level) with satisfactory oxygenation.

Circulation: Hemorrhage Control

Control of obvious external hemorrhage immediately follows securing the airway and initiating oxygen therapy and ventilatory support, or it is performed simultaneously with these steps, if sufficient assistance is present. If the hemorrhage is clearly life threatening and a rapid initial survey reveals that the patient is breathing, then efforts to control the hemorrhage can take priority. Early recognition and control of external bleeding in the trauma patient help preserve the patient's blood volume and RBCs and ensure continued perfusion of

tissues. Even a small trickle of blood can add up to substantial blood loss if it is ignored for a long period. Thus, in the multisystem trauma patient, *no bleeding is minor, and every red blood cell counts* toward ensuring continued perfusion of the body's tissues.

External hemorrhage steps in the field management of external hemorrhage include:

- Hand held direct pressure
- Compression dressings
  - Elastic wrap
  - Air splint
- Tourniquet—extremities
- Hemostatic agent—torso

Control of external hemorrhage should proceed in a stepwise fashion, escalating if initial measures fail to control bleeding.

Pressure

Direct hand pressure, applied over a bleeding site, is the initial technique employed to control external hemorrhage. The ability of the body to respond to and control bleeding from a lacerated vessel is a function of (1) the size of the vessel, (2) the pressure within the vessel, (3) the presence of clotting factors, and (4) the ability of the injured vessel to go into spasm. Vessels, especially arteries, that are completely divided (transected) often retract and go into spasm. There is often less hemorrhage from the stump of an extremity with a complete amputation than from an extremity with severe trauma but with blood vessels that are damaged but not completely transected. For damaged blood vessels, the rate of blood loss is directly related to the size of the hole in the blood vessel and the *transmural pressure* (difference between the pressure inside the vessel and the pressure outside the vessel). As previously discussed in this chapter, this relationship was first described in an equation developed by Bernoulli. The specifics of the equation are not as important as understanding the underlying principle—the size of the hole and the transmural pressure relate to hemorrhage—and direct pressure (hand held or a pressure dressing) controls blood loss.

Direct pressure over the site of hemorrhage increases the extraluminal pressure and, therefore, reduces the transmural (internal vs. external) pressure, helping to slow or stop bleeding. Direct pressure also serves a second and equally important function. Unlike the pipes inside a home discussed earlier, blood vessels are compressible. Compressing the sides of the torn vessel reduces the size (area) of the opening and further reduces blood flow out of the vessel. Even if blood loss is not completely stemmed, it may be diminished to the point that the blood-clotting system can stop the hemorrhage. This is why direct pressure is almost always successful at controlling bleeding. Multiple studies involving hemorrhage from femoral artery puncture sites after cardiac catheterization have documented that direct pressure is an effective technique.[9–12]

Following the leaky pipe analogy, if there is a small hole in the pipe, simply putting one's finger over the hole will stop the leak temporarily. Tape can then be wrapped around the pipe for a short term fix of the leak. The same concept applies to the hemorrhaging patient. Direct pressure on the open wound is followed by a pressure dressing.

In other words, the rate of fluid loss is controlled by several factors: the pressure inside of the lumen, the pressure outside of the lumen, and the size of the hole in the tubular structure.

From a vascular and patient perspective, this means that the mean arterial pressure (intraluminal) and the pressure in the tissue surrounding the vessel (extraluminal pressure) have a direct relationship in controlling the rate of blood loss from the vessel as well as the size of the hole in the vessel.

Of note, when a patient's blood pressure has been reduced by blood loss, it is appropriate not to increase it to back to normal levels, but rather to allow it to remain at a level in which perfusion is maintained, but blood loss is not ongoing. This generally occurs when the patient's systolic blood pressure is between 80mm and 90mm Hg. This means avoiding over-infusion of IV fluids into the patient.

The steps in managing hemorrhage are, therefore, to (1) increase external pressure (hand-pressure dressing) which decreases the size of the hole in the lumen of the blood vessel and decreases the differential between internal and external pressure, both of which contribute to retarding blood flow out of the injured vessel; and (2) use the technique of hypotensive resuscitation to assure that the intraluminal pressure is not raised extensively.

Three additional points about direct pressure should be emphasized. First, when managing a wound with an impaled object, pressure should be applied on either side of the object rather than over the object. Impaled objects should not be removed in the field because the object may have damaged a vessel, and the object itself could be tamponading the bleeding. Removal of the object could result in uncontrolled internal hemorrhage. Second, if hands are required to perform other lifesaving tasks, a pressure (compression) dressing can be created using gauze pads and an elastic roller bandage or a blood pressure cuff inflated until hemorrhage stops. This dressing is placed directly over the bleeding site. Third, applying direct pressure to exsanguinating hemorrhage takes precedence over insertion of intravenous (IV) lines and fluid resuscitation. It would be a serious error to deliver a well-packaged trauma victim to the receiving facility with two IV lines inserted and neatly taped in place, but who is dying from the hemorrhage of a wound that has only trauma dressings taped in place and no direct pressure applied.

Tourniquets

In the past, emphasis has been placed on elevation of an extremity and compression on a pressure point (proximal to the bleeding site) as intermediate steps in hemorrhage control. No research has been published on whether or not elevation of a bleeding extremity slows hemorrhage. If a bone in the extremity is fractured, this maneuver could potentially result in converting a closed fracture to an open one or in causing increased internal hemorrhage. Similarly, the use of pressure points for hemorrhage control has not been studied. Thus, in the absence of compelling data, these interventions can no longer be recommended for situations in which direct pressure or a pressure dressing has failed to control hemorrhage.

If external bleeding from an extremity cannot be controlled by pressure, application of a tourniquet is the reasonable next step in hemorrhage control (Figure 8-18). Tourniquets had fallen out of favor because of concern about potential complications, including damage to nerves and blood vessels and potential loss of the limb if the tourniquet is left on too long. None of these have been proven and, in fact, data from the Iraq and Afghanistan wars have demonstrated just the opposite.[13,14] Although there is a small risk that all or part of a limb may be sacrificed, given the choice between losing a limb or saving the patient's life, the obvious decision is to preserve life. Data from the military experience suggest that appropriately applied tourniquets could potentially have prevented 7 of 100 combat deaths.[15,16] Tourniquet control of exsanguinating hemorrhage is 80% or better. Tourniquets occluding arterial inflow have been widely used in the operating room (OR) by surgeons for many years with satisfactory results. *Used properly, tourniquets are not only safe, but also lifesaving.*[17]

For hemorrhage from locations not amenable to placement of a tourniquet, such as on the torso or neck, it is reasonable to use hemostatic agents. As of this publication date, the US Army Surgical Research Institute recommends Combat Gauze as the preferred third-generation product. This may change over time. Please watch the PHTLS website (phtls.org) for the latest information.

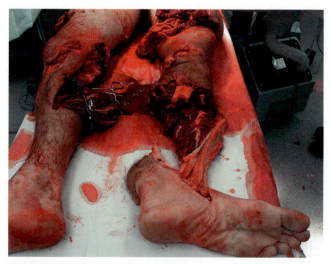

FIGURE 8-18 A fisherman who was run over by a motorboat suffered severe damage to his lower extremities. His life was saved by first responders who applied tourniquets to both thighs.

Device Options. Traditionally, a tourniquet has been devised from a cravat folded into a width of about 4 inches (10 cm) and wrapped twice around the extremity—the "Spanish windlass." A knot is tied in the bandage, a metal or wooden rod is placed on top of the knot, and a second knot is tied. The rod is twisted until hemorrhage ceases, and the rod is then secured in place. Tourniquets that are narrow and band-like should be avoided. Wider tourniquets are more effective at controlling bleeding, and they control hemorrhage at a lower pressure. An inverse relationship exists between tourniquet width and the pressure required to occlude arterial inflow. In addition, a very narrow band is also more likely to result in damage to arteries and superficial nerves. A blood pressure cuff represents another alternative that can be used as a tourniquet, although air may leak out of the cuff, diminishing its effectiveness.

Because of the US military's interest in an effective, easy-to-use tourniquet (especially one that a soldier could apply with one hand if the other arm was injured), many commercial tourniquets have been developed and marketed. Three products were 100% effective in occluding distal arterial blood flow in a laboratory study: the Combat Application Tourniquet (C-A-T, Phil Durango, Golden, Colorado), the Emergency Military Tourniquet (EMT, Delfi Medical Innovations, Vancouver, Canada), and the Special Operations Force Tactical Tourniquet (SOFTT, Tactical Medical Solutions, Anderson, South Carolina).[18] Of these, the Committee on Tactical Combat Casualty Care (COTCCC) currently recommends use of the C-A-T. Again, this recommendation may change over time, and the latest updates from the COTCCC and PHTLS will appear on the PHTLS website.

Application Site. A tourniquet should be applied just proximal to the hemorrhaging wound. If one tourniquet does not stop completely the hemorrhage, then another one should be applied just proximal to the first. Once applied, the tourniquet site should not be covered so that it can be easily seen and monitored for recurrent hemorrhage.

Application Tightness. A tourniquet should be applied tight enough to block arterial flow and occlude the distal pulse. A device that only occludes venous outflow from a limb will actually increase hemorrhage from a wound. A direct relationship exists between the amount of pressure required to control hemorrhage and the size of the limb. Thus, on average, a tourniquet will need to be placed more tightly on a leg to achieve hemorrhage control than on an arm.

Time Limit. Arterial tourniquets have been used safely for up to 120 to 150 minutes in the OR without significant nerve or muscle damage. Even in suburban or rural settings, many EMS transport times are significantly less than this period. In general, a tourniquet placed in the prehospital setting should remain in place until the patient reaches definitive care at the closest appropriate hospital. Military use has not shown significant deterioration with prolonged application times.[13] If application of a tourniquet is required, the patient

will most likely need emergency surgery to control hemorrhage. Thus, the ideal receiving facility for such a patient is one with surgical capabilities. A tourniquet can be painful for a conscious patient to tolerate, and pain management should be considered, provided that the patient does not have signs of Class III or IV shock (see Chapter 13). Figure 8-19 provides a sample protocol for tourniquet application. Another study from the military in Iraq and Afghanistan showed a marked difference in survival when the tourniquet was applied before the patient decompensated into shock compared to if it was applied after blood pressure had dropped.[19]

Topical Hemostatic Agents

The US Food and Drug Administration (FDA) has approved a number of topical hemostatic agents for use. These agents are designed to be applied topically, enhance clotting, and promote control of life-threatening hemorrhage that cannot be stopped with direct pressure alone in areas of the body that are not amenable to tourniquet placement. These agents generally come in two forms: 1) A powder that is poured onto the wound; or 2) A gauze impregnated with the hemostatic material that is applied to or packed into the wound. It is important to note that these agents should be used with the simultaneous application of direct pressure on the bleeding site. Hemostatic agents also have a number of reported complications, including heat-generating reactions that have produced burn injury, as well as embolization of the hemostatic granules into the systemic circulation in cases of open vascular injuries.

As of the writing of this chapter, Combat Gauze was the product recommended for use by the COTCCC based on research done both by the US Navy and Army surgical research lab.

FIGURE 8-19 Protocol for Tourniquet Application

1. Attempt to control hemorrhage with direct pressure or pressure dressing must fail.
2. A commercially manufactured tourniquet, blood pressure cuff, or "Spanish windlass" is applied to the extremity just proximal to the bleeding wound.
3. The tourniquet is tightened until hemorrhage ceases, and then it is secured in place.
4. The time of tourniquet application is written on a piece of tape and secured to the tourniquet ("TK 21:45" indicates that the tourniquet was applied at 9:45 pm).
5. The tourniquet should be left uncovered so that the site can be seen and monitored for recurrent hemorrhage. If bleeding continues after application and tightening of the initial tourniquet, a second tourniquet can be applied just above the first.
6. Pain management should be considered unless the patient is in Class III or IV shock.
7. The patient should ideally be transported to a facility that has surgical capability.

Internal Hemorrhage

Internal hemorrhage from fracture sites should also be considered. Rough handling of an injured extremity not only may convert a closed fracture to an open one, but also may significantly increase internal bleeding from bone ends, adjacent muscle tissue, or damaged vessels. All suspected extremity fractures should be immobilized in an effort to minimize this hemorrhage. Time may be taken to splint several fractures individually if the patient has no evidence of life-threatening conditions. If the primary survey identifies threats to the patient's life, however, the patient should be immobilized rapidly on a long backboard, thereby immobilizing all of the extremities in an anatomic manner, and transported to a medical facility. For patients with suspected intra-abdominal hemorrhage or a suspected pelvic fracture, the PASG (Figure 8-20) has been shown to tamponade internal hemorrhage just as other pressure dressings control hemorrhage. Pelvic binders have been shown to splint and approximate the fractures of the pelvic bone, but no studies have been done to show any change in outcome if used in the prehospital setting.

Disability

There are no unique, specific interventions for altered mental status in the shock patient. If the patient's abnormal neurologic status is the result of cerebral hypoxia and poor perfusion, efforts to restore perfusion throughout the body should result in improved mental status. In assessing a patient's prognosis after traumatic brain injury, an "initial" Glasgow Coma Scale (GCS) score is typically considered the score following adequate resuscitation and restoration of cerebral perfusion. Assessing a patient's GCS score while still in shock may result in an overly grim prognosis.

Body Exposure and Environment

Maintaining the patient's body temperature within a normal range is important. Hypothermia results from exposure to colder environments by convection, conduction, and other physical means (see Environmental Chapter 21) and from loss of energy production with anaerobic metabolism. Hypothermia is detrimental and worsens myocardial dysfunction, coagulopathy, hyperkalemia, vasoconstriction, and a host of other problems that negatively affect a patient's chance of survival.[25] Although cold temperatures preserve tissue for a short time, the temperature drop must be very rapid and very low for preservation to occur. Such a rapid change has not been proven effective for the patient in shock after trauma.

In the prehospital setting, increasing the core temperature once hypothermia has developed can be difficult; therefore, all steps that can be taken in the field to preserve normal body temperature should be initiated. Once exposed and examined, the patient must be protected from the environment and body temperature maintained. Any wet clothing,

---

FIGURE 8-20   **Pneumatic Antishock Garment**

The PASG remains one of the most controversial devices ever introduced to prehospital care. One large study from the Houston EMS system failed to demonstrate a benefit of using the PASG in hypotensive trauma patients in an urban setting with brief transport times to trauma centers with in-house trauma surgeons.[20] The PASG is mainly a device for controlling blood loss and not for resuscitation.

PHYSIOLOGY

Pressure applied by the PASG to the legs and abdomen is transmitted directly through the skin, fat, muscle, and other soft tissues to the blood vessels themselves. This effect controls hemorrhage in similar fashion as any other compression device or bandage.

USE IN HEMORRHAGIC SHOCK

In the following three conditions, the PASG may have significant benefit in patients with shock from blood loss:

1. *Suspected pelvic fractures with hypotension* (systolic blood pressure of 90 mm Hg). Pelvic fractures may result in severe hemorrhage into the pelvic soft tissues and retroperitoneal space. Inflation of the entire PASG decreases the volume of the pelvis and results in tamponade of the associated hemorrhage.[21]

2. *Suspected intraperitoneal hemorrhage with hypotension.* Inflation of the entire PASG compresses intraperitoneal organs. This may result in a slowing or cessation of hemorrhage (tamponade) from the solid organs, such as the liver and spleen, and the mesenteric vessels. Several studies have demonstrated improved survival in animals receiving the PASG in models of uncontrolled intra-abdominal hemorrhage.[22]

3. *Suspected retroperitoneal hemorrhage with hypotension.* Inflation of the entire device compresses the retroperitoneal organs. Because of the increased pressure, the device may cause tamponade bleeding from the kidneys, aorta, and venae cavae.[23]

The PASG is probably significantly *less effective* than direct pressure or a pressure dressing with gauze and an elastic bandage for control of external hemorrhage from the extremities.

Contraindications

■ *Penetrating thoracic trauma.* Application and inflation of the PASG increase the rate of hemorrhage from damaged blood vessels in the upper half of the body (outside the confines of the device) as the patient's blood pressure significantly increases. In the Houston PASG study, hypotensive patients with penetrating thoracic trauma clearly had a higher mortality rate when the PASG was used.[24]

■ *Splinting of lower extremity fractures.* The PASG could be thought of as a large air splint, and its use has been suggested to immobilize fractures of the femur, tibia, and fibula. A traction splint is a much better immobilization device for fractures of the midshaft femur because it reduces the bone ends back into anatomic alignment and treats pain by combating the severe muscle spasm that develops in the thigh. The PASG has been associated with the development of compartment syndromes in the calf, especially when fractures are present. Use of the PASG solely as a splint for isolated lower extremity fractures in which shock is not present is not recommended.

■ *Evisceration of abdominal organs*

■ *Impaled objects in the abdomen*

■ *Pregnancy*

■ *Traumatic cardiopulmonary arrest*

■ *Co-existing medical conditions*
   ■ *Congestive heart failure (CHF)*
   ■ *Pulmonary edema*

DEFLATION

Prehospital deflation of the PASG should *not* be done except in extreme circumstances, such as evidence of a ruptured diaphragm. Application and inflation of the device results in herniation of abdominal organs into the thoracic cavity, leading to marked respiratory distress. This may mimic the development of a tension pneumothorax; however, patient deterioration will occur almost immediately after inflation of the device.

The decision to deflate the PASG should be made in consultation with online medical direction. Except in the unusual circumstances in which inflation of the device resulted in rapid deterioration of the patient's condition, the PASG should not be deflated unless the patient's vital signs are within normal limits. Even when vital signs are within normal ranges, the patient's blood volume might still be significantly depleted. The inflated PASG may have reduced the size of the patient's container (vessels) to match the available blood volume. As the PASG is deflated, the patient's container size will increase. Unless a sufficient amount of fluid is infused, cardiac preload and SVR may drop dramatically, resulting in severe hypotension and profound shock.

including that saturated with blood, is removed from the patient because wet clothing increases heat loss. The patient is covered with warm blankets. An alternative involves covering the patient with plastic sheets, such as heavy, thick garbage bags. They are inexpensive, easily stored, disposable, and effective devices for heat retention. Heated, humidified oxygen, if available, may help preserve body heat, especially in intubated patients.

Once assessed and packaged, the shock patient is moved into the warmed patient compartment of the ambulance. Ideally, the patient compartment of an ambulance is kept at 85°F (29°C) or more when transporting a severely injured trauma patient. The patient's rate of heat loss into a cold compartment is very high. The conditions must be ideal for the patient, not for the providers, because the patient is the most important person in any emergency. A good rule of thumb to follow is that if the provider is comfortable in the patient compartment, it is too cold for the patient.

Patient Transport

Effective treatment of a patient in severe hemorrhagic shock requires a surgeon with access to an OR and blood. Because neither is routinely available in the prehospital trauma setting, rapid transportation to a facility that is capable of managing the patient's injuries is extremely important. Rapid transport does not mean disregarding or neglecting the treatment modalities that are important in patient care (doing the old-fashioned "scoop and run"). However, it does mean that the prehospital care provider quickly institutes key, potentially lifesaving measures, such as airway management, ventilatory support, and hemorrhage control. Time must not be wasted on an inappropriate assessment or with unnecessary immobilization maneuvers. When caring for a critically injured patient, many steps, such as warming the patient, starting IV therapy, and even performing the secondary survey, are accomplished in the ambulance while en route.

Patient Positioning

In general, trauma patients who are in shock should be transported in the supine position, immobilized on a long backboard. Special positioning, such as the Trendelenburg position (placed on an incline with the feet elevated above the head) or the "shock" position (head and torso supine with legs elevated), although used for 150 years, has not been proven to be effective. The Trendelenburg position may aggravate already impaired ventilatory function by placing the weight of the abdominal organs on the diaphragm and may increase intracranial pressure in patients with traumatic brain injury. More importantly, patients who are in severe hypovolemic shock are, generally, maximally vasoconstricted.[26,27]

Vascular Access

Intravenous Route

Intravenous access is obtained in a trauma patient who has known or suspected serious injuries so that the provider can initiate volume resuscitation if appropriate. Except in unusual circumstances in which a patient is undergoing extrication from a vehicle or prehospital care providers are awaiting the arrival of a helicopter, IV access should be obtained after the patient has been placed in the ambulance and transportation has been initiated to the closest appropriate facility, as this does not delay transport to the hospital for the severely injured patient.

Although volume resuscitation of a trauma patient in shock makes empiric sense, no research has demonstrated improved survival rates of critically injured trauma patients when IV fluid therapy was initiated in the prehospital setting. In fact, one physiologic computer model of prehospital IV fluid administration found that IV fluid is only beneficial when three conditions exist: (1) the patient is bleeding at a rate of 25 to 100 ml/minute; (2) the IV fluid administration rate is equal to the bleeding rate; and (3) the scene time and transport time exceed 30 minutes.[28] Therefore, *transport of the trauma patient should never be delayed to initiate IV lines.* One study has demonstrated that there was no benefit to the use of IV fluids before the hemorrhage was controlled.[29] Unfortunately, there have been no good studies that randomized the use of fluid resuscitation in patients with uncontrolled hemorrhage versus controlled hemorrhage. All of the studies that have been done mix both types of patients. Until such a study is done, the use of anecdotal and mixed studies will be the basis for the recommended practice.

For patients in shock or with potentially serious injuries, two large-bore (14- or 16-gauge), short (1-inch) IV catheters should be inserted by percutaneous puncture. The rate of fluid administration is directly proportional to the fourth power of the radius of the catheter and inversely proportional to its length (meaning more fluid will rapidly flow through a shorter, larger-diameter catheter than through a longer, smaller-diameter catheter). The preferred site for percutaneous access is a vein of the forearm. Alternative sites for IV access are the veins of the antecubital fossa, the hand, and the upper arm (cephalic vein). If two attempts at percutaneous access are unsuccessful in a child, inserting an intraosseous line should be considered. Central venous lines or venous cutdowns are not generally considered appropriate venous access in the prehospital setting and are rarely needed.

Intraosseous Route

Another alternative for vascular access in adults is the intraosseous route.[20,30] The intraosseous route of giving IV fluids is not new and was described by Dr. Walter E. Lee in 1941. This method of vascular access can be accomplished in a number of ways. It can inserted via the sternal technique, using appropriately designed devices[31,32] (e.g., F.A.S.T.1, Pyng Medical Corporation, Richmond, British Columbia). Specially designed devices such as the Bone Injection Gun ("BIG," WaisMed, Houston, Texas) and the EZ-IO (Vidacare Corp., San Antonio, Texas) may also be used to establish access through sites in the distal tibia above the ankle (Figure 8-21).[33] Such techniques are becoming commonly used in the prehospital setting, but the focus should be on rapid transport rather than IV fluid administration. For delayed or prolonged transport to definitive care, intraosseous vascular access may have a role in adult trauma patients.

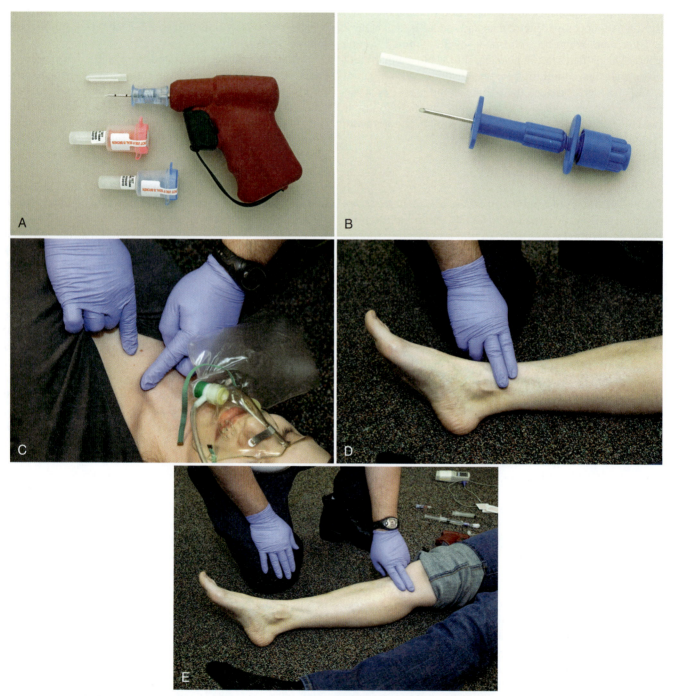

FIGURE 8-21 **A.** EZ IO device. **B.** IO Needle for manual insertion. **C.** Sternal insertion site in the manubrium below the suprasternal notch. **D.** Distal tibial insertion site above the ankle. **E.** Proximal tibial insertion site below the knee.

Volume Resuscitation

There are five fluid resuscitation strategies that have been used in the last 50 years for the management of trauma patients. These are the administration of:

- Blood
  - Whole blood
  - Reconstituted whole blood as blood products
- Large volumes of crystalloid
- Hypertonic fluid
  - 7% saline
  - 3% saline
  - Colloid solutions
- Hypotensive or restricted fluid
- Blood substitutes (only investigational use)

Each of these has both good and bad points.

Blood

Because of its ability to transport oxygen, blood or various blood products remain the fluid of choice for the resuscitation of a patient in severe hemorrhagic shock. Unfortunately, blood is impractical for use in the prehospital setting because of issues related to blood typing and because blood and its subcomponents are perishable if not kept refrigerated or frozen until the moment of use.

Intravenous Solutions

Alternative solutions for volume resuscitation fall into one of four categories: (1) isotonic crystalloids, (2) hypertonic crystalloids, (3) synthetic (artificial) colloids, and (4) blood substitutes.

Isotonic Crystalloid Solutions. Isotonic crystalloids are balanced salt solutions comprised of electrolytes (substances that separate into charged ions when dissolved in solutions). They act as effective volume expanders for a short time, but they possess no oxygen-carrying capacity. Immediately after infusion, crystalloids fill the vascular space that was depleted by blood loss, improving preload and cardiac output. *Lactated Ringer's* (LR) solution remains the isotonic crystalloid solution of choice for the management of shock because its composition is most similar to the electrolyte composition of blood plasma. It contains specific amounts of sodium, potassium, calcium, chloride, and lactate ions. *Normal saline* (NS, 0.9% sodium chloride [NaCl] solution) remains an acceptable alternative, although hyperchloremia (a marked increase in the blood chloride level) may occur with massive volume resuscitation with NS administration. Solutions of dextrose in water (e.g., D_5W) are not effective volume expanders and have no place in the resuscitation of trauma patients.

Within 30 to 60 minutes after administration of a crystalloid solution, only about ¼ to ⅓ remains in the cardiovascular system. The rest has shifted into the interstitial space because both the water and the electrolytes in the solution can freely cross the capillary membranes. The lost fluid becomes edema in the soft tissues and organs of the body. This extra fluid causes difficulties with the onloading and offloading of oxygen to the RBCs. The rule of thumb (the 3:1 rule) is that most patients with hemorrhagic shock generally achieve adequate crystalloid resuscitation when about 300 ml of crystalloid solution has been infused for every 100 ml of lost blood volume. If possible, IV fluids should be warmed to about 102°F (39°C) before infusion. Infusion of large amounts of room temperature or cold IV fluid contributes to hypothermia and increased hemorrhage.

Hypertonic Crystalloid Solutions. Hypertonic crystalloid solutions have extremely high concentrations of electrolytes compared to blood plasma. The most commonly used experimental model is *hypertonic saline,* a 7.5% NaCl solution, which is more than eight times the concentration of NaCl in NS. This is an effective plasma expander, especially in that a small, 250-ml infusion often produces the same effect as infusing 2 to 3 liters of isotonic crystalloid solution.[34,35] An analysis of several studies of hypertonic saline failed to demonstrate improved survival rates over the use of isotonic crystalloids.[36] This solution is not FDA approved for patient care in the United States. Lesser concentrations such as 3.0% are approved for patient care and are frequently used in intensive care units.

Synthetic Colloid Solutions. Proteins are large molecules produced by the body comprised of amino acids. They have countless functions; however, one type of protein found in the blood, *albumin,* helps maintain fluid in the intravascular space. Intravenous administration of human albumin is costly and has been associated with the transmission of infectious diseases, such as hepatitis. When administered to a patient in hemorrhagic shock, synthetic colloid solutions draw fluid from the interstitial and intracellular spaces into the intravascular space, thereby producing expansion of the blood volume. As with crystalloids, colloid plasma expanders do not transport oxygen.

Gelofusine is a 4% gelatin solution produced from bovine protein and is occasionally used in Europe and Australia for fluid resuscitation. It is moderately expensive and carries a risk of severe allergic reactions. A small infusion of gelofusine produces expansion of the intravascular volume for several hours.

Hetastarch (Hespan) and dextran (Gentran) are synthetic colloids that have been created by linking numerous starch (amylopectin) or dextrose molecules together until they are similar in size to an albumin molecule. These solutions are also moderately expensive compared to crystalloids and have been associated with allergic reactions and impairment of blood typing.

The use of crystalloids versus colloids has been a longstanding debate in the management of trauma patients.[37] A study of almost 7000 patients admitted to intensive care units demonstrated no difference in outcome when patients were resuscitated with colloid (albumin) versus normal saline.[38] A single study presented at the 2009 American Association for the Surgery of Trauma (AAST) meeting identified a greater survival with Hextend than with saline; however, more information needs to be available before its routine use can be recommended. Hextend is a colloid solution that has been used in military situations as a volume expander. The benefits are that it is a smaller and lighter package, which is more easily carried, it improves perfusion without overloading the patient with crystalloid, and it appears to be effective.

Virtually no research exists involving the use of these synthetic colloid solutions in the prehospital setting, and no data exist from their use in the hospital that shows them to be superior to crystalloid solutions. These products are not recommended for the prehospital management of shock.

Blood Substitutes. Blood has several undesirable qualities, including the need to type and crossmatch, a short shelf life, perishability when not refrigerated, a potential for transmission of infectious disease, and an increasing shortage of donated units. This has led to intense research in blood substitutes during the last two decades. The military has played a central role in this research because a blood substitute that would not need refrigeration and did not require blood typing could be carried to a wounded soldier on the battlefield and infused rapidly to combat shock.

Perfluorocarbons (PFCs) are synthetic compounds that have high oxygen solubility. These inert materials can dissolve approximately 50 times more oxygen than can blood plasma. PFCs contain no hemoglobin or protein; they are completely free of biologic materials, thereby greatly reducing the threat of infectious agents being found in them; and oxygen is transported by dissolving in the plasma portion. First-generation PFCs experienced limited usefulness because of numerous problems, including a short half-life and the need for a concurrent high-Fio_2 administration. Newer PFCs have fewer of these disadvantages, but their role as oxygen carriers remains undetermined.

Most *hemoglobin-based oxygen carriers* (HBOCs) use the same oxygen-carrying molecule (hemoglobin) found in human, bovine, or porcine blood cells. The major difference between HBOCs and human blood is that the hemoglobin in HBOCs is not contained within a cell membrane. This removes the need for conducting type and crossmatch studies because the antigen-antibody risk is removed. Additionally, many of these HBOCs can be stored for long periods, making them the ideal solution for mass-casualty incidents. Early problems with hemoglobin-based oxygen-carrying solutions included toxicity from hemoglobin. As of 2010, none of those experimental solutions have been found to be safe or effective in humans.

Warming Intravenous Fluids. Any IV fluid given to a patient in shock should be warm, not room temperature or cold. The ideal temperature for such fluids is 102°F (39°C). Most ambulances do not have conventional rapid fluid warmers, but other steps can keep fluids at an adequate temperature. A convenient storage area for fluids is in a box in the engine compartment. Wrapping heat packs around the bag can also warm fluid. Commercially available fluid-warmer units for the patient care compartment provide an easy and reliable means to keep fluids at the correct temperature. These units are costly but justifiable for prolonged transports.

Managing Volume Resuscitation

As noted earlier, significant controversy surrounds prehospital fluid administration for a trauma patient who is in shock. When Prehospital Trauma Life Support (PHTLS) was first introduced in the United States, prehospital care providers adopted the approach used by emergency physicians and surgeons in most hospitals and trauma centers: administer an IV crystalloid solution until the vital signs had returned to normal (typically, pulse <100 beats/minute and systolic blood pressure >100 mm Hg). When sufficient crystalloid solution is infused to restore vital signs to normal, the patient's perfusion should be improved. Experts believed that such rapid intervention would clear lactic acid and restore energy production in the cells of the body and also decrease the risk of developing irreversible shock and kidney failure. However, no study of trauma patients in the prehospital setting has shown that the administration of IV fluid decreases complications and death.

A major contribution of PHTLS over the past two decades has been to establish the conceptual change that, in the critically injured trauma patient, *transportation should never be delayed while IV lines are placed and fluid is infused.* These actions can be performed in the back of the ambulance en route to the closest appropriate facility. The critically injured trauma patient who is in shock generally requires blood and surgical intervention to control internal hemorrhage, neither of which can be accomplished in the field.

Research, primarily in experimental models of shock, has shown that IV volume resuscitation may have detrimental side effects when administered before surgical control of the source of hemorrhage. In experimental animals, internal hemorrhage often continues until the animal is hypotensive, at which point bleeding slows and a blood clot (thrombus) typically forms at the site of injury. In one sense, this hypotension is protective in that it is associated with a dramatic slowing or cessation of internal hemorrhage. When aggressive IV fluids were administered to the animals in an attempt to restore perfusion, internal hemorrhage started again, and the thrombus was disrupted. In addition, crystalloid infusions may also dilute coagulation factors. These animals often had a worse outcome compared to animals that received resuscitation *after* surgical control of the injury site.[39-41] In a similar animal model, improved survival was noted with "hypotensive resuscitation," in which the blood pressure was purposefully kept low until hemorrhage was controlled, then resuscitation took place.[42-44]

Clearly, these studies have potential implications on fluid resuscitation in the prehospital setting. Theoretically, aggressive volume resuscitation could return the blood pressure to normal. This, in turn, may dislodge blood clots that formed at bleeding sites in the peritoneal cavity or elsewhere and may result in renewed hemorrhage that cannot be controlled until the patient reaches the OR. On the other hand, withholding IV fluid from a patient in profound shock only leads to further tissue hypoxia and failure of energy production. A single clinical study conducted in an urban prehospital setting demonstrated a worse outcome in trauma patients who received crystalloid solutions before control of internal hemorrhage (mortality rate of 62% vs. 70% in the delayed-treatment group).[26] The findings of this single study have not been replicated in other prehospital systems, and the findings cannot be generalized to rural EMS systems. In a survey of trauma surgeons, fewer than 4% opted for an approach that involved withholding IV fluid from a patient in Class III shock. Almost two-thirds of the surgeons recommended that such a patient be maintained in a relatively hypotensive state during transport.[45]

Prehospital volume resuscitation should be tailored to the clinical situation (Figure 8-22 A & B).

Uncontrolled Hemorrhage. For patients with suspected internal hemorrhage in their chest, abdomen, or retroperitoneum (pelvis), sufficient IV crystalloid solution should be titrated to maintain a systolic blood pressure in the range of 80 to 90 mm Hg or MAP of 60 to 65 mm Hg. This should maintain adequate perfusion to the kidneys with less risk of worsening internal hemorrhage. A fluid bolus should not be administered because this may "overshoot" the target blood pressure range, resulting in recurrent intrathoracic, intra-abdominal, or retroperitoneal bleeding.

The current philosophy of restricted crystalloid administration in the prehospital setting and during the initial hospital care has been called by several names including permissive hypotension, hypotensive resuscitation and "balanced" resuscitation, meaning that a balance must be struck between the amount of fluid administered and the degree of blood pressure elevation. Once the patient arrives to the hospital, fluid administration continues by giving plasma and blood (1:1 ratio) until the hemorrhage is controlled. Blood pressure is then returned to normal values with ongoing 1:1 (plasma to blood) transfusion with restricted crystalloid administration in most trauma centers.

Central Nervous System Injuries. Hypotension has been associated with increased mortality in the setting of traumatic brain injury (TBI). Patients with certain conditions (e.g., TBIs) appear to benefit from a more aggressive fluid resuscitation.[46] Guidelines published by the Brain Trauma Foundation recommend maintaining the systolic blood pressure (SBP) above 90 mm Hg in patients with suspected TBI.[47] Consensus guidelines focusing on the management of acute spinal cord injury not only recommend avoiding hypotension (SBP <90 mm Hg), but also recommend maintaining a MAP of at least 85 to 90 mm Hg in hopes of improving spinal cord perfusion. To accomplish this goal, more aggressive volume resuscitation may be required, increasing the risk of recurrent bleeding from associated internal injuries.[48]

Controlled Hemorrhage. Patients with significant external hemorrhage that has been controlled can be managed with a more aggressive volume resuscitation strategy, provided the prehospital care provider has no reason to suspect associated intrathoracic, intra-abdominal, or retroperitoneal injuries. Examples include a large scalp laceration or a wound in an extremity involving major blood vessels, but with the bleeding controlled with a pressure dressing or tourniquet. Adult patients who fall in this category and present in Class II, III, or IV shock should receive an initial rapid bolus of 1 to 2 liters of warmed crystalloid solution, preferably LR. Pediatric patients should receive a bolus of 20 ml/kg of warmed crystalloid solution. As noted previously, this should always occur during transport to the closest appropriate facility. Vital signs—including pulse and ventilatory rates, as well as blood pressure—should be monitored to assess the patient's response to the initial fluid therapy. In most urban settings, the patient will be delivered to the receiving facility before the initial fluid bolus is completed.

The initial fluid bolus elicits three possible responses, as follows:

1. *Rapid response.* The vital signs return to and remain normal. This typically indicates that the patient has lost less than 20% of blood volume and that the hemorrhage has stopped.
2. *Transient response.* The vital signs initially improve (pulse slows and blood pressure increases); however, during continued assessment, these patients show deterioration with recurrent signs of shock. These patients have typically lost between 20% and 40% of their blood volume.
3. *Minimal or no response.* These patients show virtually no change in the profound signs of shock after a 1- to 2-liter bolus.

Patients who have a rapid response are candidates for continued volume resuscitation, until vital signs have returned to normal and all clinical indicators of shock have resolved. Patients who fall into either the transient response or minimal/no response groups have ongoing hemorrhage that is probably internal. These patients are then best managed in a state of relative hypotension, and IV fluid should be titrated to SBP in the range of 80 to 90 mm Hg (MAP of 60–65 mm Hg).

Prolonged Transport

During prolonged transport, it is important that perfusion is maintained to the vital organs. Airway management should

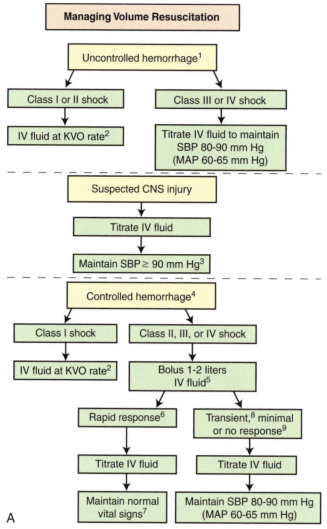

FIGURE 8-22 **A.** Algorithm for managing volume resuscitation.

[1] Suspected intrathoracic, intraabdominal or retroperitoneal hemorrhage
[2] KVO = keep vein open (about 30 mL/hr)
[3] Consider MAP 85-90 mm Hg for spinal cord injury
[4] External hemorrhage controlled with pressure dressing, topical hemostatic agent, or tourniquet
[5] Warmed crystalloid solution (102°F if possible)
[6] Rapid response = vital signs return to normal
[7] HR < 120/min; SBP > 90 mm Hg for adult
[8] Transient response = vital signs initially improve, then deteriorate
[9] Minimal or no response = little or no change in vital signs

be optimized before a long transport, and endotracheal intubation is performed if there is any question regarding airway patency. Ventilatory support is provided, with care taken to ensure that ventilations are of a reasonable tidal volume and rate so as not to compromise a patient with already tenuous perfusion. Pulse oximetry should be monitored continuously. Capnography provides information regarding the position of the endotracheal tube, as well as information on the patient's perfusion status. A marked drop in $ETCO_2$ indicates that the airway has become dislodged or that the

patient has experienced a significant drop in perfusion. A suspected tension pneumothorax is decompressed, or the equipment is kept at the bedside should the patient develop hypotension.

Direct pressure by hand is impractical during a long transport, so significant external hemorrhage should be controlled with pressure dressings. If these efforts fail, a tourniquet should be applied. In situations in which a tourniquet has been applied and transport time is expected to exceed 4 hours, attempts should be made to remove the tourniquet

SHOCK MANAGEMENT ALGORITHM

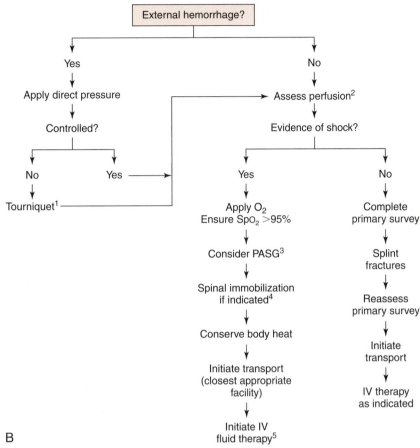

B

FIGURE 8-22—contd.   B. Algorithm for managing shock.

Notes:
[1]A manufactured tourniquet, blood pressure cuff, or cravat should be placed just proximal to the bleeding site and tightened until bleeding stops. The application time is marked on the tourniquet.

[2]Assessment of perfusion includes, presence, quality, and location of pulses; skin color, temperature, and moisture; and capillary refilling time.

[3]PASG should be considered for decompensated shock (SBP <90 mm Hg), and suspected pelvic, intraperitoneal, or retroperitoneal hemorrhage, and in patients with profound hypotension (SBP <60 mm Hg). PASG is contraindicated in penetrating thoracic trauma, abdominal evisceration, pregnancy, impaled object in the abdomen, and traumatic cardiopulmonary arrest, or for splinting the lower extremity fractures.

[4]See Indications for Spinal Immobilization algorithm (p. 235).

[5]Initiate two large-bore (14- or 16-guage) IV catheters en route. See Managing Volume Resuscitation algorithm (p. 188).

after more aggressive attempts at local hemorrhage control. The tourniquet should be slowly loosened while observing the dressing for signs of hemorrhage. If bleeding does not reoccur, the tourniquet is completely loosened but left in place in case hemorrhage recurs. Conversion of a tourniquet back to a dressing should not be attempted in the following situations: (1) presence of Class III or IV shock; (2) complete amputation; (3) inability to observe the patient for reoccurrence of bleeding; and (4) tourniquet in place longer than 6 hours.[15] Internal hemorrhage control should be optimized by splinting all frac-

tures and applying the PASG or pelvic binder, as indicated for intra-abdominal or retroperitoneal hemorrhage.

Techniques for maintaining normal body temperature, as previously described, are even more important in the setting of prolonged transport time. In addition to a warmed patient compartment, the patient should be covered with blankets or materials that preserve body heat; even large, plastic garbage bags help prevent loss of heat. Intravenous fluids should be warmed before administration. In prolonged-transport circumstances, vascular access for fluid administration may be critical, and two large-bore IV lines should be established. For both children and adults, inability to obtain vascular percutaneous venous access may necessitate use of the IO route even for adults, as described previously. For patients with suspected ongoing hemorrhage, maintaining SBP in the range of 80 to 90 mm Hg or MAP of 60 to 65 mm Hg can usually accomplish the goal of maintaining perfusion to vital organs with less risk of renewing internal hemorrhage. Patients with suspected TBIs or spinal cord injuries should have SBP maintained above 90 to 100 mm Hg.

Vital signs should be reassessed frequently to monitor response to resuscitation. The following should be documented at serial intervals: ventilation rate, pulse rate, blood pressure, skin color and temperature, capillary refill, GCS score, SpO_2, and $ETCO_2$, if available.

Although insertion of a urinary catheter is not usually required in rapid transport circumstances, monitoring urine output is an important tool that can help guide decisions regarding the need for additional fluid therapy during prolonged transport. Insertion of a urinary catheter, if local protocols permit, should be considered so that urine output can be monitored. Adequate urine outputs include 0.5 ml/kg/hour for adults, 1 ml/kg/hour for pediatric patients, and 2 ml/kg/ hour for infants younger than 1 year. Urine output of less than these amounts may be a key indicator that the patient requires further volume infusion.

If time and local protocols permit during prolonged transport, placement of a nasogastric (NG) catheter should be considered for all intubated patients, unless fractures of the patient's midface are suspected. In the latter case, placement of an orogastric (OG) catheter should be considered. Gastric distension may cause unexplained hypotension and dysrhythmias, especially in children. Placement of an NG or OG tube may also decrease the risk of vomiting and aspiration.

During prolonged transport, assessing the patient's clinical status and response to resuscitation is key to determining outcome. There are encouraging reports supporting the use of the Life Support for Trauma and Transport (LSTAT, Integrated Medical Systems) for monitoring critically injured patients during transport. This "mobile ICU" has shown promising results in the military for transport of critically injured patients, as well as in the transfer of critically injured patients in civilian practice.[49] Disadvantages of using such devices are the cost and weight. If these obstacles could be overcome, there may be a wider application for these devices when prolonged transport of the critically injured trauma patient is necessary.

SUMMARY

- Shock causes a state of generalized hypoperfusion, resulting in cellular hypoxia, anaerobic metabolism, loss of energy production, lactic acidosis, hypothermia, and death if not appropriately treated.
- In the trauma patient, hemorrhage is the most common cause of this shock state.
- Care of the patient in shock or one that may go into shock begins with appropriate and complete assessment of the patient beginning with a history of the event and a quick visual examination of the patient looking for obvious signs of shock and blood loss.
- The primary goal of therapy is to identify the likely source of hemorrhage and treat it specifically, if possible. In the prehospital setting, this approach is most effective when the bleeding source is external. Internal hemorrhage can be treated definitively only in the hospital environment, so rapid transport of the patient to the appropriate hospital is essential.
- External hemorrhage should be controlled with direct pressure, followed by application of a pressure dressing.

- If this is ineffective, a tourniquet may be applied to the extremity proximal to the bleeding site. On the torso, a topical hemostatic agent may be used.
- In some cases, nonhemorrhagic sources of shock in the trauma patient (e.g., tension pneumothorax) can be temporarily corrected.
- However, all trauma patients in shock, in addition to maintenance of adequate oxygenation, require rapid extrication and expeditious transport to a definitive care institution where the cause of the shock can be specifically identified and treated.
- Transport should not be delayed for institution of such measures as IV access and volume infusion. These interventions should be done in the ambulance during transport.
- Overaggressive fluid infusion should be avoided to minimize further bleeding and edema formation in the patient with hemorrhagic shock after trauma.

SCENARIO SOLUTION

Based on the mechanism, you should have a high suspicion for thoracic and abdominal injuries leading to hemorrhagic shock in the male patient and significant blood loss from the female patient's leg. No c-spine immobilization is required in these patients. You apply hand-pressure dressings to the hemorrhaging leg of the female and anticipate using a tourniquet if the bleeding is not controlled. An occlusive dressing is placed on the wounds that are visibly bubbling air from the male patient's chest and a saline-moistened dressing is placed over the eviscerated bowel. Both patients should be loaded into the ambulance and transported as quickly as possible to the trauma center. If

time permits, venous access should be obtained en route to the hospital. Transportation should not be delayed to start the IV. High oxygen concentration should be delivered to the most appropriate airway device based on the level of consciousness and ability to maintain a secure airway after suctioning the airway.

The major focus of management is rapid extrication and transport to the trauma center, where definitive control of hemorrhage would prevent progression through the various stages of shock, leading to death or complications of hypoperfusion, such as renal failure, respiratory failure, and multi-organ dysfunction syndrome. ■

References

1. Gross SD. *A system of surgery: pathological, diagnostic, therapeutic, and operative,* Philadelphia, 1859, Blanchard and Lea.

2. Thal AP. *Shock: A physiologic basis for treatment,* Chicago, 1971, Yearbook Medical Publishers.

3. McClelland RN, Shires GT, Baxter CR, et al. Balanced salt solutions in the treatment of hemorrhagic shock. *JAMA* 199:830, 1967.

4. J.C. Duchesne, J.P. Hunt and G. Wahl, et al: Review of current blood transfusions strategies in a mature level I trauma center: Were we wrong for the last 60 years? *J Trauma* 65(2):272–276, 2008; discussion 276–278.

5. Holcomb, John B.; Jenkins, Don; Rhee, Peter; et al: Damage Control Resuscitation: Directly Addressing the Early Coagulopathy of Trauma. *J Trauma* 62(2):307–310, 2007.

6. Marshall JC, Cook DJ, Christou NV, et al: The multiple organ dysfunction score: A reliable descriptor of a complex clinical syndrome. *Crit Care Med* 23:1638, 1995.

7. Pepe PE, Raedler C, Lurie KG, et al. Emergency ventilatory management in hemorrhagic states: Elemental or detrimental? *J Trauma* 54:1048, 2003.

8. Pepe PE, Roppolo LP, Fowler RL: The detrimental effects of ventilation during low-blood-flow states. Curr *Opin Crit Care* 11:212, 2005.

9. Koreny M, Riedmuller E, Nikfardjam M, et al: Arterial puncture closing devices compares with standard manual compression after cardiac catheterization: Systematic review and meta analysis. *JAMA* 291:350, 2004.

10. Walker SB, Cleary S, Higgins M: Comparison of the FemoStop device and manual pressure in reducing groin puncture site complications following coronary angioplasty and coronary stent placement. *Int J Nurs Pract* 7:366, 2001.

11. Simon A, Baumgarner B, Clark K, et al: Manual versus mechanical compression for femoral artery hemostasis after cardiac catheterization. *Am J Crit Care* 7:308, 1998.

12. Lehmann KG, Heath-Lange SJ, Ferris ST: Randomized comparison of hemostasis techniques after invasive cardiovascular procedures. *Am Heart J* 138:1118, 1999.

13. Beekley, AC, Sebesta, JA, Blackbourne, Lorne H, et al: Prehospital tourniquet use in Operation Iraqi Freedom: Effect on hemorrhage control and outcomes. *J Trauma* 64(2):S28–S37, 2008.

14. Kragh, JF Jr, Walters, TJ, Baer DG, etal: Practical use of emergency tourniquets to stop bleeding in major limb trauma. *J Trauma* 64(2):S38–S50, 2008.

15. Bellamy RF: The causes of death in conventional land warfare: Implications for combat casualty care research. *Mil Med* 149:55, 1984.

16. Mabry RL, Holcomb JB, Baker AM, et al: United States Army Rangers in Somalia: An analysis of combat casualties on an urban battlefield. *J Trauma* 49:515, 2000.

17. Walters TJ, Mabry RL: Use of tourniquets on the battlefield: A consensus panel report. *Mil Med* 170:770, 2005.

18. Walters TL, Wenke JC, Kauvar DS, et al: Laboratory evaluation of battlefield tourniquets in human volunteers. US Army Institute of Surgical Research (unpublished).

19. Kragh JF Jr, Littrel ML, Jones JA, et al: Battle casualty survival with emergency tourniquet use to stop limb bleeding. *J Emerg Med,* 2009. (Epub ahead of print)

20. Deboer S, Seaver M, Morissette C: Intraosseous infusion: Not just for kids anymore. *J Emerg Med Serv* 34:54, 2005.

21. Flint LM, Brown A, Richardson JD, et al: Definitive control of bleeding from severe pelvic fractures. *Ann Surg* 189:709, 1979.

22. McSwain NE Jr: Pneumatic antishock garment: State of the art. *Ann Emerg Med* 17:506, 1988.

23. Ali J, Purcell C, Vanderby B: The effect of intra-abdominal pressure and saline infusion on abdominal aortic hemorrhage. *J Cardiovasc Surg* 32:653, 1991.

24. Mattox KL, Bickell WH, Pepe PE, et al: Prospective MAST study in 911 patients. *J Trauma* 29:1104, 1986.

25. Gentilello LM: Advances in the management of hypothermia. *Surg Clin North Am* 75:2, 1995.

26. Marino PL: *The ICU Book,* ed 2, Baltimore, 1998, Williams & Wilkins.

27. Johnson S, Henderson SO, Myth L: The Trendelenburg position improves circulation in cases of shock. *Can J Emerg Med* 6:48, 2004.

28. Lewis FR: Prehospital intravenous fluid therapy: Physiologic computer modeling. *J Trauma* 26:804, 1986.

29. Bickell WH, Wall MJ Jr, Pepe PE, et al: Immediate versus delayed fluid resuscitation for hypotensive patients with penetrating torso injuries. *N Engl J Med* 331:1105, 1994.

30. Glaeser PW, Hellmich TR, Szewczuga D, et al: Five-year experience in prehospital intraosseous infusions in children and adults. *Ann Emerg Med* 22:1119, 1993.

31. Sawyer RW, Bodai BI, Blaisdell FW, et al: The current status of intraosseous infusion. *J Am Coll Surg* 179:353, 1994.

32. Macnab A, Christenson J, Findlay J, et al: A new system for sternal intraosseous infusion in adults. *Prehosp Emerg Care* 4:173, 2000.

33. Hubble MW, Trigg DC: Training prehospital personnel in saphenous vein cut down and adult intraosseous techniques. *Prehosp Emerg Care* 5(2):181, 2001.

34. Vassar MJ, Fischer RP, Obrien PE, et al: A multicenter trial of resuscitation of injured patients with 7.5% sodium chloride: The effect of added dextran 70. *Arch Surg* 128:1003, 1993.

35. Vassar MJ, Perry CA, Holcroft JW: Prehospital resuscitation of hypotensive trauma patients with 7.5% NaCl versus 7.5% NaCl with added dextran: A controlled trial. *J Trauma* 34:622, 1993.

36. Wade CE, Kramer GC, Grady JJ: Efficacy of hypertonic 7.5% saline and 6% dextran in treating trauma: A meta analysis of controlled clinical trials. *Surgery* 122:609, 1997.

37. Rizoli SB: Crystalloids and colloids in trauma resuscitation: A brief overview of the current debate. *J Trauma* 54:S82, 2003.

38. SAFE Study Investigators: A comparison of albumin and saline for fluid resuscitation in the intensive care unit. *N Engl J Med* 350:2247, 2004.

39. Solomonov E, Hirsh M, Yahiya A, et al: The effect of vigorous fluid resuscitation in uncontrolled hemorrhagic shock after massive splenic injury. *Crit Care Med* 28:749, 2000.

40. Krausz MM, Horn Y, Gross D: The combined effect of small volume hypertonic saline and normal saline solutions in uncontrolled hemorrhagic shock. *Surg Gynecol Obstet* 174:363, 1992.

41. Bickell WH, Bruttig SP, Millnamow, et al: The detrimental effects of intravenous crystalloid after aortotomy in swine. *Surgery* 110:529, 1991.

42. Kowalenko T, Stern S, Dronen SC, et al: Improved outcome with hypotensive resuscitation of uncontrolled hemorrhagic shock in a swine model. *J Trauma* 33:349, 1992.

43. Sindlinger JF, Soucy DM, Greene SP, et al: The effects of isotonic saline volume resuscitation in uncontrolled hemorrhage. *Surg Gynecol Obstet* 177:545, 1993.

44. Capone AC, Safar, Stezoski W, et al: Improved outcome with fluid restriction in treatment of uncontrolled hemorrhagic shock. *J Am Coll Surg* 180:49, 1995.

45. Salomone JP, Ustin JS, McSwain NE, et al: Opinions of trauma practitioners regarding prehospital interventions for critically injured patients. *J Trauma* 58:509, 2005.

46. York J, Abenamar A, Graham R, et al: Fluid resuscitation of patients with multiple injuries and severe closed head injury: Experience with an aggressive fluid resuscitation strategy. *J Trauma* 48(3):376, 2000.

47. Brain Trauma Foundation: *Guidelines for prehospital management of traumatic brain injury,* New York, 2000, The Foundation.

48. American Association of Neurological Surgeons and Congress of Neurological Surgeons Joint Section on Disorders of the Spine and Peripheral Nerves: Blood pressure management after acute spinal cord injury. In: Guidelines for the management of acute cervical spine and spinal cord injuries. *Neurosurgery* 50:S58, 2002.

49. Velmahos GC, Demetriades D, Ghilardi M, et al: Life Support for Trauma and Transport: A mobile ICU for safe in-hospital transport of critically injured patients. *J Am Coll Surg* 199:62, 2004.

Suggested Reading

American College of Surgeons Committee on Trauma: Shock. In *Advanced trauma life support for doctors, student course manual,* ed 7, Chicago, 2004, ACS.

Allison KP, Gosling P, Jones S, et al: Randomized trial of hydroxyethyl starch versus gelatine for trauma resuscitation. *J Trauma* 47:1114, 1999.

Moore EE: Blood substitutes: the future is now. *J Am Coll Surg* 196:1, 2003.

Novak L, Shackford SR, Bourgenignon P, et al: Comparison of standard and alternative prehospital resuscitation in uncontrolled hemorrhagic shock and head injury. *J Trauma* 47(5):834, 1999.

Proctor KG: Blood substitutes and experimental models of trauma. *J Trauma* 54:S106, 2003.

Revell M, Greaves I, Porter K: Endpoints for fluid resuscitation in hemorrhagic shock. *J Trauma* 54:S637, 2003.

Trunkey DD: Prehospital fluid resuscitation of the trauma patient: an analysis and review. *Emerg Med* 30(5):93, 2001.

SPECIFIC SKILLS

Intraosseous Vascular Access

Principle: To establish a vascular access site for fluids and medications when traditional IV access is unobtainable.

This technique may be performed in both adult and pediatric patients, using a variety of commercially available devices.

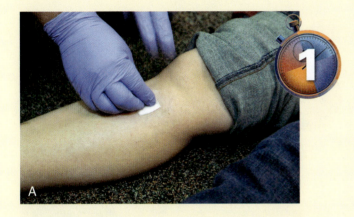

1 Assemble the equipment, which includes IO infusion needle, syringe filled with at least 5 ml of sterile saline, antiseptic, IV fluid and tubing, and tape. Assure proper body substance isolation, or BSI. Place the patient in a supine position.

The choice of insertion site may be the anterior tibia, in children or adults, or the sternum, which is used only in adults. For tibial insertion in adult patients, the insertion site is usually located at the anterior-medial distal tibia. For pediatric patients, the insertion site is the anterior-medial proximal tibia just below the tibial tuberosity. The provider identifies the insertion site and landmarks. If the tibia is the insertion site, the lower extremity is stabilized by another provider. Clean the insertion site area with an antiseptic.

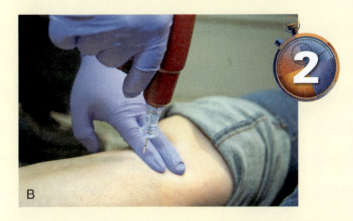

2 Holding the drill and needle at a 90-degree angle to the selected bone, activate the drill and insert the rotating needle through the skin and into the bone cortex. A "pop" will be felt upon entering the bone cortex.

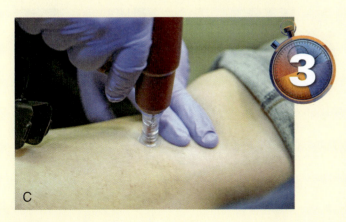

3 When you feel a lack of resistance against the needle, release the trigger of the drill. While holding the needle, remove the drill from the needle.

SPECIFIC SKILLS

Release and remove the trocar from the center of the needle.

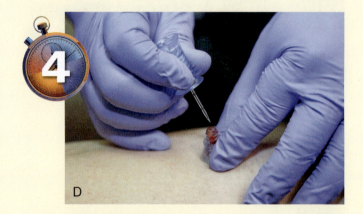

Attach the syringe with saline to the needle hub. Draw back with the syringe plunger slightly, looking for fluid from the marrow cavity to mix with the saline. "Dry" taps are not uncommon.

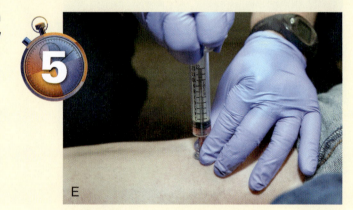

Next inject 5 ml of the saline, observing for signs of infiltration. If there are no signs of infiltration, remove the syringe from the needle hub, attach the IV tubing, and set the flow rate. Secure the needle and IV tubing.

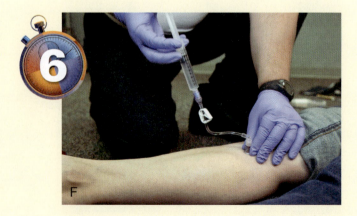

Tourniquet Application: Israeli Trauma Bandage

Principle: To provide mechanical circumferential pressure and dressing to an open wound of an extremity with uncontrolled hemorrhage.

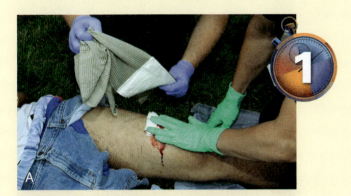

Assure proper BSI and place the dressing pad over the wound.

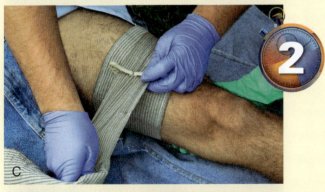

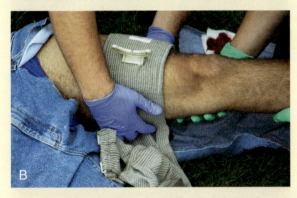

Wrap the elastic bandage around the extremity at least once.

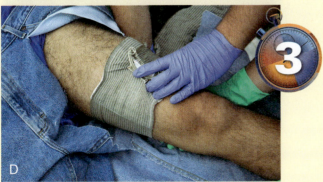

Loop the elastic bandage through the bar.

SPECIFIC SKILLS

Wrap the bandage tightly around the wounded extremity in the opposite direction applying enough pressure to control the bleeding.

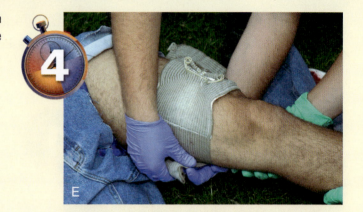

Continue wrapping the bandage around the extremity.

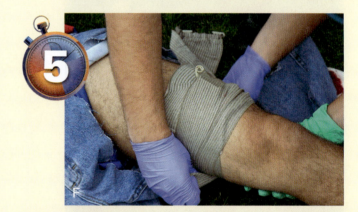

Secure the distal end of the bandage to maintain continued pressure to control the hemorrhage.

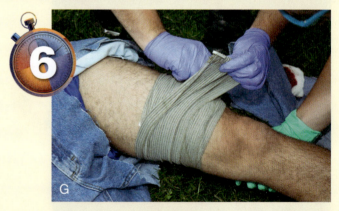

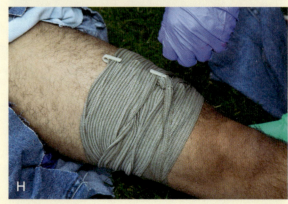

CHAPTER 9

Head Trauma

CHAPTER OBJECTIVES

At the completion of this chapter, the reader will be able to do the following:

- ✓ Relate the kinematics of trauma to the potential for traumatic brain injury (TBI).

- ✓ Incorporate the recognition of pathophysiologic manifestations and historical data significant for TBI into assessment of the trauma patient to formulate a field impression.

- ✓ Formulate a plan of field intervention for both short and prolonged transport times for patients with TBI.

- ✓ Compare and contrast the pathophysiology, management, and potential consequences of specific types of primary TBI and secondary brain injury.

- ✓ Identify criteria for patient care decisions with regard to mode of transport, level of prehospital care, and hospital resources needed for the appropriate management of the TBI patient.

- ✓ Understand the role of hyperventilation in the TBI patient.

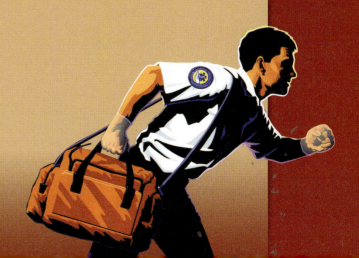

SCENARIO

You and your partner are dispatched to an alleyway where a 30-year-old male was found lying unconscious and bleeding from the head. Bystanders state that he was assaulted by another man who ran away after striking the patient with a 2' x 4' piece of wood. They report he was unconscious for about 5 minutes but has now awakened. The scene appears safe. The primary survey reveals that the patient is maintaining his airway and breathing normally. A $3\frac{1}{4}$-inch (8-cm) laceration on the right side of his scalp is bleeding copiously but is readily controlled with direct pressure and a pressure dressing. His pulse rate is 116 beats/minute, and his skin is warm, pink, and well perfused. He opens his eyes spontaneously and follows commands; however, he does not recall the events leading up to the assault. He exhibits some confusion as he attempts to answer questions (GCS 14). You apply oxygen using a nonrebreather mask. During spinal immobilization, he speaks incomprehensible words and now only opens his eyes and withdraws his extremities to painful stimuli (GCS 9).

How should you alter your care based on the change in the patient's level of consciousness? What injury is most likely present given the patient's presenting signs? What are your management priorities at this point? What actions may you need to take to combat increased intracranial pressure and maintain cerebral perfusion during a prolonged transport?

Approximately 1.4 million emergency department (ED) visits for traumatic brain injury (TBI) occur each year in the United States.[1] Although 80% of these patients are categorized as having only mild injuries, approximately 235,000 patients are hospitalized annually and about 50,000 patients with TBI die as a result of their injury.[1] TBI contributes significantly to the death of about half of all trauma victims. Moderate to severe brain injuries are identified in about 100,000 trauma patients annually. Mortality rates for moderate and severe brain injuries are about 10% and 30%, respectively. Of those who survive moderate and severe brain injuries, between 50% and 99% have some degree of permanent neurologic disability.

Motor vehicle crashes (MVCs) remain the leading cause of TBI in those between the ages of 5 and 65 years of age, and falls are the leading cause of TBI in pediatric patients up to the age of 4 years and the elderly population. The head is the most frequently injured part of the body in patients with multisystem injuries. The incidence of gunshot wounds to the brain has increased in recent years in urban areas, and up to 60% of these victims die from their injury.

Patients with TBI represent some of the most challenging trauma patients to treat. They may be combative, and attempts to intubate can be extremely difficult because of clenched jaw muscles and vomiting. Intoxication with drugs or alcohol or the presence of shock from other injuries can hinder assessment. Occasionally, serious intracranial injuries can be present with only minimal external evidence of trauma. Skilled care in the prehospital setting focuses on ensuring the adequate delivery of oxygen and nutrients to the brain and rapidly identifying patients at risk for herniation and elevated intracranial pressure. This approach can not only decrease mortality from TBI, but also reduce the incidence of permanent neurologic disability.

Anatomy

Knowledge of head and brain anatomy is essential to understand the pathophysiology of TBI. The scalp is the outermost covering of the head and offers some protection to the skull and brain. The scalp is comprised of several layers, including skin, connective tissue, galea aponeurotica, and the periosteum of the skull. The galea is important because it provides the structural support to the scalp and is the key to its integrity. The scalp and soft tissues overlying the face are highly vascular.

The skull, or cranium, is composed of a number of bones that fuse into a single structure during childhood. Several small openings (*foramina*) through the base of the skull provide pathways for blood vessels and cranial nerves. One large opening, the foramen magnum, is located on the caudal aspect of the skull base and serves as a passageway for the brainstem to the spinal cord (Figure 9-1). In infants, "soft spots" (*fontanelles*) can often be identified between the bones. The infant has no bony protection over these portions of the brain until the bones fuse, typically by 2 years of age.

Although most of the bones forming the cranium are thick and strong, the skull is especially thin in the temporal and ethmoid regions, which are more prone to fracture. The cranium provides significant protection to the brain, but the interior surface of the skull base is rough and irregular (see Figure 9-1). When exposed to a blunt force, the brain may slide across these irregularities, producing cerebral contusions or lacerations.

Three separate membranes, the *meninges,* cover the brain (Figure 9-2). The outermost layer, the *dura mater,* is composed of tough fibrous tissue and is applied to the inner table, or inside, of the skull. Under normal circumstances, the space between the dura and the inside of the skull—the epidural space—does not exist; it is a potential space. The dura is

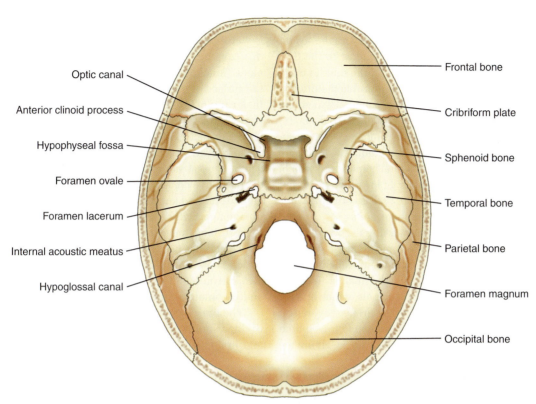

Optic canal
Anterior clinoid process
Hypophyseal fossa
Foramen ovale
Foramen lacerum
Internal acoustic meatus
Hypoglossal canal

Frontal bone
Cribriform plate
Sphenoid bone
Temporal bone
Parietal bone
Foramen magnum
Occipital bone

FIGURE 9-1 Internal view of the base of the skull.

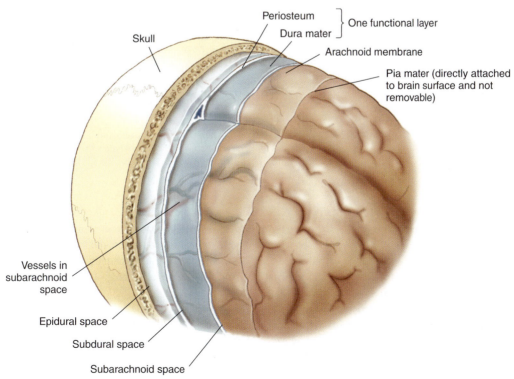

Skull
Periosteum
Dura mater
One functional layer
Arachnoid membrane
Pia mater (directly attached to brain surface and not removable)

Vessels in subarachnoid space
Epidural space
Subdural space
Subarachnoid space

FIGURE 9-2 Meninges: Meningeal coverings of the brain.

applied to the skull similar to a laminate. The middle meningeal arteries are located in grooves in the temporal bones on either side of the head, outside the dura. A blow to the thin temporal bone can create a fracture and tear the middle meningeal artery, the common etiology for epidural hematomas.

Unlike the epidural space, which is a potential space, the subdural space is an actual space between the dura and the brain. This space is spanned in places by veins, which create a vascular communication between the skull and brain. The traumatic rupture of these veins often creates subdural hematomas, which, unlike epidural hematomas, are venous, of lower pressure, and often associated with brain injury. Injury to these bridging veins accounts for the morbidity of subdural hematomas.

On the other side of the subdural space lies the brain, which is closely covered with two additional meningeal layers, the arachnoid and the pia. The *pia mater* is closely adhered to the brain, again similar to a laminate, and is the final brain covering. On top of the pia run cerebral blood vessels, which emerge from the base of the brain and then cover its surface. Layered on top of these blood vessels is the *arachnoid membrane,* which more loosely covers the brain and its blood vessels, giving the appearance of a "cellophane wrap" around the brain when it is viewed from the subdural space. Before cellophane existed, this covering was thought to resemble a spider web, thus the name "arachnoid." Because the cerebral blood vessels run on the surface of the brain but beneath the arachnoid membrane, their rupture (usually from trauma or a ruptured cerebral aneurysm) will result in bleeding into the subarachnoid space, causing a subarachnoid bleed. This blood normally does not enter the subdural space but is contained beneath the arachnoid; it can be seen at surgery as a thin layer of blood on the surface of the brain, contained beneath this translucent membrane. Unlike epidural and subdural hematomas, subarachnoid blood does not normally create mass effect but can be symptomatic of other serious injury to the brain.

The brain also is surrounded by *cerebrospinal fluid* (CSF), which is produced in the ventricular system of the brain and also surrounds the spinal cord. CSF helps cushion the brain and is contained in the subarachnoid space as well.

The brain occupies about 80% of the cranial vault and is divided into three main regions: the cerebrum, cerebellum, and brainstem (Figure 9-3). The *cerebrum* consists of right

---

FIGURE 9-3   The Brain

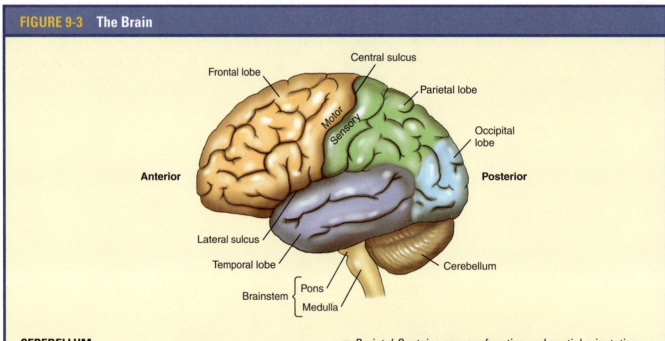

CEREBELLUM
Controls coordination and balance.

CEREBRUM
The cerebrum is composed of the right and left cerebral hemispheres. The dominant hemisphere is the one that contains the language center. This is the left hemisphere in virtually all right-handed individuals and about 85% of left-handed individuals. The cerebrum is composed of the following lobes:

- *Frontal.* Contains emotions, motor function, and expression of speech on the dominant side.

- *Parietal.* Contains sensory function and spatial orientation.
- *Temporal.* Regulates certain memory functions; contains the area for speech reception and integration in all right-handed and the majority of left-handed individuals.
- *Occipital.* Contains vision.

BRAINSTEM

- *Midbrain and upper pons.* Contain the reticular activating system (RAS), which is responsible for arousal and alertness.
- *Medulla.* Contains the cardiorespiratory centers.

and left hemispheres that can be subdivided into several lobes. The cerebrum houses sensory functions, motor functions, and higher intellectual functions such as intelligence and memory. The *cerebellum* is located in the posterior fossa of the cranium, behind the brainstem and beneath the cerebrum, and coordinates movement. The *brainstem* contains the medulla, an area that controls many vital functions, including breathing and heart rate. Much of the reticular activating system (RAS), the portion of the brain responsible for arousal and alertness, is also found in the brainstem. Blunt trauma can impair the RAS, leading to a transient loss of consciousness. The tentorium cerebelli, a portion of the dura mater, lies between the cerebrum and the cerebellum and contains an opening, the tentorial incisura, at the level of the midbrain.

The 12 cranial nerves originate from the brain and brainstem (Figure 9-4). The oculomotor nerve, cranial nerve III, controls pupillary constriction and provides an important tool in the assessment of a patient with a suspected brain injury.

Physiology

Cerebral Blood Flow

It is critical that the brain's neurons receive a constant flow of blood in order to provide oxygen and glucose. This constant cerebral blood flow is maintained by ensuri pressure (cerebral perfusion pressure) to fo head and (2) a regulatory mechanism (auto ensures a constant blood flow by varying blood flow as the perfusion pressure changes.

Mean Arterial Pressure

The heart is a cyclic pump, and thus the pressure created by the heart is represented as two pressures. The *diastolic pressure* is the baseline pressure that is maintained within the circulatory system when the heart is resting and not pumping, and the *systolic pressure* is the maximum pressure generated at the peak of cardiac contraction. Because such a dynamic characterization of the pressures generated by the heart can be difficult to work with, for the purposes of discussing cerebral blood flow and perfusion pressure, we use an average pressure for the entire cardiac cycle—the *mean arterial pressure* (MAP)—to characterize the pressure driving blood into the head.

Calculation of the MAP assumes that cardiac contraction (systole) takes up one-third of the cardiac cycle and that the remaining two-thirds of the cycle, the systemic pressure, remain at baseline (diastole). The MAP is therefore calculated by (1) averaging the additional pressure added to the system during cardiac contraction, or systole, over the entire cardiac cycle and (2) adding it to the diastolic pressure. This is done by calculating the additional pressure added to the system during systole, the *pulse pressure,* dividing

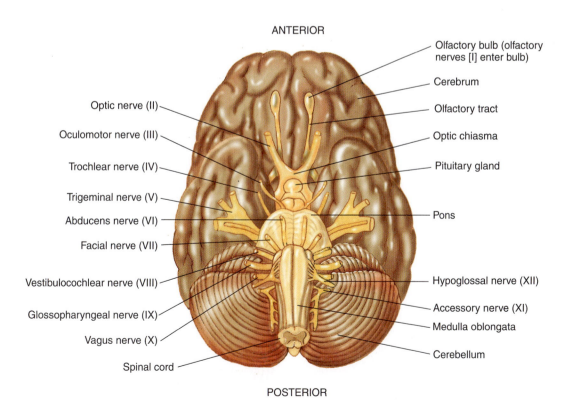

ANTERIOR

Optic nerve (II)
Oculomotor nerve (III)
Trochlear nerve (IV)
Trigeminal nerve (V)
Abducens nerve (VI)
Facial nerve (VII)
Vestibulocochlear nerve (VIII)
Glossopharyngeal nerve (IX)
Vagus nerve (X)
Spinal cord

Olfactory bulb (olfactory nerves [I] enter bulb)
Cerebrum
Olfactory tract
Optic chiasma
Pituitary gland
Pons
Hypoglossal nerve (XII)
Accessory nerve (XI)
Medulla oblongata
Cerebellum

POSTERIOR

FIGURE 9-4   Inferior surface of the brain showing the origins of the cranial nerves.

it by 3, and adding this number to the diastolic pressure, as follows:

Pulse pressure = Systolic pressure − Diastolic pressure

and

MAP = Diastolic pressure + ⅓ Pulse pressure

Most blood pressure monitors report the MAP with a much more accurate method of calculation that uses the actual blood pressure waveform. Because the percentage of time the heart spends in systole increases as the heart rate increases, the assumption that systole is one-third of diastole becomes less and less accurate as the patient becomes more tachycardic. Therefore, the blood pressure monitor, in the vast majority of patients being transported for neurologic injury, will more accurately represent the MAP than the preceding calculation. The value in learning the calculation lies in the insights it provides into the nature of the MAP.

Cerebral Perfusion Pressure

Cerebral perfusion pressure is the amount of pressure it takes to push blood through the cerebral circulation and, thus, maintain blood flow and oxygen and glucose delivery to the energy demanding cells of the brain. This relates directly to the amount of pressure inside the cranial vault, or intracranial pressure (ICP). Because the space inside the skull is fixed, anything that occupies additional space within the cranial vault will cause the intracranial pressure to start to increase. As the ICP increases, the amount of pressure needed to push blood through the brain also increases. If the MAP cannot keep up with the increase in ICP or if treatment to decrease the ICP is not rapidly instituted, the amount of blood flowing through the brain will start to decrease, leading to ischemic brain damage. All of this is expressed by the following formula:

Cerebral perfusion pressure (CPP) is the MAP minus the pressure in the head, the *intracranial pressure* (ICP) or

CPP = MAP − ICP

Normal MAP ranges from about 85 to 95 mm Hg, and ICP is normally below 15 mm Hg. Therefore, CPP is normally about 70 to 80 mm Hg.

Autoregulation of CBF

The most important factor for the brain, however, is not CPP itself, but rather cerebral blood flow (CBF). The brain works very hard at keeping its cerebral blood flow constant over a wide range of changing conditions. This is known as autoregulation. Autoregulation is crucial to the brain's normal function.

To understand autoregulation, we need to remember that for any flowing system:

Pressure = Flow × Resistance

In the case of the brain, this translates into:

Cerebral perfusion pressure =
Cerebral blood flow × Cerebral vascular resistance
CPP = CBF × CVR

Because the brain's principle concern is CBF, it is useful to rewrite this equation as:

CBF = CPP/CVR

Looking at this equation, it is evident how the brain keeps blood flow constant. If a person changes position from lying down to standing up, the CPP will fall. The only way to keep CBF constant is to also have the cerebral vascular resistance (CVR) drop as well. The brain accomplishes this decline in CVR by dilating the cerebral vasculature. The process of changing the caliber of the cerebral blood vessels to adjust CVR to compensate for changes in CPP is how the brain accomplishes its *autoregulation.*

In people who stand up too quickly and faint, their autoregulatory mechanisms simply did not react quickly enough to their change in position, resulting in a temporary but dramatic loss of cerebral blood flow and, therefore, brain function.

To function normally, the autoregulatory mechanism must have a certain minimum pressure. Clearly, at a pressure of 0 mm Hg, no amount of vasodilation will cause blood to flow, and there are limits to how much the blood vessels in the head can dilate. Therefore, below a CPP of about 50 mm Hg, the autoregulatory mechanisms can no longer compensate for the decreased CPP, and CBF starts to decrease. Cerebral function declines as CBF begins to fall, and the risk of permanent cerebral injury from ischemia increases.

To make matters worse, injured brains often require higher-than-normal CPPs to activate the autoregulatory mechanisms and keep CBF adequate. Although each individual patient probably has his or her own CPP threshold above which CBF is adequate, there is no way to determine this threshold in the field. Therefore, the best estimate of an adequate CPP is 60 to 70 mm Hg.

Unfortunately, the best ways to measure CBF are not very convenient; therefore, CPP is used to estimate the adequacy of CBF. Measuring CPP requires both a blood pressure monitor and an ICP monitor. In the absence of an ICP monitor, the best practice is simply to try and maintain a high normal MAP. Because most literature on outcomes from TBI has used *systolic blood pressure* (SBP) instead of MAP to measure blood pressure, SBP is the value used to monitor the adequacy of cerebral perfusion in settings without ICP monitoring. Best evidence suggests that an SBP greater than 90 mm Hg is desirable for neurologically injured patients.[2–6]

Hyperventilation

Hyperventilation reduces ICP but also impacts CBF. In fact, data suggest that hyperventilation more reliably reduces CBF than ICP. Hyperventilation reduces ICP by reducing the arterial carbon dioxide partial pressure ($PaCO_2$) by increasing the rate at which CO_2 is blown off by the lungs. This reduced $PaCO_2$ (hypocapnia) changes the acid-base balance in the brain, resulting in vasoconstriction. This cerebral vasoconstriction reduces the intravascular volume of the brain, reducing cerebral blood volume and, therefore, often ICP.[7,8]

Under normal circumstances, autoregulation ensures adequate CBF by making sure that CVR is correct for the available CPP to ensure continuing adequate CBF. It is important to note that hyperventilation of a patient is bypassing autoregulation. Therefore, hyperventilation causes cerebral vasoconstriction, which may reduce cerebral blood volume enough to reduce ICP, but it also increases CVR, whether or not CPP is adequate to maintain CBF. As a result, hyperventilation can reduce CBF, placing the injured brain at risk for ischemic injury. A $PaCO_2$ less than 35 mm Hg increases the risk of cerebral ischemia, and a $PaCO_2$ greater than the normal range of 35 to 45 mm Hg (hypercapnia) leads to dilation of cerebral arterioles, thus increasing CBF and potentially also increasing ICP. (Management of TBI using hyperventilation is discussed later.)

Pathophysiology

TBI can be divided into two categories: primary and secondary.

Primary Brain Injury

Primary brain injury is the direct trauma to the brain and associated vascular structures that occur at the time of the original insult. It includes contusions, hemorrhages, and lacerations and other direct mechanical injury to the brain, its vasculature, and coverings. Because neural tissue does not regenerate well, there is minimal expectation of recovery of the structure and function lost due to primary injury. Also, little possibility exists for repair.

Secondary Brain Injury

Secondary brain injury refers to the ongoing injury processes that are set in motion by the primary injury. At the time of injury, pathophysiologic processes are initiated that continue to injure the brain for hours, days, and weeks after the initial insult. The primary focus in the management of TBI is to identify and limit or stop these secondary injury mechanisms.

Before computed tomography (CT) was available, the principle secondary injury mechanism was "unidentified intracranial bleeds." The literature referred to "talk and die" patients, or those who were initially lucid after a traumatic insult but then lapsed into a coma and died as an unidentified intracranial hematoma expanded, leading to fatal herniation. Clearly, in these patients, if the initiated pathologic process could be interrupted, the patient's life could be saved.[9–11]

Pathologic mechanisms related to intracranial mass effect, elevated ICP, and herniation still are concerns as causes of secondary injury, but their management has been revolutionized by CT, ICP monitoring, and immediate surgery. In the prehospital environment, the identification of patients at high risk for herniation from mass effect and their rapid transport to a hospital with the facilities to address these issues are still the key priorities.

With the advent of CT, it became easier to identify and treat these hematomas. However, it also became clear that other mechanisms were present and continued to injure the brain after injury. Large studies in the late 1980s demonstrated that unrecognized and untreated hypoxia and hypotension were as damaging to the injured brain as elevated ICP. Subsequent observations have shown that impaired delivery of oxygen or energy substrate (e.g., glucose) to the injured brain has a much more devastating impact than in the normal brain. Therefore, in addition to hematoma, two other sources of secondary injury are hypoxia and hypotension.[5,6,12–14]

Ongoing research in the laboratory is revealing a fourth class of secondary injury mechanisms, those occurring at the cellular level. Studies have identified multiple destructive cellular mechanisms that are initiated by injury. The ability to understand, manipulate, and stop these mechanisms may lead to new therapies to limit brain injury, perhaps even a prehospital "cocktail." At present, the study of these mechanisms is limited to the laboratory.

Secondary injury mechanisms include the following:

1. Mass effect and the subsequent elevated ICP and mechanical shifting of the brain, which can lead to herniation and significant morbidity and mortality if not addressed.
2. Hypoxia, which results from inadequate delivery of oxygen to the injured brain caused by ventilatory or circulatory failure or mass effect.
3. Hypotension and inadequate CBF, which can cause inadequate oxygen delivery to the brain. Low CBF also reduces delivery of substrate (e.g., glucose) to the injured brain and results in inadequate substrate (e.g., glucose).
4. Cellular mechanisms, including energy failure, inflammation, and "suicide" cascades, which can be triggered at the cellular level and can lead to cell death, called *apoptosis.*

Intracranial Causes

Mass Effect and Herniation. The secondary injury mechanisms most often recognized are those related to mass effect. These mechanisms are the result of the complex interactions described by the Monro-Kellie doctrine.[15] The brain is encased in a space that is fixed in size once the fontanelles are closed. All of the space within the cranium is taken up by brain, blood, or CSF. If any other mass, such as a hematoma, cerebral swelling, or a tumor, occupies any space within the

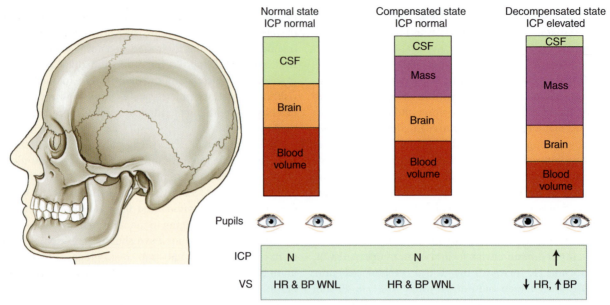

	Normal state ICP normal	Compensated state ICP normal	Decompensated state ICP elevated
	CSF Brain Blood volume	CSF Mass Brain Blood volume	CSF Mass Brain Blood volume
Pupils	👁 👁	👁 👁	👁 👁
ICP	N	N	↑
VS	HR & BP WNL	HR & BP WNL	↓ HR, ↑ BP

FIGURE 9-5 Monro-Kellie doctrine: intracranial compensation for expanding mass. The volume of the intracranial contents remains constant. If the addition of a mass such as a hematoma results in the squeezing out of an equal volume of cerebrospinal fluid *(CSF)* and venous blood, the intracranial pressure *(ICP)* remains normal. However, when this compensatory mechanism is exhausted, an exponential increase occurs in ICP for even a small additional increase in the volume of the hematoma.

cranial vault, some other structure needs to be forced out (Figure 9-5).

The dynamics of forcing blood, CSF, or brain out of the cranial vault in response to an expanding mass effect are the second part of the Monro-Kellie doctrine. At first, in response to the expanding mass, the volume of CSF surrounding the brain is reduced. The CSF naturally circulates within and around the brain, brainstem, and spinal cord; however, as the mass expands, more CSF is forced out of the head, and the total CSF volume within the skull is reduced. Blood volume in the cranial vault is also reduced in a similar manner, with venous blood the principle volume reduced in the head.

As a result of the reduction of CSF and blood volumes, the pressure in the head does not rise during the early phases of the expansion of intracranial masses. During this phase, if the growing mass is the only intracranial pathology, patients can appear to be asymptomatic. Once the ability to force out CSF and blood has been exhausted, however, the pressure inside the cranium—the ICP—starts to rise rapidly and causes brain shift and various herniation syndromes, which can compress vital centers and jeopardize arterial blood supply to the brain. The consequences of this movement toward the foramen magnum are described as the various herniation syndromes.

If the expanding mass is along the convexity of the brain, as in the typical position for a temporal lobe epidural hematoma, the temporal lobe will be forced toward the center of the brain at the tentorial opening. This movement forces the medial portion of the temporal lobe, the *uncus,* into the third nerve, the motor tract, and the brainstem and RAS on that side. This is called *uncal herniation* and results in malfunc-

tion of the third cranial nerve, causing a dilated or blown pupil on the side of the herniation (Figure 9-6). It also results in loss of function of the motor tract on the same side, which causes weakness on the opposite of the body from the lesion. In the last stages of uncal herniation, the RAS is affected, and the patient lapses into coma, an event associated with a much poorer prognosis.

Some convexity masses lead to *cingulate herniation,* either in conjunction with uncal herniation or in isolation. In cingulate herniation, the cingulate gyrus along the medial surface of the cerebral hemispheres is forced under the falx, the dural division between the two hemispheres. This can cause injury to the medial cerebral hemispheres and the midbrain.

Another type of herniation, called *tonsillar herniation,* occurs as the brain is pushed down toward the foramen magnum and pushes the cerebellum and medulla ahead of it. This can ultimately result in the most caudal part of the cerebellum, the cerebellar tonsils, and the medulla becoming wedged in the foramen magnum, with the medulla subsequently being crushed. Injury to the lower medulla results in cardiac and respiratory arrest, a common final event for

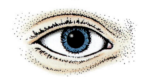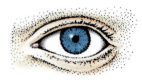

FIGURE 9-6 Suspect injury to the brain whenever a patient's pupils are unequal in size.

patients with herniation. The process of forcing the posterior fossa contents into the foramen magnum is referred to as "coning"[16] (Figure 9-7).

Clinical Herniation Syndromes. Clinical features of the herniation syndromes can help identify a patient who is herniating. Traditionally, as just mentioned, uncal herniation will often result in dilation or sluggishness of the ipsilateral pupil, referred to as a "blown pupil." Abnormal motor findings can also accompany herniation. Contralateral weakness may be associated with uncal herniation. More extensive herniation can result in destruction of structures in the brainstem known as the red nucleus or the vestibular nuclei. This can result in *decorticate posturing,* which involves flexion of the upper extremities and rigidity and extension of the lower extremities. A more ominous finding is *decerebrate posturing,* in which all extremities are extended and arching of the spine may occur. Decerebrate posturing occurs with injury and damage to the brainstem. After herniation, a terminal event may ensue and the extremities become flaccid, and motor activity is absent.[17,18]

In the final stages, herniation often produces abnormal ventilatory patterns or apnea, with worsening hypoxia and significantly altered blood CO_2 levels. *Cheyne-Stokes ventilations* are a repeating cycle of slow, shallow breaths that become deeper and more rapid and then return to slow, shallow breaths. Brief periods of apnea may occur between cycles. *Central neurogenic hyperventilation* refers to consistently rapid, deep breaths, and *ataxic breathing* refers to erratic ventilatory efforts that lack any discernible pattern. Spontaneous respiratory function ceases with compression of the brainstem, a common final pathway for herniation.[16]

As tissue hypoxia develops in the brain, reflexes are activated in an effort to maintain cerebral oxygen delivery. To overcome rising ICP, the autonomic nervous system is activated to increase systemic blood pressure, and therefore the MAP, to maintain a normal CPP. Systolic pressures can reach up to 250 mm Hg. However, as the baroreceptors in the carotid arteries and aortic arch sense a greatly increased blood pressure, messages are sent to the brainstem to activate the parasympathetic nervous system. A signal then travels via the tenth cranial nerve, the vagus nerve, to slow the heart rate. *Cushing's phenomenon* refers to this ominous combination of greatly increased arterial blood pressure and the resultant bradycardia that can occur with severely increased ICP.

Ischemia and Herniation. The herniation syndromes describe how the swelling brain, because it is contained in a fully enclosed space, can sustain mechanical damage. However, elevated ICP from cerebral swelling can also cause injury to the brain by creating cerebral ischemia as well as the resulting decreased oxygen delivery. As cerebral swelling increases, ICP also increases. Because CPP = MAP − ICP, as ICP increases, CPP decreases. Increases in ICP, therefore, threaten CBF. In addition to mechanical injury to the brain, cerebral swelling also can cause ischemic injury to the brain, compounding the ischemic insults the brain might sustain from other causes, such as systemic hypotension.

To complicate matters further, as these mechanical and ischemic insults create injury to the brain, they create more cerebral swelling. In this way, cerebral edema can cause injury that creates more cerebral edema, which in turn leads to further injury and edema in a downward spiral that can lead to herniation and death if not interrupted. Limiting this secondary injury and breaking this cycle of injury is the principle goal of TBI management.

Cerebral Edema. Cerebral edema (brain swelling) often occurs at the site of a primary brain injury. Injury to the neuronal cell membranes allows intracellular fluid to collect within damaged neurons, leading to cerebral edema. In addition, injury can lead to inflammatory responses that injure the neurons and the cerebral capillaries, leading to fluid collection within the neurons as well as within the interstitial spaces, both leading to cerebral edema. As the edema develops, the mechanical and ischemic injury previously described occurs, which aggravates these processes and leads to further edema and injury.

Cerebral edema can occur in association with or as a result of intracranial hematomas, as a result of injury to the brain parenchyma in the form of cerebral contusion, or as a result of diffuse brain injury from hypoxia or hypotension.

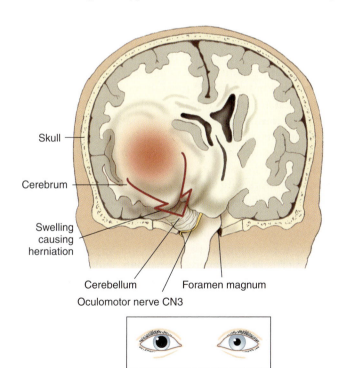

Skull

Cerebrum

Swelling causing herniation

Cerebellum   Foramen magnum

Oculomotor nerve CN3

FIGURE 9-7 The skull is a large, bony structure that contains the brain. The brain cannot escape the skull if it expands because of edema or if there is hemorrhage in the skull that presses on the brain.

Intracerebral Hematomas. In trauma, mass effect results from actual accumulation of blood in the intracranial space. Intracranial hematomas, such as epidural, subdural, or intracerebral hematomas, are major sources of mass effect. Because the mass effect from these hematomas is caused by their size, rapid removal of these hematomas can break the cycle of edema and injury described earlier. Unfortunately, these hematomas often have associated cerebral edema, and other means in addition to removing the hematoma are required to stop the cycle of injury and edema. (Specific cerebral hematomas are described later.)

Intracranial Hypertension. Intracranial hypertension results because cerebral edema occurs in an enclosed space. ICP is measured as a way to quantify and assess the degree of cerebral edema. ICP monitors are placed to allow providers to quantify the cerebral swelling, assess the risk of herniation, and monitor the effectiveness of therapies designed to combat cerebral edema. In this sense, elevated ICP is a sign of cerebral swelling.

Because elevated ICP, or intracranial hypertension, is part of the cycle previously described, it also causes cerebral injury in the form of mechanical compression of the brain and ischemic and hypoxic injury to the brain. For this reason, ICP is often discussed, correctly, both as a symptom and as a cause of cerebral edema.

ICP monitoring is not routinely available in the prehospital environment, but understanding it and the reasons for its control can help prehospital care providers with decision making for the brain-injured patient.

Extracranial Causes

Hypotension. As long known, brain ischemia is common in head injury. Evidence of ischemia is found in 90% of the patients who die of TBI, and even many of the survivors have evidence of ischemic injury.[19] Therefore, the impact of low CBF on the outcome from TBI has been a primary focus for limiting secondary injury after TBI.

In the national TBI database, the two most significant predictors of poor outcome from TBI were the amount of time spent with an ICP greater than 20 mm Hg and with an SBP less than 90 mm Hg. In fact, a single episode of SBP less than 90 mm Hg can lead to a poorer outcome.[20] Several studies have confirmed the profound impact of low SBP on the outcome after TBI.

Many patients with TBI sustain other injuries, often involving hemorrhage and subsequent low blood pressure. Aggressive fluid resuscitation of these injuries in a focused effort to keep SBP greater than 90 mm Hg is essential to limiting the secondary injury to the brain that can result from failing to meet this goal.

In addition to hemorrhage, a second factor threatens CBF after TBI, especially in the most severe injuries. A typical cortical CBF is 50 ml/100g of brain/minute. After severe TBI, this value can drop to 30 ml or even as low as 20 ml/100g/minute in the most severe injuries. Exactly why this occurs is not clear. This decline in CBF may be caused by loss of autoregulation, or it may be a protective mechanism to try to downregulate the entire brain in response to injury. Whatever the cause, this effect—added to the impact of hemorrhagic shock—compounds the ischemic threat to the brain.[8,8,20,21]

In addition, as noted earlier, autoregulation in the injured brain is deranged. As a result, higher CPP is required to maintain adequate CBF. Severely injured areas of the brain can lose almost all ability to autoregulate. In these areas, the blood vessels become dilated, causing hyperemia and shunting blood toward the most severely injured brain areas and possibly away from areas that could still be saved by adequate perfusion.[22,23] Lastly, aggressive hyperventilation can further threaten CBF and compound the ischemic threat by constricting blood vessels.

This combination of physiologic downregulation, shunting, and hemorrhagic shock creates multiple ischemic threats to the brain and makes the aggressive management of hypotension an essential part of the management of TBI. For this reason, an aggressive approach in the prehospital environment, with fluid resuscitation aimed at keeping the SBP above 90 mm Hg, is essential to limit secondary injury in the brain-injured patient.

Hypoxia. One of the most critical substrates delivered to the injured brain by the circulation is oxygen. Irreversible brain damage can occur after only 4 to 6 minutes of cerebral anoxia. Studies have also demonstrated a significant impact of an oxygen saturation less than 90% in TBI patients.[2,5,14] A significant number of TBI patients are not adequately resuscitated in the field.[14] In addition, several studies have demonstrated that significant numbers of TBI victims present with low or inadequate O_2 saturation.[13] The emphasis on prehospital airway management and oxygen delivery for brain-injured patients has partly been the result of these studies.

Elegant work with brain-tissue-oxygen monitors has demonstrated the impact of hemorrhagic shock on oxygen delivery to the brain. Limiting hypotension is a key component in ensuring that the brain receives an adequate supply of oxygen during the postinjury phase.[24]

Hemorrhage is common in patients with TBI, resulting not only in shock, but also in loss of blood and, therefore, hemoglobin.

For oxygenated blood to be delivered to the brain, the lungs must be properly functioning, which they often are not after trauma. Patients with an inadequate airway, aspiration of blood or gastric contents, pulmonary contusions, or pneumothoraces have pathology that will interfere with good respiratory function and the ability to transfer oxygen from the atmosphere to the blood. In addition to ensuring oxygen transport to the brain through adequate hemoglobin and circulation, providers must ensure adequate oxygenation through an adequate airway and with adequate ventilation.

As with hypotension, aggressive limitation of cerebral hypoxia with appropriate management of airway, breathing, and circulation is essential for limiting secondary brain injury.

Anemia. Also critical to the delivery of oxygen to the brain is the oxygen-carrying capacity of the blood, which is determined by the amount of hemoglobin it contains. A 50% drop in hemoglobin has a much more profound effect on oxygen delivery to the brain than a 50% drop in PO_2. For this reason, anemia can impact the outcome of TBI.

Hypocapnia and Hypercapnia. As discussed earlier in this chapter, both hypocapnia (decreased $PaCO_2$) and hypercapnia (increased $PaCO_2$) can worsen brain injury. When cerebral blood vessels constrict, as results from significant hypocapnia, CBF is compromised, leading to a decrease in oxygen delivery to the brain. Hypercapnia can result from hypoventilation from many causes, including drug or alcohol intoxication and abnormal ventilation patterns seen in patients with increased ICP. Hypercapnia causes cerebral vasodilation, which can further increase ICP.

Hypoglycemia and Hyperglycemia. Hypotension makes it highly likely that CBF is also low. As CBF falls, oxygen delivery to the brain also falls, as does delivery of glucose and other necessary brain metabolites. The epidemiologic effects of low SBP and the physiology of low oxygen delivery to the brain have been well studied. However, the injured brain's use of glucose and the impact of glucose utilization and delivery on the injured brain are still the subjects of research.

The research available, however, offers a fascinating look into the brain's response to injury. It appears that after head injury, cerebral glucose metabolism can become deranged in complex ways. Some compelling evidence indicates that glucose metabolism and, therefore, cerebral glucose requirements actually increase after severe head injury, threatening a mismatch between glucose delivery and utilization.[25–27]

On the other hand, good clinical and laboratory data in stroke patients show that patients whose serum glucose is allowed to remain elevated for long periods in the intensive care unit (ICU) may have larger areas of infarction and less effective resuscitation of salvageable brain than patients whose glucose is better controlled. Limited studies seem to indicate that these same factors are present in the ischemia that occurs after head injury. Elevated blood glucose levels in patients with TBI have also been associated with poorer neurologic outcome.

Both elevations (hyperglycemia) and decreases (hypoglycemia) in blood sugar can jeopardize ischemic brain tissue. The disastrous impact of significant hypoglycemia on the nervous system, during injury and at other times, is well known. Neurons are unable to store sugar and require a continual supply of glucose to carry out cellular metabolism. In the absence of glucose, ischemic neurons can be permanently damaged. However, it is also true that a prolonged serum glucose level greater than 150 mg/dl, and probably greater than 200 mg/dl, may be harmful to the injured brain and should be avoided.[28,29]

In the prehospital environment the emphasis should be on avoiding hypoglycemia because the physiologic threat from low sugar is much more immediate than from elevated serum glucose. Blood-glucose measurement should be performed in the field, if available, in all patients with altered mentation and, if found to be below normal values, treated with glucose administration. In addition, any induced hyperglycemia is likely to be transient, and the tight glucose control required to manage these patients properly will be established upon admission to the hospital.

Seizures. A patient with acute TBI is at risk for seizures for several reasons. Hypoxia from either airway or breathing problems can induce generalized seizure activity, as can hypoglycemia and electrolyte abnormalities. Ischemic or damaged brain tissue can serve as an irritable focus to produce grand mal seizures or status epilepticus. Seizures, in turn, can aggravate pre-existing hypoxia caused by impairment of respiratory function. Additionally, the massive neuronal activity associated with generalized seizures rapidly depletes oxygen and glucose levels, further worsening cerebral ischemia.

Assessment

A quick survey of the kinematics of the injury, combined with a rapid primary survey, will help identify potential life-threatening problems in a patient with a suspected TBI.

Kinematics

As with all trauma patients, assessment must include consideration of the mechanism of injury. Because many patients with severe TBI have an altered level of consciousness (LOC), key data about the kinematics will frequently come from observation of the scene or from bystanders. The windshield of the patient's vehicle may have a "spider web" pattern, suggesting an impact with the patient's head, or a bloody object may be present that was used as a weapon during an assault. A lateral impact on the side of the head can cause fracture of the skull with injury to the underlying middle meningeal artery leading to epidural hematoma or may cause a coup/contrecoup injury with venous damage and subdural hemorrhage. This important information should be reported to personnel at the receiving facility because it may be essential for proper diagnosis and management of the patient.

Primary Survey

Airway

The patency of the patient's airway should be examined and assured. In unconscious individuals, the tongue may completely occlude the airway. Noisy ventilations indicate partial obstruction by either the tongue or foreign material. Emesis, hemorrhage, and swelling from facial trauma are common causes of airway compromise in patients with TBI.

Breathing

Evaluation of respiratory function must include an assessment of the rate, depth, and adequacy of breathing. As noted previously, several different breathing patterns can result from severe brain injury. In multisystem trauma patients, thoracic injuries can further impair both oxygenation and ventilation. Cervical spine fractures occur in about 2% to 5% of patients with TBI and may result in spinal cord injuries that significantly interfere with ventilation.

Adequate oxygen delivery to the injured brain is an essential part of the effort to limit secondary brain injury. Failure to keep the oxygen saturation of hemoglobin (SpO_2) above 90% appears to result in poorer outcomes for brain-injured patients; maintaining SpO_2 above 90% is critical. Assessing for adequate airway and ventilatory effort is crucial in the early stages of managing TBI.

Circulation

As noted previously, maintaining an SBP greater than 90 mm Hg is critical for limiting secondary brain injury in the victims of TBI. Therefore, the control of hemorrhage and the prevention and treatment of shock are critical. The prehospital care provider will note and quantify evidence of external bleeding, if possible. In the absence of significant external blood loss, a weak, rapid pulse in a victim of blunt trauma suggests life-threatening internal hemorrhage in the pleural spaces, peritoneum, retroperitoneum, or soft tissues surrounding long-bone fractures. In an infant with open fontanelles, sufficient blood loss can occur inside the cranium to produce hypovolemic shock. A slow, forceful pulse may result from intracranial hypertension and indicate impending herniation (Cushing's phenomenon). In a patient with potentially life-threatening injuries, transport should not be delayed to measure blood pressure but should be performed en route as time permits.

Disability

During the primary survey and after the initiation of appropriate measures to treat problems identified in the airway, breathing, and circulation assessments, a baseline Glasgow Coma Scale (GCS) score should be calculated to assess the patient's LOC accurately (Figure 9-8). As described in Chapter 6, the GCS score is calculated by using the best response noted when evaluating the patient's eyes, verbal response, and motor response. Each component of the score should be recorded individually, rather than just providing a total, so

FIGURE 9-8 Glasgow Coma Scale

Evaluation	Points
EYE OPENING	
Spontaneous eye opening	4
Eye opening on command	3
Eye opening to painful stimulus	2
No eye opening	1
BEST VERBAL RESPONSE	
Answers appropriately (oriented)	5
Gives confused answers	4
Inappropriate response	3
Makes unintelligible noises	2
Makes no verbal response	1
BEST MOTOR RESPONSE	
Follows command	6
Localizes painful stimuli	5
Withdrawal to pain (nonlocalizing movement to pain)	4
Responds with abnormal flexion to painful stimuli (decorticate)	3
Responds with abnormal extension to pain (decerebrate)	2
Gives no motor response	1

Note that the lowest possible score is 3 and the highest possible score is 15.

that specific changes can be noted over time. If a patient lacks spontaneous eye opening, a verbal command (e.g., "Open your eyes") should be used. If the patient does not respond to a verbal stimulus, a painful stimulus, such as nail bed pressure with a pen or squeezing of anterior axillary tissue, should be applied.

The patient's verbal response can be examined using a question such as, "What happened to you?" If fully oriented, the patient will supply a coherent answer. Otherwise, the patient's verbal response is scored as confused, inappropriate, unintelligible, or absent. If the patient is intubated, the score is calculated from only the eye and motor scales, and a "T" is added to note the inability to assess the verbal response, such as "8T."

The last component of the GCS is the motor score. A simple, unambiguous command should be given to the patient, such as, "Hold up two fingers" or "Show me a hitchhiker's sign." A patient who squeezes the finger of a prehospital care provider may simply be demonstrating a grasping reflex as opposed to following a command purposefully. A painful stimulus is used if the patient fails to follow a command, and the patient's *best* motor response scored. A patient who attempts to push away a painful stimulus is considered to be "localizing." Other possible responses to pain include withdrawal from the stimulus, abnormal flexion (decorticate) or extension (decerebrate) of the upper extremities, and absence of a motor function.

The pupils are examined quickly for symmetry and response to light. A difference of greater than 1 mm in pupil size is considered abnormal. A significant portion of the population has *anisocoria,* inequality of pupil size that is either congenital or acquired as the result of ophthalmic trauma. It is not always possible in the field to distinguish between pupillary inequality caused by trauma and congenital or preexisting posttraumatic anisocoria. Pupillary inequality should always be treated as secondary to the acute trauma until the appropriate workup has ruled out cerebral edema or motor or ophthalmic nerve injury.[30]

Expose/Environment

Patients who have sustained a TBI frequently have other injuries, which threaten life and limb as well as the brain. All such injuries must be identified. The entire body should be examined for other potentially life-threatening problems.

Secondary Survey

Once life-threatening injuries have been identified and managed, a thorough secondary survey should be completed if time permits. The patient's head and face should be palpated carefully for wounds, depressions, and crepitus. Any drainage of clear fluid from the nose or ear canals may be CSF. When placed on a gauze pad or cloth, CSF may diffuse out from blood, producing a characteristic yellowish "halo." Although a positive halo is not always caused by CSF, this is an excellent test to use in the field if time permits, because it alerts the provider that a CSF leak may be present.[31]

The pupillary size and response should be rechecked at this time. Because of the incidence of cervical spine fractures in patients with TBI, as noted previously, the neck should be examined for tenderness and bony deformities.

In a cooperative patient, a more thorough neurologic examination should also be performed. This will include assessing the cranial nerves, sensation, and motor function in all extremities. Neurologic deficits, such as hemiparesis (weakness) or hemiplegia (paralysis), present on only one side of the body, are considered "lateralizing signs," and tend to be indicative of TBI.

History

A SAMPLE history can be obtained from the patient, family members, or bystanders (*s*ymptoms, *a*llergies, *m*edications, *p*ast history, *l*ast meal, *e*vents). Diabetes mellitus, seizure dis-

orders, and drug or alcohol intoxication can mimic TBI. Any evidence of drug use or overdose should be noted. The patient may have a history of prior head injury and may complain of persistent or recurring headache, visual disturbances, nausea and vomiting, or difficulty speaking.[32]

Serial Examinations

About 3% of patients with apparently mild brain injury (GCS 14 or 15) may experience an unexpected deterioration in their mentation. During transport, both the primary survey and assessment of the GCS should be repeated at frequent intervals. Patients whose GCS deteriorates by more than 2 points during transport are at particularly high risk for an ongoing pathologic process.[30,33,34] These patients need rapid transport to an appropriate facility. The receiving facility will use GCS trends during transport in the patient's early management. Trends in the GCS or vital signs should be reported to the receiving facility and documented on the patient care report. Responses to management should also be recorded.[35]

Specific Head and Neck Injuries

Scalp

As noted in the anatomy section, the scalp is composed of multiple layers of tissue and is highly vascular; even a small laceration may result in copious hemorrhage. More complex injuries, such as a degloving injury in which a large area of the scalp is torn back from the skull, can result in hypovolemic shock and even exsanguination (Figure 9-9). These types of injury often occur in an unrestrained front-seat occupant

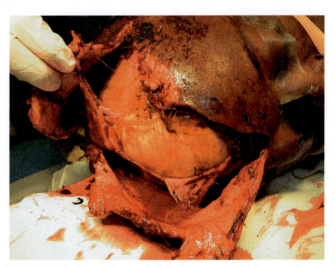

FIGURE 9-9 Extensive scalp injuries may result in massive external hemorrhage.

of a vehicle whose head impacts the windshield, as well as in workers whose long hair becomes caught in machinery. A serious blow to the head may result in the formation of a scalp hematoma, which may be confused with a depressed skull fracture while palpating the scalp.

Skull Fractures

Fractures of the skull can result from either blunt or penetrating trauma. *Linear fractures* account for about 80% of skull fractures; however, a powerful impact may produce a *depressed* skull fracture, in which fragments of bone are driven toward or into the underlying brain tissue (Figure 9-10). Although simple linear fractures can be diagnosed only with a radiographic study, depressed skull fractures can often be palpated during a careful physical examination. A closed, nondepressed skull fracture by itself is of little clinical significance, but its presence increases the risk of an intracranial hematoma. Closed, depressed skull fractures may require neurosurgical intervention. Open skull fractures can result from a particularly severe impact or from a gunshot wound and serve as an entry site for bacteria, predisposing the patient to meningitis. If the dura mater is torn, brain tissue or CSF may leak from an open skull fracture. Because of the risk of meningitis, these wounds require immediate neurosurgical evaluation.

Basilar skull fractures (fractures of the floor of the cranium) should be suspected if CSF is draining from the nostrils or ear canals. Periorbital ecchymosis ("raccoon eyes") and

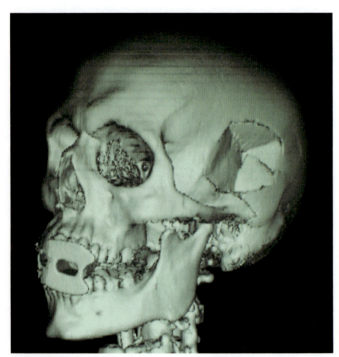

FIGURE 9-10 A 3-D reconstruction of a depressed skull fracture after an assault.

Battle's sign, in which ecchymosis is noted over the mastoid area behind the ears, often occur with basilar skull fractures, although they may take several hours after injury to become apparent.

Facial Injuries

Injuries to the face range from minor soft tissue trauma to severe injuries associated with airway compromise or hypovolemic shock. The airway may be compromised by either structural changes resulting from the trauma or from fluid or other objects in the airway itself. Structural changes may result from deformities of the fractured facial bones or from hematomas that develop in the tissues. Because the head has a high concentration of blood vessels, many injuries to this region result in significant hemorrhage. Blood and blood clots may interfere with the patency of the airway. Facial trauma is often associated with alterations in consciousness and even severe trauma to the brain. Trauma to the face may result in fractures or displacement of teeth into the airway lumen. TBIs and swallowed blood from facial injuries may lead to vomiting, which also leads to airway obstruction.

Trauma to the Eye and Orbit

Injury to the structures of the orbit and eye are not uncommon and often result from direct trauma to the face, either from intentional (assault) or unintentional causes. Although injury of the globe (eyeball) itself is not often encountered, it must be considered whenever trauma to the face and orbit is noted, as proper management of a globe injury may result in salvage of the patient's vision.

Eyelid Laceration. In the prehospital setting, laceration of an eyelid must cause consideration of the possibility that the globe has been penetrated. Field treatment consists of immediately covering the eye with a protective rigid shield (NOT a pressure patch) that is placed over the bony orbit. The primary consideration is to avoid any pressure on the eye that might do further harm by forcing intraocular contents out through a corneal or scleral laceration.

Corneal Abrasion. A corneal abrasion is disruption of the protective epithelial covering of the cornea. This abrasion results in intense pain, tearing, light sensitivity (photophobia), and increased susceptibility to infection until the defect has healed (usually in 2 to 3 days). There is typically a history of antecedent trauma or contact lens wear. Prehospital management for this disorder in the urban setting is to cover the eye with a patch, shield, or sunglasses to reduce the discomfort caused by light sensitivity.

Subconjunctival Hemorrhage. Subconjunctival hemorrhage is a bright red area over the sclera of the eye that results from bleeding between the conjunctiva and the sclera (Figure 9-11). It is easily visible without the use of a slit lamp. This injury is

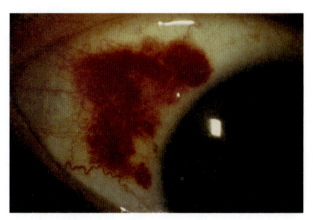

FIGURE 9-11   Subjunctival hemorrhage.

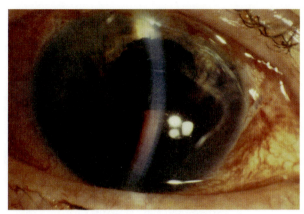

FIGURE 9-12   Hyphema.

innocuous and resolves over a period of several days to several weeks without treatment. In the presence of antecedent trauma, one should be alert for another, more serious injury. In particular, if hemorrhage results in massive swelling of the conjunctiva (chemosis), an occult globe rupture should be suspected. Prehospital management of this disorder consists solely of transporting the patient to the hospital so that the diagnosis can be confirmed and other associated disorders ruled out.

Hyphema. The term hyphema is defined as blood in the anterior chamber of the globe between the iris and the cornea. This is usually seen in the setting of acute trauma. The eye should be examined with the victim sitting upright. If enough blood is present, it collects at the bottom of the anterior chamber and is visible as a layered hyphema (Figure 9-12). This may not be appreciated if the victim is examined while in a supine position or if the amount of blood is very small. Hyphema patients should have a protective shield placed over the eye and be transported to the hospital in a sitting position (if there is no other contraindication) so that a complete eye examination can be performed.

Open Globe. If there is a history of trauma and penlight inspection of the eye reveals an obvious open globe, the examination should be discontinued and a protective shield placed onto the bony orbit over the eye. Do NOT apply a pressure patch or instill any topical medication. There are two primary concerns in the management of this condition. The first is to minimize manipulation of or additional trauma to the eye that might raise intraocular pressure and result in expulsion of intraocular contents through the corneal or scleral defect. The second is to prevent development of posttraumatic endophthalmitis, an infection of the aqueous and vitreous humors of the eye. This typically has devastating visual results, with only 30% of victims in one study retaining visual acuity greater than or equal to 20/400. Expeditious transport to the hospital is warranted for ophthalmologic evaluation and surgical repair.

A penetrating injury to the eye or a ruptured globe may not always be obvious. Clues to occult rupture include large subconjunctival hemorrhage with chemosis, dark uveal tissue (the colored iris) present at or protruding through the limbus (junction of the cornea and the sclera), distorted pupil, leak from a linear or punctate corneal epithelial defect, mechanism of injury (hammering metal on metal, impaling injury, etc.), or decrease in vision. If an occult globe rupture is suspected, the victim should be treated as described previously for an obvious open globe. The relatively less severe appearance of the injury does not eliminate the threat of endophthalmitis, so again rapid transport to the hospital is warranted.

Nasal Fractures

Fracture of the nasal bones is the most common fracture in the face. Indications that a nasal fracture is present include ecchymosis, edema, nasal deformity, swelling, and epistaxis. On palpation, bony crepitus may be noted.

Midface Fractures

Midfacial fractures can be categorized as follows (Figure 9-13):

- *Le Fort I fracture* involves a horizontal detachment of the maxilla from the nasal floor. Although air passage through the nares may not be affected, the oropharynx may be compromised by a blood clot or edema in the soft palate.
- *Le Fort II fracture,* also known as a *pyramidal fracture,* includes the right and left maxillae, the medial portion of the orbital floor, and the nasal bones. The sinuses are well vascularized, and this fracture may be associated with airway compromise from significant hemorrhage.
- *Le Fort III fracture* involves the facial bones being fractured off the skull (craniofacial disjunction). Because of the forces involved, this injury may be associated with airway compromise, presence of TBI, injuries to the tear ducts, malocclusion of teeth, and CSF leakage from the nares.

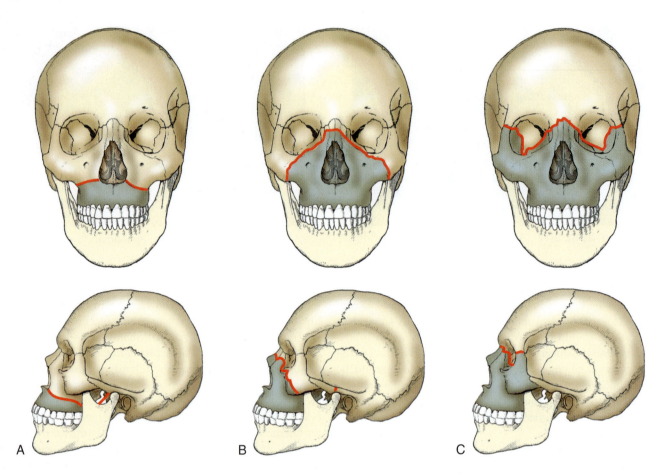

FIGURE 9-13 Types of Le Fort fractures of the midface. **A.** Le Fort I fracture. **B.** Le Fort II fracture. **C.** Le Fort III fracture. (Modified from Sheehy S: *Emergency nursing,* ed 3, St. Louis, 1992, Mosby.)

Patients with a midface fracture generally have loss of normal facial symmetry. The face may appear flattened, and the patient may be unable to close the jaws or teeth. If conscious, the patient may complain of facial pain and numbness. On palpation, crepitus may be noted over fracture sites.

Mandibular Fractures

Following fractures of the nasal bones, mandibular fractures are the second most common type of facial fracture. In more than 50% of cases, the mandible is broken in more than one location. The most common complaint of a patient with a mandibular fracture is malocclusion of the teeth; that is, the upper and lower teeth no longer meet in usual alignment. On palpation, a "step-off" type of deformity and crepitance may be noted.

In a supine patient with a mandible fracture, the tongue may occlude the airway as the bony support structure of the tongue is no longer intact.

Laryngeal Injuries

Fractures of the larynx typically result from a blunt blow to the anterior neck, or a motorcycle or bicycle rider's anterior neck may be struck by an object. The patient may complain of a change in voice (usually lower in tone). On inspection, the provider may note a neck contusion or loss of the prominence of the thyroid cartilage (Adam's apple). A fracture of the larynx may result in the development of subcutaneous emphysema in the neck, which may be detected on palpation. Endotracheal intubation is generally contraindicated in the presence of a laryngeal fracture because this procedure may dislodge fracture segments. If a patient with a suspected laryngeal fracture has a compromised airway, a surgical cricothyrotomy may be lifesaving.

Injuries to Cervical Vessels

A carotid artery and internal jugular vein traverse the anterior neck on either side of the trachea. The carotid arteries supply blood to the majority of the brain, and the internal jugular veins drain this region. Injury to one of these vessels can produce profound hemorrhage. An added danger from internal jugular vein injuries is air embolism. If a patient is sitting up or the head is elevated, venous pressure may fall below atmospheric pressure during inspiration, permitting air to enter the venous system. A large air embolus can be fatal because it can interfere with both cardiac function and cerebral perfusion.

Brain Injuries

Cerebral Concussion

The diagnosis of a "concussion" is made when an injured patient shows any transient alteration in neurologic function. Although most people associate a loss of consciousness with the diagnosis of concussion, loss of consciousness is not required to make a diagnosis of concussion; rather, posttraumatic amnesia is the hallmark of concussion. Other neurologic changes include the following:

- Vacant stare (befuddled facial expression)
- Delayed verbal and motor responses (slow to answer questions or follow instructions)
- Confusion and inability to focus attention (easily distracted and unable to follow through with normal activities)
- Disorientation (walking in the wrong direction; unaware of time, date, and place)
- Slurred or incoherent speech (making disjointed or incomprehensible statements)
- Lack of coordination (stumbling, inability to walk tandem/straight line)
- Inappropriate emotions to the circumstances (distraught, crying for no apparent reason)
- Memory deficits (exhibited by patient repeatedly asking the same question that has already been answered)
- Inability to memorize and recall (e.g., 3 of 3 words or 3 of 3 objects in 5 minutes)[36]

In all patients with only a simple concussion, head CT will be normal.

Severe headache, dizziness, and nausea and vomiting frequently accompany a concussion. Although most of these findings last several hours to a couple days, some patients experience a postconcussive syndrome with headaches, dizziness, and difficulty concentrating for weeks, and even months, after a severe concussion. Patients exhibiting signs of concussion and especially patients with nausea, vomiting, or neurologic findings on secondary survey should be immediately transported for further evaluation.

Intracranial Hematoma

Intracranial hematomas are divided into three general types: epidural, subdural, and intracerebral. Because the signs and symptoms of each of these have significant overlap, specific diagnosis in the prehospital setting (as well as the ED) is almost impossible, although the prehospital care provider may suspect an epidural hematoma based on the characteristic clinical presentation. Even so, a definitive diagnosis can only be made after a CT scan is performed at the receiving facility. Because these hematomas occupy space inside the rigid skull, they may produce rapid increases in ICP, especially if they are sizable.

Epidural Hematoma. Epidural hematomas account for about 2% of TBIs that require hospitalization. These hematomas often result from a low-velocity blow to the temporal bone, such as the impact from a punch or baseball. A fracture of this thin bone damages the middle meningeal artery, which results in arterial bleeding that collects between the skull and dura mater (Figure 9-14). This high-pressure arterial blood can start to dissect or peal the dura off of the inner table of the skull, creating an epidural space full of blood. Such an

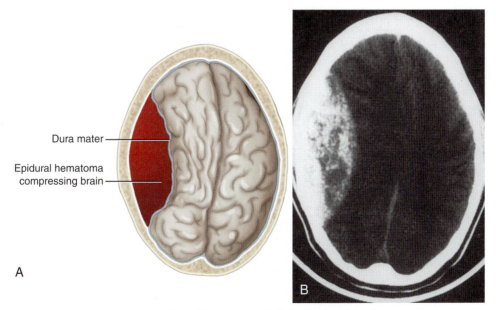

Dura mater

Epidural hematoma compressing brain

A

B

FIGURE 9-14 **A.** Epidural hematoma. **B.** CT scan of epidural hematoma.
(**B** from Cruz J: *Neurologic and neurosurgical emergencies,* Philadelphia, 1998, Saunders.)

epidural hematoma has a characteristic lens shape, as seen on the CT scan, created by the dura holding the hematoma against the inner table of the skull. The principle threat to the brain is from the expanding mass of blood displacing the brain and threatening herniation. For this reason, patients whose epidural hematoma is rapidly evacuated often have excellent recoveries.

The classic history for an epidural hematoma is a patient experiencing a brief loss of consciousness, then regaining consciousness, and then experiencing a rapid decline in consciousness. During the period of consciousness, the *lucid interval,* the patient may be oriented, lethargic, or confused or may complain of a headache. Only about one-third of patients with epidural hematomas actually experience this "lucid interval," however, and it may also occur with other types of intracranial hemorrhages, making it nonspecific for epidural hematoma. Nonetheless, a patient who experiences a "lucid interval," followed by a decline in GCS, is at risk for a progressive intracranial process and needs emergency evaluation.

As a patient's LOC worsens, examination may reveal a dilated and sluggish or nonreactive pupil on the side of the herniation (ipsilateral side). Because motor nerves cross over to the other side above the spinal cord, hemiparesis or hemiplegia typically occurs on the side opposite the impact (contralateral side). The mortality rate for an epidural hematoma is about 20%; however, with rapid recognition and evacuation, the mortality rate can be as low as 2%. This is because an epidural hematoma is usually a "pure" space-occupying lesion, with little injury to the brain beneath. Once the hematoma is removed, the pathologic effect is also removed, and the patient can make an excellent recovery. Such rapid removal reduces not only mortality, but also subsequent, significant neurologic morbidity. Epidural hematomas often occur in young people, who are just beginning their careers, emphasizing the societal value as well as the human value of their rapid identification and removal.

Subdural Hematoma. Subdural hematomas account for about 30% of severe brain injuries. In addition to being more common than epidural hematomas, they also differ in etiology, location, and prognosis. Unlike the epidural hematoma caused by arterial hemorrhage, a subdural hematoma generally results from a venous bleed from bridging veins that are torn during a violent blow to the head. In this injury, the blood collects in the subdural space, between the dura mater and the arachnoid membrane (Figure 9-15).

Subdural hematomas present in two different ways. In some patients who have just experienced significant trauma, the disruption of the bridging veins results in relatively rapid accumulation of blood in the subdural space, with rapid onset of mass effect. Adding to this morbidity is injury to the brain parenchyma beneath the subdural hematoma, which occurs as part of the injury leading to the venous disruption. As a result, unlike that of epidural hematomas, the mass effect of subdural hematomas is often caused by both the accumulated blood and the swelling of the injured brain beneath. Patients presenting with such acute mass effect will have an acutely depressed mental status and will need emergency ICP monitoring and management and possibly surgery.

In some patient populations, however, clinically occult subdural hematomas can occur. In elderly or debilitated patients, such as those with chronic disease, the subdural space is enlarged secondary to brain atrophy. In such patients,

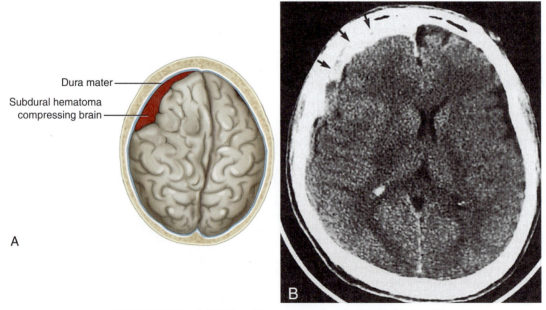

FIGURE 9-15 **A.** Subdural hematoma. **B.** CT scan of subdural hematoma.
(**B** from Cruz J: *Neurologic and neurosurgical emergencies,* Philadelphia, 1998, Saunders.)

blood may accumulate in the subdural space without inducing mass effect and, thus, may be clinically occult. Such subdural hematomas can occur during falls in elderly persons or during apparently minor trauma. At particular risk are patients receiving anticoagulants such as warfarin (Coumadin). Because these falls are minor, patients often do not present for evaluation, and the bleeds are not identified. Many patients in whom chronic subdural hematoma is eventually identified cannot recall the traumatic event.

In some patients in whom occult subdural hematoma *is* eventually identified, however, the subdural blood liquefies but is retained in the subdural space. Over time, through a mechanism that includes repeated small bleeds into the liquid hematoma, the now-chronic subdural hematoma can expand and slowly start to exert mass effect on the brain. Because the onset of the mass effect is slow, the patient will not have the dramatic presentation associated with an acute subdural hematoma and is more likely to present with headache, visual disturbances, personality changes, difficulty speaking (dysarthria), and hemiparesis or hemiplegia of a slowly progressive nature. Only when some of these symptoms become pronounced enough to prompt the patient or caregiver to seek help is the chronic subdural hematoma discovered. On CT scan, a chronic subdural hematoma has a distinct appearance compared with the more emergent, acute subdural hematoma. Often the event precipitating transport for evaluation and care is the most recent of the small, repetitive subdural bleeds that create chronic subdural hematomas, and a small amount of acute blood may be found in a larger collection of chronic blood. The need for and the urgency of surgery are determined by the patient's symptoms, the amount of mass effect, and the patient's overall medical condition.

Prehospital personnel frequently encounter these patients when called to facilities that care for chronically ill populations. Because the symptoms are nonspecific, diagnosing a chronic subdural hematoma in the field is rarely possible, and the symptoms may be confused with those of a stroke, infection, or even a generalized decline in the patient.

Although many subdural hematomas in these patients will be chronic, patients taking Coumadin, after an apparently insignificant trauma, may have a subdural hematoma that expands over several hours and progresses to herniation resulting from the patient's inability to clot. These patients can have a benign presentation and then deteriorate several hours after arrival. Elderly patients, and especially patients receiving Coumadin, who have experienced apparently minor falls should be managed with a heightened sense of urgency and care.

Cerebral Contusions. Damage to the brain itself may produce cerebral contusions and, if this damage includes injury to the blood vessels within the brain, actual bleeding into the substance of the brain, or *intracerebral hematomas*. Cerebral contusions are relatively common, occurring in about 20% to 30% of severe brain injuries and in a significant percentage of moderate head injuries as well. Although typically the result of blunt trauma, these injuries may also occur from penetrating trauma, such as a gunshot wound to the brain. In blunt trauma, cerebral contusions may be numerous. Cerebral contusions result from a complex pattern of transmission and reflection of forces within the skull. As a result, contusions often occur in locations remote from the site of impact, often on the opposite side of the brain, the familiar "contrecoup" injury.

Cerebral contusions often take 12 to 24 hours to appear on CT scans, and thus, a patient with a cerebral contusion may have an initially normal head CT scan. The only clue to its presence may be a depressed GCS, with many patients showing moderate head injuries (GCS 9–13). As the contusion evolves after injury, it not only becomes more apparent on head CT, but also can cause increased mass effect and create increasing headache, or cause moderate head injuries to deteriorate to severe head injuries in about 10% of patients.[37]

Subarachnoid Hemorrhage. Subarachnoid hemorrhage is bleeding beneath the arachnoid membrane, which lies under the subdural space covering the brain. Blood in the subarachnoid space cannot enter the subdural space. Many of the brain's blood vessels are located in the subarachnoid space, so injury to these vessels will cause subarachnoid bleeding, a layering of blood beneath the arachnoid membrane on the surface of the brain. This layering of blood is thin and rarely causes mass effect.

Subarachnoid hemorrhage is usually thought to be associated with ruptured cerebral aneurysms. In fact, posttraumatic subarachnoid hemorrhage is the most common cause of subarachnoid bleeding. Because subarachnoid bleeding rarely causes mass effect, it does not require surgery for decompression. It is a marker for potentially severe brain injury, however, and its presence increases the risk for other space-occupying lesions. Patients with traumatic subarachnoid hemorrhage (tSAH) have a 63% to 73% increased risk of a cerebral contusion, and 44% will develop subdural hematomas. Patients with tSAH have an increased risk of elevated ICP and intraventricular hemorrhage. Patients with large amounts of tSAH (>1 cm of blood thickness, blood in suprasellar or ambient cisterns) have a positive predictive value of 72% to 78% for a poor outcome, and in the Trauma Coma Data Bank, the presence of tSAH doubled the incidence of death in brain-injured patients.[38,39]

Management

Effective management of a patient with TBI begins with orderly interventions focused on treating any life-threatening problems identified in the primary survey. Once these problems are addressed, the patient should be rapidly packaged and transported to the nearest facility capable of caring for TBI.

Airway

Patients with a depressed LOC may be unable to protect their airway, and adequate oxygenation of the injured brain is critical to preventing secondary injury. As noted earlier, facial injuries can be associated with hemorrhage and edema that may compromise the airway. Hematomas in the floor of the mouth or in the soft palate may occlude the airway. The essential skills are appropriate initial airway interventions (see Chapter 7). Both oral and nasal airways may become occluded by edema or blood clots, and intermittent suctioning may be necessary. Patients with facial fractures and laryngeal or other neck injuries will typically assume a position that maintains their airway. Attempts to force a patient to lie supine or wear a cervical collar may be met with extreme combativeness if they become hypoxic as a result of positional airway impairment. In these situations, airway patency takes precedence over spinal immobilization, and patients may be transported in a sitting or semisitting position, as tolerated.

Cervical collars may be deferred if thought to compromise the airway while manual stabilization is performed. Conscious patients can often assist in managing their airway by suctioning when they feel it is needed; the provider can allow them to hold and use the suction device. Facial trauma, including those injuries caused by GSWs, is not a contraindication to ET intubation.

An early study showed that victims of TBI who were intubated appeared to do better.[40] Recent studies, however, have yielded mixed results in TBI casualties intubated in the field.[41–46] The specific explanation for these conflicting data awaits further study. However, poorly performed intubation appears be more harmful than no intubation at all. Several studies have shown that patients intubated in the field may have unrecognized episodes of hypoxia or hypotension, thus leading to poorer outcomes.[47] The deciding factors on whether or not to intubate a patient may be operator skill and length of transport. In urban settings, short transport times allow patients to be fairly urgently delivered to and intubated in an ED setting. Patients intubated in the field may do worse because of prolonged field times and a less experienced provider performing the intubation. Similarly, intubation in a system in which providers perform only a few intubations a year may be more detrimental than other means of airway support during transport. Conversely, in systems with longer transport times, intubation may be more beneficial than no intubation at all, even when done by a less experienced operator. Future studies should help determine the best practice in the prehospital environment.

With these qualifiers in mind, all patients with a severe TBI (GCS $\leq$ 8) should be considered for intubation. Because this can be extremely challenging due to the patient's combativeness, clenched jaw muscles (trismus), vomiting, and the need to maintain in-line cervical spine stabilization, intubation should be performed by the most skilled operator who can be available in a timely manner. It is essential that the patient's oxygen saturation be monitored throughout the performance of intubation and that hypoxia (oxygen saturation less than 90%) be avoided. The use of neuromuscular blocking agents as part of a rapid-sequence intubation (RSI) protocol may facilitate successful intubation.[48] Blind nasotracheal intubation (BNTI) can serve as an alternative technique, but the presence of midface trauma is a relative contraindication for this procedure. Concern has often been voiced about the possibility of inadvertent cranial and cerebral penetration with nasotracheal intubation in patients who have sustained head trauma. Review of the medical literature reveals that this complication has only been reported twice in head trauma patients.[49,50]

Suction equipment should be readily available. If initial attempts at intubation are unsuccessful, prolonged laryngoscopy should be avoided, especially with a short transport time. An oropharyngeal airway with bag-mask ventilation or a percutaneous transtracheal ventilation (PTV) are reasonable alternatives. Patients with severe facial injuries and obvious airway compromise may require PTV or a surgical cricothyroidotomy.

Breathing

All patients with suspected TBI should receive supplemental oxygen. As mentioned previously in this chapter, the use of pulse oximetry is strongly recommended because hypoxia can worsen neurologic outcome. Oxygen concentration can be titrated when using pulse oximetry; SpO_2 should be at least 90%, with 95% or higher as optimal. If pulse oximetry is not available, oxygen should be provided via a nonrebreather facemask for a spontaneously breathing patient. For intubated patients, an oxygen concentration of 100% (FiO_2 of 1.0) should be maintained with a bag-mask device. If hypoxia persists despite oxygen therapy, the provider should attempt to identify and treat all likely etiologies, including aspiration and tension pneumothoraces. Use of positive end-expiratory pressure (PEEP) valves, if available, may be considered to improve oxygenation; however, levels of PEEP greater than 15 cm H_2O may increase ICP.[51,52]

Because both hypocapnia and hypercapnia can aggravate TBI, control of ventilatory rate is important. When arterial blood gases (ABGs) are available, $PaCO_2$ should be maintained in the range of 35 to 40 mm Hg. In the hospital setting, end-tidal carbon dioxide ($ETCO_2$) can be used to estimate serum $PaCO_2$ in hemodynamically stable patients. Because the measured values for $ETCO_2$ and $PaCO_2$ vary widely from patient to patient, each in-hospital patient must have a unique "offset" between $PaCO_2$ and $ETCO_2$ determined by comparison with an ABG to obtain acceptable accuracy from the use of $ETCO_2$. New ABGs are obtained each time the patient's condition changes.

In the prehospital environment, $PaCO_2$ is not routinely available to determine its "offset" with $ETCO_2$. In addition, other patient factors, such as changes in pulmonary perfusion, in cardiac output, and in patient temperature, all cause changes in $ETCO_2$, which cannot be distinguished from $ETCO_2$ changes that result from changes in $PaCO_2$. Because physiologic changes occur rapidly in the prehospital phase as patients are resuscitated and warmed as well as ventilated, they are rarely stable enough to allow $ETCO_2$ to be used with any accuracy. Although $ETCO_2$ is an excellent tool for monitoring ventilation, it is not accurate enough to guide hyperventilation therapy meaningfully in the prehospital setting.[53–61]

It is simpler simply to judge the degree of ventilation by counting breaths per minute.

Normal ventilatory rates should be used when assisting ventilation in patients with TBI: 10 breaths/minute for adults, 20 breaths/minute for children, and 25 breaths/minute for infants. Overaggressive hyperventilation produces cerebral vasoconstriction, which in turn leads to a decrease in cerebral oxygen delivery. Routine prophylactic hyperventilation has been shown to worsen neurologic outcome and should not be used. A subgroup analysis of patients enrolled in the San Diego Paramedic RSI trial showed that both hyperventilation and severe hypoxia in the prehospital setting were associated with an increase in mortality. For adult patients, ventilating with a tidal volume of 350 to 500 ml at a rate of 10 breaths/minute should be sufficient to maintain adequate oxygenation without inducing hypocarbia.[62]

Hyperventilation of a patient in a controlled fashion may be considered in the specific circumstance of signs of herniation. These signs include asymmetric pupils, dilated and nonreactive pupils, extensor posturing or no response on motor examination, or progressive neurologic deterioration defined as a decrease in the GCS of more than 2 points in patient whose initial GCS was 8 or less. In such cases, mild, controlled hyperventilation in the field may be performed during the prehospital phase of care. Mild hyperventilation is defined as an ETCO2 of 30–35 mm Hg as measured by capnography or by careful control of the breathing rate (20 breaths/minute for adults, 25 breaths/minute for children, and 30 breaths/minute for infants less than 1 year of age).[63]

Circulation

Both anemia and hypotension are important causes of secondary brain injury, so efforts should be taken to prevent or treat these conditions. Hemorrhage control is essential. Direct pressure or pressure dressings should be applied to any external hemorrhage. Complex scalp wounds can produce significant external blood loss. Several gauze pads held in place by an elastic roller bandage create an effective pressure dressing to control bleeding. If this fails to control bleeding, it can often be controlled by applying direct pressure along the wound edges, thereby compressing the scalp vasculature between the skin and soft tissues and the galea. Dramatic bleeding can often be controlled with this maneuver. A pressure dressing should not be applied to a depressed or open skull fracture unless significant hemorrhage is present, because it may aggravate brain injury and lead to an increase in ICP. Direct gentle pressure may also limit the size of extracranial (scalp) hematomas. Gentle handling and immobilization to a long backboard in anatomic alignment can minimize interstitial blood loss around fractures.

Hemorrhage from the carotid arteries and internal jugular veins may be massive. In most circumstances, direct pressure will control such external hemorrhage. Injuries to these vessels from penetrating trauma may be associated with internal bleeding, presenting as an expanding hematoma. These hematomas may compromise the airway, and endotracheal intubation may be necessary. However, attempts to intubate a conscious patient with an expanding neck hematoma but no external bleeding may stimulate a cough, which may be sufficient to disrupt a clot that may have formed at a knife or bullet wound, resulting in massive external hemorrhage.

Because hypotension further worsens brain ischemia, standard measures should be employed to combat shock. In patients with TBI, the combination of hypoxia and hypotension is associated with a mortality rate of about 75%. If shock is present and major internal hemorrhage is suspected, prompt transport to a trauma center takes priority over brain injuries. Hypovolemic and neurogenic shock are aggressively treated by resuscitation with isotonic crystalloid solutions; however, transport should not be delayed to establish intravenous (IV) access. Although assessing blood volume is extremely difficult in the prehospital setting, the patient should be returned to a state of normal circulating blood volume (euvolemia) if possible. To preserve cerebral perfusion, attempts should be made to maintain an SBP of at least 90 to 100 mm Hg. For adult TBI patients with normal vital signs and no other suspected injuries, IV fluid at a rate of no more than 125 ml/hour should be administered and adjusted if signs of shock develop.[64] A randomized trial of patients with severe TBI showed that those who received prehospital resuscitation with hypertonic saline had almost identical neurologic functioning 6 months after injury compared to those treated with crystalloid.[65] Because of its increased cost and lack of benefit compared to normal saline or lactated Ringer's solution, hypertonic saline is not recommended for routine prehospital volume replacement.

Disability

Assessment of the GCS should be integrated into the routine evaluation of all trauma patients after circulation is addressed. Use of the GCS helps evaluate the patient's status and may impact transport and triage decisions, depending on the system in which the provider is working.

Prehospital management of TBI patients primarily consists of measures aimed at reversing and preventing factors that cause secondary brain injury. Prolonged or multiple grand mal seizures can be treated with IV administration of a benzodiazepine, such as diazepam, lorazepam, or midazolam. These drugs should be cautiously titrated because hypotension and ventilatory depression may occur.

Because of the significant incidence of cervical spine fractures, patients with suspected TBI should be placed in spinal immobilization. Some degree of caution must be exercised when applying a cervical collar to a patient with TBI. Some evidence suggests that a tightly fitted cervical collar can impede venous drainage of the head, thereby increasing ICP. *Application of a cervical collar is not mandatory as long as the head and neck are sufficiently immobilized.*

Transportation

To achieve the best possible outcome, patients with moderate and severe TBI should be transported directly to a trauma center that can perform a CT scan and ICP monitoring and provide prompt neurosurgical intervention. If such a facility is not available, aeromedical transport from the scene to an appropriate trauma center should be considered.[35]

The patient's pulse rate, blood pressure, SpO_2, and GCS should be reassessed and documented every 5 to 10 minutes during transport. PEEP valves may be used cautiously if persistent hypoxia exists because, as noted, levels of PEEP greater than 15 cm H_2O may increase ICP. The patient's body heat should be preserved during transport.

Controversy exists regarding the optimal position for a patient with TBI. In general, patients with TBI should be transported in a supine position because of the presence of other injuries.[66] Although elevating the head on the ambulance stretcher or long backboard (reverse Trendelenburg position) may decrease ICP, cerebral perfusion pressure may also be jeopardized, especially if the head is elevated higher than 30 degrees.

The receiving facility should be notified as early as possible so that appropriate preparations can be made before the patient's arrival. The radio report should include information regarding the mechanism of injury, initial GCS score and any changes en route, focal signs (e.g., motor exam asymmetry, unilaterally or bilaterally dilated pupils) and vital signs, other serious injuries, and response to management.[35]

Prolonged Transport

As with all patients with suspected TBI, efforts should focus on preventing secondary brain injury. A prolonged transport time may lower the threshold for performing endotracheal intubation. RSI may be used in this setting, especially if aeromedical transport is considered, because a combative patient

in the confines of a helicopter threatens the crew, pilot, and himself. Efforts to control the airway should be performed while cervical spine stabilization is being applied. Oxygenation should be administered to maintain an appropriate SpO_2 level. Because of the risk of developing pressure ulcers from lying on a hard backboard, the patient may be placed on a padded long backboard, especially if the anticipated transport time is lengthy. Patients should be attached to continuous pulse oximetry, and serial vital signs, including ventilations, pulse, blood pressure, and GCS score, should be measured. Pupils should be periodically checked for response to light and symmetry.

When there is a delay in transport or a prolonged transport time to an appropriate facility, additional management options can be considered. For patients with an abnormal GCS score, the blood glucose level should be checked. If the patient is hypoglycemic, a 50% dextrose solution can be administered intravenously until the blood sugar is restored to a normal level. Benzodiazepines may be titrated intravenously if recurrent or prolonged seizures occur.

External hemorrhage should be controlled, and volume resuscitation is administered if signs of shock are apparent. Fluids should be titrated to maintain the SBP greater than 90 mm Hg. Associated injuries should be managed while en route to the receiving facility. Fractures should be appropriately splinted to control both internal hemorrhage and pain.

Appropriate management of increased ICP in the prehospital setting is extremely challenging because the ICP is not monitored in the field unless the patient is undergoing interfacility transfer and an ICP monitor or ventriculostomy has been placed at the referring center. Although a declining GCS score may represent increasing ICP, it may also be the result of worsening cerebral perfusion from hypovolemic shock. Warning signs of possible increased ICP and herniation include the following:

- Decline in GCS score of two points or more
- Development of a sluggish or nonreactive pupil
- Development of hemiplegia or hemiparesis
- Cushing's phenomenon

The decision to intervene and manage increased ICP is based on written protocol or made in consultation with medical control at the receiving facility. Possible temporizing management options include sedation, chemical paralysis, osmotherapy (the use of osmotically active agents that may assist in the treatment of intracranial hypertension), and controlled hyperventilation. Small doses of benzodiazepine sedatives should be titrated cautiously because of the potential side effects of hypotension and ventilatory depression. Use of a long-acting neuromuscular blocking agent, such as vecuronium, may be considered if the patient is intubated. If the cervical collar is believed to be too tight, it may be loosened slightly or removed, provided that the head and neck are adequately immobilized with other measures.

Osmotherapy with mannitol (0.25–1.0 g/kg) can be given intravenously. However, aggressive diuresis may produce hypovolemia, which can worsen cerebral perfusion. Mannitol should be avoided for patients in whom systemic resuscitation has not been achieved—that is, patients with SBP less than 90 mm Hg. If an osmotic agent is used, the patient should be maintained in a euvolemic state. In addition, a Foley catheter should be placed if transport will be extremely prolonged.

Controlled, mild therapeutic hyperventilation (ETCO2 = 30–35 mm Hg) may be considered for obvious signs of herniation. The following ventilatory rates should be used: 20 breaths/minute for adults, 25 breaths/minute for children, and 30 breaths/minute for infants. *Prophylactic hyperventilation has no role in TBI, and therapeutic hyperventilation, if instituted, should be stopped if signs of intracranial hypertension resolve.* Steroids have not been shown to improve the outcome of patients with TBI and should not be administered.

The primary focus for the TBI patient during prolonged transport or in austere environments is the best possible maintenance of cerebral oxygenation and perfusion and the best efforts possible to control cerebral edema.

Brain Death and Organ Donation

The diagnosis of brain death is made when there is no clinical evidence of neurologic function in a patient who is warm, whose mental status is not impacted by sedating or paralyzing medications, and who is completely resuscitated with an SBP greater than 90 mm Hg and SpO_2 greater than 90%.

Assessment for clinical evidence of neurologic function consists of ensuring that there is no evidence of cortical function, followed by an assessment of midbrain and brainstem function down to the respiratory center in the lower medulla. This assessment consists of establishing the absence of response to deep pain, followed by the midbrain and brainstem assessment for nonreactive pupils, absence of a corneal reflex, and absence of response to cold caloric stimulation. A few patients can safely be tested for the absence of an oculocephalic reflex. In addition, absence of a gag reflex, absence of a cough reflex, and, finally, absence of any effort to breathe, with $PaCO_2$ greater than 60 mm Hg and adequate PO_2, are all determined. This last observation is obtained with an apnea test. In the absence of any activity on these tests, the patient can be declared clinically "brain dead."

Many clinical protocols and some state statutes also require that brain death be confirmed by an ancillary test, such as radionucleotide CBF studies or electroencephalography (EEG).

The physiologic definition of brain death just described is the definition typically used in the United States. Philosophical, ethical, and legal issues remain about how much of the brain must be dead before "personhood" is lost, and thus, the definition of brain death varies throughout the world. In addition, various hospitals and systems have differing methods for declaring brain death, and the states have varying legal statutes defining who may declare death and brain death and how it is to be declared. Those interested should ask within their local system.

It must be emphasized, however, that brain death is not the same as a "hopeless prognosis." Brain death is a *physiologic* event in which the brain dies while the heart and lungs are still functioning, usually through artificial support. As noted, how much brain must die before declaring brain death is debatable, but the fact that it is a physiologic event is not debatable.

In contrast, a hopeless prognosis is a medical judgment that a good outcome is not possible from the current injuries. This distinction is often blurred by health care providers, with the resulting confusion resulting in a loss of credibility on the part of the health care system.

This credibility is critical because the victim of TBI that progresses to brain death provides an important source of organs for transplantation. In 1999, TBI was the cause of brain death for more than 40% of individuals from whom organs were procured, with the majority of organs coming from those between 18 and 49 years of age. Despite the presence of a fatal brain injury, an individual's heart, lungs, liver, kidneys, pancreas, and corneas may benefit others with chronic illnesses. Enlisting the trust and support of the public in obtaining these organs is critical to ensuring their availability to those who so desperately need them. To gain this trust, the families of TBI victims first need to be sure that the resuscitation of the injured brain has been the first priority of the treating team, and second, when that resuscitation has failed, they need to understand the issues surrounding physiologic brain death versus a futile situation. A clear understanding of these issues empowers families to make good decisions for themselves and their loved one, decisions that they can live with as they gain more information in the aftermath of the event. Blurring or confusing these issues erodes the trust of the family and the credibility of the health care and organ-procurement communities. It is essential that health care providers clearly understand the issues surrounding brain death and effectively communicate these issues to the family members of the victims of TBI. In most cases, approaching a family concerning possible organ donation should occur only after all of the medical interventions have been attempted and completed and the contact made by trained representatives of the hospital or organ recovery team (Figure 9-16).

MANAGEMENT OF SUSPECTED TRAUMATIC BRAIN INJURY

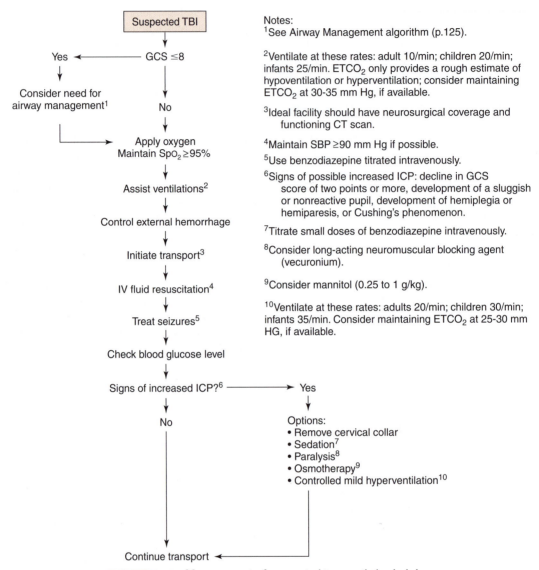

Notes:
[1]See Airway Management algorithm (p.125).

[2]Ventilate at these rates: adult 10/min; children 20/min; infants 25/min. $ETCO_2$ only provides a rough estimate of hypoventilation or hyperventilation; consider maintaining $ETCO_2$ at 30-35 mm Hg, if available.

[3]Ideal facility should have neurosurgical coverage and functioning CT scan.

[4]Maintain SBP ≥90 mm Hg if possible.

[5]Use benzodiazepine titrated intravenously.

[6]Signs of possible increased ICP: decline in GCS score of two points or more, development of a sluggish or nonreactive pupil, development of hemiplegia or hemiparesis, or Cushing's phenomenon.

[7]Titrate small doses of benzodiazepine intravenously.

[8]Consider long-acting neuromuscular blocking agent (vecuronium).

[9]Consider mannitol (0.25 to 1 g/kg).

[10]Ventilate at these rates: adults 20/min; children 30/min; infants 35/min. Consider maintaining $ETCO_2$ at 25-30 mm HG, if available.

FIGURE 9-16 Management of suspected traumatic brain Injury.

SUMMARY

- Preventing the development of or recognizing and treating hypoxia and reduced cerebral blood flow in the field can make the difference between a good and an unacceptable outcome.
- The severity of TBI may not be immediately apparent; therefore, serial neurologic evaluations of the patient, including Glasgow Coma Scale scores and pupillary response are necessary to recognize changes in the patient's condition.
- TBI is often found in association with multisystem trauma, so all problems are addressed in the appropriate order of

priority. Not only are airway, breathing, and circulation always the priorities of patient care, but they are specifically important in the management of TBI in preventing secondary brain injury.

- Prehospital management of the TBI patient involves controlling hemorrhage from other injuries, maintaining a systolic blood pressure of at least 90 mm Hg, and providing oxygen to maintain oxygen saturation of at least 90%.
- Hyperventilation of patients is performed only when objective signs of herniation are noted.

SCENARIO SOLUTION

The rapid decrease in this patient's GCS score is extremely worrisome, so you need to transport the patient to a facility with neurosurgical coverage immediately on completion of spinal immobilization. Given the lucid interval demonstrated by this patient, suspect the presence of an epidural hematoma. Examination of the eyes may reveal an enlarged, sluggishly reactive pupil on the right side, and weakness or paralysis may develop on the left side of the body. A CT scan at the receiving trauma center can confirm the diagnosis.

Once en route, re-evaluate the patient's airway and breathing and apply a pulse oximeter. If his SpO_2 is less than 90%, you supply supplemental oxygen and assist ventilations, as necessary with a bag-mask device. If the GCS score further deteriorates, also consider intubating this patient, preferably using a rapid-sequence technique while assuring adequate oxygenation throughout the procedure. Reassess the scalp wound to ensure that hemorrhage is adequately controlled and start two large-bore IV lines. Measure the patient's vital signs and take a blood pressure reading. Perform a complete secondary survey to rule out additional injuries, and determine blood glucose level. During transport, you frequently assess the patency of the patient's airway, measure his vital signs, and check his GCS score and papillary response. Notify the receiving facility of the patient's condition and update it if any significant changes occur.

Consider controlled hyperventilation if signs of herniation are present. When combined with appropriate neurosurgical intervention, aggressive prehospital care should improve the outcome of patients with moderate to severe TBI. ■

References

1. Centers for Disease Control: What is traumatic brain injury? http://www.cdc.gov/ncipc/tbi/TBI.htm. Accessed March 10, 2010.
2. Chestnut RM, Marshall LF, Klauber MR, et al: The role of secondary brain injury in determining outcome from severe head injury. *J Trauma* 34:216, 1993.
3. Fearnside MR, Cook RJ, McDougall P, et al. The Westmead Head Injury Project outcome in severe head injury: A comparative analysis of prehospital, clinical, and CT variables. *Br J Neurosurg* 7:267, 1993.
4. Gentleman D. Causes and effects of systemic complications among severely head-injured patients transferred to a neurosurgical unit. *Int Surg* 77:297, 1992.
5. Marmarou A, Anderson RL, Ward JL, et al. Impact of ICP instability and hypotension on outcome in patients with severe head trauma. *J Neurosurg* 75:S59, 1991.
6. Miller JD, Becker DP. Secondary insults to the injured brain. *J R Coll Surg Edinb* 27:292, 1982.
7. Obrist WD, Gennarelli TA, Segawa H, et al. Relation of cerebral blood flow to neurological status and outcome in head injured patients. *J Neurosurg* 51:292, 1979.
8. Obrist WD, Langfitt TW, Jaggi JL, et al. Cerebral blood flow and metabolism in comatose patients with acute head injury. *J Neurosurg* 61:241, 1984.
9. Marshall LF, Toole BM, Bowers SA. Part 2: Patients who talk and deteriorate: Implications for treatment. *J Neurosurg* 59:285, 1983.
10. Reilly PL, Adams JH, Graham DI, et al. Patients with head injury who talk and die. *Lancet* 2:375, 1975.
11. Rose J, Valtonen S, Jennett B: Avoidable factors contributing to death after head injury. *BMJ* 2:615, 1977.
12. Miller JD, Sweet RC, Narayan RK, et al: Early insults to the injured brain. *JAMA* 240:439, 1978.
13. Silverston P: Pulse oximetry at the roadside: A study of pulse oximetry in immediate care. *BMJ* 298:711, 1989.
14. Stochetti N, Furlan A, Volta F: Hypoxemia and arterial hypotension at the accident scene in head injury. *J Trauma* 40:764, 1996.
15. Kellie G: An account of the appearances observed in the dissection of two of three individuals presumed to have perished in the storm of the 3rd, and whose bodies were discovered in the vicinity of Leith on the morning of the 4th of November 1821 with some reflections on the pathology of the brain. *Trans Med Chir Sci Edinb* 1:84, 1824.
16. Plum F: *The diagnosis of stupor and coma*, ed 3, New York, 1982, Oxford University Press.
17. Langfitt TW, Weinstein JD, Kassell NF, et al: Transmission of increased intracranial pressure. I. Within the craniospinal axis. *J Neurosurg* 21:989, 1964.
18. Langfitt TW: Increased intracranial pressure. *Clin Neurosurg* 16:436, 1969.
19. Graham DI, Ford I, Adams JH, et al: Ischeaemic brain damage is still common in fatal non-missile head injury. *J Neurol Neurosurg Psychiatry* 52:346, 1989.

20. Marmarou A, Anderson RL, Ward JL, et al: Impact of ICP instability and hypotension on outcome in patients with severe head trauma. *J Neurosurg* 75:S59, 1991.

21. Obrist WD, Wilkinson WE: Regional cerebral blood flow measurement in humans by xenon-133 clearance. *Cerebrovasc Brain Metab Rev* 2:283, 1990.

22. Darby JM, Yonas H, Marion DW, et al: Local "inverse steal" induced by hyperventilation in head injury. *Neurosurgery* 23:84, 1988.

23. Marion DW, Darby J, Yonas H: Acute regional cerebral blood flow changes caused by severe head injuries. *J Neurosurg* 74:407, 1991.

24. Manley GT, Pitts LH, Morabito D, et al: Brain tissue oxygenation during hemorrhagic shock, resuscitation, and alterations in ventilation. *J Trauma Injury Infect Crit Care* 46:261, 1999.

25. Caron MJ, Hovda DA, Mazziotta JC, et al: The structural and metabolic anatomy of traumatic brain injury in humans: A computerized tomography and positron emission tomography analysis. *J Neurotrauma* 10(suppl 1):S58, 1993.

26. Caron MJ, Mazziotta JC, Hovda DA, et al: Quantification of cerebral glucose metabolism in brain-injured humans utilizing positron emission tomography. *J Cereb Blood Flow Metab* 13(suppl 1): S379, 1993.

27. Caron MJ: PET/SPECT imaging in head injury. In Narayan RK, Wilberger JE, Povlishock JT, editors: *Neurotrauma,* New York, 1996, McGraw-Hill.

28. Lam AM, Winn HR, Cullen BF, et al: Hyperglycemia and neurological outcome in patients with head injury. *J Neurosurg* 75:545, 1991.

29. Young B, Ott L, Dempsey R, et al: Relationship between admission hyperglycemia and neurologic outcome of severely brain-injured patients. *Ann Surg* 210:466, 1989.

30. Brain Trauma Foundation: Glasgow Coma Score. In Gabriel EJ, Ghajar J, Jagoda A, et al: *Guidelines for prehospital management of traumatic brain injury,* New York, 2000, The Foundation.

31. Dula DJ, Fales W: The "ring sign:" Is it a reliable indicator for cerebral spinal fluid? *Ann Emerg Med* 22:718, 1993.

32. American College of Surgeons: *Advanced trauma life support,* Chicago, 2004, The College.

33. Servadei F, Nasi MT, Cremonini AM: Importance of a reliable admission Glasgow Coma Scale score for determining the need for evacuation of posttraumatic subdural hematomas: A prospective study of 65 patients. *J Trauma* 44:868, 1998.

34. Winkler JV, Rosen P, Alfrey EJ: Prehospital use of the Glasgow Coma Scale in severe head injury. *J Emerg Med* 2:1, 1984.

35. Brain Trauma Foundation: Hospital transport decisions. In Gabriel EJ, Ghajar J, Jagoda A, et al: *Guidelines for prehospital management of traumatic brain injury,* New York, 2000, The Foundation.

36. American Academy of Neurology: The management of concussion in sports (summary statement). *Neurology* 48:581, 1997.

37. Rimel RW, Giordani B, Barth JT: Moderate head injury: Completing the clinical spectrum of brain trauma. *Neurosurgery* 11:344, 1982.

38. Brain Trauma Foundation: CT scan features. In Bullock MR, Chesnut RM, Clifton GL, et al: *Management and prognosis of severe traumatic brain injury,* ed 2, New York, 2000, The Foundation.

39. Kihtir T, Ivatury RR, Simon RJ, et al: Early management of civilian gunshot wounds to the face. *J Trauma* 35:569, 1993.

40. Winchell RJ, Hoyt DB: Endotracheal intubation in the field improves survival in patients with severe head injury. *Arch Surg* 132:592, 1997.

41. Davis DP, Hoyt DB, Ochs M, et al: The effect of paramedic rapid sequence intubation on outcome in patients with severe traumatic brain injury. *J Trauma Injury Infect Crit Care* 54:444, 2003.

42. Bochicchio GV, Ilahi O, Joshi M, et al: Endotracheal intubation in the field does not improve outcome in trauma patients who present without an acutely lethal traumatic brain injury. *J Trauma Injury Infect Crit Care* 54:307, 2003.

43. Davis DP, Peay J, Sise MJ, et al: The impact of prehospital endotracheal intubation in moderate to severe traumatic brain injury. *J Trauma* 58:933, 2005.

44. Bulger EM, Copass MK, Sabath DR, et al: The use of neuromuscular blocking agents to facilitate prehospital intubation does not impair outcome after traumatic brain injury. *J Trauma* 58:718, 2005.

45. Wang HE, Peitzman AB, Cassidy LD, et al: Out-of-hospital endotracheal intubation and outcome after traumatic brain injury. *Ann Emerg Med* 44:439, 2004.

46. Chi JH, Knudson MM, Vassar MJ, et al: Prehospital hypoxia affects outcome in patients with traumatic brain injury: A prospective multi-center study. *J Trauma* 61:1134, 2006.

47. Dunford JV, Davis DP, Ochs M, et al: Incidence of transient hypoxia and pulse rate reactivity during paramedic rapid sequence intubation. *Ann Emerg Med* 42:721, 2003.

48. Davis DP, Ochs M, Hoyt DB, et al: Paramedic-administered neuromuscular blockade improves prehospital intubation success in severely head-injured patients. *J Trauma Injury Infect Crit Care* 55:713, 2003.

49. Marlow TJ, Goltra DD, Schabel SI: Intracranial placement of a nasotracheal tube after facial fracture: A rare complication. *J Emerg Med* 15:187, 1997.

50. Horellou MD, Mathe D, Feiss P: A hazard of nasotracheal intubation. *Anaesthesia* 22:78, 1978.

51. Cooper KR, Boswell PA, Choi SC: Safe use of PEEP in patients with severe brain injury. *J Neurosurg* 63:552, 1985.

52. McGuire G, Crossley D, Richards J, et al: Effects of varying levels of positive end-expiratory pressure on intracranial pressure and cerebral perfusion pressure. *Crit Care Med* 25:1059, 1997.

53. Christensen MA, Bloom J, Sutton KR: Comparing arterial and end-tidal carbon dioxide values in hyperventilated neurosurgical patients. *Am J Crit Care* 4:116, 1995.

54. Grenier B, Dubreuil M: Noninvasive monitoring of carbon dioxide: end-tidal versus transcutaneous carbon dioxide. *Anesth Analg* 86:675, 1998.

55. Grenier B, Verchere E, Mesli A, et al: Capnography monitoring during neurosurgery: Reliability in relation to various intra-operative positions. *Anesth Analg* 88:43, 1999.

56. Isert P: Control of carbon dioxide levels during neuroanaesthesia: Current practice and an appraisal of our reliance upon capnography. *Anaesth Intensive Care* 22:435, 1994.

57. Kerr ME, Zempsky J, Sereika S, et al: Relationship between arterial carbon dioxide and end-tidal carbon dioxide in mechanically ventilated adults with severe head trauma. *Crit Care Med* 24:785, 1996.

58. Mackersie RC, Karagianes TG: Use of end-tidal carbon dioxide tension for monitoring induced hypocapnia in head-injured patients. *Crit Care Med* 18:764, 1990.

59. Russell GB, Graybeal JM: Reliability of the arterial to end-tidal carbon dioxide gradient in mechanically ventilated patients with multisystem trauma. *J Trauma Injury Infect Crit Care* 36:317, 1994.

60. Sanders AB: Capnometry in emergency medicine. *Ann Emerg Med* 18:1287–1290, 1989.

61. Sharma SK, McGuire GP, Cruise CJE: Stability of the arterial to end-tidal carbon dioxide difference during anaesthesia for prolonged neurosurgical procedures. *Can J Anaesthesiol* 42:498, 1995.

62. Davis DP, Dunford JV, Poste JC, et al: The impact of hypoxia and hyperventilation on outcome after paramedic rapid sequence intubation of severely head injured patients. *J Trauma* 57:1, 2004.

63. Badjatia N, Carney N, Crocco TJ, et al: Treatment: Cerebral Herniation. In Gabriel EJ, Ghajar J, Jagoda A, et al: *Guidelines for prehospital management of traumatic brain injury,* New York, 2000, The Foundation.

64. Brain Trauma Foundation: Treatment: fluid resuscitation. In Gabriel EJ, Ghajar J, Jagoda A, et al: *Guidelines for prehospital management of traumatic brain injury,* New York, 2000, The Foundation.

65. Cooper DJ, Myles PS, McDermott FT, et al: Prehospital hypertonic saline resuscitation of patients with hypotension and severe traumatic brain injury: A randomized controlled trial. *JAMA* 291:1350, 2004.

66. Feldman Z, Kanter MJ, Robertson CS: Effect of head elevation on intracranial pressure, cerebral perfusion pressure and cerebral blood flow in head-injured patients. *J Neurosurg* 76:207, 1992.

Suggested Reading

American College of Surgeons Committee on Trauma: Head trauma. In *Advanced trauma life support for doctors, student course manual,* ed 7, Chicago, 2004, ACS.

Atkinson JLD: The neglected prehospital phase of head injury: Apnea and catecholamine surge. *Mayo Clin Proceed* 75:37, 2000.

Bertz JE: Maxillofacial injuries. *Clin Symp* 33:2, 1981.

Chi JH, Nemani V, Manley GT: Prehospital treatment of traumatic brain injury. *Sem Neurosurg* 14:71, 2003.

Guidelines for the determination of brain death. *JAMA* 246:2184, 1981.

Kolb JC, Summer RL, Galli L: Cervical collar–induced changes in intracranial pressure. *Am J Emerg Med* 17:135, 1999.

Muizelaar JP, Marmarou A, Ward JD, et al: Adverse effects of prolonged hyperventilation in patients with severe brain injury: A randomized clinical trial. *J Neurosurg* 75:731, 1991.

Rosner MJ, Coley IB: Cerebral perfusion pressure, intracranial pressure and head elevation. *J Neurosurg* 65:636, 1986.

Teasdale G, Jennett B: Assessment of coma and impaired consciousness: A practical scale. *Lancet* 2:81, 1974.

Valadka AB: Injury to the cranium. In Mattox KL, Feliciano DV, Moore EE: *Trauma,* ed 4, Norwalk, Conn, 2000, Appleton & Lange.

CHAPTER 10

Spinal Trauma

CHAPTER OBJECTIVES

At the completion of this chapter, the reader will be able to do the following:

- ✓ Describe the epidemiology of spinal injuries.

- ✓ Compare and contrast the most common mechanisms that produce spinal injury in adults with those in children.

- ✓ Recognize patients with the potential for spinal trauma.

- ✓ Relate the signs and symptoms of spinal injury and neurogenic shock with their underlying pathophysiology.

- ✓ Integrate principles of anatomy and pathophysiology with assessment data and principles of trauma management to formulate a treatment plan for the patient with obvious or potential spinal injury.

- ✓ Describe the indications for spinal immobilization.

- ✓ Discuss factors associated with prehospital findings and interventions that may affect spinal injury morbidity and mortality.

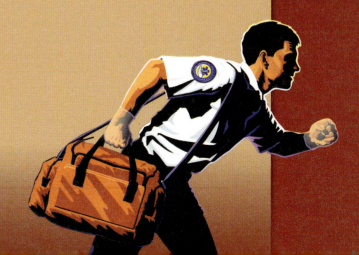

SCENARIO

You have been dispatched to the scene of a gymnastics event. On arrival, you find a 19-year-old female, lying supine on a gym mat underneath exercise bars. The scene is safe. Her gymnastics coach is sitting next to her trying to talk to her, but she is not responding.

As you begin your primary survey, you find an unresponsive female patient who fell while performing her gymnastics routine. She has abrasions on her forehead and an obvious deformity of the right wrist. Her airway is open, and she is breathing regularly. She shows no obvious signs of external blood loss. Her skin appears dry and warm with normal color. As you are performing your primary assessment, she begins to awaken, but remains confused as to what happened.

What pathologic processes explain the patient's presentation? What intermediate interventions and further assessments are needed? What are the management goals for this patient?

Spinal trauma, if not recognized and properly managed, can result in irreparable damage to the spinal cord and leave a patient paralyzed for life. Some patients sustain immediate spinal cord damage as a result of trauma. Others sustain an injury to the spinal column that does not initially damage the cord; cord damage may result later with movement of the spine. Because the central nervous system (CNS) is incapable of regeneration, a severed spinal cord cannot be repaired. The consequences of inappropriately moving a patient with a spinal column injury, or allowing the patient to move, can be devastating. Failure to detect and immobilize a fractured spine properly may produce a much worse outcome than, for example, failure to immobilize a fractured femur properly. Conversely, spinal immobilization of the patient who has no indications of injury also has consequences and should not be done without careful consideration of the risks versus the benefits.

Spinal cord injury can have profound effects on human physiology, lifestyle, and financial circumstances. Human physiology is affected because the use of extremities or other areas is severely limited or completely impaired as a result of cord damage. Lifestyle is affected because spinal cord injury usually results in profound changes to daily activity levels and independence. Spinal cord injury also impacts the financial circumstances of the patient as well as the population in general.[1] A patient with this injury requires both acute and long-term care. The lifetime cost of this care is estimated at approximately $1.35 million per patient for a permanent spinal cord injury.[2]

About 32 people per 1 million of population will sustain some type of spinal cord injury annually. An estimated 250,000 to 400,000 people live with spinal cord injuries in the United States. Spinal cord injury can occur at any age; however, it usually occurs in those 16 to 35 years of age because this age group is involved in the most violent and high-risk activities. Most trauma patients are 16 to 20 years

of age. The second largest group of patients is 21 to 25 years, and the third largest group is 26 to 35 years of age. Common causes are motor vehicle crashes (48%), falls (21%), penetrating injuries (15%), sports injuries (14%), and other injuries (2%). Overall, approximately 11,000 people sustain spinal cord injuries annually in the United States.[3]

Sudden violent forces acting on the body can force the spine beyond its normal limits of motion by either impacting on the head or neck or driving the torso out from under the head. The following four concepts help clarify the possible effect of energy on the spine when evaluating the potential for injury:

1. The head is similar to a bowling ball perched on top of the neck, and its mass often moves in a different direction from the torso, resulting in strong forces being applied to the neck (cervical spine, spinal cord).
2. Objects in motion tend to stay in motion, and objects at rest tend to stay at rest.
3. Sudden or violent movement of the upper legs displaces the pelvis, resulting in forceful movement of the lower spine. Because of the weight and inertia of the head and torso, force in an opposite (contra) direction is applied to the upper spine.
4. Lack of neurologic deficit does not rule out bone or ligament injury to the spine or conditions that have stressed the spinal cord to the limit of its tolerance.

Some trauma patients with neurologic deficit will have a temporary or permanent spinal cord injury. Other patients have neurologic deficit caused by either a peripheral nerve injury or an extremity injury not associated with spinal cord injury. It should be assumed that any patient who has sustained any of the following injuries has a potential spinal injury:

- Any blunt mechanism that produced a violent impact on the head, neck, torso, or pelvis

- Incidents that produce sudden acceleration, deceleration, or lateral bending forces to the neck or torso
- Any fall from a height, especially in elderly persons
- Ejection or a fall from any motorized or otherwise powered transportation device
- Any victim of a shallow-water diving incident[4,5]

Any such patient should be manually stabilized in a neutral in-line position (unless contraindicated) until the need for spinal immobilization has been assessed.

Anatomy and Physiology

Vertebral Anatomy

The spinal column is composed of 33 bones called *vertebrae,* which are stacked on top of one another. Except for the first (C1) and second (C2) vertebrae (cervical) at the top of the spine and the fused sacral and coccygeal vertebrae at the lower spine, all the vertebrae are almost alike in form, structure, and motion (Figure 10-1). The largest part of each vertebra is the anterior part called the *body.* Each vertebral body bears most of the weight of the vertebral column and torso superior to it. Two curved sides called the *neural arches* are formed by the pedicle and posteriorly by the lamina. The posterior part of the vertebra is a tail-like structure called the *spinous process.* In the lower five cervical vertebrae, this posterior process points directly posterior; in the thoracic and lumbar vertebrae, it points slightly downward in a caudad direction (toward the feet).

Most vertebrae also have similarly styled protuberances called *transverse processes* at each side near their anterior lateral margins. The transverse and spinous processes serve as points for muscle attachment and are, therefore, fulcrums for movement. The neural arches and the posterior part of each vertebral body form a near-circular shape with an opening in the center called the *vertebral foramen* (spinal canal). The spinal cord passes through this opening. The cord is protected somewhat from injury by the bony vertebrae surrounding it. Each vertebral foramen lines up with that of the vertebrae above and the vertebrae below to form the hollow spinal canal through which the spinal cord passes.

Vertebral Column

The individual vertebrae are stacked in an S-like shape (Figure 10-2). This organization allows extensive multidirectional movement while imparting maximum strength. The spinal column is divided into five individual regions for reference. Beginning at the top of the spinal column and descending downward, these regions are the cervical, thoracic, lumbar, sacral, and coccygeal regions. Vertebrae are identified by the first letter of the region in which they are

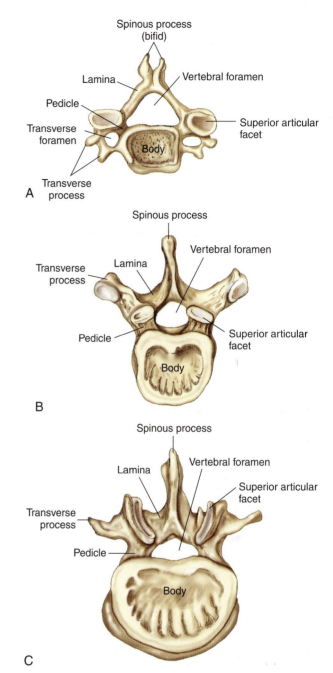

FIGURE 10-1 Except for the fused sacral and coccygeal vertebrae, each vertebra has the same parts as the other vertebrae. The body (anterior portion) of each vertebra becomes larger and stronger because it must support more weight nearing the pelvis. **A.** Fifth cervical vertebra. **B.** Thoracic vertebra. **C.** Lumbar vertebra.

found and their sequence from the top of that region. The first cervical vertebra is called *C1,* the third thoracic vertebra *T3,* the fifth lumbar vertebra *L5,* and so on throughout the entire spinal column. Each vertebra supports increasing body weight as the vertebrae progress down the spinal column. Appropriately, the vertebrae from C3 to L5 become

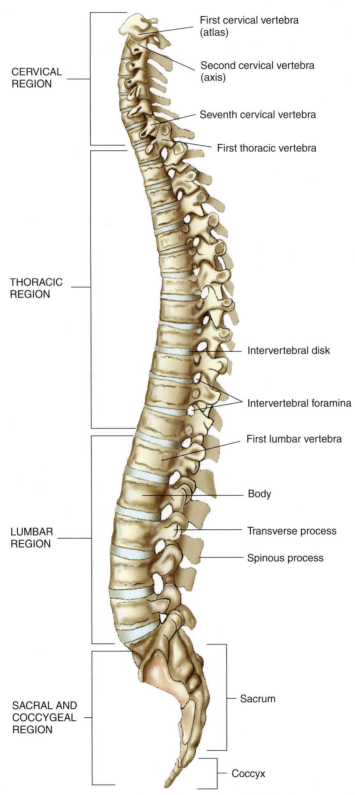

CERVICAL
REGION

First cervical vertebra
(atlas)

Second cervical vertebra
(axis)

Seventh cervical vertebra

First thoracic vertebra

THORACIC
REGION

Intervertebral disk

Intervertebral foramina

First lumbar vertebra

Body

LUMBAR
REGION

Transverse process

Spinous process

SACRAL AND
COCCYGEAL
REGION

Sacrum

Coccyx

FIGURE 10-2 The vertebral column is not a straight rod, but a series of blocks that are stacked to allow for several bends or curves. At each of the curves, the spine is more vulnerable to fractures, thus the origin of the phrase "breaking the S in a fall."

progressively larger to accommodate the increased weight and workload (see Figure 10-1).

Located at the top end of the spinal column are the seven *cervical* vertebrae that support the head. The cervical region is flexible to allow for total movement of the head. Next are 12 *thoracic* vertebrae. Each pair of ribs connects posteriorly to one of the thoracic vertebrae. Unlike the cervical spine, the thoracic spine is relatively rigid with less movement. Below the thoracic vertebrae are the five *lumbar* vertebrae. These are the most massive of all the vertebrae. The lumbar area is also flexible, allowing for movement in several directions. The five *sacral* vertebrae are fused, forming a single structure known as the *sacrum.* The four *coccygeal* vertebrae are also fused, forming the *coccyx* (tailbone). Approximately 55% of spinal injuries occur in the cervical region, 15% in the thoracic region, 15% at the thoracolumbar junction, and 15% in the lumbosacral area.

Ligaments and muscles tether the spine from the base of the skull to the pelvis. These ligaments and muscles form a web that sheathes the entire bony part of the spinal column, holding it in normal alignment and allowing for movement. If these ligaments and muscles are torn, excessive movement of one vertebra in relation to another occurs. In the presence of torn spinal ligaments, this excessive movement may result in dislocation of the vertebrae, which can compromise the space inside the spinal canal and, thus, damage the spinal cord.

The anterior and posterior longitudinal ligaments connect the vertebral bodies anteriorly and inside the canal. Ligaments between the spinous processes provide support for flexion-extension (forward and backward) movement, and those between the lamina provide support during lateral flexion (side bending). (Figure 10-3)

The head balances on top of the spine, and the spine is supported by the pelvis. The skull perches on the ring-shaped first cervical vertebra (C1), referred to as the *atlas.* The *axis,* C2, is also basically ring shaped but has a spur (the odontoid process) that protrudes upward similar to a tooth, located just behind the anterior arch of the atlas (Figure 10-4). The axis allows the head approximately a 180-degree range of rotation.

The human head weighs between 16 and 22 pounds (7–10 kg), somewhat more that the average weight of a bowling ball. The weight and position of the head atop the thin and flexible neck, the forces that act on the head, the small size of the supporting muscle, and the lack of ribs or other bones help make the cervical spine particularly susceptible to injury. At the level of C3, the spinal cord occupies approximately 95% of the spinal canal (the spinal cord occupies approximately 65% of the spinal canal area at its end in the lumbar region), and only 3 mm of clearance exists between the cord and the canal wall. Even a minor dislocation at this point can produce compression of the spinal cord. The

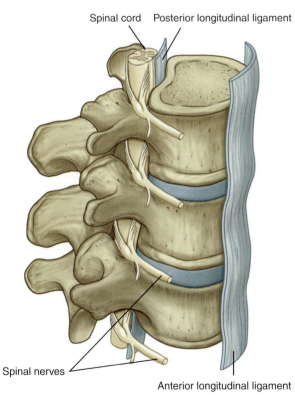

FIGURE 10-3   Anterior and posterior longitudinal ligaments of vertebral column.

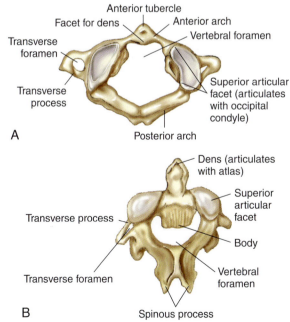

FIGURE 10-4   The first and second cervical vertebrae are uniquely shaped. **A.** Atlas (C1). **B.** Axis (C2).

posterior neck muscles are strong, permitting up to 60% of the range of flexion and 70% of the range of extension of the head without any stretching of the cord. However, when sudden violent acceleration, deceleration, or lateral force is applied to the body, the significant weight of the head on the narrow cervical spine can amplify the effects of sudden movement. An example of this would be a rear-end collision without the headrest properly adjusted.

The *sacrum* is the base of the spinal column, the platform on which the spinal column rests. The sacrum supports between 70% and 80% of the body's total weight. The sacrum is a part of both the spinal column and the pelvic girdle, and it is joined to the rest of the pelvis by immovable joints.

Spinal Cord Anatomy

The spinal cord is continuous with the brain and starts from the base of the brainstem, passing through the foramen magnum (the hole at the base of the skull) and through each vertebra to the level of the second lumbar (L2) vertebra. Blood is supplied to the spinal cord by the vertebral and spinal arteries.

The spinal cord is surrounded by cerebrospinal fluid (CSF) and is encased in a dural sheath. This dural sheath covers the brain and continues down to the second sacral vertebra to a saclike reservoir (the great cistern). CSF produced by the brain passes around the cord and is absorbed in this cistern. CSF performs the same function for the cord as for the brain, acting as a cushion against injury during rapid and severe movement.

The spinal cord itself consists of gray matter and white matter. The white matter contains the anatomic spinal tracts. Spinal tracts are divided into two types: ascending and descending (Figure 10-5).

Ascending nerve tracts carry sensory impulses from body parts through the cord up to the brain. Ascending nerve tracts can be further divided into tracts that carry the different sensations of pain and temperature; touch and pressure; and sensory impulses of motion, vibration, position, and light touch. The nerve tracts that carry pain and temperature sensation "cross over" in the body, meaning that the nerve root with that information from the right side of the body crosses over to the left side of the spinal cord and then goes up to the brain. In contrast, the nerve tract that carries the sensory information for position, vibration, and light touch does *not* cross over in the spinal cord. Thus, this sensory information is carried up to the brain on the same side of the spinal cord as the nerve roots.

Descending nerve tracts are responsible for carrying motor impulses from the brain through the cord down to the body, and they control all muscle movement and muscle tone. These descending tracts also do not cross over in the spinal cord. Therefore the motor tract on the right side of the cord controls motor function on the right side of the body. These motor tracts *do* cross over in the brainstem, however, so the left side of the brain controls motor function on the right side of the body, and vice versa.

As the spinal cord continues to descend, pairs of nerves branch off from the cord at each vertebra and extend to the various parts of the body (Figure 10-6). The spinal cord has 31 pairs of spinal nerves, named according to the level from which they arise. Each nerve has two roots on each side.

The *dorsal root* is for sensory impulses, and the *ventral root* is for motor impulses. Neurologic stimuli pass between the brain and each part of the body through the cord and particular pairs of these nerves. As they branch from the spinal cord, these nerves pass through a notch in the inferior lateral side of the vertebra, posterior to the vertebral body, called the *intervertebral foramen*. Cartilage-like intervertebral discs lie

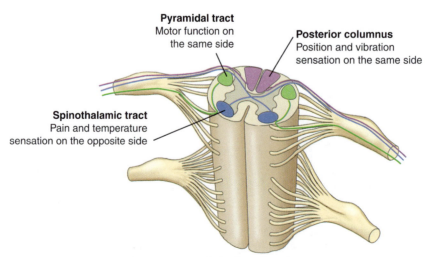

Pyramidal tract
Motor function on the same side

Posterior columnus
Position and vibration sensation on the same side

Spinothalamic tract
Pain and temperature sensation on the opposite side

FIGURE 10-5 Spinal cord tracks.

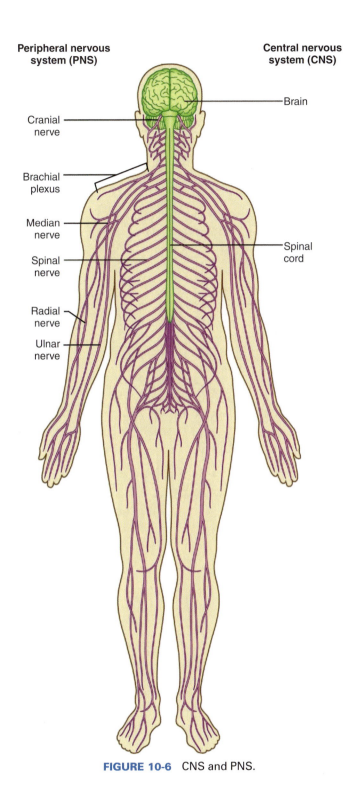

Peripheral nervous system (PNS)

Central nervous system (CNS)

Cranial nerve

Brachial plexus

Median nerve

Spinal nerve

Radial nerve

Ulnar nerve

Brain

Spinal cord

FIGURE 10-6   CNS and PNS.

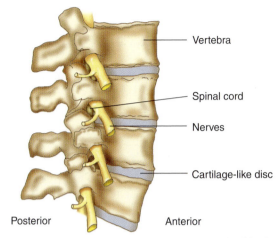

Vertebra

Spinal cord

Nerves

Cartilage-like disc

Posterior   Anterior

FIGURE 10-7   The cartilage between each vertebral body is called the *intervertebral disc*. These discs act as shock absorbers. If damaged, the cartilage may protrude into the spinal canal, compressing the cord or the nerves that come through the intervertebral foramina.

between the body of each vertebra and act as shock absorbers (Figure 10-7).

These nerve branches have multiple control functions, and their level in the spinal cord is represented by dermatomes. A *dermatome* is the sensory area on the body for which a nerve root is responsible. Collectively, dermatomes allow the body areas to be mapped out for each spinal level (Figure 10-8). Dermatomes help determine the level of a spinal cord injury. Two landmarks to keep in mind are the *nipple level*, which is the T4 dermatome, and the *umbilicus level*, which is the T10 dermatome.

The process of inhalation and exhalation requires both chest excursion and proper changes in the shape of the diaphragm. The diaphragm is innervated by the phrenic nerves, which originate from the nerves arising from the cord between levels C2 and C5. If the cord above the level of C2 or the phrenic nerves are cut or the nerve impulses are otherwise disrupted, a patient will lose the ability to breathe spontaneously. A patient with this injury may asphyxiate before the arrival of providers unless bystanders initiate rescue breathing. Positive-pressure ventilation will need to be continued during transport.

Pathophysiology

The bony spine can normally withstand forces of up to 1000 foot-pounds (1360 joules) of energy. High-speed travel and contact sports can routinely exert forces on the spine well in excess of this amount. Even in a low- to moderate-speed vehicle crash, the body of an unrestrained 150-pound (68-kg) person can easily place 3000 to 4000 foot-pounds (4080–5440 joules) of force against the spine as the head is suddenly stopped by the windshield or roof. Similar force can occur when a motorcyclist is thrown over the front of the motorcycle or when a high-speed skier collides with a tree.

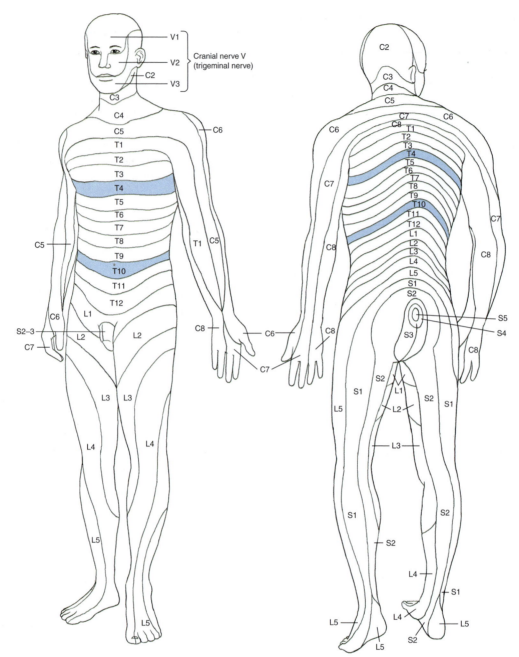

FIGURE 10-8 Dermatome map shows the relationship between areas of touch sensation on the skin and the spinal nerves that correspond to these areas. Loss of sensation in a specific area may indicate injury to the corresponding spinal nerve.

Skeletal Injuries

Various types of injuries can occur to the spine, including the following:

- Compression fractures that produce wedge compression or total flattening of the body of the vertebra.
- Fractures that produce small fragments of bone that may lie in the spinal canal near the cord.
- *Subluxation,* which is a partial dislocation of a vertebra from its normal alignment in the spinal column.
- Overstretching or tearing of the ligaments and muscles, producing instability between the vertebrae. [6]

Any of these skeletal injuries may immediately result in the irreversible transection of the cord, or the injury may compress or stretch the cord. In some patients, however, damage to the vertebrae or ligaments results in an *unstable* spinal column injury but does not produce an immediate spinal cord injury. In addition, patients who have cervical spine injuries also have a 10% chance of having another spinal fracture.

Therefore, the entire spine must be immobilized in patients who have indications for cervical spinal immobilization.

A lack of neurologic deficit does not rule out a bony fracture or an unstable spine. Although the presence of good motor and sensory responses in the extremities indicates that the cord is currently intact, it does not exclude a damaged vertebra or associated bony or soft tissue injury. A significant percentage of patients with spine fractures have no neurologic deficit. A full assessment is required to determine the need for immobilization.

Specific Mechanisms of Injury That Cause Spinal Trauma

Axial loading can occur in several ways. Most often, this compression of the spine occurs when the head strikes an object and the weight of the still-moving body bears against the stopped head, such as when the head of an unrestrained occupant strikes the windshield or when the head strikes an object in a shallow-water diving incident. Compression and axial loading also occur when a patient sustains a fall from a substantial height and lands in a standing position. This drives the weight of the head and thorax down against the lumbar spine while the sacral spine remains stationary. About 20% of falls from a height greater than 15 feet involve an associated lumbar spine fracture. During such an extreme energy exchange, the spinal column tends to exaggerate its normal curves, and fractures and compressions occur at such areas. The spine is S shaped; therefore, it can be said that the compressive forces tend to "break the patient's S." These forces compress the concave side and open the convex side of the spine.

Excessive flexion (hyperflexion), excessive extension (hyperextension), and *excessive rotation (hyper-rotation)* can cause bone damage and tearing of muscles and ligaments, resulting in impingement on or stretching of the spinal cord.

Sudden or excessive lateral bending requires much less movement than flexion or extension before injury occurs. During lateral impact, the torso and the thoracic spine are moved laterally. The head tends to remain in place until it is pulled along by the cervical attachments. The center of gravity of the head is above and anterior to its seat and attachment to the cervical spine; therefore, the head will tend to roll sideways. This movement often results in dislocations and bony fractures.

Distraction (over-elongation of the spine) occurs when one part of the spine is stable and the rest is in longitudinal motion. This pulling apart of the spine can easily cause stretching and tearing of the cord. Distraction injury is a common mechanism in children's playground injuries and in hangings.

Although any one of these types of violent movements may be the dominant cause of spinal injury in a given patient, one or more of the others will usually also be involved.

Spinal Cord Injuries

Primary injury occurs at the time of impact or force application and may cause cord compression, direct cord injury (usually from sharp unstable bony fragments or projectiles), and interruption of the cord's blood supply. Secondary injury occurs after the initial insult and can include swelling, ischemia, or movement of bony fragments.[7]

Cord concussion results from the temporary disruption of the spinal cord functions distal to the injury. *Cord contusion* involves bruising or bleeding into the tissues of the spinal cord, which may also result in a temporary loss of cord functions distal to the injury (spinal "shock"). Spinal shock is a neurologic phenomenon that occurs for an unpredictable and variable amount of time after spinal cord injury, resulting in temporary loss of all sensory and motor function, flaccidity and paralysis, and loss of reflexes below the level of the spinal cord injury. Cord contusion is usually caused by a penetrating type of injury or movement of bony fragments. The severity of injury resulting from the contusion is related to the amount of bleeding into the spinal cord tissue. Damage to or disruption of the spinal blood supply can result in local cord tissue ischemia. *Cord compression* is pressure on the spinal cord caused by swelling, but also may occur from traumatic disc rupture and bone fragments. Compression may result in tissue ischemia and in some cases may require decompression to prevent a permanent loss of function. *Cord laceration* occurs when cord tissue is torn or cut. Neurologic deficits may be reversed if the cord has sustained only slight damage; however, spinal cord injury usually results in permanent disability if some or all spinal tracts are disrupted.

Spinal cord transection can be categorized as complete or incomplete. In *complete cord transection,* all spinal tracts are interrupted, and all cord functions distal to the site are lost. Because of the additional effects of swelling, determination of the extent of loss of function may not be accurate until 24 hours after the injury. Most complete cord transections result in either paraplegia or quadriplegia, depending on the level of the injury. In *incomplete cord transection,* some tracts and motor/sensory functions remain intact. Prognosis for recovery is greater in these cases than with complete transections. Types of incomplete cord injuries include the following:

- *Anterior cord syndrome* is a result of bony fragments or pressure on spinal arteries (Figure 10-9). Symptoms include loss of motor function and pain, temperature, and light touch sensations. However, some light touch, motion, position, and vibration sensations are spared.
- *Central cord syndrome* usually occurs with hyperextension of the cervical area (Figure 10-10). Symptoms include weakness or paresthesia in the upper extremities but normal strength in the lower extremities. This syndrome causes varying degrees of bladder dysfunction.

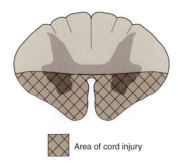

FIGURE 10-9 Anterior cord syndrome.

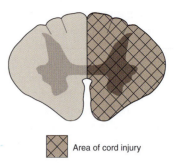

FIGURE 10-11 Brown-Séquard syndrome.

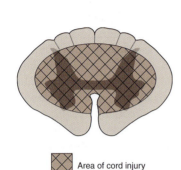

FIGURE 10-10 Central cord syndrome.

■ *Brown-Séquard syndrome* is caused by penetrating injury and involves hemi-transection of the cord, involving only one side of the cord (Figure 10-11). Symptoms include complete cord damage and loss of function on the affected side (motor, vibration, motion, and position) with loss of pain and temperature sensation on the side opposite the injury. [8]

Neurogenic "shock" secondary to spinal cord injury represents a significant additional finding. When the cord is disrupted, the body's sympathetic control mechanism is lost and cannot maintain constriction of the muscles in the walls of the blood vessels below the point of disruption. These arteries and arterioles dilate, enlarging the size of the vascular container and producing relative hypovolemia and partial loss of systemic vascular resistance (SVR). As a result, the blood pressure will decrease. The skin, however, will be warm and dry. Instead of the tachycardia usually associated with hypovolemic shock, this type of injury is associated with a normal heart rate or a slight bradycardia. Although the patient may be hypotensive, neurogenic "shock" often does not cause impairment in oxygen delivery to peripheral tissues (see Chapter 8). High spinal cord injuries (C5 or above) are more likely to require cardiovascular interventions such as vasopressors and pacemakers. [9] A recent consensus statement recommends prompt correction of hypo-

tension (SBP <90 mm Hg) in the setting of acute spinal cord injury. Ideally, the blood pressure of patients with suspected spinal cord injury should be maintained in a normal range (MAP 85–90 mm Hg). [10]

Assessment

Spinal injury, as with other conditions, should be assessed in the context of other injuries and conditions present. The primary survey is the first priority. However, often the patient first needs to be moved in order to assure the safety of all individuals at the scene. Therefore, a rapid scene assessment and history of the event should determine if the possibility of a spinal injury exists, in which case the patient's spine must be manually protected. The patient's head is brought into a neutral in-line position, unless contraindicated (see discussion on page 259). The head is maintained in that position until the assessment reveals no indication for immobilization, or the manual stabilization is replaced with a spine immobilization device, such as a half-spine board, long backboard, or vest-type device.

Neurologic Examination

In the field, a rapid neurologic examination is performed to identify obvious deficits related to a spinal cord injury. The patient is asked to move the arms, hands, and legs, and any inability to do so is noted. Then the patient is checked for the presence or absence of sensation, beginning at the shoulders and moving down the body to the feet. A complete neurologic examination does not need to be performed in the prehospital setting as it will not provide additional information that will affect the decisions about needed prehospital care and only serves to expend precious time on scene and delay transport.

The rapid neurologic examination should be repeated after the patient has been immobilized, any time the patient is moved, and upon arrival to the receiving facility. This will help identify any changes in patient condition that may have occurred after the initial assessment.

Using Mechanism of Injury to Assess Spinal Cord Injury

Traditionally, prehospital care providers have been taught that suspicion for a spinal injury is based solely on the mechanism of injury and that spinal immobilization is required for any patient with a suggestive mechanism of injury. This generalization has caused a lack of clear clinical guidelines for assessment of spinal cord injuries. However, assessment of the neck for spinal immobilization should also include assessment of the motor and sensory function, presence of pain or tenderness, and patient reliability as predictors of spinal cord injury. In addition, the patient may not complain of pain in the spinal column because of pain associated with a more distracting painful injury, such as a fractured femur.[9] Alcohol or drugs that the patient may have ingested may also blunt the patient's perception of pain and mask serious injury.

The primary focus of care should be to recognize the indications for spinal immobilization rather than to attempt to clear the spine.[11–18] Because many patients do not have spinal injury, a more selective approach to performing spinal immobilization is appropriate, especially since spinal immobilization has been shown to produce adverse effects in healthy volunteers, including increases in respiratory effort, skin ischemia, and pain.[18] Providers should focus on appropriate indications for performing spinal immobilization.

If no indications are present after a careful and thorough examination, there may be no need for spinal immobilization. The cornerstone to proper spinal care is the same as with all trauma care: superior assessment, with appropriate and timely treatment.

Blunt Trauma

Major causes of spinal injury in adult patients include the following:

1. Motor vehicle crashes (MVCs)
2. Shallow-water incidents
3. Motorcycle crashes
4. Falls
5. Sports injuries

Major causes of spinal injury in pediatric patients include the following:

1. Falls from heights (generally two to three times the patient's height)
2. Falls from a tricycle or bicycle
3. Being struck by a motor vehicle

As a guideline, the provider should assume the presence of spinal injury and an unstable spine with the following situations, and an assessment of the spine should be conducted to determine the need for immobilization:

- Any blunt mechanism that produced a violent impact on the head, neck, torso, or pelvis (e.g., assault, entrapment in a structural collapse).
- Incidents that produce sudden acceleration, deceleration, or lateral bending forces to the neck or torso (e.g., moderate- to high-speed MVCs, pedestrians struck by vehicle, involvement in explosion).
- Any fall, especially in elderly persons.
- Ejection or a fall from any motorized or otherwise powered transportation device (e.g., scooters, skateboards, bicycles, motor vehicles, motorcycles, recreational vehicles).
- Any victim of a shallow-water incident (e.g., diving, body surfing).

Other situations often associated with spinal damage include the following:

- Head injuries with any alteration in level of consciousness
- Significant helmet damage
- Significant blunt injury to the torso
- Impacted or other deceleration fractures of the legs or hips
- Significant localized injuries to the area of the spinal column

These mechanisms of injury should mandate a thorough and complete examination to determine if indications are present to necessitate spinal immobilization.

The wearing of proper seat belt restraints has proven to save lives and reduce head, face, and thoracic injuries. However, the use of proper restraints does not rule out the possibility of spinal injury. In significant frontal-impact collisions when sudden severe deceleration occurs, the restrained torso stops suddenly, but the unrestrained head attempts to continue its forward movement. Held by the strong posterior neck muscles, the head can move forward only slightly. If the force of deceleration is strong enough, the head then rotates down until the chin strikes the chest wall, frequently rotating across the diagonal strap of the shoulder restraint. Such rapid, forceful hyperflexion and rotation of the neck can result in compression fractures of the cervical vertebrae, "jumped" facets (dislocation of the articular processes), and stretching of the spinal cord. Different mechanisms can also cause spinal trauma in restrained victims of rear or lateral collisions. The amount of damage to the vehicle and the patient's other injuries are the key factors in determining if a patient needs to be immobilized.

The patient's ability to walk should not be a factor in determining whether a patient needs to be treated for spinal injury. A significant number of patients who require surgical repair of unstable spinal injuries were found "walking around" at the scene or walked into the emergency department at the hospital.

Penetrating Trauma

Penetrating injury represents a special consideration regarding the potential for spinal trauma.[20] In general, if a patient did not sustain definite neurologic injury at the moment that the trauma occurred, there is little concern for subsequent development of a spinal cord injury. This is because of the mechanism of injury and the kinematics associated with the force involved. Penetrating objects generally do not produce unstable spinal fractures because penetrating trauma produces minimal risk of unstable ligamentous or bony injury, unlike blunt injury. A penetrating object causes injury along the path of penetration. If the object did not directly injure the spinal cord as it penetrated, the patient is unlikely to develop a spinal cord injury. Numerous studies have shown that unstable spinal injuries rarely occur from penetrating trauma to the head, neck, or torso[22–27] and that penetrating injuries are **not** indications for spinal immobilization. Because of the very low risk of an unstable spinal injury and because the other injuries created by the penetrating trauma often require a higher priority in management, patients with penetrating trauma need not undergo spinal immobilization. In fact, one recent retrospective study utilizing the National Trauma Data Bank documented that patients with penetrating trauma who received spinal immobilization in the field possessed a higher overall mortality rate than those who did not.[28]

Indications for Spinal Immobilization

The mechanism of injury can be used as an aid to determine indications for spinal immobilization (Figure 10-12). The key point always is that a complete physical assessment coupled with good clinical judgment will guide decision making, and *if in doubt, immobilize.*

Patients with a penetrating injury (e.g., gunshot or stab wounds) to the head, neck, or torso should be considered to have a concerning mechanism of injury when they complain of neurologic symptoms or display such findings as numbness, tingling, and loss of motor or sensory function or actual loss of consciousness. However, if patients with penetrating injury have no neurologic complaints, secondary mechanism of injury, or findings, the spine does not need to be immobilized (although the backboard may still be used for lifting and transport purposes).

In the patient with blunt trauma, the following conditions should mandate spinal immobilization:

1. *Altered level of consciousness* (LOC), with Glasgow Coma Scale (GCS) score less than 15. Any factor that alters the patient's perception of pain will hinder the responder's assessment for injury; this includes the following:

   - Traumatic brain injury (TBI)
   - Altered mental status (AMS) other than TBI. For example, patients with psychiatric illness, with Alzheimer's disease, or under the influence of intoxicants may have impaired pain perception.
   - Acute stress reactions (ASRs) may cause "pain masking."

2. *Spinal pain or tenderness.* This includes pain or pain on movement, point tenderness, and deformity and guarding of the spinal area.

3. *Neurologic deficit or complaint.* This includes bilateral paralysis, partial paralysis, paresis (weakness), numbness, prickling or tingling, and neurogenic spinal shock below the level of the injury. In males, a continuing erection of the penis (priapism) may be an additional indication of spinal cord injury.

4. *Anatomic deformity of the spine.* This includes any deformity noted on physical examination of the patient.

However, the absence of these signs does not rule out bony spinal injury (Figure 10-13).

When a patient has a concerning mechanism of injury in the absence of the conditions just listed, the reliability of the patient must be assessed. A reliable patient is calm, cooperative, and has a completely normal mental status. An unreliable patient may exhibit any of the following:

- *Intoxication.* Patients who are under the influence of drugs or alcohol are immobilized and managed as if they had spinal injury until they are calm, cooperative, and sober.
- *Distracting painful injuries.* Injuries that are severely painful may prevent the patient from giving reliable responses during the assessment.[9] Examples include a fractured femur or a large burn (see Figure 10-12).
- *Communication barriers.* Communication problems include language barriers, deafness, very young patients, or patients who for any reason cannot communicate effectively.

The patient should be continually rechecked for reliability at all phases of an assessment. If at any time the patient exhibits these signs or symptoms or the reliability of the examination is in question, it should be assumed that the patient has a spinal injury, and full immobilization management techniques should be implemented.

In many situations the mechanism of injury is not suggestive of neck injury (e.g., falling on outstretched hand and producing Colles' fracture). In these patients, in the presence of a normal examination and proper assessment, spinal immobilization is not indicated.

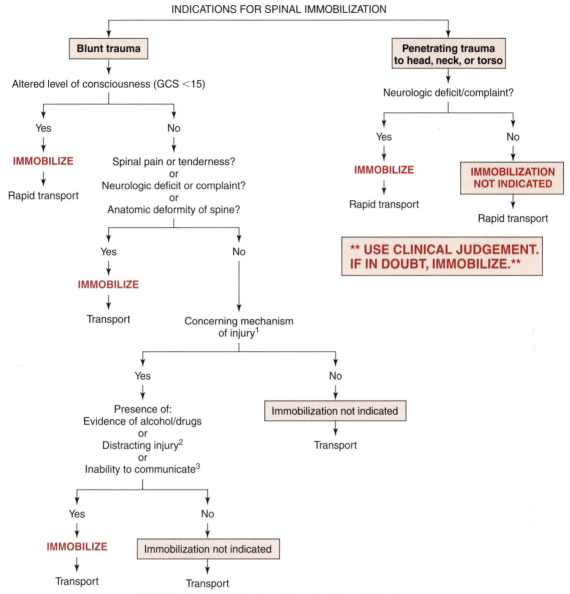

FIGURE 10-12 Indications for spinal immobilization.

Notes:

[1]Concerning mechanisms of injury
- Any mechanism that produced a violent impact to the head, neck, torso, or pelvis (e.g., assault, entrapment in structural collapse, etc.)
- Incidents producing sudden acceleration, deceleration, or lateral bending forces to the neck or torso (e.g., moderate- to high-speed MVC, pedestrian struck, involvement in an explosion, etc.)
- Any fall, especially in elderly persons
- Ejection or fall from any motorized or otherwise-powered transportation device (e.g., scooters, skateboards, bicycles, motor vehicles, motorcycles, or recreational vehicles)
- Victim of shallow-water diving incident

[2]Distracting injury
Any injury that may have the potential to impair the patient's ability to appreciate other injuries. Examples of distracting injuries include a) long bone fracture; b) a visceral injury requiring surgical consultation; c) a large laceration, degloving injury, or crush injury; d) large burns, or e) any other injury producing acute functional impairment.
(Adapted from Hoffman JR, Wolfson AB, Todd K, Mower WR: Selective cervical spine radiography in blunt trauma: methodology of the National Emergency X-Radiography Utilization Study [NEXUS], *Ann Emerg Med* 461, 1998.)

[3]Inability to communicate. Any patient who, for reasons not specified above, cannot clearly communicate so as to actively participate in their assessment. Examples: speech or hearing impaired, those who only speak a foreign language, and small children.

FIGURE 10-13   **Signs and Symptoms of Spinal Trauma**

- Pain in the neck or back
- Pain on movement of the neck or back
- Pain on palpation of the posterior neck or midline of the back
- Deformity of the spinal column
- Guarding or splinting of the muscles of the neck or back
- Paralysis, paresis, numbness, or tingling in the legs or arms at any time after the incident
- Signs and symptoms of neurogenic shock
- Priapism (in male patients)

Management

In the United States, the management for a potentially unstable spine is to immobilize the patient in a supine position, usually on a rigid long backboard in a neutral in-line position. In many other countries, a full-body vacuum mattress splint is often used instead of the backboard. The head, neck, torso, and pelvis should each be immobilized in a neutral in-line position to prevent any further movement of the unstable spine that could result in damage to the spinal cord. Spinal immobilization follows the common principle of fracture management: immobilizing the joint above and the joint below an injury. Because of the anatomy of the spine, this principle of immobilization must be extended beyond just the joint above and below a suspected vertebral injury. The joint above the spine means the head, and the joint below means the pelvis.

Moderate anterior flexion or extension of the arms may cause significant movement of the shoulder girdle. Any movement or angulation of the pelvis results in movement of the sacrum and of the vertebrae attached to it. For example, lateral movement of both legs together can result in angulation of the pelvis and lateral bending of the spine.

Fractures of one area of the spine are often associated with fractures of other areas of the spine.[27] Therefore, the entire weight-bearing spine (cervical, thoracic, lumbar, and sacral) should be considered as one entity, and the entire spine immobilized and supported to achieve proper immobilization. The supine position is the most stable position to ensure continued support during handling, carrying, and transporting a patient. It also provides the best access for further examination and additional resuscitation and management of a patient. When the patient is supine, the airway, mouth and nose, eyes, chest, and abdomen can be accessed simultaneously.

Patients usually present in one of four general postures: sitting, semi-prone, supine, or standing. The patient's spine needs to be protected and stabilized immediately and continuously from the time the patient is discovered until the patient is mechanically secured to a long backboard. Techniques and equipment, such as manual stabilization, half-spine boards, immobilization vests, standing take-down, scoop stretchers, proper logroll methods, and rapid extrication with full manual stabilization, are interim techniques used to protect a patient's spine. These techniques allow for a patient's safe movement from the position in which the patient was found until full supine immobilization on a rigid long backboard can be implemented. A recent study suggests that one type of scoop stretcher currently manufactured may be as effective as a standard rigid long backboard.[29]

Often, too much focus is placed on particular immobilization devices without an understanding of the principles of immobilization and how to modify these principles to meet individual patient needs. Specific devices and immobilization methods can be safely used only with an understanding of the anatomic principles that are generic to all methods and equipment. Any inflexible, detailed method for using a device will not meet the varying conditions found in the field. Regardless of the specific equipment or method used, the management of any patient with an unstable spine should follow the general steps described in the next section.

General Method

When the decision is made to immobilize a trauma patient, follow these principles:

1. Move the patient's head into a proper neutral in-line position (unless contraindicated; see next section). Continue manual support and in-line stabilization without interruption.
2. Evaluate the patient by performing the primary survey, and provide any immediately required intervention.
3. Check the patient's motor ability, sensory response, and circulation in all four extremities, if the patient's condition allows.
4. Examine the patient's neck, and measure and apply a properly fitting, effective cervical collar.
5. Depending on the situation, position a shortboard or vest-type device on the patient, or place the patient on a long backboard.
6. Immobilize the patient's torso to the device so that it cannot move up, down, left, or right.
7. Evaluate and pad behind the adult patient's head or pediatric patient's chest as needed.
8. Immobilize the patient's head to the device, maintaining a neutral in-line position.
9. Once the patient is on the long backboard (if a short device is used), immobilize the legs so that they cannot move anteriorly or laterally.
10. Fasten the patient's arms to the backboard.
11. Re-evaluate the primary survey and reassess the patient's motor ability, sensory response, and circulation in all four extremities, if the patient's condition allows.

Manual In-line Stabilization of the Head

Once it has been determined from the mechanism of injury that an injured spine potentially exists, the first step is to provide manual in-line stabilization. The patient's head is grasped and carefully moved into a neutral in-line position unless contraindicated (see below). A proper neutral in-line position is maintained without any significant traction on the head and neck. Only enough pull should be exerted on a sitting or standing patient to cause *axial unloading* (taking the weight of the head off the axis and the rest of the cervical spine). The head should be constantly maintained in the manually stabilized, neutral in-line position until mechanical immobilization of the torso and head is completed or the examination reveals no need for spinal immobilization. In this way, the patient's head and neck are immediately immobilized and remain so until after examination at the hospital. Moving the head into a neutral in-line position presents less risk than if the patient were carried and transported with the head left in an angulated position. In addition, both immobilization and transport of the patient are much simpler with the patient in a neutral position.

Movement of the patient's head into a neutral in-line position is contraindicated in a few cases. If careful movement of the head and neck into a neutral in-line position results in any of the following, *the movement must be stopped:*

- Resistance to movement is noted
- Neck muscle spasm
- Increased pain
- Commencement or increase of a neurologic deficit, such as numbness, tingling, or loss of motor ability
- Compromise of the airway or ventilation

Neutral in-line movement should not be attempted if a patient's injuries are so severe that the head presents with such misalignment that it no longer appears to extend from the midline of the shoulders. In these situations, the patient's head must be immobilized in the position in which it was initially found. Fortunately, such cases are rare.

Rigid Cervical Collars

Rigid cervical collars alone do not provide adequate immobilization; they simply aid in supporting the neck and promote a lack of movement. Rigid cervical collars limit flexion by about 90% and limit extension, lateral bending, and rotation by about 50%. A rigid cervical collar is an important adjunct to immobilization but must always be used with manual stabilization or mechanical immobilization provided by a suitable spine-immobilization device. A soft cervical collar is of no use as an adjunct to spinal immobilization in the field.

The unique primary purpose of a cervical collar is to protect the cervical spine from compression. Prehospital methods of immobilization (using a vest, shortboard, or a long backboard device) still allow some slight movement of the patient and the spine because these devices only fasten externally to the

patient, and the skin and muscle tissue move slightly on the skeletal frame even when the patient is extremely well immobilized. Most rescue situations involve some movement of the patient and spine when extricating, carrying, and loading the patient. This type of movement also occurs when an ambulance accelerates and decelerates in normal driving conditions.

An effective cervical collar sits on the chest, posterior thoracic spine and clavicle, and trapezius muscles, where the tissue movement is at a minimum. This still allows movement at C6, C7, and T1 but prevents compression of these vertebrae. The head is immobilized under the angle of the mandible and at the occiput of the skull. The rigid collar allows the unavoidable loading between the head and the torso to be transferred from the cervical spine to the collar, eliminating or minimizing the cervical compression that could otherwise result.

Even though it does not fully immobilize, a cervical collar aids in limiting head movement. The rigid anterior portion of the collar also provides a safe pathway for the lower head strap across the neck.

The collar must be the correct size for the patient. A collar that is too short will not be effective and will allow significant flexion; a collar that is too large will cause hyperextension or full motion if the chin is inside of it. Also, a collar must be applied properly. A collar that is too loose will be ineffective in limiting head movement and can accidentally cover the anterior chin, mouth, and nose, obstructing the patient's airway; a collar that is too tight can compress the veins of the neck, causing increased intracranial pressure.

A collar should be applied after bringing the patient's head into a neutral in-line position. If the head cannot be returned to a neutral in-line position, use of any collar is difficult and should not be considered. In this case, the use of an improvised blanket or towel roll may assist in stabilization. A collar that does not allow the mandible to move down and the mouth to open without motion of the spine will produce aspiration of gastric contents into the lungs if the patient vomits and, therefore, should not be used. Alternative methods to immobilize a patient when a collar cannot be used may include use of such items as blankets, towels, and tape. In the prehospital setting, the care provider may need to be creative when presented with these types of patients. Whatever method is used, the basic concepts of immobilization should be followed (Figure 10-14).

FIGURE 10-14 Guidelines for Rigid Cervical Collars

Rigid cervical collars:
- Do not adequately immobilize by their use alone
- Must be properly sized for each patient
- Must not inhibit a patient's ability to open the mouth or the prehospital care provider's ability to open the patient's mouth if vomiting occurs
- Should not obstruct or hinder ventilation in any way

Immobilization of Torso to the Board Device

Regardless of the specific board device used, the patient must be immobilized so that the torso cannot move up, down, left, or right. The rigid device is strapped to the torso and the torso to the device. The device is secured to the patient's torso so that the head and neck will be supported and immobilized when affixed to it. The patient's torso and pelvis are immobilized to the device so that the thoracic, lumbar, and sacral sections of the spine are supported and cannot move. **The torso should be immobilized to the device before the head is secured.** In this way, any movement of the device that may occur when fastening the torso straps is prevented from angulating the cervical spine.

Many different methods exist for immobilizing the device to the torso. Protection against movement in any direction—up, down, left, or right—should be achieved at both the upper torso (shoulders or chest) and the lower torso (pelvis) to avoid compression and lateral movement of the vertebrae of the torso. Immobilization of the upper torso can be achieved with several specific methods; an understanding of the basic anatomic principles common to each method must be applied. Cephalad movement of the upper torso is prohibited by use of a strap on each side, fastened to the board inferior to the upper margin of each shoulder, which then passes over the shoulder and is fastened at a lower point. Caudad movement of the torso can be prohibited by use of straps that pass snugly around the pelvis and legs.

In one method, two straps (one going from each side of the board over the shoulder, then across the upper chest and through the opposite armpit, to fasten to the board on the armpit side) produce an X, which stops any upward, downward, left, or right movement of the upper torso. The same immobilization can be achieved by fastening one strap to the board and passing it through one armpit, then across the upper chest and through the opposite armpit, to fasten to the second side of the board. A strap, or cravat, is then added to each side and passed over the shoulder to fasten it to the armpit strap, similar to a pair of suspenders.

Immobilization of the upper torso of a patient with a fractured clavicle is accomplished by placing backpack-type loops around each shoulder through the armpit and fastening the ends of each loop in the same handhold. The straps remain near the lateral edges of the upper torso and do not cross the clavicles. With any of these methods, the straps are over the upper third of the chest and can be fastened tightly without producing the ventilatory compromise typically produced by tight straps placed lower on the thorax.

Immobilization of the lower torso can be achieved by use of a single strap fastened tightly over the pelvis at the iliac crests. If the long backboard will have to be upended or carried on stairs or over a distance, a pair of groin loops will provide stronger immobilization than the single strap across the iliac crests.

Lateral movement or anterior movement away from the rigid device at the midtorso can be prevented by use of an additional strap around the midtorso. Any strap that surrounds the torso between the upper thorax and the iliac crests should be snug but not so tight that it inhibits chest excursion, impairing ventilatory function, or causes a significant increase in intra-abdominal pressure.

Maintenance of Neutral In-line Position of the Head

In many patients, when the head is placed in a neutral in-line position, the posterior-most portion of the occipital region at the back of the head is between ½ and 3½ inches anterior to the posterior thoracic wall (Figure 10-15A). Therefore, in most adults, a space exists between the back of the head and the device when the head is in a neutral in-line position, so suitable padding should be added before securing the head to the board device (Figure 10-15B). To be effective, this padding must be made of a material that does not readily compress. Firm, semi-rigid pads designed for this purpose or folded towels can be used. The amount of padding needed must be individualized for each patient; a few individuals require none. If too little padding is inserted or if the padding is of an unsuitable spongy material, the head will be hyperextended when head straps are applied. If too much padding is inserted, the head will be moved into a flexed position. Both

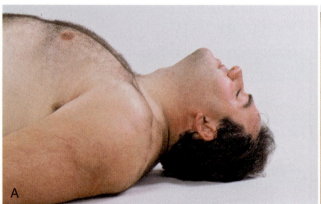
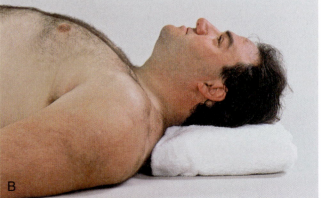

FIGURE 10-15 **A.** In some patients, pulling the skull back to the level of the backboard can produce severe hyperextension. **B.** Padding is needed between the back of the head and the backboard to prevent such hyperextension.

hyperextension and flexion of the head can increase spinal cord damage and are contraindicated.

The same anatomic relationship between the head and back applies when most people are supine, whether on the ground or on a backboard. When most adults are supine, the head falls back into a hyperextended position. On arrival, the head should be moved into a neutral in-line position and manually maintained in that position, which in many adults will require holding the head up off the ground. Once the patient is placed on the long backboard and the head is about to be fastened to the board, proper padding (as described) should be inserted between the back of the head and the board to main-

tain the neutral position. These principles should be used with all patients, including athletes with shoulder pads and patients with abnormal curvature of the spine (Figure 10-16).

In small children, generally those with the body size of a 7-year-old or younger, the size of the head is much larger relative to the rest of the body than it is in adults, and the muscles of the back are less developed.[29] When a small child's head is in a neutral in-line position, the back of the head usually extends 1 to 2 inches (2.5–5 cm) beyond the posterior plane of the back. Therefore, if a small child is placed directly on a rigid surface, the head will be moved into a position of flexion (Figure 10-17A).

FIGURE 10-16 Athletic Equipment Removal

A number of recent publications, including a position paper, have advocated the immobilization of helmeted athletes to a long backboard with the helmet in place.[30–37] A search of the medical literature for supporting evidence reveals that these recommendations are based on, at best, Class III research. Studies criticizing the practice of helmet removal have primarily been done in cadavers. These studies report that extreme hyperextension of the cervical spine occurs when the helmet alone is removed and the shoulder pads are left in place; however, all the studies were done without the placement of appropriate padding under the head to prevent it from falling back onto the backboard. Adherence to proper spinal precautions and application of treatment principles will best accomplish the task of spinal immobilization whether or not the helmet or shoulder pads are removed.

Athletic equipment should be removed by personnel trained and experienced in the removal of sports equipment. Historically, these trained and experienced personnel generally have been those individuals, usually athletic trainers, present at the athletic event site. Emergency medical services (EMS) responders,

however, need to receive training in such removal, because access to the airway, if needed, can be accomplished only by appropriate access to the patient's face and head, which requires removal of the facemask at a minimum and the helmet in many cases. If the decision is made *not* to remove the equipment at the scene, someone knowledgeable in sports equipment removal should accompany the patient to the hospital.

While special care for helmeted athletes is needed, the general principles of spinal immobilization taught in Prehospital Trauma Life Support (PHTLS) courses are appropriate and need to be followed. Ideally, the helmet and shoulder pads should be removed as one unit. However, it is still possible to immobilize a player to a long backboard without causing hyperextension of the cervical spine when the helmet alone is removed. This is accomplished by the appropriate use of padding behind the head to maintain the head in neutral alignment with the rest of the spine if the shoulder pads are not removed. EMS responders must determine the specific medical needs for an injured athlete and take appropriate steps to meet those needs, which may often include immediate removal of the athletic equipment.

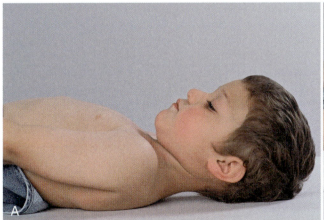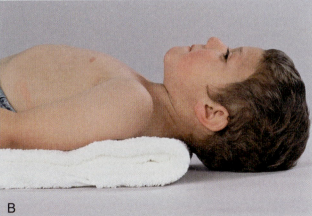

FIGURE 10-17 **A.** The larger size of a child's head relative to body size, combined with the reduced development of the posterior thoracic muscles, produces hyperflexion of the head when a child is placed on a backboard. **B.** Padding beneath the shoulders and torso will prevent this hyperflexion.

The placement of small children on a standard long backboard results in unwanted flexion of the head and neck. The long backboard needs to be modified by either creating a recess in the board or inserting padding under the torso to maintain the head in a neutral position (Figure 10-17B). The padding placed under the torso should be of the appropriate thickness so that the head lies on the board in a neutral position; too much will result in extension, too little in flexion. The padding under the torso must also be firm and evenly shaped. Use of irregularly shaped or insufficient padding, or placing it under only the shoulders, can result in movement and misalignment of the spine.

Completing Immobilization

Head

Once the patient's torso has been immobilized to the rigid device and appropriate padding inserted behind the head as needed, the head should be secured to the device (only after securing the torso). Because of its rounded shape, the head cannot be stabilized on a flat surface with only straps or tape. Use of these alone will still allow the head to rotate and move laterally. Also, because of the angle of the forehead and the slippery nature of moist skin and hair, a simple strap over the forehead is unreliable and can easily slide off. Although the human head weighs about the same as a bowling ball, it has a significantly different shape. The head is ovoid, longer than it is wide with almost completely flat lateral sides, resembling a bowling ball with about 2 inches (5 cm) cut off to form left and right sides. Adequate external immobilization of the head, regardless of method or device, can be achieved only by placing pads or rolled blankets on these flat sides and securing them with straps or tape. In the case of vest-type devices, this is accomplished with hinged side flaps that are part of the vest.

The side supports, whether they are preshaped foam blocks or rolled blankets, are placed next to both sides of the head. The sidepieces should be at least as wide as the patient's ears, or larger, and be at least as high as the level of the patient's eyes. Two straps or pieces of tape surrounding these headpieces draw the sides together. When it is packaged between the blocks or blankets, the head now has a flat posterior surface that can be realistically fixed to a flat board. The upper forehead strap is placed tightly across the front of the lower forehead (across the supraorbital ridge) to help prevent anterior movement of the head. This strap should be pulled tightly enough to indent the blocks or blankets and rest firmly on the forehead. Sandbags are not recommended for use as side supports because of the weight that may be placed on the head and neck when the immobilized patient is turned on his side.[38]

The use of chin cups or straps encircling the chin prevents opening of the mouth to vomit, so these devices should not be used. The device that holds the head, regardless of type, also requires a lower strap to help keep the sidepieces firmly pressed against the lower sides of the head and to anchor the device further and prevent anterior movement of the lower head and neck. The lower strap passes around the sidepieces and across the anterior rigid portion of the cervical collar. This strap should not place too much pressure on the front of the collar, which could produce an airway or venous return problem at the neck. Use of sandbags secured to the long backboard on the sides of the head and neck represents a dangerous practice. Regardless of how well they are secured, these heavy objects can shift and move. Should the need arise to rotate the patient and board to the side, such as when the patient needs to vomit, the combined weight of the sandbags can produce localized lateral pressure against the cervical spine. Raising or lowering the head of the board when moving and loading the patient, or any sudden acceleration or deceleration of the ambulance, can also produce shifting of the bags and movement of the head and neck.

Legs

Significant outward rotation of the legs may result in anterior movement of the pelvis and movement of the lower spine; tying the feet together eliminates this possibility. Placing a rolled blanket or piece of padding between the legs will increase comfort for the patient.

The patient's legs are immobilized to the board with two or more straps: one strap proximal to the knees at about midthigh and one strap distal to the knees.

The average adult measures 14 to 20 inches (35–50 cm) from one side to the other at the hips and only 6 to 9 inches (15–23 cm) from one side to the other at the ankles. When the feet are placed together, a V shape is formed from the hips to the ankles. Because the ankles are considerably narrower than the board, a strap placed across the lower legs can prevent anterior movement but will not prevent the legs from moving laterally from one edge of the board to the other. If the board is angled or rotated, the legs will fall to the lower edge of the board, which can angulate the pelvis and produce movement of the spinal column.

One way to hold the patient's lower legs effectively in place is to encircle them several times with the strap before attaching it to the board. The legs can be kept in the middle of the board by placing blanket rolls between each leg and the edges of the board before strapping. It is important to assure that the straps are not so tight as to impair distal circulation.

Arms

For safety, the patient's arms should be secured to the board or across the torso before moving the patient. One way to achieve this is with the arms placed at the sides on the board with the palms in, secured by a strap across the forearms and torso. This strap should be snug but not so tight as to compromise the circulation in the hands.

The patient's arms should not be included in the strap at the iliac crests or in the groin loops. If the straps are tight enough to provide adequate immobilization of the lower torso, they can compromise the circulation in the hands. If the straps are loose, they will not provide adequate immobilization of the torso or arms. Use of an additional strap exclusively to hold the arms allows the strap to be opened for taking a blood pressure measurement or starting an intravenous line once the patient is in the ambulance without compromising the immobilization. If the arm strap is also a torso strap, loosening it to free just an arm has the side effect of loosening the torso immobilization as well.

Most Common Mistakes

The following are the four most common immobilization errors:

1. *Inadequate immobilization.* The torso can move significantly up or down on the board device or the head can still move excessively.
2. *Immobilization with the head hyperextended.* The most common cause is a lack of appropriate padding behind the head.
3. *Immobilizing the head before the torso or readjusting the torso straps after the head has been secured.* This causes movement of the device relative to the torso, which results in movement of the head and cervical spine.

4. *Inadequate padding.* Failure to fill the voids under a patient can allow for inadvertent movement of the spine with additional injury as well as increased discomfort for the patient.

Complete spine immobilization is generally not a comfortable experience for the patient. As the degree and quality of the immobilization increase, the patient's comfort decreases. Spine immobilization is a balance between the need to protect and immobilize the spine completely and the need to make it tolerable for the patient. This is why proper evaluation of the need for spinal immobilization is indicated (Figure 10-18).

Obese Patients

With the increasing size of the current U.S. population, care of the *bariatric* (overweight, obese) patient is becoming more common. Transport of a 400-pound (182-kg) patient is becoming an everyday occurrence, and special bariatric transport cots have been developed for this purpose. However, a review of commercially available backboards shows that most long backboards measure 16 × 72 inches, with a few measuring 18 inches wide. The weight limit for these long backboards varies from 250 pounds (113 kg) to 600 pounds (272 kg). When using backboards on bariatric trauma patients, special care is needed to ensure that the safe operating limits are not exceeded. Also, additional personnel must be used to lift and extricate bariatric patients, without further injury

---

FIGURE 10-18 Criteria for Evaluating Immobilization Skills

Practice is needed using immobilization skills in hands-on sessions using mock patients before use with real patients. At least one study has shown that appropriate immobilization was not performed in a significant number of patients with potential spinal injury.[39] When practicing or when evaluating new methods or equipment, the following criteria will serve as good tools for measuring how effectively the "patient" has been immobilized:

1. Initiate manual in-line stabilization immediately and maintain until it is replaced mechanically.
2. Check neurologic function distally.
3. Apply an effective, properly sized cervical collar.
4. Secure the torso before the head.
5. Prevent movement of the torso up or down the board device.
6. Prevent movement of the upper and lower torso left or right on the board device.
7. Prevent anterior movement of the torso off the rigid device.
8. Assure ties crossing the chest do not inhibit chest excursion or result in ventilatory compromise.
9. Effectively immobilize the head so that it cannot move in any direction, including rotation.

10. Provide padding behind the head, if necessary.
11. Maintain the head in a neutral in-line position.
12. Assure that nothing inhibits or prevents the mouth from being opened.
13. Immobilized the legs so that they cannot move anteriorly, rotate, or move from side to side, even if the board and patient are rotated to the side.
14. Maintain the pelvis and legs in a neutral in-line position.
15. Assure that the arms are appropriately secured to the board or torso.
16. Assure that any ties or straps do not compromise distal circulation in any limb.
17. Re-evaluate the patient if bumped, jostled, or in any way moved in a manner that could compromise an unstable spine while the device was being applied.
18. Complete the procedure within an appropriate time frame.
19. Recheck distal neurologic function.

Many methods and variations can meet these objectives. The selection of a specific method and specific equipment will be based on the situation, the patient's condition, and available resources.

to the patient or provider. This subgroup of trauma patients presents challenges of safe packaging and moving procedures balanced against short scene times normally recommended in the critically injured trauma patients.

Use of Steroids

A series of studies suggested that high doses of methylprednisolone improve the neurologic outcome of patients with acute spinal cord injuries resulting from blunt trauma, when started within 8 hours of the injury.[39–41] In many centers, it has become common for patients with such injuries to receive a bolus of 30 mg/kg of methylprednisolone followed by an infusion of 5.4 mg/kg/hour for up to 48 hours, depending upon when the medication was initiated. Spinal cord injuries in children or those resulting from penetrating trauma were not studied and steroids are not indicated for neurologic deficits resulting from stab or gunshot wounds. Because steroids have known adverse effects, including suppression of adrenal glands and immune functioning, and because of concerns regarding the scientific validity of these studies, administration of steroids to patients with spinal cord injuries has become increasingly controversial.[38] In fact, the complications associated with steroid administration may significantly outweigh any benefit they may confer. Numerous publications no longer recommend steroid use for spinal injury, either in the field or in the hospital.[42–46] The decision to administer steroids ultimately remains a local choice and should be left to the trauma surgeons, orthopedic surgeons, or neurosurgeons ultimately caring for the patient.

Prolonged Transport

As with other injuries, the prolonged transport of patients with suspected or confirmed spinal and spinal cord injuries presents special considerations. Keeping in mind the goal to move patients with a suspected spinal cord injury only once, care should be taken to pad a long backboard prior to securing the patient. Cervical spine stabilization and spinal movement precautions should be utilized as the patient is moved to the padded backboard. Such efforts should help reduce the risk for the development of pressure ulcers in a patient with spinal cord injury. Any areas where there could be pressure on the patient's body, especially over bony prominences, should be sufficiently padded.

Patients who are immobilized to long backboards are at risk for aspiration should they regurgitate. In the event the patient begins to vomit, the backboard and patient should immediately be tipped onto the side. Suction should be kept near the head of the patient so it is readily accessible should vomiting occur. Insertion of a gastric tube (either nasogastric or orogastric) and the judicious use of antiemetic medications may help reduce this risk.

Patients with high spinal cord injuries may have involvement of their diaphragm and accessory respiratory muscles (i.e., intercostal muscles) predisposing them to respiratory failure. Impending respiratory failure may be aggravated and hastened by straps placed for spinal immobilization that further restrict respiration. Prior to initiating a prolonged transport, double check to make sure that the patient's torso is secured at the shoulder girdle and at the pelvis, and that any straps do not limit chest wall excursion.

As described in the text, patients with high spinal cord injuries may experience hypotension from loss of sympathetic tone (neurogenic "shock"). Although these patients rarely suffer from widespread hypoperfusion of their tissues, crystalloid boluses are generally sufficient to restore their blood pressure to normal. Vasopressors are rarely, if ever, necessary to treat neurogenic shock. Another hallmark of a high cervical spine injury is bradycardia. If associated with significant hypotension, bradycardia may be treated with intermittent doses of atropine, 0.5 to 1.0 mg administered intravenously.

The presence of tachycardia combined with hypotension should raise suspicion for the presence of hypovolemic, rather than neurogenic, shock. Careful assessment may pinpoint the source of hemorrhage, although intra-abdominal sources and pelvic fractures are most likely. Insertion of a urinary catheter will allow urine output to be used as another guide to tissue perfusion. In an adult, a urine output of greater than 30 to 50 ml/hour generally indicates satisfactory end-organ perfusion. The loss of sensation that accompanies a spinal cord injury may prevent a conscious patient from perceiving peritonitis or other injuries below the level of the sensory deficit.

Patients with spinal injuries may have significant back pain or pain from associated fractures. As described in Chapter 13, pain may be managed with small doses of intravenous narcotics titrated until pain is relieved. Narcotics may exaggerate the hypotension associated with neurogenic shock. Padding the backboard as described above may also provide some comfort for spinal fractures.

Patients with spinal cord injuries lose some ability to regulate body temperature, and this effect is more pronounced with higher injuries. Thus, these patients are sensitive to the development of hypothermia, especially when they are in a cold environment. Patients should be kept warm (normothermic), but remember that covering them with too many blankets may lead to hyperthermia.

Spine and spinal cord injuries are best managed at facilities that have excellent orthopedic or neurosurgical service and are experienced in the management of these injuries. All Level I and II trauma centers should be capable of managing the spinal cord injury and any associated injuries. Some facilities that specialize in the management of spine and spinal cord injuries may directly accept a patient who has suffered only a spinal cord injury (i.e., a shallow water diving injury with no evidence of aspiration).

SCENARIO SOLUTION

The patient's vital signs are: pulse 66, respirations 14, and blood pressure 96/70. As you continue your examination, you note that the patient is not moving her arms or legs. This patient is exhibiting signs of neurogenic shock. Interruption of the sympathetic nervous system and unopposed parasympathetic influence on the vascular system below the point of spinal injury result in an increased size of the vascular container and a relative hypovolemia. The patient's response to the spinal cord injury is a low blood pressure and bradycardia.

The first priorities of care are to continue to maintain a patent airway and oxygenation and assist ventilation as necessary to ensure an adequate minute volume while concurrently providing manual stabilization of the cervical spine. Immobilize the patient effectively and efficiently on a long backboard and transport the patient to an appropriate facility. Manage hypotension caused by neurogenic shock with intravenous fluids. Splint the fractured arm while en route.

The goals of prehospital management for this patient are to prevent additional spinal cord trauma, maintain tissue perfusion, and care for extremity trauma en route, and transport without delay to a trauma center for definitive care. ■

SUMMARY

- The vertebral column is composed of 24 separate vertebrae plus the sacrum and coccyx stacked on top of one another.
- The major functions of the spinal column are to support the weight of the body and allow movement.
- The spinal cord is enclosed within the vertebral column and is vulnerable to injury from abnormal movement and positioning. When support for the vertebral column has been lost as a result of injury to the vertebrae or to the muscles and ligaments that help hold the spinal column in place, injury to the spinal cord can occur.
- Because the cord does not regenerate, permanent neurologic injury, often involving paralysis, can result. The presence of spinal trauma and the need to immobilize the patient may be indicated by other injuries that could occur only with sudden, violent forces acting on the body or by specific signs and symptoms of vertebral or spinal cord injury.
- Damage to the bones of the spinal column is not always evident. If an initial injury to the cord has not occurred, neurologic deficit will not be present, even though the spinal column is unstable. Immobilization of spinal fractures, as with other fractures, requires immobilization of the joint above and the joint below the injury. For the spine, the joints above are the head and neck, and the joint below is the pelvis. The device selected should immobilize the head, chest, and pelvis areas in a neutral in-line position without causing or allowing movement.

References

1. DeVivo MJ. Causes and costs of spinal cord injury in the United States. *Spinal Cord* 35:809, 1997.
2. Spinal Cord Injury Information Pages. http://www.sci-info-pages.com/facts.html Accessed November 15, 2009.
3. Jackson AB, Dijkers M, Devivo MJ, Poczatek RB. A demographic profile of new traumatic spinal cord injuries: Change and stability over 30 years. *Arch Phys Med Rehabil* 85:1740, 2004.
4. Meldon SW, Moettus LN. Thoracolumbar spine fractures: Clinical presentation and the effect of altered sensorium and major injury. *J Trauma* 38:1110, 1995.
5. Ross SE, O'Malley KF, DeLong WG, et al. Clinical predictors of unstable cervical spine injury in multiply-injured patients. *Injury* 23:317, 1992.
6. Lindsey RW, Gugala Z, Pneumaticos SG. Injury to the vertebrae and spinal cord. In Feliciano DV, Mattox KL, Moore EE, editors: *Trauma*, New York, 2008, McGraw Hill, pp. 479-510.
7. Tator CH, Fehlings MG. Review of the secondary injury theory of acute spinal cord trauma with special emphasis on vascular mechanisms. *J Neurosurg* 75:15, 1991.
8. Tator CH. Spinal cord syndromes: Physiologic and anatomic correlations. In Menezes AH, Sonntag VKH, editors: *Principles of spinal surgery*, New York, 1995, McGraw-Hill.
9. Bilello JP, Davis JW, Cunningham MA, et al. Cervical spinal cord injury and the need for cardiovascular intervention. *Arch Surg* 138:1127, 2003.
10. Section on Disorders of the Spine and Peripheral Nerves of the American Association of Neurologic Surgeons/Congress of Neurologic Surgeons. Blood pressure management after acute spinal cord injury. *Neurosurgery* 50:S58, 2002.
11. Ullrich A, Hendey GW, Geiderman J, et al: Distracting painful injuries associated with cervical spinal injuries in blunt trauma. *Acad Emerg Med* 8:25, 2001.

12. Domeier RM, Evans RW, Swor RA, et al: Prospective validation of out-of-hospital spinal clearance criteria: A preliminary report. *Acad Emerg Med* 4:643, 1997.

13. Domeier RM, Swor RA, Evans RW, et al: Multicenter prospective validation of prehospital clinical spinal clearance criteria. *J Trauma* 53:744, 2002.

14. Hankins DG, Rivera-Rivera EJ, Ornato JP, et al: Spinal immobilization in the field: Clinical clearance criteria and implementation. *Prehosp Emerg Care* 5:88, 2001.

15. Stroh G, Braude D: Can an out-of-hospital cervical spine clearance protocol identify all patients with injuries? An argument for selective immobilization. *Ann Emerg Med* 37:609, 2001.

16. Dunn TM, Dalton A, Dorfman T, et al: Are emergency medical technician-basics able to use a selective immobilization of the cervical spine protocol? A preliminary report. *Prehosp Emerg Care* 8:207, 2004.

17. Domeier RM, Frederiksen SM, Welch K: Prospective performance assessment of an out-of-hospital protocol for selective spine immobilization using clinical spine clearance criteria. *Ann Emerg Med* 46:123, 2005.

18. Domeier RM, National Association of EMS Physicians Standards and Practice Committee: Indications for prehospital spinal immobilization. *Prehosp Emerg Care* 3:251, 1997.

19. Kwan I, Bunn F: Effects of prehospital spinal immobilization: A systematic review of randomized trials on healthy subjects. *Prehosp Disast Med* 20:47, 2005.

20. Connell RA, Graham CA, Munro PT: Is spinal immobilization necessary for all patients sustaining isolated penetrating trauma? *Injury* 34:912, 2003.

21. Kennedy FR, Gonzales P, Beitler A, et al: Incidence of cervical spine injuries in patients with gunshot wounds to the head. *Southern Med J* 87:621, 1994.

22. Chong CL, Ware DN, Harris JH: Is cervical spine imaging indicated in gunshot wounds to the cranium? *J Trauma* 44:501, 1998.

23. Kaups KL, Davis JW: Patients with gunshot wounds to the head do not require cervical spine immobilization and evaluation. *J Trauma* 44:865, 1998.

24. Lanoix R, Gupta R, Leak L, Pierre J: C-spine injury associated with gunshot wounds to the head: Retrospective study and literature review. *J Trauma* 49:860, 2000.

25. Barkana Y, Stein M, Scope A, et al: Prehospital stabilization of the cervical spine for penetrating injuries of the neck: Is it necessary? *Injury* 34:912, 2003.

26. Cornwell EE, Chang, DC, Boner JP, et al: Thoracolumbar immobilization for trauma patients with torso gunshot wounds—is it necessary? *Arch Surg* 136:324, 2001.

27. American College of Surgeons Committee on Trauma: *Advanced trauma life support for doctors, student course manual*, ed 7, Chicago, 2004, American College of Surgeons.

28. Haut ER, Kalish BT, Efron DT, et al. Spine immobilization in penetrating trauma: More harm than good? *J Trauma* 68:115-121, 2010.

29. DeBoer SL, Seaver M: Big head, little body syndrome: What EMS providers need to know. *Emerg Med Serv* 33:47, 2004.

30. Donaldson WF, Lauerman WC, Heil B, et al: Helmet and shoulder pad removal from a player with suspected cervical spine injury: A cadaveric model. *Spine* 23:1729, 1998.

31. Gastel JA, Palumbo MA, Hulstyn MJ, et al: Emergency removal of football equipment: A cadaveric cervical spine injury model. *Ann Emerg Med* 32:411, 1998.

32. Kleiner DM, Almquist JL, Bailes J, et al: *Prehospital care of the spine-injured athlete: A Document from the Inter-Association Task Force for Appropriate Care of the Spine-Injured Athlete*, Dallas, 2001, National Athletic Trainers' Association.

33. Palumbo MA, Hulstyn MJ: The effect of protective football equipment on the alignment of the injured cervical spine. *Am J Sports Med* 24:446, 1996.

34. Prinsen RKE, Syrotuik DG, Reid DC: Position of the cervical vertebrae during helmet removal and cervical collar application in football and hockey. *Clin J Sport Med* 5:155, 1995.

35. Swenson TM, Lauerman WC, Blanc RO, et al: Cervical spine alignment in the immobilized football player: Radiographic analysis before and after helmet removal. *Am J Sports Med* 25:226, 1997.

36. Waninger KN: Management of the helmeted athlete with suspected cervical spine injury. *Am J Sports Med* 32:1331, 2004.

37. Waninger KN: On-field management of potential cervical spine injury in helmeted football players: Leave the helmet on! *Clin J Sport Med* 8:124, 1998.

38. Nesathurai S: Steroids and spinal cord injury: Revisiting the NASCIS 2 and NASCIS 3 trials. *J Trauma* 45:1088, 1998.

39. Bracken MB, Shepard MJ, Collins, et al: A randomized, controlled trial of methylprednisolone or naloxone in the treatment of acute spinal-cord injury. Results of the Second National Acute Spinal Cord Injury Study. *N Engl J Med* 322(20):1405–1411, 1997.

40. Bracken MB, Shepard MJ, Collins WF Jr et al: Methylprednisolone or naloxone treatment after acute spinal cord injury: 1-year follow-up data. Results of the second National Acute Spinal Cord Injury Study. *J Neurosurg* 76(1):23–31, 1992.

41. Otani K, Abe H, Kadoya S, et al: Beneficial effect of methyl-prednisolone sodium succinate in the treatment of acute spinal cord injury, *Sekitsui Sekizui J* 7:633–647, 1996.

42. Bledsoe BE, Wesley AK, Salomone JP: High-dose steroids for acute spinal cord injury in emergency medical services. *Prehosp Emerg Care* 8:313, 2004.

43. Spine and Spinal Cord Trauma. In ACS Committee on Trauma: *Advanced Trauma Life Support for Doctors*, Chicago, 2008, American College of Surgeons.

44. Short DJ, El Masry WS, Jones PW: High Dose methylprednisolone in the management of acute spinal cord injury—A systematic review from the clinical perspective. *Spinal Cord* 38:273, 2000.

45. Coleman WP, Benzel D. Cahill DW, et al: A critical appraisal of the reporting of the National Acute Spinal Cord Injury Studies (II and III) of methylprednisolone in acute spinal cord injury. *J Spinal Disord* 13:185, 2000.

46. Hurlbert RJ: The role of steroids in acute spinal cord injury: An evidence-based analysis. *Spine* 26:S39, 2001.

Suggested Reading

American College of Surgeons Committee on Trauma: *Advanced trauma life support for doctors, student course manual*, ed 7, Chicago, 2004, ACS.

Pennardt AM, Zehner WJ: Paramedic documentation of indicators for cervical spine injury. *Prehosp Disaster Med* 9:40, 1994.

SPECIFIC SKILLS

Spine Management

Cervical Collar Sizing and Application

Principle: To select and apply an appropriate sized cervical collar to assist in providing neutral alignment and stabilization of the patient's head and neck.

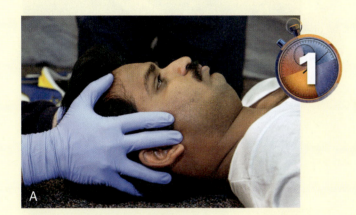

First provider provides manual neutral in-line stabilization of the patient's head and neck.

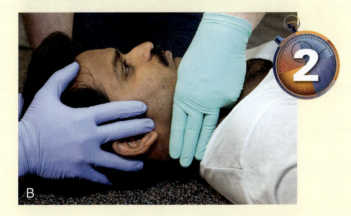

Second provider uses his or her fingers to measure the patient's neck between the patient's lower jaw and shoulder.

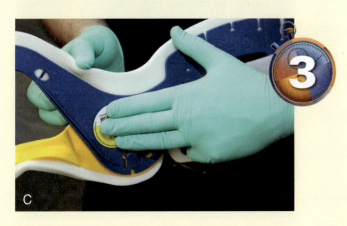

Second provider uses this measurement to select a proper sized collar or adjust an adjustable collar to the correct size.

SPECIFIC SKILLS

If an adjustable collar is utilized, make sure the collar is locked into the proper size.

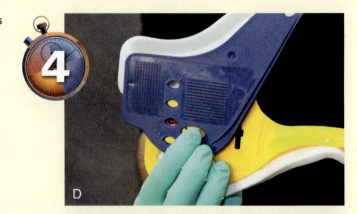

The second provider applies the properly sized collar while the first provider continues to maintain the neutral in-line head and neck stabilization.

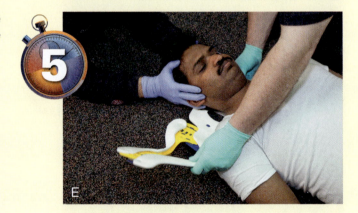

After applying and securing the cervical collar, manual in-line stabilization of the head and neck is maintained until the patient is secured to an immobilization device.

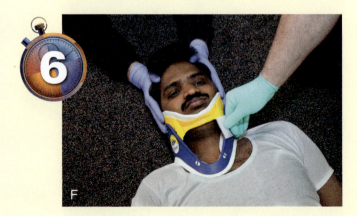

Logroll

Principle: To turn a patient while maintaining manual stabilization with minimal movement of the spine. The logroll is indicated for (1) positioning a patient onto a long backboard or other device to facilitate movement of the patient and (2) turning a patient with suspected spinal trauma to examine the back.

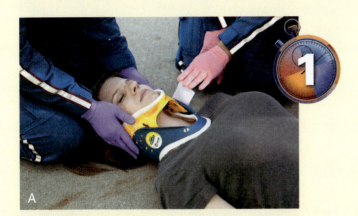

A. Supine Patient

While one prehospital care provider maintains neutral in-line stabilization at the patient's head, a second provider applies a properly sized cervical collar.

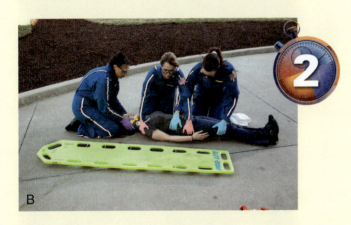

While one provider maintains neutral in-line stabilization, a second provider kneels at the patient's midthorax, and a third provider kneels at the level of the patient's knees. The patient's arms are straightened and placed palms-in next to the torso while the patient's legs are brought into neutral alignment. The patient is grasped at the shoulder and hips in such a fashion as to maintain a neutral in-line position of the lower extremities. The patient is "logrolled" slightly onto his or her side.

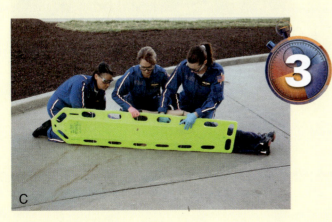

The long backboard is placed with the foot end of the board positioned between the patient's knees and ankles (the head of the long backboard will extend beyond the patient's head). The long backboard is held against the patient's back and the patient is logrolled back onto the long backboard, and the board is lowered to the ground with the patient.

SPECIFIC SKILLS

Once on the ground, the patient is grasped firmly by the shoulders, the pelvis, and the lower extremities.

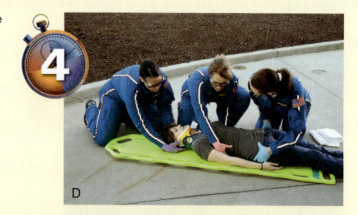

The patient is moved upward and laterally onto the long backboard. Neutral in-line stabilization is maintained without pulling on the patient's head and neck.

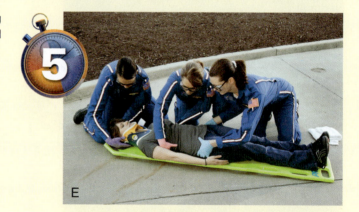

The patient is positioned onto the long backboard with the head at the top of the board and the body centered.

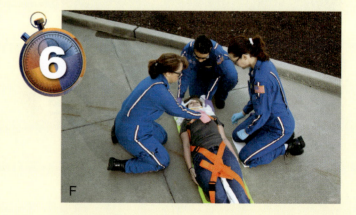

B. Prone or Semi-prone Patient

When a patient presents in a prone or semi-prone position, a stabilization method similar to that used for the supine patient can be used. The method incorporates the same initial alignment of the patient's limbs, the same positioning and hand placement of the prehospital care providers, and the same responsibilities for maintaining alignment.

The patient's arms are positioned in anticipation of the full rotation that will occur. When using the semi-prone logroll method, a cervical collar can be safely applied only after the patient is in an in-line position and supine on the long backboard, not before.

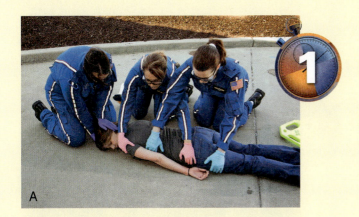

Whenever possible, the patient should always be rolled away from the direction in which the patient's face initially points. One provider establishes in-line manual stabilization of the patient's head and neck. Another provider kneels at the patient's thorax and grasps the patient's opposite shoulder and wrist and pelvis area. A third provider kneels at the patient's knees and grasps the patient's wrist and pelvis area and lower extremities.

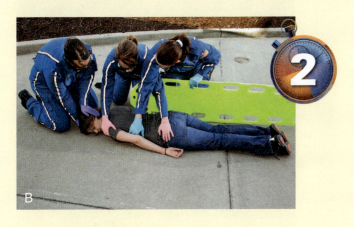

The long backboard is placed on the lateral edge and brought into position between the patient and the providers.

SPECIFIC SKILLS

The board is placed with the foot of the board between the patient's knees and ankles, and the patient is logrolled onto his or her side. The patient's head rotates less than the torso, so by the time the patient is on his or her side (perpendicular to the ground), the head and torso have come into proper alignment.

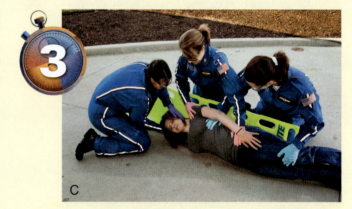

C

Once the patient is supine on the long backboard, the patient is moved upward and toward the center of the board. The prehospital care providers should take care not to pull the patient but to maintain neutral in-line stabilization. Once the patient is positioned properly on the long backboard, a properly sized cervical collar can be applied, and the patient can be secured to the backboard.

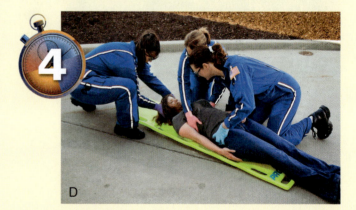

D

Standing Long Backboard Application

Principle: To fully immobilize a standing patient to a long backboard while maintaining the head and neck in a neutral position and minimizing the risk of additional injury.

This application is indicated for spinal immobilization of a trauma patient who is ambulatory but is found to have an indication for spinal immobilization (see Figure 10-12).

Two general methods exist for immobilizing a standing patient to a long backboard. The first method involves securing the standing patient's torso and head to the board before lowering the board to the ground. This method causes some discomfort to the patient and may not allow the patient to be lowered to the ground without movement. The second method involves manual stabilization of the patient to the board while lowering the board and patient to the ground and then securing the patient to the board. This second method is the preferred method and can be accomplished with two or three rescuers.

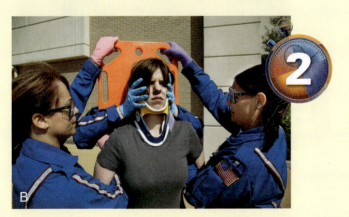

A. Three or More Providers

Prehospital care providers can apply manual in-line stabilization from either behind the patient or in front of the patient. Once manual in-line stabilization of the patient's head and neck is applied, a properly sized, rigid cervical collar can be applied. A long backboard is placed behind the patient from the side and pressed against the patient. Manual in-line stabilization is maintained throughout the procedure until the patient is secured to the long backboard.

Two prehospital care providers stand on either side of the patient, turned slightly toward the patient. Each provider inserts the hand closest to the patient under the patient's armpit and grasps the nearest handhold of the backboard without moving the patient's shoulders. The other hand grasps a higher handhold on the board. While manual in-line stabilization is maintained, the patient and backboard are lowered to the ground.

SPECIFIC SKILLS

As the patient is lowered to the ground, the provider behind the patient providing the manual stabilization must rotate his or her hands to maintain the stabilization.

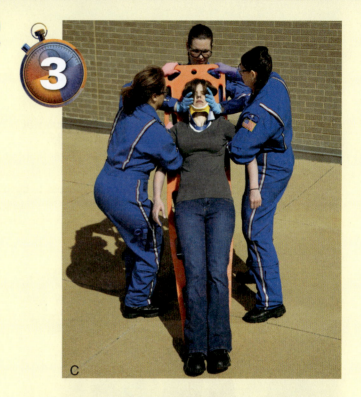

C

As the patient is lowered to the ground each provider on the side of the patient—one at a time—will need to release their holds on the upper portion of the board and reposition their hand under the provider's arm maintaining manual stabilization of the patient's head and neck.

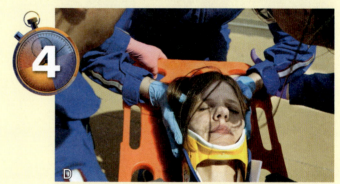

D

Once the patient and board are on the ground, the patient is secured to the long backboard.

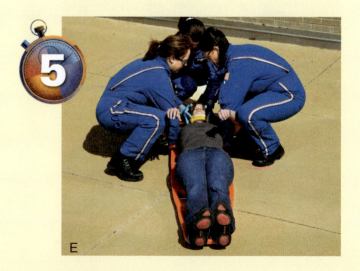

E

B. Two Providers

When three or more prehospital care providers are not available, two providers can still achieve immobilization. The first provider establishes and maintains manual stabilization of the patient's head and neck while the second provider measures and applies an appropriate sized cervical collar. Once the collar has been applied, the second provider places a backboard behind the patient and in front of the first provider.

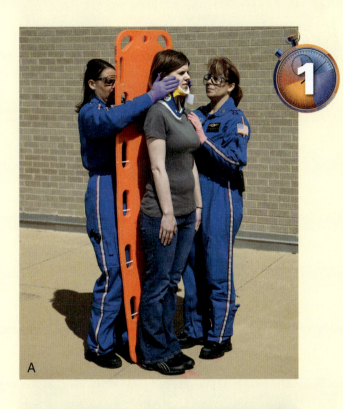

A

The second provider holds the backboard with the hand closest to the board. The second provider now places the other hand, palm surface with fingers extended, on the patient's head and applies light pressure to assist in maintaining manual stabilization.

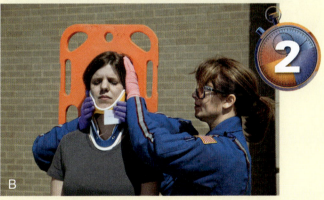

B

The first provider now can release the patient's head with the hand closest to the second provider. With his or her other hand, the provider repositions it to the side of the patient's head to apply lateral pressure while moving to the patient's side and grasping the backboard at the level of the patient's head or higher.

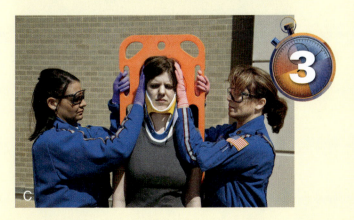

C

SPECIFIC SKILLS

The patient and backboard are lowered to the ground while both providers maintain manual stabilization with equal lateral pressure against the side of the patient's head. The prehospital care providers need to work together during this move to ensure maximum manual stabilization.

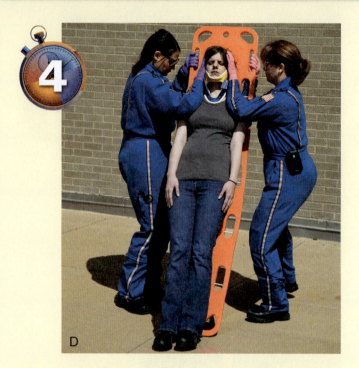

D

Once the patient and backboard are on the ground, manual in-line stabilization can be maintained by one provider from above the patient's head until the patient is secured to the long backboard.

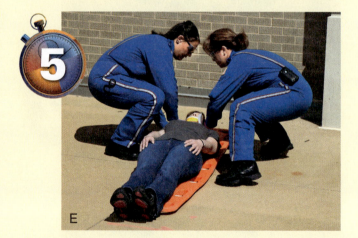

E

Sitting Immobilization (Vest-Type Extraction Device) 💿

Principle: To immobilize a trauma patient without critical injuries before moving the patient from a sitting position.

This type of immobilization is used when spinal stabilization is indicated for a sitting trauma patient without life-threatening conditions. Several brands of vest-type extrication devices are available. Each model is slightly different in design, but any model can serve as a general example. The **Kendrick Extrication Device (KED)** is used in this demonstration. The details (but not the general sequence) are modified when using a different model or brand of extrication device. Also, during this demonstration, the windshield of the vehicle has been removed for clarification purposes.

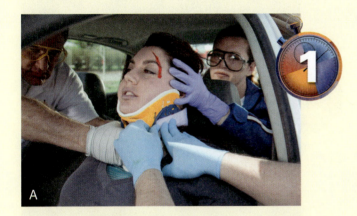

Manual in-line stabilization is initiated and a properly sized cervical collar applied.

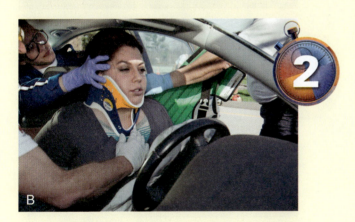

The patient is maintained in an upright position slightly forward to provide an adequate amount of space between the patient's back and the vehicle seat for placement of the vest-type device. *Note:* Before placing the vest-type device behind the patient, the two long straps (groin straps) are unfastened and placed behind the vest device.

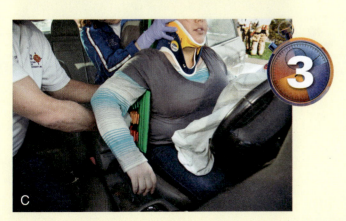

After placing the vest device behind the patient, the side flaps are placed around the patient and moved until the side flaps are touching the patient's armpits.

SPECIFIC SKILLS

The torso straps are positioned and fastened, starting with the middle chest strap and followed by the lower chest strap. Each strap is tightened after attachment. Use of the upper chest strap at this time is optional. If the upper chest strap is used, the provider should ensure that it is not so tight that it impedes the patient's ventilations. The upper chest strap should be tightened just before moving the patient.

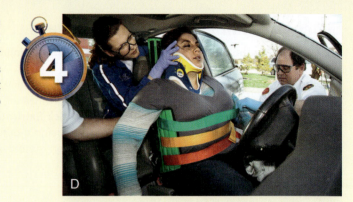

Each groin strap is positioned and fastened. Using a back-and-forth motion, each strap is worked under the patient's thigh and buttock until it is in a straight line in the intergluteal fold from front to back. Each groin strap is placed under the patient's leg and attached to the vest on the same side as the strap's origin. Once in place, each groin strap is tightened. The patient's genitalia should not be placed under the straps but to the side of each strap.

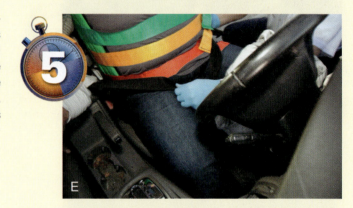

Padding is placed between the patient's head and the vest to maintain neutral alignment.

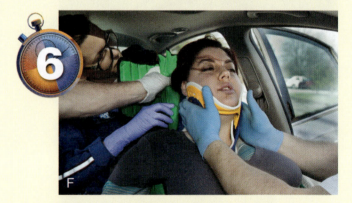

The patient's head is secured to the head flaps of the vest device. The provider should be careful not to seat the patient's mandible or obstruct the airway. *Note:* The torso straps should be evaluated and readjusted as needed.

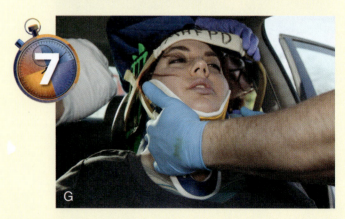

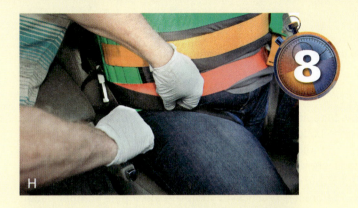

All straps should be rechecked before moving the patient. If the upper chest strap has not been secured, it should be attached and tightened.

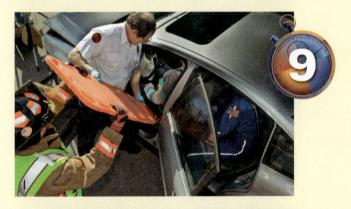

If possible, the ambulance cot with a long backboard should be brought to the opening of the vehicle door. The long backboard is placed under the patient's buttocks so that one end is securely supported on the vehicle seat and the other end on the ambulance cot. If the ambulance cot is not available or the terrain will not allow the placement of the cot, other prehospital care providers can hold the long backboard while the patient is rotated and lifted out of the vehicle.

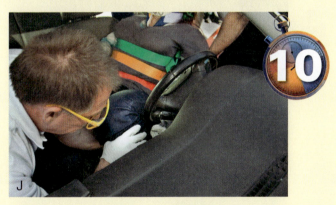

While rotating the patient, the patient's lower extremities must be elevated onto the seat. If the vehicle has a center console, the patient's legs should be moved over the console one at a time.

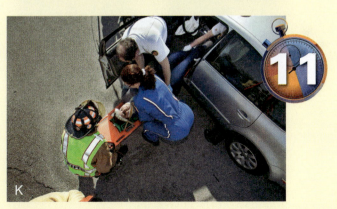

Once the patient is rotated with his or her back to the center of the long backboard, the patient is lowered to the board while keeping the legs elevated. After placing the patient onto the long backboard, the two groin straps are released and the patient's legs are lowered. The patient is positioned by moving him or her up on the board with the vest device in place. The provider should consider releasing the upper chest strap at this time.

Once the patient is positioned on the long backboard, the vest device is left secured in place to continue to immobilize the patient's head, neck, and torso. The patient and vest device are secured to the long backboard. The patient's lower extremities are immobilized to the board, and the long backboard is secured to the ambulance cot.

SPECIFIC SKILLS

Rapid Extrication

Principle: To manually stabilize a patient with critical injuries before and during movement from a sitting position.

A. Three or More Providers

Sitting patients with life-threatening conditions and indications for spinal immobilization (see Figure 10-12) can be rapidly extricated. Immobilization to an interim device before moving the patient provides more stable immobilization than when using only the manual (rapid extrication) method. However, it requires an additional 4 to 8 minutes to complete. The prehospital care provider will use the vest or halfboard methods when (1) the scene and patient's condition are stable and time is not a primary concern, or (2) a special rescue situation involving substantial lifting or technical rescue hoisting exists, and significant movement or carrying of the patient is involved before it is practical to complete the supine immobilization to a long backboard.

Rapid extrication is indicated in the following situations:

■ When the patient has life-threatening conditions identified during the primary survey that cannot be corrected where the patient is found.
■ When the scene is unsafe and clear danger to the prehospital care provider and patient exists, necessitating rapid removal to a safe location.
■ When the patient needs to be moved quickly to access other, more seriously injured patients.

Note: Rapid extrication is only selected when life-threatening conditions are present and not on the basis of personal preference.

Once the decision is made to extricate a patient rapidly, manual in-line stabilization of the patient's head and neck in a neutral position is initiated. This is best accomplished from behind the patient. If a provider is unable to get behind the patient, manual stabilization can be accomplished from the side. Whether from behind the patient or the side, the patient's head and neck are brought into a neutral alignment, a rapid assessment of the patient is performed, and a properly sized cervical collar is applied.

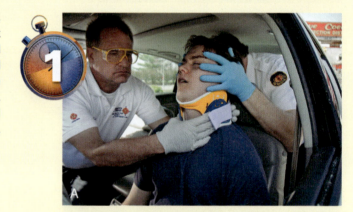

While manual stabilization is maintained, the patient's upper torso and lower torso and legs are controlled. The patient is rotated in a series of short, controlled movements.

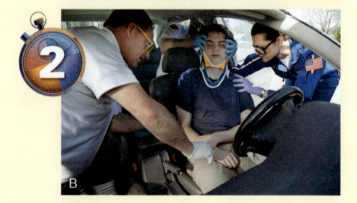

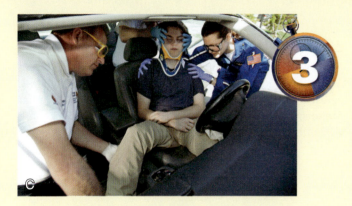

3 If the vehicle has a center console, the patient's legs should be moved one at a time over the console.

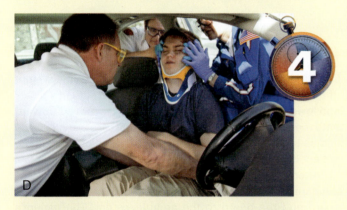

4 The provider continues to rotate the patient in short controlled movements until control of manual stabilization can no longer be maintained from behind and inside the vehicle. A second provider assumes manual stabilization from the first provider while standing outside of the vehicle.

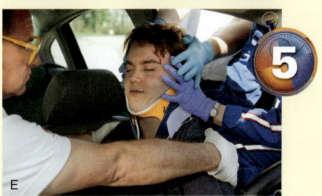

5 The first provider can now move outside the vehicle and reassume manual stabilization from the second provider.

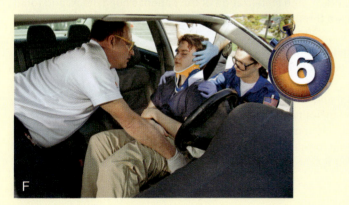

6 The rotation of the patient is continued until the patient can be lowered out of the vehicle door opening and onto the long backboard.

SPECIFIC SKILLS

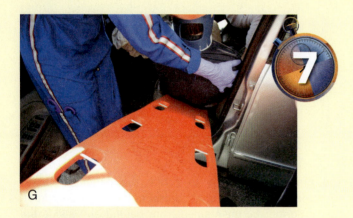

7

The long backboard is placed with the foot end of the board onto the vehicle seat and the head end on the ambulance cot. If the cot cannot be placed next to the vehicle, other prehospital care providers can hold the long backboard while the patient is lowered onto it.

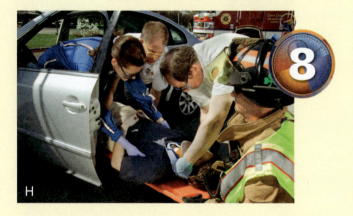

8

Once the patient's torso is down on the board, the weight of the patient's chest is controlled while the patient's pelvis and lower legs are controlled. The patient is moved upward onto the long backboard. The prehospital care provider who is maintaining manual stabilization is careful not to pull the patient but to support the patient's head and neck.

After the patient is positioned onto the long backboard, the prehospital care providers can secure the patient to the board and the board to the ambulance cot. The patient's upper torso is secured first, then the lower torso and pelvis area, then the head. The patient's legs are secured last. If the scene is unsafe, the patient should be moved to a safe area before being secured to the board or cot.

Note: This represents only one example of rapid extrication. Because very few field situations are ideal, prehospital care providers may need to modify the steps for extrication for the particular patient and situation. The principle of rapid extrication should remain the same regardless of the situation: maintain manual stabilization throughout the extrication process without interruption, and maintain the entire spine in an in-line position without unwarranted movement. Any positioning of the prehospital care providers that works can be successful. However, numerous position changes and hand position takeovers should be avoided because they invite a lapse in manual stabilization.

The rapid extrication technique can effectively provide manual in-line stabilization of the patient's head, neck, and torso throughout a patient's removal from a vehicle. The following are three key points of rapid extrication:

1. One prehospital care provider maintains stabilization of the patient's head and neck at all times, another rotates and stabilizes the patient's upper torso, and a third moves and controls the patient's lower torso, pelvis, and lower extremities.
2. Maintaining manual in-line stabilization of the patient's head and neck is impossible if attempting to move the patient in one continuous motion. The prehospital care providers need to limit each movement, stopping to reposition and prepare for the next move. Undue haste will cause delay and may result in movement of the spine.
3. Each situation and patient may require adaptation of the principles of rapid extrication. This can only work effectively if the maneuvers are practiced. Each provider needs to know the actions and movements of the other providers.

B. Two Providers

In some situations an adequate number of providers may not be available to extricate a critical patient rapidly. In these situations a two-provider technique is useful.

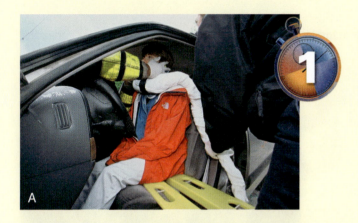

One prehospital care provider initiates and maintains manual in-line stabilization of the patient's head and neck. A second provider places a properly sized cervical collar on the patient and places a prerolled blanket around the patient. The center of the blanket roll is placed at the patient's midline on the rigid cervical collar. The ends of the blanket roll are wrapped around the cervical collar and placed under the patient's arms.

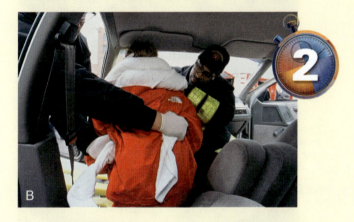

The patient is turned using the ends of the blanket roll and until the patient's back is centered on the door opening.

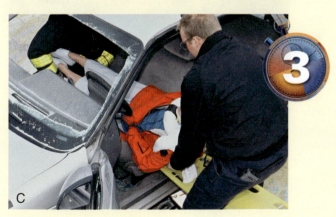

The first provider takes control of the blanket ends, moving them under the patient's shoulders, and moves the patient by the blanket while the second provider moves and controls the patient's lower torso, pelvis, and legs.

SPECIFIC SKILLS

Infant Child Seat

Principle: To provide spinal immobilization to an infant with suspected spinal injuries while remaining seated in a car seat.

Inspect car seat to rule out structural damage. If structure damage is noted, *do not immobilize patient in seat.* Move the patient onto an immobilization device.

First provider stabilizes the child's head and neck in a neutral position.

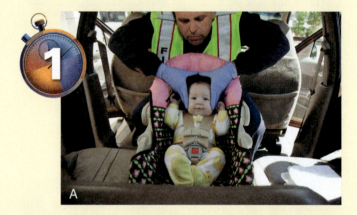

Second provider uses folded towels and/or blankets to fill all voids between the child and the car seat while the first provider maintains manual stabilization of the patient's head and neck.

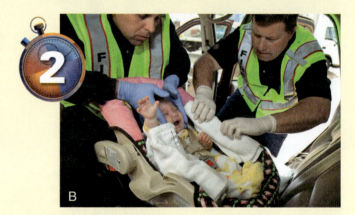

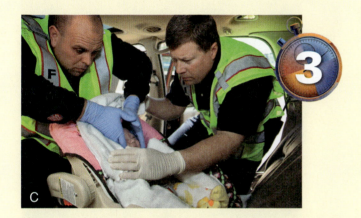

After the voids around the patient's torso have been filled, pad around the patient's head and neck.

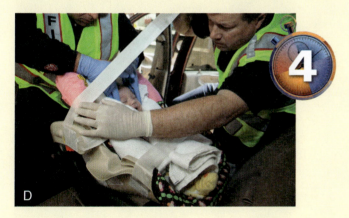

After all voids have been identified and filled, the second provider secures the patients torso to the seat with tape and/or straps while the first provider maintains manual stabilization of the patient's head and neck. After the patient's torso has been secured, the second provider secures the patient's head to the seat.

SPECIFIC SKILLS

Child Immobilization Device

Principle: To provide spinal immobilization to a child with a suspected spinal injury.

The first provider kneels above the patient's head and provides manual in-line stabilization of the patient's head and neck. The second provider sizes and applies a cervical collar while the first provider maintains neutral in-line stabilization. The second provider straightens the patient's arms and legs, if needed.

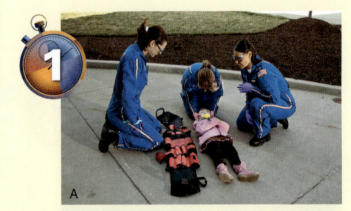

The second provider now kneels at the patient's side between their shoulders and knees. The second provider grasps the patient at the shoulder and hips in such a fashion as to maintain a neutral in-line position of the lower extremities. On command from the first provider, the patient is logrolled slightly onto his or her side.

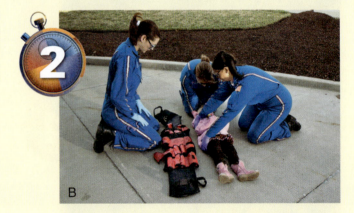

A third provider positions the immobilization device behind the patient and holds it in place.

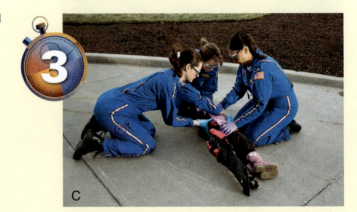

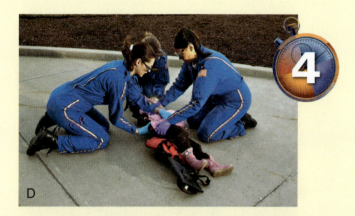

The device is held against the patient's back and the patient is logrolled onto the device, and the device is lowered to the ground with the patient.

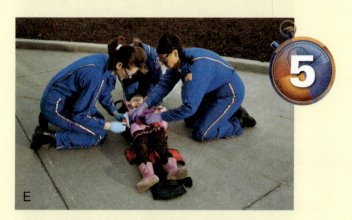

The patient is now secured to the immobilization device by the second and third provider while the first provider maintains head and neck stabilization.

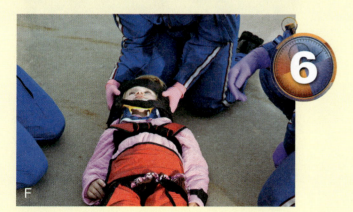

After securing the patient's torso and lower extremities to the immobilization device, the patient's head is secured to the immobilization device.

SPECIFIC SKILLS

Helmet Removal 💿

Principle: To remove a safety helmet while minimizing the risk of additional injury.

Patients who are wearing full-face helmets must have the helmet removed early in the assessment process. This provides immediate access for the prehospital care provider to assess and manage a patient's airway and ventilatory status. Helmet removal ensures that hidden bleeding is not occurring into the posterior helmet and allows the provider to move the head (from the flexed position caused by large helmets) into neutral alignment. It also permits complete assessment of the head and neck in the secondary survey and facilitates spinal immobilization when indicated (see Figure 10-12). The prehospital care provider explains to the patient what will occur. If the patient verbalizes that the provider should not remove the helmet, the provider explains that properly trained personnel can remove it by protecting the patient's spine. Two providers are required for this maneuver.

One provider takes position above the patient's head. With palms pressed on the sides of the helmet and fingertips curled over the lower margin, the first provider stabilizes the helmet, head, and neck in as close to a neutral in-line position as the helmet allows. A second provider kneels at the side of the patient, opens or removes the face shield if needed, remove eyeglasses if present, and unfastens or cuts the chin strap.

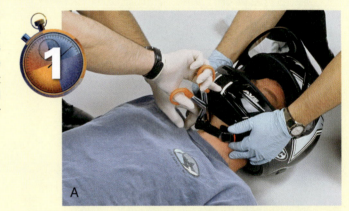

The patient's mandible is grasped between the thumb and the first two fingers at the angle of the mandible. The other hand is placed under the patient's neck on the occiput of the skull to take control of manual stabilization. The provider's forearms should be resting on the floor or ground or on the provider's thighs for additional support.

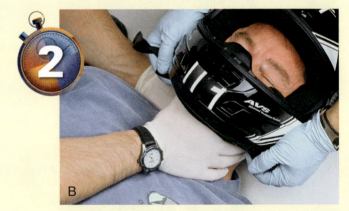

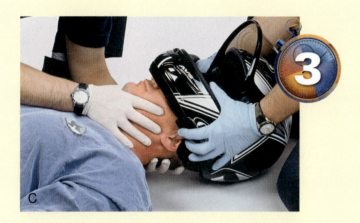

The first provider pulls the sides of the helmet slightly apart, away from the patient's head, and rotates the helmet with up-and-down rocking motions while pulling it off of the patient's head. Movement of the helmet is slow and deliberate. The provider takes care as the helmet clears the patient's nose.

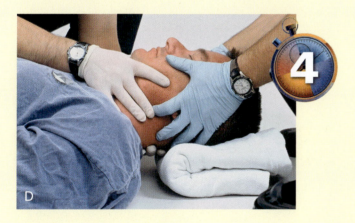

Once the helmet is removed, padding should be placed behind the patient's head to maintain a neutral in-line position. Manual stabilization is maintained, and a properly sized cervical collar is placed on the patient.

Note: Two key elements are involved in helmet removal, as follows:

1. While one provider maintains manual stabilization of the patient's head and neck, the other provider moves. At no time should both providers be moving their hands.
2. The provider rotates the helmet in different directions, first to clear the patient's nose and then to clear the back of the patient's head.

CHAPTER 11

Thoracic Trauma

CHAPTER OBJECTIVES

At the completion of this chapter, the reader will be able to do the following:

- ✓ Discuss the normal anatomy and physiology of the thoracic organs.
- ✓ Describe the alterations in anatomy and physiology that result from thoracic injury.
- ✓ Discuss the relationships among the kinematics of trauma, thoracic anatomy and physiology, and various assessment findings, leading to an index of suspicion for various injuries.
- ✓ Differentiate between patients in need of rapid stabilization and transport and patients in whom further on-scene assessment and management is warranted or appropriate.
- ✓ Discuss the impact of an urban or suburban and rural or austere setting on assessment and management of thoracic injury.
- ✓ Describe the signs, symptoms, pathophysiology, and management of the following specific thoracic injuries:
    - ✓ Rib fractures
    - ✓ Flail chest
    - ✓ Pulmonary contusion
    - ✓ Pneumothorax (simple, open, and closed)
    - ✓ Tension pneumothorax
    - ✓ Hemothorax
    - ✓ Blunt cardiac injury
    - ✓ Cardiac tamponade
    - ✓ Commotio cordis
    - ✓ Traumatic aortic disruption
    - ✓ Tracheobronchial disruption
    - ✓ Traumatic asphyxia
    - ✓ Diaphragmatic rupture

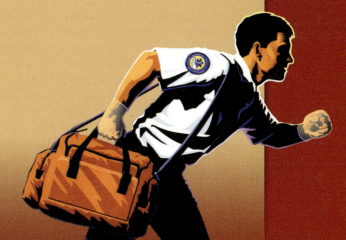

SCENARIO

You are dispatched to a scene of a stabbing at a residence. While en route, you receive additional information that the patient is a male with a single stab wound to his chest. Police are noted to be on scene and that the scene is secure. Your anticipated response time is less than 5 minutes.

Upon arrival, you enter a house to the sounds of a woman yelling at police about being handcuffed coming from a back room. An officer points you to a male patient seated shirtless on a couch, handcuffed, who begins yelling at you to do something because his chest hurts. As you approach and attempt to calm the patient, you notice a small wound to his left anterior chest just medial to the nipple. Your partner places oxygen on the patient and begins to assess vital signs, while you note that the patient is diaphoretic, and tachypneic, between yelling at you and the police. He appears to have jugular venous distension even sitting up, and you note a small area of crepitus in the chest wall surrounding the wound. Lung sounds are present but diminished on the left, and it is difficult to assess heart sounds. You note no abdominal injuries or tenderness, and he is moving all his extremities without apparent difficult.

Is this patient in respiratory distress? Does he have life-threatening injuries? What interventions should you undertake in the field? What modality should be used to transport this patient? How would a different location (e.g., rural) impact your management and plans during prolonged transport? What other injuries do you suspect based on the above information?

As with other forms of injury, thoracic trauma can result from blunt or penetrating mechanisms. Blunt force applied to the thoracic cage in motor vehicle crashes, high falls, beatings, or crush injuries can cause disruption of the normal anatomy and physiology of the thoracic organs. Similarly, penetrating wounds from gunshots, knives, or impalement on objects such as rebar can injure the thorax. Definitive management of most thoracic injuries does not require *thoracotomy* (opening the chest cavity operatively). In fact, only 15% to 20% of all chest injuries require thoracotomy. The remaining 85% are well managed with relatively simple interventions, such as supplemental oxygen, ventilatory support, analgesia, and tube *thoracostomy* (chest tube placement) when necessary.[1–3]

Nevertheless, these injuries can be quite significant. The thoracic organs are intimately involved in the maintenance of oxygenation, ventilation, and oxygen delivery. Injury to the chest, especially if not promptly recognized and appropriately managed, can lead to significant morbidity. *Hypoxia* (inadequate amounts of oxygen in the blood), *hypercarbia* (excessive carbon dioxide in the blood), *acidosis* (excessive acid in the blood), and *shock* (inadequate amounts of oxygen reaching the body's organs and tissues) can result from inadequate management of chest injury in the short term and thereby contribute to late complications, such as multisystem organ failure. This accounts for the 25% of trauma deaths that result from thoracic injury.[1–3]

Anatomy

The chest is roughly a hollow cylinder formed by its bony and muscular structures. There are 12 paired ribs. The upper 10 pairs attach to the spinal column in the back and either the sternum or the rib above in the front. The lower two pairs of ribs only attach in back to the spine. In the front they are free and thus referred to as "floating ribs." This bony cage provides a great deal of protection to the internal organs of the chest cavity. In fact, the lower ribs also shield the organs of the upper abdomen (most notably the spleen and liver). This bony cage is reinforced with muscle. The *intercostal muscles* lie between and connect the ribs to one another. A number of muscle groups move the upper extremity and are part of the chest wall, including the major and minor pectoral muscles, anterior and posterior serratus muscles, and latissimus dorsi muscles, along with the various muscles of the back. All this "padding" means that it takes a considerable amount of force to injure the internal organs.

There are also muscles involved in the process of breathing (ventilation), including the intercostal muscles; the *diaphragm*, which is a dome-shaped muscle attached around the lower aspect of the chest; and muscles in the neck that attach to upper ribs. An artery, vein, and nerve course along the lower edge of each rib and provide blood and stimulation to the intercostal muscles.

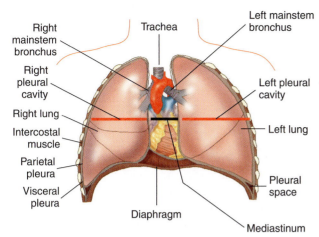

FIGURE 11-1 The thoracic cavity, including the ribs, intercostal muscles, diaphragm, mediastinum, lungs, heart, great vessels, bronchi, trachea, and esophagus.

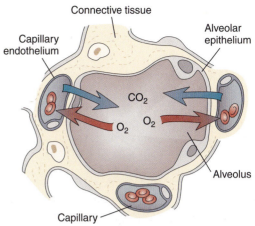

FIGURE 11-2 The capillaries and alveolus lie in close proximity; therefore, oxygen *(O₂)* can easily diffuse through the capillary, alveolar walls, capillary walls, and red blood cells. Carbon dioxide *(CO₂)* can diffuse back in the opposite direction.

Lining the cavity formed by these structures is a thin membrane called the *parietal pleura.* A matching thin membrane covers the other organs of the chest cavity, called the *visceral pleura.* There is normally no space between these two membranes. In fact, they are adhered to one another by a small amount of fluid between them that holds them together, much as a thin layer of water will hold two sheets of glass together. This pleural fluid creates a surface tension, which serves to oppose the elastic nature of the lungs, preventing their otherwise natural tendency to collapse.

The lungs occupy the right and left sides of the chest cavity (Figure 11–1). Between them and enveloped by them is a space called the *mediastinum,* which contains the trachea, the main bronchi, the heart, the major arteries and veins to and from the heart, as well as the esophagus.

Physiology

The two components of chest physiology that are most likely to be impacted by injury are *breathing* and *circulation.*[1–3] Both these processes need to be working properly for oxygen to reach the body's organs, tissues, and ultimately cells and to expel carbon dioxide. To best understand what happens to patients when their chests are injured and how to manage their injuries, it is important to understand the physiology of these two processes.

Ventilation

The lay terms "breathing" and "respiration" actually refer to the physiologic process of ventilation. *Ventilation* is the mechanical act of drawing air through the mouth and nose into the trachea and bronchi and then into the lungs, where it arrives in small air sacs known as *alveoli. Respiration* is ventilation plus the delivery of oxygen to the cells. The process of drawing air in is called *inhalation.* Oxygen in that air is transported across the lining membrane of the alveoli, into adjacent small blood vessels known as *capillaries,* where it attaches to hemoglobin in the red blood cells for transport to the body. This process is known as *oxygenation.* Simultaneously, carbon dioxide (CO₂), which is dissolved in the blood, diffuses out into the air within the alveoli for expulsion when that air is blown out again in the process of *exhalation* (Figure 11–2). *Cellular respiration* is the use of oxygen by the cells to produce energy (see Chapter 7).

Inhalation is brought about by contraction of the muscles of respiration (primarily the intercostals and the diaphragm), which results in a lifting and separating of the ribs and downward motion of the diaphragm. This action increases the size of the thoracic cavity and creates a negative pressure within the chest cavity compared with the air pressure outside the body, resulting in flow of air into the lungs (Figures 11–3 and 11–4). *Expiration* is achieved by relaxing the intercostals and diaphragm, resulting in the return of the ribs and diaphragm to their resting positions. This return causes the pressure within the chest to exceed the pressure outside the body, and air from the lungs is emptied through the bronchi, trachea, mouth, and nose to the outside.

Ventilation is under the control of the respiratory center of the brainstem. The brainstem controls ventilation through monitoring of the partial pressure of arterial carbon dioxide (PaCO₂) and oxygen (PaO₂) by specialized cells known as *chemoreceptors.* Chemoreceptors are located in the brain stem and in the aorta and carotid arteries. If the chemoreceptors detect increased PaCO₂, they stimulate the respiratory center to increase the depth and frequency of breaths, eliminating more CO₂ and returning PaCO₂ to normal (Figure 11–5). This process is very efficient and can increase the volume of

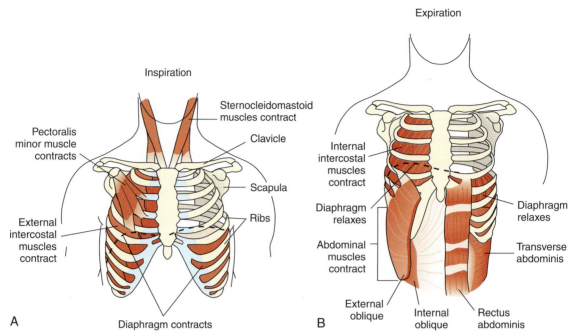

FIGURE 11-3 **A.** During inspiration, the diaphragm contracts and flattens. Accessory muscles of inspiration—such as the external intercostal, pectoralis minor, and sternocleidomastoid muscles—lift the ribs and sternum, which increases the diameter and volume of the thoracic cavity. **B.** In expiration during quiet breathing, the elasticity of the thoracic cavity causes the diaphragm and ribs to assume their resting positions, which decreases the volume of the thoracic cavity. In expiration during labored breathing, muscles of expiration—such as the internal intercostal and abdominal muscles—contract, causing the volume of the thoracic cavity to decrease more rapidly.

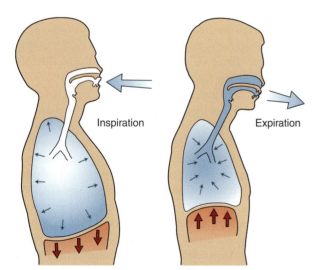

FIGURE 11-4 When the diaphragm is relaxed and the glottis is open, the pressure inside and outside the lungs is equal. When the chest cavity expands, the intrathoracic pressure decreases and air goes in the lungs.

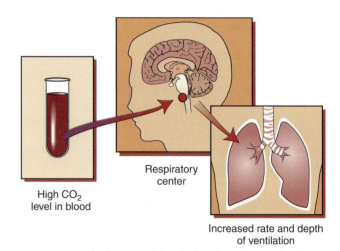

FIGURE 11-5 An increased level of carbon dioxide is detected by nerve cells sensitive to this change, which stimulates the lung to increase both depth and rate of ventilation.

air moved in and out of the lungs per minute by a factor of 10. Mechanoreceptors, found in the airways, lungs, and chest wall, measure the degree of stretch in these structures and also provide feedback to the brainstem.

In certain lung diseases, such as emphysema, or chronic obstructive pulmonary disease (COPD), the lungs are not able to eliminate CO_2 as effectively. This results in a chronic elevation of the CO_2 level in the blood. The chemoreceptors become insensitive to changes in $PaCO_2$. As a result, the chemoreceptors in the aorta and carotid arteries stimulate breathing when the partial pressure of arterial oxygen (PaO_2) falls. Similar to when the brainstem chemoreceptors detect

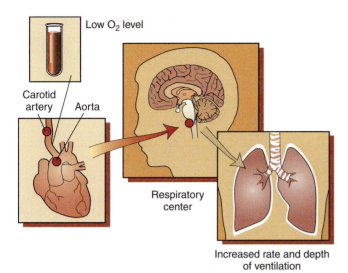

Low O₂ level

Carotid
artery   Aorta

Respiratory
center

Increased rate and depth
of ventilation

FIGURE 11-6   Receptors located in the aorta and carotid arteries are sensitive to the oxygen level and will stimulate the lungs to increase air movement into and out of the alveolar sacs.

FIGURE 11-7   Pulmonary Volumes and

Dead space: Amount of air brought into the lungs that does not have the opportunity to exchange oxygen and carbon dioxide with the blood in the alveolar capillaries (e.g., air in trachea and bronchi).

Minute ventilation (V_E): Total volume of air moved into and out of the lungs in 1 minute.

Tidal volume (V_6): Amount of air that is inhaled then exhaled during a normal breath (0.4–0.5 liters).

Total lung capacity (TLC): Total volume the lungs contain when maximally inflated. This volume declines with age from 6.0 liters in young adults to approximately 4.0 liters in elderly persons.

Work of breathing: Physical work or effort performed in moving the chest wall and diaphragm to breathe. This work increases with rapid breathing, increasing minute ventilation, and when the lungs are abnormally stiff.

---

an increase in $PaCO_2$ and stimulate increased respirations to lower the CO_2 level, the oxygen chemoreceptors send feedback to the respiratory center that stimulate the respiratory muscles to be more active, increasing the respiratory rate and depth to raise the PaO_2 to more normal values (Figure 11–6). This mechanism is often referred to as "hypoxic drive" as it is related to falling levels of oxygen in the blood.[4]

Figure 11–7 defines several terms that are important in discussing and understanding the physiology of ventilation.[5]

Circulation

The other major physiologic process that may be affected after thoracic injury is circulation. Chapter 8 covers this topic more extensively, but the following discussion sets the stage for the pathophysiology of chest injury.

The heart, which lies in the center of the chest within the mediastinum, functions as a biologic pump. For a pump to work, it must be primed with fluid. For the heart, this priming function is provided by the return of blood through two large veins, the *superior vena cava* (SVC) and the *inferior vena cava* (IVC). The heart then normally contracts 70 to 80 times per minute, ejecting blood out to the body through the aorta.

Processes that interfere with the return of blood to the heart through the SVC and IVC (e.g., loss of blood through hemorrhage, increased pressure in chest cavity from tension pneumothorax) cause the output of the heart and thus the blood pressure to decrease. Similarly, processes that injure the heart itself (e.g., blunt cardiac injury) may make the heart a less efficient pump, causing the same physiologic abnormalities. Just as chemoreceptors recognize changes in CO_2 or O_2 levels, *baroreceptors* recognize changes in blood pressure

and direct the heart to change the rate and forcefulness of its beating to return to the blood pressure to normal.

Pathophysiology

As mentioned earlier, both blunt and penetrating mechanisms may disrupt the physiologic processes just described. There are common elements in the disturbances created by these mechanisms.

Penetrating Injury

In these injuries, objects of varying size transgress the chest wall, enter the thoracic cavity, and possibly injure the organs within the thorax. Normally, no space exists between the pleural membranes. However, when a penetrating wound creates a communication between the chest cavity and the outside world, air tends to rush into the pleural space through the wound during inspiration when the pressure inside the chest is lower than that outside, and because the resistance to airflow through the wound is often less than that through the airways. Air in the pleural space *(pneumothorax)* disrupts the adherence between the pleural membranes created by the thin film of pleural fluid. All these processes together allow the lung to collapse, preventing effective ventilation. Penetrating wounds result in an open pneumothorax only when the size of the chest wall defect is large enough that the surrounding tissues do not close the wound at least partially during inspiration and/or expiration. Wounds of the lung by a penetrating object also allow air to escape from the lung into the pleural space and also result in collapse of the lung. In either case, the patient becomes short of breath. To make up for the lost ventilation capacity, the respiratory center will stimulate more rapid breathing. This increases the work of breathing. The patient may be able to tolerate the increased workload for a time, but if not recognized and treated, the patient is at risk for ventilatory failure, which will be manifested by increasing respiratory distress as the CO_2 levels in the blood rise and the O_2 levels fall.

If there is continued entry of air into the chest cavity without any exit, pressure will begin to build in the pleural space, leading to tension pneumothorax. This will further impede the patient's ability to ventilate. It also will begin to impact circulation negatively as venous return to the heart is reduced by the increasing intrathoracic pressure, and shock may then ensue. In extreme cases with displacement of the mediastinal structures into the opposite side of the chest, venous return is highly compromised leading to decreased blood pressure and jugular venous distension, and the classic finding of tracheal shift may be detected.

Lacerated tissues and torn blood vessels bleed. Penetrating wounds to the chest may result in bleeding into the pleural space *(hemothorax)* from the chest wall muscles, the intercostal vessels, and the lungs. Penetrating wounds to the major vessels in the chest result in catastrophic bleeding. Each pleural space can accommodate approximately 3000 ml of fluid. Thoracic bleeding into the pleural space may not be readily apparent externally, but it may be of sufficient magnitude to create a shock state. The presence of large volumes of blood in the pleural space will also impede the patient's ability to breathe; the blood in the pleural space prevents expansion of the lung on that side.

Wounds of the lung may also result in bleeding into the lung tissue itself. This blood floods the alveoli, preventing them from filling with air. Alveoli filled with blood cannot participate in gas exchange. The more alveoli that are flooded, the more the patient's ventilation and oxygenation may be compromised.

Blunt Force Injury

Blunt force applied to the chest wall is transmitted through the chest wall to the thoracic organs, especially the lungs. This wave of energy can tear lung tissue, which may result in bleeding into the alveoli. In this setting the injury is called a *pulmonary contusion.* The impact on oxygenation and ventilation is the same as with penetrating injury.

If the force applied to the lung tissue also tears the parietal pleura, air may escape from the lung into the pleural space, creating a pneumothorax and the potential for a tension pneumothorax, as previously described. Blunt force trauma to the chest can also break ribs, which can then lacerate the lung, resulting in pneumothorax as well as hemothorax (both caused by bleeding from the broken ribs as well as from the torn lung and intercostal muscles). Blunt force injury may also cause shearing or rupture of the major blood vessels in the chest, particularly the aorta, leading to catastrophic hemorrhage. Finally, in some cases, blunt force can disrupt the chest wall, leading to instability of the chest wall and compromise of the changes in intrathoracic pressure leading to impaired ventilation.

Assessment

As in all aspects of medical care, assessment involves taking a history and performing a physical examination. In trauma situations, we speak of an *SAMPLE history,* in which the patient's **s**ymptoms, **a**ge and **a**llergies, **m**edications, **p**ast history, time of the **l**ast meal, and the **e**vents surrounding the injury are elucidated.[6]

Besides the overall mechanism that resulted in injury, patients are asked about any symptoms they may be experiencing if they are conscious and able to communicate. Victims of chest trauma will likely be experiencing chest pain, which may be sharp, stabbing, or constricting. Frequently, the pain is worse with respiratory efforts or movement. The patient may report a sense of being short of breath or being unable to take in an adequate breath. The patient may feel apprehensive or lightheaded if shock is developing. It is important to remember that the absence of symptoms does not equate to the absence of injury.

The next step in assessment is the performance of a physical examination. There are four components to the physical examination: observation, palpation, percussion, and auscultation. The assessment should also include a determination of vital signs. Placement of a pulse oximeter to assess arterial oxygen saturation is a useful adjunct in the assessment of the injured patient.[6,7]

- **Observation.** The patient is observed for pallor of the skin and sweating, which may indicate the presence of shock. The patient may also appear apprehensive. The presence of *cyanosis* (bluish discoloration of skin, especially around mouth and lips) may be evident in advanced hypoxia. The frequency of respirations and whether the patient appears to be having trouble breathing (gasping, contractions of the accessory muscles of respiration in the neck, nasal flaring) should be noted. Is the trachea in the midline, or deviated to one side or the other? Are the jugular veins distended? The chest is examined for contusions, abrasions, lacerations, and whether the chest wall expands symmetrically with breathing. Does any portion of the chest wall move paradoxically with respiration (instead of moving out during inspiration, does it collapse inward, and vice versa, during exhalation)?
- **Auscultation.** The entire chest is evaluated. Decreased breath sounds on one side compared to the other may

indicate pneumothorax or hemothorax on the examined side. Pulmonary contusions may result in abnormal breath sounds (crackles). Although often difficult to discern in the field, muffled heart sounds and murmurs may also be noted on auscultation of the heart.

- **Palpation.** By gently pressing the chest wall with hands and fingers, assessment for the presence of tenderness, crepitus (either bony or subcutaneous emphysema), and bony instability of the chest wall is performed.
- **Percussion.** This examination technique is difficult to perform in the field because the environment is often noisy, making evaluation of the percussion note difficult. A finger is placed flat on the chest wall, then that finger is struck sharply with a finger of the opposite hand. This produces a sound wave in the percussed structure. A *dull* percussion note over the chest may indicate underlying pulmonary contusion or hemothorax. A *resonant* percussion note may indicate the presence of a pneumothorax.
- **Pulse Oximetry.** This should be performed to assess the level of oxygen bound to hemoglobin and followed to indicate changes in the patient's condition and responses to therapy.
- **Wave form capnography.** Whether by sidestream assessment with a nasal probe, mask, or by in-line assessment in an intubated patient, capnography is used to assess the level of carbon dioxide in expired air, and followed to indicate changes in the patient's condition and responses to therapy.

Repeat determinations of the respiratory rate may be the most important assessment tool. As patients become hypoxic and compromised, an early clue to this change is a gradual increase in the respiratory rate.

Management of Specific Injuries

Rib Fractures

Despite the ribs being fairly well protected by overlying musculature, rib fractures are a common occurrence in thoracic trauma. The upper ribs are broad, thick, and particularly well protected by the shoulder girdle and muscles.[1-3] Because it requires great energy to fracture the upper ribs, this patient is at risk for harboring other significant injuries, such as traumatic disruption of the aorta. Rib fractures occur most often in ribs 4 to 8 laterally, where they are thin and have less overlying musculature. The broken ends of the ribs may tear muscle, lung, and blood vessels, with the possibility of an associated pulmonary contusion.[1,3,8] Simple rib fractures, though

rarely life threatening in adults, may be deadly in the elderly patient. Compression of the lung may rupture the alveoli and lead to pneumothorax as discussed above.

Fracture of the lower ribs[8-10] may be associated with injuries of the spleen and liver and may indicate the potential for other intra-abdominal injuries. These injuries may also present with signs of blood loss or shock.[1,3,8]

Assessment

Patients with simple rib fractures may have few symptoms. Most often they will complain of chest pain and difficulty breathing. They may have labored respirations, chest wall tenderness, and crepitus. The prehospital care provider assesses vital signs, paying particular attention to the respiratory rate and depth of breathing. Pulse oximetry also should be performed, as well as capnography if available.[1,12,13]

Management

Pain relief is a primary goal in the initial management of patients with rib fractures. This may involve reassurance and positioning of the patient's arms using a sling and swath. It is important to reassure and continuously reassess the patient, keeping in mind the potential for deterioration in ventilation and the development of shock. Establishing intravenous (IV) access should be considered, depending on the patient's condition and anticipated transport time. Administration of small doses of IV narcotic analgesics may be appropriate in some situations for advanced units with appropriate medical control. The patient is encouraged to take deep breaths and cough to prevent the collapse of the alveoli *(atelectasis)* and the potential for pneumonia and other complications. Rigid immobilization of the rib cage with tape or straps should be avoided because these interventions predispose to the development of atelectasis and pneumonia.[1,3] Administration of oxygen and assisting ventilations may be necessary.

Flail Chest

Flail chest occurs when two or more adjacent ribs are fractured in more than one place along their length. This produces a segment of chest wall that is no longer in continuity with the remainder of the chest. The significant force necessary to produce such a lesion is generally transmitted to the underlying lung resulting in a pulmonary contusion. The patient thus may have two mechanisms to compromise ventilation and gas exchange, the flail segment and the underlying pulmonary contusion (which is the bigger problem when it comes to compromising ventilation). When the respiratory muscles contract to raise the ribs up and out and lower the diaphragm, the flail segment paradoxically moves inward in response to the negative pressure being created within the thoracic cavity (Figure 11–8). Similarly, when these muscles relax, the segment may move outward as pressure inside the chest increases. This paradoxical motion of the flail segment makes ventilation less efficient. The degree of inefficiency is directly

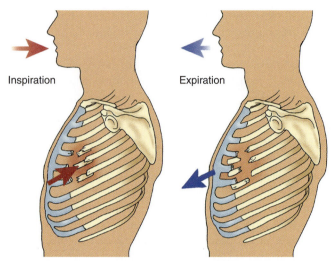

Inspiration   Expiration

FIGURE 11-8 Paradoxical motion. If stability of the chest wall has been lost by ribs fractured in two or more places, in which case intrathoracic pressure decreases during inspiration, the external air pressure forces the chest wall inward. When intrathoracic pressure increases during expiration, the chest wall is forced outward.

related to the size of the flail segment. As described earlier, the pulmonary contusion does not allow for gas exchange in the contused portion of the lung because of alveolar flooding with blood.

Assessment

As with a simple rib fracture, assessment of flail chest will reveal a patient in pain. The pain is typically more severe, however, and the patient usually appears to be in distress. The respiratory rate is elevated, and the patient does not take deep breaths. Hypoxia may be present, as demonstrated by pulse oximetry or cyanosis. Paradoxical motion may or may not be evident or easily recognized. Initially, the intercostal muscles will be in spasm and tend to stabilize the flail segment. As these muscles fatigue, the paradoxical motion becomes increasingly evident. The patient will have tenderness and potentially bony crepitus over the injured segment. The instability of the segment may also be appreciated on palpation.

Management

Management of flail chest is directed toward pain relief, ventilatory support, and monitoring for deterioration. The respiratory rate may be the most important parameter to follow. Pulse oximetry, if available, is also useful to detect hypoxia.[7] Oxygen should be administered. Intravenous access may be obtained, except in cases of extremely short transport times. Support of ventilation with bag-mask assistance, CPAP, or endotracheal intubation and positive-pressure ventilation may be necessary (particularly with prolonged transport times).[12] Efforts to stabilize the flail segment with sandbags or

other means that may further compromise chest wall motion and, thus, ventilation are contraindicated.[1]

Pulmonary Contusion

When lung tissue is lacerated or torn by blunt or penetrating mechanisms, bleeding into the alveolar air spaces can result in pulmonary contusion. This prevents gas exchange because no air enters these alveoli from the terminal airways. Blood and edema fluid in the tissue between the alveoli further impedes gas exchange in the alveoli that are ventilated. Pulmonary contusion is almost always present in the patient with a flail segment and is a common—and potentially lethal—complication of thoracic injury.[3,8] Deterioration to the point of frank respiratory failure may occur over the first 24 hours after injury.

Assessment

Assessment findings of the patient are variable depending on the severity of the contusion (percentage of involved lung). Early assessment may reveal no respiratory compromise. A high index of suspicion is necessary, particularly in the presence of a flail segment.

Management

Management is directed toward support of ventilation. Supplemental oxygen should be administered with a goal of maintaining oxygen saturation in the normal range. The prehospital care provider should repeatedly reassess the respiratory rate and any sign of respiratory distress. Continuous pulse oximetry and capnography, if available, should be utilized. Supplemental oxygen should be provided to all patients with suspected pulmonary contusion. Continuous positive airway pressure (CPAP) can be used to improve oxygenation in patients in whom supplemental oxygen alone proves to be inadequate for maintaining acceptable oxygen saturation levels.[14] Support of ventilation with bag-mask or endotracheal intubation may be necessary.[13] In the absence of hypotension (systolic BP < 90 mm Hg), aggressive IV fluid administration may further increase edema and compromise ventilation and oxygenation. Instead, fluids should be administered to maintain normal pulse and blood pressure. Pulmonary contusion is another example in which fluid resuscitation must be balanced with the patient's other needs. (See Shock, Chapter 8, balanced resuscitation).

Pneumothorax

Pneumothorax is present in up to 20% of severe chest injuries.[9] The three types of pneumothorax represent increasing levels of severity: simple, open, and tension.

Simple pneumothorax is the presence of air within the pleural space. As the amount of air in the pleural space increases, the lung on that side collapses (Figure 11–9). *Open pneumothorax* ("sucking chest wound") involves a

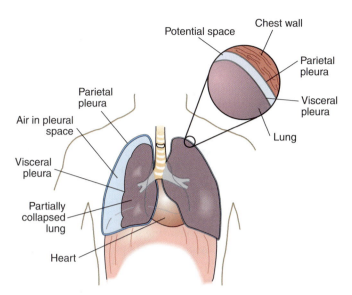

FIGURE 11-9 Air in the pleural space forces the lung in, decreasing the amount that can be ventilated and, therefore, decreasing oxygenation of the blood leaving the lung.

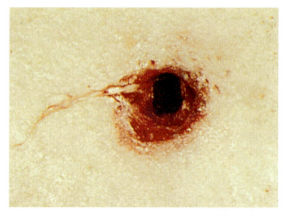

FIGURE 11-10 A gunshot or stab wound to the chest produces a hole in the chest wall through which air can flow both into and out of the pleural cavity.

pneumothorax associated with a defect in the chest wall that allows air to enter and exit the pleural space from the outside with ventilatory effort. *Tension pneumothorax* occurs when air continues to enter and is trapped in the pleural space with gradual increase in intrathoracic pressure. This leads to shift of the mediastinum and results in decreased venous blood return to the heart and compromised circulatory function.

Simple Pneumothorax

Assessment. Assessment in simple pneumothorax is likely to demonstrate findings similar to those in rib fracture. The patient frequently complains of pleuritic chest pain and may exhibit varying symptoms and signs of respiratory dysfunction. The classic findings are decreased breath sounds on the side of injury and a tympanitic percussion note. Any patient with respiratory distress and diminished breath sounds should be assumed to have a pneumothorax.

Management. The provider administers supplemental oxygen, obtains IV access, and prepares to treat shock if it develops. Monitoring of pulse oximetry and waveform capnography, if available, is essential to expectant management of the patient. [9–13,15,16] If spinal immobilization is not necessary, the patient may be more comfortable in a semi-recumbent position. Rapid transport is essential. [10,13,15] If the provider is functioning at the basic level, rendezvous with an advanced life support (ALS) unit should be considered. A key point in management is the recognition that a simple pneumothorax may quickly evolve into a tension pneumothorax. The patient needs to be continuously monitored for development of ten-

sion pneumothorax so that timely intervention can occur before there is a serious compromise of circulation.

Open Pneumothorax

Open pneumothorax, as with simple pneumothorax, involves air entering the pleural space, causing the lung to collapse. A defect in the chest wall that results in a communication between the outside air and the pleural space is the hallmark of an open pneumothorax. When the patient attempts to inhale, air crosses the wound and enters the pleural space because of the negative pressure created in the thoracic cavity as the muscles of respiration contract. In larger wounds, there may be free flow of air in and out of the pleural space with the different phases of respiration (Figure 11–10). Noise is created as air travels in and out of the hole in the chest wall; this has been referred to as a "sucking chest wound." Because air flow follows the path of least resistance, this abnormal airflow through the chest wall may occur preferentially to the normal flow through the upper airways into the lung, especially if a defect is similar or larger in size than the glottic opening to the lower airway. Resistance to flow through a wound decreases as the defect size increases. Effective ventilation is then inhibited both by collapse of the lung on the injured side and with preferential flow of air into the pleural space rather than into alveoli of the lung. Though the patient is breathing, oxygen is prevented from entering the circulatory system.

Mechanisms leading to open pneumothorax include gunshot wounds, shotgun blasts, stabbings, impalements, and occasionally blunt trauma.

Assessment. Assessment of the patient with open pneumothorax generally reveals obvious respiratory distress. The patient will be anxious and tachypneic. The pulse rate will be elevated and potentially thready. Observation of the chest wall will reveal the wound, which may make audible sucking sounds during inspiration, with bubbling during expiration.

Management. Initial management of an open pneumothorax involves sealing the defect in the chest wall and administering supplemental oxygen. Airflow through the wound into the pleural cavity is prevented by applying an occlusive dressing. Unlike plain gauze, Vaseline or petroleum gauze, aluminum foil, or plastic wrap do not allow airflow through them. A patient with an open pneumothorax virtually always has an injury to the underlying lung, allowing for two sources of air leak, the hole in the chest wall and the hole in the lung. Even if an injury to the chest wall is sealed with an occlusive dressing, air leakage into the pleural space can continue from the injured lung, setting the stage for a tension pneumothorax (Figure 11–11). The traditional teaching has been that for an open pneumothorax, the occlusive dressing is secured on three sides.[1] This prevents airflow into the chest cavity during inspiration while allowing air to escape through the loose side of the dressing during exhalation (Figure 11–12). Several devices are marketed for management of open pneumothoraces (Asherman chest seal, etc); however, no data has been published demonstrating that devices are superior to a simple occlusive dressing (aluminum foil or Vaseline gauze). Thus, the added cost is probably not justified. In addition, taping the occlusive dressing on all four sides has been advocated as preferable to taping only on three sides; however, no definitive answer to this issue has been conclusively determined.

If these measures fail to support the patient adequately, endotracheal intubation and positive-pressure ventilation may be necessary.[12] If positive pressure is utilized, the provider needs to monitor the patient carefully for the development of tension pneumothorax. If signs of increasing respiratory distress develop, the dressing over the wound should be removed to allow for decompression of any accumulating tension. If this is ineffective, needle decompression and positive-pressure ventilation should be considered if not already employed.[11]

Tension Pneumothorax

Tension pneumothorax is a life-threatening emergency. As air continues to enter the pleural space without any release, intrathoracic pressure builds up. As intrathoracic pressure rises, ventilatory compromise increases and venous return to the heart decreases. The decreasing cardiac output coupled with worsening gas exchange results in profound shock. The increasing pressure on the injured side of the chest may eventually push the structures in the mediastinum toward the other side of the chest (Figure 11–13). This distortion of anatomy may further impede venous return to the heart through the kinking of the inferior vena cava. Additionally, inflation of the lung on the uninjured side is increasingly restricted and respiratory compromise results.

Any patient with thoracic injury is at risk for development of tension pneumothorax. Patients at particular risk are those who likely have a pneumothorax (e.g., patient with signs of rib fracture), those who have a known pneumothorax (e.g., patient with a penetrating wound to the chest), and those with chest injury who are undergoing positive-pressure ventilation. Such patients must be continuously monitored and rapidly transported to an appropriate facility.

Assessment. The findings during assessment depend on how much pressure has accumulated in the pleural space (Fig-

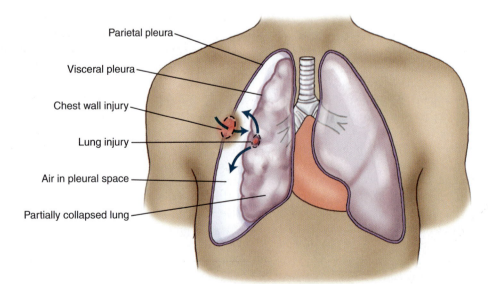

Parietal pleura

Visceral pleura

Chest wall injury

Lung injury

Air in pleural space

Partially collapsed lung

FIGURE 11-11 Because of the proximity of the chest wall to the lung, it would be extremely difficult for the chest wall to be injured by penetrating trauma and the lung not to be injured. Stopping the hole in the chest wall does not necessarily decrease air leakage into the pleural space; leakage can come from the lung just as easily.

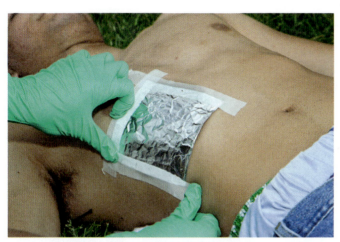

FIGURE 11-12 Taping a piece of foil or plastic to the chest wall on three sides creates a flutter-valve effect, allowing air to escape from the pleural space but not enter into it.

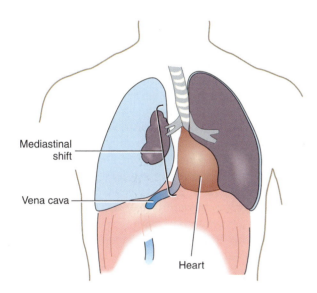

FIGURE 11-13 Tension pneumothorax. If the amount of air trapped in the pleural space continues to increase, not only is the lung on the affected side collapsed, but the mediastinum is also shifted to the opposite side. The lung on the opposite side then collapses and intrathoracic pressure increases, which decreases capillary blood flow and kinks the vena cava.

FIGURE 11-14   Signs of Tension Pneumothorax

Although the following signs are frequently discussed with a tension pneumothorax, many may not be present or are difficult to identify in the field.

OBSERVATION:

■ *Cyanosis* may difficult to see in the field. Poor lighting, variation in skin color, and dirt and blood associated with trauma often render this sign unreliable.

■ *Distended neck veins* are described as a classic sign of tension pneumothorax. However, since a patient with a tension pneumothorax may also have lost a considerable amount of blood, distended neck veins may not be prominent.

PALPATION:

■ *Percussion of the chest* for the hypertympany associated with pneumothorax is an excellent method for determining the status of the chest cavity in the relative quiet of a hospital. In the noisy prehospital environment, this sound is much more difficult to detect. Given the difficulty in obtaining this sign and the time and environment necessary with which to perform it, it is not recommended for field diagnosis of tension pneumothorax.

■ *Tracheal deviation* is usually a late sign. Even when it is present, it can be difficult to diagnose by physical examination. In the neck, the trachea is bound to the cervical spine by fascial and other supporting structures; thus, the deviation of the trachea is more of an intrathoracic phenomenon, although deviation may be palpated in the jugular notch if it is severe. Tracheal deviation is not often noted in the prehospital environment.

AUSCULTATION:

■ *Decreased breath sounds on the injured side.* The most helpful part of the physical examination is checking for decreased breath sounds on the side of the injury. However, to use this sign the prehospital care provider must be able to distinguish between normal and decreased sounds. Such differentiation requires a great deal of practice. Listening to breath sounds during every patient contact will help.

---

ure 11–14). Initially, patients will exhibit apprehension and discomfort. They will generally complain of chest pain and difficulty in breathing. As the tension worsens, they will exhibit increasing agitation and respiratory distress. In severe cases, cyanosis and apnea may occur. The classic findings are tracheal deviation away from the side of injury, diminished breath sounds on the side of injury, and a tympanitic percussion note. It is difficult to detect diminished breath sounds in the field environment. Constant practice with auscultation of all patients will hone the provider's skill and make detection of this important finding more likely. Detection of a tympanitic percussion note in the field is basically impossible, but the finding is mentioned for the sake of completeness. Other physical findings that may be evident are jugular venous distension, chest wall crepitus, and cyanosis. Tachycardia and tachypnea become increasingly prominent as the intrathoracic pressure builds, culminating in hypotension and uncompensated shock.

Management. The priority in management involves decompressing the tension pneumothorax.[11] Decompression should be performed when three findings are present: (1) worsening respiratory distress or difficulty ventilating with a bag-mask device; (2) unilateral decreased or absent breath sounds; and (3) decompensated shock (systolic blood pressure <90 mm Hg).[11,16]

Depending upon the clinical setting and the training level of the prehospital care provider, several options for pleural decompression exist. If decompression is not an option (BLS only available and no occlusive dressing to remove), rapid transport to an appropriate facility while administering high-concentration oxygen ($FiO_2 \geq 85\%$) is imperative. Positive-pressure ventilatory assistance should be used only if the patient is hypoxic and fails to respond to supplemental oxygen, as this may rapidly worsen the tension pneumothorax. Assisting ventilations may result in air accumulating more rapidly in the pleural space. If ALS intercept is an option, this should be accomplished if faster than delivery to an appropriate facility.

Removal of an Occlusive Dressing

In the patient with an open pneumothorax, if an occluding dressing has been applied, it should be briefly removed. This should allow the tension pneumothorax to decompress through the wound with a rush of air. This procedure may need to be repeated periodically during transport if symptoms of tension recur. If removing the dressing for several seconds is ineffective or if there is no open wound, an ALS provider may proceed with a needle thoracostomy.

Needle Decompression

Insertion of a needle into the pleural space of the affected side permits accumulated air, under pressure, to escape. The immediate improvement in oxygenation and in ease of ventilation may be lifesaving. Needle decompression has been shown to be effective in an animal model.[17] If a patient with suspected tension pneumothorax was intubated, the position of the endotracheal tube should be assessed prior to performing needle decompression. If an endotracheal tube has slipped from the trachea into one of the main stem bronchi (usually the right), breath sounds and chest wall excursion may be markedly diminished on the opposite site as that lung is not being ventilated.

Needle decompression is performed though the second or third intercostal space in the midclavicular line of the involved side of the chest (Figure 11–15). This location is chosen because of ease of access for the prehospital care provider transporting a patient who likely has been "packaged for transport" on a backboard with cervical collar, with arms down along the sides (making access difficult to the midaxillary line, where chest tubes are usually placed). Once placed, the catheter is less likely to be displaced from the chest wall in the midclavicular line. The lung on the affected side is

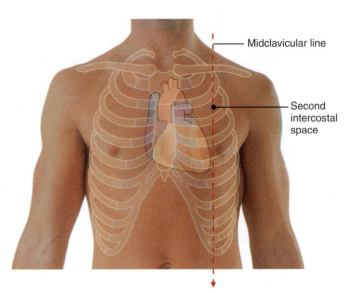

Midclavicular line

Second intercostal space

FIGURE 11-15 Needle decompression of the thoracic cavity is most easily accomplished and produces the least chance for complication if it is done at the midclavicular line through the second intercostal space.

collapsed and shifted to the contralateral side; thus, it is unlikely to be injured during the procedure. The needle and catheter should be advanced until the return of a rush of air is achieved and advanced no farther. Once the decompression is achieved, the catheter is taped to the chest to prevent dislodgement. Improper placement (location or depth) may result in injuries to the lungs, heart, or great vessels.[18]

Decompression is performed with a large bore (10- to 16-gauge) intravenous needle that is at least 8 cm in length. In some cases, needle decompression may not be effective, especially when using a standard IV catheter that is too short to penetrate the chest wall or because the catheter kinked after removal of the needle, blocking further air escape.[19–21] Recent research has focused on the length of the catheter necessary to reach the pleural space.[21]

This procedure converts the tension pneumothorax into a negligible open pneumothorax. The relief to respiratory effort far outweighs the negative effect of the open pneumothorax. Because the diameter of the decompression catheter is significantly smaller than the patient's airway, it is unlikely that any air movement through the catheter will significantly compromise ventilatory effort. Thus, creation of a one-way valve (Heimlich valve) is probably unnecessary from a clinical standpoint. Using a manufactured valve is costly, and fashioning a valve from a glove is time consuming, Continued provision of supplemental oxygen, as well as ventilatory support as needed, is appropriate.

As a general rule, bilateral tension pneumothorax is exceedingly rare in patients who are not intubated and ventilated with positive pressure. The first step in reassessing the patient is to confirm the location of the endotracheal (ET) tube, ensure that it has no kinks or bends causing compression of the tube, and ensure that the tube has not inadvertently moved down into a main stem bronchus. Extreme caution should be exercised with bilateral needle decompression in patients who are not being ventilated with positive-pressure ventilation. If the provider's assessment is in error, the creation of bilateral pneumothoraces can cause severe respiratory distress.

The patient should be rapidly transported to an appropriate facility. Intravenous access should be obtained unless transport time is particularly short. The patient must be closely observed for deterioration. Repeat decompression and endotracheal intubation may become necessary.

Tube Thoracostomy (Chest Tube)

In general, chest tubes (tube thoracostomy) are not inserted in the prehospital setting because of concerns of time, procedural complications, infection, and training issues. Needle decompression can be accomplished in a fraction of the time of performing a tube thoracostomy because fewer steps are necessary. Published complication rates with tube thoracostomy range from 2.8% to 21%[22, 23] and include damage to the heart or lungs

and malposition in the subcutaneous tissues of the chest wall or in the peritoneal cavity. This procedure requires a sterile field, which is challenging to create in the field. A break in sterile technique, such as contamination of the chest tube or instruments may result in the development of an empyema (collection of pus in the pleural space), requiring surgical intervention and drainage. Significant training is required to develop this skill and ongoing practice is required to maintain skill proficiency.

Patients being transported with a chest tube in place are still at risk for the development of a tension pneumothorax, particularly if they are undergoing positive-pressure ventilatory assistance. If signs of a tension pneumothorax begin to manifest, first ensure that there are no kinks in the chest tube or connecting tubing. Next, insure that the connecting tubing is correctly connected to a water seal and drainage device. Even with no identified problems, the patient with signs of an increasing tension pneumothorax may require needle decompression. Do not delay just because there is already a chest tube in place (Figure 11–16).

FIGURE 11-16   Troubleshooting Tube Thoracostomy

THREE BASIC COMPONENTS OF CHEST TUBE DRAINAGE SYSTEMS

1. Seal—allows air to escape pleural space but not return. Generally water seal, bubbles as air escapes pleural space and rises with inspiratory negative pressure.
2. Collecting system—collects and measures output. Observe for changes in volume of output and nature.
3. Suction—provides negative pressure to assist drainage and expansion.
   Ensure suction is appropriately attached and functioning. Review the basic operation of any drainage system with care team prior to transfer of patient.

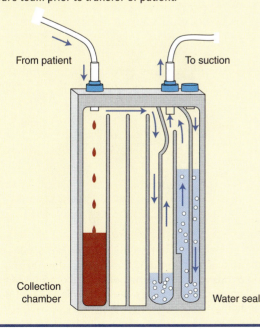

From patient   To suction

Collection chamber   Water seal

CHANGES IN RESPIRATORY STATUS IN PATIENTS WITH CHEST TUBES

- Assess vital signs including pulse oximetry.
- Assess lung sounds.
- Assess ventilatory effort.
- Assess circulation.
- Assess levels of consciousness.

TROUBLESHOOTING STEPS

- Assess dressing and tune site to ensure tube has not been dislodged during transfers.
- Tubing all tightly connected and unobstructed—no kinks or clamps?
- Seal intact and functioning—bubbling and/or variation with ventilations.
- Tube fogging and/or drainage continuing?
- Suction functioning—continuous bubbling or negative pressure indicator throughout ventilation cycle?
- If patient's ventilatory status continues to deteriorate, assess closely for signs of developing tension pneumothorax. If indicated, disconnect the chest tube from the drainage system, which should allow release of tension if chest tube is properly placed and unobstructed. If this does not relieve the condition, consider needle decompression and contact on-line medical control.

Hemothorax

Hemothorax occurs when blood enters the pleural space. Because this space can accommodate a large volume of blood (2500–3000 ml), hemothorax can represent a source of significant blood loss. In fact, the loss of circulating blood volume from bleeding into the pleural space represents a greater physiologic insult to the patient with chest injury than the collapse of the lung that the hemothorax produces (Figure 11–17). It is rare that enough blood accumulates to create a "tension hemothorax." The mechanisms resulting in hemothorax are the same as those causing the various types of pneumothorax. The bleeding may come from the chest wall musculature, the intercostal vessels, the lung parenchyma, pulmonary vessels, or the great vessels of the chest.

Assessment

Assessment reveals a patient in some distress. Chest pain and shortness of breath are again prominent features, generally with signs of significant shock. The prehospital care provider monitors the patient for signs of shock: tachycardia, tachypnea, confusion, pallor, and hypotension. Breath sounds on the side of the injury are diminished or absent, but the percussion note is dull (compared to tympanitic for a pneumothorax). Pneumothorax may be present in conjunction with hemothorax, increasing the likelihood for cardiorespiratory compromise. Because of loss of circulating blood volume, distended neck veins often are not present.

Management

Management includes constant observation to detect physiologic deterioration while providing appropriate support. High-concentration oxygen should be administered and ventilation supported if necessary with bag-mask or endotracheal intubation if available and indicated. Hemodynamic status is closely monitored. Intravenous access should be obtained and appropriate fluid therapy provided with a goal of maintaining adequate perfusion without large volumes indiscriminately administered. Rapid transport to an appropriate facility capable of immediate surgical intervention completes the management algorithm for hemothorax.

Blunt Cardiac Injury

Cardiac injury most often results from application of force to the anterior chest, especially in a deceleration event such as an MVC with violent frontal impact.[1,2,24] The heart is then compressed between the sternum anteriorly and the spinal column posteriorly (Figure 11–18). This compression of the heart causes an abrupt increase in the pressure within the ventricles to several times normal, which results in cardiac contusion, sometimes valvular injury, and rarely cardiac rupture, as follows:

- *Cardiac contusion.* The most common result of cardiac compression is cardiac contusion. The heart muscle is bruised, with varying amounts of injury to the myocardial cells. This most often results in abnormal heart rhythms, such as sinus tachycardia.[24] Of greater concern, but less common, are premature ventricular contractions (PVCs) or nonperfusing rhythms such as ventricular tachycardia (VT) and ventricular fibrillation (VF). If the septal region of the heart is injured, the electrocardiogram (ECG) may demonstrate intraventricular conduction abnormalities, such as right bundle branch block (RBBB). If a sufficient volume of myocardium is injured, the contractility of the heart may be impaired, and cardiac output falls, resulting in cardiogenic shock. Unlike the other forms of shock usually encountered in the trauma setting, this shock does not improve with fluid administration and may actually worsen.

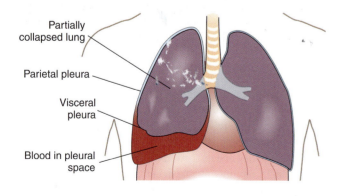

FIGURE 11-17 Hemothorax. The amount of blood that can accumulate in the thoracic cavity (leading to hypovolemia) is a much more severe condition than the amount of lung compressed by this blood loss.

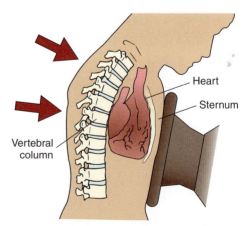

FIGURE 11-18 The heart can be compressed between the sternum (as the sternum stops against the steering column or dashboard) and the posterior thoracic wall (as the wall continues its forward motion). This can contuse the myocardium.

- *Valvular rupture.* Rupture of the supporting structures of the heart valves or the valves themselves typically renders the valves incompetent. The patient will present in varying degrees of shock with symptoms and signs of congestive heart failure (CHF), such as tachypnea, rales, and new-onset heart murmur.
- *Blunt cardiac rupture.* A rare event, blunt cardiac rupture occurs in less than 1% of patients with blunt chest trauma.[24–26] Most of these patients will die at the scene from exsanguination or fatal cardiac tamponade. The surviving patients will typically present with cardiac tamponade.

Assessment

Assessment of the patient with the potential for blunt cardiac injury reveals a mechanism that imparted a frontal impact to the center of the patient's chest. A bent steering column accompanied by bruising over the sternum implies such a mechanism. As with other chest injuries, the patient is likely to complain of chest pain and/or shortness of breath. If a dysrhythmia is present, the patient may complain of palpitations. Physical findings of concern are bruising over the sternum, crepitus over the sternum, and sternal instability. With a floating sternum *(flail sternum),* the ribs on either side of the sternum are broken, allowing it to move paradoxically with respirations, similar to flail chest, as described earlier. If valvular disruption has occurred, a harsh murmur may be detectable over the precordium along with signs of acute CHF, such as hypotension, jugular venous distension, and abnormal breath sounds. ECG monitoring may demonstrate tachycardia, PVCs, other rhythm disturbances, or ST-segment elevation.

Management

The key management strategy is correct assessment that blunt cardiac injury may have occurred and transmission of that concern along with the clinical findings to the receiving hospital. In the meantime, high-concentration oxygen is administered and IV access established for judicious fluid therapy.

The patient should be placed on a cardiac monitor to detect dysrhythmias and ST-segment elevations, if present. If dysrhythmias are present and ALS providers are present, standard antidysrhythmic pharmacotherapy should be instituted. There is no data to support prophylactic dysrythmics in blunt cardiac injury. As always, ventilatory support measures should be implemented as indicated.

Cardiac Tamponade

Cardiac tamponade occurs when a wound of the heart allows fluid to acutely accumulate between the pericardial sac and the heart.[1,25] The pericardial sac is composed of a fibrous, inelastic tissue. Normally, there is very little fluid in the pericardial sac, similar to the pleural space, as described earlier. Because the pericardium is inelastic, pressure begins to rise rapidly within the pericardial sac as fluid accumulates within it. This rising pericardial pressure impedes venous return to the heart and leads to diminished cardiac output and blood pressure. With each contraction of the heart, additional fluid may enter the pericardial sac, further impeding the ability of the heart to fill in preparation for the next contraction (Figure 11–19). This can become profound enough to precipitate *pulseless electrical activity* (PEA), a life-threatening injury requiring coordinated response by providers in all phases of care to achieve an optimal outcome. The normal adult pericardium may be able to accommodate as much as 300 ml of fluid before pulselessness occurs, but as little as 50 ml is usually enough to impede cardiac return and, thus, cardiac output.[1]

Most often, cardiac tamponade is caused by a stab wound to the heart. This may result in penetration into one of the cardiac chambers or just a laceration of the myocardium. In either event, bleeding into the pericardial sac occurs. The rising pressure within the pericardium results in the cardiac tamponade physiology. At the same time, the increased pressure within the pericardium may temporarily tamponade further bleeding from the cardiac wound, allowing for survival. In the case of gunshot wounds to the heart, the damage to the heart and pericardium is usually so severe that the pericardium cannot

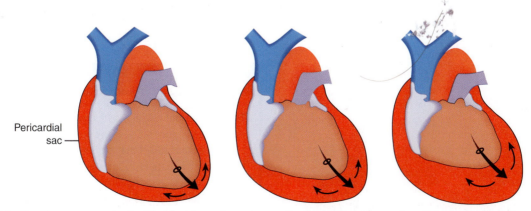

FIGURE 11-19 Cardiac tamponade. As blood courses from the cardiac lumen into the pericardial space, it limits expansion of the ventricle. Therefore, the ventricle cannot fill completely. As more blood accumulates in the pericardial space, less ventricular space is available to accumulate blood, and cardiac output is reduced.

contain the hemorrhage, resulting in rapid exsanguination. The same is true in the case of impalements. Blunt rupture of a cardiac chamber can result in cardiac tamponade but more often causes exsanguinating hemorrhage.

Cardiac tamponade should be kept in mind as a possibility when evaluating any patient with a thoracic penetration. This index of suspicion should be raised to the level of "present until proven otherwise" posture when the penetrating injury is within a rectangle (the cardiac box) formed by drawing a horizontal line along the clavicles, vertical lines from the nipples to the costal margins, and a second horizontal line connecting the points of intersection between the vertical lines and the costal margin (Figure 11–20). The presence of such a wound should be communicated to the receiving institution as soon as it is recognized.

Assessment

Assessment involves quickly recognizing the presence of at-risk wounds, as previously described, in combination with an appreciation for the physical findings of pericardial tamponade. *Beck's triad* is a constellation of findings indicative of cardiac tamponade: (1) distant or muffled heart sounds (the fluid around the heart makes it difficult to hear the sounds of the valves closing); (2) jugular venous distension (caused by the increasing pressure in the pericardial sac backing blood up into the neck veins); and (3) low blood pressure. Another physical finding described in cardiac tamponade is paradoxical pulse (Figure 11–21).

Detection of some of these signs is difficult in the field, especially muffled heart tones and paradoxical pulse. Thus, the field provider needs to maintain a high index of suspicion, based on the location of the wounds and hypotension, and implement therapy accordingly.

Management

Management requires rapid, monitored transport to a facility that can perform immediate surgical repair.[10,13,27–31] The prehospital care provider first needs to recognize that car-

diac tamponade likely exists and to inform the receiving facility so that preparations can be made for emergent surgical intervention. Oxygen in high concentration should be administered. Intravenous access should be obtained and judicious fluid therapy initiated, because this can augment central venous pressure and, thus, improve cardiac filling for a time. The provider should strongly consider endotracheal intubation and positive-pressure ventilation if the patient is hypotensive.[15,29,30]

Definitive therapy requires release of the tamponade and repair of the cardiac injury. A patient with a suspected cardiac tamponade should be transported directly to a facility capable of immediate surgical intervention, if available. Draining some of the pericardial fluid by pericardiocentesis is often an effective temporizing maneuver. Risks of pericardiocentesis include injury to the heart and coronary arteries, resulting in increased tamponade and injury to the lung, great vessels, and liver. In rare cases, resuscitative thoracotomy has been performed in the field by physicians in systems in which they respond to field emergencies.[32,33] Use of the pneumatic anti-shock garment (PASG) has been demonstrated to be detrimental in these patients.[34]

Commotio Cordis

The term *commotio cordis* refers to the clinical situation in which an apparently innocuous blow to the anterior chest results in sudden cardiac arrest.[35,36] Commotio cordis is believed to account for about 20 deaths per year in the United States, predominantly in children and adolescents (mean age about 13 years). Most experts theorize that commotio cordis results from a relatively minor, nonpenetrating blow to the precordium (area over the heart), occurring at an electrically vulnerable portion of the cardiac cycle, whereas some believe that coronary artery vasospasm may play a role in its development. Whichever the mechanism, the terminal result is a cardiac dysrhythmia resulting in ventricular fibrillation and sudden cardiac arrest.

This condition most frequently occurs during amateur sporting events in which the victim is struck by a projectile, such as a baseball (most common), ice hockey puck, lacrosse ball, or softball. However, commotio cordis has also been

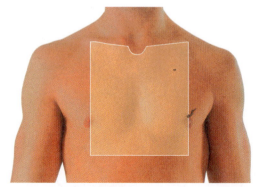

FIGURE 11-20 In a series of 46 patients with penetrating cardiac injuries, 40 had a wound within the "cardiac box." (From Richardson JD, Flint LM: *Trauma: Pathophysiology and clinical care,* Chicago, 1987, Yearbook Medical.)

FIGURE 11-21 Paradoxical Pulse

The paradoxical pulse, also known as pulsus paradoxus, is actually an accentuation of the normal, slight drop in systolic blood pressure (SBP) that occurs during inspiration. As the lungs expand, there is preferential filling and ejection of blood from the right side of the heart at the expense of the left side. Thus, peripheral blood pressure falls. This decrease in SBP is usually less than 10 to 15 mm Hg. A greater decrease in SBP constitutes the so-called paradoxical pulse.

reported after bodily impacts (e.g., karate blows), a low-velocity MVC, and the collision of two outfielders trying to catch a baseball. After the impact, victims have been known to walk a step or two and then drop to the ground in cardiac arrest. Typically, no injury is noted to the ribs, sternum, or heart at autopsy. Most victims have no known history of heart disease. The condition may be prevented through the use of equipment such as safety baseballs.[37]

Assessment

Patients who have sustained commotio cordis are found to be in cardiopulmonary arrest. In some victims, a minor bruise is noted over the sternum. Ventricular fibrillation (VF) is the most common rhythm, although complete heart block and left bundle branch block (LBBB) with ST-segment elevations have also been seen.

Management

Once cardiac arrest is confirmed, cardiopulmonary resuscitation (CPR) is initiated. Commotio cordis is managed in a manner similar to cardiac arrests resulting from myocardial infarction rather than those resulting from trauma. The cardiac rhythm should be determined as expeditiously as possible, with rapid defibrillation administered if VF is identified. Prognosis is poor, with chance of survival at 15% or less.[36] Virtually all survivors of this condition received both rapid, bystander-initiated CPR and immediate defibrillation, often with an automatic external defibrillator (AED). Precordial thumps have not been shown to terminate VF. If immediate attempts at defibrillation are unsuccessful, the airway is secured and IV access initiated. Epinephrine and antidysrhythmics may be administered as outlined in cardiac arrest protocols.

Traumatic Aortic Disruption

Traumatic aortic disruption results from a deceleration/acceleration mechanism of significant force.[38] Examples include high-speed frontal-impact MVCs and high falls in which the patient lands flat.

The aorta arises from the upper portion of the heart in the mediastinum. The heart and the aortic arch are relatively mobile within the chest cavity. As the arch of the aorta becomes the descending aorta, the aorta becomes adherent to the vertebral column and is relatively immobile. When there is a sudden deceleration of the body, such as occurs in a high-speed frontal impact, the heart and the aortic arch continue to move forward relative to the fixed (immobile) descending aorta. This produces shear forces in the aortic wall at the junction between these two segments of the aorta.[38] Thus, the typical location for a traumatic aortic injury is just distal to the takeoff of the left subclavian artery. This shear force can disrupt the wall of the aorta in varying degrees (Figure 11–22). When the tear extends through the full thickness of the aortic wall, the patient rapidly exsanguinates into their pleural cavity. However, if the tear is only partially through the wall, leaving the outer layer (adventitia) intact, the patient may survive for a variable length of time, making rapid identification and treatment essential for a successful outcome.[38]

Assessment

Assessment of aortic disruption hinges on index of suspicion. A high index should be maintained in situations involving high-energy deceleration/acceleration. Ironically, for such a devastating injury, there may be little external evidence of chest injury. Nevertheless, the prehospital care provider needs to assess the adequacy of the airway and breathing. Careful auscultation and palpation should be undertaken. Careful examination may demonstrate that the pulse quality may be different between the two upper extremities (pulse stronger in the right arm than the left) or between the upper (brachial artery) and lower extremities (femoral artery). Blood pressures, if measured, may be higher in the upper extremities than the lower extremities, comprising the signs of a pseudo-coarctation of the aorta.

Definitive diagnosis requires radiographic imaging in the hospital. Plain chest radiographs may demonstrate a variety of signs indicating the injury may be present. The most reliable of these is widening of the mediastinum. The injury can be definitively demonstrated with aortography, computed tomography (CT) of the chest, and transesophageal echocardiography.[38]

Management

Management of traumatic aortic disruption in the field is supportive. A high index of suspicion for its presence is maintained when the appropriate mechanism exists. High-concentration supplemental oxygen is administered and intravenous access is obtained, except in cases of extremely short transport times. Communication with the receiving facility about the mechanism and suspicion for aortic disruption should occur at the earliest opportunity. Strict blood pressure control is imperative to the successful outcome of these injuries (Figure 11–23). Traumatic aortic disruption represents another situation in which balanced resuscitation is clinically useful. Fluid resuscitation that results in normal or elevated blood pressure may result in rupture of the remaining tissue of the aorta and rapid exsanguination. If transport times are longer, blood pressure management should be guided by the highest blood pressure obtained, typically in the right arm. Control of both blood pressure and contractile force may be accomplished with the administration of beta-blockers.[39]

Tracheobronchial Disruption

Tracheobronchial disruption is an uncommon, but potentially highly lethal, entity.[40] All lacerations of the lung involve disruption of airways to some degree, however, in these cases, the intrathoracic portion of the trachea itself or one of the main stem or secondary bronchi is disrupted. This results in high flow of air through the injury into the

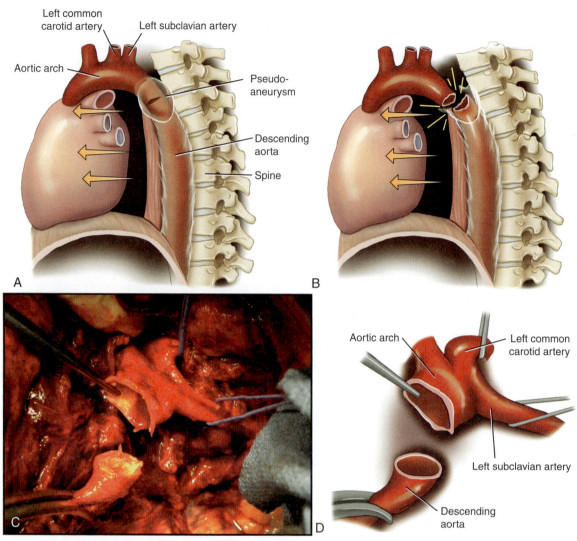

FIGURE 11-22 **A.** The descending aorta is a fixed structure that moves with the thoracic spine. The arch, aorta, and heart are freely movable. Acceleration of the torso in a lateral-impact collision or rapid deceleration of the torso in a frontal-impact collision produces a different rate of motion between the arch-heart complex and the descending aorta. This motion may result in a tear of the inner lining of the aorta that is contained within the outermost layer, producing a pseudoaneurysm. **B.** Tears at the junction of the arch and descending aorta may also result in a complete rupture, leading to immediate exsanguination in the chest. **C** and **D.** Operative photograph and drawing of a traumatic aortic tear.

FIGURE 11-23   Blood Pressure Maintenance

Caution: When performing inter-hospital transfer of patients with suspected aortic disruption, it is important not to raise the patient's blood pressure aggressively because this may lead to exsanguinating hemorrhage (see Chapter 8). Many of these patients may be given infusions of medications, such as beta blockers (e.g., esmolol, metoprolol), to maintain the blood pressure at a lower level, typically a mean arterial pressure of 70 mm Hg or less. Such therapy typically requires invasive monitoring, such as insertion of an arterial line, so that blood pressure can be monitored much more carefully.

mediastinum or pleural space. Pressure rapidly accumulates, resulting in tension pneumothorax or even tension pneumomediastinum, which is similar to cardiac tamponade. Unlike the usual situation in tension pneumothorax, needle thoracostomy may result in continuous flow of air through the catheter and may fail to relieve the tension (Figure 11–24). This is caused by the ongoing high flow of air across these major airways into the pleural space. Respiratory function may be significantly impaired because of preferential airflow across the lesion as well as the pressure. Positive pressure may worsen the tension. Penetrating trauma is more likely to cause this injury than blunt trauma. However, blunt injury of high energy may also cause tracheobronchial disruption.[40]

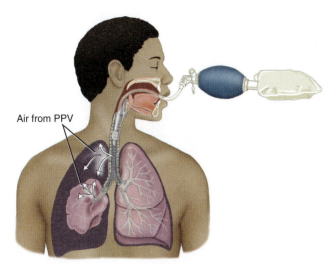

FIGURE 11-24 Tracheal or bronchial rupture. Positive-pressure ventilation *(PPV)* can directly force large amounts of air through the trachea or bronchus, rapidly producing a tension pneumothorax.

Assessment

Assessment demonstrates a patient in obvious distress, who may be pale and diaphoretic. The patient with tracheobronchial disruption will demonstrate signs of respiratory distress, such as use of accessory muscles of respiration, grunting, and nasal flaring. Extensive subcutaneous emphysema, especially in the upper chest and neck, may be identified. Although traditionally taught as important findings, jugular venous distension may be obscured by subcutaneous emphysema, and/or deviation of the trachea may only be noted upon palpation of the trachea in the jugular notch. Respiratory rate will be elevated, and oxygen saturation may be diminished. The patient may or may not be hypotensive and may cough up blood (hemoptysis). The hemorrhage associated with penetrating trauma may not be present in the blunt cases, but hemothorax is a possibility in both penetrating and blunt trauma.

Management

Successful management of tracheobronchial disruption requires administration of supplemental oxygen and judicious use of ventilatory assistance. If assisted ventilation makes the patient more uncomfortable, only oxygen is administered and the patient is transported as quickly as possible to an appropriate facility. Continuous monitoring for signs of progression toward a tension pneumothorax is imperative, and rapid needle decompression should be attempted if these signs present. Complex advanced airway management, such as selective main stem intubation, are difficult to accomplish in the field and have the potential for worsening a major bronchial injury.

Traumatic Asphyxia

Traumatic asphyxia is so named because the victims physically resemble strangulation patients. They exhibit the same bluish discoloration of the face and neck (and in the case of traumatic asphyxia, upper chest) as patients who have been strangled. Unlike strangled patients, however, traumatic asphyxia patients do not suffer from true asphyxia (cessation of air and gas exchange). The similarity in appearance with strangulation patients results from the impaired venous return from the head and neck that is present in both groups of patients.

The mechanism for traumatic asphyxia is an abrupt, significant increase in thoracic pressure resulting from a crush to the torso (e.g., car falling off a jack onto the patient's chest). This results in blood being forced back out of the heart and into the veins in a retrograde direction. Because the veins of the arms and lower extremities contain valves, this limits backward flow into the extremities. On the other hand, the veins of the neck and head lack such valves, and blood is preferentially forced into these areas. Subcutaneous venules and small capillaries rupture, resulting in the purplish discoloration of the skin. Rupture of small vessels in the brain and retina may result in brain and eye dysfunction. Traumatic asphyxia is reported to be a marker for blunt cardiac rupture.[41]

Assessment

The hallmark of traumatic asphyxia is plethora, or the bodily condition characterized by an excess of blood and turgescence, or swelling and distension of blood vessels, with a reddish coloration of the skin. This appearance is most prominent above the level of the crush (Figure 11–25). The skin below the level of injury is normal. Because of the force applied to the chest necessary to cause this injury, many of the injuries already discussed in this chapter may be present, as well as injures to the spine and spinal cord.

Management

Management is supportive. High-concentration oxygen is administered, IV access obtained, and judicious ventilatory support provided, if indicated. The reddish-purple discoloration typically fades within a week in survivors.

Diaphragmatic Rupture

Small lacerations of the diaphragm may occur in penetrating injuries to the thoracoabdominal region.[1] Because the diaphragm rises and falls with respiration, any penetration that is below the level of the nipples anteriorly or the level of the scapular tip posteriorly is at risk for having traversed the diaphragm. Generally, these lesions do not present any acute problems on their own, but they should be repaired because of the risk for herniation and strangulation of abdominal contents through the defect in the future. Significant injuries to thoracic or abdominal organs may accompany these otherwise apparently innocuous injuries.

Blunt diaphragmatic injury results from the application of sufficient force to the abdomen to increase abdominal pressure acutely, abruptly, and sufficiently to disrupt the diaphragm. Unlike the small tears that usually accompany penetrating injury, the tears resulting from blunt mechanisms are frequently

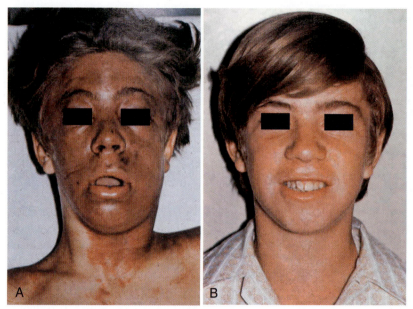

FIGURE 11-25 Traumatic asphyxia. **A.** The patient on admission to the hospital. **B.** The patient 3 weeks after injury. (From Moore JD, Mayer JH, Gago O: Traumatic asphyxia. *Chest* 62(5), 1972.)

large and allow acute herniation of the abdominal viscera into the chest cavity.[1] Respiratory distress results from the pressure of the herniated organs on the lungs, preventing effective ventilation, as well as from contusion of the lungs. This impairment of ventilation may be life threatening (Figure 11–26). In addition to the ventilatory dysfunction, rib fractures, hemothorax, and pneumothorax may occur. Injury of intra-abdominal organs may also accompany the injury to the diaphragm, including injuries to the liver, spleen, stomach, or intestines, as these organs are forced through the tear in the diaphragm into the pleural cavity. These patients are frequently in acute distress and require rapid intervention to recover.

Assessment

Assessment frequently reveals a patient in acute respiratory distress who may appear anxious, tachypneic, and pale. The patient may have contusions of the chest wall, bony crepitus, or subcutaneous emphysema. Breath sounds on the affected side may be diminished, or bowel sounds may be auscultated over the chest. The abdomen may be scaphoid if enough of the abdominal contents have herniated into the chest.

Management

Prompt recognition that diaphragmatic rupture may be present is necessary. Supplemental oxygen in high concentration should be administered and ventilation supported as necessary. The patient should be rapidly transported to an appropriate facility. Use of a PASG is contraindicated in patients with suspected diaphragmatic rupture as inflation of the abdominal compartment may push intra-abdominal organs through the tear in the diaphragm. Thus, these patients typically exhibit increased distress when the abdominal compartment of the PASG is inflated.[1]

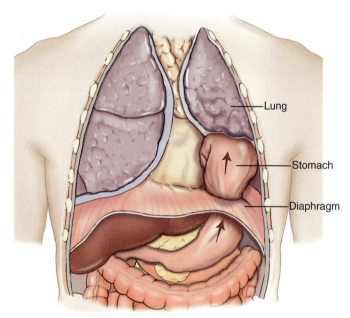

FIGURE 11-26 Diaphragmatic rupture may cause the bowel or other structures to herniate through the tear, causing partial compression of the lung and respiratory distress.

Prolonged Transport

Priorities for managing patients with known or suspected thoracic injuries during prolonged transport remain fundamental, including managing the airway, supporting ventilation and oxygenation, controlling hemorrhage, and providing appropriate volume resuscitation. When faced with a prolonged transport, prehospital care personnel may have a lower threshold for securing the airway with endotracheal intubation. Indications for performing endotracheal intubation include increasing respiratory distress or impending respiratory failure (after exclusion or treatment of a tension pneumothorax), a flail chest, open pneumothorax, or multiple rib fractures. Oxygen should be provided to maintain oxygen saturation at 95% or greater.

Ventilations should be assisted as necessary. Pulmonary contusions worsen over time, and the use of CPAP, positive end-expiratory pressure (PEEP) with a transport ventilator, or PEEP valves with bag-mask device may facilitate oxygenation. Any patient with significant thoracic trauma may have a tension pneumothorax, and ongoing assessment should look for the hallmark signs. In the presence of decreased or absent breath sounds, worsening respiratory distress, difficulty squeezing the bag-mask device, increasing peak inspiratory pressures in patients on a ventilator, and hypotension, pleural decompression should be performed. A tube thoracostomy (chest tube) may be performed by authorized personnel, typically air medical flight crews, if the patient requires needle decompression or is found to have an open pneumothorax.

Intravenous access should be secured and IV fluids administered judiciously. Patients with suspected intrathoracic, intra-abdominal, or retroperitoneal hemorrhage should be maintained with SBP in the range of 80 to 90 mm Hg. Overaggressive volume resuscitation may significantly worsen pulmonary contusions, as well as lead to recurrent internal hemorrhage (see Chapter 8). Patients with severe pain from multiple rib fractures may benefit from small doses of narcotics titrated intravenously. If narcotic administration results in hypotension and respiratory failure, volume resuscitation and ventilatory support should be provided.

Patients with cardiac dysrhythmias associated with blunt cardiac injury may benefit from the use of antidysrhythmic medications. Any interventions performed should be carefully documented on the patient care record (PCR) and the receiving facility must be made aware of the procedures.

SUMMARY

- Chest injuries are particularly significant because of the potential for compromise of respiratory and circulatory function and because thoracic injuries are frequently associated with multisystem trauma.
- Patients with chest injury need to be managed aggressively and transported quickly to definitive care.
- Particular attention should be paid to the administration of supplemental high-concentration oxygen and the need for ventilatory support in any patient suspected of having chest trauma.
- The use of pulse oximetry and sidestream or in-line waveform capnography is a useful adjunct for assessing ventilatory status and responses to therapy.
- Signs of tension pneumothorax should be carefully sought because treatment in the field with needle decompression may prevent this possible, rapidly fatal problem.
- Because of the high risk of multisystem trauma in patients with blunt chest trauma, spinal immobilization is considered and hemorrhage is controlled.
- Intravenous access should be obtained en route to the medical facility, and fluid therapy administered with appropriate goals in mind.
- ECG monitoring may suggest blunt cardiac injury.
- Although many thoracic injuries can be managed without surgical intervention, the patient with a chest injury must still be evaluated and managed at an appropriate medical facility.

SCENARIO SOLUTION

The scene report, patient complaints, and examination lead you to suspect that this patient may have serious and potentially life-threatening injuries. He is awake and speaking coherently, indicating that he has a stable airway. He is experiencing severe respiratory distress. The location of the wound, the crepitus, and decreased breath sounds indicate a possible pneumothorax. The presence of distended neck veins may indicate impending tension pneumothorax or pericardial tamponade. Move quickly to provide the patient with supplemental oxygen and consider ventilatory assistance with a bag-mask device. The first priorities in this scenario are to recognize the seriousness of the injuries, stabilize the patient, and initiate transfer to an appropriate facility. Given this patient's respiratory distress and findings, he is at significant risk for complications. Transportation to the closest trauma center is appropriate. Intravenous access should be obtained en route. There is risk for respiratory deterioration, and the patient's ventilatory status needs to be monitored closely. Signs of progressing circulatory compromise and respiratory distress should prompt the prehospital care provider to perform needle decompression. If transport time will be extended, air transport should be considered. ■

References

1. American College of Surgeons: Thoracic trauma. In ACS Committee on Trauma: *Advanced trauma life support for doctors, student course manual*, Chicago, 2008, ACS.
2. Wall MJ, Huh J, Mattox KL: Thoracotomy. In Mattox KL, Feliciano DV, Moore EE: *Trauma*, ed 5, New York, 2004, McGraw-Hill.
3. Livingston DH, Hauser CJ: Trauma to the chest wall and lung. In Mattox KL, Feliciano DV, Moore EE: *Trauma*, ed 5, New York, 2004, McGraw-Hill.
4. Harwood-Nuss A, Wolfson AB, Linden H, et al: *The Clinical Practice of Emergency Medicine*, ed 3, Philadelphia, 2001, Lippincott, Williams & Wilkins.
5. Wilson RF: Pulmonary physiology. In Wilson RF: *Critical care manual: Applied physiology and principles of therapy*, ed 2, Philadelphia, 1992, Davis.
6. American College of Surgeons (ACS): Initial assessment. In ACS Committee on Trauma: *Advanced trauma life support for doctors*, Chicago, 2004, ACS.
7. Silverston P: Pulse oximetry at the roadside: A study of pulse oximetry in immediate care. *BMJ* 298:711, 1989.
8. Richardson JD, Adams L, Flint LM: Selective management of flail chest and pulmonary contusion. *Ann Surg* 196:481, 1982.
9. Di Bartolomeo S, Sanson G, Nardi G, et al: A population-based study on pneumothorax in severely traumatized patients. *J Trauma* 51(4):677, 2001.
10. Regel G, Stalp M, Lehmann U, et al: Prehospital care: Importance of early intervention outcome. *Acta Anaesthesiol Scand Suppl* 110:71, 1997.
11. Eckstein M, Suyehara DL: Needle thoracostomy in the pre-hospital setting. *Prehosp Emerg Care* 2:132, 1998.
12. Barone JE, Pizzi WF, Nealon TF, et al: Indications for intubation in blunt chest trauma. *J Trauma* 26:334, 1986.
13. Mattox KL: Prehospital care of the patient with an injured chest. *Surg Clin North Am* 69(1):21, 1989.
14. Simon B, Ebert J, Bokhari F, et al: Practice management guideline for "pulmonary contusion—flail chest." Charleston (SC): Eastern Association for the Surgery of Trauma (EAST); 2006 Jun. 74 pages.

[100 references]. http://www.guideline.gov/summary/summary. aspx?ss=15&doc_id=10167&nbr=5352. Accessed November 16, 2009.
15. Cooper C, Militello P: The multi-injured patient: The Maryland Shock Trauma protocol approach. *Semin Thorac Cardiovasc Surg* 4(3):163, 1992.
16. Barton ED, Epperson M, Hoyt DB, et al: Prehospital needle aspiration and tube thoracostomy in trauma victims: A six-year experience with aeromedical crews. *J Emerg Med* 13:155, 1995.
17. Holcomb JB, McManus JG, Kerr ST, Pusateri AE: Needle versus tube thoracostomy in a swine model of traumatic tension hemopneumothorax. Prehosp Emerg Care. 2009 Jan-Mar; 13(1):18-27.
18. Butler KL, Best IM, Weaver WL, et al: Pulmonary artery injury and cardiac tamponade after needle decompression of a suspected tension pneumothorax. *J Trauma* 54:610, 2003.
19. Cullinane DC, Morris JA, Bass JG, et al: Needle thoracostomy may not be indicated in the trauma patient. *Injury* 32:749, 2001.
20. Givens ML, Ayotte K, Manifeld C: Needle thoracostomy: Implications of computed tomography chest wall thickness. *J Acad Emerg Med* 11:211, 2004.
21. Marinaro JL, Kenny CV, Smith SR, et al: Needle thoracostomy in trauma patients: What catheter length is adequate? *Acad Emerg Med* 10(5):495, 2003.
22. Davis DP, Pettit K, Rum CD, et al: The safety and efficacy of prehospital needle and tube thoracostomy by aeromedical personnel. *Prehosp Emerg Care* 9:191, 2005.
23. Etoch SW, Bar-Natan MF, Miller FB, et al: Tube thoracostomy: Factors related to complications. *Arch Surg* 130:521, 1995.
24. Newman PG, Feliciano DV: Blunt cardiac injury. *New Horizons* 7(1):26, 1999.
25. Ivatury RR: The injured heart. In Mattox KL, Feliciano DV, Moore EE: *Trauma*, ed 5, New York, 2004, McGraw-Hill, p 555.
26. Symbas NP, Bongiorno PF, Symbas PN: Blunt cardiac rupture: The utility of emergency department ultrasound. *Ann Thorac Surg* 67(5):1274, 1999.

27. Ivatury RR, Nallathambi MN, Roberge RJ, et al: Penetrating thoracic injuries: In-field stabilization versus prompt transport. *J Trauma* 27:1066, 1987.

28. Bleetman A, Kasem H, Crawford R: Review of emergency thoracotomy for chest injuries in patients attending a UK Accident and Emergency department. *Injury* 27(2):129, 1996.

29. Durham LA III, Richardson RJ, Wall MJ Jr, et al: Emergency center thoracotomy: Impact of prehospital resuscitation. *J Trauma* 32(6):775, 1992.

30. Honigman B, Rohweder K, Moore EE, et al: Prehospital advanced trauma life support for penetrating cardiac wounds. *Ann Emerg Med* 19(2):145, 1990.

31. Lerer LB, Knottenbelt JD: Preventable mortality following sharp penetrating chest trauma. *J Trauma* 37(1):9, 1994.

32. Wall MJ Jr, Pepe PE, Mattox KL: Successful roadside resuscitative thoracotomy: case report and literature review, *J Trauma* 36(1):131, 1994.

33. Coats TJ, Keogh S, Clark H, et al: Prehospital resuscitative thoracotomy for cardiac arrest after penetrating trauma: Rationale and case series. *J Trauma* 50(4):670, 2001.

34. Honigman B, Lowenstein SR, Moore EE, et al: The role of the pneumatic antishock garment in penetrating cardiac wounds. *JAMA* 266:2398, 1991.

35. Zangwill SD, Strasburger JF: Commotio cordis. *Pediatr Clin North Am* 51(5):1347–1354, 2004.

36. Perron AD, Brady WJ, Erling BF: Commodio cordis: An underappreciated cause of sudden cardiac death in young patients: assessment and management in the ED. *Am J Emerg Med* 19(5):406–409, 2001.

37. Madias C, Maron BJ, Weinstock J, et al. Commotio cordis—sudden cardiac death with chest wall impact. *J Cardiovasc Electrophysiol* 18(1):115–122, 2007.

38. Mattox KL, Wall MJ, Lemaire SA: Injury to the thoracic great vessels. In Mattox KL, Feliciano DV, Moore EE: *Trauma,* ed 5, New York, 2004, McGraw-Hill.

39. Fabian TC: Roger T. Sherman Lecture, Advances in the management of blunt thoracic aortic injury: Parmley to the present. *Am Surg* 75(4):273–278, 2009.

40. Riley RD, Miller PR, Meredith JW: Injury to the esophagus, trachea, and bronchus. In Mattox KL, Feliciano DV, Moore EE: *Trauma,* ed 5, New York, 2004, McGraw-Hill.

41. Rogers FB, Leavitt BJ: Upper torso cyanosis: A marker for blunt cardiac rupture. *Am J Emerg Med* May 15(3):275, 1997.

Suggested Reading

Bowley DM, Boffard KD: Penetrating trauma of the trunk. *Unfallchirurg* 104(11):1032, 2001.

Brathwaite CE, Rodriguez A, Turney SZ, et al: Blunt traumatic cardiac rupture: A 5-year experience. *Ann Surg* 212(6):701, 1990.

Callaham M: Pericardiocentesis in traumatic and nontraumatic cardiac tamponade. *Ann Emerg Med* 13:924, 1984.

Deakin CD: Morbidity in 624 patients requiring prehospital chest tube decompression. *J Trauma* 44(1):98, 1998.

Gervin AS, Fischer RF: The importance of prompt transport in salvage of patients with penetrating heart wounds. *J Trauma* 22:443, 1982.

Helm M, Schuster R, Hauke J: Tight control of prehospital ventilation by capnography in major trauma victims. *Br J Anaesth* 90(3):327, 2003.

Kulshrestha P, Das B, Iyer KS, et al: Cardiac injuries: A clinical and autopsy profile. *J Trauma* 30(2):203, 1990.

Lateef F: Commotio cordis: An underappreciated cause of sudden death in athletes. *Sports Med* 30:301, 2000.

Luna GK, Eddy AC, Copass M: The sensitivity of vital signs in identifying major thoracoabdominal hemorrhage. *Am J Surg* 157(5):512, 1989.

Papadopoulos IN, Bukis D, Karalas E, et al: Preventable prehospital trauma deaths in a Hellenic urban health region: An audit of prehospital trauma care. *J Trauma* 41(5):864, 1996.

Rozycki GS, Feliciano DV, Oschner MG, et al: The role of ultrasound in patients with possible penetrating cardiac wounds: A prospective multicenter study. *J Trauma* 46:542, 1999.

Ruchholtz S, Waydhas C, Ose C, et al: Prehospital intubation in severe thoracic trauma without respiratory insufficiency: A matched-pair analysis based on the Trauma Registry of the German Trauma Society. *J Trauma* 52(5):879, 2002.

Schmidt U, Stalp M, Gerich T, et al: Chest tube decompression of blunt chest injuries by physicians in the field: Effectiveness and complications. *J Trauma* 44(1):98, 1998.

Streng M, Tikka S, Leppaniemi A: Assessing the severity of truncal gunshot wounds: A nation-wide analysis from Finland. *Ann Chir Gynaecol* 90(4):246, 2001.

SPECIFIC SKILLS

Thoracic Trauma Skills

Needle Decompression

Principle: To decease intrathoracic pressure from a tension pneumothorax affecting the patient's breathing, ventilation, and circulation.

In patients with increasing intrathoracic pressure from a developing tension pneumothorax, the side of the thoracic cavity that has the increased pressure should be decompressed. If this pressure is not relieved, it will progressively limit the patient's ventilatory capacity and cause inadequate venous return, producing inadequate cardiac output and death.

In patients in whom an open pneumothorax has been treated by the use of an occlusive dressing and a tension pneumothorax develops, decompression can usually be achieved through the wound, which provides an existing opening into the thorax. Opening the occlusive dressing over the wound for a few seconds should initiate a rush of air out of the wound as increased pressure in the thorax is relieved.

Once this pressure has been released, the wound is resealed with the occlusive dressing to allow for proper alveolar ventilation and to stop air from "sucking" into the wound. The patient should be monitored carefully and, if any signs of tension recur, the dressing should be "burped" again to release the intrathoracic pressure.

Decompression in a closed-tension pneumothorax is achieved by providing an opening—a thoracostomy—in the affected side of the chest. Different methods for performing a thoracostomy exist. Because needle thoracostomy is the most rapid method and does not require special equipment, it is the preferred method for use in the field.

Needle decompression carries minimal risk and can greatly benefit the patient by improving oxygenation and circulation. Needle decompression should be performed when the following three criteria are met:

1. Evidence of worsening respiratory distress or difficulty with a bag-mask device
2. Decreased or absent breath sounds
3. Decompensated shock (SBP <90 mm Hg)

Necessary equipment for needle chest decompression includes a needle, a syringe, $1/2$-inch adhesive tape, and alcohol swabs. The needles should be large-bore, over-the-needle IV catheters between 10 and 14 gauge, at least 8 cm in length. A 16-gauge catheter can be used if a larger bore is not available.

One prehospital care provider attaches the needle to the syringe while a second provider auscultates the patient's chest to confirm which side has the tension pneumothorax, which is indicated by absent or diminished breath sounds.

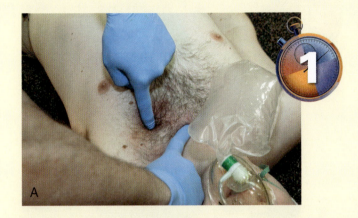

After confirmation of a tension pneumothorax, the anatomic landmarks are located on the affected side (midclavicular line, second or third intercostal space).

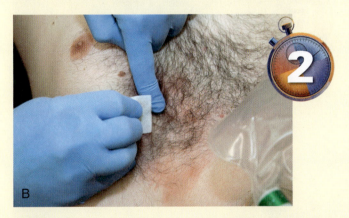

The site is swabbed with an antiseptic wipe.

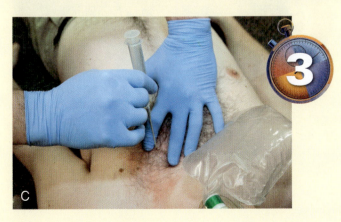

The skin over the site is stretched between the fingers of the non-dominate hand. The needle and syringe is placed for placement over the top of the rib.

SPECIFIC SKILLS

Once the needle enters into the thoracic cavity, air will escape into the syringe and the needle should not be advance further.

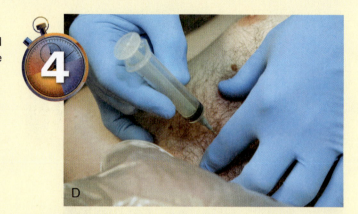

The catheter should be left in place and the needle removed, with care not to kink the catheter. As the needle is removed, a rush of air from the hub of the catheter should be heard. If no air escapes, the catheter should be left in place to indicate that needle decompression of the chest was attempted.

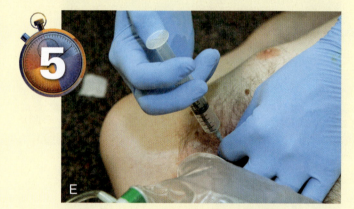

After the needle is removed, the catheter is taped in place with adhesive tape. After securing the catheter, the chest is auscultated to check for increased breath sounds. The patient is monitored and transported to an appropriate facility. The provider does not waste time applying a one-way valve. Needle decompression may need to be repeated if the catheter becomes occluded with a blood clot and tension pneumothorax reoccurs.

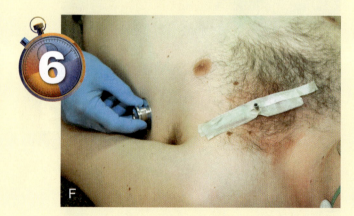

CHAPTER 12

Abdominal Trauma

CHAPTER OBJECTIVES

At the completion of this chapter, the reader will be able to do the following:

- ✓ Analyze scene assessment data to determine the level of suspicion for abdominal trauma.

- ✓ Recognize the secondary survey assessment findings indicative of intra-abdominal bleeding.

- ✓ Relate external signs of abdominal injury to the potential for specific abdominal organ injuries.

- ✓ Anticipate the pathophysiologic effects of a blunt or penetrating injury to the abdomen based on assessment data obtainable by a prehospital care provider.

- ✓ Identify the indications for rapid intervention and transport in the context of abdominal trauma.

- ✓ Understand appropriate field management decisions for patients with suspected abdominal trauma, including those with impaled objects, evisceration, and external genital trauma.

- ✓ Relate the anatomic and physiologic changes associated with pregnancy to the pathophysiology and management of trauma.

- ✓ Describe the effects of maternal trauma on the fetus and the priorities of management.

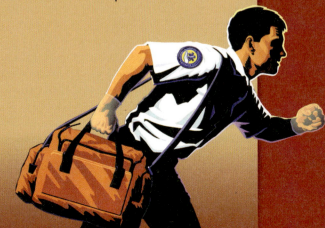

SCENARIO

You have just arrived at an apartment where a male patient in his mid-20s requested assistance. He states that he was out walking his dog when he suffered a near-syncopal episode. The patient notes moderate pain over his lower left ribcage when he takes deep breaths and complains of mild difficulty in breathing. He smells vaguely of alcohol. Upon further questioning, you learn that he and friends spent the evening playing pool and drinking beer at a neighborhood pub. At one point during the evening, he and a friend began boxing and he recalls suffering a blow to his left lower ribs. Soon thereafter, he came home and fell asleep until his dog woke him about 6 hours later. While taking his dog for a walk, the patient became profoundly lightheaded and weak. He managed to return to his apartment and summon help.

The patient is laying supine on a couch. He has a patent airway, a ventilatory rate of 28 breaths/minute, a heart rate of 124 beats/minute, and a blood pressure of 94/58 mm Hg. The patient's skin is pale and diaphoretic. He has tenderness on palpation of the left lower ribs. His abdomen is nondistended and soft to palpation, but he has tenderness and voluntary guarding in the left upper quadrant. No ecchymosis or subcutaneous emphysema is present.

What are the patient's possible injuries? What are the priorities in the care of this patient? Are signs of peritonitis present?

Unrecognized abdominal injury is one of the major causes of death in the trauma patient. Because of the limitations of prehospital assessment, patients with suspected abdominal injuries are best managed by prompt transportation to the closest appropriate facility.

Early deaths from severe abdominal trauma typically result from massive blood loss caused by either penetrating or blunt injuries. Any patient with unexplained shock should be assumed to have an intra-abdominal hemorrhage until proven otherwise (in the hospital). Complications and death may occur from liver, spleen, colon, small intestine, stomach, or pancreatic injuries that were not initially detected. The absence of local signs and symptoms does not rule out the possibility of abdominal trauma, especially in the patient whose level of consciousness is altered by alcohol, drugs, or traumatic brain injury. Consideration of the kinematics will raise the index of suspicion of the alert prehospital care provider to possible abdominal trauma and intra-abdominal hemorrhage. A prehospital care provider should not be as concerned with pinpointing the exact extent of abdominal trauma as with treating the clinical findings.

Anatomy

The abdomen contains the major organs of the digestive, endocrine, and urogenital systems and major vessels of the circulatory system. The abdominal cavity is located below the diaphragm; its boundaries include the anterior abdominal wall, the pelvic bones, the vertebral column, and the muscles of the abdomen and flanks. The abdominal cavity is divided into two regions. The *peritoneal cavity* (the "true" abdominal cavity) contains the spleen, liver, gallbladder, stomach, portions of the large intestine (transverse and sigmoid colon), most of

the small intestines (primarily the jejunum and ileum), and female reproductive organs (uterus and ovaries) (Figure 12-1). The *retroperitoneal space* (potential space behind the "true" abdominal cavity) contains the kidneys, ureters, inferior vena cava, abdominal aorta, pancreas, much of the duodenum, ascending and descending colon, and rectum (Figure 12-2). The urinary bladder and male reproductive organs (penis, testes, and prostate) lie inferior to the peritoneal cavity.

A significant portion of the abdomen lies in the lower thorax. This superior portion of the abdomen, referred to by trauma surgeons as the thoracoabdomen, is protected in front and along the flanks by the ribs and in back by the vertebral column. The thoracoabdomen contains the liver, gallbladder, spleen, and stomach anteriorly and the lower lobes of the lungs posteriorly, separated by the diaphragm. Because of their location, the same forces that fracture ribs may injure the underlying lungs, liver, or spleen. The relationship of these abdominal organs to the lower portion of the thoracic cavity changes with the respiratory cycle. At peak expiration, the dome of the relaxed diaphragm rises to level of the fourth intercostal space (nipple level in the male), providing greater protection to abdominal organs from the rib cage. Conversely, at peak inspiration, the dome of the contracted diaphragm lies at the level of the sixth intercostal space, the inflated lungs almost fill the thorax and largely push these abdominal organs out from under the ribcage. Thus, the organs injured by penetrating trauma to the thoracoabdomen may differ depending upon which phase of respiration the patient is in when injured (Figure 12-3). The most inferior portion of the abdomen is protected on all sides by the pelvis. This area contains the rectum, a portion of the small intestine (especially when the patient is upright), the urinary bladder, and in the female, the reproductive organs. Retroperitoneal hemorrhage associated with a fractured pelvis is a major concern in this portion of the abdominal cavity. The abdomen between the

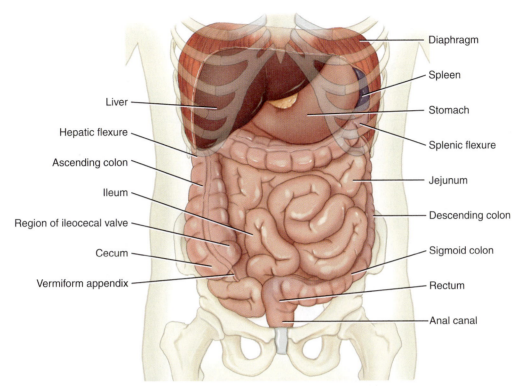

FIGURE 12-1 The organs inside the peritoneal cavity frequently produce peritonitis when injured. Organs in the peritoneal cavity include solid organs (spleen and liver), hollow organs of the gastrointestinal tract (stomach, small intestine, and colon), and the reproductive organs.

rib cage and the pelvis is only protected by the abdominal muscles and other soft tissues anterior and laterally. Posteriorly, the lumbar vertebrae and the thick, strong paraspinal and psoas muscles provide more protection (Figure 12-4).

For purposes of patient assessment, the surface of the abdomen is divided into four quadrants. These quadrants are formed by drawing two lines: one in the middle from the tip of the xiphoid to the symphysis pubis and one perpendicular to this midline at the level of the umbilicus (Figure 12-5). Knowledge of anatomic landmarks is important because of the high correlation of organ location to pain response. The right upper quadrant (RUQ) includes the liver and gallbladder, the left upper quadrant (LUQ) contains the spleen and stomach, and the right lower quadrant (RLQ) and left lower quadrant (LLQ) contain primarily the intestines. A portion of the intestinal tract exists in all four quadrants. The urinary bladder is midline between the lower quadrants.

Pathophysiology

Dividing the abdominal organs into hollow, solid, and vascular (blood vessel) groups helps explain manifestations of injury to these structures. When injured, solid organs and blood vessels (liver, spleen, aorta, vena cava) bleed, whereas hollow organs (intestine, gallbladder, urinary bladder) primarily spill their contents into the peritoneal cavity or ret-

roperitoneal space. Loss of blood into the abdominal cavity, regardless of its source, can contribute to or can be the primary cause of the development of hypovolemic shock. The release of acids, digestive enzymes, or bacteria from the gastrointestinal (GI) tract into the peritoneal cavity results in *peritonitis* (inflammation of the peritoneum or the lining of the abdominal cavity) and *sepsis* (massive infection) if not promptly treated by surgical intervention. Because urine and bile are generally sterile (do not contain bacteria) and do not contain digestive enzymes, perforation of the gallbladder or urinary bladder does not produce peritonitis as quickly as material spilled from the intestine. Similarly, because it also lacks acids, digestive enzymes, and bacteria, blood in the peritoneal cavity does not cause peritonitis for a number of hours. Bleeding from intestinal injury is typically minor, unless the larger blood vessels in the mesentery are damaged.

Injuries to the abdomen can be caused by either penetrating or blunt trauma. Penetrating trauma, such as a gunshot or stab wound, is more readily visible than blunt trauma. Multiple organ damage can occur in penetrating trauma, although it is less likely with a stab wound than with a gunshot wound. A mental visualization of the potential trajectory of a missile, such as a bullet or the path of a knife blade, can help identify possible injured internal organs.

The diaphragm extends superiorly to the fourth intercostal space anteriorly, the sixth intercostal space laterally, and the eighth intercostal space posteriorly during maximum

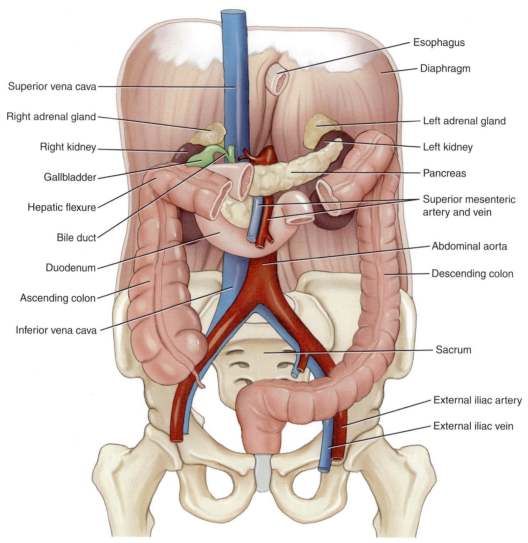

FIGURE 12-2 The abdomen is divided into two spaces: peritoneal cavity and retroperitoneal space. The retroperitoneal space includes the portion of the abdomen behind the peritoneum. Because the retroperitoneal organs are not within the peritoneal cavity, injury to these structures generally does not produce peritonitis.

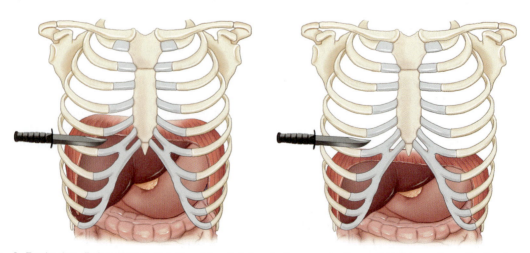

FIGURE 12-3 **A.** Expiration. **B.** Inhalation. Relationship of abdominal organs to thorax in phases of respiration in a patient with a stab wound.

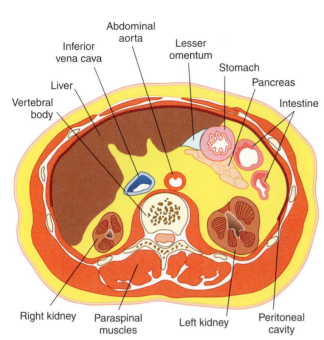

FIGURE 12-4 labels: Abdominal aorta, Inferior vena cava, Lesser omentum, Stomach, Pancreas, Liver, Intestine, Vertebral body, Right kidney, Paraspinal muscles, Left kidney, Peritoneal cavity

FIGURE 12-4 This transverse section of the abdominal cavity provides an appreciation of the organ's positions in the anteroposterior direction.

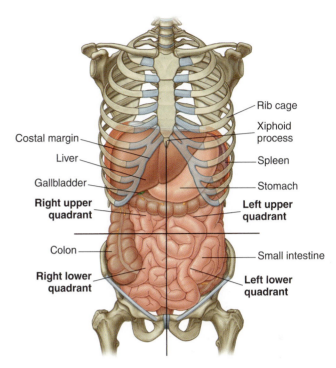

FIGURE 12-5 labels: Rib cage, Xiphoid process, Spleen, Stomach, Left upper quadrant, Small intestine, Left lower quadrant, Costal margin, Liver, Gallbladder, Right upper quadrant, Colon, Right lower quadrant

FIGURE 12-5 As with any part of the body, the better the description of pain, tenderness, guarding, and other signs, the more accurate the diagnosis. The most common system of identification divides the abdomen into four quadrants: left upper, right upper, left lower, and right lower.

expiration (see Figure 12-3). Patients with penetrating injury to the thorax below this line may also have an abdominal injury. Penetrating wounds of the flanks and buttocks may involve organs in the abdominal cavity as well. These penetrating injuries may cause bleeding from a major vessel or solid organ and perforation of a segment of the intestine, the most frequently injured organ in penetrating trauma.

Blunt trauma injuries are often more challenging to diagnose than those caused by penetrating trauma. These injuries to abdominal organs result from either compression or shear forces. In *compression* incidents, the organs of the abdomen are crushed between solid objects, such as between the steering wheel and spinal column. *Shear forces* create rupture of the solid organs or rupture of blood vessels in the cavity because of the tearing forces exerted against their supporting ligaments. The liver and spleen can shear and bleed easily, and blood loss can occur at a rapid rate. Increased intra-abdominal pressure produced by compression can rupture the diaphragm, causing the abdominal organs to move upward into the pleural cavity (see Chapters 4 and 11). The intra-abdominal contents forced into the chest cavity can compromise lung expansion and affect both respiratory and cardiac function (Figure 12-6). Although rupture of each half of the diaphragm is now believed to occur equally, rupture of the left hemidiaphragm is diagnosed more often.

Pelvic fractures may be associated with the loss of large volumes of blood caused by damage to the many smaller arteries and veins adjacent to the pelvis. Other injuries associated with pelvic fractures include damage to the urinary bladder and the rectum, as well as injuries to the urethra in the male and the vagina in the female.

Assessment

The assessment of abdominal injury can be difficult, especially with the limited diagnostic capabilities of the prehospital setting. An index of suspicion for abdominal injury should develop from a variety of sources of information, including kinematics, findings from the physical examination, and input from the patient or bystanders.

Kinematics

As with other types of trauma, knowledge of the mechanism of injury plays an important role in shaping the prehospital care provider's index of suspicion for abdominal trauma. Abdominal trauma may result from numerous types of trauma, including both penetrating and blunt forces.

Penetrating trauma. Most penetrating trauma in the civilian setting results from stab wounds and gunshot wounds from handguns. These low to moderate kinetic energy forces lacer-

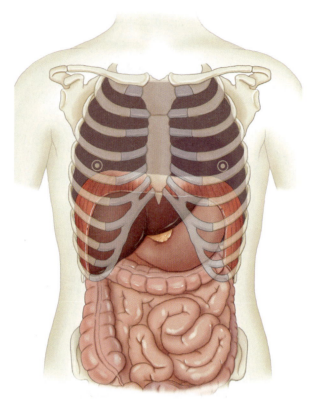

FIGURE 12-6 With increased pressure inside the abdomen, the diaphragm can rupture allowing intrabdominal organs such as the stomach or small intestine to herniate into the chest.

ate or cut abdominal organs along the pathway of the knife or projectile. High velocity injuries, such as those created by high-powered rifles and assault weapons, tend to create more serious injuries because of the larger temporary cavities created as the projectile moved through the peritoneal cavity. Projectiles may strike bones (ribs, spine, or pelvis) resulting in fragments that may also perforated internal organs. Stab wounds are less likely to penetrate the peritoneal cavity than projectiles fired from a handgun, rifle, or shotgun.

When the peritoneum is penetrated, stab wounds are most likely to injure the liver (40%), small bowel (30%), diaphragm (20%), and colon (15%), whereas gunshot wounds most commonly damage the small bowel (50%), colon (40%), liver (30%), and abdominal vessels (25%).[1] Because of the thicker musculature of the back, penetrating trauma to the back is less likely to result in injuries of intraperitoneal structures than wounds to the anterior abdominal wall. Overall, only about 15% of patients with stab wounds to the abdomen will require surgical intervention, whereas about 85% of patients with gunshot wounds will need surgery for definitive management of their abdominal injuries. Tangential gunshot wounds may pass through subcutaneous tissues but never enter the peritoneal cavity. Explosive devices may also propel fragments that penetrate the peritoneum and injure internal organs.

Blunt trauma. Numerous mechanisms lead to the compression and shear forces that may damage abdominal organs. A patient may experience considerable deceleration or compression forces when involved in motor vehicle and motorcycle crashes, when struck or run over by a vehicle, or after falling from a significant height. Although abdominal organs are most often injured in events associated with significant kinetic injury, such as those with rapid deceleration or severe compression, abdominal injuries may result from more innocuous-appearing mechanisms, such as assaults, falls down a flight of stairs, and sporting activities (e.g., being tackled in football). Any protective devices or gear used by the patient should be noted, including seat belts, air bags, or sports padding.

Compression of a solid organ may result in splitting of its structure (e.g., hepatic laceration), whereas such forces applied to a hollow structure, such as a loop of bowel, may cause the structure to burst open ("rupture"). Shearing forces may result in tears of structures at sites of tethering to other structures, such as where the more mobile small bowel joins the ascending colon, which is fixed in the retroperitoneum. The organs most commonly injured following blunt trauma to the abdomen include the spleen (40–55%), liver (35–45%), and small bowel (5–10%). Not all injuries to solid organs require surgical intervention (Figure 12-7).

History

History may be obtained from the patient, family, or bystanders and should be documented on the patient care report (PCR) and relayed to the receiving facility. In addition to the components of the SAMPLE history (**s**ymptoms, **a**llergies and **a**ge, **m**edications, **p**ast medical/surgical history, **l**ast meal, **e**vents preceding injury), other questions should be tailored to the type of injury. Those related to motor vehicle crashes (MVCs) include the following:

- Type of collision and position of patient in the vehicle
- Extent of vehicle damage, including compromise of the passenger compartment, steering wheel deformity, and requirement for prolonged extrication
- Use of safety devices, including seat belts, deployment of air bags, and presence of child safety seats

Questions related to penetrating injury include the following:

- Type of weapon (handgun vs. rifle, caliber, length of knife)
- Number of times the patient was shot or stabbed
- Amount of blood at the scene

Physical Examination

Primary Survey

Most severe abdominal injuries will present as abnormalities identified in the primary survey, primarily in the evaluation of breathing and circulation. Unless there are associated injuries,

patients with abdominal trauma generally present with a patent airway. The alterations found in the breathing, circulation, and disability assessments generally correspond to the degree of shock present. Patients with early, compensated shock may have a mild increase in their respiratory rate, whereas those with severe hypovolemic shock demonstrate marked tachypnea. Rupture of a hemidiaphragm often compromises respiratory function, and bowel sounds may be heard over the thorax when breath sounds are auscultated. Similarly, shock from intra-abdominal hemorrhage may range from mild tachycardia, with few other findings, to severe tachycardia, marked hypotension and pale, cool, clammy skin.

The most reliable indicator of intra-abdominal bleeding is the presence of hypovolemic shock from an unexplained source.[1] When assessing disability, the prehospital care provider may note only subtle signs, such as mild anxiety or agitation, in the patient with compensated shock from abdominal trauma, whereas patients with life-threatening hemorrhage may have serious depression in their mental status. When abnormalities are found in the assessment of these systems and while preparing for immediate transport, the abdomen should be exposed and examined for evidence of trauma, such as bruising or penetrating wounds.

Secondary Survey

During the secondary survey the abdomen is examined in greater detail. This examination primarily involves inspection and palpation of the abdomen and should be approached systematically. Figure 12-8 lists physical findings consistent with the presence of peritonitis.

Inspection. The abdomen is examined for soft tissue injuries and distension. Intra-abdominal injury may be suspected when soft tissue trauma is noted over the abdomen, flanks, or back. Such injuries may include contusions, abrasions, stab or gunshot wounds, obvious bleeding, and unusual findings such as evisceration, impaled objects, or tire marks. The "seat belt" sign (ecchymosis or abrasion across the abdomen, resulting from compression of the abdominal wall against the shoulder harness or lap belt) indicates that significant force was applied to the abdomen (Figure 12-9). Although the incidence of intra-abdominal injuries in adult patients with seat belt signs is about 20%, the incidence may approach 50% in

---

FIGURE 12-7 Nonoperative Management of Solid Organ Injuries

Suspected injuries of the spleen, liver, or kidney no longer mandate surgical exploration in the modern trauma center. Experience has shown that many of these injuries will stop bleeding prior to the development of shock and then heal without the need for surgical repair. Research in the last 15 years has shown that even significant solid organ injuries may be safely observed, provided the patient is not in hypovolemic shock or has peritonitis. Patients are admitted to the hospital for close monitoring of their vital signs, blood count, and abdominal exam, initially in the intensive care unit. The advantage of this approach is that it prevents the patient from undergoing a potentially unnecessary operation. Since the spleen performs an important role in fighting infections, removal of the spleen (splenectomy) predisposes to certain bacterial infections, especially in children. Successful nonoperative management of these injuries was first reported for splenic injuries in children, but this approach is now often applied to adult patients, as well as to injuries to the liver and kidney. Following blunt trauma, recent data indicates that about 50% of splenic injuries and about 67% of liver injuries can be managed in this manner, with reported success rates ranging from 70% to over 90%.[13]

The risk of failure of this technique (rebleeding with the development of shock requiring surgical intervention) is greatest in the first 7–10 days following injury. Prehospital care providers should be aware of this approach, as they may be called to see patients who have experienced rebleeding after discharge from the hospital.

FIGURE 12-8 Findings from the Physical Examination that Support a Diagnosis of Peritonitis

Peritoneal signs
- Significant abdominal tenderness on palpation or with coughing (either localized or generalized)
- Involuntary guarding
- Percussion tenderness
- Diminished or absent bowel sounds

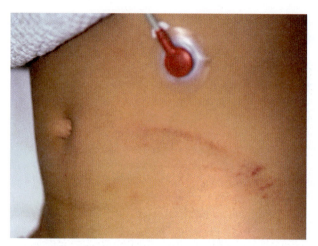

FIGURE 12-9 An abdominal "seat belt sign" resulting from the patient decelerating against a lap belt.

children. The injuries associated with restraints are typically to the bowel and its supporting mesentery, and often present in a delayed fashion. *Grey-Turner's sign* (ecchymosis involving the flanks) and *Cullen's sign* (ecchymosis around the umbilicus) indicate retroperitoneal bleeding; however, these signs may not be seen in the first few hours after injury.

The contour of the abdomen should be noted, assessing if it is flat or distended. Distension of the abdomen may indicate significant internal hemorrhage; however, the adult peritoneal cavity can hold up to 1.5 liters of fluid before showing any signs of distension. Abdominal distension may also be the result of a stomach filled with air, as can occur during artificial ventilation with a bag-mask device. Although these signs may indicate intra-abdominal injury, some patients with substantial internal injury may lack these findings.

Palpation. Palpation of the abdomen is undertaken to identify areas of tenderness. Ideally, palpation is begun in an area in which the patient does not complain of pain. Then, each of the abdominal quadrants is palpated. While palpating a tender area, the provider may note that the patient "tenses up" the abdominal muscles in that area. This reaction, called *voluntary guarding,* serves to protect the patient from the pain resulting from palpation. *Involuntary guarding* represents rigidity or spasm of the abdominal wall muscles in a response to peritonitis. Unlike voluntary guarding, involuntary guarding remains when the patient is distracted (e.g., with conversation) or the abdomen is surreptitiously palpated (e.g., with pressure on the stethoscope while appearing to auscultate bowel sounds). Although the presence of *rebound tenderness* has long been considered an important finding indicating peritonitis, many surgeons now consider that this maneuver—pressing deeply on the abdomen and then quickly releasing the pressure—causes excessive pain. If rebound tenderness is present, the patient will note more severe pain when the abdominal pressure is released.

Deep or aggressive palpation of an obviously injured abdomen should be avoided because palpation may dislodge blood clots and restart hemorrhage and may spill contents from the GI tract if perforations are present. Great care during palpation should also be exercised if there is an impaled object in the abdomen. Although tenderness is an important indicator of intra-abdominal injury, several factors may confound the assessment of tenderness. Patients with altered mental status, such as those with a traumatic brain injury (TBI) or under the influence of drugs or alcohol, may have an *unreliable* examination; that is, the patient may not report tenderness or respond to palpation even when significant internal injuries are present. Pediatric and geriatric patients are more likely to have unreliable abdominal examinations because of impaired pain responses. Conversely, patients with lower rib fractures or a pelvic fracture may have an *equivocal* examination, with tenderness resulting from either the associated fractures or internal injuries. If the patient has distracting pain from injuries, such as extremity or spinal fractures, abdominal pain may not be elicited on palpation.

The pelvis should be gently palpated for instability and tenderness. This is evaluated in three steps by (1) pressing inward on the iliac crests, (2) pulling outward on the iliac crests, and (3) pressing posteriorly on the symphysis pubis. If instability is noted, no further palpation of the pelvis should take place as this may result in significant additional internal hemorrhage.

Auscultation. Hemorrhage and spillage of intestinal contents in the peritoneal cavity may result in an ileus, a condition in which the peristalsis of the bowel ceases. This results in a "quiet" abdomen as bowel sounds are diminished or absent. Auscultation of bowel sounds is generally not a helpful prehospital assessment tool. Time should not be wasted trying to determine their presence or absence because this diagnostic sign will not alter the prehospital management of the patient. If bowel sounds are heard over the thorax during auscultation of breath sounds, however, the presence of a diaphragmatic rupture may be considered.

Percussion. Although percussion of the abdomen may reveal tympanitic or dull sounds, this information does not alter prehospital management of the trauma patient. Significant tenderness on percussion or pain when the patient is asked to cough represents a key finding of peritonitis. Peritoneal signs are summarized in Figure 12-8.

Special Examinations and Key Indicators

Surgical evaluation and, in many cases, intervention remains a key need for most abdominal injuries; time should not be wasted in attempts to determine the exact details of injury. In many patients, identification of specific organ injury will not be revealed until the abdomen is further evaluated by computed tomography (CT) scanning or surgical exploration.

In the emergency department, ultrasound has become the primary bedside modality used to assess a trauma patient for intra-abdominal hemorrhage.[1–5] The *focused assessment sonography in trauma* (FAST) involves three views of the peritoneal cavity and a fourth view of the pericardium to assess for the presence of fluid, presumably blood (Figure 12-10).

FIGURE 12-10 Focused Assessment Sonography in Trauma (FAST)*

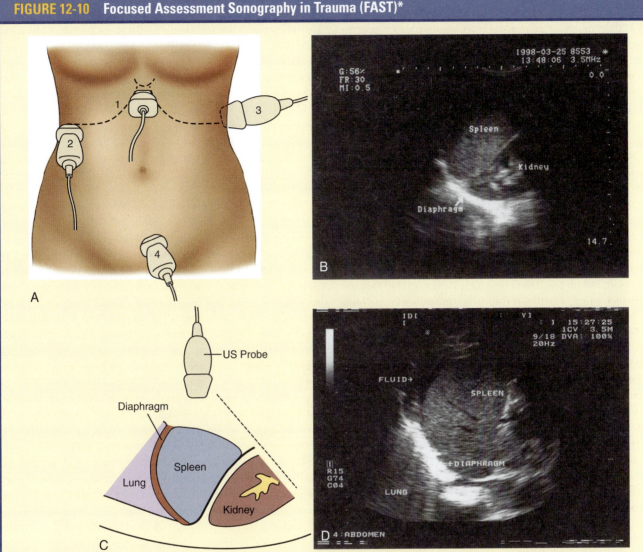

A. Four views constituting the FAST examination. **B.** Normal splenorenal view. **C.** Normal splenorenal view identifying organs. **D.** Abnormal view demonstrating the presence of fluid (blood) (*black stripe* next to spleen).

The FAST examination has value in the trauma patient because most significant intra-abdominal injuries are associated with hemorrhage into the peritoneal cavity. Although ultrasound cannot differentiate the type of fluid present, any fluid in the trauma patient is presumed to be blood.

TECHNIQUE
- Four acoustic windows (views) are imaged, three of which evaluate the peritoneal cavity:
  1. Pericardial
  2. Perihepatic (Morrison's pouch)
  3. Perisplenic
  4. Pelvic
- Accumulated fluid appears anechoic (sonographically black)
- Presence of fluid in one or more of the areas indicates a positive scan

ADVANTAGES
- Can be rapidly performed
- Can be done at the bedside
- Does not interfere with resuscitation
- Is noninvasive
- Is less costly than CT

DISADVANTAGES
- Results compromised in patients who are obese, who have subcutaneous air, or who have had previous abdominal surgery
- Skill at imaging is operator dependant

*FAST has been studied in several prehospital systems.[8–11]

Because fluid does not reflect the ultrasound waves back to the device, fluid appears anechoic (sonographically black). Presence of fluid in one or more areas is worrisome; however ultrasonography cannot differentiate blood from other fluids (ascites, urine, etc.) Compared to other techniques used to evaluate the peritoneal cavity, the FAST can be rapidly performed at the patient's bedside, does not interfere with resuscitation, is noninvasive, and is much less costly than CT scanning. The primary disadvantage of FAST is that it does not definitively diagnose injury, but only indicates the presence of fluid that may represent blood. Other disadvantages are that imaging is dependent upon the performer's skill and experience and its utility is compromised in patients who are obese, have subcutaneous air, and have had previous surgery.

Because of ease of use and improved ultrasound technology, some ground and air emergency medical services and military teams have explored the use of FAST in the prehospital setting. The FAST exam has been shown to be feasible in the field, but no published data have demonstrated that use of this technology results in improved outcomes for patients with abdominal trauma.[6–10] Thus, use of FAST is not recommended for routine prehospital care, especially in that it may delay transport to the receiving facility.

Despite all these different components, the assessment of abdominal injury can be difficult. The following are key indicators for establishing the index of suspicion for abdominal injury:

- Obvious signs of trauma (e.g., soft tissue injuries, gunshot wounds)
- Presence of hypovolemic shock without an obvious cause
- Degree of shock greater than can be explained by other injuries (e.g., fractures, external hemorrhage)
- Presence of peritoneal signs

Management

The key aspects of prehospital management of abdominal trauma are to recognize the presence of potential injury and initiate rapid transport to the closest appropriate facility that is capable of managing the patient.

Abnormalities in vital functions identified in the primary survey are supported during transport. Supplemental oxygen is administered to maintain saturation at 95% or greater, and ventilations are assisted as needed. External hemorrhage is controlled with direct pressure or a pressure dressing. If the patient has suffered blunt trauma, immobilization to a long backboard is performed. Victims of penetrating trauma to the torso do not need spinal immobilization.

The patient is rapidly packaged and transport is initiated. Because patients with abdominal trauma often require surgical intervention to control internal hemorrhage and repair injuries, patients should be transported to facilities that have immediate surgical capability, such as a trauma center, if available, when the following findings are noted: evidence of abdominal trauma associated with hypotension or peritoneal signs; or the presences of an evisceration or impaled object. Taking a patient with intra-abdominal injuries to a facility that does not have an available operating room (OR) and a surgical team defeats the purpose of rapid transportation. In a rural setting where there is no hospital with general surgeons on staff, consideration should be given to direct transfer to a trauma center, either by ground or air. Early surgical intervention is the key to survival of the unstable patient with abdominal trauma.

During transport, intravenous (IV) access is obtained. The decision to administer crystalloid fluid replacement en route depends on the patient's clinical presentation. Abdominal trauma represents one of the key situations in which balanced resuscitation is indicated. As discussed in Chapter 8, aggressive administration of IV fluid may result in recurrence of bleeding that had ceased because of blood clotting and hypotension. Thus, prehospital care providers must achieve a delicate balance: maintenance of a blood pressure that provides perfusion to vital organs without restoring blood pressure to normal (which may reinitiate bleeding sites in the abdomen). In the absence of TBI, the target systolic blood pressure is 80 to 90 mm Hg (mean arterial pressure [MAP] of 60–65 mm Hg). For patients with suspected intra-abdominal bleeding and a TBI, the systolic blood pressure is maintained at least 90 mm Hg.

When managing a patient with suspected abdominal trauma or pelvic fracture during a prolonged transport, the pneumatic antishock garment can be considered when decompensated shock is present (see Chapter 8). Inflation of the abdominal compartment is contraindicated in patients with obvious respiratory compromise, presence of an evisceration, impalement, or suspected diaphragmatic rupture and in pregnancy.

Special Considerations

Impaled Objects

Because removal of an impaled object may cause additional trauma and because the object's distal end may be actively controlling (tamponading) the bleeding, removal of an impaled object in the prehospital environment is contraindicated (Figure 12-11). The prehospital care provider should neither move nor remove an object impaled in a patient's abdomen. In the hospital, these objects are not removed until their shape and location have been identified by radiographic evaluation and until blood replacement and a surgical team are present and ready. Often these objects are removed in the

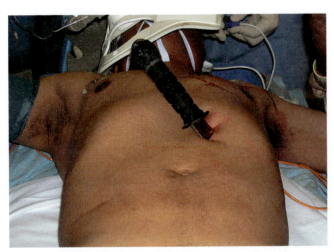

FIGURE 12-11 Knife impaled in the abdomen.

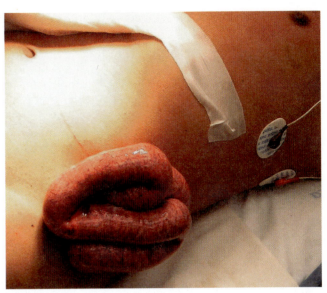

FIGURE 12-12 Bowel eviscerated through a wound in the abdominal wall.

OR. A prehospital care provider may stabilize the impaled object, either manually or mechanically, to prevent any further movement in the field and during transport. In some circumstances the impaled object may need to be cut in order to free that patient and permit transport to the trauma center. If bleeding occurs around it, direct pressure should be applied around the object to the wound with the palm of the hand. Psychological support of the patient is important, especially if the impaled object is visible to the patient.

The abdomen should not be palpated or percussed in these patients because these actions may produce additional organ injury from the distal end of the object. Further examination is unnecessary because the presence of impaled objects indicates the need for management by a surgeon.

Evisceration

In an abdominal evisceration, a section of intestine or other abdominal organ is displaced through an open wound and protrudes externally outside the abdominal cavity (Figure 12-12). The tissue most often visualized is the fatty omentum that lies over the intestines. Attempts should not be made to replace the protruding tissue in the abdominal cavity. The viscera should be left on the surface of the abdomen or protruding as found. Efforts should focus on protecting the protruding segment of intestine or other organ from further damage. Most of the abdominal contents require a moist environment. If the intestine or some of the other abdominal organs become dry, cell death will occur. Therefore, the eviscerated abdominal contents should be covered with clean or sterile dressing that has been moistened with saline (normal saline IV fluid can be used). These dressings should be periodically remoistened with saline to prevent them from

drying out. Wet dressings may be covered with a large, dry dressing to keep the patient warm.

Psychological support is extremely important for patients with an abdominal evisceration, and care should be taken to keep the patient calm. Any action that increases pressure within the abdomen, such as crying, screaming, or coughing, can force more of the organs outward. These patients should be expeditiously transported to a facility that has surgical capability.

Trauma in the Obstetrical Patient

Anatomic and Physiologic Changes

Pregnancy causes both anatomic and physiologic changes to the body's systems. These changes can affect the patterns of injuries seen and make the assessment of an injured pregnant patient especially challenging. The prehospital care provider is dealing with two or more patients and must be aware of the changes that have occurred to the mother's anatomy and physiology throughout the pregnancy.

A human pregnancy typically last about 40 weeks from conception to birth, and this period is divided into three sections, or trimesters. The first trimester ends about the 12th week of gestation, and the second trimester is slightly longer than the other two, ending about week 28.

Following conception and implantation of the fetus, the uterus continues to enlarge through the 38th week of pregnancy. Until about the 12th week, the growing uterus remains protected by the bony pelvis. By the 20th week of gestation, the top of the uterus (fundus) is at the umbilicus, and the fundus approaches the xiphoid process by the 38th week. This anatomic change makes the uterus and its contents more susceptible to both blunt and penetrating injury (Figure 12-13). Injury to

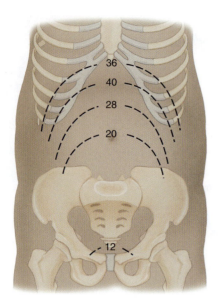

FIGURE 12-13 Fundal height.

the uterus can include rupture, penetration, abruptio placentae (when a portion of the placenta is pulled away from the uterine wall), and premature rupture of the membranes (Figure 12-14). The placenta and gravid uterus are highly vascular; injuries to these structures can result in profound hemorrhage. Because the hemorrhage can also be concealed inside the uterus or peritoneal cavity, it may not be externally visible.

Although a marked protuberance of the abdomen is obvious in late pregnancy, abdominal organs remain essentially unchanged, with the exception of the uterus. Intestine that is displaced superiorly is shielded by the uterus in the last two trimesters of pregnancy. The increased size and weight of the uterus alter the patient's center of gravity and increase the risk of falls. Because of its prominence, the gravid abdomen is often injured in a fall.

In addition to these anatomic changes, physiologic changes also occur throughout pregnancy. The mother's heart rate normally increases throughout pregnancy by 15 to 20 beats/minute above normal by the third trimester. This makes the interpretation of tachycardia more difficult. Systolic and diastolic blood pressures normally drop 5 to 15 mm Hg during the second trimester but often return to normal at term. By the 10th week of pregnancy, the mother's cardiac output increases by 1 to 1.5 liters/minute. By term, the mother's blood volume has increased by about 50%. *Because of these increases in cardiac output and blood volume, the pregnant patient may lose 30% to 35% of her blood volume before signs and symptoms of hypovolemia become apparent.* Hypovolemic shock may induce premature labor in patients in the third trimester. Oxytocin, which is released along with antidiuretic hormone (ADH) in response to loss of circulating blood volume, stimulates uterine contractions.

Some women may have significant hypotension when supine. This supine hypotension of pregnancy typically occurs in the third trimester and is caused by the compression of the vena cava by the uterus. This dramatically decreases venous return to the heart, and because there is less filling, cardiac output and blood pressure fall (Figure 12-15).

The following maneuvers may be used to relieve supine hypotension:

1. The woman may be placed on her left side (left lateral decubitus position), or if spinal immobilization is indicated, 4 to 6 inches (10 to 15 cm) of padding should be placed under the right side of the long backboard (Figure 12-16).
2. If the patient cannot be rotated, the patient's right leg should be elevated to displace the uterus to the left.
3. The uterus may be manually displaced toward the patient's left side.

These three maneuvers reduce compression on the vena cava, increasing venous return to the heart and improving cardiac output.

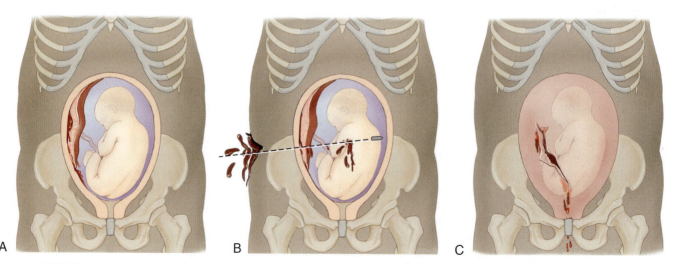

FIGURE 12-14 Diagram of uterine trauma: **A.** Abruptio placentae, **B.** Gunshot to the uterus, **C.** Ruptured uterus.

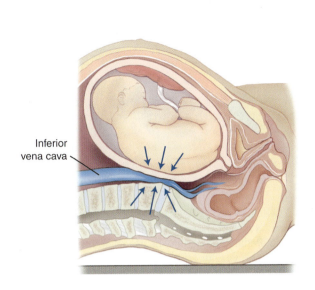

FIGURE 12-15 Full-term uterus compressing the vena cava.

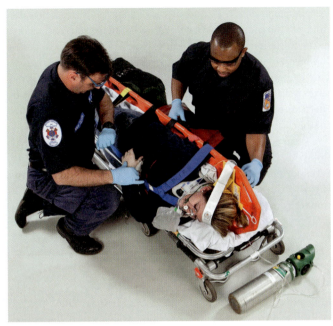

FIGURE 12-16 Photo of immobilized pregnant patient tilted to side.

During the third trimester, the diaphragm is elevated and may be associated with mild dyspnea, especially when the patient is supine. Peristalsis (propulsive, muscular movements of intestines) is slower during pregnancy, so food may remain in the stomach many hours after eating. Therefore, the pregnant patient is at greater risk for vomiting and subsequent aspiration.

Toxemia of pregnancy (also known as eclampsia) is a late complication of pregnancy. Whereas *pre-eclampsia* is characterized by edema and hypertension, *eclampsia* is characterized by mental status changes and seizures, thus mimicking TBI. A careful neurologic assessment and asking about complications of pregnancy and other medical conditions are important.[11,12]

Assessment

Pregnancy typically does not alter the mother's airway, but significant respiratory distress may occur when a patient in her third trimester is placed supine on a long backboard. The decrease in peristalsis of the GI tract makes vomiting and aspiration more likely. Airway patency and pulmonary function are assessed, including auscultation of breath sounds and monitoring of pulse oximetry.

As with hemoperitoneum from other sources, intra-abdominal bleeding associated with uterine injury may not produce peritonitis for hours. More likely, blood loss from any injury may be masked by the pregnant female's increased cardiac output and blood volume. Therefore, a high index of suspicion and assessment for subtle changes (e.g., skin color) may provide important clues. In general, the condition of the fetus often depends on the condition of the mother; however, the fetus may be in jeopardy while the mother's condi-

tion and vital signs appear hemodynamically normal. This occurs because the body shunts blood away from the uterus (and fetus) to the vital organs. Neurologic changes should be noted and documented, although the exact etiology may not be identifiable in the prehospital setting.

As with the nonpregnant patient, auscultation of bowel sounds is generally not helpful in the prehospital setting. Similarly, spending valuable minutes searching for fetal heart tones at the scene is also not useful; their presence or absence will not alter prehospital management. The external genitalia should be checked for evidence of vaginal bleeding, and the patient should be asked about the presence of contractions and fetal movement. Contractions may indicate that premature labor has begun, whereas a decrease in fetal movement may be an ominous sign.

Management

With an injured pregnant patient, the survival of the fetus is best ensured by focus on the mother's condition. In essence, for the baby to survive, usually the mother needs to survive. It is wise to anticipate vomiting and have suction nearby. Priority is given to ensuring an adequate patent airway and supporting ventilatory function. Sufficient oxygen should be administered to maintain a pulse oximetry reading of 95% or higher. Ventilations may need to be assisted, especially in the later stages of pregnancy.

The goals of shock management are essentially the same as for any patient and include IV fluid administration, especially if evidence of decompensated shock is present. Any evidence of vaginal bleeding or a rigid, board-like abdomen with external bleeding in the last trimester of pregnancy may indicate abruptio placentae or a ruptured uterus. These conditions threaten not only the life of the fetus, but also that of the mother because exsanguination can occur rapidly. No good data exist to define the best target blood pressure for an injured pregnant patient. However, restoration of normal systolic and mean blood pressures will most likely result in better fetal perfusion, despite the risk of promoting additional internal hemorrhage in the mother.

Transport of the pregnant trauma patient should not be delayed. Every pregnant trauma patient should be rapidly transported—even those who appear to have only minor injuries—to the closest appropriate facility. An ideal facility is one that has both surgical and obstetric capabilities immediately available. Adequate resuscitation of the mother is the key to survival of the mother and fetus.

Genitourinary Injuries

Injuries to the kidneys, ureters, and bladder most often present with hematuria. This sign will not be noted unless the patient has a urinary catheter inserted. Because the kidneys receive a significant portion of cardiac output, blunt or penetrating injuries to these organs may result in life-threatening retroperitoneal hemorrhage. Pelvic fractures may be associated with lacerations of the urinary bladder and the walls of the vagina or the rectum walls. Open pelvic fractures, such as those with deep groin or perineal lacerations may result in severe external hemorrhage.

Trauma to the external genitalia may occur from multiple mechanisms, although injuries resulting from ejection from a motorcycle or motor vehicle, an industrial accident, gunshot wounds, or sexual assault typically predominate. Because of the numerous nerve endings in these organs, such inju-

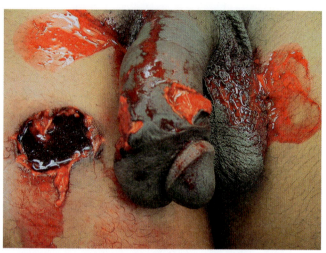

FIGURE 12-17   Gunshot wound through penis and into right thigh. Penile injuries may be associated with significant hemorrhage.

ries are associated with significant pain and psychological concern. These organs also contain numerous blood vessels, and copious amounts of blood may be seen (Figure 12-17). In general, such bleeding can be controlled with direct pressure or a pressure dressing. Dressings should not be inserted into the vagina or the urethra to control bleeding, particularly in pregnant women. If direct pressure is not required to control hemorrhage, these injuries should be covered with moist, clean, saline-soaked gauze. Any amputated parts should be managed as described in Chapter 13. Further evaluation of all genital injuries should occur at the hospital.

SUMMARY

- Intra-abdominal injuries are often life threatening because of internal hemorrhage and spillage of gastrointestinal contents into the peritoneal cavity.
- The extent of internal injuries is not identifiable in the prehospital setting; therefore mechanism of injury in combination with signs of abdominal trauma should increase the provider's index of suspicion.
- Management of the patient with abdominal trauma includes oxygenation, hemorrhage control, and rapid packaging for transport. Spinal immobilization is not necessary for penetrating torso trauma.
- Balanced resuscitation with crystalloid solutions permits perfusion of vital organs while potentially minimizing the risk of aggravating internal hemorrhage.

- As emergent surgical intervention may be lifesaving, a patient with abdominal trauma should be transported to a facility with immediate surgical capability.
- The PASG may be useful for prolonged transport of patients with decompensated shock and suspected abdominal or pelvic hemorrhage.
- The anatomic and physiologic changes of pregnancy have implications for the pattern of injury, presentation of signs and symptoms of trauma, and management of the pregnant trauma patient.
- Management of potential fetal compromise caused by trauma is accomplished through effective resuscitation of the mother.

SCENARIO SOLUTION

The patient is tender over his left lower ribs and left upper quadrant. These findings can represent either injuries to the thorax, intra-abdominal organs, or both. His vital signs are consistent with compensated hypovolemic shock, and a hemothorax or intra-abdominal bleeding must be considered. More likely, the tenderness over the lower ribs may indicate fractured ribs with an associated laceration of the spleen, resulting in intraperitoneal hemorrhage. Oxygen should be administered and the patient packaged for transport. En route to the trauma center, intravenous access is obtained; however given the patient's blood pressure, crystalloid fluid should be administered sparingly as aggressive fluid infusion may raise his blood pressure and lead to increased bleeding. ■

References

1. American College of Surgeons Committee on Trauma: Abdominal trauma. In ACS Committee on Trauma: *Advanced trauma life support for doctors, student course manual,* ed 8, pp. 111–126, Chicago, 2008, ACS.

2. Rozycki GS, Ochsner MG, Jaffin JH, et al: Prospective evaluation of surgeons' use of ultrasound in the evaluation of trauma patients. *J Trauma Injury Infect Crit Care* 34(4):516, 1993.

3. Rozycki GS, Ochsner MG, Schmidt JA, et al: A prospective study of surgeon-performed ultrasound as the primary adjuvant modality for injured patient assessment. *J Trauma Injury Infect Crit Care* 39(3):492, 1995.

4. Rozycki GS, Ochsner MG, Feliciano DV, et al: Early detection of hemoperitoneum by ultrasound examination of the right upper quadrant: a multicenter study. *J Trauma Injury Infect Crit Care* 45(5):878, 1998.

5. Rozycki GS, Ballard RB, Feliciano DV, et al: Surgeon-performed ultrasound for the assessment of truncal injuries: Lessons learned from 1540 patients. *Ann Surg* 228(4):557, 1998.

6. Polk JD, Fallon WF Jr: The use of focused assessment with sonography for trauma (FAST) by a prehospital air medical team in the trauma arrest patient. *Prehosp Emerg Care* 4(1):82, 2000.

7. Melanson SW, McCarthy J, Stromski CJ, et al: Aeromedical trauma sonography by flight crews with a miniature ultrasound unit. *Prehosp Emerg Care* 5(4):399, 2001.

8. Walcher F, Kortum S, Kirschning T, et al: Optimized management of polytraumatized patients by prehospital ultrasound. *Unfall-chirurg* 105(11):986, 2002.

9. Strode CA, Rubal BJ, Gerhardt RT, et al: Wireless and satellite transmission of prehospital focused abdominal sonography for trauma. *Prehosp Emerg Care* 7(3):375, 2003.

10. Heegaard WG, Ho J, Hildebrandt DA: The prehospital ultrasound study: Results of the first six months (abstract). *Prehosp Emerg Care* 13(1):139, 2009.

11. American College of Surgeons Committee on Trauma: Trauma in women. In ACS Committee on Trauma: *Advanced trauma life support for doctors, student course manual,* ed 7, pp. 259–268, Chicago, 2004, ACS.

12. Knudson MM, Rozycki GS, Paquin MM: Reproductive system trauma. In Moore EE, Feliciano DV, Mattox KL, editors: *Trauma,* ed 5, New York, 2004, McGraw-Hill.

13. Pachter HL, Hofstetter SR: The current status of nonoperative management of adult blunt hepatic injuries. *Am J Surg* 169:442–454, 1995.

Suggested Reading

Berry MJ, McMurray RG, Katz VL: Pulmonary and ventilatory responses to pregnancy, immersion and exercise. *J Appl Physiol* 66(2):857, 1989.

Coburn M: Genitourinary trauma. In Moore EE, Feliciano DV, Mattox KL, editors: *Trauma,* ed 5, New York, 2004, McGraw-Hill, p 809.

Esposito TJ: Trauma during pregnancy. *Emerg Med Clin North Am* 12:167, 1994.

Frame SB, Timberlake GA, Rosh DS, et al: Penetrating injuries of the abdominal aorta. *Am Surg* 56(10):651, 1990.

Hill DA, Delaney LM, Duflou J: A population-based study of outcome after injury to car occupants and to pedestrians. *J Trauma* 40(3):351, 1996.

Pearlman MD, Tintinalli JE, Lorenz RP: Blunt trauma during pregnancy. *N Engl J Med* 323:1606, 1991.

Schoenfeld A, Ziv E, Stein L, et al: Seat belts in pregnancy and the obstetrician. *Obstet Gynecol Surv* 42(5):275, 1987.

Timberlake GA, McSwain NE Jr: Trauma in pregnancy: A 10-year perspective. *Am Surg* 55(3):151, 1989.

Tso EL, Beaver BL, Haller JA Jr: Abdominal injuries in restrained pediatric passengers. *J Pediatr Surg* 28(7):915, 1993.

CHAPTER 13

Musculoskeletal Trauma

CHAPTER OBJECTIVES

At the completion of this chapter, the reader will be able to do the following:

- ✓ List the three categories used to classify patients with extremity injuries, and relate this classification to priority of care.

- ✓ Describe the primary and secondary surveys as related to extremity trauma.

- ✓ Discuss the significance of hemorrhage in both open and closed fractures of the long bones, pelvis, and ribs.

- ✓ List the five major pathophysiologic problems associated with extremity injuries that may require management in the prehospital setting.

- ✓ Explain the management of extremity trauma as an isolated injury and in the presence of multisystem trauma.

- ✓ Given a scenario involving an extremity injury, select an appropriate splint and splinting method.

- ✓ Describe the special considerations involved in femur fracture management.

- ✓ Describe the management of amputations.

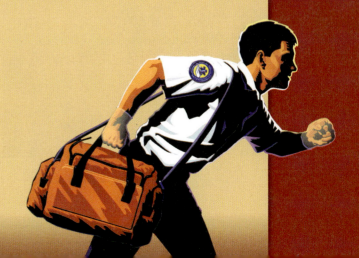

SCENARIO

You are called to a construction site where a worker is complaining of pain to his right thigh after a fork lift pinned him against a container. Once you determined the scene was safe to enter, you discover the patient lying on the ground. He is able to describe the sequence of events leading up to his injury but appears tired, is in a great deal of pain, and he is diaphoretic and pale. You've determined that his airway is open and he is breathing without difficulty or obstruction at a rate of 24 breaths/minute. The patient complains only of pain to the right thigh and loss of sensation and the ability to move beyond the injury. He has a pulse of 120 and blood pressure is 104/76. On exposing the right leg you note swelling midthigh and shortening of the limb which is rotated outward.

What do the kinematics of this event tell you about the potential injuries for this patient? What type of injury does this patient have and what would your management priorities be?

Musculoskeletal injury, although common in trauma patients, rarely poses an immediate life-threatening condition. Skeletal trauma can be life threatening, however, when it produces severe blood loss (hemorrhage), either externally or from internal bleeding into the extremity or the retroperitoneum (in the case of the pelvis).

When caring for a critical trauma patient, the prehospital care provider has three primary considerations with regard to extremity injuries:

1. Maintain assessment priorities. Do not be distracted by dramatic, non-life-threatening musculoskeletal injuries (Figure 13-1).
2. Recognize potentially life-threatening musculoskeletal injuries.
3. Recognize the kinematics that created the musculoskeletal injuries and the potential for other life-threatening injuries caused by that energy transfer.

If a life-threatening or potentially life-threatening condition is discovered anywhere in the body during the primary survey (initial assessment), the secondary survey (detailed history and physical examination) should not be started. Any problems found during the primary survey should be corrected in ABC order before moving to the secondary survey (see later discussion). This may mean delaying the secondary survey until the patient is en route or even until arrival at the emergency department (ED).

Critical trauma patients should be transported on longboards to allow for resuscitation and treatment of both critical and noncritical injuries. Use of a longboard allows for immobilization of the entire patient and all of his or her injuries on a single platform that makes it possible to move the victim without disturbing the splinting. Although some injuries are more obvious than others, the prehospital care provider should treat every painful musculoskeletal injury as a possible fracture and immobilize it to limit the potential for further injury and to provide some comfort and reduction of pain.

Anatomy and Physiology

Understanding the gross anatomy and physiology of the human body is an important piece of the prehospital care provider's fund of knowledge. Anatomy and physiology are the foundations on which assessment and management are based. Without a good grasp of the structures of the bones and muscles, one will not be able to relate kinematics and superficial injuries to injuries that are internal. Although this textbook does not discuss all the anatomy and physiology of the musculoskeletal system, it reviews some of the basics.

The mature human body has approximately 206 bones separated into categories by shape: long, short, flat, sutural, and sesamoid. *Long bones* include the femur, humerus, ulna, radius, tibia, and fibula. *Short bones* include metacarpals,

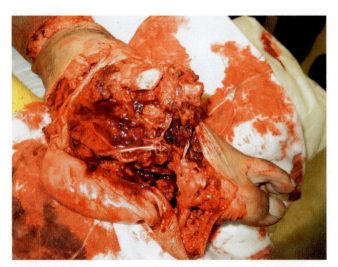

FIGURE 13-1 Some extremity injuries, although dramatic in appearance, are not life threatening.

metatarsals, and phalanges. *Flat bones* are usually thin and compact, such as the sternum, ribs, and scapulae. *Sutural bones* are part of the skull and are located between the joints of certain cranial bones. *Sesamoid bones* are bones located within tendons; the patella is the largest sesamoid bone (Figure 13-2).

The human body has more than 700 individual muscles, which are categorized by function. The muscles that are specific to this chapter are the voluntary, or skeletal, muscles.

They are termed *skeletal* because they move the skeletal system. Muscles in this category voluntarily move the structures of the body (Figure 13-3).

Other important structures discussed in this chapter are tendons and ligaments. A *tendon* is a band of tough, inelastic, fibrous tissue that connects a muscle to bone. It is the white part at the end of a muscle that directly attaches a muscle to the bone that it will move. A *ligament* is a band of tough, fibrous tissue connecting bone to bone; its function is to hold joints together.

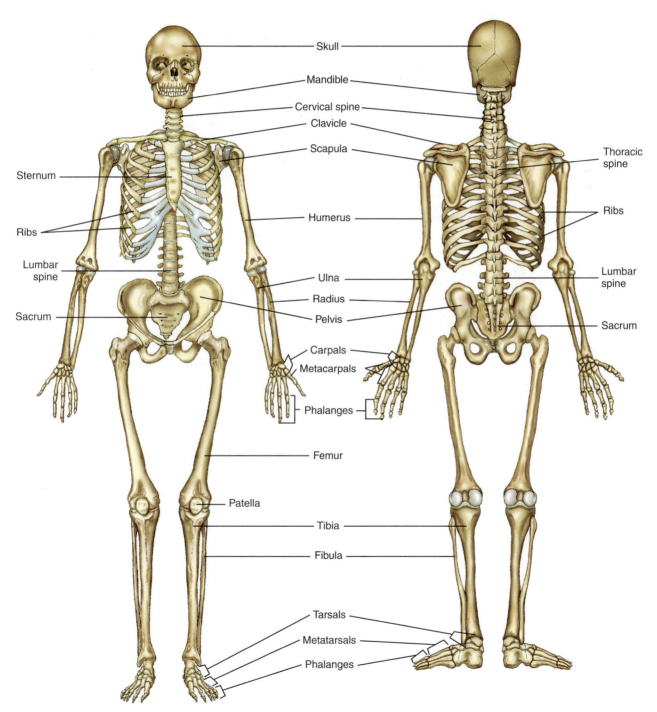

FIGURE 13-2   The human skeleton.

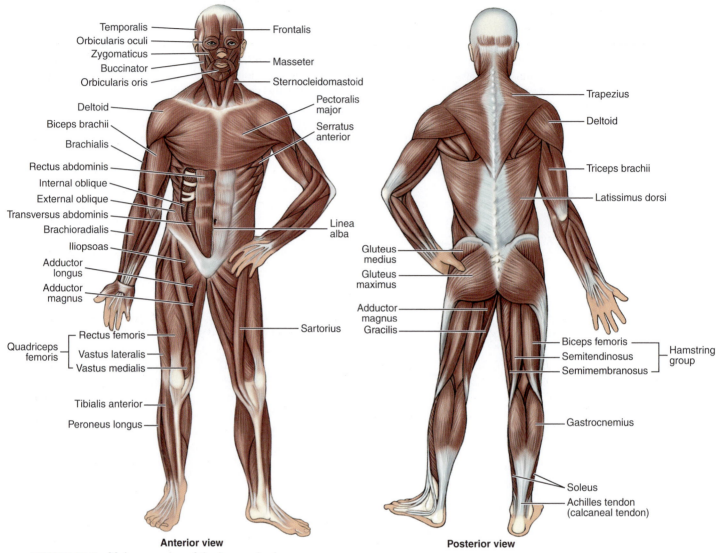

FIGURE 13-3 Major muscles of the human body.
(From Herlihy B, Maebius NK: *The human body in health and illness,* ed 2, St. Louis, 2003, Saunders.)

Assessment

Musculoskeletal trauma can be categorized into the following three main types:

1. Life-threatening injuries resulting from musculoskeletal trauma, such as external hemorrhage, or internal hemorrhage associated with pelvic or femur fractures with life-threatening blood loss.
2. Non-life-threatening musculoskeletal trauma associated with multisystem life-threatening trauma (life-threatening injuries plus limb fractures).
3. Isolated non-life-threatening musculoskeletal trauma (isolated limb fractures).

The purpose of the primary survey is to identify and treat life-threatening injuries. The presence of a non-life-threatening musculoskeletal injury can be an indicator of possible multisystem trauma and should not distract the prehospital care provider from performing a complete primary assessment. Although the presence of musculoskeletal trauma should not distract from the care of more life-threatening conditions, the injuries should be looked at as possible indicators for potential life-threatening conditions. Evaluating the kinematics that created the obvious injuries may point to occult serious injuries.

Kinematics

Understanding the kinematics involved in an injury is one of the most important functions of the assessment and management of a trauma patient. Rapidly determining the kinematics and whether it involved low-energy versus high-energy transference (e.g., falling from a bike vs. being thrown from a motorcycle) will lead the prehospital care provider to the recognition of most critical injuries. The best source for determining the kinematics is directly from the patient. If the patient is unresponsive, details of the injury mechanism can be obtained from witnesses. Often a "best guess" approach to the events based on injuries can be used if no one was present at the incident. This information should be reported to the receiving facility and documented on the patient care record.

Based on the kinematics, the prehospital care provider may develop a high index of suspicion for the injuries that a patient might have sustained. Consideration of the kinematics may bring to mind additional injuries for which the provider should assess, given knowledge of various injury patterns. For example:

- If a patient jumps out of a window feet first, the primary injury suspicion would be fractures of the calcaneus, tibia, fibula, femur, pelvis, and spine and aortic shear injuries. However, secondary injuries might include abdominal injury or head injury from tumbling forward after hitting the ground.
- If a patient is involved in a motorcycle collision with a telephone pole and hits his or her head on the pole, primary injuries will include head, cervical spine, and thoracic injury. A secondary injury might include a femur fracture from "striking" the femur on the handlebars.

Another example involves a patient riding in the passenger side of a vehicle that sustains a side-impact collision. As discussed in Chapter 4, Newton's first law of motion states that a body in motion will stay in motion until acted on by an equal but opposite force. The vehicle is the moving object until acted on by the other vehicle. The door of the target vehicle is pushed against the upper arm, which can then be pushed into the chest wall, producing rib fractures, lung contusion, and possibly a fractured humerus. Given the kinematics of this crash, suspicion for musculoskeletal injury would include humerus, pelvis, and femur fractures. Further injury suspicion would include rib fractures, chest wall muscle injury, and lung and heart injuries. Another secondary injury to consider is abrasion from a deployed air bag.

Another possible injury from a side-impact collision results from an unrestrained passenger becoming a missile (object) inside the vehicle. The other vehicle striking the passenger side sets the passenger in motion until he or she is stopped by another object, such as the driver. However, near-side injuries are more severe than far-side injuries In this case, the kinematics to consider for the driver is the energy delivered by the unrestrained passenger's body.

A basic understanding of kinematics guides the provider's assessment for the less obvious injuries.

Primary and Secondary Surveys

Primary Survey

The first step of any assessment is to ensure scene safety and evaluate the situation. Once the scene is safe, the patient can be assessed. The primary survey addresses the immediately life-threatening conditions that are identified. Although angulated fractures or partial amputations may draw the provider's attention, life-threatening conditions should take priority. Airway, breathing, circulation, disability, and exposure (ABCDE) remain the most important parts of assessment. For a patient with life-threatening conditions identified in the primary survey, management of musculoskeletal trauma is delayed until those problems are corrected; however external hemorrhage is included in the primary survey and must be controlled when deemed life threatening. If the patient has no life-threatening injuries, the prehospital care provider proceeds to the secondary survey.

Secondary Survey

Assessment of the extremities occurs during the secondary survey. To facilitate examination, the provider considers removing any clothing that was not removed during the primary survey, as allowed by the environment. If the mechanism of injury is not obvious, the patient or bystanders can be questioned about how the injuries occurred. The patient should also be queried about the presence of pain in the extremities. Most patients with significant musculoskeletal injuries have pain, unless a spinal cord or peripheral nerve injury is present. Assessment of the extremities also includes evaluating the pain, weakness, or abnormal sensations in the extremities, such as:

- Bones and joints. This evaluation is accomplished by inspecting for deformities that may represent fractures or dislocations (Figure 13-4) and palpating the extremity for tenderness and crepitus. *Crepitus* is the grinding feeling that bones make when the fractured ends rub against one another. Crepitus can be elicited by palpating the site of injury and by movement of the extremity. Crepitus sounds like a "snap, crackle, and pop" or the popping of plastic "bubble wrap" used for packing. This feeling of bones grating against one another during the assessment of a patient can produce further injury, and therefore, once the crepitus is noted, no additional or repetitive steps should be taken to produce it. Crepitus is a distinct feeling that is not easily forgotten.
- Soft tissue injuries. The provider visually inspects for swelling, lacerations, abrasions, hematomas, skin color, and wounds. Any wound adjacent to a fracture may indicate the presence of an open fracture. Firmness and tenseness of the soft tissues may indicate presence of a compartment syndrome.
- Perfusion. This is accomplished by palpating distal pulses (radial or ulnar in the upper extremity and dorsalis pedis

FIGURE 13-4   Common Joint Dislocation Deformities

Joint	Direction	Deformity
Shoulder	Anterior	Squared off
	Posterior	Locked in internal rotation
Elbow	Posterior	Olecranon prominent posteriorly
Hip	Anterior	Flexed, abducted, externally rotated
	Posterior	Flexed, adducted, internally rotated
Knee	Anteroposterior	Loss of normal contour, extended
Ankle	Lateral is most common	Externally rotated, prominent medial malleolus
Subtalar joint	Lateral is most common	Laterally displaced os calcis

(From: American College of Surgeons Committee on Trauma: *Advanced Trauma Life Support,* ed 8, Chicago, 2009, ACS.)

fracture is suspected, do not ask the patient to move the extremity, as such movement can induce significant pain and possibly convert a closed fracture to an open fracture. For most situations in the prehospital setting, evaluating gross neurologic functioning is sufficient.

- Motor function can be assessed by first asking the patient if any weakness is noted. Motor function in the upper extremity is evaluated by having the patient open and close a fist and by testing grip strength (the patient squeezes the providers fingers), while lower extremity motor function is tested by having the patient wiggle their toes.
- Sensory function is evaluated by asking about the presence of any abnormal sensations or numbness and testing to see if the patient feels the provider touching various locations on the extremities, including the fingers and toes. Figures 13-5 and 13-6 provide information on performing more detailed evaluations of motor and sensory function of the extremities.

Repeat evaluation of extremity perfusion and neurologic functioning should be performed after any splinting procedure.

or posterior tibial in the lower extremity) and noting capillary refill time in the fingers or toes. Absence of distal pulses in the extremities can indicate disruption of an artery, compression of the vessel by a hematoma or bone fragment, or a compartment syndrome. Large or expanding hematomas may indicate the presence of an injury to a large vessel.
- Neurologic function. The provider assesses both motor and sensory function in the extremities. If a long bone

Associated Injuries

While performing the secondary survey, clues to the kinematics may be uncovered and an injury pattern may be suspected. Such injury patterns can prompt the provider to assess for occult injuries associated with specific fractures. An example would be a thoracic injury associated with a shoulder injury. Thorough examination of the entire body will ensure injuries are not missed. Figure 13-7 provides some examples of associated injuries.

FIGURE 13-5   Peripheral Nerve Assessment of Upper Extremities

Nerve	Motor	Sensation	Injury
Ulnar	Index finger abduction	Little finger	Elbow injury
Median distal	Thenar contraction with opposition	Index finger	Wrist dislocation
Median, anterior interosseous	Index tip flexion		Supracondylar fracture of humerous (children)
Musculocutaneous	Elbow tip flexion	Lateral forearm	Anterior shoulder dislocation
Radial	Thumb, finger metacarpophalangeal extension	First dorsal web space	Distal humeral shaft, anterior shoulder dislocation
Axillary	Deltoid	Lateral shoulder	Anterior shoulder dislocation, proximal humerous fracture

(From: American College of Surgeons Committee on Trauma, *Advanced Trauma Life Support,* ed 8, Chicago, 2009, ACS.)

FIGURE 13-6   **Peripheral Nerve Assessment of Lower Extremities**

Nerve	Motor	Sensation	Injury
Femoral	Knee extension	Anterior knee	Pubic rami fractures
Obturator	Hip adduction	Medial thigh	Obturator ring fractures
Posterior tibial	Toe flexion	Sole of foot	Knee dislocation
Superficial peroneal	Ankle eversion	Lateral dorsum of foot	Fibular neck fracture, knee dislocation
Deep peroneal	Ankle/toe dorsiflexion	Dorsal first to second web space	Fibular neck fracture, compartment syndrome
Sciatic nerve	Plantar dorsiflexion	Foot	Posterior hip dislocation
Superior gluteal	Hip abduction	—	Acetabular fracture
Inferior gluteal	Gluteus maximus hip extension	—	Acetabular fracture

(From: American College of Surgeons Committee on Trauma, *Advanced Trauma Life Support,* ed 8, Chicago, 2009, ACS.)

Specific Musculoskeletal Injuries

Injuries to the extremities result in two primary problems that require management in the prehospital setting: hemorrhage and instability (fractures and dislocations).

Hemorrhage

Bleeding can be dramatic or subtle. Whether it is the capillary ooze of a large abrasion, the dark red blood flowing from a superficial laceration, or the bright red spurting of an open artery, the amount of blood lost and the rate of its loss will determine the patient's ability to compensate or descend into shock. A good rule to remember is, "No bleeding is minor; every red blood cell counts." Even a small trickle of blood can add up to substantial blood loss if it is ignored for a long period.

External arterial bleeding should be identified during the primary survey. Generally, this type of bleeding is easily recognized, but assessment can be difficult when blood is hidden under a patient or in heavy or dark clothing. Ideally, obvious hemorrhage is controlled while the patient's airway and breathing are being managed, if sufficient assistance is present; otherwise, it is controlled when identified during assessment of circulation or when the patient's clothing is removed. Estimation of external blood loss is extremely difficult. Although less experienced individuals tend to overestimate the amount of external hemorrhage, underestimation is also possible as overt signs of external blood loss may not always be apparent. A recent study suggested that prehospital estimates of blood loss were inaccurate and not clinically beneficial.[1] The reasons for these inaccurate blood loss estimates are many and include that the patient may have been moved from the site of injury, or lost blood may have been absorbed by clothing or soil or washed away in water or by rain.

FIGURE 13-7   **Injuries Associated with Musculoskeletal Injuries**

Injury	Missed/Associated Injury
Clavical fracture Scapular fracture Fracture and/or dislocation of shoulder	Major thoracic injury, especially pulmonary contusion and rib fractures
Displaced thoracic spine fracture	Thoracic aortic rupture
Spine fracture	Intraabdominal injury
Fracture/dislocation of elbow	Brachial artery injury Median, ulnar, and radial nerve injury
Major pelvic disruption (motor vehicle occupant)	Abdominal, thoracic, or head injury
Major pelvic disruption (motorcyclist or pedestrian)	Pelvic vascular hemorrhage
Femur fracture	Femoral neck fracture Posterior hip dislocation
Posterior knee dislocation	Femoral fracture Posterior hip dislocation
Knee dislocation or displaced tibial plateau fracture	Popliteal artery and nerve injuries
Calcaneal fracture	Spine injury or fracture Fracture-dislocation of hindfoot Tibial plateau fracture
Open fracture	70% incidence of associated nonskeletal injury

(From: American College of Surgeons Committee on Trauma, *Advanced Trauma Life Support,* ed 8, Chicago, 2009, ACS.)

Internal hemorrhage is also common with musculoskeletal trauma. It may result from damage to major blood vessels, from disrupted muscle, and from the bone marrow of fractured bones. Continued swelling of an extremity or a cold, pale, pulseless extremity could indicate internal hemorrhage from major arteries or veins. Significant internal blood loss can be associated with fractures (Figure 13-8). The prehospital care provider considers both the potential internal and the external blood loss associated with extremity trauma. This will help the provider anticipate the development of shock, prepare for the possibility of systemic deterioration, and intervene appropriately to minimize its occurrence.

Management

The initial management of external hemorrhage involves the application of direct pressure. As discussed in Chapter 8, elevation of an extremity has not been shown to slow hemorrhage, and in musculoskeletal trauma, it may aggravate injuries that are present. If hemorrhage is not controlled with direct pressure or a pressure dressing, a tourniquet should be applied, following the principles described in Chapter 8. A recommended topical hemostatic agent can be considered for hemorrhage that is not amenable to use of a tourniquet, such as in the groin or axilla. Such agents may also be utilized for prolonged-transport situations.

After controlling bleeding in patients with life-threatening hemorrhage from an extremity, prehospital care providers can reassess the primary survey and focus on resuscitation and rapid transport to the facility that can best treat the condition. During transport, administration of oxygen and initiation of intravenous (IV) fluid resuscitation for patients with shock can begin, keeping in mind that when internal hemorrhage is suspected, the target systolic blood pressure is 80–90 mm Hg (mean BP 60–65 mm Hg.) For patients with more minor bleeding and no signs of shock or other life-threatening problems, bleeding can be controlled with direct pressure and the secondary survey performed.

FIGURE 13-8 Approximate Internal Blood Loss Associated with Fractures

Bone fractured	Internal blood loss (ml)
Rib	125
Radius or ulna	250–500
Humerus	500–750
Tibia or fibula	500–1000
Femur	1000–2000
Pelvis	1000–massive

Instability (Fractures and Dislocations)

Tears of the supporting structures of a joint, fracture of a bone, and major muscle or tendon injury affect the ability of an extremity to support itself. The two injuries that cause instability of bones or joints are fractures and dislocations.

Fractures

If a bone is fractured, immobilizing it will reduce the potential for further injury and pain. Movement of the sharp ends of the fractured bone may damage blood vessels, resulting in internal and external hemorrhage. Additionally, fractures can damage muscle tissue and nerves.

In general, fractures are classified as either closed or open. In a *closed fracture,* the skin is not punctured by the bone ends, whereas in an *open fracture,* the integrity of the skin has been interrupted (Figure 13-9A). Orthopedic surgeons may classify fractures by their pattern (e.g., greenstick, comminuted), but these types cannot be differentiated without an x-ray, and knowledge of the fracture pattern really does not alter field management.

Closed fractures are fractures in which the bone has been broken but the patient has no loss of skin integrity (i.e., the skin is not broken) (Figure 13-9B). Signs of a closed fracture include tenderness, deformity, hematomas, swelling, and crepitus, although in some patients, tenderness may be the only finding. Pulses, skin color, and motor and sensory function should be assessed distal to the suspected fracture site. Asking a patient to move the fractured extremity could result in an open fracture. It is not always true that an extremity is not fractured because the patient can voluntarily move it; adrenalin from a traumatic event may motivate patients to do things they normally would not tolerate. Additionally, some patients have a remarkably high pain tolerance.

Open fractures usually occur when a sharp bone end penetrates the skin from the inside or an injury lacerates the skin and muscle down to a fracture site (Figure 13-9C). When a bone punctures the skin, the end can be contaminated with bacteria from the skin or environment. This can lead to the serious complication of a bone infection *(osteomyelitis),* which can interfere with healing of the fracture. Although the skin wound associated with an open fracture often is not associated with significant hemorrhage, persistent bleeding may come from the marrow cavity of the bone or as a hematoma deep inside the tissue decompresses through the skin opening. Any open wound near a possible fracture needs to be considered an open fracture and treated as such. A protruding bone or bone end should generally not be intentionally replaced; however, the bones occasionally return to a near-normal position when realigned or by the muscle spasms that usually occur with fractures. Inadequate splinting or rough handling of a fractured extremity may convert a closed fracture into an open one. Open fractures may be easy to locate on a trauma patient. Although bone protruding from a wound is pretty obvious, soft tissue injuries in proximity to a fracture/deformity may have resulted from a bone end that

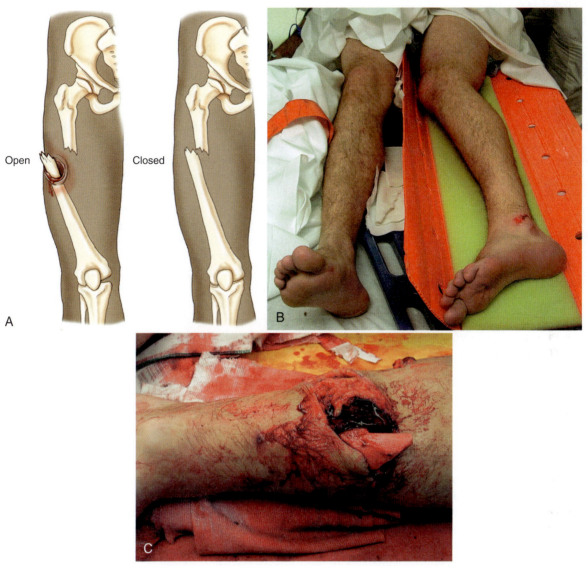

FIGURE 13-9 **A.** Open versus closed fracture. **B.** Closed fracture of the femur. Note the internal rotation and shortening of the left leg. **C.** Open fracture of the tibia.

broke through the surface of the skin only to recede back into the tissue.

As noted earlier, fractures may result in significant internal hemorrhage into the tissue planes surrounding the fracture. The two most common fractures associated with the greatest hemorrhage are femur and pelvic fractures. An adult can lose 1000 to 2000 ml of blood per thigh. Thus, internal hemorrhage associated with bilateral femur fractures may be sufficient to result in death from hypovolemic shock.

Pelvic fractures also are a common cause of significant hemorrhage (Figure 13-10). Multiple small arteries and veins lie adjacent to the pelvis and may be torn by bone ends or as the sacroiliac joints fracture or open up. Overaggressive palpation or manipulation of the pelvis (pelvic rock) can signifi-

cantly increase blood loss when an unstable pelvic fracture is present. To assess the pelvis, gentle palpation is acceptable but should only be performed once. Gentle manual pressure anterior to posterior and from the sides may identify crepitus or instability. The area around the pelvis is a "potential space" because it can expand and accommodate a huge amount of blood. Because of the amount of space in the pelvic cavity, hemorrhage may occur with few external signs of compromise. Open fractures of the pelvis, often resulting when a pedestrian is struck by a car or when an occupant is ejected from a motor vehicle, are particularly deadly. Falls can also result in pelvic fracture, so it is important to consider pelvic fracture with any mechanism that involves energy absorbed by the pelvis or complaints of pain around the pelvis. Often,

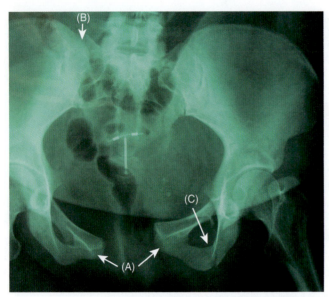

FIGURE 13-10 Radiograph of a severe anterior-posterior compression fracture of the pelvis. There is marked widening of the symphysis pubis (**A**), disruption of the sacroiliac joint (**B**), and fractures of the pubic rami (**C**).

massive external—rather than internal—hemorrhage results, and bone ends may lacerate the rectum or vagina, resulting in severe pelvic infection.

Management.

Open and Closed Fracture. The first consideration in managing fractures is to control hemorrhage and treat for shock. Direct pressure and pressure dressings will control virtually all external hemorrhage encountered in the field. Open wounds or exposed bone ends should be covered with a sterile dressing moistened with sterile normal saline or water. Internal hemorrhage is primarily controlled by immobilization, which has the added benefit of providing pain relief. If the bone ends of an open fracture retract into the wound during splinting, this information must be documented on the patient care record and reported to ED personnel. There is little to be gained from administering IV antibiotics to patients with open fractures in the field, especially in the urban or suburban setting, but this may be important with prolonged transport times.

An injured extremity should be moved as little as possible, both during the secondary survey and application of a splint. Prior to splinting, an injured extremity should generally be returned to normal anatomical position, including the use of gentle traction to restore an extremity to its normal length. The two primary contraindications for doing this include either significant pain or resistance to movement experienced during an attempt to normal anatomic position. Traditional teaching was to splint a suspected fracture "in the position found;" however, there is good rationale for restoring normal anatomic position. First, a "reduced fracture," one that is returned to normal anatomic alignment, is easier to splint.

Secondly, reducing a fracture may alleviate compression on arteries or nerves and result in improved perfusion and neurologic functioning. Reduction of fractures also decreases hemorrhage. If the fracture is open and bone is exposed, the bone end should be gently rinsed with sterile water or normal saline to remove obvious contamination prior to an attempt to restore normal anatomic position. It is not of major concern if the bone ends retract back into the skin during this manipulation, as open fractures require irrigation and debridement in the operating room regardless. However, the fact that the bone was exposed prior to reduction is key information that should be passed on during the patient report at the receiving facility. No more than two attempts should be made to restore an extremity to normal position, and, if unsuccessful, the extremity should be splinted "as is."

The primary objective of splinting is to prevent movement of the body part. This will help decrease the patient's pain and prevent further soft tissue damage and hemorrhage. To immobilize any long bone in an extremity effectively, the entire limb should be immobilized. To do this, the injured site should be supported manually while the joint and bone above (proximal to) and the joint and bone below (distal to) the injury site are immobilized. Numerous types of splints are available and most can be used with both open and closed fractures (Figure 13-11). With virtually all splinting techniques, further inspection of the extremity is limited, and a thorough assessment should be performed before splinting.

Four additional points are important to remember when applying any type of splint are:

1. Pad rigid splints to prevent movement of the extremity inside the splint, to help increase the patient's comfort, and to prevent pressure sores.
2. Remove jewelry and watches so that these objects will not inhibit circulation as additional swelling occurs. Lubrication with lotion or a water-soluble jelly may facilitate removal of tight rings.
3. Assess neurovascular functions distal to the injury site before and after applying any splint and periodically thereafter. A pulseless extremity indicates either a vascular injury or a compartment syndrome, and rapid transport to an appropriate facility becomes even more of a priority.
4. After splinting, consider elevating the extremity, if possible, to decrease edema and throbbing. Ice or cold packs can also be used to decrease pain and swelling and may be placed on the splinted extremity near the suspected fracture site.

Femur Fractures. Femur fractures represent a unique splinting situation because of the musculature of the thigh. In addition to providing key structural support for the lower extremity, the femur also provides resistance to the powerful thigh muscles, keeping them out to length. When the femur is fractured

FIGURE 13-11   Types of Splints

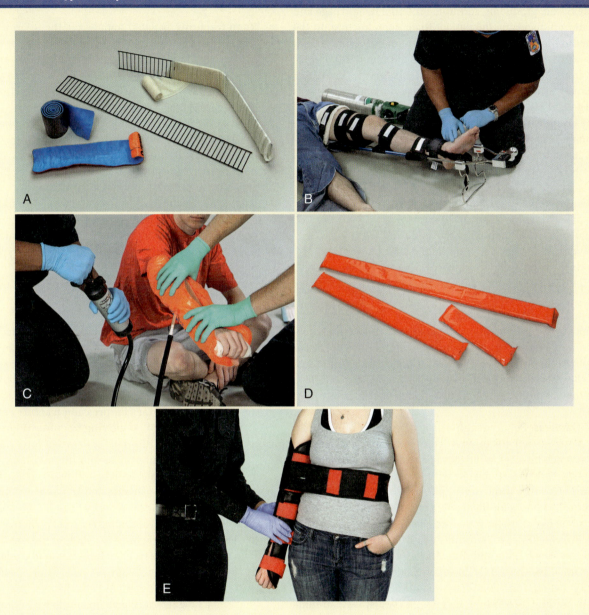

Various splints and splinting materials are available, including the following:

- **Rigid splints** cannot be changed in shape. They require that the body part be positioned to fit the splint's shape. Examples of rigid splints include board splints (wood, plastic, or metal), fracture packs, and inflatable "air splints." This group of splints also includes the long backboard. Rigid splints are best used for long bone injuries.

- **Formable splints** can be molded into various shapes and combinations to accommodate the shape of the injured extremity. Examples of formable splints include vacuum splints, pillows, blankets, cardboard splints, wire-ladder splints, and foam-covered moldable metal splints. Formable splints are best used for ankle, wrist, and longbone injuries.
- **Traction splints** are designed to maintain mechanical in-line traction to help realign fractures. Traction splints are most often used to stabilize femur fractures.

A. Formable splint. **B.** Traction splint. **C.** Vacuum splint. **D.** Board splint. **E.** Fracpac. (**B** and **C** from Sanders, MJ: Mosby's Paramedic Textbook, ed 3, St. Louis, 2006, Mosby.)

in the midshaft area, this resistance to contraction is removed. As these muscles contract, the sharp bone ends tear through muscle tissue, producing additional internal hemorrhage and pain and predisposing the patient to an open fracture. In the absence of life-threatening conditions, a *traction splint* should be applied to stabilize suspected midshaft femoral fractures. The application of traction, both manually and by the use of a mechanical device, will help decrease internal bleeding as well as decrease the patient's pain. One study of prehospital use of traction splints documented that almost 40% of the patients had an injury that either complicated or contraindicated use of a traction splint.[2] Contraindications to the use of a traction splint include the following:

- Suspected pelvic fracture
- Suspected femoral neck (hip) fracture
- Avulsion or amputation of the ankle and foot
- Suspected fractures adjacent to the knee (A traction splint may be used as a rigid splint in this situation, but traction should not be applied.)

When midshaft femoral fractures are encountered in a patient with additional injuries that are life threatening, time should not be taken to apply a traction splint. Instead, attention should be focused on the critical problems, and the suspect lower extremity fractures will be sufficiently stabilized when the patient is immobilized to a long backboard.

Pelvic Fractures. Pelvic fractures can range from minor, relatively insignificant fractures to complex injuries associated with massive internal and external hemorrhage. Fractures of the **pelvic ring** are associated with overall mortality of 6%, whereas mortality from open fractures may exceed 50%. Blood loss accounts for the leading cause of death in patients with pelvic fractures; the remaining deaths are from traumatic brain injury (TBI) and multiple organ failure. Because the pelvis is a strong bone and difficult to fracture, patients with pelvic fractures frequently have associated injuries, including TBIs (51%), long bone fractures (48%), thoracic injuries (20%), urethral disruption in men (15%), splenic trauma (10%), and liver and kidney trauma (7% each). Examples of pelvic fractures include:

- **Rami fractures.** Isolated fractures of the inferior or superior rami are generally minor and do not require surgical stabilization. Individuals who fall forcibly on their perineum may fracture all four rami ("straddle" injury). These fractures typically are not associated with significant internal hemorrhage.
- **Acetabular fractures.** These fractures occur when the head of the femur is driven into the acetabulum of the pelvis. Surgical intervention is generally needed to optimize normal hip function. These injuries may be associated with significant internal hemorrhage.
- **Pelvic ring fractures.** Fractures of the pelvic ring are typically classified into three categories. Life-threatening hemorrhage is probably most common with vertical shear fractures, but it may be associated with each type of pelvic ring fracture. The prehospital care provider may palpate crepitus and note bony instability with each of these ring fractures.

1. **Lateral compression fractures** account for the majority of pelvic ring fractures (Figure 13-12A). These injuries may occur when forces are applied to the lateral aspects of the pelvis (e.g., pedestrian is struck by a car). The volume of the pelvis is decreased in these fractures.
2. **Anterior-posterior compression fractures** account for about 15% of pelvic ring fractures (Figure 13-12B). These injuries occur when forces are applied in an anteroposterior direction (e.g., person pinned between a vehicle and wall). These injuries are also known as "open book" pelvic fractures because usually the symphysis pubis is separated and the volume of the pelvis greatly increased.
3. **Vertical shear fractures** account for the smallest proportion of pelvic ring fractures but tend to cause the highest mortality (Figure 13-12C). They occur when a vertical force is applied to the hemi-pelvis (e.g., fall from a height, landing on one leg first). Because one

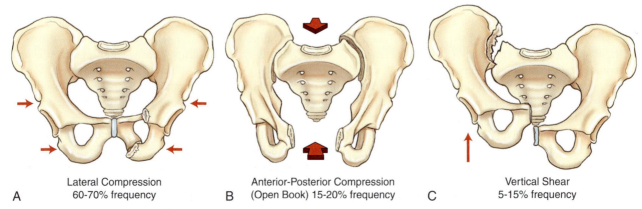

| A | Lateral Compression 60-70% frequency | B | Anterior-Posterior Compression (Open Book) 15-20% frequency | C | Vertical Shear 5-15% frequency |

FIGURE 13-12 Pelvic fractures. **A.** Lateral compression. **B.** Anterior-posterior compression. **C.** Vertical shear.

half of the pelvis is sheared off the remaining portion, blood vessels are often torn, resulting in severe internal hemorrhage.

Severe pelvic fractures present two challenging problems for prehospital care providers. The greatest concern is internal hemorrhage, which can be very difficult to manage. Some data suggest that a PASG can be useful in compressing the pelvis and presumably can tamponade internal hemorrhage.[3,4] If available, use of the PASG can be considered for decompensated (Class III or IV) shock. Another option includes wrapping a bed sheet tightly around the lower aspect of the pelvis and tying it as a sling. The lower extremities should also be adducted and internally rotated and secured in that position. Several companies manufacture "pelvic binders," designed to stabilize certain types of pelvic fractures. When used on appropriate types of fractures in the hospital, these devices can close a disrupted pelvic ring and decrease the volume of the pelvis. For numerous reasons, pelvic binders are not recommended for use when pelvic fractures have not been confirmed by x-ray, such as during transport from the scene of a motor vehicle crash to the trauma center. However, if a pelvic fracture has been diagnosed by x-ray, and the fracture type is amenable to management with a binder, consideration should be given to applying a binder prior to an inter-facility transfer (i.e., from a nontrauma center to a trauma center), especially if the patient is in shock (Figure 13-13). At present, there are no published studies of prehospital use of pelvic binders.

A second related concern is that patients with grossly unstable pelvic fractures may be difficult to move, and even turning the patient using a modified logroll procedure can shift bone fragments, causing additional hemorrhage. The best way to move a patient with an unstable fracture identified on palpation may be with a scoop stretcher. If a scoop stretcher is not available, the patient should be turned using a modified logroll procedure only enough to slide a long backboard under the patient. This action should be carried out expeditiously.

Dislocations

Joints are held together by ligaments. The bones are attached to muscles by tendons. Movement of an extremity is accomplished by the contraction (shortening) of muscles. This reduction of muscle length pulls the tendons that are attached to a bone and moves the extremity at a joint. A *dislocation* is a separation of two bones at the joint, resulting from significant disruption to the ligaments that normally provide stability at a joint (Figures 13-14 and 13-15). A dislocation, similar to a fracture, produces an area of instability that the prehospital care provider needs to secure. Dislocations can produce great pain. A dislocation can be difficult to distinguish from a fracture and may be associated with fractures as well (fracture-

---

FIGURE 13-13 Pelvic Binders

As noted in the text, at least three pelvic binders are commercially available: Pelvic Binder (Pelvic Binder, Dallas, Texas); Sam Sling (Sam Products, Newport, Oregon); and TPOD (BioCybernetics International, LaVerne, California).

RATIONALE

Some pelvic ring fractures are associated with an increase in the pelvic volume (e.g., anteroposterior [AP] compression fracture), permitting large amounts of intra-abdominal hemorrhage. Because the volume is increased, there is less tissue surrounding the pelvis to tamponade bleeding. Before the development of pelvic binders, patients with these injuries and hemodynamic instability (shock) would undergo external fixation of the pelvis to decrease the pelvic volume and increase the likelihood of tamponade of hemorrhage. Although external fixation seemed to decrease blood requirements, minimal published data exist to suggest external fixation lowered mortality from these fractures.

PROBLEMS

Several potential problems exist with the use of pelvic binders in the prehospital setting:

1. Pelvic fractures are difficult to diagnose in the absence of an x-ray film. No published data show that prehospital care personnel can reliably diagnose a pelvic fracture based on clinical examination. Furthermore, not all pelvic fractures benefit from compression. Although AP compression fractures may benefit, lateral compression fractures already have a decreased pelvic volume.

2. Limited data exist on efficacy. Only a few retrospective case series have reported on patients with in-hospital use of pelvic binders. Although some demonstrate that the pelvic volume is significantly decreased, few address transfusion requirements, and none has shown a decrease in mortality in those treated with a pelvic binder.

3. No published research exists on the use of pelvic binders in the prehospital setting, and therefore no data show improved outcome.

4. There is significant cost for this single-use device.

POTENTIAL USE

One conceivable use for the pelvic binder in the out-of-hospital setting would be the inter-facility transfer of a patient with an AP compression fracture, confirmed by x-ray film, and associated Class II, III, or IV shock. In these patients, the device could be applied before transfer, especially to those in decompensated shock. The decision to use the device should be made in conjunction with medical control.

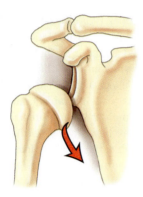

FIGURE 13-14 A dislocation is a separation of a bone from a joint.
(From McSwain NE Jr, Paturas JL: *The basic EMT: Comprehensive prehospital patient care,* ed 2, St. Louis, 2001, Mosby.)

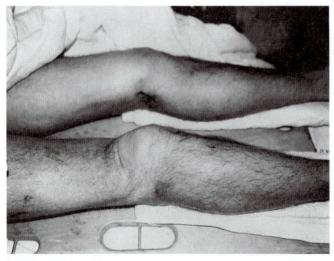

FIGURE 13-15 Right anterior knee dislocation with overriding tibia on the femur.
(From Ferrera PC, Colucciello SA, Marx JA, et al: *Trauma management: An emergency medicine approach,* St. Louis, 2001, Mosby.)

dislocation). Individuals with prior dislocations have more lax ligaments and may be prone to more frequent dislocations unless the problem is corrected surgically. Unlike those sustaining a dislocation for the first time, these patients are often familiar with their injury and can help in assessment and stabilization. Deformity of a joint provides a clue to the type of dislocation.

Management. As a general rule, suspected dislocations should be splinted in the position found. Gentle manipulation of the joint can be done to try to return blood flow when the pulse is absent or weak. When faced with a brief transport time to the hospital, however, the better decision may be to initiate transport rather than attempt manipulation. This manipulation will cause the patient great pain, so the patient should be pre-

pared before moving the extremity. A splint should be used to immobilize the injury. Documentation of how the injury was found and of the presence of pulses, movement, sensation, and color before and after splinting is important. During transport, ice or cold packs can be used to decrease pain and swelling. Analgesia should also be provided to reduce pain.

A position paper from the National Association of EMS Physicians (NAEMSP) recommends reduction of dislocations when transport time is prolonged.[5] The rationale is that joints are more difficult to reduce if they are left in a dislocated position for a prolonged period. Attempted reduction of a dislocation should only be undertaken when permitted by written protocols or online medical control, and when the provider has been properly trained in the appropriate techniques. All attempts at reduction of a dislocation should be properly documented.

Special Considerations

Critical Multisystem Trauma Patient

Adherence to the primary assessment priorities in patients with multisystem trauma that includes injured extremities does not imply that extremity injuries should be ignored or that injured extremities should not be protected from further harm. Rather, it means that *life takes precedence over limb* when faced with a critically injured trauma patient with extremity injuries that are not bleeding. The focus should be on maintaining vital functions through resuscitation, and only limited measures should be taken to address the extremity injuries, regardless of how dramatic the injuries appear. By properly immobilizing a patient to a long backboard, all extremities are essentially splinted in an anatomic position. A secondary survey need not be completed if the life-threatening problems identified in the primary survey require ongoing interventions and if transport time is short. If a secondary survey is deferred for this reason, the prehospital care provider can simply document the findings that precluded performing the secondary survey.

Pain Management

Analgesia should be considered in patients with isolated extremity trauma and hip fractures.[6] Basic interventions that provide effective pain relief should be attempted first (i.e., immobilization of suspected fractures and ice packs), as well as good communication skills with the patient to decrease anxiety. Protocols for analgesia use should be in place with clear indications and contraindications. Examples of acceptable pharmaceutical intervention include morphine sulfate, fentanyl, nitrous oxide, and nonsteroidal anti-inflammatory drugs (NSAIDs). The patient must be monitored with proper documentation before and after administration of the analgesic and any pain management protocol should include ensuring that naloxone is immediately available if reversal of the side effects of narcotic analgesics is needed. Appropriate monitoring includes continuous pulse oximetry and serial vital signs, including pulse, respiratory rate, and blood pressure. Continuous capnography may provide early warning signs that a patient is becoming overmedicated ("narcotized").[7]

Analgesics are recommended for isolated joint and limb injuries but are generally not advocated in multisystem trauma patients. Once the fracture or dislocation is stabilized and splinted, the patient should experience a great reduction in pain. Stabilizing the affected extremity decreases the amount of movement of the area, thus decreasing the amount of discomfort. The patient should be observed for signs of alcohol or drug use if he or she does not appear to be in much pain with significant injuries.

Pain medications should be used judiciously and as tolerated by the patient. Analgesics should not be administered when (1) the patient presents with or develops signs and symptoms of shock, (2) pain is significantly relieved with stabilization and splinting, or (3) the patient appears under the influence of drugs or alcohol. Medication should not be administered without understanding the potential complications.

Moderate to severe pain may be treated with an NSAID, such as ketorolac, administered intravenously, while severe pain is typically treated with narcotics (opiates). Morphine and fentanyl are the most commonly used narcotics. Respiratory depression, even apnea, is the greatest concern of the possible detrimental effects of narcotics. Another worrisome adverse effect is that narcotics are vasodilators. This is of particular concern for trauma patients because patients who are in a compensated state of shock (Class II) may have their hypovolemia "unmasked" by the narcotic, and profound hypotension may occur. In patients with potential compensated shock, the lowest possible dose should be administered, intravenously (IV), and slowly titrated upward until satisfactory pain relief is noted. Narcotics are best given IV in trauma patients because intramuscular (IM) doses may be absorbed erratically if hypoperfusion is present. Other possible adverse reactions for all narcotics include nausea and emesis, dizziness, sedation, and euphoria. For this reason, these agents should be used with caution in patients with head injuries because intracranial hypertension may be exaggerated. Data suggest that the analgesic and adverse affects of morphine and fentanyl are comparable.[8]

Morphine

Morphine is for use in patients with moderate to severe pain. Dosage should be titrated to the patient's response to the pain and physiologic status. It can be given IV, IM, or subcutaneously (SQ). Adult IV dosage is typically 2.5 to 15 mg, administered slowly over several minutes while monitoring the patient for relief and complications. For IM or subcutaneous (SQ) administration, the adult dose is 10 mg/70 kg body weight.

Fentanyl

Fentanyl has properties that make it attractive for prehospital trauma patients. Fentanyl has rapid onset and does not cause an increase in the release of histamine (as morphine does), which can exacerbate hypotension in hypovolemic patients. As with all narcotics, the dose should be titrated to patient relief and overall physiologic status. Typical adult dose is 50 to 100 mcg; 1 to 2 mcg/kg is the typical dose for children. The adverse effects are similar to morphine, but specific contraindications include allergy to fentanyl, traumatic brain injury (TBI) with possible increased intracranial pressure (ICP), respiratory depression, and loss of airway control.

Relief of Anxiety (Anxiolysis)

Treating pain in trauma patients involves both the physical pain and the anxiety about the pain and the situation in which patients find themselves. Analgesics manage the pain, and sedatives address the anxiety. Benzodiazepines such as diazepam (Valium®), midazolam (Versed®), lorazepam (Ativan®), and alprazolam (Xanax®) are the best known and have the added benefit of antegrade amnesia. The patients often will not remember details of what happened after the drug is administered. The use of a narcotic and benzodiazepine together can have a synergistic effect that can be of added benefit in relieving pain and anxiety; however, extreme caution must be used when administering simultaneous doses of both a benzodiazepine and a narcotic. Ketamine, a dissociative agent, is commonly used in the prehospital setting in Europe for its sedative effects and limited impact on respiratory drive.

Amputations

When tissue has been totally separated from an extremity, the tissue is completely without nutrition and oxygenation. This type of injury is termed amputation or avulsion. An *amputation* is the loss of part or all of a limb, and an *avulsion* involves the tearing away of soft tissue. Initially, bleeding may be severe with these injuries; however, vessels at the injured site may constrict, and clotting may combine to diminish the blood loss. Movement may disrupt the blood clot, and bleeding can recur. All amputations may be accompanied by significant bleeding but more so with partial amputations. This is because when vessels are completely transected, they retract and constrict and blood clots may form, decreasing or stopping hemorrhage. On the other hand, when a vessel is only partially transected, the two ends cannot retract and blood continues to pour out of the hole.

Amputations are often evident on the scene (Figure 13-16). This type of injury receives great attention from bystanders, and the patient may or may not know that the extremity is

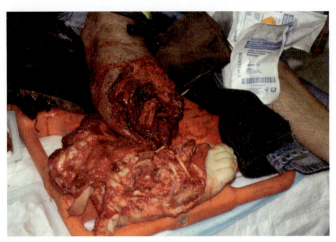

FIGURE 13-16   Complete amputation of the right leg after it became entangled in machinery.

FIGURE 13-17   **Phantom Pain**

In some circumstances, the patient may complain of pain distal to the amputation. This *phantom pain* is the sensation that pain exists in a missing extremity. The reason for phantom pain is not understood completely, but the brain may not realize that the extremity is not present. This is usually not present at the time of the initial injury.

---

missing. Psychologically, the prehospital care provider needs to deal with this injury cautiously (Figure 13-17). The patient may not be ready to confront the loss of a limb and should be told after being assessed and treated. The missing extremity should be located for possible reattachment. Even if it is not possible to regain complete function of the extremity, the patient may regain partial function. The primary survey should be performed before looking for a missing extremity. The appearance of an amputation may be horrifying, but if the patient is not breathing, the loss of the limb is secondary. Amputations are very painful. Pain management should be employed once life-threatening problems have been excluded in the primary survey (Figure 13-18).

Principles of managing an amputated part include the following:

1. Clean the amputated part by gentle rinsing with lactated Ringer's (LR) solution.
2. Wrap the part in sterile gauze moistened with LR solution and place it in a plastic bag or container.
3. After labelling the bag or container, place it in an outer container filled with crushed ice.

4. *Do not* freeze the part by placing it directly on the ice or by adding another coolant such as dry ice.
5. Transport the part along with the patient to the closest appropriate facility. [9]

The longer the amputated portion is without oxygen, the less likely that it can be replaced successfully. Cooling the amputated body part, without freezing it, will reduce the metabolic rate and prolong this critical time. However, replantation is not a guarantee of successful attachment or ultimate function. Because lower extremity prostheses generally allow the patient to resume a near-normal life, lower extremities are rarely considered for replantation. Furthermore, only cleanly separated amputations in otherwise healthy, younger individuals are usually considered for replantation. Smokers are less likely to have successful replantation because the nicotine in tobacco is a potent vasoconstrictor and may compromise blood flow to the replanted segment. Patients who are candidates for replantation of fingers or a hand/forearm should be transported to a Level I trauma center because Level II and III facilities often lack replantation capability.

Transport of a patient should not be delayed to locate a missing amputated part. If the amputated part is not readily found, law enforcement officials or other responders should remain at the scene to search for it. When the amputated part is transported in a separate vehicle from the patient, the prehospital care provider ensures that the transporters of the amputated part understand clearly where the patient is being transported and how to handle the part once it is located. The receiving facility should be notified as soon as the part is located, and transportation of the part should be initiated as soon as possible.

Field Amputation

In general, many extremities that appear hopelessly entrapped can be released with additional extrication expertise. If the patient has the extremity entangled in a machine, an often-overlooked expert is the maintenance person who repairs the machine. This person often has the technical knowledge for expeditiously removing parts from a machine, thereby facilitating extrication. But, on rare occasions, a patient may have an entrapped extremity for which a field amputation may be the only reasonable option. [10] Although formal field amputation is not considered part of the scope of practice of prehospital care providers in the United States, some entrapped extremities may be connected by only a small strand of tissue. The decision to cut this tissue or wait for a physician to arrive at the scene must be made in consultation with medical oversight. If a substantial amputation is necessary, it should ideally be performed by a surgeon because of the anatomic knowledge and technical expertise required (Figure 13-19). Significant sedation may need to be administered for the procedure, including intubation.

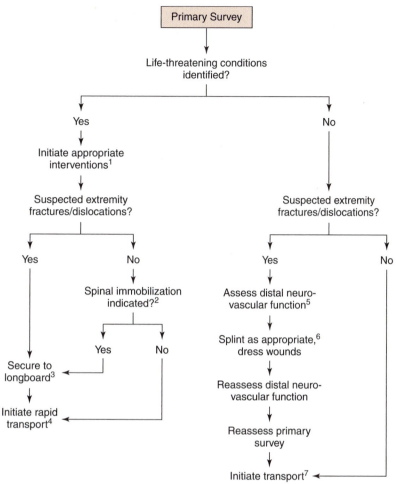

FIGURE 13-18 Primary survey algorithm.

[1] Airway management, ventilatory support, shock therapy.

[2] See Indications for Spinal Immobilization algorithm (p. 257).

[3] Injured extremities are immobilized in anatomic position by securing to longboard.

[4] Transport to closest appropriate facility (trauma center, if available); assess distal neurovascular function and apply traction splint (if suspected femur fracture) as time permits.

[5] Assess perfusion (pulses and capillary refilling) and neurologic function (motor and sensory) distal to the suspected fracture or dislocation.

[6] Use appropriate splinting technique to immobilize suspected fracture or dislocation; if suspected midshaft femur fracture, apply traction splint.

[7] Transport to closest appropriate facility.

Compartment Syndrome

Compartment syndrome refers to a limb-threatening condition in which the blood supply to an extremity is compromised by increased pressure in that limb. The muscles of extremities are enveloped by dense connective tissue called *fascia*. This fascia forms numerous compartments in the extremities in which the muscles are contained. The forearm has three compartments, and the lower leg (calf) has four. Muscle fascia has minimal stretch, and any force that increases the pressure inside the compartments may result in a compartment syndrome. The two most common causes of compartment syndrome are hemorrhage from a fracture or vascular injury and third-space edema that forms when ischemic muscle tissue is reperfused after a period of diminished or absent blood flow. However, a splint or cast that is applied too tightly may

FIGURE 13-19   Field Amputation Set

An amputation set can be assembled and maintained in a medical director's or supervisor's vehicle in case a field amputation is ever necessary.

Medical instruments:

Curved Mayo scissors	1 each
Curved hemostats	4 each
Kelly clamps, regular	2 each
Needle holder, regular	2 each
Towel clamps	4 each
Forceps with teeth, regular	1 each
Rake retractor, six prong, sharp	2 each
Gigli saw handles	2 each
Gigli saw wire	3 each
Amputation knife	1 each
Bone cutter	1 each

Disposable materials:
Surgical gowns, sterile
Surgical gloves, sterile
Scalpel, #10 blade
Sterile towels (4 pack)
Lap pads (10 pack)
Drapes
Bone wax

Suture:
2–0 silk ties
0 silk ties
0 silk on atraumatic needle
2–0 silk on GI needle, multipack
3–0 silk on GI needle, multipack

Dressing supplies:
Roller gauze
ABD pads, large
Elastic bandages, 4 inch
Elastic bandage, 6 inch

Medications:
Neuromuscular blocking agents (succinylcholine, vecuronium, etc.)
Ketamine
Fentanyl

Airway management (if not on EMS units):
Intubation tray
Endotracheal tubes

also produce a compartment syndrome. As the pressure in the compartment increases beyond that of capillary pressure (about 30 mm Hg), flow is impaired to the capillaries. The tissue served by these vessels then becomes ischemic. The pressure may continue to build to the point that even arterial flow is compromised by compression in the arteries.

The two earliest signs of a developing compartment syndrome are pain and paresthesia. Pain is often described as out of proportion to the injury. This pain may be dramatically increased on passive movement of a finger or toe in that extremity. Nerves are extremely sensitive to their blood supply, and any compromised blood flow soon manifests as paresthesia. Because these symptoms may be normally associated with a fracture, this underscores the need for baseline circulatory, motor, and sensory examinations and repeated serial examinations so that the prehospital care provider can identify changes.

The other three "classic" signs of compartment syndrome—pulselessness, pallor, and paralysis—are late findings and indicate a clear compartment syndrome and a limb in jeopardy of muscle death (necrosis). Pulselessness is an uncommon finding, because it indicates the presence of a vascular injury or that pressure in the compartment which contains that blood vessel has exceeded systolic pressure. Compartments may also be extremely tense and firm to palpation, although it is difficult to judge the compartment pressures

by physical examination alone. In the hospital, compartment pressures are measured in extremities in which compartment syndrome is suspected.

Compartment syndrome can be definitively managed only in the hospital. Only basic maneuvers can be attempted in the field. Any tightly applied splint or dressings should be removed and distal perfusion reassessed. Because compartment syndrome may develop during a long-distance transfer, serial examinations are essential for early identification of this problem. In the hospital, compartment syndrome is managed with surgical intervention (fasciotomy), with an incision through the skin into the affected compartments to decompress the compartment syndrome.

Crush Syndrome

Crush syndrome, also known as *traumatic rhabdomyolysis*, is a clinical entity characterized by renal failure and death after severe muscle trauma. Crush syndrome was first described in World War I in German soldiers rescued from collapsed trenches, then again in World War II in patients of the London Blitz. In World War II, crush syndrome had a mortality rate in excess of 90%. During the Korean War, mortality was 84%, but after the advent of hemodialysis, mortality decreased to 53%. In the Vietnam War, the mortality rate was approximately the same at 50%.

The importance of crush syndrome, however, should not be limited to historical or military interest. Approximately 3% to 20% of the survivors of earthquakes have sustained a crush injury, and approximately 40% of survivors from collapsed buildings will have crush injuries.[11,12] In 1978, an earthquake near Beijing, China, injured more than 350,000 persons, with 242,769 deaths. More than 48,000 of these people died from crush syndrome. More commonly, mechanisms of crush syndrome include prolonged entrapment from a trench collapse, construction collapse, or motor vehicle collision.

Crush syndrome arises from a crushing-type injury to large muscle masses, commonly involving the thigh or calf. Crush syndrome occurs when destruction of muscle releases the molecule known as myoglobin. *Myoglobin* is a protein found in muscle that is responsible for giving meat its characteristic red color. The function of myoglobin in muscle tissue is to serve as an intracellular storage site for oxygen. When myoglobin is released from damaged muscle, however, it is capable of causing damage to the kidneys and acute renal failure (ARF).

Patients with crush syndrome are identified by the following:

- Prolonged entrapment
- Traumatic injury to muscle mass
- Compromised circulation to the injured area

Traumatic injury to the muscle causes release of not only myoglobin but also potassium. Once the patient has been extricated, the affected limb becomes reperfused with new blood, but the old blood with elevated levels of myoglobin and potassium is washed out of the injured area and into the rest of the body. Elevated potassium can result in life-threatening cardiac dysrhythmias, and free myoglobin will produce tea- or cola-colored urine and will eventually result in renal failure.

The key in improving outcomes in crush syndrome is early and aggressive fluid resuscitation. It is important for the prehospital care provider to remember that toxins are accumulating within the entrapped limb during the extrication. Once the entrapped limb is freed, the accumulated toxins wash into the central circulation, similar to a bolus of poison. Therefore, success will depend on minimizing the toxic effects of accumulated myoglobin and potassium before release of the limb. Resuscitation needs to occur before extrication.[13] Some authors have advocated that final extrication be delayed until the patient has been adequately resuscitated.[14] A delay in fluid resuscitation will result in renal failure in 50% of the patients, and a delay of 12 hours or more produces renal failure in almost 100% of the patients. A poorly resuscitated patient may go into cardiac arrest during extrication because of the sudden release of metabolic acid and potassium into the blood stream when the compression on the extremity is released.[15] Fluid resuscitation should proceed with normal saline at a rate of up to 1500 ml per hour. LR solution is avoided because of the presence of potassium. The addition of one ampule (50 mEq) of sodium bicarbonate and 10 grams of mannitol to each liter of fluid used during the extrication period may help decrease the incidence of renal failure. Once the patient has been extricated, the normal saline fluids can be slowed to 500 ml per hour, alternating with 5% dextrose in water (D5W), with one ampule of sodium bicarbonate per liter.[16]

Once the blood pressure is stabilized and volume status restored, attention is turned toward prophylaxis against hyperkalemia and the toxic effects of serum myoglobin. Hyperkalemia in the field will be recognized by the development of peaked T waves on the cardiac monitor. Treatment of the increased potassium follows standard protocols for hyperkalemia including intravenous sodium bicarbonate administration, inhaled beta-agonists (albuterol), administration of dextrose and insulin (if available), and if life-threatening cardiac dysrhythmias occur, intravenous calcium chloride. Alkalinization of the urine will provide some degree of protection to the kidneys; however, the key is maintain increased urine output (typically in the range of 50–100 ml/hr).

Mangled Extremity

A "mangled extremity" refers to a complex injury resulting from high-energy transfer in which significant injury occurs to two or more of the following: (1) skin and muscle, (2) tendons, (3) bone, (4) blood vessels, and (5) nerves (Figure 13-20). Common mechanisms producing mangled extremities include motorcycle crashes, ejection from a motor vehicle crash (MVC), and a pedestrian struck by an automobile. When encountered, patients may be in shock from either external blood loss or hemorrhage from associated injuries, which are common because of the high-energy mechanism. Most mangled extremities involve severe open fractures, and amputation may be necessary in 50% to 75% of patients. Limb salvage is possible in some patients, typically involving six to eight procedures, and success often depends on the experience of the trauma and orthopedic surgeons.

Even with a mangled extremity, the focus is still on the primary survey to rule out or address life-threatening conditions. Hemorrhage control, including the use of a tourniquet, may be required. The mangled extremity should be splinted, if the patient's condition allows. These patients are probably best cared for at high-volume, Level I trauma centers.

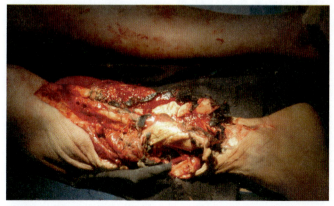

FIGURE 13-20 Mangled extremity resulting from crushing injury between two vehicles. The patient has fractures and extensive soft tissue injury.

Sprains

A *sprain* is an injury in which ligaments are stretched or torn. Sprains are caused by a sudden twisting of the joint beyond its normal range of motion. They are characterized by significant pain, swelling, and possible hematoma. Externally, sprains may resemble a fracture or dislocation. Definitive differentiation between a sprain and a fracture is accomplished only through a radiographic study. In the prehospital setting, it is reasonable to splint a suspected sprain in case it turns out to be a fracture or dislocation. An ice or cold pack may help relieve pain, as well as use of narcotic pain medication.

Management

The general management for suspected extremity injury includes the following steps:

1. Identify and treat any and all life-threatening injuries found in the primary assessment.
2. Stop any bleeding and treat the patient for shock.
3. Evaluate for distal neurovascular function.
4. Support the area of injury.
5. Immobilize the injured extremity, including the joint above and the joint below the injury site.
6. Re-evaluate the injured extremity after immobilization for changes in distal neurovascular function.
7. Provide pain management as appropriate.

Prolonged Transport

Patients with extremity trauma often have coexisting injuries. Ongoing internal blood loss may be from abdominal or thoracic injuries, and during a prolonged transport, the primary survey will need to be assessed frequently to ensure that all life-threatening conditions are identified and no new ones have emerged. Vital signs should be obtained at regular intervals. Intravenous crystalloid solutions should be administered at a rate to maintain normal vital signs, unless significant internal hemorrhage is suspected in the pelvis, abdomen, or thorax.

During long transports, the prehospital care provider needs to focus greater attention on extremity perfusion. In limbs with compromised vascular supply, the provider can attempt to restore normal, anatomic positioning to optimize the chance for improved blood flow. Similarly, dislocation with impaired distal circulation should be considered for reduction in the field. Distal perfusion, including pulses, color, and temperature, as well as motor and sensory function, should be examined in a serial manner. Compartments should be palpated for the development of potential compartment syndromes.

Measures to ensure patient comfort should be taken. Splinting devices should be comfortable and well padded. The limbs should be assessed for any potential points inside the splint where pressure could contribute to the creation of an ulcer, especially in an extremity with compromised perfusion. Parenteral narcotic analgesia should be given at regular intervals, with monitoring of respiratory rate, blood pressure, pulse oximetry, and capnography, if available. If properly trained personnel are present, nerve blocks may be particularly comforting to the patient, such as a femoral nerve block for a midshaft femoral fracture.

Contaminated wounds should be flushed with normal saline irrigation so that gross particulate matter (e.g., soil, grass) is removed. If the transport will take longer than 120 minutes, and if protocols allow and appropriate personnel are present, antibiotics may be administered for patients with open fractures. A first-generation cephalosporin, cefazolin, is sufficient for minor open fractures, whereas a broader-spectrum agent, such as cefoxitin, might be administered for a more serious open fracture. If a body part has been amputated, it should also be periodically assessed so that it remains cool but does not freeze or become macerated by soaking in water.

SUMMARY

- In patients with multisystem trauma, attention is directed toward the primary survey and the identification and management of all life-threatening injuries, including internal or external hemorrhage in the extremities.
- Prehospital care providers must be careful not to be distracted from addressing life-threatening conditions by the gross, dramatic appearance of any noncritical injuries or by the patient's request for their management.
- Once the patient has been fully assessed and found to have only isolated injuries without systemic implication, those noncritical injuries should be addressed.

- Musculoskeletal injuries, in the order of their threat to life, should be immobilized in order to prevent further injury and provide comfort as well as some relief from pain.
- When the mechanism of injury indicates sudden, violent changes in motion, multisystem trauma, or spinal trauma, potential systemic decline needs to be anticipated and the patient's age, physical condition, and medical history included in the evaluation.

SCENARIO SOLUTION

With your partner's help, you were able to apply a traction splint to the midshaft femur fracture of the right leg. After securing your patient to the backboard, you were able to move the patient to the ambulance for transport to the hospital. Once in the ambulance, oxygen via mask was administered and an IV was established. The patient's vital signs remained unchanged throughout the transport. ■

References

1. Williams B, Boyle M: Estimation of external blood loss by paramedics: Is there any point? *Prehosp Disaster Med* 22(6):502–506, 2007.
2. Wood SP, Vrahas M, Wedel S: Femur fracture immobilization with traction splints in multisystem trauma patients. *Prehosp Emerg Care* 7:241, 2003.
3. Flint LM, Brown A, Richardson JD, et al: Definitive control of bleeding from severe pelvic fractures. *Ann Surg* 189:709, 1979.
4. Flint L, Babikian G, Anders M, et al: Definitive control of mortality from severe pelvic fracture. *Ann Surg* 211:703, 1999.
5. Goth P, Garnett G: Clinical guidelines for delayed or prolonged transport: II. Dislocations. Rural Affairs Committee, National Association of Emergency Medical Services Physicians. *Prehosp Disaster Med* 8(1):77, 1993.
6. Alonso-Serra HM, Wesley K: Prehospital pain management. *Prehosp Emerg Care* 7:842, 2003.
7. Hatlestad D: Capnography in sedation and pain management. *J Emerg Med Serv*, 34:65, 2005.
8. Galinski M, Dolveck F, Borron SW, et al: A randomized, double-blind study comparing morphine with fentanyl in prehospital analgesia. *Am J Emerg Med* 23:114, 2005.
9. Seyfer AE: *Guidelines for management of amputated parts,* Chicago, 1996, American College of Surgeons Committee on Trauma.
10. Pagliery J. Surgery at crash scene rescues trapped Miami police officer. http://www.miamiherald.com/1374/story/1191078.html. Accessed September 25, 2009.
11. Pepe E, Mosesso VN, Falk JL: Prehospital fluid resuscitation of the patient with major trauma. *Prehosp Emerg Care* 6:81, 2002.
12. Better OS: Management of shock and acute renal failure in casualties suffering from crush syndrome. *Ren Fail* 19:647, 1997.
13. Michaelson M, Taitelman U, Bshouty Z, et al: Crush syndrome: Experience from the Lebanon war, 1982. *Isr J Med Sci* 20:305, 1984.
14. Pretto EA, Angus D, Abrams J, et al: An analysis of prehospital mortality in an earthquake. *Prehosp Disaster Med* 9:107, 1994.
15. Collins AJ, Burzstein S: Renal failure in disasters. *Crit Care Clin* 7:421, 1991.
16. Sever MS, Vanholder R, Lameire N: Management of crush-related injuries after disasters. *N Engl J Med* 354:1052, 2006.

Suggested Reading

American College of Surgeons Committee on Trauma: Musculoskeletal trauma. In ACS Committee on Trauma: *Advanced trauma life support,* ed 8, Chicago, 2009, ACS, pp 187–203.

Ashkenazi I, Isakovich B, Kluger Y, et al: Prehospital management of earthquake casualties buried under rubble. *Prehosp Disast Med* 20:122, 2005.

Coppola PT, Coppola M: Emergency department evaluation and treatment of pelvic fractures. *Emerg Med Clin North Am* 18(1):1, 2003.

Gregory RT, Gould RJ, Peclet M, et al: The mangled extremity syndrome: A severity grading system for multisystem injury of the extremity. *J Trauma* 25:1147, 1985.

Howe HR, Poole GV, Hansen KJ, et al: Salvage of lower extremities following combined orthopedic and vascular trauma: A predictive salvage index. *Am Surg* 53:205, 1987.

McSwain NE Jr, Paturas JL, editors: *The basic EMT: Comprehensive prehospital patient care,* ed 2, St. Louis, 2001, Mosby.

Roessler MS, Wisner DH, Holcroft JW: The mangled extremity: When to amputate? *Arch Surg* 126:1243, 1991.

CHAPTER 14

Burn Injuries

CHAPTER OBJECTIVES

At the completion of this chapter, the reader will be able to do the following:

- ✓ Define various depths of burns.
- ✓ Define the zones of burn injuries.
- ✓ Understand how ice can deepen the depth of burns.
- ✓ Estimate burn size using the "rule of nines."
- ✓ Calculate fluid resuscitation using the Parkland formula.
- ✓ Define the additional fluid needs in children with burns.
- ✓ Describe appropriate burn dressings for prehospital care.
- ✓ Discuss the unique concerns of electrical injuries.
- ✓ Discuss the management concerns in patients with circumferential burns.
- ✓ Discuss the three elements of smoke inhalation.
- ✓ Apply principles of various zones in hazardous material (hazmat) scenes.
- ✓ Discuss criteria for the transfer of patients to burn centers.

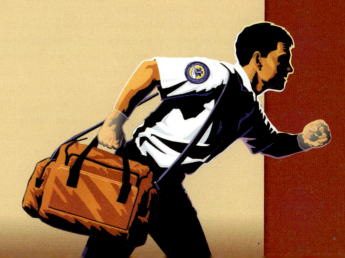

SCENARIO

You are called to a residential structure fire. When your unit arrives, you witness a two-story house that is fully involved with fire and with thick black smoke pouring out of the roof and windows. You are directed to a victim (patient 1) that is being care for by the first responders. They tell you that the patient re-entered the burning building in an attempt to rescue his dog, and he was carried out unconscious by fire fighters. When you arrive at the side of the patient you find a male who is likely in his thirties. The majority of his clothes have been burned off. He has obvious burns to his face and his hair has been singed. He is unconscious; he is breathing spontaneously, but labored. The first responders have placed the patient on oxygen with a nonrebreather mask. On exam, his airway is patent with assistance; he ventilates easily. The sleeves of his shirt have been burned off. His arms have circumferential burns, but his pulse is easily palpable. His heart rate is 118 beats/minute, blood pressure 148/94 mm Hg, respirations 22 breaths/minute, and the pulse oximeter is reading an SpO^2 of 92%. On examination, you determine that the patient is burned on his entire head, anterior chest and abdomen, and his entire right and left arm and hand. Several feet away is the patient's brother (patient 2), who is frantic about the condition of his brother (patient 1). From where you are, you can see that patient 2 has burns to his entire right arm and hand, from the tips of the finger to his shoulder.

What is the extent of burns for each patient? What are the initial steps for managing these patients? How does the prehospital care provider recognize an inhalation injury?

Many people consider burns to be the most frightening and dreaded of all injuries. In the course of our daily lives, we have all sustained a burn of some degree and have experienced the intense pain and anxiety associated with even a small burn. Burns are common in industrialized and agricultural cultures and in civilian and military settings. Burns can range from small to catastrophic injuries covering large regions of the body. Regardless of size, all burns are serious. Even minor burns can result in serious disability.

A common misconception is that burn injuries are isolated to the skin. On the contrary, large burns can be extensive, multisystem injuries capable of life-threatening effects involving the heart, lungs, kidneys, gastrointestinal (GI) tract, and immune system. The most common cause of death in a fire victim is not from the direct complications of the burn wound, but from complications of respiratory failure.

Although considered a form of trauma, burns have some significant differences from other types of trauma that merit consideration. After a trauma, such as a motor vehicle crash (MVC) or a fall, the victim's physiologic response is to initiate several adaptive mechanisms to preserve life. These responses can include the shunting of blood to vital organs, increase in cardiac output, and increase in production of various protective serum proteins. In contrast, after a burn, the patient's body essentially attempts to shut down, go into shock, and die. A substantial portion of initial burn care is directed at reversal of this initial shock. In patients who have traumatic injuries as well as burns, actual mortality of these combined injuries is much greater than the combined predicted mortality of each injury individually.

Consideration of the etiology of burns will prevent the rescuer from sustaining unnecessary injury, as well as provide optimal care for the victim. The circumstances in which the burn occurred should also be considered, because a large percentage of burns in both children and adults result from an intentional injury.

Smoke inhalation is a life-threatening injury that is often more dangerous than the burn injury. Inhalation of toxic fumes from smoke is a greater predictor of burn mortality than the age of the patient or the size of the burn.[1] A victim need not inhale a large quantity of smoke to predispose the patient to a severe injury, and often life-threatening complications may not manifest for several days.

Approximately 20% of all burn victims are children, and 20% of these children are the victims of intentional injury or child abuse.[2,3] Most health care providers are surprised to learn that intentional burn injury is second only to beating in the forms of physical violence inflicted on children. Burns as a form of abuse are not limited to children. It is common to see women burned in cases of domestic violence, as well as elderly persons in cases of elder abuse.

Anatomy of Skin

The skin serves several complex functions, including protection from the external environment, regulation of fluids, thermoregulation, sensation, and metabolic adaptation (Figure 14-1). The skin covers about 1.5 to 2.0 square meters in the average adult. It is made up of two layers, the epidermis

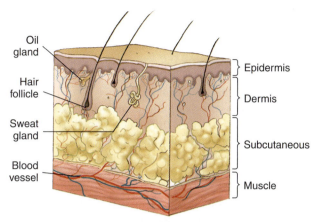

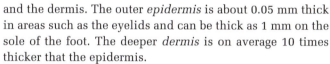

FIGURE 14-1   Normal skin. The skin in composed of three tissue layers—epidermis, dermis, and subcutaneous layer—and associated muscle. Some layers contain structures such as glands, hair follicles, blood vessels, and nerves. All these structures are interrelated to the maintenance, loss, and gain or body temperature.

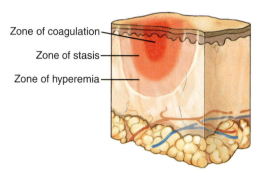

FIGURE 14-2   Three zones of burn injury.

and the dermis. The outer *epidermis* is about 0.05 mm thick in areas such as the eyelids and can be thick as 1 mm on the sole of the foot. The deeper *dermis* is on average 10 times thicker that the epidermis.

The skin of males is thicker than the skin of females, and the skin of children and elderly persons is thinner than that of the average adult. These facts explain how an individual can suffer burns of varying depths when exposed to a singular burning agent, and how a child might experience a deep burn while an adult with the same exposure has only a superficial injury.

Burn Characteristics

The creation of a burn is analogous to frying an egg. When one breaks an egg into a hot skillet, the egg is initially liquid and transparent. As the egg is exposed to the high temperatures, it rapidly becomes opaque and solidifies. A virtually identical process occurs when a patient is burned. In the case of the egg, the proteins of the egg change shape and are destroyed in a process known as *denaturation*. When a burn occurs to patients, the elevated or freezing temperature, radiation, or chemical agent causes the proteins in the skin to be severely damaged, resulting in protein denaturation. Injury to the skin can occur in two phases: immediate and delayed. Skin is capable of tolerating temperatures of 40 degrees Centigrade (104 degrees Fahrenheit) for brief periods of time. However, once temperatures exceed this point there is a logarithmic increase in the magnitude of tissue destruction.[4]

A full-thickness burn has three zones of tissue injury[5] (Figure 14-2). The central zone is known as the *zone of coagulation*, and this is the region of greatest tissue destruction. This zone is necrotic and is not capable of tissue repair.

Adjacent to the zone of necrosis is a region of lesser injury, the *zone of stasis*. The cells in this zone are injured, but not irreversibly. If they are subsequently deprived of the delivery of oxygen or blood flow, these viable cells will die and become necrotic. This zone is referred to as the zone of stasis because immediately after injury, the blood flow to this region is stagnant. Timely and appropriate burn care will preserve blood flow and oxygen delivery to these injured cells. Resuscitation of the patient will eliminate this stasis and re-establish delivery of oxygen to the injured and susceptible cells. Failure to resuscitate the patient appropriately results in death of the cells in the injured tissue, and a partial-thickness burn then converts to a full-thickness burn. A common error that results in damage to this area is the application of ice by a well-meaning bystander or provider. When ice is used to stop the burning process, the ice causes vasoconstriction, preventing re-establishment of blood flow. It is now argued that when ice is applied to a burn, the patient will experience some reduction in pain; however, the analgesia will be at the expense of additional tissue destruction. For these reasons, ongoing burning should be arrested with the use of ambient or room-temperature water, and analgesia should be provided with oral or parenteral medications.

The outermost zone is known as the *zone of hyperemia*. This zone has minimal cellular injury and is characterized by increased blood flow secondary to an inflammatory reaction initiated by the burn injury.

Burn Depth

Estimation of burn depth can be deceptively difficult to even the most experienced provider. Often, a burn that appears to be second degree will prove to be third degree in 24 to 48 hours.

The surface of a burn may appear to be a first- or second-degree burn at first glance, but on debridement, the superficial epidermis separates off, revealing a white, third-degree burn eschar. Because the burn may evolve over time, it is often wise to withhold final judgment of burn depth for up to 48 hours after injury. Often it is best simply to tell patients that the injury is either superficial or deep and that time is required to determine ultimate burn depth.

First-Degree Burns

First-degree burns involve only the epidermis and are characterized as being red and painful (Figure 14-3). These are also referred to as *superficial* burns. These are rarely clinically significant, with the exception of large areas of sunburn, in which the patient has significant pain and risks dehydration without attention to appropriate oral hydration. These wounds heal typically within a week, and the patients will not scar.

Second-Degree Burns

Second-degree burns, also known as *partial-thickness burns*, are those that involve the epidermis and varying portions of the underlying dermis (Figure 14-4). Second-degree burns can be further classified as either *superficial* or *deep*. Second-degree burns will appear as blisters (Figure 14-5) or as denuded,

burned areas with a glistening or wet-appearing base. These wounds will be painful. Because remnants of the dermis survive, these burns are often capable of healing in 2 to 3 weeks. In partial-thickness burns the zone of necrosis involves the entire epidermis and varying depths of the superficial dermis. If not well cared for, the zone of stasis in these injuries can progress to necrosis, making these burns larger and perhaps converting the wound to a third-degree burn. A superficial second-degree burn will heal with vigilant wound care. Deep second-degree burns may require surgery.

Third-Degree Burns

Third-degree burns may have several appearances (Figure 14-6). Most often these wounds will appear as thick, dry, white, leathery burns, regardless of race or skin color (Figure 14-7). In severe cases, the skin will have a charred appearance with visible thrombosis of blood vessels (Figure 14-8). This burn injury is also called *full-thickness* as it involves the entire

---

FIGURE 14-5   Blisters

Much discussion has been generated about blisters, including whether or not to debride them and how to approach the blister associated with partial-thickness burn. A blister occurs when the epidermis separates off of the underlying dermis and fluid that is leaking from nearby vessels fills the blister. The presence of osmotically active proteins in the blister fluid draws additional fluid into the blister space, causing the blister to continue to enlarge. As the blister enlarges, it creates pressure on the injured tissue of the wound bed, which increases the patient's pain. Many think that the skin of the blister acts as a dressing and prevents contamination of the wound. However, the skin of the blister is not normal and, therefore, cannot serve as a protective barrier. Additionally, maintaining the blister intact prevents one from applying topical antibiotics directly on the injury. For these reasons, most burn specialists open and debride blisters after arrival of the patient to the hospital.[6]

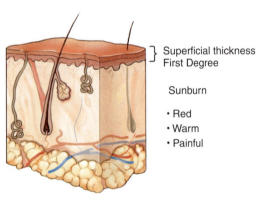

} Superficial thickness
First Degree

Sunburn

• Red
• Warm
• Painful

FIGURE 14-3   First-degree burn.

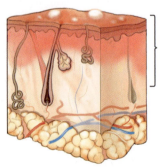

Partial thickness
Second Degree

• Blistering
• Painful
• Glistening wound bed

FIGURE 14-4   Second-degree burn.

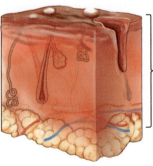

Full thickness
Third Degree

• Leathery
• White to charred
• Dead tissue
• Victims will have pain from burned
  areas adjacent to the third
  degree burn.

FIGURE 14-6   Third-degree burn.

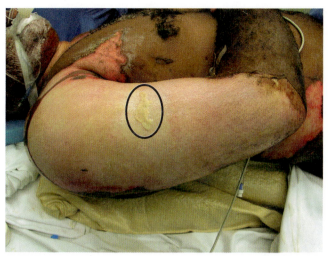

FIGURE 14-7 This patient has suffered from partial-thickness and a full-thickness burn, characterized as white and leathery in appearance.

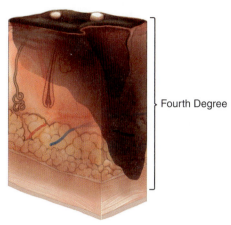

Fourth Degree

FIGURE 14-9 Fourth-degree burn.

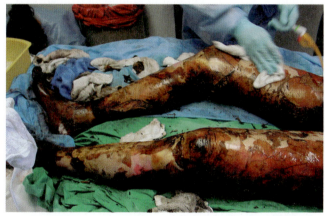

FIGURE 14-8 Example of deep, full-thickness burn with charring of the skin and visible thrombosis of blood vessels.

thickness of the skin. People have generally been taught, erroneously, that full-thickness burns are not painful because the full-thickness nature of the burns destroys the nerve ending in the burned tissue. It is a misperception that third-degree burns are pain free. Patients with third-degree burns have pain. Third-degree burns are typically surrounded by areas of partial- and superficial-thickness burns. The nerves in these areas are intact and continue to transmit pain sensations from the damaged tissues. Burns of this depth can be disabling and life threatening. Prompt surgical excision and intensive rehabilitation at a specialized center will be required.

Fourth-Degree Burns

Fourth-degree burns are those that not only burn all layers of the skin, but also burn underlying fat, muscles, bone, or internal organs (Figure 14-9, Figure 14-10).

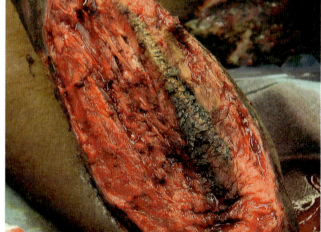
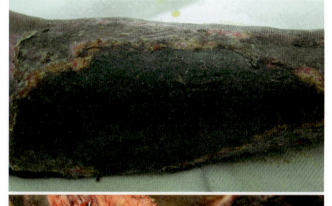

FIGURE 14-10 Fourth-degree burns to the arm, with burns not only to the skin but also to the subcutaneous fat, muscle, and bone.

Burn Assessment and Management

Primary Survey and Resuscitation

The goal of the primary assessment is to systematically evaluate and treat life-threatening disorders in order of importance to preserve life. The ABCDE method of trauma care applies to the management of the burn patient, although burn patients provide unique challenges in every step of the resuscitation.

Major burns are often a very lethal injury. However, aside from burn-related compromise of the airway or breathing, burns by themselves are not typically an immediately life-threatening injury. The overall appearance of the burns can be dramatic and even grotesque. The sophisticated provider will be mindful that the patient may also have suffered from a mechanical trauma and have less apparent, internal injuries that are more rapidly lethal.

Airway

Preservation of the patency of the airway is the highest priority in caring for a burn victim. The heat from the fire can cause edema of the airway above the level of the vocal cords and can occlude the airway. Therefore, careful initial, as well as continuous, evaluation is required. It is a mistake to believe that once one has completed the ABC assessment, the box for doing so has been checked and, therefore, all is well with the airway. Those providers who are likely to experience prolonged transport times need to be particularly vigilant with airway assessment. For example, a burned patient might well have a patent airway on the first airway evaluation. In the time that follows, the face, as well as the airway, will likely swell. As a result, an airway that was satisfactory initially may become critically narrowed 30 or 60 minutes later. The airway can narrow to the degree that the airway becomes obstructed and air cannot pass down the trachea. A more likely scenario is related to the physiological effect of a narrowed, but not obstructed, airway. Narrowing of the trachea from swelling of the mucosa decreases the flow of the inhaled gases which is the same physiologically as increasing the resistance to the flow. An increase in airway resistance produces an increase in the work of breathing for the patient. An increase in the work of breathing from a swollen airway can contribute or produce respiratory arrest even when the patient has a patent airway. To avoid catastrophic airway narrowing or occlusion, early control of the airway is prudent. Intubation of these patients is often difficult and hazardous because of the distorted anatomy. Often, patients are the individuals best suited to manage their own airway by assuming a position that maintains an open airway and allows for comfortable respiration. In those instances in which intervention is required, the airway should be managed by the most experienced person available. In addition, pharmacologic interventions will suppress the patient's ability to manage the airway, necessitating airway intervention and maintenance by the providers.

If the patient is intubated, special precautions must be taken when securing the endotracheal (ET) tube and preventing inadvertent dislodgement or extubation. Following a burn, the skin of the face will often peel or weep fluid. With face burns, adhesive tapes are not suitable for securing the ET tube. The tube can be secured using two umbilical tapes or pieces of IV tubing wrapped around the head. One piece should be draped over the ear and the second under the ear. Commercially available cloth and Velcro® devices are also suitable.

Breathing

As with any trauma patient, breathing can be adversely affected by such problems as fractured ribs, pneumothoraces, and open chest wounds. In the event of circumferential chest wall burns, chest wall compliance progressively decreases to such an extent that it inhibits the patient's ability to inhale. Following a burn injury, the burned skin will start to harden and contract while the deeper, soft tissues will simultaneously swell. The net result is that the burns constrict the chest wall similarly to having several leather belts tighten around the patient's chest wall. As time progresses, the patient cannot move the chest wall to breath. When attempting to ventilate patients with circumferential chest wall burns, the bag-mask device may become difficult or impossible to compress. In such cases, prompt escharotomies of the chest wall will allow re-establishment of ventilation. An escharotomy is a surgical procedure that involves making an incision through the hardened burn eschar, allowing the burn and chest to expand and move with the patient's respiratory movements.

Circulation

Evaluation and management of circulation includes the measurement of blood pressure, evaluation of circumferential burns, and establishment of IV catheters. Accurate measurement of blood pressure becomes difficult or impossible with burns to the extremities, and if a blood pressure can be obtained, it may not correctly reflect systemic arterial blood pressure because of full-thickness burns and edema of the extremities. Even if the patient has adequate arterial blood pressure, distal limb perfusion may be critically reduced because of circumferential injuries. Burned extremities should be elevated during transport to reduce the degree of swelling in the affected limb.

Establishment of two large-caliber IV catheters capable of the rapid flow rate needed for large-volume resuscitation is a requirement for burns that involve more than 20% of the total body surface area. Ideally, the IV catheters should not be placed through or adjacent to burned tissue; however, placement through the burn is appropriate if no alternative sites are available. When the catheter is placed in or near a burn, special measures must be taken to ensure the catheter does not inadvertently fall out. Adhesive tapes and dressings typically used to secure IV catheters will be ineffective when applied on or adjacent to burned tissue. Alternative means to secure the lines include wrapping the site with Kerlix™ or Coban™ rolls. In some patients, the provider may not be able to obtain venous access. Intraosseous (IO) access is an alternative and reliable method to administer intravenous fluids as well as narcotics.

Disability

Burn patients are trauma patients and may have sustained injuries other than the thermal injuries. Burns are obvious and sometimes intimidating injuries, but it is vital to assess for other, less obvious internal injuries that may be more immediately life threatening than the burn injuries. In attempts to escape being burned, patients will leap from the windows of buildings; elements of the burning structure may collapse and fall on the patient; or the victim may be trapped in the burning wreckage of an MVC. Evaluate the patient for neurologic and motor deficits. Identify and splint fractures of long bones. Perform spinal immobilization if you suspect a potential spine injury. A source of life-threatening neurological disability that is unique to burn victims is the effect of inhaled toxins such as carbon monoxide and hydrogen cyanide gas.

Exposure/Environment

The next priority is to expose the patient completely. Every square inch of the patient should be exposed and inspected. All clothing and jewelry should be promptly removed. In the victim of mechanical trauma, all of the patient's clothes are removed in order to identify injuries that might be concealed by the clothing. In a burn victim, removal of the clothing can potentially have a therapeutic benefit. As noted earlier, clothing and jewelry can retain residual heat which may continue to injure the patient. Following chemical burns, the clothing may be soaked with the agent that burned the patient. Therefore, improper handling of the victim's clothing that has been saturated with a potentially hazardous material can result in injury to both the patient and providers.

Controlling the environmental temperature is critical when caring for patients with large burns. Burn patients are not able to retain their own body heat and are extremely susceptible to hypothermia. Make every effort to preserve body temperature. Apply several layers of blankets. Keep the passenger compartment of the transporting ambulance or aircraft warm, regardless of the time of year. As a general rule, if you as a prehospital care provider are comfortable, then ambient temperature is not warm enough for the patient.

Secondary Survey

After completing the primary assessment, the next objective is completion of the secondary assessment. The secondary assessment of a burn patient is no different than that of any other trauma patient. The provider should complete a head-to-toe evaluation, attempting to identify additional injuries or medical conditions. The appearance of the burns can be dramatic; however, these wounds are not typically immediately life threatening. A thorough and systematic evaluation needs to be performed the same as for any other trauma patient.

Burn Size Estimation (Assessment)

Estimation of burn size is necessary to resuscitate the patient appropriately and prevent the complications associated with hypovolemic shock from burn injury. Burn size determination is also used as a tool for stratifying injury severity and triage. The most widely applied method is known is the "rule of nines." This method applies the principle that major regions of the body in adults are considered to be 9% of the total body surface area (Figure 14-11). The perineum, or genital area, represents 1%.

Children have different proportions than adults. Children's heads are proportionally larger than adults' heads, and children's legs are shorter in proportion than adults' legs. Because these proportions vary with differing age groups, it is not appropriate to apply the rule of nines to pediatric patients.

The *Lund-Browder chart* is a diagram that takes into account age-related changes in children. Using these charts, a provider maps the burn and then determines burn size based on an accompanying reference table (Figure 14-12).

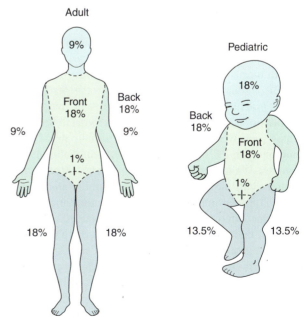

FIGURE 14-11   Rule of nines.

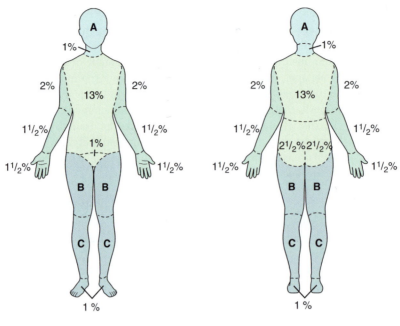

Area	Age 0	1	5	10	15	Adult
A - ¹/₂ of head	9¹/₂%	8¹/₂%	6¹/₂%	5¹/₂%	4¹/₂%	3¹/₂%
B - ¹/₂ of one thigh	2 ³/₄%	3¹/₄ %	4%	4¹/₄%	4¹/₂%	4¹/₄%
C - ¹/₂ of one leg	2¹/₂%	2¹/₂%	2³/₄%	3%	3¹/₄%	3¹/₂%

FIGURE 14-12 Lund-Browder chart.

This method requires drawing a map of the burns and then converting the map to a calculated burned surface area. The complexity of this method makes it difficult to use in a prehospital situation.

Small burns can be assessed using the Rule of Palms. The use of the patient's palm has been a widely accepted and long-standing practice for the estimation of size of smaller burns. There has not been uniform acceptance as what defines a palm and how large it is.[7] The average area of the palm alone (not including extended fingers) is 0.5% BSA in males and 0.4% in females. When one includes the palmar aspect of all five extended digits along with the palm, then the area increases to 0.8% TBSA for males and 0.7% TBSA for females.[7] Aside from gender differences of palm size, the size of the palm also varies with body weight of the patient. As the patient's body mass index (BMI) increases, the total skin surface area of the body increases and the percent body surface area of the palm decreases.[8] Therefore, in most cases, the palm plus the fingers of the patient can be considered to be approximately 1% of the patient's BSA.

Dressings

Before transport, the wounds should be dressed. The goal of the dressings is to prevent ongoing contamination and prevent airflow over the wounds which will help with pain control.

Dressings in the form of a sterile sheet or towel are sufficient before transporting the patient. Several layers of blankets are then placed over the sterile burn sheets to help the patient maintain body heat. Topical antibiotics should not be applied until the patient has been evaluated by the burn center.

Transportation

Patients who have multiple injuries in addition to their burns should first be transported to a trauma center, where immediately life-threatening injuries can be identified and surgically treated, if necessary. Once stabilized at a trauma center, the patient with burns can then be transported to a burn center for definitive burn care and rehabilitation. The American Burn Association and the American College of Surgeons have identified criteria for transport or transfer of burn patients to a burn center, as outlined in Figure 14-13. In those geographic

---

| **FIGURE 14-13** | **Injuries Requiring Burn Unit Care** |

Patients with serious burns should receive care at centers that have special expertise and resources. Initial transport or early transfer to a burn unit should result in a lower mortality rate and fewer complications. A burn unit may treat adults, children, or both. The Committee on Trauma of the American College of Surgeons recommends referral to a burn unit for patients with burn injuries who meet the following criteria:

1. Inhalation injury.
2. Partial-thickness burns over greater than 10% of the total body surface area (TBSA).
3. Full-thickness (third-degree) burns in any age group.
4. Burns that involve the face, hands, feet, genitalia, perineum, or major joints.

5. Electrical burns, including lightning injury.
6. Chemical burns.
7. Burn injury in patients with pre-existing medical disorders that could complicate management, prolong recovery, or affect mortality.
8. Any patients with burns and concomitant trauma (e.g., fractures) in which the burn injury poses the greatest risk of morbidity or mortality; if trauma poses the greater immediate risk, the patient may be initially stabilized in a trauma center before transfer to a burn unit.
9. Burned children in hospitals without qualified personnel or equipment for the care of children.
10. Burn injury in patients who will require special social, emotional, or long-term rehabilitative intervention.

(From the American College of Surgeons (ACS) Committee on Trauma: *Resources for optimal care of the injured patient: 1999,* Chicago, 1998, ACS.)

areas without easy access to a burn center, local medical direction will determine the preferred choice of destination for such cases.

Management

Initial Burn Care

The initial step in the care of a burn patient is to stop the burning process. The most effective and appropriate method of terminating the burning is irrigation with copious volumes of room-temperature water. Use of cold water or ice is contraindicated. As previously mentioned, the application of ice will stop the burning and provide analgesia, but it also will increase the extent of tissue damage in the zone of stasis. Remove all clothing and jewelry; these items maintain residual heat and will continue to burn the patient. In addition, jewelry may constrict digits or extremities as the tissues begin to swell.

A potentially controversial topic is the practice of burn cooling. Several investigators have evaluated the effect of various cooling methods on the microscopic appearance of the burned tissue, as well as the impact on wound healing. Experimental scald burns of 10% body surface area in animals treated with cooling had less cellular damage than those that were not cooled. In one study, the researchers concluded that burn cooling had a beneficial effect on the experimental burn wound.[9] Not all methods of burn cool-

ing are equivalent. Cooling that is too aggressive will lead to tissue damage. If delayed, it is not likely to be beneficial. In patients with large burns, burn wound cooling is likely to induce hypothermia. Investigators have been able to directly measure the impact of cooling on the temperature of the burned dermis, the microscopic structure of the tissue, and wound healing. Another study evaluated the outcomes of various cooling methods. These investigators compared burns cooled with tap water (15° C) to application of Melaleuca Alternifolia hydrogel. Each of these methods was applied immediately after the burns as well as after a 30 minute delay. Immediate tap water cooling was almost twice as effective in reducing the temperature within the burned tissue. In this trial, wounds that were cooled had better microscopic appearance and wound healing at 3 weeks after injury.[10] Over aggressive cooling with ice is harmful and will increase the injury to the tissue already damaged by the burn. This was demonstrated in an animal model—cooling the burn immediately by the application of ice is more harmful than application of tap water or no treatment at all.[11] The application of ice water at a temperature of 1° to 8° C (34° to 46° F) results in more tissue destruction than in burns that received no cooling treatment at all. In contrast, cooling with tap water at a temperature of 12° to 18° C (54° to 64° F) had less tissue necrosis and a faster rate of healing than wounds not cooled.[12] A potential complication of cooling is the development of systemic hypothermia. An important consideration is that the research on cooling was performed on experimental animals, and the burns were very limited in size. Ten percent total body surface area was the largest burn size evaluated. Cooling large burns could potentially produce hypothermia. Another potential hazard of cooling a burn is that in the patient with both burns and mechanical trauma, systemic hypothermia has predictable and detrimental effects on the ability of blood to form clot.

Effective dressing of the recent burn is the application of sterile, nonadherent dressings. Cover the area with a clean sheet. If a sheet is not readily available, substitute a sterile surgical gown, drapes, or towels. The dressing will prevent ongoing environmental contamination while helping to prevent the patient from experiencing pain from air flowing over the exposed nerve endings (Figure 14-14).

Prehospital providers have often been unsatisfied and frustrated with the simple application of sterile sheets to a burn. However, topical ointments and conventional topical antibiotics should *not* be applied because they prevent a direct inspection of the burn. Such topical ointments and antibiotics are removed on admission to the burn center to allow direct visualization of the burn and determination of burn severity. Also, some topical medications may complicate the application of tissue-engineered products used to aid wound healing.

High-concentration antimicrobial-coated dressings (e.g., Silverlon™ or Acticoat™) have become the mainstay of wound care in burn centers (Figure 14-15). These dressings are coated with silver, which is time-released over several days when applied to an open burn wound. The released silver provides rapid antimicrobial coverage of the common organisms contaminating and infecting wounds. Recently, these dressings have been adapted from burn center use to prehospital applications. These large antimicrobial sheets can be rapidly applied to the burn and can eradicate any contaminating organisms. This method of wound care allows prehospital providers to apply a nonpharmaceutical device that greatly reduces burn wound contamination within 30 minutes after application.[13–15] An advantage of these dressings in frontier and military application is their compact size and light weight. An entire adult can be covered with antibiotic dressings that can be stored in the volume of a manila envelope with minimal weight.

Fluid Resuscitation

Administration of large amounts of intravenous (IV) fluids is needed over the course of the first day postburn to prevent a burn patient from going into hypovolemic shock. After a burn, the victim loses a substantial amount of intravascular fluid in the form of obligatory whole-body edema, as well as evaporative losses at the site of the burn. Massive fluid shifts will occur, even though total body water may remain unchanged. Evaporative losses can be enormous. However, excessive fluid administration is harmful. Therefore, although large fluid requirements are needed to treat burn shock, too much fluid will complicate the patient's management and even worsen the patient's wounds.

The resuscitation of burn shock is aimed not only at restoration of the loss of intravascular volume, but also replacement of anticipated intravascular losses at a rate that mimics those losses as they occur (Figure 14-16). In trauma patients, the prehospital care provider is replacing the volume that the patient has already lost from hemorrhage from an open fracture or bleeding viscera. In contrast, when treating the burn patient, the objective is to calculate and replace the fluids that the patient has already lost as well as replace the volume that the provider anticipates the patient will lose over the first 24 hours after the burn injury.

Intravenous access should be considered for those situations involving long transport time to the hospital. In urban settings with short transport times, the need for obtaining IV access is based, not upon the burn, but rather as other conditions warrant.

Adult Patient

The use of IV fluids, especially Lactated Ringer's (LR) solution, is the best way initially to manage a burn patient. The amount of fluids administered in the first 24 hours after injury is typically 2 to 4 ml per kilogram of body weight/% area burn (using only the total of second and third degree burn). There are several formulas that guide fluid resuscitation in the burned patient. The most notable is the *Parkland formula* which delivers 4 ml/kg/% area burn. Half of this fluid needs to be administered in the first 8 hours after injury, and the remaining half of the volume from hours 8 to 24. Importantly, the first half of the

---

FIGURE 14-14 Prevent Airflow Over Patient's Burn

Most of us have experienced the pain associated with a dental cavity. The pain is intensified when we inhale air over the exposed nerve. With a partial-thickness burn, thousands of the nerves are exposed, and the air currents in the environment produce pain in the patient when the currents come into contact with the exposed nerves of the wound bed. Therefore, by keeping burns covered, the patient will experience less pain.

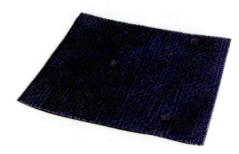

FIGURE 14-15 Acticoat dressing.
(Courtesy Smith & Nephew Wound Management.)

FIGURE 14-16 Resuscitating a Burn Patient

Resuscitating a burn patient can be compared to a filling a leaking bucket. The bucket is leaking water at a constant rate. The bucket has a line drawn in the inside near the top of the bucket. Your objective is to keep that water at the level of the line. Initially, when one comes to the bucket, the water depth will be very low. The longer the bucket has been unattended, the lower the water level, and the greater the amount of fluid that will need to be replaced. The container will continue to leak, so once the bucket has been filled to an appropriate level, fluids will need to be continuously added at a constant rate to maintain the desired level.

The longer the burn patient is not resuscitated or under-resuscitated, the more hypovolemic the patient becomes. Therefore, greater amounts of fluids are required to establish a "level" of homeostasis. Once the patient has been resuscitated, the vascular space continues to leak in the same manner as the bucket. To maintain equilibrium with this homeostatic point, additional fluids need to be provided to replace the ongoing losses.

fluid is administered within 8 hours from the time the patient was *injured*, not from the point the provider started to resuscitate the patient. This is especially important in frontier or military settings, in which there may be an initial delay in treatment. For example, if the patient presents for emergency care 3 hours after the injury with no or little fluid administration, the first half of the calculated total needs to be administered over 5 hours. In this way, the patient will have received the target volume by hour 8 after injury. Lactated Ringers is preferred to 0.9% Normal Saline for burn resuscitation. Burn patients typically require large volumes of intravenous fluids. Patients who receive large amounts of normal saline in the course of burn resuscitation will often develop a condition known as hyperchloremic acidosis because of the large amounts of chloride in the normal saline solution.

Calculation of Fluid Resuscitation Measures

For example, consider an 80-kg man who has sustained 30% third-degree burns and is managed on scene shortly after the injury. The fluid resuscitation volume would be calculated as follows:

24-hour fluid total = 4 ml/kg/% TBSA burn
= 4 ml/kg/% TBSA burn × 80 kg × 30% TBSA burn
= 9600 ml

Note that in this formula, the units of kilograms and percent cancel out so that only ml are left in the calculation, thus making it 4 ml × 80 × 30 = 9600 ml.

Once the 24-hour total is calculated, divide that number by 2:

Amount of fluid to be given from time of injury to hour 8 = 9600 ml/2 = 4800 ml

To determine the hourly rate for the first 8 hours, divide this total by 8:

Fluid rate for the first 8 hours = 4800 ml/8 hours = 600 ml/hour

The fluid requirement for the next period (hours 8–24) is calculated as follows:

Amount of fluid to be given from hours 8 to 24 = 9600 ml/2 = 4800 ml

To determine the hourly rate for the final 16 hours, divide this total by 16:

Fluid rate for final 16 hours = 4800 ml/16 hours = 300 ml/hour

The Rule of 10 for Burn Resuscitation

In an effort to simplify the process of calculating fluid requirements for butn patients in the prehospital setting, researchers from the U.S. Army Institute of Surgical Research developed the "Rule of 10" to help guide initial fluid resuscitation.[16] The percent of BSA burned is calculated and rounded to the nearest 10. For example a burn of 37% would be rounded to 40%. The percent burn is then multiplied by 10 to get the number of mL per hour of crystalloid. Thus, in the previous example, the calculation would be 40 x 10 equals 400 mL per hour. This formula is used for adults weighing 40 to 70 kg. For each 10 kg in body weight over 70 kg, an additional 100 mL per hour is given.

Pediatric Patient

Children require relatively larger volumes of IV fluids than adults with similar-size burns. Also, children have less metabolic reserves of the molecule glycogen in their livers to maintain adequate blood glucose during the periods of burn resuscitation. For these reasons, children should receive 5% dextrose containing IV fluids (D5LR) at a standard maintenance rate in addition to burn resuscitation fluids.

Smoke Inhalation—Fluid Management Considerations

The patient with both thermal burns and smoke inhalation will require significantly more fluid than the burn patient without smoke inhalation.[17] In an attempt to "protect the lungs," providers will often administer less fluid than calculated. Withholding fluids actually increases the severity of the pulmonary injury.

Special Considerations

Electrical Burns

Electrical injuries are devastating injuries that can easily be underappreciated. In many cases the extent of apparent tissue damage does not accurately reflect the magnitude of the injury. Tissue destruction and necrosis are excessive compared to the visually apparent trauma because most of the destruction occurs internally as the electricity is conducted through the patient. The patient will have external burns at the points of contact with the electrical source as well as grounding points (Figure 14-17). As the electricity courses through the patient's body, deep layers of tissue are destroyed despite seemingly minor injuries on the surface.

Electrical and crush injuries share many similarities. In both injuries, there is massive destruction of large muscle groups with resultant release of both potassium and myoglobin (see Chapter 12). The release of muscle *potassium* causes a significant increase in the serum level, which can result in cardiac dysrhythmias. Elevated potassium levels can make use of the depolarizing muscle relaxant succinylcholine prohibitively dangerous. *Myoglobin* is a molecule found in the muscle that assists the muscle tissue in transportation of oxygen. When released into the bloodstream in considerable amounts, the myoglobin is toxic to the kidneys and can cause kidney failure. This condition, *myoglobinuria,* is evidenced by tea- or cola-colored urine (Figure 14-18).

Prehospital providers are commonly called upon to provide inter-hospital transfers of patients after electrical injuries. Patients with electrical burns should be transported with a urinary catheter in place. These patients require an aggressive urine output of greater than 100 ml/hour in adults or 1 mL/kg/hour in children to avoid renal failure. Sodium bicarbonate is administered in some cases to make the myoglobin more soluble in urine and reduce the likelihood of renal injury.

The electrical burn patient may have associated injuries as well. Approximately 15% of patients with electrical injuries will also have traumatic injuries. This is a rate that is twice that seen in patients burned by other mechanisms.[18] Tympanic membranes may rupture, resulting in hearing difficulties. Intense and sustained muscle contraction *(tetany)* can result in compression fractures of multiple levels of the spine as well as long bones. Patients with electrical injury should have their spine immobilized. Long-bone fractures should be splinted when detected or suspected. Intracranial bleeds and cardiac dysrhythmias may also occur.

Electrical flash burns are the result of superheated air. Nevertheless, because of the catastrophic and occult nature of conduction injuries, it is imperative that providers maintain a high index of suspicion for the presence of a transmission type of injury.

Circumferential Burns

Circumferential burns of the trunk or limbs are capable of producing a life- or limb-threatening condition. Circumferential burns of the chest can constrict the chest wall to such a degree that the patient suffocates from inability to take a breath. Circumferential burns of the extremities create a tourniquet-like effect that can render an arm or leg pulseless. Therefore, all circumferential burns should be handled as an emergency and patients transported to a burn center or to the local trauma center, if a burn center is not available. *Escharotomies* are surgical incisions made through the burn eschar to allow expansion of the deeper tissues and decompression of previously compressed and often occluded vascular structures (Figure 14-19).

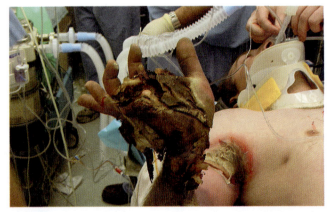

FIGURE 14-17 Patient after electrical injury from high-tension wires.

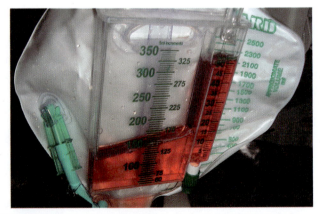

FIGURE 14-18 Urine of patient after electrical injury from high-tension wires. The patient has myoglobinuria after extensive muscle destruction.

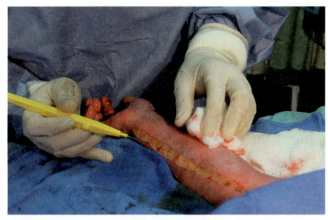

FIGURE 14-19 Escharotomies are performed to release the constricting effect of circumferential burns.

FIGURE 14-20 Signs and Symptoms of Smoke Inhalation
■ Burn in a confined space ■ Confusion or agitation ■ Burns to face or chest ■ Singing of eyebrows or nasal hair ■ Soot in the sputum ■ Hoarseness, loss of voice, or stridor

Smoke Inhalation Injuries

The leading cause of death in fires is not thermal injuries but the inhalation of toxic smoke. Any patient with a history of exposure to smoke in an enclosed space should be considered at risk of having an inhalation injury. Any patient with burns to the face or soot in the sputum is at risk for a smoke-inhalation injury; however, the absence of these signs does not exclude the diagnosis of a toxic inhalation (Figure 14-20). Maintaining a high index of suspicion is vitally important because signs and symptoms may not manifest for days after the exposure.

There are three elements of smoke inhalation: thermal injury, asphyxiation, and delayed toxin-induced lung injury. Dry air is a poor conductor of heat; the inhalation of heated air associated with a structure fire rarely induces thermal injury to the airways below the level of the vocal cords. The large surface area of the nasopharynx acts effectively as a heat exchanger and cools the inhaled, heated air to about body temperature by the time the air reaches the level of the vocal cords. When heated dry air at 300° C (572° F) is inhaled, the air is cooled to 50° C (122° F) by the time it is at the level of the trachea.[19] The vocal cords provide additional protection by reflexively moving into an adduction, or closed position.[20] The exception to this is the inhalation of steam. Steam has 4000 times the heat-carrying capacity of dry heat and is capable of burning the distal airways and bronchioles.[19]

Asphyxiants

Two gaseous products that are clinically important as asphyxiants are *carbon monoxide* (CO) and *cyanide gas* (CN). Both molecules are classified as asphyxiants and, thus, cause cell death by cellular hypoxia or asphyxia. Patients with asphyxia from smoke containing one or both of these compounds will have inadequate delivery of oxygen to tissues despite an adequate blood pressure or pulse oximeter reading. Carbon monoxide binds to hemoglobin with greater affinity than oxygen. The symptoms of CO inhalation depend on the duration or severity and resultant serum levels. Symptoms can range from mild headache to coma and death. Traditional teaching is that patients poisoned with CO develop "classic" cherry red skin coloration. Unfortunately, this is often a late sign and should not be relied on to consider the diagnosis.

Portable Pulse CO-Oximeters™ (Figure 14-21) that noninvasively measure the amount of carbon monoxide in the bloodstream are available for use in the prehospital settings. These monitors look and work similar to pulse oximeters. Treatment of CO toxicity is removal of the patient from the source and administration of oxygen. When breathing room air (21% oxygen), the body will eliminate half the CO in 250 minutes.[21] When the patient is placed on 100% oxygen, the half-life of the CO-hemoglobin complex is reduced to 40 to 60 minutes.[22]

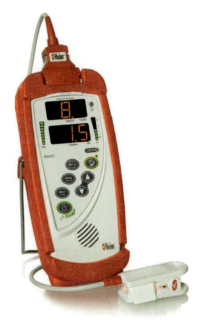

FIGURE 14-21 Masimo prehospital CO monitor, Rad-57. (Courtesy of Masimo Corporation.)

Cyanide gas is produced from the burning of plastics or polyurethane. Cyanide poisons cellular machinery, preventing the body's cells from using oxygen. The patient can die from asphyxia despite having adequate oxygen in the blood. Symptoms of cyanide toxicity include altered level of consciousness, dizziness, headache, and tachycardia or tachypnea. Patients with carbon monoxide toxicity from a structure fire should also be considered to be at risk for cyanide poisoning. The treatment of cyanide poisoning has traditionally been rapid transport to an emergency center capable of providing the patient with the antidote therapy. However, a commercially available antidote kit, widely used in Europe for many years and recently available in the United States, allows for field treatment of CN toxicity. The preferred antidote for cyanide poisoning is a medication that directly binds to the cyanide molecule, rendering it harmless. *Hydroxocobalamin* (Cyanokit™) detoxifies the cyanide by directly binding to it and forming cyanocobalamin (vitamin B12), which is non-toxic. Hydroxocobalamin is available for prehospital use in Europe and in the United States. A second chelating agent that has been used in Europe for cyanide poisoning is *dicobalt edetate.* If this medication is administered in the absence of cyanide poisoning, however, cobalt toxicity is a risk.

The "Lilly kit" or "Pasadena kit" has been the traditional cyanide antidote kit used in the United States and may still be utilized in some settings. This method of treating cyanide poisoning was developed in the 1930s and found to be effective in detoxifying animals poisoned with 21 times the lethal dose of cyanide.[23] The goal of this antidote therapy is to induce the formation of a second poison in the patient's blood. This therapeutically induced poison binds with the cyanide and allows the body to slowly detoxify and excrete the cyanide. The "Lilly kit" contains several medications. The first agent to be administered is a nitrate, either amyl nitrate or sodium nitrate. Amyl nitrate comes in an ampule that is broken open and the fumes inhaled, and sodium nitrate is given intravenously (IV) which is the preferred method of administration. The nitrate medications change the patient's hemoglobin into a form called methemoglobin, which attracts the CN away from the site of toxic action in the mitochondria of the cell. Once the CN binds with the methemoglobin, the mitochondria can once again begin to produce energy for the cell. Unfortunately, methemoglobin is toxic because it does not carry oxygen to cells as well as hemoglobin does. This decrease in oxygen delivery can further exacerbate the tissue hypoxia associated with increased CO levels that the victim may also have as a result of smoke inhalation exposure.[24,25] The third medication in the kit is sodium thiosulfate, which is given intravenously after the nitrate. The thiosulfate and CN from the methemoglobin are metabolized to thiocyanate, which is safely excreted in the patient's urine. Because of the toxicity of methemoglobin and the time needed to administer the full "Lilly" kit, hydroxocobalamin has become the preferred antidote for the treatment of cyanide poisoning.

Toxin-Induced Lung Injury

The thermal and asphyxiant components of an inhalation injury are usually apparent at the time of the rescue. In contrast, the signs and symptoms of toxin-induced lung injury typically do not manifest for several days. The first several days after a smoke inhalation injury are often described as the "honeymoon period." During this period the patient may appear deceptively stable with little or no pulmonary dysfunction. The severity of this lung injury is largely dependent on two factors: the composition of the smoke and the duration of exposure.[26]

In simplified terms, smoke is the product of incomplete combustion—that is, chemical dust. The chemicals in the smoke react with the lining of the trachea and lungs and damage the cells lining the airways and lungs.[27–29] Compounds such as ammonia, hydrogen chloride, and sulfur dioxide form corrosive acids and alkalis when inhaled.[30] These poisons cause necrosis of the cells lining the trachea and bronchioles. Normally, these cells have tiny hair-like structures called cilia. On these cilia is a blanket of mucus that captures and transports normally inhaled debris to the oropharynx, where the debris is swallowed into the gastrointestinal tract. Several days after an inhalation injury, these cells die. The debris from these necrotic cells and the debris these cells typically capture are capable of flooding the lungs. The result is an increase in secretions, plugging of the airways with mucus and cellular debris, and an increased rate of life-threatening pneumonia.

Prehospital Management

The initial and most important element of caring for a patient with smoke exposure is determining the need for orotracheal intubation. Whenever patency of the patient's airway is in doubt, the prehospital care provider can proceed with securing the airway using orotracheal intubation.[31,32] Continuous re-evaluation of airway patency is required. Change in the character of the voice, difficulty handling secretions, or drooling are signs of pending airway occlusion.

Patients with smoke inhalation should be transported to burn centers even in the absence of surface burns. Burn centers treat a greater volume of patients with smoke inhalation and offer unique modes of mechanical ventilation.

Child Abuse

Approximately 20% of all child abuse is the result of intentional burning. The majority of the children intentionally burned are 1 to 3 years of age.[33]

The most common form of burn child abuse is forcible immersion. These injuries typically occur when an adult places a child in hot water, often as a punishment related to toilet training. Factors that determine the severity of injury include age of the patient, temperature of the water, and duration of exposure. The child may sustain deep second- or third-degree burns of the hands or feet in a glove-like or stocking-like pattern. This is especially suspicious when the burns are sym-

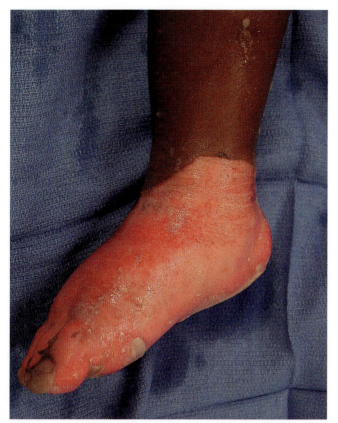

FIGURE 14-22 Stocking-type scald of child's foot indicative of intentional immersion burn injury consistent with child abuse.

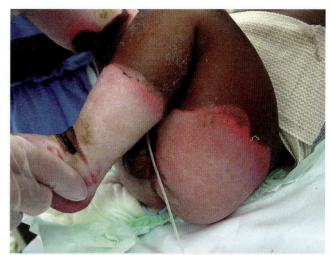

metric and lack splash patterns[34] (Figures 14-22 and 14-23). In cases of intentional scalding, the child will tightly flex the arms and legs into a defensive posture because of fear or pain. The resultant burn pattern will spare the flexion creases of the popliteal fossa, the antecubital fossa, and the groin. Sharp lines of demarcation will also be seen between burned and unburned tissue, essentially indicating a dip[35,36] (Figure 14-24).

In accidental scald injuries, the burns will have variable burn depth, irregular margins, and smaller burns remote from the large burns, indicating splash.[37]

Contact Burns

Contact burns are the second most common mechanism of burn injury in children, whether accidental or intentional. All body surfaces have some degree of curvature. When an accidental contact burn occurs, the burning agent makes contact with the curved body surface area. The burning instrument is deflected off the curved surface, or the victim of the burn withdraws from the hot object. The resultant injury has an irregular burn edge and depth. When a child receives an intentional contact burn, the inflicting implement is pressed onto the child's skin. The resultant injury has sharp lines of demarcation between burned and unburned tissue and uniform depth.[36]

Many jurisdictions require health care providers to report such cases of suspected child abuse.

FIGURE 14-23 The straight lines of the burn pattern and absence of splash marks indicate that this burn is the result of abuse.

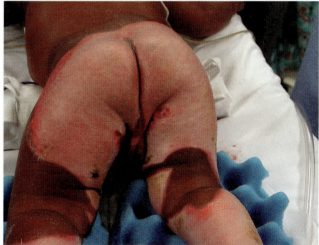

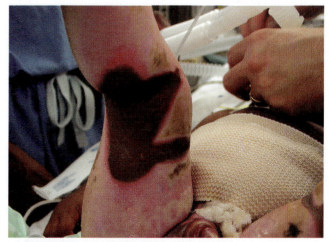

FIGURE 14-24 The sparing of the areas of flexion and the sharp lines of demarcation between burned and unburned skin indicate that this child was in a tightly flexed, defensive position before injury. Such a posture indicates that the scald is not accidental.

Radiation Burns

The severity of burns produced from various forms of radiation is a product of the amount of energy absorbed by the target tissue. The various forms of radiation include electromagnetic, x-rays, gamma rays, and particulate radiation. The different forms of radiation are able to transfer varying degrees of energy to tissue. Additionally, some forms of radiation (e.g., electromagnetic) can pass through tissue or an individual, resulting in no damage. In contrast, other forms of radiation (e.g., neutron exposure) are absorbed by the target tissue and result in significant injury. It is the absorption of the radiation that results in damage to the absorbing tissue. The absorption capacity of the radiation is more damaging than the actual dose of radiation. Equivalent doses of different forms of radiation will have dramatically different effects on an individual.

The typical exposure to radiation occurs in the setting of an industrial or occupational incident. However, with the increasing threat of global terrorism, the detonation of a small, hybrid, nuclear device (i.e., "dirty nuke") is a real possibility.

The detonation of a nuclear weapon in a metropolitan area would injure and kill by three mechanisms: thermal burns from the initial firestorm, supersonic destructive blast, and production of radiation. Mortality from a combination of thermal and radiation burns is greater than that from either thermal or radiation burns alone of equal magnitude. The combination of thermal and radiation burns has a synergistic effect on mortality.[38]

A nuclear attack would result in massive loss of life and casualties capable of overwhelming medical providers and facilities. An attack on a population center would destroy medical facilities, kill medical providers, and cripple supply lines. Prehospital providers would likely be required to care for victims over a long period.

Radiation is a hazardous material, and many of the initial priorities are the same as for any patient with a hazardous material exposure. The initial priorities are to remove the patient from the source of contamination, remove contaminated clothing, and irrigate the patient with water. Remember that any removed clothing should be considered contaminated and should be handled with caution. Irrigation is done carefully to remove any radioactive debris or particles from contaminated areas without spreading the injury to uncontaminated body surfaces. Continue with irrigation until contamination has been minimized to a steady state, as determined by a Geiger counter.[39] The exception to this approach is the patient who has sustained major trauma in addition to their radiation injury. In these cases, clothing should be removed immediately, and then the traumatic injury is dealt with and the patient stabilized. Patients with burns should undergo fluid resuscitation similar to any burn patient. Irradiated patients may experience vomiting and diarrhea, which will necessitate an increase in resuscitation fluids.

The physiologic consequences of whole-body radiation are termed *acute radiation syndrome* (ARS). The initial symptoms of ARS typically appear within hours of exposure. The cells of the body that are most sensitive to the effects of radiation are those that typically undergo rapid division. These rapidly dividing cells are found in the skin, GI tract, and bone marrow; therefore, these tissues manifest the first signs of ARS. Within a few hours after radiation exposure, the patient will experience nausea, vomiting, and cramping abdominal pain. Aggressive fluid management is required to prevent the development of renal failure. Over the following days, the patient may develop bloody diarrhea, ischemia of the bowel, and overwhelming infection and may die. The bone marrow is extremely sensitive to the effects of radiation. The bone marrow will stop production of white blood cells needed to fight infections and platelets needed to make blood clots. The resultant infections and bleeding complications are often fatal.

After a nuclear event, IV supplies, infusion pumps, and receiving medical facilities may be in short supply. If unable to provide the patient with IV resuscitation, the prehospital care provider can resuscitate the patient with oral fluids. A cooperative patient should be encouraged to drink a balanced salt solution to maintain a large urine output; alternatively, fluids can be delivered by nasogastric or nasoenteric tubes. Oral balanced salt solutions include Moyer's solution (4 grams sodium chloride [0.5 teaspoon of salt] and 1.5 grams sodium bicarbonate [0.5 teaspoon baking soda] in 1 liter water) and World Health Organization oral rehydration solution (WHO ORS). Animal research has shown encouraging results with such resuscitation strategies in patients with burns as large as 40% total body surface area. Administration of balanced salt solution to the GI tract at a rate of 20 ml/kg provided resuscitation equivalent to standard IV fluid resuscitation.[40]

Chemical Burns

Regardless of practice location or type, all prehospital providers need to be familiar with the basics of treating chemical injuries. Providers in urban settings may be called to a chemical incident at an industrial setting, whereas a rural provider may be summoned to an occurrence with agents used in agriculture. Tons of hazardous materials are transported through urban and rural settings daily by both highways and rail systems. Military providers may treat casualties of chemical burns caused by weapons, incendiary devices, chemicals used to fuel or maintain equipment, or chemical spills after damage to civilian installations.

Injuries from chemicals are often the result of prolonged exposure to the offending agent. This is contrasted with thermal injuries, in which the duration of exposure is usually very brief. The severity of chemical injury is determined by four factors: nature of the chemical, concentration of the chemical, duration of contact, and mechanism of action of the chemical.

Chemical agents are classified as acid, base, organic, or inorganic. *Acids* are chemicals with a pH between 7 (neutral) and 0 (strong acid). *Bases* are agents with a pH between 7 and 14. Acids damage tissue by a process called *coagulative necrosis;* the damaged tissue transforms into a barrier that prevents deeper penetration of the acid. In contrast, alkali burns destroy the tissue by *liquefaction necrosis;* the base liquefies the tissue, which allows the chemical to penetrate more deeply and cause increasingly deeper damage.

Treatment

The greatest priority in the care of a chemically exposed patient, as in any emergency, is personal and scene safety. Always protect yourself first. If there is any question of a chemical hazard, ensure scene safety and determine if any special garment or breathing apparatus is required. Avoid contamination of your equipment and emergency vehicles; a contaminated vehicle creates a risk of exposure to other, unsuspecting individuals wherever that vehicle travels. Attempt to obtain identification of the offending agent as soon as possible.

Remove all clothing from the patient. Clothing will be contaminated with either liquid or powder chemical. The contaminated clothing needs to be discarded with care. If any particulate substance is on the skin, it should be brushed away. Next, wash (lavage) the patient with copious amounts of water. Lavage will dilute the concentration of the injurious agent and wash away any remaining reagent. The key to lavage is to use large amounts of the water. A common error is to rinse 1 or 2 liters of water across the patient, then stop the lavage process once the water starts to pool and accumulate on the floor. When lavaged with only small amounts of fluid, the offending agent is only spread across the patient's surface area and not flushed away.[41,42] Failure to provide adequate runoff and drainage of lavage fluid may cause injury to previously unexposed and uninjured areas of the body as the contaminated lavage accumulates. One simple way of promoting runoff in a prehospital setting is to place the patient on a backboard and then tilt it with cribbing or other means to elevate an end. At the lower end of the board, tuck a large plastic garbage bag to contain the contaminated runoff.

Neutralizing agents for chemical burns are typically avoided. Often in the neutralizing process the agents give off heat in an exothermic reaction. Therefore, a well-meaning provider may create a thermal burn in addition to the chemical burn. Most commercially available decontamination solutions are made for the purpose of decontaminating equipment, not people.

Injuries to the eye caused by exposure to alkali may be encountered. A small exposure to the eye can result in a vision-threatening injury. The eyes should be irrigated with large amounts of irrigation fluid. If possible, ocular decontamination with continuous irrigation using a Morgan lens is performed (Figure 14-25). Application of an ophthalmic local anesthetic such as proparacaine will simplify the patient's care for the provider.

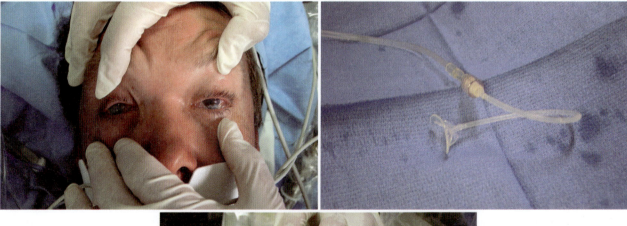

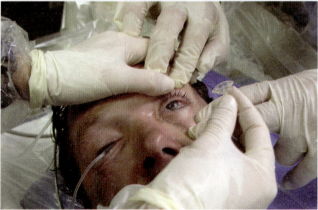

FIGURE 14-25 Eyes that have sustained a chemical injury require prompt irrigation with copious amounts of saline. A Morgan lens can be placed on the eye to provide appropriate ocular irrigation.

Specific Chemical Exposures

Cement is an alkali that may be retained on the clothing or in the footwear of individuals. The powdered cements will react with the victim's sweat in a reaction that gives off heat and excessively dries, or *desiccates,* the skin. These injuries typically present with a burn injury hours or the day after contact with the cement.

Fuels such as gasoline and kerosene can cause contact burns after prolonged exposure. These organic hydrocarbons can dissolve cell membranes, resulting in skin necrosis.[43] An exposure of sufficient duration or severity also may result in systemic toxicity. Decontamination of the patient covered with fuel is accomplished by irrigation with large volumes of water.

Hydrofluoric acid is a dangerous substance widely used in domestic, industrial, and military settings. The real danger of this chemical is the fluoride ion, which produces profound alterations in the exposed electrolytes, especially calcium and magnesium.[44] Left untreated, hydrofluoric acid will liquefy tissues and leach the calcium from bones. Initial treatment for hydrofluoric acid exposure is irrigation with water, followed by application of calcium gluconate gel at an emergency center. Patients with hydrofluoric acid burns should be promptly transferred to a burn center for additional treatment.

Injuries from phosphorus are often seen in military settings. *White phosphorus* (WP) is a powerful incendiary agent used in the production of munitions. It burns violently when exposed to air, producing brilliant flames. It will continue to burn until all of the agent has been consumed or is deprived of oxygen. The initial treatment is to deprive the WP of access to oxygen. All the clothing needs to be rapidly removed because it may contain some retained phosphorus particles that could ignite the clothing. Keep the affected areas immersed in water or saline-soaked dressings, and remoisten the dressings during transport. If the dressings dry out, any retained WP will reignite and could ignite the dressings and continue to burn the patient.

Hypochlorite solutions are often used to produce household bleaches and industrial cleaners. These solutions are strong alkalis; the commonly available solutions are 4% to 6% and are not usually lethal unless large areas of the body are involved. In greater concentrations, however, small volumes are potentially lethal. About 30 ml of a 15% solution is considered a life-threatening exposure.

Sulfur and nitrogen mustards are compounds that are classified as *vesicants or blister agents.* These agents have been used as chemical weapons and are recognized as a threat in chemical terrorism. These chemicals will burn and blister skin on exposure. These agents not only are irritants to the skin but also cause irritation to the lungs and the eyes. After exposure, patients will complain of a burning sensation of the throat and eyes. The skin involvement develops several hours later as redness is followed by blistering in the exposed or contaminated areas. After intense exposure, the victims will develop full-thickness necrosis and respiratory failure.[45–47] The principle treatment required from the prehospital care provider is decontamination.

In caring for victims of vesicant exposure, providers must wear appropriate gloves, garments, and breathing equipment. The patients must be decontaminated and irrigated with water or saline. Other agents used to decontaminate victims, used by specially trained personnel, include dilute hypochlorite solution and Fuller's earth powder. Additional specialized treatment is required when the patient arrives at a specialty center.

Tear gas and similar chemicals are known as "riot control agents." These agents will rapidly and briefly disable those exposed by causing irritation to the skin, lungs, and eyes. The extent of the injury is determined by the magnitude of exposure to the agent. The duration of the irritation typically lasts 30 to 60 minutes. Treatment consists of removing those exposed from the source of the exposure, removing contaminated clothing, and irrigating the skin and eyes.

Hazmat Scene Control Zones

To limit the spread of a hazardous material (hazmat), the National Institute of Occupational Safety and Health (NIOSH) and the Environmental Protection Agency (EPA) have developed and advocated the use of control zones. The objective of this concept is to perform specific activities in specific zones. By adherence to such principles, the likelihood of spread of contamination and injury to rescue personnel and bystanders is reduced.

The zones are three concentric circles. The innermost zone is the *hot zone.* This is the region immediately involved with and adjacent to the hazmat incident. Personnel entering this area must be fully protected, in most cases using Level A PPE, against the potential hazard. The task of rescuers in the hot zone is to evacuate injured patients without decontamination or patient care. The next zone is the *warm zone,* where decontamination of patients, personnel, and equipment occurs, again by personnel using appropriate protective equipment. In this zone, the only patient care administered is primary assessment and spine immobilization. The outermost zone is the *cold zone,* where equipment and personnel are staged. Once the patient is evacuated to the cold zone, providers can then deliver definitive care without the need for chemical PPE.

If a patient arrives to your hospital or aid station from a hazmat scene and the patient has not been decontaminated, you should follow the concepts of these hazmat zones.

SCENARIO SOLUTION

Patient 1: This patient has sustained critical injuries. Given that the patient was found collapsed in a burned building with burns to the face and labored respirations, you must be concerned that the patient has inhaled a large amount of smoke.

Evaluate and re-evaluate for airway edema and an inhalation injury. Airway patency needs to be a concern; however, the patient currently is managing his own airway. Keeping in mind that often the best person to manage an airway is the patient, you need to balance the time required to transport the patient with the difficulties of airway management in a patient with an edematous airway. If transport will be prolonged or delayed, secure the airway by tracheal intubation. The patient clearly needs 100% oxygen given the exposure to smoke and concerns about asphyxiants. If you elect to intubate this patient, be careful to secure the endotracheal tube. Anchor the tube with two pieces of umbilical tape or IV tubing placed above and below the ears. A portable carbon monoxide monitor placed on the patient reports a carboxyhemoglobin level of 16%, which is already being treated since the patient is on 100% oxygen. You consult the local protocol regarding management of smoke inhalation with potential cyanide poisoning.

Both upper extremities have deep, third-degree burns. You are not able to identify any veins to establish an intravenous line. Neither leg is burned nor is there evidence of any fractures. An intraosseous line is started in the left tibia and an infusion of Lactated Ringers (LR) is begun.

The patient is burned on the face, both upper extremities, and the anterior trunk. Each limb is approximately 9% of total body surface area (TBSA), the anterior trunk is 9%, and the face is approximately 4%. Therefore, the estimated burn surface area is approximately 31%. The patient weighs approximately 80 kg. Estimate the patient's fluid needs using the Parkland formula, as follows:

31% TBSA burn × 80 kg × 4 ml/kg/TBSA burn = 9920 ml to be administered in first 24 hours

Half this fluid total is administered in the first 8 hours after injury. Therefore, the hourly rate for the first 8 hours is:

9920 ml/2 = 4960 ml to be administered in first 8 hours

Calculate the hourly fluid rate:

4960 ml/8 = 620 ml per hour for hours 0 to 8

Patient 2: This patient is at risk for smoke inhalation based on the historical information provided. He has serious burns to his arm and hand. The patient is spontaneously managing his airway and ventilation. The burns of the entire arm and hand comprise 9% of the total body surface area. You cool the burns with ambient temperature water and then cover the burn with sterile towels. The circumferential nature of these burns makes this a potentially limb threatening injury that will require prompt surgical attention. Since the size of the burns is less than 20% total body surface area, a formal burn or Parkland resuscitation is not indicated. You start a peripheral IV with LR at a maintenance rate and administer a narcotic analgesic for pain relief.

SUMMARY

- All burns are serious, regardless of their size.
- Potentially life-threatening burns include large thermal burns, electrical injuries, and chemical burns.
- Unlike in mechanical trauma (e.g., penetrating, blunt), the body has little to no adaptive mechanisms to survive a burn injury.
- Burn injuries are not isolated to the skin; these are systemic injuries of unparalleled magnitude. Patients with major burn injury will experience dysfunction of the cardiovascular, pulmonary, GI, renal, and immune systems.
- Failure to provide appropriate fluid resuscitation will lead to refractory shock, multiorgan dysfunction, and even deepening of the burns. The role of the prehospital care provider is, therefore, crucial in optimizing survival after a burn injury. Although complicated and dangerous, burns are rarely rapidly fatal. A patient with severe smoke inhalation and large thermal burns may take several hours or days to die. Burn patients also are likely to have other mechanical trauma.
- Dramatic burns may focus the prehospital provider's attention away from other, potentially life-threatening injuries. Performing primary and secondary assessments will reduce the likelihood of missing these injuries (e.g., pneumothorax, pericardial tamponade, splenic rupture).
- Constant vigilance is required to avoid becoming a victim oneself. Often the injuring agent still poses a risk for injuring the providers.
- Even small burns in areas of high function (hands, face, joints, perineum) may result in long-term impairment from scar formation.
- Familiarity with burn center transport criteria will help ensure that all patients can achieve maximal function recovery after burn injury.
- The leading cause of death in burn patients is complications from smoke inhalation: asphyxiation, thermal injury, and delayed toxic-induced lung injury. Frequently, patients do not develop symptoms of respiratory failure for 48 hours or longer. Even without burns to the skin, victims of smoke inhalation should be transported to burn centers.
- Victims of burn injury from hazardous materials, such as chemicals or radioactive agents, should undergo decontamination to avoid inadvertent spread of the material to care providers.

References

1. Tredget EE, Shankowsky HA, Taerum TV, et al: The role of inhalation injury in burn trauma: A Canadian experience. *Ann Surg* 212:720, 1990.
2. Herndon D, Rutan R, Rutan T: Management of the pediatric patient with burns. *J Burn Care Rehabil* 14(1):3, 1993.
3. Rossignal A, Locke J, Burke J: Pediatric burn injuries in New England, USA. *Burns* 16(1):41, 1990.
4. Mortiz AR, Henrique FC Jr: Studies of thermal injury: The relative importance of time and surface temperature in the causation of cutaneous burn injury. *Am J Pathol* 1947, 23: 695.
5. Robinson MC, Del Becarro EJ: Increasing dermal perfusion after burning by decreasing thromboxane production. *J Trauma* 20:722, 1980.
6. Heggers JP, Ko F, Robson MC, et al: Evaluation of burn blister fluid. *Plast Reconstr Surg* 65:798, 1980.
7. Rossiter, N. D., P. Chapman, et al. (1996). "How big is a hand?" *Burns* 22(3):230–231.
8. Berry, M. G., D. Evison, et al. (2001). "The influence of body mass index on burn surface area estimated from the area of the hand." *Burns* 27(6):591–594.
9. de Camara DL, Robinson MC: Ultrastructure aspects of cooled thermal injury. *J Trauma* 21: 911–919, 1981.
10. Jandera V, Hudson DA, de Wet PM, Innes PM, Rode H: Cooling the burn wound: Evaluation of different modalities." *Burns* 26:265–270, 2000.
11. Sawada Y, Urushidate S, Yotsuyanagi T, Ishita K: Is prolonged and excessive cooling of a scalded wound effective?" *Burns* 23(1):55–58, 1977.
12. Venter TH, Karpelowsky JS, Rode H: Cooling of the burn wound: The ideal temperature of the coolant. *Burns* 33:917–922, 2007.
13. Dunn K, Edwards-Jones VT: The role of Acticoat with nanocrystalline silver in the management of burns. *Burns* 30(suppl):S1, 2004.
14. Wright JB, Lam K, Burrell RE: Wound management in an era of increasing bacterial antibiotic resistance: A role for topical silver treatments. *Am J Infect Control* 26:572, 1998.
15. Yin HQ, Langford R, Burrell RE: Comparative evaluation of the antimicrobial activity of Acticoat antimicrobial dressing. *J Burn Care Rehabil* 20:195, 1999.
16. Chung KK, Salinas J, Renz EM, et al. Simple derivation of the initial fluid rate for the resuscitation of severely burned adult combat casualties: In silico validation of the rule of 10. *J Trauma,* 2010;69:S49–S54.
17. Navar PD, Saffle JR, Warden GD: Effect of inhalation injury on fluid resuscitation requirements after thermal injury. *Am J Surg* 150:716, 1985.
18. Layton TR, McMurty JM, McClain EJ, Kraus DR, Reimer BL. Multiple spine fractures from electrical injuries. *J Burn Care Rehabil* 5:373–375, 1984.
19. Moritz AR, Henriques FC, McClean R: The effects of inhaled heat on the air passages and lungs. *Am J Pathol* 21:311, 1945.

20. Peters WJ: Inhalation injury caused by the products of combustion. *Can Med Assoc J* 125:249, 1981.

21. Forbes WH, Sargent F, Roughton FJW: The rate of carbon monoxide uptake by normal men. *Am J Physiol* 143:594, 1945.

22. Mellins RB, Park S: Respiratory complications of smoke inhalation in victims of fires. *J Pediatr* 87:1, 1975.

23. Chen KK, Rose CL, Clowes GH: Comparative values of several antidotes in cyanide poisoning. *Am J Med Sci* 188:767, 1934.

24. Feldstein M, Klendshoj NJ: The determination of cyanide in biological fluids by microdiffusion analysis. *J Lab Clin Med* 44:166, 1954.

25. Vogel SN, Sultan TR: Cyanide poisoning. *Clin Toxicol* 18:367, 1981.

26. Crapo R: Smoke inhalation injuries. *JAMA* 246:1694, 1981.

27. Herndon DN, Traber DL, Niehaus GD, et al: The pathophysiology of smoke inhalation in a sheep model. *J Trauma* 24:1044, 1984.

28. Till GO, Johnson KJ, Kunkel R, et al: Intravascular activation of complement and acute lung injury. *J Clin Invest* 69:1126, 1982.

29. Thommasen HV, Martin BA, Wiggs BR, et al: Effect of pulmonary blood flow on leukocyte uptake and release by dog lung. *J Appl Physiol Respir Environ Exerc Physiol* 56:966, 1984.

30. Trunkey DD: Inhalation injury. *Surg Clin North Am* 58:1133, 1978.

31. Haponik E, Summer W: Respiratory complications in the burned patient: Diagnosis and management of inhalation injury. *J Crit Care* 2:121, 1987.

32. Cahalane M, Demling R: Early respiratory abnormalities from smoke inhalation. *JAMA* 251:771, 1984.

33. Hight DW, Bakalar HR, Lloyd JR: Inflicted burns in children: Recognition and treatment. *JAMA* 242:517, 1979.

34. Chadwick DL: The diagnosis of inflicted injury in infants and young children. *Pediatr Ann* 21:477, 1992.

35. Adronicus M, Oates RK, Peat J, et al: Nonaccidental burns in children. *Burns* 24:552, 1998.

36. Purdue GF, Hunt JL, Prescott PR: Child abuse by burning: An index of suspicion. *J Trauma* 28:221, 1988.

37. Lenoski EF, Hunter KA: Specific patterns of inflicted burn injuries. *J Trauma* 17:842, 1977.

38. Brooks JW, Evans EI, Ham WT, Reid JD: The influence of external body radiation on mortality from thermal burns. *Ann Surg* 136:533, 1953.

39. American Burn Association: Radiation injury. In ABA: *Advanced burn life support course,* 1999, American Burn Association, p 66.

40. Michell MW, Oliveira HM, Vaid SU, et al: Enteral resuscitation of burn shock using intestinal infusion of World Health Organization oral rehydration solution (WHO ORS): A potential treatment for mass casualty care. *J Burn Care Rehabil* 25:S48, 2004.

41. Bromberg BF, Song IC, Walden RH: Hydrotherapy of chemical burns. *Plast Reconstr Surg* 35:85, 1965.

42. Leonard LG, Scheulen JJ, Munster AM: Chemical burns: Effect of prompt first aid. *J Trauma* 22:420, 1982.

43. Mozingo DW, Smith AD, McManus WF, et al: Chemical burns. *J Trauma* 28:642, 1998.

44. Mistry D, Wainwright D: Hydrofluoric acid burns. *Am Fam Physician* 45:1748, 1992.

45. Willems JL. Clinical management of mustard gas casualties. *Ann Med Milit Belg* 3S:1, 1989.

46. Papirmeister B, Feister AJ, Robinson SI, et al: The sulfur mustard injury: Description of lesions and resulting incapacitation. In Papirmeister B, Feister A, Robinson S, Ford R: *Medical defense against mustard gas,* Boca Raton, Fla, 1990, CRC Press, p 13.

47. Sidell FR, Takafuji ET, Franz DR: *Medical aspects of chemical and biological warfare,* Washington, DC, 1997, Office of the Surgeon General.

CHAPTER 15

Pediatric Trauma

CHAPTER OBJECTIVES

At the completion of this chapter, the reader will be able to do the following:

- ✓ Identify the anatomical and physiologic differences in children that account for unique pediatric injury patterns.

- ✓ Demonstrate an understanding of the special importance of managing the airway and restoring adequate tissue oxygenation in pediatric patients.

- ✓ Identify the quantitative vital signs for children.

- ✓ Demonstrate an understanding of management techniques for the various injuries found in pediatric patients.

- ✓ Calculate the Pediatric Trauma Score.

- ✓ Identify the signs of pediatric trauma suggestive of nonaccidental trauma.

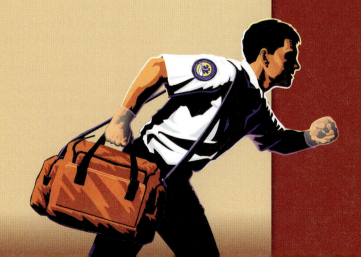

SCENARIO

You are called to the scene of a motor vehicle crash on a heavily travelled highway. Two vehicles have been involved in a frontal offset collision. One of the vehicle's occupants was a child who had been placed in—but not properly restrained in—a child car seat. No weather-related factors are involved on this average spring afternoon.

On arrival at the scene, you see that the police have secured and blocked traffic from the area around the crash. As your partner and the other arriving crew are assessing the other patients, you approach the child, you see a young boy, approximately 2 years of age, sitting in the car seat slightly turned at an angle, there is blood on the back of the headrest of the seat in front of him. You also note that, despite numerous abrasions and minor bleeding from the head, face, and neck, the child appears very calm.

Your primary and secondary surveys reveal a 2-year-old boy who repeats weakly "ma-ma, ma-ma." He has central and distal pulses at a rate of 180 beats/minute, with the radial pulse weaker than the carotid; his blood pressure is 50 mm Hg by palpation; and his ventilatory rate is 18 breaths/minute, slightly irregular, but without abnormal sounds. As you continue to assess him, you note that he has stopped saying "ma-ma" and seems to just stare into space. You also note that his pupils are slightly dilated, and his skin is pale and sweaty. A woman who identifies herself as the family's nanny tells you that the mother is en route and that you should wait for her.

What are the management priorities for this patient? What are the most likely injuries in this child? Where is the most appropriate destination for this child?

A nnual data reporting from the Center for Disease Control continues to show that, although the leading cause of death continues to vary by age group, injury is the most common cause of death for children in the United States. More than 8.7 million children are injured annually, and approximately every 30 minutes a child dies as a result of injuries.[1,2] Tragically, as many as 80% of these deaths may be avoidable, either by effective injury-prevention strategies or by ensuring proper care in the acute injury phase.[3]

As with all aspects of pediatric care, proper assessment and management of an injured child requires a thorough understanding of not only the unique characteristics of childhood growth and development (including their immature anatomy and developing physiology) but also their unique mechanisms of injury.

Thus, the adage holds true that "children are not just little adults." Children have distinct, reproducible patterns of injury, different physiologic responses, and special treatment needs, based on their physical and psychosocial development at the time of injury.

This chapter first describes the special characteristics of the pediatric trauma patient, then reviews optimal trauma management and its rationale. Although the unique characteristics of pediatric injury are important for the prehospital care provider to understand, the fundamental basic and advanced life support treatment approach using the primary and secondary surveys are the same for every patient, regardless of age or size.

The Child as Trauma Patient

Demographics of Pediatric Trauma

The unique needs and characteristics of pediatric patients require special attention when assessing the acutely injured child. The incidence of blunt (versus penetrating) trauma is highest in the pediatric population. As did its predecessor, the National Pediatric Trauma Registry (NPTR), the National Trauma Data Bank (NTDB) of the American College of Surgeons (ACS) continues to identify blunt trauma as the most common mechanism of injury, with penetrating injury accounting for only 10% of cases. The consequences of penetrating trauma are relatively predictable, but blunt trauma mechanisms have a greater potential for multisystem injury.

Falls, pedestrians struck by autos, and occupant injury as a result of motor vehicle crashes are the most common causes of pediatric injury in the United States, with falls alone accounting for more than 2.5 million injuries a year.[2] According to statistics, injury is "unintentional" in 87% of cases, sports-related in 4%, and the result of assault in 5%. For a variety of reasons, to be discussed throughout this chapter, multisystem involvement is the rule rather than the exception in major pediatric trauma. Although there may only be minimal external evidence of injury present, potentially life-threatening internal injury may still exist and must be evaluated for at a definitive treatment center.

Kinematics of Pediatric Trauma

A child's size produces a smaller target to which forces from fenders, bumpers, and falls are applied. Because of minimal cushioning body fat, increased elasticity of connective tissue, and proximity of the viscera to the surface of the body, these forces are not as easily dissipated as in the adult, and therefore, energy is more readily transmitted to underlying organs. Additionally, the skeleton of a child is incompletely calcified, contains multiple active growth centers, and is more resilient than that of an adult. Consequently, the skeleton of a child is less able to absorb the kinetic forces applied during a traumatic event, allowing significant force to be transmitted to underlying organs. As a result, there may be significant internal injuries without obvious evidence of external trauma. For example, in a pediatric patient with blunt thoracic trauma, the chest wall might appear intact without evidence of rib fractures, though significant underlying pulmonary contusion might still exist.

Common Patterns of Injury

The unique anatomic and physiologic characteristics of the pediatric patient combined with the age-specific common mechanisms of injury, produce distinct, but predictable, patterns of injury (Figure 15-1). Improper seat belt usage or placement in the vehicle with resulting impact with airbags can lead to significant injury in the pediatric patient (Figure 15-2). Trauma is frequently a time-critical illness and familiarity with these patterns will assist the prehospital provider in optimizing management decisions for the injured child in an expeditious manner. For example, blunt pediatric trauma involving closed-head injury results in apnea, hypoventilation, and hypoxia much more commonly than hypovolemia and hypotension. Therefore, clinical care guidelines for pediatric trauma patients should include greater emphasis on aggressive management of the airway and breathing.

Thermal Homeostasis

The ratio between a child's body surface area (BSA) and body mass is highest at birth and diminishes throughout infancy and childhood. Consequently, more surface area exists through which heat can quickly be lost, not only providing additional stress to the child, but also complicating the child's physiologic responses to concomitantly occurring metabolic derangements and shock. Profound hypothermia can result in severe coagulopathy and potentially irreversible cardiovascular collapse. In addition, many of the clinical signs of hypothermia are similar to those of impending decompensated shock, thereby potentially complicating the prehospital provider's clinical assessment.

Psychosocial Issues

The psychological ramifications of caring for an injured child also present a major challenge. Particularly with a very young child, regressive psychological behavior may result when stress, pain, or other perceived threats impair the child's ability to compensate for the surrounding events. A child's ability

FIGURE 15-1   **Common Patterns of Injury Associated with Pediatric Trauma**

Type of trauma	Patterns of injury
Motor vehicle crash (child is passenger)	*Unrestrained:* Multiple trauma, head and neck injuries, scalp and facial lacerations *Restrained:* Chest and abdomen injuries, lower spine fractures *Side impact:* Head, neck, and chest injuries; extremity fracture *Deployed air bag:* Head, face, chest injuries; upper extremity fractures
Motor vehicle crash (child is pedestrian)	*Low speed:* Lower extremity fractures *High speed:* Multiple trauma, head and neck injuries, lower extremity fractures
Fall from a height	*Low:* Upper extremity fractures *Medium:* Head and neck injuries, upper and lower extremity fractures *High:* Multiple trauma, head and neck injuries, upper and lower extremity fractures
Fall from bicycle	*Without helmet:* Head and neck lacerations, scalp and facial lacerations, upper extremity fractures *With helmet:* Upper extremity fractures *Striking handlebar:* Internal abdominal injuries

(Modified from American College of Surgeons Committee on Trauma: Pediatric trauma. In ACS Committee on Trauma: *Advanced trauma life support for doctors, student course manual*, ed 8, Chicago, 2008, ACS.)

It may only consist of simple words of compassion, or great lengths of patience, but you cannot be an effective provider for the pediatric patient if you are ignorant of the parents/caregivers needs. When you include the parents/caregivers in the process, they can often act as functional members of their child's emergency care team.

Recovery and Rehabilitation

Another problem unique to the pediatric trauma patient is the effect that even minor injury may have on subsequent growth and development. Unlike an anatomically mature adult, a child must not only recover from the injury but also continue their normal growth. The effect of injury on this process, especially in terms of permanent disability, growth deformity, or subsequent abnormal development, cannot be overestimated. Children sustaining even minor traumatic brain injury may have prolonged disability in cerebral function, psychological adjustment, or other regulated organ systems. As many as 60% of children who have sustained severe multiple trauma have personality changes, and 50% are left with subtle cognitive or physical handicaps. The reach of these injuries does not stop there, as these disabilities can have a substantial effect on siblings and parents, resulting in a high incidence of family dysfunction, including divorce. The direct and indirect costs of correcting these problems are staggering and lifelong.

The effects of inadequate or suboptimal care in the acute injury phase may have far reaching consequences not only on the child's immediate survival but also, perhaps more importantly, on the long term quality of the child's life. Therefore, it is extremely important to maintain a high index of suspicion for injury and to use clinical "common sense" when caring and making transport decisions for the acutely injured child.

Pathophysiology

The final outcome for the injured child may be determined by the quality of care rendered in the first moments following an injury. During this critical period, a coordinated, systematic primary survey is the best strategy to avoid overlooking a potentially fatal injury or one that may cause unnecessary morbidity. As in the adult patient, the three most common causes of immediate death in the child are hypoxia, massive hemorrhage, and overwhelming central nervous system (CNS) trauma. Lack of expedient triage, stabilizing emergency medical treatment, and transport to the most appropriate center for treatment can compound these problems or even eliminate the potential for a meaningful recovery.

Hypoxia

The first priority in prehospital care is always to maintain a patent airway, whether by basic supportive measures or

to interact with unfamiliar individuals in strange surroundings is usually limited and makes history-taking, examination, and treatment an arduous task. An understanding of these characteristics and a willingness to soothe and comfort an injured child are frequently the most effective means of achieving good rapport and obtaining a comprehensive assessment of the child's physiologic state.

The child's parents, or caregivers, also frequently have unique needs and issues that, if addressed, may assist the prehospital care provider in caring for the child successfully; however, if ignored, these needs and issues can present significant obstacles to effective care. Whenever a child is sick or injured, the caregivers are also affected and should be considered your patients as well. The treatment of all patients begins with effective communication, but this becomes even more important when dealing with these "parent-patients."

through advanced techniques. Confirming that a child has an open and functioning airway does not preclude the need for supplemental oxygen and assisted ventilation, especially when CNS injury, hypoventilation, or hypoperfusion is present. Well-appearing, injured children can rapidly deteriorate from mild tachypnea to a state of total exhaustion and apnea. Once an airway is established, the rate and depth of ventilation should be carefully evaluated to confirm adequate ventilation. If ventilation is inadequate, merely providing an excessive concentration of oxygen will not prevent ongoing or worsening hypoxia.

The effects of even transient hypoxia on the traumatically injured brain can be particularly devastating and, hence, deserve special attention. A child may have significant alteration in level of consciousness (LOC) but retain an excellent potential for a complete functional recovery if cerebral hypoxia is avoided. Patients who require aggressive airway management should be pre-oxygenated before attempting to place an advanced airway device. This simple maneuver may not only begin the reversal of existing hypoxia, but also provide sufficient reserves to improve the margin of safety when placement of an advanced airway is performed. A period of hypoxia during multiple or prolonged attempts at placing an advanced airway may be more detrimental to the child than simply ventilating the child with a bag-mask and providing for rapid transport.[4,5,6] In light of recent data, the risks of attempting advanced airway management must be carefully considered if the child is adequately ventilated and oxygenated using good basic life support skills, such as bag-mask ventilation.

Hemorrhage

Most pediatric injuries do not cause immediate exsanguination. Unfortunately, however, children who sustain injuries that result in major blood loss frequently die within moments of the injury or shortly after arrival at a receiving facility. These fatalities frequently have multiple internal organs injured and have at least one significant injury associated with acute blood loss. This bleeding may be minor, such as a simple laceration or contusion, or it may be a life-threatening hemorrhage, such as a ruptured spleen, lacerated liver, or avulsed kidney.

As in adults, the injured child compensates for hemorrhage by increasing systemic vascular resistance (SVR); however, this is at the expense of peripheral perfusion. In fact, children are physiologically more adept at this response because their ability for vasoconstriction is not limited by pre-existing peripheral vascular disease. Utilizing blood pressure measurements alone is an inadequate strategy to identify the early signs of shock. Tachycardia, although it may be the result of fear or pain, should be considered to be secondary to hemorrhage or hypovolemia until proven otherwise. A narrowing pulse pressure and increasing tachycardia may be the first subtle signs of impending shock. Furthermore, the prehospital provider must pay close attention to signs of ineffective organ perfusion as evidenced by a decreased level

of consciousness and diminished skin perfusion (decreased temperature, poor color, delayed capillary refill). Unlike in the adult, these early signs of hemorrhage in the child may be subtle and difficult to identify, leading to a deceptive presentation of shock. If the prehospital care provider misses these early signs, a child may lose enough circulating blood volume that compensatory mechanisms fail. When this happens, cardiac output plummets, organ perfusion decreases, and the child can rapidly decompensate, often leading to irreversible, fatal hypotension and shock. Therefore, every child who sustains blunt trauma should be carefully monitored to detect these subtle signs that might signal that there is ongoing hemorrhage, long before there are vital sign abnormalities.

A major reason for the rapid transition to decompensated shock is the loss of red blood cells (RBC) and their corresponding oxygen-carrying capacity. Restoration of lost intravascular volume with crystalloid solutions will provide a transient increase in blood pressure, but circulating volume will dissipate quickly as the fluid shifts across capillary membranes. It is generally thought that when replacing the intravascular volume with isotonic crystalloid solutions, a 3:1 ratio of crystalloid to the suspected blood loss is needed to compensate for this fluid shift. As blood is lost and intravascular volume is replaced with crystalloids, the remaining RBCs are diluted in the bloodstream, reducing the blood's ability to carry oxygen to the tissues. Therefore, it should be assumed that any child who requires more than one 20-ml/kg bolus of crystalloid solution may be rapidly deteriorating and needs not only intravascular volume resuscitation with crystalloid solution, but will likely also require a transfusion of RBCs so that oxygen-delivery capacity is restored in parallel to the intravascular volume.

However, once vascular access has been secured, there is a tendency to inadvertently over-resuscitate an injured child who is not in frank shock. In the child with moderate bleeding, no evidence of end-organ hypoperfusion, and normal vital signs, fluid resuscitation should be limited to no more than one or two boluses of 20 ml/kg. The intravascular component of one bolus represents approximately 25% of a child's blood volume. Therefore, if more than two boluses are required, the prehospital provider must take care to reassess the child for sources of previously undetected ongoing bleeding.

Given the high incidence of traumatic brain injury (TBI) with associated blunt trauma and the relatively low incidence of severe hemorrhagic shock, it was once thought that aggressive fluid resuscitation of a child with a TBI might actually worsen or hasten the development of cerebral edema. Currently, no evidence supports withholding fluid from a child with TBI to reduce cerebral edema.[7] In fact, there is more evidence in the literature to support aggressive resuscitation to prevent hypotension, a known and preventable secondary insult to head injury.[8,9] The cerebral perfusion pressure is the difference between the intracranial pressure (the pressure inside the skull) and the mean arterial pressure (the pressure driving blood into the skull). Traumatic brain injury can cause increases in intracranial pressures and so, even if the blood is adequately oxygenated but does not reach the brain because of low blood pressure, hypoxic brain injury can still occur. There is even some research to show that a *single* episode of hypotension can increase mortality by as much as 150%.[10] Additionally, careful assessment of the child's vital signs and frequent re-evaluation of any therapeutic interventions are the primary considerations immediately after the injury.

Isotonic crystalloid solutions should be the fluid of choice for resuscitation of the child with TBI, because *hypotonic* crystalloid solutions (e.g., dextrose in water) are known to increase cerebral edema. Furthermore, although *hypertonic* crystalloid solutions (e.g., hypertonic saline) may be useful for treatment of cerebral edema in the pediatric intensive care unit where there is extensive monitoring, there is no evidence to date that shows that it is safe or that it improves the outcome of pediatric trauma patients when administered in the field.

Central Nervous System Injury

The pathophysiologic changes after CNS trauma begin within minutes. Early and adequate resuscitation is the key to increased survival of children with CNS trauma. Although a subset of CNS injuries are instantaneous and overwhelmingly fatal, many children may present with the appearance of a devastating neurological injury only to go on to a complete and functional recovery, but only if there is a coordinated and deliberate effort to prevent secondary injury. This is achieved through the prevention of subsequent episodes of hypoperfusion, hypoventilation, hyperventilation, and ischemia. Adequate ventilation and oxygenation (while avoiding hyperventilation) are as critical in the management of TBIs as the avoidance of hypotension.[9] Thus, in traumatic brain injury, care must be taken with every child to prevent secondary brain injury from hypotension, hypoxia, and other insults.

For given degrees of injury severity, children have lower mortality and a higher potential for survival than their adult counterparts. However, the addition of injuries outside the brain lessens the child's chances of survival. This fact illustrates the potentially negative effect of associated injuries and of shock from CNS trauma on the outcome.

Children with TBI frequently present with an alteration in consciousness, and they may have sustained a period of unconsciousness not recorded during the initial evaluation. A history of loss of consciousness is one of the most important prognostic indicators of potential CNS injury, and should be investigated and recorded for every case. In the event that the injury was not witnessed, amnesia to the event is commonly used as a surrogate for a loss of consciousness. Similarly, complete documentation of baseline neurologic status is important, including the following:

1. Glasgow Coma Scale score (modified for pediatrics)
2. Pupillary reaction
3. Response to sensory stimulation
4. Motor function

These are essential steps in the initial pediatric trauma assessment for neurological injury. The absence of an adequate baseline assessment makes ongoing follow-up and evaluation of the effectiveness of any interventions extremely imprecise and difficult.

Attention to detail in history-taking is especially important in patients with possible cervical spine injury. A child's skeleton is incompletely calcified and has multiple active growth centers, so minimal, if any, radiographic evidence may exist of a mechanism causing stretch, contusion, or blunt injury to the spinal cord (spinal cord injury without radiographic abnormality, or SCIWORA). A transient neurologic deficit may be the only indicator of a potentially significant spinal cord injury.

Assessment

Primary Survey

The small and variable size of the pediatric patient (Figure 15-3), the diminished caliber and size of the blood vessels and circulating volume, and the unique anatomic characteristics of the airway frequently make the standard procedures used in basic life support extremely challenging and technically difficult. Effective pediatric trauma resuscitation mandates the availability of appropriately sized airways, laryngoscope blades, ET tubes, nasogastric tubes, blood pressure cuffs, oxygen masks, bag-mask resuscitators, and associated equipment. Attempting to place an overly large intravenous catheter or an inappropriately sized airway can do more harm than good, not only because of the potential physical damage to the patient, but also because it may delay transport to the appropriate facility. Therefore, a color-coded, length-based resuscitation tape was devised that will be discussed later.[11]

Airway

As in the injured adult, the immediate priority and focus in the acutely injured child is on airway management. However, there are several anatomic differences that complicate the care of the injured child. Children have a relatively large occiput, tongue, and anterior position of the airway. Additionally, the smaller the child, the greater the size discrepancy between the cranium and the midface. Therefore, the relatively large occiput forces passive flexion of the cervical spine (Figure 15-4). These factors all predispose children to a higher risk of anatomical airway obstruction than adults. In the absence of trauma, the pediatric patient's airway is best protected by a slightly superior-anterior position of the midface, known as the *sniffing position* (Figure 15-5). In the presence of trauma, however, the *neutral position* best protects the cervical spine while ensuring adequate airway opening. Thus, in the pedi-

FIGURE 15-3 **Height and Weight Range for Pediatric Patients**

| Group | Age | Range of mean norms | |
		Average height (cm/in)	Average weight (kg/lbs)
Newborn	Birth–6 weeks	51–63/20–25	4–5/8–11
Infant	7 weeks–1 year	56–80/22–32	4–11/8–24
Toddler	1–2 years	77–91/30–36	11–14/24–30
Preschool	2–6 years	91–122/36–48	14–25/30–55
School age	6–13 years	122–165/48–66	25–63/55–138
Adolescent	13–16 years	165–182/66–72	62–80/138–176

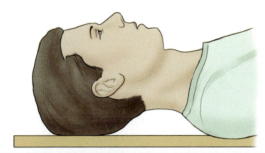

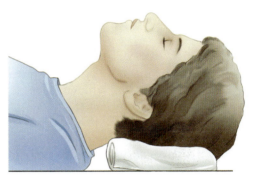

FIGURE 15-5 Sniffing position.

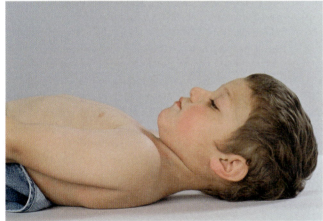

FIGURE 15-4 Compared to an adult (above), a child has a larger occiput and more shoulder musculature. When placed on a flat surface, these factors result in flexion of the neck.

atric trauma patient, the neck should be kept immobilized to prevent the flexion at the fifth and sixth cervical vertebrae (C5-C6) and the extension at C1-C2 that occurs with the sniffing position. Placing a pad or blanket of 2 to 3 cm in thickness under the child's torso will lessen the acute flexion of the neck and help keep the airway patent. Manual stabilization of the cervical spine is done during airway management and maintained until the child is immobilized on a long backboard with an appropriate cervical immobilization device, whether it is commercially purchased or a simple solution such as towel rolls.

Bag-mask ventilation with high flow (at least 15 liters per minute) 100% oxygen probably represents the best choice when the injured child requires assisted ventilation, whether for failure to ventilate, failure to oxygenate, or anticipated course.[4] If the child is unconscious, an oropharyngeal airway (OPA) may sometimes be safely placed, but it is likely to cause vomiting in the child with an intact gag reflex. This is also true of the laryngeal mask airway (LMA), and King LT airways, both of which are supraglottic airways which, when sized appropriately, are acceptable advanced airways for use in pediatric trauma patients. However, in comparison to that of the adult, the child's larynx is smaller in size and is slightly more anterior and cephalad (forward and toward the head), making it more difficult to visualize the vocal cords during intubation attempts (Figure 15-6). Tracheal intubation, despite being the most reliable means of ventilation in the child with airway compromise, is therefore reserved for those situations in which bag-mask ventilation is ineffective or results in excessive gastric insufflation, or when nonvisualized advanced airway devices have failed. Nasotracheal intubation should only be attempted as a last resort in the child. This is because it requires a spontaneously breathing patient, blind passage around the relatively acute posterior nasopharyngeal angle, and can cause severe bleeding. Additionally, in the patient

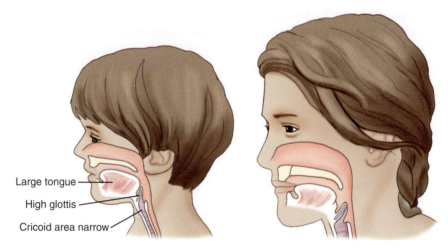

Large tongue —
High glottis —
Cricoid area narrow —

FIGURE 15-6 Comparison of the adult and child airways.

with a basilar skull fracture, it can even inadvertently penetrate the cranial vault. A child with craniofacial injuries that cause upper airway obstruction should be considered for percutaneous transtracheal jet ventilation with a large angiocatheter. This is only a temporary measure to improve oxygenation, but it does not improve ventilation and, hence, increasing hypercarbia dictates that a more definitive airway should be established as soon as safely possible. Surgical cricothyroidotomy is usually not indicated in the care of the pediatric trauma patient, though it may be considered in the larger child (usually at the age of 12).[12]

Breathing

As in all trauma patients, a significantly traumatized child typically needs an oxygen concentration of 85% to 100% (FiO$_2$ of 0.85–1.0). This is accomplished by the use of supplemental oxygen and an appropriately sized, *clear plastic,* pediatric mask. When hypoxia occurs in the small child, the body compensates by increasing the ventilatory rate (tachypnea) and by a strenu-

ous increase in ventilatory effort, including increased thoracic excursion efforts and the use of accessory muscles in the neck and abdomen. This increased metabolic demand can produce severe fatigue and result in ventilatory failure, as an increasing percentage of the patient's cardiac output becomes devoted to maintaining this respiratory effort. Ventilatory distress can rapidly progress from a compensated ventilatory effort to ventilatory failure, then respiratory arrest, and ultimately a hypoxic cardiac arrest. Central (rather than peripheral) cyanosis is a fairly late and often inconsistent sign of respiratory failure and should not be depended on to recognize developing respiratory failure.

Evaluation of the child's ventilatory status with early recognition of the signs of distress and the provision of ventilatory assistance are key elements in the management of the pediatric trauma patient. The normal ventilatory rate of infants and children younger than 4 years is typically two to three times that of adults (Figure 15-7).

Tachypnea with signs of increased effort or difficulty may be the first manifestations of respiratory distress and shock. As distress increases, additional signs and symptoms include

FIGURE 15-7 Ventilatory Rates for Pediatric Patients

Group	Age	Ventilatory rate (breaths/minute)	Ventilatory rate (breaths/minute) that indicates possible need for ventilatory assistance with bag-valve-mask
Newborn	Birth–6 weeks	30–50	<30 or >50
Infant	7 weeks–1 year	20–30	<20 or >30
Toddler	1–2 years	20–30	<20 or >30
Preschool	2–6 years	20–30	<20 or >30
School age	6–13 years	(12–20)–30	<20 or >30
Adolescent	13–16 years	12–20	<12 or >20

shallow breathing or minimal chest movement. Breath sounds may be weak or infrequent, and air exchange at the nose or mouth may be reduced or minimal. Ventilatory effort becomes more labored and may include the following:

- Head bobbing with each breath
- Gasping or grunting
- Flared nostrils
- Stridor or snoring respirations
- Suprasternal, supraclavicular, subcostal, or intercostal retractions
- Use of accessory muscles, such as neck and abdominal wall muscles
- Distension of the abdomen when the chest falls (seesaw effect between the chest and abdomen)

The effectiveness of a child's ventilation should be evaluated using the following indicators:

- Rate and depth (minute volume) and effort indicate adequacy of ventilation.
- Pink skin may indicates adequate ventilation.
- Dusky, gray, cyanotic, or mottled skin indicates insufficient oxygenation and perfusion.
- Anxiety, restlessness, and combativeness can be early signs of hypoxia.
- Lethargy, depressed LOC, and unconsciousness are probably advanced signs of hypoxia.
- Breath sounds evaluate the depth of exchange.
- Wheezing, rales, or rhonchi may indicate inefficient oxygenation.
- Declining pulse oximetry and/or declining capnography indicate respiratory failure.

A rapid evaluation of ventilation includes assessment of the patient's ventilatory rate (particularly tachypnea), ventilatory effort (degree of labor, nostril flaring, accessory muscle use, retraction, and seesaw movement), auscultation (air exchange, bilateral symmetry, and pathologic sounds), skin color, and mental status.

In the child initially presenting with tachypnea and increased ventilatory effort, normalization of the ventilatory rate and apparent lessening of the respiratory effort should not be immediately interpreted as a sign of improvement as it may indicate exhaustion or impending failure. As with any change in the patient's clinical status, frequent reassessment is necessary to determine if this is an improvement or deterioration in physiologic status. Ventilatory assistance should be given to those children in acute ventilatory distress. Because the main problem is one of inspired volume rather than concentration of oxygen, assisted ventilation is best given by use of a bag-mask device, supplemented with an oxygen reservoir attached to high-concentration oxygen (FiO_2 of 0.85–1.0). Because a child's airway is so small, it is prone to obstruction from increased secretions, blood/body fluids, and for-

eign materials; therefore, early and periodic suctioning may be necessary. In infants, who are obligate nose breathers, the nostrils should also be suctioned.

When obtaining a mask seal in infants, caution should be exercised to avoid compressing the soft tissues underneath the chin because this pushes the tongue against the soft palate and increases the risk of occluding the airway. Pressure on the uncalcified, soft trachea should also be avoided. One or two hands can be used to obtain a mask seal, depending on the size and age of the child.

Use of the correct size bag-mask is essential for obtaining a proper mask seal, providing the proper tidal volume, and ensuring that the risks of hyperinflation and barotrauma are minimized. Ventilating a child too forcefully or with too large a tidal volume can lead to gastric distension. In turn, *gastric distension* can result in regurgitation, aspiration, and prevention of adequate ventilation by limiting diaphragmatic excursion. Hyperinflation can lead to a *tension pneumothorax* that can result in both severe respiratory distress and sudden cardiovascular collapse, as the mediastinum is more mobile in the child. This protects the child from traumatic aortic injuries but increases the susceptibility to tension pneumothorax. The more mobile mediastinum compresses easily, allowing for earlier respiratory compromise and cardiovascular collapse than occurs in an adult.

Changes in a child's ventilatory status can be subtle, but ventilatory effort can rapidly deteriorate until ventilation is inadequate and hypoxia ensues. The patient's breathing should be evaluated as part of the primary survey and carefully and periodically reassessed to ensure its continued adequacy. Pulse oximetry should also be monitored, and efforts should be made to keep oxygen saturation (SpO_2) at greater than 95% (at sea level).

Whenever a child is manually ventilated, it is important to carefully control the rate at which ventilations are being administered. It is relatively easy to inadvertently hyperventilate the patient, which will decrease the CO_2 level in the blood and cause cerebral vasoconstriction. This can lead to poorer outcomes in patients with traumatic brain injury.

Circulation

The survival rate from immediate exsanguinating injury is low in the pediatric population. Fortunately, the incidence of this type of injury is also low. External hemorrhage should be quickly identified and controlled by direct manual pressure during the primary survey. Injured children usually present with at least some circulating blood volume and should respond appropriately to volume replacement. As in the assessment of the airway, a single measurement of heart rate (HR) or blood pressure (BP) does not equate with physiologic stability. Serial measurements and changing trends of vital signs are critical in gauging a child's evolving hemodynamic state in the acute injury phase. Close monitoring of vital signs is absolutely essential to recognizing the signs of impending shock, so that the appropriate interventions can be performed

FIGURE 15-8 Pulse Rate for Pediatric Patients

Group	Age	Pulse rate (beats/minute)	Pulse rate (beats/minute) that indicates a possible serious problem*
Newborn	Birth–6 weeks	120–160	<100 or >160
Infant	7 weeks–1 year	80–140	<80 or >150
Toddler	1–2 years	80–130	<60 or >140
Preschool	2–6 years	80–120	<60 or >130
School age	6–13 years	(60–80)–100	<60 or >120
Adolescent	13–16 years	60–100	<60 or >100

*Bradycardia or tachycardia.

to prevent clinical deterioration. Figures 15-8 and 15-9 provide the normal ranges for pulse rate and BP, respectively, for different pediatric age groups.

If the primary survey suggests hypotension, the most likely cause is blood loss through a major external wound that is readily observable (large scalp laceration, open femur fracture), an intrathoracic wound (identifiable by diminished ventilatory mechanics and auscultatory findings), or a major intra-abdominal injury. Because blood is not a compressible medium, blood loss from a major intra-abdominal injury can produce abdominal distension and increasing abdominal girth. However, increased abdominal girth in the young pediatric trauma patient can also commonly be caused by gastric distension from crying and air swallowing. Gastric decompression through a nasogastric or orogastric tube can help to distinguish between these causes of distension, although it is best to assume that a distended abdomen is a sign of potentially significant abdominal injury.

A major consideration in the assessment of a pediatric patient is compensated shock. Because of their increased physiologic reserve, children with hemorrhagic injury frequently present with only slightly abnormal vital signs. Initial tachycardia may be not only the result of hypovolemia but also the effect of psychological stress, pain, and fear. All injured children should have their HR, ventilatory rate, and overall CNS status monitored closely. An accurate BP reading may be difficult to obtain in the prehospital setting and focus should be placed on other signs of perfusion. If measured, a small patient may have a systolic BP that, although considered alarmingly low for an adult, may be within the normal range for a healthy child.

A child with hemorrhagic injury can maintain adequate circulating volume by increasing peripheral vascular resistance (PVR) to maintain mean arterial pressure (MAP). Clinical evidence of this compensatory mechanism includes prolonged capillary refill, peripheral pallor or mottling, cool peripheral skin temperature, and decreased intensity of the peripheral pulses. In the child, signs of significant hypotension develop with the loss of approximately 30% of the circulating volume. If initial resuscitation is inadequate, circulating volume will eventually diminish to a point below which increased PVR cannot maintain arterial pressure. The concept of evolving shock must be of paramount concern in the initial management of an injured child and is a major indication for transport to an appropriate facility for expeditious evaluation and treatment.

FIGURE 15-9 Blood Pressure (BP) for Pediatric Patients

Group	Age	Expected BP range (mm Hg)	Lower limit of systolic BP (mm Hg)
Newborn	Birth–6 weeks	74–100 50–68	>60
Infant	7 weeks–1 years	84–106 56–70	>70
Toddler	1–2 years	98–106 50–70	>70
Preschool	2–6 years	98–112 64–70	>75
School age	6–13 years	104–124 64–80	>80
Adolescent	13–16 years	118–132 70–82	>90

*Top numbers represent systolic range; bottom numbers represent diastolic range.

Disability

After assessment of airway, breathing, and circulation, the primary survey must include an assessment of neurologic status. Although the *AVPU scale* (**A**lert, responds to **V**erbal stimulus, responds to **P**ainful stimulus, **U**nresponsive) remains a simple, rapid assessment tool for the child's neurological status, it remains less informative than the Glasgow Coma Scale. It should be combined with a careful examination of the pupils to determine whether they are equal, round, and reactive to light. As in adults, the GCS provides a more thorough assessment of neurologic status and should be calculated for each pediatric trauma victim. The scoring for the verbal section for children under 4 years of age must be modified because of developing communication skills in this age group, and the child's behavior should be observed carefully (Figure 15-10).

The GCS score should be repeated frequently and used to document progression or improvement of neurologic status during the postinjury period (refer to Chapters 6 and 9 for a review of the GCS). A more thorough assessment of motor and sensory function should be performed in the secondary survey if time permits.

Expose/Environment

Children should be examined for other potentially life-threatening injuries; however, they may be frightened at attempts to remove their clothes. In addition, because of children's high BSA, they are more prone to developing hypothermia. Therefore, once the examination to identify other injuries is complete, the patient should be covered to preserve body heat and prevent further heat loss.

Pediatric Trauma Score

The decision as to which child requires what level of care must proceed from a careful and rapid evaluation of the entire child. Overlooking potential organ system injury and inadequately managing the patient are two common problems. For this reason, the Pediatric Trauma Score (PTS) has been developed to provide a reliable and simple protocol for assessment that is predictive of outcome; however, the PTS is not used in the field triage algorithm as physiologic, anatomic, and mechanistic considerations have been considered adequate in the initial field assessment (Figure 15-11). To calculate the PTS, six components of pediatric injury are graded and then added together to produce a score predictive of injury severity and potential for mortality. The system is based on an analysis of pediatric injury patterns and is designed to provide a protocol checklist to ensure that all the major injury factors related to injury outcome are considered in the initial evaluation of the child. The PTS is different than the Revised Trauma Score (RTS), which only considers the BP, ventilatory rate, and GCS score.

Size is the first component because it is readily observed and is a major consideration in the infant/toddler group. The airway is assessed next, because the functional status and the level of care required to provide adequate ventilation and oxygenation must be considered.

The most important historical factor in initial assessment of the CNS is LOC. Because children frequently sustain transient loss of consciousness during an injury, the obtunded grade (+1) is applied to any child with loss of consciousness, no matter how fleeting. This grade identifies children at higher risk of developing potentially fatal, yet frequently treatable, intracranial injuries that may lead to secondary brain injury.

FIGURE 15-10 Pediatric Verbal Score

Verbal response	Verbal score
Appropriate words or social smile; fixes and follows	5
Crying but consolable	4
Persistently irritable	3
Restless, agitated	2
No response	1

Component	+2	+1	−1
Size	Child/adolescent >20 kg	Toddler 11-20 kg	Infant <10 kg
Airway	Normal	Assisted: O$_2$ mask, cannula	Intubated: ETT, cricothyroidotomy
Consciousness	Awake	Obtunded, lost consciousness	Coma, unresponsive
Systolic blood pressure	90 mm Hg Good peripheral pulses, perfusion	51-90 mm Hg Carotid, femoral pulse palpable	<50 mm Hg Weak or no pulses
Fracture	None seen or suspected	Single closed fracture anywhere	Open or multiple fractures
Cutaneous	No visible injury	Contusion, abrasion, laceration <7 cm not through fascia	Tissue loss, any gun shot wound or stab through fascia

FIGURE 15-11 Pediatric Trauma Score (PTS) is primarily designed to function as a checklist. Each component can be assessed by basic physical examination. Airway evaluation is designed to reflect intervention required for effective care. An open fracture is graded −1 for fracture and −1 for cutaneous injury. As clinical observation and diagnostic evaluation continue, further definition and reassessment will establish a trend that predicts severity of injury and potential outcome.

FIGURE 15-12 **Pediatric Vital Signs and Quantitative Norms**

The term *pediatric or child* includes a vast range of physical development, emotional maturity, and body sizes. The approach to the patient and the implications of many injuries vary greatly between an infant and an adolescent.

In most anatomic and therapeutic dosage considerations, a child's weight (or specific height or length) serves as a more accurate indicator than exact chronologic age.[11] Figure 15-3 lists the average height and weight for healthy children of varying ages.

The acceptable ranges of vital signs vary for the different ages within the pediatric population. Adult norms cannot be used as guidelines in smaller children. An adult ventilatory rate of 30 breaths/minute is tachypneic, and an adult heart rate of 120 beats/minute is tachycardic. Both are considered alarmingly high in an adult and are significant pathologic findings. However, the same findings in an infant may be within the normal ranges.

Normal ranges of vital signs for different age groups may not be consistent across all pediatric references. In an injured child without a previous history of normal vital signs, borderline vital signs may be viewed as pathologic, even though in that individual child the signs may be physiologically acceptable. The guidelines in Figures 15-7, 15-8, and 15-9 can aid in evaluating vital signs. These tables present statistically common ranges into which most children in these age groups will fall.

Several commercially available items serve as rapid reference guides for pediatric vital signs and equipment size. These include the length-based resuscitation tape (Broselow tape) and several slide-rule–type plastic scales.

The following guideline formulas can also be used to estimate the expected finding for any age:

Weight (kg) = 8 + (2 x Child's age [years])
Lowest acceptable systolic blood pressure (mm Hg) =
70 + (2 x Child's age [years])
Total vascular blood volume (ml) =
80 ml x Child's weight (kg)

Quantitative vital signs in children, although important, are only one piece of information used in making an assessment. A child with a normal set of vital signs can rapidly deteriorate into either critical ventilatory difficulty or decompensated shock. Vital signs should be considered along with mechanism of injury and other clinical findings.

Systolic blood pressure (SBP) is used to identify children in whom evolving preventable shock may occur (SBP 51–90 mm Hg; +1). Regardless of size, a child whose SBP is less than 50 mm Hg (-1) is in obvious jeopardy (Figure 15-12). A child whose SBP exceeds 90 mm Hg (+2) falls into a better outcome category. If the appropriately sized BP cuff is not available, SBP is assessed as (+2) if the radial or pedal pulse is palpable, (+1) if only the carotid or femoral pulse is palpable, and (−1) if no pulse is palpable.

Because of the high incidence of skeletal injury in the pediatric population and its potential contribution to mortality and disability, the presence of a long-bone fracture is included in the PTS as a component. Finally, the skin is assessed for open wounds and penetrating injury.

By nature of its design, the PTS serves as a straightforward checklist that ensures all components necessary to identify a critically injured child are considered. As a predictor of injury, the PTS has a statistically significant, direct linear relationship with the Injury Severity Score (ISS) and an inverse linear relationship with patient mortality. There is a threshold score of 8, below which injured children should be taken to an appropriate pediatric trauma center because they have the greatest potential for preventable mortality and morbidity. Although research has shown that other scores, such as the RTS, the unresponsive element (U) of the AVPU score, and a best motor response of "1" from the GCS, predict mortality at least as well as the PTS, the PTS remains the only score that includes size, skeletal injury, and open wounds. Although the PTS is a readily available assessment and triage tool, it has not been universally accepted. Other methods of triage may be used in many areas.

Secondary Survey (Detailed Physical Examination)

The secondary survey of the child should follow the primary survey only after life-threatening conditions have been identified and managed. The head and neck should be examined for obvious deformities, contusions, abrasions, punctures, burns, tenderness, lacerations, or swellings. The thorax should be re-examined. Potential pulmonary contusions may become evident after volume resuscitation, manifested by respiratory distress or abnormal lung sounds. Trauma patients are infrequently "NPO" (fasting) at the time of their injuries, so insertion of a nasogastric or orogastric tube may be indicated, if local protocols allow. This is especially true for children who are obtunded or who have post-traumatic seizure activity.

Examination of the abdomen should focus on distension, tenderness, discoloration, ecchymoses, and presence of a mass. Careful palpation of the iliac crests may suggest an unstable pelvic fracture and increase the suspicion for possible retroperitoneal or urogenital injury as well as increased risk for hidden blood loss. An unstable pelvis should be noted, but repeated examinations of the pelvis should not be performed, as this may result in further injury and increased blood loss. The patient should be appropriately immobilized on a longboard and prepared for transfer to a pediatric trauma facility.

Each extremity should be inspected and palpated to rule out tenderness, deformity, diminished vascular supply, and neurologic deficit. A child's incompletely calcified skeleton with its multiple growth centers increases the possibility of epiphyseal (growth plate) disruption. Accordingly, any area of edema, pain, tenderness, or diminished range of motion should be treated as if it were fractured until evaluated by radiographic examination. In children as in adults, a missed orthopedic injury in an extremity may have little effect on mortality but may lead to long-term deformity and disability.

Management

The keys to pediatric trauma survival are rapid cardiopulmonary assessment, age-appropriate aggressive management, and transport to a facility capable of managing pediatric trauma. A color-coded, length-based resuscitation tape was devised to serve as a guide that allows for rapid identification of a patient's height with a correlated estimation of weight, size of equipment to be used, and appropriate dosages of potential resuscitative drugs. In addition, most prehospital systems have a guideline for selecting appropriate destination facilities for pediatric trauma patients.

Airway

Ventilation, oxygenation, and perfusion are as essential to an injured child as to an adult. Thus, the primary goal of the initial resuscitation of an injured child is restoration of adequate tissue oxygenation as quickly as possible. The first priority of assessment and resuscitation is the establishment of a patent airway.

A patent airway should be ensured and maintained with suctioning, manual maneuvers, and airway adjuncts. As in the adult, initial management in the child includes in-line cervical spine stabilization. Unless a specialized pediatric spine board that has a depression at the head is used, adequate padding

(2–3 cm) should be placed under the torso of the small child so that the cervical spine is maintained in a straight line rather than forced into slight flexion because of the disproportionately large occiput (Figure 15-13). When adjusting and maintaining airway positioning, compressing the soft tissues of the neck and trachea should be avoided. Once manual control of the airway is achieved, an oropharyngeal airway can be placed if no gag reflex is present. The device should be inserted carefully and gently, parallel to the course of the tongue rather than turned 90 or 180 degrees in the posterior oropharynx as in the adult. Use of a tongue blade to depress the tongue can be helpful. Orotracheal intubation under direct visualization of the trachea is the preferred method of definitive airway control during long transports (Figure 15-14). One study suggests, however, that during short transports, there is no improved survival or neurologic outcome in pediatric trauma patients intubated early in the field versus those who underwent bag-mask ventilation.[4] A more recent study in a rural setting found that multiple prehospital intubation attempts were associated with significant complications (Figure 15-15).[13] Although the Combitube™ has been a proven rescue airway device for adult trauma victims,[40] its large size and lack of smaller sizes makes it inadequate as a rescue device for small children (under 4 feet in height). The laryngeal mask airway (LMA) and now the smaller sizes of the King LT airways have been shown to provide a safe rescue airway in children and are reasonable alternatives to endotracheal intubation in certain situations.[41]

Thus, the risks and benefits of orotracheal intubation must be carefully weighed before attempting the procedure, especially in the pediatric patient in which bag-mask ventilation is providing adequate ventilation and oxygenation. This is increasingly important as additional nonvisualized advanced airway devices come into use.

Breathing

The patient's minute volume and ventilatory effort should be evaluated carefully. Because of the potential for rapid deterioration from mild hypoxia to ventilatory arrest, ventilation should be assisted if dyspnea and increased ventilatory effort are observed. A properly sized bag-mask device with a reservoir and

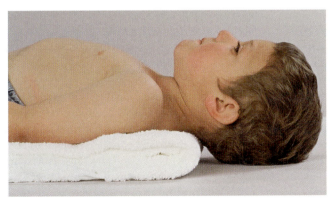
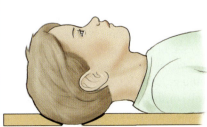

FIGURE 15-13   Provide adequate padding under the child's torso or use a spine board with a cut-out for the child's occiput.

FIGURE 15-14   Pediatric Endotracheal Intubation

Endotracheal intubation of an injured child should include careful attention to cervical spine immobilization. One person should maintain the patient's spine in a neutral position while another person intubates. The narrowest portion of the pediatric airway is the cricoid ring, creating a "physiologic cuff," so uncuffed tracheal tubes should always be used in children less than 8 years of age. The appropriate size for a tracheal tube can be estimated by using the diameter of the child's fifth finger, external nares, or by using the formula (16 + Age)/4. A slight amount of cricoid pressure frequently brings the anterior structures of the child's larynx into better view and will passively obstruct the esophagus, thus diminishing gastric insufflation. However, pediatric tracheal rings are relatively soft and pliable, and overzealous cricoid pressure may completely occlude the airway. Pharmacologically assisted intubation, or rapid-sequence intubation (RSI), should always include the use of atropine sulfate to prevent vagal induced bradycardia. Heart rate is a major determinant of perfusion in pediatric patients.

A common error that occurs during intubation of children under emergency circumstances is aggressive advancement of the tracheal tube resulting in its placement into the right mainstem bronchus. The tube should never be advanced more than three times the tube size (in centimeters). For example, a 3.0 cm endotracheal tube should rest at a depth no greater than 9 cm. The chest and epigastrium should always be auscultated after the tracheal tube is placed and $ETCO_2$ capnometry used when available. Tube placement should be frequently reassessed, especially after any movement of the patient. In addition to confirming endotracheal tube placement, auscultation may rule out the possibility of other pulmonary injury. The child with a compromised airway and a pulmonary injury who has been successfully intubated may be in greater jeopardy for the development of a tension pneumothorax as a result of positive pressure ventilation.

FIGURE 15-15   Prehospital Pediatric Intubation: The Great Debate

It would almost seem intuitive that providing a tracheal tube as early as possible in the management of the child with traumatic brain injury (TBI) would be of benefit. A retrospective review showed improved survival in adult patients with TBI who were intubated prior to arrival at the receiving hospital.[34] Subsequent studies evaluated rapid-sequence intubation (RSI), demonstrating its improved efficiency and success rate in intubation of adults and children.[35,36] However, many retrospective and prospective case-control studies found that prehospital intubation compared with bag-mask ventilation did not improve survival or neurologic outcome and even might have been detrimental.[5,37,38] A prospective randomized trial in children comparing endotracheal intubation versus bag-mask ventilation in an urban area with short transport times demonstrated no difference in survival or neurologic outcome between the two groups but an increased incidence of complications in the intubated group.[4]

Prolonged periods of hypoxia are often associated with the intubation process, as well as periods of overaggressive ventilation following intubation in patients transported to the trauma center.[6]

Data supporting prehospital pediatric tracheal intubation are limited and ambiguous. In the spontaneously breathing child, intubation with or without pharmacologic assistance should be initiated with extreme caution. EMS programs that perform pediatric prehospital intubation should include at least the following:[39]

1. Close medical direction and supervision.
2. Training and continuing education, including hands-on operating room (OR) experience.
3. Resources for patient monitoring, drug storage, and tube placement confirmation.
4. Standardized RSI protocols.
5. Availability of backup rescue airway such as a LMA or King LT airway.
6. Intensive continuing quality assurance/quality control and performance review program.

high-flow oxygen to provide an oxygen concentration of between 85% and 100% (FiO_2 of 0.85–1.0) should be used. Continuous pulse oximetry serves as an adjunct for ongoing assessment of airway and breathing. The SpO_2 should be kept at greater than 95% (at sea level). In the intubated child with a closed head injury, endotracheal tube placement should be confirmed in multiple fashions, including directly visualizing the tube pass through the vocal folds, the presence of equal bilateral breath sounds, and the absence of sounds over the epigastrium when ventilated. Continuous end-tidal carbon dioxide ($ETCO_2$) monitoring, when available, should be used to document continuing appropriate endotracheal tube placement and avoid extremes of hypercarbia and hypocarbia, both of which can be just as detrimental to recovery from a closed head injury as hypoxia. $ETCO_2$ should be targeted at 30 to 40 mm Hg.[6]

Children are more susceptible than adults to acute cardiovascular collapse from a tension pneumothorax. Most children with tension pneumothoraces will present with acute cardiac decompensation secondary to decreased venous return before any detectable changes in oxygenation and ventilation have occurred. Any child, who acutely decompensates, especially after initiation of positive-pressure ventilation by bag-mask or advanced airway placement, should be emergently assessed for tension pneumothorax. Jugular venous distension may be difficult to determine because an extrication collar has been applied or because of the presence of hypovolemia from hemorrhage. Tracheal shift is a late sign and may only be determined by palpating the trachea in the jugular notch. In these children, unilateral absent breath sounds, in association with cardiovascular compromise, represent an indication for emergency needle decompression. In the intubated patient, diminished sounds on the left may indicate a right mainstem intubation, but when associated with acute cardiac decompensation, these sounds may represent tension pneumothorax. Careful reassessment of the patient's airway and respiratory status is needed to distinguish these subtle differences in the presentation. Needle decompression is performed using the same landmarks as in the adult, but it is often more immediately effective in the child because the mediastinum rapidly shifts back to its normal position and venous return is quickly restored.

Circulation

Once the patient's external hemorrhage is controlled, perfusion should be evaluated. Controlling external hemorrhage involves applying direct manual pressure on the bleeding point, the use of advanced hemostatic dressings, and the selective use of tourniquets in extreme cases in which other measures have failed; it is *not* just covering the bleeding site with layer after layer of absorbent dressing. If the initial dressing does become saturated in blood, it is best to add an additional dressing rather than to replace it, as the removal may dislodge any clot that has begun to form, while at the same time performing additional interventions to stop the ongoing hemorrhage. The pediatric vascular system is usually able to maintain a normal BP until severe collapse occurs, at which point it is often unresponsive to resuscitation. Therefore, fluid resuscitation should be started whenever signs of compensated hypovolemic shock are present and *must* be immediately started in patients who present with decompensated shock. Lactated Ringer's (LR) or normal saline (NS) solution in 20 ml/kg boluses should be used. For pediatric trauma patients who display any signs of hemorrhagic shock or hypovolemia, key factors to survival are appropriate volume resuscitation and rapid initiation of transport to a suitable facility. Transportation should not be delayed to obtain vascular access or administer intravenous (IV) fluid.

Vascular Access

Fluid replacement in a child with severe hypotension or signs of shock must deliver adequate fluid volume to the right atrium to avoid further reduction in cardiac preload. The most appropriate initial sites for IV access are the antecubital fossa and the saphenous vein at the ankle. Access through the external jugular vein is another possibility, but airway management takes priority in such a small space and spinal immobilization makes the neck poorly accessible.

In the unstable or potentially unstable patient, attempts at peripheral access should be limited to two in 90 seconds. If peripheral access is unsuccessful, intraosseous access should be considered (Figure 15-16).

FIGURE 15-16 Pediatric Intraosseous Infusion

Intraosseous (IO) infusion can provide an excellent alternative site for resuscitative volume replacement in injured children of all ages. This is an effective route for infusion of medications, blood, or high-volume fluid administration.

The most accessible site for IO infusion is the anterior tibia just inferior and medial to the tibial tuberosity. After preparing the skin antiseptically and securing the leg adequately, a site is chosen on the anterior portion of the tibia, 1 to 2 cm below and medial to the tibial tuberosity. Specially manufactured IO infusion needles are optimal for the procedure, but spinal or bone marrow needles may also be used. Spinal needles that are 18- to 20-gauge work well because they have a trocar to prevent the needle from being obstructed as it passes through the bony cortex into the marrow. Any 14- to 20-gauge needle can be used in an emergency. There are a variety of commercially available devices that ease the difficulty of placing an IO needle, using various mechanical devices. For example, the EZ-IO uses a high speed drill to insert a specially designed IO needle. The needle is placed at a 90-degree angle to the bone and advanced firmly through the cortex into the marrow. Evidence that the needle is adequately within the marrow includes the following:

1. A soft "pop" and lack of resistance after the needle has passed through the cortex.
2. Aspiration of bone marrow into the needle.
3. Free flow of fluid into the marrow without evidence of subcutaneous infiltration.
4. The needle is secure and does not appear loose or wobbly.

IO infusion should be considered during initial resuscitation if percutaneous venous cannulation has been unsuccessful. Because the flow rate is limited by the bone marrow cavity, the administration of fluids and medications should normally be done under pressure, and the IO route alone will seldom be sufficient after initial resuscitation.

Placement of a subclavian or internal jugular catheter in an injured child should be performed only under the most controlled circumstances within the hospital; this should not be attempted in the prehospital environment.

The determination of which pediatric patients should have intravascular access depends on the severity of injury, the experience of the involved personnel, and transport times among other factors. If uncertainty exists as to which patients need intravascular access, or if fluid replacement is needed during transport, online medical direction should be obtained.

Fluid Therapy

Lactated Ringer's solution, or NS solution if LR solution is unavailable, is the initial resuscitation fluid of choice for a hypovolemic child. As discussed in the Shock chapter, the time that a crystalloid fluid remains in the intravascular space is relatively short, which is why a 3:1 ratio of crystalloid fluid to blood lost has been recommended. An initial fluid bolus for an injured child is 20 ml/kg, which is approximately 25% of the normal circulating blood volume of the child. Considering the 3:1 ratio, as much as 40–60 ml/kg may be required to achieve adequate and rapid initial replacement in response to significant blood loss. Any injured child who does not show at least a minor improvement in hemodynamic status with the first 20-ml/kg fluid bolus and stabilization after the second 20-ml/kg bolus should receive a blood transfusion. The crystalloid bolus may temporarily restore cardiovascular stability as it transiently fills and then leaks from the circulatory system. However, until circulating RBCs are replaced and oxygen transport is restored, hypoxic injury will continue.

Pain Management

As with adults, pain management should be considered for children in the prehospital setting. Indications for analgesia include isolated limb injury and suspected spinal fracture. Small doses of a narcotic analgesia that are appropriately titrated should not compromise the neurologic or abdominal examination. Both morphine and fentanyl are acceptable choices, but they should be administered only according to written prehospital care guideline or with orders from online medical control. Because of the side effects of hypotension and hypoventilation, all patients receiving IV narcotics should be monitored with pulse oximetry and serial vital signs. In general, benzodiazepines should not be administered in combination with narcotics because of their synergistic effects on respiratory depression or even respiratory arrest.

Transport

Because timely arrival at the most appropriate facility may be the *key* element in the patient's survival, *triage* is an important consideration of management.

The tragedy of preventable pediatric traumatic death has been documented in multiple studies reported over the past three decades. It is estimated that as many as 80% of pediatric trauma deaths can be classified as preventable or potentially preventable. These statistics have been one of the primary motivations for the development of regionalized pediatric trauma centers, where continuous, coordinated, high-quality, sophisticated care can be provided.

Many urban areas have both pediatric trauma centers and adult trauma centers. Ideally, the pediatric multisystem trauma patient will benefit from the initial resuscitation capability and definitive care available at a pediatric trauma center because of its specialization in treating traumatized children. Thus, bypassing an adult trauma center in favor of transport to a pediatric trauma center is justifiable. For many communities, however, the nearest specialized pediatric trauma center may be hours away. In these cases, the seriously traumatized child should be transported to the nearest adult trauma center because early resuscitation and evaluation before transport to a pediatric facility may improve survival.[23] In areas where no specialized pediatric trauma center is nearby, personnel working in adult trauma centers should be experienced in the resuscitation and treatment of both adult and pediatric trauma patients. In areas where neither facility is readily close, the seriously injured child should be transported to the nearest appropriate hospital capable of caring for trauma victims, according to local prehospital triage guidelines. Aeromedical transport may be considered in rural areas to expedite transport. There is little evidence that aeromedical transport provides any benefit in urban areas in which ground transport to a pediatric trauma center is almost as quick.[24] It is becoming increasingly evident that utilizing aeromedical transport exposes both the patient and the crew to a significant amount of risk. These concerns must be carefully weighed when deciding whether to utilize this resource.

Review of more than 15,000 records in the NPTR indicates that 25% of children are injured severely enough to require triage to a designated pediatric trauma center. Use of the PTS can help with appropriate triage. Many emergency medical services (EMS) and trauma systems use other pediatric triage criteria, which may be dictated by state, regional, or local guidelines. All prehospital care providers need to be familiar with the triage protocols in place within their own systems.

Specific Injuries

Traumatic Brain Injury

Traumatic brain injury (TBI) is the most common cause of death in the pediatric population. Of the fatalities included in the first 40,000 patients in the NPTR, 89% had a CNS injury as either the primary or the secondary contributor to mortality. Although many of the most severe injuries are treatable only by prevention, initial resuscitative measures may minimize secondary brain injury and, consequently, the severity of the child's injury. Adequate ventilation, oxygenation, and perfusion are needed to prevent secondary morbidity. The outcome of children sustaining severe TBI is typically better than in adults, except in the subset of children younger than 3 years in which it is worse than that of older children.

The results of the initial neurologic assessment are useful for prognosis. Even with a normal initial neurologic evaluation, however, any child who sustains a head injury may be susceptible to cerebral edema, hypoperfusion, and secondary insults. These conditions can result even from a mechanism that appears minor.

A baseline GCS score should be assessed and frequently repeated during transport. Supplemental oxygen should be administered, and if possible, pulse oximetry should be monitored. Although vomiting is common after a concussion, persistent or forceful projectile vomiting is of concern and requires further evaluation.

As with hypoxia, hypovolemia may dramatically worsen the original TBI. External hemorrhage must be controlled and the patient's fractured extremities immobilized to limit internal blood loss associated with these injuries. An attempt should be made to keep these children in a euvolemic state with IV volume resuscitation. On rare occasions, infants less than about 6 months of age may become hypovolemic as a result of intracranial bleeding because they have open cranial sutures and fontanelles. The infant with an open fontanelle may better tolerate an expanding intracranial hematoma but may not become symptomatic until rapid decompensation occurs. An infant with a bulging fontanelle should be considered to have a more severe TBI.

Children with a GCS score of 8 or less may benefit from endotracheal (ET) intubation. However, adequate oxygenation and ventilation should be the goal at all times, not the placement of an ET tube. Prolonged attempts at securing an endotracheal airway may increase periods of hypoxia and delay transport to an appropriate facility. The *best* airway for a child is the one that is both safest and most effective. Ventilation with a bag-mask device while being prepared to suction emesis, should it occur, may be safer than intubation and is often the best airway for the child with TBI.[4,5,6]

A child with signs and symptoms of intracranial hypertension or increased intracranial pressure (ICP), such as a sluggishly reactive or nonreactive pupil, systemic hypertension, bradycardia, and abnormal breathing patterns, may benefit from temporary mild hyperventilation to lower ICP. However, this effect of hyperventilation is transient and also decreases overall oxygen delivery to the CNS actually causing additional secondary brain injury.[15] It is strongly recommended that this strategy not be used unless the child is exhibiting signs of active herniation or lateralizing signs. ETCO$_2$ monitoring should guide management in the intubated child, with the target range about 35 mm Hg. Hyperventilation to an ETCO$_2$ of less than 25 mm Hg has been associated with worse neurologic

outcome.[6] If capnography is not available, a ventilation rate of 30 breaths/minute for children and 35 breaths/minute for infants should be used.[7]

During prolonged transports, small doses of mannitol (0.5–1 g/kg body weight) may benefit children with evidence of intracranial hypertension, if local protocols permit. However, use of mannitol in the setting of insufficient volume resuscitation may result in hypovolemia and worsening shock. Mannitol should not be given in the field without discussing this option with online medical control, unless permitted by standing orders or protocol. Brief seizures may occur soon after TBI and, aside from ensuring patient safety, oxygenation, and ventilation, often do not require specific treatment by prehospital care personnel. However, recurrent seizure activity is worrisome and may require IV boluses of a benzodiazepine, such as diazepam (0.1–0.2 mg/kg/dose). Depending on protocol, midazolam or lorazepam may also be used, but all benzodiazepines should be used with extreme caution because of the potential side effects of ventilatory depression and hypotension, as well as their ability to cloud the neurological exam.

Spinal Trauma

The indication for spinal immobilization in a pediatric patient is based on the mechanism of injury and physical findings; the presence of other injuries that suggest violent or sudden movement of the head, neck, or torso; or the presence of specific signs of spine injury, such as deformity, pain, or a neurologic deficit. As with adult patients, the correct prehospital management of a suspected spine injury is in-line manual stabilization followed by the use of a properly fitting cervical collar and immobilization of the patient to a long backboard so that the head, neck, torso, pelvis, and legs are maintained in a neutral in-line position. This should be achieved without impairing the patient's ventilation, ability to open the mouth, or any other resuscitative efforts. The threshold for performing spinal immobilization is lower in young children because of their inability to communicate or otherwise participate in their own assessment. No studies have validated the safety of clinically clearing a child's spine in the field. The same immaturity previously discussed also contributes to children's fear and lack of cooperation with immobilization. A child who strongly fights attempts at immobilization may actually be at increased risk of worsening any existing spinal injuries. It may be valid to decide not to restrain such a patient if the child can be persuaded to lie quietly without restraints. However, any decision to stop immobilization attempts in the interest of patient safety must be supported by careful and thorough documentation of the reason as well as serial assessment of neurologic status during and immediately after transport. Ideally, this decision would be made in concert with online medical control.

When most small children are placed on a rigid surface, the relatively larger size of the child's occiput will result in passive neck flexion. Unless you are using a specialized pediatric spine board that has a depression at the head to accommodate the occiput, sufficient padding (2–3 cm) should be placed under the patient's torso to elevate it and allow the head to be in a neutral position. The padding should be continuous and flat from the shoulders to the pelvis and extend to the lateral margins of the torso to ensure that the thoracic, lumbar, and sacral spine are on a flat, stable platform without the possibility of anterior-posterior movement. Padding should also be placed between the lateral sides of the child and the edges of the board to ensure that no lateral movement occurs when the board is moved or if the patient and board need to be rotated to the side to avoid aspiration during vomiting episodes.

Various new pediatric immobilization devices are available. The prehospital care provider needs to regularly practice and be familiar with any specialized equipment used in the provider's system as well as the required adjustments necessary when immobilizing a child using adult-sized equipment. If a vest-type device is used on a child, adequate immobilization while at the same time preventing respiratory compromise must be assured. The provider also needs to be familiar with the techniques of immobilizing a young child in a car safety seat.[16,17] Additionally, in some instances, it may be better to transport the child immobilized in their child safety seat rather than to extricate and immobilize them on a long spine board.

Thoracic Injuries

The extremely resilient rib cage of a child often results in less injury to the bony structure of the thorax, but more risk for pulmonary injury, such as pulmonary contusion, pneumothorax, or hemothorax. Although rib fractures are rare in childhood, they are associated with a high risk of intrathoracic injury when present. Crepitus may be appreciated on examination and may be a sign of pneumothorax. The risk of mortality increases with the number of ribs fractured. A high index of suspicion is the key to identifying these injuries. Every child who sustains trauma to the chest and torso should be carefully monitored for signs of respiratory distress and shock. Abrasions or contusions over the child's torso after blunt force trauma may be the only clues to the provider that the child has suffered thoracic trauma.

Additionally, when transporting a child who has sustained a high-impact blunt thoracic injury, the patient's cardiac rhythm should be monitored once the child is en route to a medical facility. In all cases, the key items in managing thoracic trauma involve careful attention to ventilation, oxygenation, and timely transport to an appropriate facility.

Abdominal Injuries

The presence of blunt trauma to the abdomen, an unstable pelvis, post-traumatic abdominal distension, rigidity or tenderness, or otherwise unexplained shock can be associated with possible intra-abdominal hemorrhage. A "seat belt sign" (or mark) across the abdomen of a child is often an indicator of serious internal injuries (Figure 15-17). The key prehospital elements in management of abdominal injuries include fluid resuscitation, supplemental high-concentration oxygen, and rapid transport to an appropriate facility with continued careful monitoring en route. There are really no definitive interventions that prehospital providers can offer to patients with intra-abdominal injuries, and, as such, there should be every effort to transport these patients rapidly to the closest, most appropriate facility.

Extremity Trauma

Compared with the adult skeleton, the child's skeleton is actively growing and consists of a large proportion of cartilaginous tissue and metabolically active growth plates. The ligamentous structures that hold the skeleton together are frequently stronger and better able to withstand mechanical disruption than the bones to which they are attached. As a result, children with skeletal trauma frequently sustain major traumatic forces before developing long-bone fractures, dislocations, or deformities. Incomplete ("greenstick") fractures are common and may be indicated only by bony tenderness and pain on use of the affected extremity.

Primary joint disruption from injury other than penetrating injury is uncommon compared with disruption of the diaphyseal or epiphyseal segments of bone. Fractures that involve the growth plate are unique in that they must be carefully identified and managed in the acute injury phase to not only ensure adequate healing, but also prevent subsequent displacement or deformity as the child continues to develop. The association of neurovascular injuries with orthopedic injuries in children should always be considered, and the distal vascular and neurological exam should be carefully evaluated. Often, the presence of a potentially debilitating injury

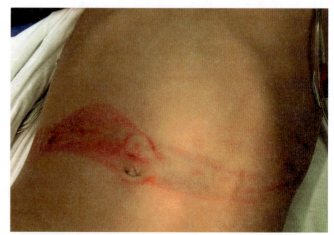

FIGURE 15-17 "Seat belt sign" in a 6-year-old patient who was found to have a ruptured spleen. Seat belt signs are often associated with serious intra-abdominal injuries.

can be determined only by radiologic study or, when the slightest suggestion of a decrease in distal perfusion exists, by arteriography.

The apparent gross deformity sometimes associated with extremity injury should not distract focus from potentially life-threatening injuries. Uncontrolled hemorrhage represents the sole life-threatening condition associated with extremity trauma. In multisystem pediatric and adult trauma patients alike, the initiation of transport to an appropriate facility without delay after completion of the primary survey, resuscitation, and rapid packaging remains paramount in reducing mortality. If basic splinting can be provided en route without detracting from the child's resuscitation, it will help to minimize bleeding and pain from long-bone fractures, but attention to life-threatening injuries should remain the primary focus.

Thermal Injuries

Following motor vehicle crashes and drowning, burns rate third as a cause of pediatric trauma deaths.[18] Caring for an injured child always poses significant physical and emotional challenges to the prehospital care provider, and these difficulties are only amplified when caring for the burned child. The burned child may have an edematous airway; IV access may be complicated by burns of the extremity; and the child may be hysterical from pain.

The primary survey should be followed as in other causes of pediatric trauma, but every step of the primary assessment may be more complicated than in a nonthermally injured child. Most deaths related to structure fires are not directly related to soft tissue burns but are secondary to smoke inhalation. When children are trapped in a structure fire, they often hide from the fire under beds or in closets. These children frequently die, and their recovered bodies often have no burns; they die from carbon monoxide or hydrogen cyanide toxicity and hypoxia. More than 50% of children less than 9 years old in structure fires have some degree of smoke-inhalation injury.

Thermally induced edema of the airway is always a concern in burn patients but especially in children. The smaller diameter of the pediatric trachea means that 1 mm of edema will produce a greater magnitude of airway obstruction than in an adult with a larger-diameter airway. Early control of the airway with endotracheal intubation should be done before the child develops signs or symptoms of respiratory compromise. A child with an edematous airway may be sitting forward and drooling, or complaining of hoarseness or voice changes. Once an ET tube is placed, it needs to be protected against inadvertent dislodgement or removal. If the patient accidentally becomes extubated, the provider may not be able to intubate the child again due to progressive edema; the results could be disastrous. Securing an ET tube in a child who has peeling facial skin and moist wounds is difficult. Securing the ET tube to the face with adhesive tape should not be attempted in children with facial burns. The ET tube

should be secured with two pieces of umbilical tape, with one piece draped above the ear and the second piece placed below the ear. An effective alternative to umbilical tape is IV tubing. If none of these are available and extra hands are, designate a provider to be solely responsible for holding the airway in place.

Rapid establishment of intravascular access is vital to prevent the development of shock. Delayed fluid resuscitation in children has been associated with significantly worse clinical outcomes and an increased mortality, especially in burned infants.

Excessive fluids can result in respiratory complications as well as excessive edema, which can complicate burn care. After securing an airway, providing adequate ventilation and oxygenation, it is critical that venous access is obtained quickly. Children have a relatively small intravascular volume, and a delay in fluid resuscitation may lead to the rapid development of hypovolemic shock. To provide the large volumes of IV fluids required in critical burns, such patients usually require two peripheral IV catheters to achieve the required IV flow rates. The insertion of a single large-bore IV catheter is often challenging, let alone two IV catheters. Burns on the extremities may make it difficult to impossible to establish enough access for an appropriate fluid resuscitation. In pediatric burn patients, as in adult burn patients, fluid needs are calculated from the time of the injury, so even a delay of 30 minutes to the beginning of fluid resuscitation can result in hypovolemic shock. Once peripheral IV access has been obtained, provisions must be made to ensure that the IV line is not inadvertently removed or dislodged. Usual techniques used to secure IV lines are often ineffective when a line is placed in or adjacent to a burn because adhesive tape and dressings may not adhere to burned tissue. If possible, the IV line is secured with a Kerlix™ dressing, though circumferential dressings must be frequently monitored as edema develops, to prevent tissue damage from the dressing becoming a constricting band.

When peripheral venous access cannot be obtained, intraosseous catheters should be used. Although previously advocated only for children less than 3 years of age, intraosseous infusions are now used in older children as well as adults.

The amount of fluids typically given to a burn patient is calculated based on the estimated percentage of body surface area burned using the "rule of nines," a rapid and imprecise method of estimating resuscitative fluid needs based on *adult* battlefield burn casualties. The premise of this method of burn size estimation is that major regions of the adult body (e.g., head, arm, anterior torso) each comprise 9% of the total body surface area (TBSA). Children's anatomic regions are proportionally different than those in adults; children have larger heads and smaller limbs. Therefore, estimation of pediatric burn size should use diagrams that are age specific, such as the Lund Browder chart, and not the rule of nines. If charts and diagrams are not available, the "rule of palms" may be utilized in which the size of the child's palm represents approximately 1% of their body surface area.

Based on the percentage of body surface area burned, the volume of IV fluids needed for resuscitation is determined (see Chapter 14). Two important pediatric considerations merit mention. First, small children have a limited reserve of glycogen. *Glycogen* is essentially glucose molecules strung together and is used for carbohydrate storage purposes. These glycogen molecules can then be mobilized in times of stress. If these limited glycogen stores become depleted, the child may rapidly develop hypoglycemia. Second, children have a large volume/surface area ratio; the general shape of an adult is a cylinder, whereas children resemble a sphere. The clinical implication is that a child will require more IV fluids. To address both these issues, in addition to the calculated resuscitative fluids, maintenance fluids containing 5% dextrose are also administered. In prolonged transports of a child with a Foley catheter, the fluids should be titrated to ensure a urine output of 1 ml/kg/hr. If the urine output is not adequate, a fluid bolus of 20 ml/kg is administered, and the rate of administration of the resuscitative fluids is increased to achieve the desired urine output.

Each year approximately 1.5 million children are abused by burning, accounting for 20% of all child abuse.[19,20] Approximately 20% to 25% of children admitted to a pediatric burn center are victims of child abuse.[21,22] An increased awareness of this problem among prehospital providers can improve detection of this cause of pediatric trauma. Careful documentation of the situation surrounding the injury, as well as of the injury patterns themselves, can aid officials in the prosecution of the offenders.

The two most common mechanisms by which these children receive burns are scalds and contact burns. Scalds are the most common source of nonaccidental burns. Scalding injuries typically are inflicted on children of toilet-training age. The usual scenario is that children soil themselves and are subsequently immersed in a tub of scalding water. These scald burns are characterized by a pattern of sharp demarcation between burned and unburned tissue and sparing of flexion creases, as the child will frequently draw their legs up to avoid the scalding water (see Chapter 14).

Contact burns are the second most common mechanism of abuse burns. Common items used to inflict contact burns are curling irons, clothing irons, and cigarettes. Cigarette burns appear as round wounds measuring slightly over 1 cm in diameter (typically 1.3 cm). To conceal these injuries, the abuser may place these in areas usually covered by clothing, above the hairline in the scalp, or even in the axillae. All the surfaces of the human body have some degree of curvature; a hot item that falls onto any body surface will have an initial point of contact, and then the hot item will deflect from the point of contact. Therefore, the resultant accidental contact burns will have irregular borders and uneven depths. In contrast, when a hot item is deliberately used to burn someone, the item is pressed onto the region of the body. The burn will then have a pattern with a sharp regular outline and uniform burn depth (see Chapter 14).

A high index of suspicion for abuse is important and *all* cases of suspected abuse should be reported. Make meticulous observations of the surroundings, such as the position of various pieces of furniture, curling irons, and depth of bath water. Record the names of individuals present at the scene. Any child suspected of being abused by burns, regardless of the size of the burns, needs to be cared for at a center experienced in pediatric burn care. Child abuse and neglect is further discussed later in this chapter.

Motor Vehicle Injury Prevention

The American Academy of Pediatrics has defined *optimal restraint* for children in motor vehicles. Children should always ride in the rear seat. Children should be in child safety seats until 4 years of age (rear facing, up to 1 year), then graduate into a belt-positioning booster seat until they are 8 to 10 years old. At that time, the standard three-point (seatbelt/shoulder harness combination, never lap belt alone) adult restraint can be used. *Suboptimal restraint* is defined as the lack of use of a child safety seat or booster seat in anyone under age 8 years, and lack of a three-point restraint for a child over age 8 years (see Figure 15-2, page 380).[28] In a recent review, when these guidelines were observed, the risk of abdominal injury in children appropriately restrained was 3.5 times less than in the suboptimally restrained pediatric population.[29] The protective benefit of the rear-seat position is such that risk of death is decreased by at least 30%, even if restrained with a lap belt only in the rear seat versus three-point restraint in the front seat.[30]

The Abused and Neglected Child

Child abuse (maltreatment or nonaccidental trauma) is a significant cause of childhood injury. As mentioned previously, almost 20% of all pediatric burns involve either child abuse or child neglect. Prehospital care providers must always consider the possibility of child abuse when circumstances warrant.

Prehospital care providers should suspect abuse or neglect if they note any of the following scenarios:

- Discrepancy between the history and the degree of physical injury, or the history changes frequently.
- Inappropriate response from the family.
- Prolonged interval between time of injury and call for medical care.
- History of the injury inconsistent with the developmental level of the child. For example, a history indicating that a newborn rolled off a bed would be suspect because newborns are developmentally unable to roll over.

Certain types of injury also suggest abuse, such as the following (Figure 15-18):

- Multiple bruises in varying stages of resolution (excluding the palms, forearms, tibial areas, and the forehead in ambulatory children, who are frequently injured in normal falls). Accidental bruises usually occur over bony prominences.
- Bizarre injuries such as bites, cigarette burns, rope marks, or any pattern injury.
- Sharply demarcated burns or scald injuries in unusual areas (see Chapter 14).

In many jurisdictions, prehospital care providers are legally mandated reporters if they identify potential child abuse. Generally, prehospital providers who act in good faith and in the best interests of the child are protected from legal action. Reporting procedures vary, so prehospital providers should be familiar with the appropriate agencies that handle child abuse cases in their location. The need to report abuse is emphasized by data suggesting that up to 50% of maltreated children are released back to their abusers because abuse was not suspected or reported (Figure 15-19).

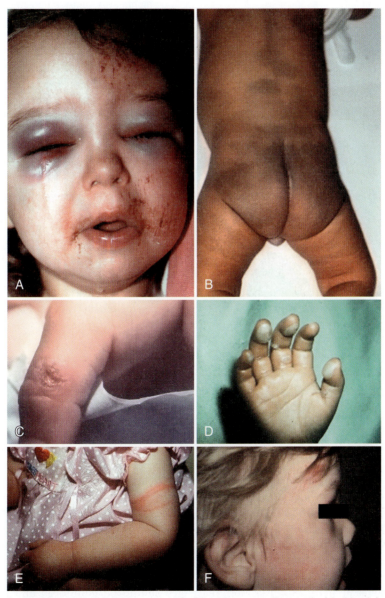

FIGURE 15-18 Indicators of possible nonaccidental trauma. **A.** "Raccoon eyes," or periorbital bruising, a possible indication of anterior fossa skull fracture. **B.** Mongolian blue spots, shown here on the trunk and buttocks of a newborn Asian infant, can be easily confused with bruising. **C.** Well-circumscribed lesions with blistering, seen here as a result of a cigarette burn. **D.** Fingertip burns caused by having the hand held forcibly against an electric stove burner. The burns are confined to the tips as she had tried to prevent her hand from being flattened against the burner. **E.** Abrasion caused by a ligature. **F.** Facial bruising from a slap to the face. The handprint can just be identified.
(Taylor S, Raffles A: *Diagnosis in color: Pediatrics,* London, 1997, Mosby-Wolfe.)

FIGURE 15-19   Documenting Nonaccidental Trauma in Children

Emergency medical technicians (EMTs) may be the only medical responders to a potential crime scene involving nonaccidental (abuse) trauma. Although EMTs are under intense pressure at an emergency scene, they are in a unique position to collect items of evidentiary importance that may assist in determining the mechanism of injury and the identification of the abuser. EMTs should ideally document 10 fundamental items when responding to a "child in need of assistance" call:

1. Document all adults and children present.
2. Document all statements and the demeanors of all persons present. As recorders of "scene" statements, EMTs must be familiar with the general requirements that allow certain statements to be used in court.
   a. Identify and document the maker of the statement.
   b. Record all statements in the official report.
   c. Record verbatim content, using quotes when appropriate.
   d. Document the time when the statement was made.
   e. Record the speaker's demeanor.
   f. Explain your job.
   g. Ask probing follow-up questions, but do not expose yourself to risk if you encounter aggression at this further questioning.
   h. Record the question. The content of an answer can often be understood only by knowing the question that was asked.
   i. List all persons present who heard the statement.
3. Document the environment. EMTs may arrive before caregivers clean up, modify, or destroy evidence.
4. Collect significant items. Preserving the potential mechanism of injury is vital to verifying a suspect's history.

5. Identify and record the child's age and developmental stage.
6. Know the signs of abuse and neglect.
   a. Signs of physical abuse: unexplained fractures, bruises, black eyes, cuts, burns, and welts; pattern injuries and bite marks; antisocial behavior; fear of adults; signs of apathy, depression, hostility, or stress; eating disorders.
   b. Signs of sexual abuse: difficulty walking or sitting, overcompliance, excessive aggressiveness, nightmares, bed-wetting, drastic change in appetite, inappropriate interest or knowledge of sexual acts, fear of a particular person.
   c. Signs of neglect: unsuitable clothing; unbathed/dirty; severe body odor; severe diaper rash; underweight; lack of food, formula, or toys; parent or child use of drugs or alcohol; apparent lack of supervision; unsuitable living conditions.
7. Assess children present at unrelated calls.
8. Evaluate children and adults with disabilities.
9. Adhere to mandatory reporting requirements and procedures.
10. Interact with the multidisciplinary team (MDT).

Nonaccidental pediatric trauma and neglect cases are wrought with difficult issues. Holding abusers responsible for their acts requires meticulous documentation; thorough, coordinated investigations; and teamwork. EMTs are uniquely positioned to observe and document vital information when assessing the possibility of child abuse.

(Modified from Rogers LL: Emergency medical professionals: assisting in identifying and documenting child abuse and neglect. *NCPCA Update Newslett* 17(7):1, 2004.)

Prolonged Transport

Occasionally a situation arises as a result of patient location, triage decisions, or environmental considerations in which transport will be prolonged or delayed and prehospital personnel need to manage the ongoing resuscitation of an injured child. Even though this may be suboptimal because of the lack of field resources (e.g., blood) and the inability to perform diagnostic and therapeutic interventions, by applying the principles discussed in this chapter in an organized fashion, the child can be safely managed until arrival at a trauma center. If radio or cellular contact with the receiving facility is possible, constant communication and feedback are crucial for both prehospital and hospital-based members of the trauma team.

Management consists of continued serial evaluation of the components of the primary survey. The child should be securely stabilized on a backboard with spine precautions. The board should be padded as well as possible to prevent pressure sores. If the airway is tenuous and the crew is well-trained in pediatric airway management, including endotracheal intubation, then airway management should be performed. Otherwise, conscientious bag-mask ventilation is still an acceptable management strategy, assuming it provides adequate oxygenation and ventilation. Pulse oximetry should be monitored and preferably $ETCO_2$ as well, especially in the child with a head injury. If signs of shock exist, 20 ml/kg boluses of LR or NS solution are administered until the child improves or is transferred to definitive care. GCS should be calculated early and followed serially. Assessment for other injuries should continue, and all efforts to keep the child normothermic should be standard practice. Fractures should be splinted and stabilized with serial neurovascular assessments. This cycle of continued assessment of the primary survey should be repeated until the child can be safely transported or transferred to definitive care.

Any change or decompensation in the child's clinical exam requires immediate reassessment of the primary survey. For example, if oxygen saturation begins to decline, is the tracheal tube still secure and in the airway? If so, has the child developed a tension pneumothorax? Is the tube now in the right mainstem bronchus? If the child has received what was thought to be sufficient fluid and is still in shock, is there now cardiac tamponade, severe cardiac contusion, or perhaps an occult source of bleeding, such as intra-abdominal injury or missed scalp laceration? Has the GCS changed? Are there now lateralizing signs suggesting progressive head injury and requiring more aggressive treatments? Is the circulation and neurologic status of the extremities still intact? Is the child normothermic? If radio contact is available, continued advice and guidance should be sought throughout the resuscitation and transport.

By paying attention to the basics and continually reassessing your patient, adequate resuscitation can be performed until the child can be transferred to a definitive care.

SUMMARY

- The initial assessment and management of the injured child in the prehospital setting requires application of standard trauma life support principles modified to account for the unique characteristics of children.
- Traumatic brain injury is the leading cause of death from trauma, as well as the most common injury for which the child requires airway management.
- Children have the ability to compensate for volume loss longer than adults, but when they decompensate, they deteriorate suddenly and severely.
- Significant underlying organ and vascular injury can occur with few or no obvious signs external injury.

- Injured children with the following signs are unstable and should be transported without delay to an appropriate facility, ideally a pediatric trauma center:
  - Respiratory compromise
  - Signs of shock or circulatory instability
  - Any period of postinjury unconsciousness
  - Significant blunt trauma to the head, thorax, or abdomen
  - Fractured ribs
  - Pelvic fracture

SCENARIO SOLUTION

You correctly identify this child as a victim of multisystem trauma who is in shock and critically injured. Because of the probable traumatic brain injury combined with the change in mentation, you have to determine the greatest threat to his survivability: the brain injury and other injuries not yet identified. You correctly identify hypotension and tachycardia, which you assume are related to hypovolemic shock, probably the result of an unrecognized intra-abdominal injury. Initially, his breathing is supported with high-concentration oxygen through a nonrebreather mask. You realize that his respiratory rate is low for a child of his age and are prepared to provide more aggressive airway control with a bag-mask if his condition deteriorates. As you consider options for airway management, you ask your partner to hold manual stabilization of the head and neck.

Because of the nature of the child's injuries, you consult with online medical control, who agrees that helicopter transport to the closest pediatric trauma center is more appropriate than ground transport to a nearby community hospital that has no pediatric critical care, neurosurgical, or orthopedic resources. Brief efforts at peripheral venous access are unsuccessful. You begin crystalloid infusion through an intraosseous line. The patient's mother arrives just as you are transferring care to the helicopter crew. ∎

References

1. WISQARS: Leading cause of Death Reports 2005. http://wepappa.cdc.gov/sasweb/ncipc/leadcaus10.html. Accessed February 10, 2009.
2. WISQARS Leading cause of Non-fatal injuries Reports 2005, http://wepappa.cdc.gov/sasweb/ncipc/nfilead2001.html, Last accessed 10 February, 2009.
3. Gaines BA, Ford HR: Abdominal and pelvic trauma in children. *Crit Care Med* 30(11 suppl):S416, 2002.
4. Gausche M, Lewis RJ, Stratton SJ, et al: Effect of out-of-hospital pediatric endotracheal intubation on survival and neurological outcome: A controlled clinical trial. *JAMA* 283(6):783, 2000.
5. Davis DP, Hoyt DB, Ochs M, et al: The effect of paramedic rapid sequence intubation on outcome in patients with severe traumatic brain injury. *J Trauma Injury Infec Crit Care* 54(3):444, 2003.
6. Davis DP, Dunford JV, Poste JC, et al: The impact of hypoxia and hyperventilation on outcome after paramedic rapid sequence intubation of severely head-injured patients. *J Trauma Injury Infect Crit Care* 57(1):1, 2004.
7. Adelson PD, Bratton SL, Carney NA, et al: Guidelines for the acute medical management of severe traumatic brain injury in infants, children, and adolescents: Chapter 4. Resuscitation of blood pressure and oxygenation and prehospital brain-specific therapies for the severe pediatric traumatic brain injury patient. *Pediatr Crit Care Med* 4(3 suppl):S12, 2003.
8. York J, Arrillaga A, Graham R, Miller R: Fluid resuscitation of patients with multiple injuries and severe closed-head injury: Experience with an aggressive fluid resuscitation strategy. *J Trauma Injury Infect Crit Care* 48(3):376, 2000.
9. Manley G, Knudson MM, Morabito D, et al: Hypotension, hypoxia, and head injury: Frequency, duration, and consequences. *Arch Surg* 136(10):1118, 2001.
10. Chesnut RM, Marshall LF, Klauber MR, et al. The role of secondary brain injury in determining outcome from severe head injury. *J Trauma* 34(2):216–222, 1993.
11. Luten R: Error and time delay in pediatric trauma resuscitation: Addressing the problem with color-coded resuscitation aids. *Surg Clin North Am* 82(2):303, 2002.
12. American College of Surgeons Committee on Trauma: Pediatric trauma. In ACS Committee on Trauma: *Advanced trauma life support for doctors, student course manual*, ed 8, Chicago, 2008, ACS, pp 225–245.
13. Ehrlich PF, Seidman PS, Atallah D, et al: Endotracheal intubation in rural pediatric trauma patients. *J Pediatr Surg* 39:1376, 2004.
14. Venkataraman ST, Thompson AE, Orr RA: Femoral vascular catheterization in critically ill infants and children. *Clin Pediatr* 36(6):311, 1997.
15. Carmona Suazo JA, Maas AI, van den Brink WA, et al: CO_2 reactivity and brain oxygen pressure monitoring in severe head injury. *Crit Care Med* 28(9):3268, 2000.
16. De Lorenzo RA: A review of spinal immobilization techniques. *J Emerg Med* 14(5):603, 1996.
17. Valadie LL: Child safety seats and the emergency responder. *Emerg Med Serv* 33(7):68, 2004.
18. National Vital Statistics System, Centers for Disease Control and Prevention: Deaths: Final data for 1997. *MMWR* 47 (19):1, 1999.
19. Heins M: The "battered child" revisited. *JAMA* 251:3295, 1984.
20. Weimer CL, Goldfarb IW, Slater H: Multidisciplinary approach to working with burn victims of child abuse. *J Burn Care Rehabil* 9:79, 1988.
21. Feldman KW, Schaller RT, Feldman JA, McMillon M: Tap water scald burns in children. *Pediatrics* 62:1, 1978.
22. Montrey JS, Barcia PJ: Nonaccidental burns in child abuse. *South Med J* 78:1324, 1985.
23. Larson JT, Dietrich AM, Abdessalam SF, Werman HA: Effective use of the air ambulance for pediatric trauma. *J Trauma Injury Infect Crit Care* 56(1):89, 2004.
24. Eckstein M, Jantos T, Kelly N, Cardillo A: Helicopter transport of pediatric trauma patients in an urban emergency medical

services system: A critical analysis. *J Trauma Injury Infect Crit Care* 53(2):340, 2002.

25. Winston FK, Durbin DR, Kallan MJ, Moll EK: The danger of premature graduation to seat belts for young children. *Pediatrics* 105(6):1179, 2000.

26. Grisoni ER, Pillai SB, Volsko TA, et al: Pediatric airbag injuries: The Ohio experience. *J Pediatr Surg* 35(2):160, 2000.

27. Durbin DR, Kallan M, Elliott M, et al. Risk of injury to restrained children from passenger air bags. *Traffic Injury Prev* 4(1):58, 2003.

28. American Academy of Pediatrics Committee on Injury and Poison Prevention. Selecting and using the most appropriate car safety seats for growing children: Guidelines for counseling parents. *Pediatrics* 109(3):550, 2002.

29. Nance ML, Lutz N, Arbogast KB, et al. Optimal restraint reduces the risk of abdominal injury in children involved in motor vehicle crashes. *Ann Surg* 239(1):127, 2004.

30. Braver ER, Whitfield R, Ferguson SA. Seating positions and children's risk of dying in motor vehicle crashes. *Injury Prev* 4(3):181, 1998.

31. Bensard DD, Beaver BL, Besner GE, Cooney DR. Small bowel injury in children after blunt abdominal trauma: Is diagnostic delay important? *J Trauma Injury Infect Crit Care* 41(3):476, 1996.

32. Allen GS, Moore FA, Cox CS Jr, et al: Hollow visceral injury and blunt trauma. *J Trauma Injury Infect Crit Care* 45(1):69, 1998.

33. Durbin DR, Kallan M, Elliott M, et al: Risk of injury to restrained children from passenger air bags. *Annu Proc Assoc Adv Auto Med* 46:15, 2002.

34. Winchell RJ, Hoyt DB: Endotracheal intubation in the field improves survival in patients with severe head injury. *Arch Surg* 132(6):592, 1997.

35. Davis DP, Ochs M, Hoyt DB, et al: Paramedic-administered neuromuscular blockade improves prehospital intubation success in severely head-injured patients. *J Trauma Injury Infect Crit Care* 55(4):713, 2003.

36. Pearson S: Comparison of intubation attempts and completion times before and after the initiation of a rapid sequence intubation protocol in an air medical transport program. *Air Med J* 22(6):28, 2003.

37. Stockinger ZT, McSwain NE Jr: Prehospital endotracheal intubation for trauma does not improve survival over bag-valve-mask ventilation. *J Trauma Injury Infect Crit Care* 56(3):531, 2004.

38. Murray JA, Demetriades D, Berne TV, et al: Prehospital intubation in patients with severe head injury. *J Trauma Injury Infect Crit Care* 49(6):1065, 2000.

39. Davis BD, Fowler R, Kupas DF, Roppolo LP: Role of rapid sequence induction for intubation in the prehospital setting: Helpful or harmful? *Curr Opin Crit Care* 8(6):571, 2002.

40. Davis DP, Valentine C, Ochs M, et al: The Combitube as a salvage airway device for paramedic rapid sequence intubation. *Ann Emerg Med* 42(5):697, 2003.

41. Martin SE, Ochsner MG, Jarman RH, et al: Use of the laryngeal mask airway in air transport when intubation fails. *J Trauma Injury Infect Crit Care* 47(2):352, 1999.

42. Hight DW, Bakalar HR, Lloyd JR: Inflicted burns in children: Recognition and treatment. *JAMA* 242:517, 1979.

Suggested Reading

Anonymous: EMSC Partnership for Children/National Association of EMS Physicians model pediatric protocols: 2003 revision. *Prehosp Emerg Care* 8(4):343, 2004.

CHAPTER 16

Geriatric Trauma

CHAPTER OBJECTIVES

At the completion of this chapter, the reader will be able to do the following:

✓ Discuss the epidemiology of trauma in the elderly population.

✓ Discuss the anatomic and physiologic effects of aging as a factor in causes of geriatric trauma and as a factor in the pathophysiology of trauma.

✓ Explain the interaction of various pre-existing medical problems with traumatic injuries in elderly patients to produce differences in the pathophysiology and manifestations of trauma.

✓ Explain the physiologic effects of specific common classes of medications on the pathophysiology and manifestations of geriatric trauma.

✓ Compare and contrast the assessment techniques and considerations used in the elderly population with those used in younger populations.

✓ Demonstrate modifications in spinal immobilization techniques for safe and effective spinal immobilization of the elderly patient with the highest degree of comfort possible.

✓ Compare and contrast the management of the elderly trauma patient with that of the younger trauma patient.

✓ Assess the scene and elderly patients for signs and symptoms of abuse and neglect.

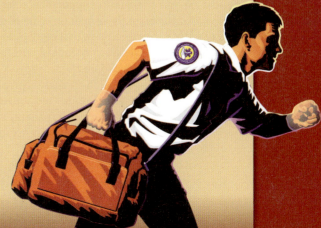

SCENARIO

Your unit is dispatched to the scene of a single-car motor vehicle crash into a tree. On your initial scene assessment, police and fire personnel have secured the scene. The vehicle is an older model car without seatbelts or airbags. The driver appears to be an elderly male who is unresponsive. Bystanders report he was driving erratically moments before the crash. While maintaining in-line stabilization of the spine, you note that the patient is unresponsive to your commands. He has a visible laceration of the forehead where he apparently impacted the windshield. He is wearing a Medic Alert bracelet that indicates that he is diabetic.

Was the injury the primary event or secondary to a medical event? Did the crash cause the change in mental status, or was there an antecedent event? How does the information that the patient is diabetic affect your level of suspicion for traumatic brain injury? How do the patient's age, medical history, and medications interact with the injuries received to make the pathophysiology and manifestations different from those in younger patients? How will you modify your approach to the management of this patient, especially in terms of stabilizing his airway? Should advanced age alone be used as an additional criterion for transport to a trauma center?

The elderly population represents the fastest-growing age group in the United States. Gerontologists (medical specialists who study and care for elderly patients) divide the term *elderly* into three specific categories, as follows:

- *Middle age:* 50 to 64 years of age
- *Late age:* 65 to 79 years of age
- *Older age:* 80 years of age and older

Although such definitions are important for epidemiologic data, it is also important to recognize that the physiologic changes of aging occur along the entire age spectrum and vary among individuals. Recovery from closed head injury starts to decline beginning in the mid-20s age group, and overall survival from trauma starts to decline in the late 30s. In addition, increasing age is often associated with multiple pre-existing medical conditions. The approach to the elderly patient includes recognition of this fact, although younger patients with comorbidities may share similar attributes.

Almost 39 million Americans (13% of the US population) are 65 years of age or older, and the size of this group has risen dramatically during the last 100 years.[1] At the same time, fertility rates have dropped, meaning that there will be fewer people under 65 years of age to support the costs of health care and living expenses of those over 65 years of age. By the year 2050, nearly 25% of Americans will be eligible for Medicare, and the population over 85 years of age will have grown from 4 million to 19 million people.[2]

The injured elderly present unique challenges in prehospital care management, second only to those encountered with infants. Sudden illness and trauma in elderly patients present a different prehospital care dimension than in younger patients. Some of the earliest data looking at the effect of age on outcome is from the Major Trauma Outcome Study by the American College of Surgeons Committee on Trauma.[3] Data

from more than 3800 patients age 65 and older were compared to almost 43,000 patients less than age 65. Mortality increased over ages 45 to 55 and doubled by age 75 years. The age-adjusted risk occurs across the spectrum of injury severity, suggesting that injuries that could be easily tolerated by younger patients may result in mortality in those of advanced age.

Because older persons are more susceptible to critical illness and trauma than the rest of the population, a wider range of complications in patient assessment and management needs to be considered. Because elderly patients access medical care through emergency systems (e.g., 911), rendering care is different than for younger patients. The range of disabilities experienced by elderly patients is enormous, and field assessment may take longer than with younger patients. Difficulties in assessment can be expected as a result of sensory deficits in hearing and vision, senility, and physiologic changes.

Advances in medicine and an increasing awareness of healthier lifestyles during the last several decades have resulted in a significant increase in the percentage of the population over 65 years of age. Although trauma occurs most frequently in young people, and geriatric emergencies are most often medical problems, a growing number of geriatric calls result from or include trauma. Trauma is the sixth leading cause of death in persons aged 55–64, and is the ninth highest cause of death in those aged 65 and above. Approximately 15% of injury-related deaths in elderly patients are classified as homicide. Trauma deaths in this age group account for 25% of all trauma deaths nationwide.[5]

Specific patterns of injury are also unique to the geriatric population.[6] Although motor vehicle crashes (MVCs) are the leading cause of death from trauma overall, falls are the predominant cause of traumatic death in patients over age 75. As with small children (age <5 years), scald injuries account for a greater percentage of burns in those over 65.

Progress in recent years has not only increased adult life expectancy but has also affected the quality of life and, therefore, the range of physical activities performed at older ages. As more people live longer and enjoy better health in their older years, more of them travel, drive, and continue active physical pursuits that can result in an associated increase in geriatric trauma. Many who could retire now continue to work despite a health problem or advancing age.

Recent social changes have increased the number of older people living in independent housing, retirement communities, and other assisted-living facilities compared with those in nursing homes or other, more guarded and limited environments. This suggests a probable increase in the incidence of simple household trauma, such as falls, in elderly persons. The past few years have also seen an increase in geriatric victims of crime in the home and on the streets. Older people are often singled out as "easy marks" and can sustain substantial trauma from crimes of seemingly limited violence, such as purse snatching, when they are struck, are knocked down, or fall.

With the growing awareness of this expanding population at risk, the prehospital care provider must understand the unique needs of an elderly trauma patient. Specifically, the aging process and the effects of coexisting medical problems on an elderly patient's response to trauma and trauma management must be understood. The special considerations outlined in this chapter should be included in the assessment and management of any trauma patient who is 65 years of age or older, physically appears elderly, or is middle-aged and has any of the significant medical problems typically associated with the elderly population.

Anatomy and Physiology of Aging

The aging process causes changes in physical structure, body composition, and organ function, and it can create unique problems during prehospital care. The aging process influences mortality and morbidity rates.

Aging, or *senescence,* is a natural biologic process and is sometimes referred to as a process of "biologic reversal" that begins during the years of early adulthood. At this time, organ systems have achieved maturation, and a turning point in physiologic growth has been reached. The body gradually loses its ability to maintain homeostasis (the state of relative constancy of the body's internal environment), and viability declines over a period of years until death occurs.

The fundamental process of aging occurs at the cellular level and is reflected in both anatomic structure and physiologic function. The period of "old age" is generally characterized by frailty, slower cognitive processes, impairment of psychological functions, diminished energy, the appearance of chronic and degenerative diseases, and a decline in sensory acuity. Functional abilities are lessened, and the well-known external signs and symptoms of older age appear, such as skin wrinkling, changes in hair color and quantity, osteoarthritis, and slowness in reaction time and reflexes (Figure 16-1).

Influence of Chronic Medical Problems

As people age, they experience the normal physiologic changes of aging and can also experience more medical problems.

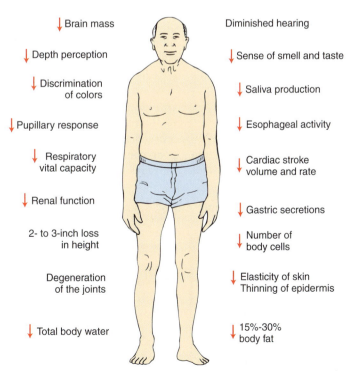

↓ Brain mass

↓ Depth perception

↓ Discrimination of colors

↓ Pupillary response

↓ Respiratory vital capacity

↓ Renal function

2- to 3-inch loss in height

Degeneration of the joints

↓ Total body water

Diminished hearing

↓ Sense of smell and taste

↓ Saliva production

↓ Esophageal activity

↓ Cardiac stroke volume and rate

↓ Gastric secretions

↓ Number of body cells

↓ Elasticity of skin Thinning of epidermis

↓ 15%-30% body fat

FIGURE 16-1   Changes caused by aging.

Although some individuals can reach an advanced age without any serious medical problems, statistically an older person is more likely to have one or more significant medical conditions (Figure 16-2). Seniors presently consume more than one-third of health care resources in the United States.[7] Usually, proper medical care can control these conditions, helping to avoid or minimize exacerbations from becoming repeated acute and often life-threatening episodes. Some older individuals have reached advanced age with minimal medical problems, whereas others may live with chronic illnesses and depend on modern medical means to survive. This latter group can deteriorate more rapidly in an emergency situation.

Repeated acute episodes of a medical problem or even the single occurrence of a significant episode can result in chronic residual effects on the body. A patient who has previously had an acute myocardial infarction sustains permanent heart damage. The resultant reduced cardiac capacity continues for the rest of the patient's life, affecting the heart and, because of the ensuing chronic impairment of circulation, other organs as well.

As a person's age advances, additional medical problems can occur. None is truly isolated because the effect on the body is cumulative. The total influence on the body usually is greater than the sum of each individual effect. As each condition progresses and reduces the quality of the body's vital functions, the individual's ability to withstand even modest anatomic or physiologic insults is greatly diminished.

Regardless of whether the patient is pediatric, middle-aged, or elderly, the priorities, intervention needs, and life-threatening conditions that usually result from serious trauma are the same. However, because of these pre-existing physical conditions, elderly patients often die from less severe injuries and die sooner than younger patients. Data support that pre-existing conditions play a role in the survival of an elderly trauma patient, and that the more conditions a trauma patient has, the higher his or her mortality rate (Figure 16-3). Certain conditions are associated with a higher mortality rate because of the way in which they interfere with an elderly patient's ability to respond to trauma (Figure 16-4).[8]

Ears, Nose, and Throat

Tooth decay, gum disease, and injury to teeth result in the need for various dental prostheses. The brittle nature of capped teeth, fixed bridges, or loose, removable bridges and dentures poses a special problem of foreign bodies that can be easily broken, aspirated, and obstruct the airway.

Changes in the contours of the face result from resorption of the mandible, in part because of absence of teeth (edentulism). The characteristic look is an infolding and shrinking of the mouth. These changes can adversely affect the ability to create an effective seal with a bag-mask device and to sufficiently visualize the airway during endotracheal intubation. The nasopharyngeal tissues become increasingly fragile; in addition to the risk this change poses during the initial trauma, interventions such as insertion of nasopharyngeal tubes may induce profuse bleeding if not placed with care.

Respiratory System

Ventilatory function declines in the elderly person partly as a result of the inability of the chest cage to expand and contract and partly from stiffening of the airway. The increased stiffness in the chest wall is associated with a reduction in the ability to expand the chest wall and a stiffening of cartilaginous connections of the ribs. As a result of these changes, the chest cage is less pliable. With declines in the efficiency of the respiratory system, the elderly person requires more exertion to carry out daily activities.

The alveolar surface area decreases with age; it is estimated to decrease by 4% for each decade after 30 years of age. A 70-year-old person, for example, would have a 16% reduction in alveolar surface area. Any alteration of the already-reduced alveolar surface decreases oxygen uptake. Additionally, as the body ages, its ability to saturate hemoglobin with oxygen decreases, leading to lower baseline oxygen saturation as a normal finding and less reserve available.[9] Because of impaired mechanical ventilation and diminished surface for gas exchange, the elderly trauma patient is less capable of compensating for physiologic losses associated with trauma.

Changes in the airway and lungs of elderly persons may not always be related to senescence alone. Cumulative chronic exposure to environmental toxins over the course of their lives may be caused by occupational hazards or tobacco smoke. Impaired cough and gag reflexes, along with poor cough strength and diminished esophageal sphincter tone, result in an increased risk of aspiration pneumonitis.

FIGURE 16-2   Percentage of Patients with Pre-Existing Disease (PED)

Age (years)	PED (%)
13–39	3.5
40–64	11.6
65–74	29.4
75–84	34.7
85+	37.3

FIGURE 16-3   Number of Pre-Existing Diseases (PEDs) and Patient Outcome

Number of PEDs	Survived	Died	Mortality rate (%)
0	6341	211	3.2
1	868	56	6.1
2	197	36	15.5
3 or more	67	22	24.7

FIGURE 16-4   Prevalence of Pre-Existing Diseases (PEDs) and Associated Mortality Rates

PED	Number of patients	PED present (%)	Total (%)	Mortality rate (%)
Hypertension	597	47.9	7.7	10.2
Pulmonary disease	286	23	3.7	8.4
Cardiac disease	223	17.9	2.9	18.4
Diabetes	198	15.9	2.5	12.1
Obesity	167	13.4	2.1	4.8
Malignancy	80	6.4	1	20
Neurologic disorder	45	3.6	0.6	13.3
Renal disease	40	3.2	0.5	37.5
Hepatic disease	41	3.3	0.5	12.2

A reduction in the number of *cilia* (hair-like projections that propel foreign particles and mucus from the bronchi) predisposes the elderly person to problems caused by inhaled particulate matter.

Another factor that affects the respiratory system is a change in the spinal curvature. Curvature changes accompanied by an anteroposterior hump (as seen in osteoporosis patients) often lead to additional ventilatory difficulty (Figure 16-5). Changes that affect the diaphragm can also contribute to ventilatory problems. Stiffening of the rib cage can cause more reliance on diaphragmatic activity to breathe. This increased reliance on the diaphragm makes an older person especially sensitive to changes in intra-abdominal pressure. Thus, a supine position or a full stomach from a large meal can provoke ventilatory insufficiency. Obesity can also play a part in diaphragm restriction, especially when fat distribution tends to be central.

Cardiovascular System

Diseases of the cardiovascular system are the primary cause of death in the elderly population. Cardiovascular disease accounts for more than 3,000 deaths per 100,000 persons over 65 years of age. In 2002, myocardial infarction accounted for 29% of deaths in the United States, with an additional 7% caused by stroke.[9]

Age-related decreases in arterial elasticity lead to increased peripheral vascular resistance. The myocardium and blood vessels rely on their elastic, contractile, and distensible properties to function properly. With aging, these properties decline, and the cardiovascular system becomes less efficient at moving circulatory fluids around the body. The cardiac output diminishes by approximately 50% from 20 to 80 years of age. Among patients over 75 years of age, as many as 10% will have some degree of overt (asymptomatic) congestive heart failure.

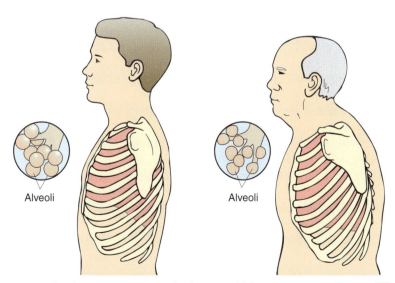

Alveoli   Alveoli

FIGURE 16-5 Spinal curvature can lead to an anteroposterior hump, which can cause ventilatory difficulties. Reduction in the alveolar surface area can also reduce the amount of oxygen that is exchanged in the lungs.

Atherosclerosis is a narrowing of the blood vessels, a condition in which the inner layer of the artery wall thickens as fatty deposits build up within the artery. These deposits, called *plaque,* protrude above the surface of the inner layer and decrease the diameter of the internal channel of the vessel. The same luminal narrowing occurs in the coronary vessels. Almost 50% of the US population has coronary artery stenosis by age 65 years.[10]

One result of this narrowing is *hypertension,* a condition that affects one of six adults in the United States. Calcification of the arterial wall reduces the ability of the vessels to change size in response to endocrine and central nervous system stimuli. The decrease in circulation can adversely affect any of the vital organs and is a common cause of heart disease. Of particular concern is that the baseline normal blood pressure of the elderly trauma patient may be higher than in younger patients. What would otherwise be accepted as normotension may indicate profound hypovolemic shock in the patient with pre-existing hypertension.[11]

With age, the heart itself shows an increase in fibrous tissue and size *(myocardial hypertrophy).* Atrophy of the cells of the conduction system results in the increased incidence of cardiac dysrhythmias. In particular, the normal reflexes in the heart that respond to hypotension diminish with age, resulting in the inability of elderly patients to increase their heart rate appropriately. Maximal heart rate also begins to decrease starting at age 40 years, calculated by the formula 220 minus the age in years. Patients with a permanent pacemaker have a fixed heart rate and cardiac output that cannot meet the demands of increased myocardial oxygen consumption accompanying the stress of trauma. Patients with hypertension taking beta blocker medications may also not have an increase in heart rate to compensate for hypovolemia.

In the elderly trauma patient, this reduced circulation contributes to cellular hypoxia. The result is cardiac dysrhythmia, acute heart failure, and even sudden death. The body's ability to compensate for blood loss or other causes of shock is significantly lowered in the elderly person because of a diminished inotropic (cardiac contraction) response to catecholamines. In addition, total circulating blood volume decreases, creating less physiologic reserve for blood loss from trauma. Diastolic dysfunction makes the patient more dependent on atrial filling to augment cardiac output, which is diminished in hypovolemic states.

The reduced circulation and circulatory-defense responses, coupled with increasing cardiac failure, produce a significant problem in managing shock in the elderly trauma patient. Fluid resuscitation needs to be carefully monitored because of the reduced compliance of the cardiovascular system and the often "stiff" right ventricle. Care must be taken when treating hypotension and shock so as not to cause volume overloading with aggressive fluid resuscitation.[12]

Nervous System

As individuals age, brain weight and the number of neurons (nerve cells) decrease. The weight of the brain reaches its peak (1.4 kg, or 3 lb) at approximately 20 years of age. By 80 years of age, the brain loses about 10% of its weight, with progressive cerebral atrophy.[13] The body compensates for the loss of size with increased cerebrospinal fluid. Although this additional space around the brain can protect it from contusion, it also allows for more brain movement in response to acceleration/deceleration injuries. The increased space in the cranial vault also explains why the elderly patient may have significant volumes of blood accumulate around the brain with minimal symptomatology.

The speed with which nerve impulses are conducted along certain nerves also decreases. These decreases result in only small effects on behavior and thinking. Reflexes are slower, but not to a significant degree. Compensatory functions can be impaired, particularly in patients with diseases such as Parkinson's disease, resulting in an increased incidence of falls. The peripheral nervous system is also affected by the slowing of nerve impulses, resulting in tremors and an unsteady gait.

General information and vocabulary abilities increase or are maintained, whereas skills requiring mental and muscular activity (psychomotor ability) may decline. The intellectual functions that involve verbal comprehension, arithmetic ability, fluency of ideas, experiential evaluation, and general knowledge tend to increase after 60 years of age in those who continue learning activities. Exceptions are those who develop senile dementia and other disorders such as Alzheimer's disease.

The normal biologic aging of the brain is not a predictor for diseases of the brain. However, decreases in the cortical structure of the brain may be involved in mental impairment. As changes occur in the brain, memory can be affected, and personality changes and other reductions in brain function can occur. These changes may involve the need for some form of mental health service. About 10% to 15% of elderly persons require professional mental health services. However, when assessing an elderly trauma patient, any impairment in mentation should be assumed to be the result of an acute traumatic insult, such as shock, hypoxia, or brain injury.

Sensory Changes
Vision and Hearing

Overall, approximately 28% of elderly persons have hearing impairment, and approximately 13% have visual impairment. Men tend to be more likely to have hearing difficulties, whereas both genders have a similar incidence of eye-related impairment.

Loss of vision is challenging at any age, and it may be even more problematic for the elderly person. The inability to read directions (e.g., on a prescription label) can lead to a disastrous effect. In addition, elderly persons experience decreases in visual acuity, ability to differentiate colors, and night vision.

The cells of the lens of the eye are incapable of restoration to their original molecular structure. One of the destructive agents over years of exposure is ultraviolet radiation. Eventually, the lens loses its capability to increase in thickness and curvature. The result is almost universal farsightedness *(presbyopia)* in persons over 40 years of age, requiring glasses for reading.

As a result of changes to the various structures of the eye, elderly persons have more difficulty seeing in dimly lit environments. Decreased tear production leads to dry eyes—itching and burning—and the inability to keep the eyes open for long periods.

With age, the lens of the eye begins to become cloudy and impenetrable to light. This gradual process results in a *cataract,* or a milky lens that blocks and distorts light that enters the eye and blurs vision. Some degree of cataract formation is present in 95% of elderly persons. This deterioration of vision increases the risk of an MVC, particularly when driving at night.[14]

A gradual decline in hearing *(presbycusis)* is also characteristic of aging. Presbycusis is usually caused by loss of conduction of sound into the inner ear; the use of hearing aids can compensate for this loss to some degree. This hearing loss is most pronounced when the person attempts to discriminate complex sounds, such as when many people are speaking at once, or with loud, ambient noise present, such as the wailing of sirens.

Pain Perception

Because of the aging process and the presence of diseases such as diabetes, elderly persons may not perceive pain normally, placing them at increased risk of injury from excesses in heat and cold exposure. Many elderly persons have conditions such as arthritis that result in chronic pain. Living with daily pain can cause an increased tolerance to pain, which may result in a patient's failure to identify areas of injury. In evaluating patients, especially those who usually "hurt all over" or who appear to have a high tolerance to pain, areas in which the pain has increased or in which the painful area has enlarged should be located. Also, it is also important to note whether the pain's characteristics or exacerbating factors have changed since the trauma occurred.

Renal System

Changes common with aging include reduced levels of filtration by the kidneys and a reduced excretory capacity. These changes should be considered when administering drugs normally cleared by the kidneys. Chronic renal inhibition typically affects elderly persons and contributes to a reduction in a patient's overall health status and ability to withstand trauma. For example, renal dysfunction may be one cause of chronic anemia, which would lower a patient's physiologic reserve.

Musculoskeletal System

Bone loses mineral as it ages. The loss of bone *(osteoporosis)* is unequal among the genders. During young adulthood, bone mass is greater in women than in men. However, bone loss is more rapid in women and accelerates after menopause. With this higher incidence of osteoporosis, older women have a greater probability of fractures, particularly of the neck of the femur (hip). Causes of osteoporosis include loss of estrogen levels, increased periods of inactivity, and inadequate intake and inefficient use of calcium.

Osteoporosis contributes significantly to hip fractures and spontaneous compression fractures of the vertebral bodies. The incidence approaches 1% per year for men and 2% for women over age 85 years.[15]

Older persons are sometimes shorter than they were in young adulthood because of dehydration of the vertebral discs. As the discs flatten, a loss of approximately 2 inches (5 cm) in height occurs between 20 and 70 years of age. *Kyphosis* (curvature of the spine) in the thoracic region can also contribute to height loss and is often caused by osteoporosis (Figure 16-6). As the bones become more porous and fragile, erosion occurs anteriorly, and compression fractures

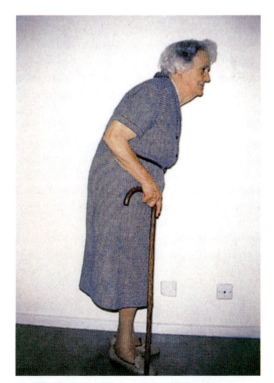

FIGURE 16-6 Kyphosis, typically caused by osteoporosis. Because of the elderly person's tendency to flex the legs, the arms appear longer.

of the vertebrae may develop. As the thoracic spine becomes more curved, the head and shoulders appear to be pushed forward. If chronic obstructive pulmonary disease (COPD), particularly emphysema, is present, the kyphosis may be more pronounced because of the increased development of the accessory muscles of breathing.

Absolute levels of growth hormones decrease with aging, in conjunction with a decline in responsiveness to anabolic hormones. The combined effect is a reduction in muscle mass of about 4% per decade after age 25 years until age 50, when the process accelerates to between 10% and 35% per decade. Muscle loss is measured microscopically by both absolute number of muscle cells and reduction in cell size.

Deficits that relate to the musculoskeletal system (e.g., inability to flex the hip or knee adequately with changes in terrain) predispose the elderly person to falls. Muscle fatigue can cause many problems that affect movement, especially falls. Changes in the body's normal posture are common, and changes in the spine make the curvature become more acute with aging. Some degree of osteoporosis is universal with aging. Because of this progressive bone resorption, the bones become less pliant, more brittle, and more easily broken. The decrease in bone strength, coupled with reduced muscle strength caused by less active exercise, can result in multiple fractures with only mild or moderate force. The most common sites of long-bone fracture in elderly persons include the proximal femur, hip, humerus, and wrist. The increased incidence of falls as a mechanism of injury results in Colles' fractures of the distal radius, as the dorsiflexed hand is outstretched.

The entire vertebral column changes with age, primarily because of the effects of osteoporosis, osteophytosis, and calcification of the supporting ligaments. This calcification results in decreased range of motion and narrowing of the spinal canal. The narrowed canal and progressive osteophytic disease put these patients at high risk for spinal cord injury with even minor trauma. The narrowing of the spinal canal is called *spinal stenosis* and increases the likelihood of cord compression without any actual break in the bony cervical spine. The thoracic and lumbar spine degenerate progressively as well, and the combined forces of osteoporosis and posture changes lead to increased falls. A high level of suspicion for spinal injury is needed during patient assessment because more than 50% of vertebral compression fractures are asymptomatic.[16]

Skin

Significant changes in the skin and connective tissues are associated with aging and result in difficulties with response to trauma as well as direct wound healing. Cell numbers decrease, tissue strength is lost, and the skin has impaired functional status. As the skin ages, sweat and sebaceous glands are lost. Loss of sweat glands reduces the body's ability to regulate temperature. Loss of sebaceous glands, which produce oil, makes the skin dry and flaky. Production of melanin, the pigment that gives color to skin and hair, declines, causing an aging pallor. The skin thins and appears translucent, primarily because of changes in connective tissue. The thinning and drying of the skin also reduce its resistance to minor injury and microorganisms, resulting in an increased infection rate from open wounds. As elasticity is lost, the skin stretches and falls into wrinkles and folds, especially in areas of heavy use, such as those overlying the facial muscles of expression.

Loss of fatty tissue can predispose the elderly person to *hypothermia*. The loss of up to 20% of dermal thickness with advanced aged and an associated loss in vascularity are also responsible for impaired thermoregulatory dysfunction. However, hypothermia should also suggest the possibility of occult sepsis, hypothyroidism, or phenothiazine overdose in the elderly population. This loss of fatty tissue also leads to less padding over bony prominences, such as the head, shoulders, spine, buttocks, hips, and heels. Prolonged immobilization without additional padding can result in tissue necrosis and ulceration as well as increased pain and discomfort during treatment and transport. Thinning of the skin also results in the potential for significant tissue loss and injury in response to relatively low energy transfers.

Nutrition and the Immune System

With aging, a reduction in lean body mass and decreases in metabolic rate cause a reduction in caloric needs. However, because of inefficient utilization mechanisms, protein needs may actually increase. These competing changes often result in pre-existing malnutrition in the elderly trauma patient. The financial status of retired individuals may also affect their choices of and access to quality nutrition.

The ability of the immune system to function decreases as it ages. Grossly, organs associated with the immune response (thymus, liver, and spleen) all decrease in size. A decrease in cell-mediated and humoral responses also results. Coupled with any pre-existing nutritional problems common in the elderly population, there is an increased susceptibility to infection. *Sepsis* is a common cause of late death after severe or even insignificant trauma in the elderly patient.

Assessment

Prehospital assessment of the elderly patient is based on the same method used for all trauma patients. Although the methodology is unchanged, the process may be altered in elderly patients. As with all trauma patients, however, the mechanism of injury should be considered first. This section discusses some special considerations in assessing an elderly trauma patient.

Kinematics

Falls

Falls are the leading cause of trauma death and disability in those over 75 years of age. Approximately one-third of community-dwelling people over 65 years of age fall each year, increasing to 50% by 80 years of age. Men and women fall with equal frequency, but women are more than twice as likely to sustain a serious injury because of more pronounced osteoporosis.

Most falls result from the inherent nature of aging, with the changes in posture and gait.[17] Declining visual acuity from cataracts, glaucoma, and loss of night vision contributes to the loss of visual clues used by elderly persons to navigate safely. Diseases of the central and peripheral nervous systems and the vascular instability of cardiovascular disease further precipitate falls. However, the most important variables contributing to falls in elderly persons are physical barriers in their environment, such as slippery floors, stairs, poorly fitting shoes, and poor lighting.

Long-bone fractures account for the majority of injuries, with fractures of the hip resulting in the greatest mortality and morbidity rates. The mortality rate from hip fractures is 20% at 1 year after the injury and rises to 33% at 2 years. Mortality is most often secondary to pulmonary embolus and the effects of decreased mobility.

Vehicular Trauma

MVCs are the leading cause of trauma death in the geriatric population between 65 and 74 years of age. An elderly patient is five times more likely to be fatally injured in an MVC than a younger driver, even though excessive speed is rarely a causative factor in the older age group.[18] For many reasons, elderly persons are often involved in collisions during daylight hours, during good weather, and close to their domicile.

These high fatality rates have been attributed to certain physiologic changes. In particular, subtle changes in memory and judgment together with impaired visual and auditory acuity can result in delayed reaction time. A common finding at crash investigations is that the elderly driver failed to yield to traffic. The National Highway Traffic Safety Administration has produced a CD-ROM program to assist physicians in assessing and counselling older drivers.

Alcohol is rarely involved, unlike with MVCs in younger persons. Only 6% of fatally injured elderly persons are intoxicated, compared with 23% for all other age categories.[18]

Elderly pedestrians represent more than 20% of all pedestrian fatalities. Because of slower walking speeds, the time allowed by traffic signals may be too short for the elderly person to traverse the crosswalk safely. This may explain the observation that more than 45% of all elderly pedestrian fatalities occur near a crosswalk.

Assault and Domestic Abuse

Abuse is defined as willful infliction of injury, unreasonable confinement, intimidation, or cruel punishment resulting in physical or psychological harm or pain, or the withholding of services that would prevent these. The elderly are highly vulnerable to crime. Violent assaults have been estimated to account for more than 10% of trauma admissions in elderly patients. The need for chronic care because of debilitation may predispose an elderly person to abuse or neglect from his or her caregivers. It is estimated that only about 15% of cases are reported to the proper authorities[19,20] (see later discussion).

Burns

Elderly patients represent 20% of burn unit admissions, with an estimated 1500 fire-related deaths per year. Burn fatalities in elderly patients occur from burns of smaller size and severity compared with other age groups. Fatality rates are seven times those of younger burn victims.

Because of impairments in visual and auditory acuity, elderly persons may have delayed recognition of house fires. Decreased pain perception can result in more significant burns. Thinning of dermal elements may result in a deeper thickness of burns.

The presence of pre-existing medical conditions, such as cardiovascular disease and diabetes, results in poor tolerance to the resuscitative care of burns. Vascular collapse and infection are the most common causes of death from burns in elderly patients.

Traumatic Brain Injury

The brain has undergone a 10% reduction in mass by 70 years of age. The dura mater adheres more closely to the skull, resulting in a loss of some brain volume. The dural bridging veins become more stretched and, thus, susceptible to tearing. This results in a lower frequency of epidural hemorrhage and a higher frequency of subdural hemorrhage. Because of brain atrophy, a fairly large subdural hemorrhage can exist with minimal clinical findings. The combination of head trauma and hypovolemic shock yields a greater fatality rate. Pre-existing medical conditions or their treatment may be a cause of altered mentation in elderly patients. When in doubt as to whether confusion represents an acute or chronic process, the injured patient should be preferentially transported to a trauma center for evaluation when possible.

Airway

Evaluation of the elderly patient begins with assessment of the airway. Changes in mentation may be associated with the tongue blocking the airway. The oral cavity should be examined for foreign bodies, such as dentures, that have become dislodged.

Breathing

Elderly patients who breathe at a rate of less than 10 or greater than 30 breaths/minute, similar to any other adult, will not have adequate minute volume and will require positive-pressure assisted ventilations. In most adults, a ventilatory rate between 12 and 20 breaths/minute is normal and confirms that an adequate minute volume is present. However, in an elderly patient, reduced tidal volume capacity and pulmonary function may result in an inadequate minute volume, even at rates of 12 to 20 breaths/minute. Breath sounds should be immediately assessed if the ventilatory rate is abnormal; however, these sounds may be harder to hear because of smaller tidal volumes.

An elderly patient's vital capacity is diminished by 50%. Kyphotic changes in the spine (anteroposterior) result in a ventilation-perfusion mismatch at rest. Hypoxia is much more likely to be a consequence of shock than in younger patients. Elderly patients also have a decreased ability for chest excursions. Lower tidal volumes and lower minute volumes are typical. Reductions in capillary oxygen and carbon dioxide exchange are significant. Hypoxemia tends to be progressive.

Circulation

Some findings can only be interpreted properly by knowing the individual patient's pre-event, or "baseline," status. Expected ranges of vital signs and other findings usually accepted as normal are not "normal" in every individual, and deviation is much more common in the elderly patient. Although the typical ranges are broad enough to include most individual adult differences, an individual of any age may vary beyond these norms; therefore, such variation in elderly patients should be expected. Medication may contribute to these changes. For example, in the average adult, a systolic blood pressure (SBP) of 120 mm Hg is considered normal and generally unimpressive. However, in the chronically hypertensive patient who normally has SBP of 150 mm Hg, a pressure of 120 mm Hg would be a concern, suggestive of hidden bleeding (or some other mechanism causing hypotension) of such a degree that decompensation has occurred. Likewise, heart rate is a poor indicator of trauma in elderly patients because of the effects of medications and the heart's poor response to circulating catecholamines (epinephrine). Quantitative information or signs should not be used in isolation from other findings. However, failing to recognize that such a change occurred or that it is a serious pathologic finding in a particular patient can produce a poor outcome for the patient.

Delayed capillary refilling time is common in the elderly because of less efficient circulation (peripheral arterial disease); therefore, it is a poor indicator of acute circulatory changes in these patients. Some degree of decreased distal motor, sensory, and circulatory ability in the extremities represents a common normal finding in elderly patients.

Disability

All findings should be viewed collectively to maintain an increased level of suspicion for neurologic injury in the elderly patient. Wide differences in mentation, memory, and orientation (to the past and present) can exist in elderly persons.

Significant neurologic trauma should be identified in light of the individual's pre-injury, normal status. Unless someone on the scene can describe this status, it should be assumed that the patient has a neurologic injury, hypoxia, or both. The ability to distinguish between a patient's chronic status and acute changes is an essential factor to prevent underreaction or overreaction to the patient's present neurologic status when evaluating his or her overall condition. However, unconsciousness remains a serious sign in all cases.

The elderly patient's orientation to time and place should be assessed by careful and complete questioning. People who work 5 days a week with weekends off usually know the day of the week. If they do not, it can be assumed that they have some level of disorientation. For those who no longer work a traditional job and who are often surrounded by others who do not, a lack of distinction between days of the week or even months of the year may not indicate disorientation but only of a lack of "calendar" importance in the structure of their lives. Similarly, people who no longer drive pay less attention to roads, town borders, locations, and maps. Although normally oriented, they may not be able to identify their present location. Confusion or the inability to recall events and details long past may be more indicative of how long ago the events occurred rather than how forgetful the individual is. Similarly, the repeated retelling of events long past and more attention paid to the far past than the immediate past often simply represent a nostalgic lingering on years and events. Such social and psychological compensations should not be considered as signs of senility or a diminished mental capacity.

Expose/Environment

Elderly persons are more susceptible to ambient environmental changes. They have a decreased ability to respond to temperature changes, decreased heat production, and a decreased ability to rid the body of excessive heat. Thermoregulatory problems are related to an imbalance of electrolytes (e.g., potassium depletion, hypothyroidism, diabetes mellitus). Other factors include a decreased basal metabolic rate, decreased ability to shiver, arteriosclerosis, and effects of drugs and alcohol. Hyperthermia may result from cerebrovascular accidents (strokes) and administration of diuretics, antihistamines, and antiparkinsonian drugs. Hypothermia is often associated with decreased metabolism, less fat, less efficient peripheral vasoconstriction, and poor nutrition.

Secondary Survey (Detailed History and Physical Examination)

The secondary survey of the elderly trauma victim is performed in the same manner as for younger patients and after urgent life-threatening conditions have been addressed. However, a number of factors may complicate assessment of the geriatric patient. Because of this, more than the average time may need to be taken when assessing elderly patients.

Communication Challenges

- *Additional patience may be needed because of the elderly patient's hearing or visual deficits.* Empathy and compassion are essential. A patient's intelligence should not be underestimated merely because communication may be difficult or absent. If the patient has close associates or relatives, they may participate in giving information or may stay nearby to help validate information. However, not all elderly patients have significant deficits. Speaking in a louder tone or slower cadence to the elderly patient may be unnecessary and insulting.
- *Assessment of the elderly patient requires different questioning tactics.* The patient should be asked for specific versus general information because elderly persons tend to respond "yes" to all questions during the assessment process. Asking open-ended questions is a useful tool in evaluating most patients. When dealing with a problem, however, providing specific details from which to choose can be helpful. For example, instead of saying, "Describe the pain in your hip," ask, "Is the pain in your hip sharp, stabbing, or dull?" or "On a scale of 1 to 10, with 10 being the most intense pain, how would you rate the pain?"
- *A significant other may need to be involved.* With the patient's permission, involving the caregiver or spouse may be necessary to gather valid information. It is important, however, to not approach elderly patients as if they were small children. A common mistake by health care professionals in both prehospital and emergency department settings is to treat the elderly in this way. Often, well-meaning relatives are so aggressive in reporting the events for an elderly loved one that they take over as the respondent to all inquiries. In such a situation, the provider can easily overlook that the clinical impression and history are from someone other than the patient and may not be correct. Not only does this increase the danger of obtaining incomplete or inaccurate information through a third party's impressions and translation, but it also discounts the patient as a mature adult. Some elderly patients may be reluctant to give information without the assistance of a relative or support person. However, the elderly patient may not want any other person present for many reasons, including abuse problems. The elderly patient may fear punishment for telling someone, in the presence of the abuser, why he or she has multiple bruise marks. Also, some problems may embarrass the elderly patient, and the person may not want any family members to know about them.
- *Pay attention to impaired hearing, sight, comprehension, and mobility capabilities.* Eye contact should be made with the patient. The patient may be hearing impaired and depend on watching your lips and other facial movements. Noise, distractions, and interruptions should be minimized. Fluency in speech, an involuntary movement, cranial nerve dysfunction, or difficulty breathing should be noted. Is the patient's movement easy, unsteady, or unbalanced?
- The patient should be addressed by his or her last name, unless otherwise told by the patient. Phrases such as, "Now, now, you'll be fine," should be avoided. Open-ended questions such as, "Describe the pain in your abdomen, is it . . . ?" should be used and such questions as, "Where does it hurt?" should be avoided.

Physiologic Changes

- *The body may not respond the same as in younger patients.* Typical findings of serious illness, such as fever, pain, or tenderness, may take longer to develop and, thus, make it more difficult to evaluate the elderly patient. In addition, many medications will alter the body's response. Often a prehospital care provider will have to depend on history alone.
- *Altered comprehension or neurologic disorders are a significant problem for many elderly patients.* These impairments can range from confusion to senile dementia of the type associated with Alzheimer's disease. Not only may these patients have difficulty in communicating, but they may also be unable to comprehend or help in the assessment. They may be restless and sometimes combative.
- *Shake the patient's hand to feel for grip strength, skin turgor, and body temperature. Look at the patient's state of nourishment.* Does the patient appear to be well, thin, or emaciated? Elderly patients have a decreased thirst response, and they also have a decreased amount of body fat (15%–30%) and total body water.
- *Elderly patients have a decrease in skeletal muscle weight, widening and weakening of bones, degeneration of joints, and osteoporosis.* They have an increased probability of fractures with minor injuries and a greatly increased risk of fractures to the vertebrae, hip, and ribs.
- *Elderly patients have degeneration of heart muscle cells and fewer pacemaker cells.* Elderly persons are prone to dysrhythmia as a result of a loss of elasticity of the heart and major arteries. Widespread use of beta blockers, calcium channel blockers, and diuretics further complicates this problem. Often after injury, elderly patients present with low cardiac output with hypoxia and have no lung injury. Cardiac stroke volume and rate decrease, as does cardiac reserve, all leading to morbidity and mortality in the elderly trauma patient. An elderly patient with a SBP of 120 mm Hg should be considered to be in hypovolemic shock until proved otherwise.

Environmental Factors

- *Look for behavioral problems or manifestations that do not fit the scene.* Look at grooming. Are the patient's attire and grooming appropriate for where and how the patient was found? The ease of rising or sitting should be observed. Is there the potential for elder abuse or neglect?

Medications

Knowledge of a patient's medications can provide key information in determining prehospital care. Pre-existing disease in the elderly trauma patient is a significant finding. The following classes of drugs are of particular interest because of their frequent use by elderly persons and their potential to affect care of the trauma patient:

- Beta blockers (e.g., propranolol, metoprolol) may account for a patient's absolute or relative bradycardia. In this situation, an increasing tachycardia as a sign of developing shock may not occur. The drug's inhibition of the body's normal sympathetic compensatory mechanisms can mask the true level of the patient's circulatory deterioration. Such patients can rapidly decompensate, seemingly without warning.
- Calcium channel blockers (e.g., verapamil) may prevent peripheral vasoconstriction and accelerate hypovolemic shock.
- Nonsteroidal anti-inflammatory agents (e.g., ibuprofen) may contribute to platelet dysfunction and increase bleeding.
- Anticoagulants (e.g., clopidogrel, aspirin, warfarin) may increase blood loss. Data suggest that use of warfarin increases the risk of isolated head injury and adverse outcome. Any bleeding from trauma will be more brisk and difficult to control when a patient is taking an anticoagulant. More importantly, internal bleeding can progress rapidly, leading to shock and death.
- Hypoglycemic agents (e.g., insulin, metformin, rosiglitazone) may be causally related to the events that caused injury and may make blood glucose therapy difficult if their use is unrecognized.
- Over the counter (OTC) medications, including herbal preparations and supplements, are frequently used by elderly persons. Their inclusion in the list of medications is often omitted by patients, who should be specifically questioned about their use. These preparations are unregulated and, thus, have unpredictable dose effects and possible drug interactions. Complications of these agents include bleeding (garlic) and myocardial infarction (ephedrine/Ma-Huang).

The difficulty in assessing the elderly trauma patient's medication list may include loss of consciousness and an extensive list of medications with difficult names. In some communities, emergency medical services (EMS) agencies have promoted programs such as the File of Life Project (www.folife.org). In this program, the patient's detailed medical history is placed in a common location in any house: the refrigerator door. The patient completes a medical history form that is then placed into a magnetic holder that is applied to the refrigerator, alerting the prehospital team to the File of Life (Figure 16-7).

Medical Conditions

Numerous medical conditions may predispose individuals to traumatic events, especially those that result in an alteration in the level of consciousness or other neurologic deficit. Common examples include seizure disorders, insulin shock from diabetes mellitus, syncopal episodes from antihypertensive medication, cardiac dysrhythmia from an acute coronary syndrome, and cerebrovascular accidents (CVA). Because the incidence of chronic medical conditions increases with age, geriatric patients are more prone to suffering trauma as the result of such a medical problem than are younger victims. The astute provider always keeps this concept in mind during the assessment and notes clues from the primary and secondary surveys that may point to a medical problem that precipitated the injury, such as:

- Bystanders may note that a victim appeared unconscious prior to a crash
- A Medic Alert bracelet that indicates the patient has diabetes
- An irregular heartbeat or cardiac dysrhythmia seen during ECG monitoring

This key information is passed on to the receiving facility.

Management

Airway

The presence of dentures, common in the elderly population, may affect airway management. Ordinarily, dentures should be left in place to maintain a better seal around the mouth with a mask. However, partial dentures (plates) may become dislodged during an emergency and may completely or partially block the airway; these should be removed.

Friable nasopharyngeal mucosal tissues and the possible use of anticoagulants put the elderly trauma patient at increased risk of bleeding from placement of a nasopharyngeal airway. This hemorrhage may further compromise the patient's airway and result in aspiration. Arthritis may affect the temporomandibular joints and cervical spine. The decreased flexibility of these areas may make endotracheal intubation more difficult.

The objective of airway management is primarily to ensure a patent airway for the delivery of adequate tissue oxygenation. Early mechanical ventilation by either bag-mask device or advanced airway interventions such as endotracheal intubation should be considered in elderly trauma patients because of their greatly limited physiologic reserve.[21]

FILE OF LIFE

KEEP INFORMATION UP TO DATE !!
Review At Least Every Six Months !
MEDICAL DATA REVIEWED AS OF___MO.___YR.

Name: _____ Sex: M F

Address: _____

Doctor: _____ Phone #: _____

Doctor: _____ Phone #: _____

EMERGENCY CONTACTS

Name: _____ Phone #: _____

Address: _____

Name: _____ Phone #: _____

Address: _____

KEEP INFORMATION UP TO DATE !!
Review At Least Every Six Months !
MEDICAL DATA REVIEWED AS OF   MO.   YR.

Name: _____ Sex: M F

Address: _____

Doctor: _____ Phone #: _____

Preferred Hospital: _____

EMERGENCY CONTACTS

Name: _____ Phone #: _____

Address: _____

Name: _____ Phone #: _____

Address: _____

MEDICAL DATA
Use pencil for ease in making changes.

Special Conditions/Remarks: _____

Medication	Dosage	Frequency

Pharmacy: _____ Phone: _____

Date of Birth: _____

Blood Type: _____ Religion: _____

Health Care Proxy on file at: _____

Living Will on file at: _____

® **FILE OF LIFE**   SEE BACK OF CARD FOR ADDITIONAL INFORMATION

Use Pencil for ease in making changes

Recent Surgery: _____ Date: _____

_____

Do you have an EMS-NO CPR Directive or a DNR form ?
YES ☐   NO ☐   Where is it located ?

MEDICAL CONDITIONS
Check all that exist

☐ No known medical conditions
☐ Abnormal EKG
☐ Adrenal Insufficiency
☐ Angina
☐ Asthma
☐ Bleeding Disorder
☐ Cancer
☐ Cardiac Dysrhythmia
☐ Cataracts
☐ Clotting Disorder
☐ Coronary Bypass Graft
☐ Dementia ☐ Alzheimer's ☐
☐ Diabetes/Insulin Dependent
☐ Eye Surgery
☐ Glaucoma
☐ Hearing Impaired
☐ Heart Valve Prosthesis
☐ Other: _____

☐ Hemodialysis
☐ Hemolytic Anemia
☐ Hepatitis-Type [   ]
☐ Hypertension
☐ Hypoglycemia
☐ Laryngectomy
☐ Leukemia
☐ Lymphomas
☐ Memory Impaired
☐ Myasthenia Gravis
☐ Pacemaker
☐ Renal Failure
☐ Seizure Disorder
☐ Sickle Cell Anemia
☐ Stroke
☐ Tuberculosis
☐ Vision Impaired

ALLERGIES

☐ Aspirin
☐ Barbiturate
☐ Codeine
☐ Demerol
☐ Horse Serum
☐ Environmental:
☐ Other:

☐ Insect Stings
☐ Latex
☐ Lidocaine
☐ Morphine
☐ Novocaine

☐ Penicillin
☐ Sulfa
☐ Tetracycline
☐ X-Rays Dyes
☐ No Known Allergies

MEDICAL INSURANCE

Med Ins Co: _____

Policy #: _____

Other Med Ins Co: _____

Policy #: _____

Medicaid #: _____ Medicare #: _____

FIGURE 16-7 File of life.

Breathing

In all trauma patients, supplemental oxygen should be administered as soon as possible. Oxygen saturation (SpO_2) should generally be kept at greater than 95%. The elderly population has a high prevalence of COPD. Even if a patient has severe COPD, it is unlikely that high-flow oxygen administration will be detrimental to the respiratory drive during routine urban or suburban transports. However, if the provider notes somnolence or a slowing of respiratory rate, ventilations can be assisted with a bag-mask device with consideration for advanced airway management.

Elderly persons experience increased stiffness of the chest wall. In addition, reduced chest-wall muscle power and stiffening of the cartilage makes the chest cage less flexible. These and other changes are responsible for reductions in lung volumes. The elderly patient may need ventilatory support by assisted ventilations with a bag-mask device earlier than younger trauma patients. The mechanical force applied to the resuscitation bag may need to be increased to overcome the increased chest wall resistance.

Circulation

Elderly persons may have poor cardiovascular reserve. Vital signs are a poor indicator of shock in the elderly patient because the patient who is normally hypertensive may be in shock with a blood pressure that is considered "normal" for a younger patient. Reduced circulating blood volume, possible chronic anemia, and pre-existing myocardial and coronary disease leave the patient with very little tolerance for even modest amounts of blood loss. Because of the laxity of skin or use of anticoagulant agents, geriatric patients are prone to the development of larger hematomas and potentially more significant internal hemorrhage. Early control of hemorrhage through direct pressure on open wounds, stabilization or immobilization of fractures, and rapid transport to a trauma center are essential. Fluid resuscitation should be guided by the index of suspicion for serious bleeding based on the mechanism of injury and an overall appearance of shock. The kidney's ability to concentrate urine is decreased, leading to dehydration even before an injury occurs. Urine output is a poor measure of perfusion in elderly persons.

Immobilization

Protection of the cervical spine, particularly in trauma patients who have sustained multisystem injury, is an expected standard of care. In the elderly population, this standard of care must apply not only in trauma situations but also during acute medical problems in which attempts to maintain airway patency is a priority. Degenerative arthritis of the cervical spine may subject the elderly patient to spinal cord injury from positioning and manipulating the neck, even if the patient has no injury to the bony spine. Another consid-

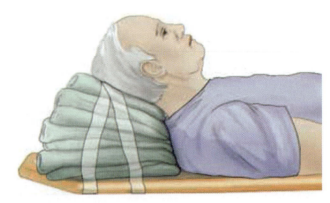

FIGURE 16-8   Immobilization of a kyphotic patient. (NOTE: Other straps and the cervical collar are not shown for clarity of illustration purposes.)

eration with improper movement of the cervical spine is the possibility of occlusion of the arteries to the brain, which can result in unconsciousness and even stroke.

A cervical collar applied to an elderly patient with severe kyphosis should not compress the airway or carotid arteries. Less traditional means of immobilization, such as a rolled towel and head block, can be considered if standard collars are inappropriate.

Padding may need to be placed under the patient's head and between the shoulders when immobilizing the kyphotic supine elderly patient (Figure 16-8). Because the thin skin and lack of adipose tissue in the frail, elderly patient, geriatric patients are more likely to develop pressure (decubitus) ulcers from lying on their back; therefore, additional padding will be required when the patient is immobilized to a long backboard. It is always a good idea to check for pressure points when the patient is resting on the board and pad appropriately. When applying the straps to secure the patient, the elderly patient may not be able to straighten the legs fully because of decreased range of motion of the hips and knees. This may require the placement of padding under the legs for comfort and security of the patient during transport.[22]

Temperature Control

The elderly patient should be monitored closely for hypothermia and hyperthermia during treatment and transportation. Although it is appropriate to expose the patient to facilitate a thorough examination, elderly persons are especially prone to heat loss. On the other hand, the effects of various medications may mean that a patient is more prone to overheating; therefore, some means of cooling the patient should be considered if the patient is unable to be moved quickly to a controlled environment. Prolonged extrication in the extremes of heat and cold may also place the elderly patient at risk and should be rapidly addressed. External methods of heating or cooling the elderly trauma patient should be balanced by the possibility of direct thermal injury to the site of application with the patient's attenuated skin structure.

Legal Considerations

Several legal distinctions can become issues when giving care to the elderly trauma patient. Recent evidence demonstrates that although mortality increases with age, 80% of discharged geriatric trauma patients return to a high functional level. Under certain circumstances, the patient or family member may forego potentially lifesaving interventions and provide comfort measures only (e.g., elderly patient with extensive burns). The most appropriate care plan for the patient can be determined by identifying a living will, advance directives, or other legal documents, if available to the providers at the scene.

In most of the United States, spouses, siblings, children, spouses of children, and parents have no legal standing in making medical decisions for an adult. Persons with power of attorney or court-appointed conservators may have authority over an individual's financial affairs, but they do not necessarily have control over that individual's personal medical decisions. Court-appointed custodians or guardians may or may not have the power to make medical decisions, depending on the local laws and the specific charge of their appointment. Such powers are considered to exist only when a guardianship of person or a durable power of attorney for health care is specified and clear documentation of such third-party powers is present.

In the midst of a trauma scene, it may be difficult to make such a fine legal distinction. Because the ambulance was summoned and a "call for help" was made, the concept of "implied consent" to care for the patient applies in cases of patients who are unconscious or have reduced mental capacity.

In many states, health care workers, including prehospital care personnel, are required to report cases of suspected elder maltreatment to authorities. Should further clarification be necessary or should anyone attempt to interfere with the prehospital care, the problem should be presented to the police officer in charge at the scene. The law generally provides a protocol for an officer to make a timely decision at the scene, with clarification to occur later at the hospital when time allows. Such events should be documented carefully and completely as a part of the run report.

Elder Maltreatment

Elder abuse is defined as any action by an elderly person's family member (any relative), associated persons who have daily household contact (housekeeper, roommate), anyone on whom the elderly person is reliant for daily needs of food, clothing, and shelter, or a professional caregiver who takes advantage of the elderly person's property or emotional state.

Reports and complaints of abuse, neglect, and other related problems among the elderly population are increasing. The exact extent of elder abuse is not known for the following reasons:

1. Elder abuse has been largely hidden from society.
2. Abuse and neglect of elderly persons have varying definitions.
3. Elders are uneasy or fearful of reporting the problem to law enforcement agencies or human and social welfare personnel. A typical victim of elder abuse may be a parent who feels ashamed or guilty because he or she raised the abuser. The abused may also feel traumatized by the situation or fear continued reprisal by the abuser.
4. Some jurisdictions lack formal reporting mechanisms. Some areas do not even have a statutory provision requiring the reporting of elder abuse.

The physical and emotional signs of abuse, such as rape, beating, or nutritional deprivation, are often overlooked or perhaps are not accurately identified. Older women in particular are not likely to report incidents of sexual assault to law enforcement agencies. Sensory deficits, senility, and other forms of altered mental status (e.g., drug-induced depression) may make it impossible or extremely difficult for the elderly patient to report the maltreatment.

Profile of the Abused

The elderly adult most likely to be abused fits into the following profile:

- Over 65 years of age, especially women over 75 years of age
- Frail
- Multiple chronic medical conditions
- Demented
- Impaired sleep cycle, sleepwalking, or loud shouting at night
- Incontinent of feces, urine, or both
- Dependent on others for activities of daily living or incapable of independent living

Profile of the Abuser

Because many elderly people live in a family environment and are typically women older than 75 years of age, that environment may provide clues. The abuser is frequently the spouse of the patient or the middle-age daughter-in-law of the patient who is caring for dependent children and dependent parents while perhaps holding full-time or part-time employment. Most of these abusers are untrained in the particular care required by the elderly and have little relief time from the constant care demands of their family.

Abuse is not restricted to the home. Other environments such as nursing, convalescent, and continuing care centers are sites where the elderly may sustain physical, chemical, or pharmacologic harm. Care providers in these environments may consider elderly persons to represent management problems or categorize them as obstinate or undesirable patients. The usual profile of the abuser includes the following signs:

- Existence of household conflict
- Marked fatigue
- Unemployment
- Financial difficulties
- Substance abuse
- Previous history of abuse

Categories of Maltreatment

Abuse can be categorized in the following ways:

1. *Physical abuse* includes assault, neglect, malnutrition, poor maintenance of the living environment, and poor personal care. The signs of physical abuse or neglect may be obvious, such as the imprint left by an item (e.g., fireplace poker) or may be subtle (e.g., malnutrition). The signs of elder abuse are similar to those of child abuse (Figure 16-9) (see Chapter 15).
2. *Psychological abuse* can take on the forms of neglect, verbal abuse, infantilization, or deprivation of sensory stimulation.
3. *Financial abuse* can include theft of valuables or embezzlement.
4. *Sexual assault and/or abuse.*
5. *Self abuse.*

Important Points

Many abused patients are terrorized into making false statements for fear of retribution. In the case of elder abuse by family members, fear of removal from the home environment can cause the elderly patient to lie about the origin of the abuse. In other cases of elder abuse, sensory deprivation or dementia may deter adequate explanation. The prehospital care provider should identify abuse and uncover any pathology reported by the patient. Any history of maltreatment or findings consistent with it should be documented on the patient care report.

Further trauma to a patient may be reduced by identifying an abusive situation. Reporting a high index of suspicion for abuse can allow for referral to and protective services from human, social, and public safety agencies (Figure 16-10).

Disposition

One of the greatest challenges with prehospital care of the injured patient is defining which patients are most likely to benefit from the surgeons and advanced treatment options available at a trauma center. For many of the reasons mentioned previously, triage criteria may be less reliable in the elderly patient because of physiologic or pharmacologic

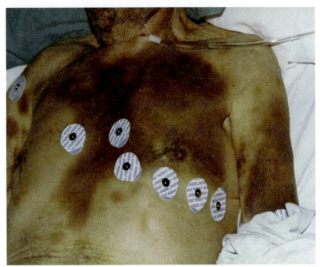

FIGURE 16-9 A 70-year-old man was brought from his caregiver's home to the emergency department by police after his daughter found him severely bruised. He had multiple contusions at varying stages of healing on his chest and arms, as well as a linear-patterned injury across his left anterior chest. The central and bilateral locations of the contusions, varying colors, and linear pattern of the bruise on his left chest are highly suggestive of physical abuse.
(From Marx J: *Rosen's Emergency Medicine*, ed 7, St. Louis, 2010, Mosby. Courtesy of Dr. D.C. Schneider.)

effects. A major recommendation in the *Guidelines for Geriatric Trauma* of the Eastern Association for the Surgery of Trauma is that prehospital providers treating trauma patients of advanced age should have a lower threshold to triage these victims directly to a trauma center.[23] Data from several states demonstrate that a disproportionate number of elderly trauma patients are receiving care at trauma centers. Furthermore, potentially preventable mortality in the geriatric trauma population is lower at trauma centers.

Prolonged Transport

The majority of care of the elderly trauma patient follows general guidelines for prehospital care of the injured patient. However, several special circumstances exist in prolonged transport scenarios. These concerns are particularly important for the recommendations to triage patients with less significant anatomic injuries directly to trauma centers.

Treatment of shock in the prehospital environment over an extended period requires careful reassessment of vital signs during transport. After control of hemorrhage with local measures, fluid resuscitation should be titrated to physiologic response to optimize resuscitation of intravascular volume status while avoiding potential volume overload in a patient with impaired cardiac function.

Immobilization on a long backboard places these patients at increased risk for pressure-related skin breakdown over

---

FIGURE 16-10   Reporting Elder Abuse and Neglect

In many states, EMS personnel are legally considered to be mandated reporters of suspected elder (or adult) abuse, neglect, and exploitation. *Abuse* is considered the deliberate infliction of pain, injury, mental anguish, unreasonable confinement, or nonconsensual sexual contact. *Neglect* involves living in conditions in which the adult or responsible caretaker is not providing care required to maintain the elderly person's physical and mental health and well-being. *Exploitation* is the illegal use of an adult's resources for another's gain or advantage. In recent years, elder abuse has been increasingly recognized. However, younger adults who have incapacitating conditions such as mental illness, mental retardation, and physical disability are also at risk for abuse and neglect.

Signs of abuse and neglect include unexplained or unusual injuries; conflicting accounts of how an injury occurred; a caregiver who prevents the adult from speaking with others; dehydration or malnutrition; depression; lack of access to medications, eyeglasses, dentures, or other aids; lack of personal hygiene; unkempt environment; and lack of adequate heating and cooling.

Mandated reporters must report directly to the social services agency responsible for investigating adult abuse, rather than relying on intermediaries such as hospital personnel. If the individual is in immediate danger or has been sexually assaulted, law enforcement must be notified as well. In the event that a death appears to have been caused by abuse or neglect, mandatory reporters generally must notify the office of the medical examiner or coroner and law enforcement. Mandatory reporters are liable for failing to report suspected abuse, neglect, and exploitation. However, they are protected against civil and criminal liability associated with reporting, they may be able to keep their identity confidential, and they are allowed to share medical information that is related to the case, although this information would be protected under the Health Insurance Portability and Accountability Act (HIPAA) in normal circumstances. Laws governing the mandatory reporting of elder abuse are enacted at the state level. All EMS providers must be aware of the laws in the state in which they work.

---

extended transports. Weakened skin structure and impaired vascular supply may lead to earlier complications than expected. Prior to a long transport, consideration should be given to clearing the spine or logrolling a patient onto an appropriately padded long backboard to protect the patient's skin. Agencies in remote regions should consider purchasing a specially designed, low-pressure backboard that immobilizes the patient while limiting the potential for skin breakdown.

Environmental control is essential in geriatric patients with a lengthy transport. Limiting body exposure and controlling ambient temperature of the vehicle may limit hypothermia. The hypothermic patient may shiver, producing anaerobic metabolism, leading to lactic acidosis, and accelerating shock.

Finally, transport of the geriatric trauma patient from remote regions may be a valid use of aeromedical transport. Transport via helicopter may limit the duration of environmental exposure, reduce the duration of shock, and ensure earlier access to hospital-based care, including early surgery and blood transfusion.

SUMMARY

- Elderly persons are living healthier, more active, and longer lives than ever before.
- Although general guidelines for care of the injured patient remain the same, several specific approaches are unique to care of the injured geriatric patient.
- Anatomic and physiologic changes associated with aging, chronic disease, and medications can make certain types of trauma more likely, complicate traumatic injuries, and cause a decreased ability to compensate for shock. Older patients have less physiologic reserve and tolerate physical insult poorly.

- Knowledge of the elderly trauma patient's medical history and medications is an essential component of care.
- Many factors in elderly trauma patients can mask early signs of deterioration, increasing the possibility of sudden, rapid decompensation without apparent warning.
- With an elderly trauma patient, more serious injury may have occurred than indicated by the initial presentation.
- A lower threshold for direct triage of these patients to trauma centers is important.

SCENARIO SOLUTION

When dealing with trauma in the elderly patient, you cannot always determine immediately whether the trauma was the primary event or whether it was secondary to a medical event, such as a stroke, myocardial infarction, or syncopal episode. However, you always need to consider the possibility that a significant medical event preceded the trauma. Your primary assessment reveals that the patient is maintaining a patent airway and is breathing at 16 times per minute. There is no major external hemorrhage and the bleeding from the forehead laceration is easily controlled with pressure. His heart rate is 84. You immobilize the patient to a longboard and provide appropriate padding underneath. Because he is a known diabetic you check his blood sugar to see if there is a correctable cause for his altered mentation. Given his age, the apparent head trauma, and the magnitude of the crash, you transport him emergently to the closest trauma center.

References

1. http://www.census.gov/Press-Release/www/releases/archives/population/013733.html. Accessed August 30, 2009.
2. Scommegna P: United States growing bigger, older, and more diverse. *Population Reference Bureau, 2005*, http://www.prb.org/.
3. Champion H et al: The Major Trauma Outcome Study: Establishing national norms for trauma care. *J Trauma* 30(11):1356, 1990.
4. National Center for Injury Prevention and Control, Centers for Disease Control and Prevention: Web-based Injury Statistics Query and Reporting System. Ten Leading Causes of Death, 1999–2004.
5. ACS Committee on Trauma: *Advanced trauma life support for doctors, student course manual,* ed 8, Chicago, 2008, ACS, pp 247–258.
6. Jacobs D: Special considerations in geriatric injury. *Curr Opin Crit Care* 9(6):535, 2003.
7. US Department of Health and Human Services, Centers for Disease Control and Prevention, National Center for Health Statistics: Access to health care: Part 3. Older adults, 2005. http://www.cdc.gov/nchs/.
8. Milzman DP, Boulanger BR, Rodriguez A, et al: Pre-existing disease in trauma patients: A predictor of fate independent of age and injury severity score. *J Trauma* 32:236, 1992.
9. Smith T: Respiratory system: Aging, adversity, and anesthesia. In McCleskey CH, editor: *Geriatric anesthesiology,* Baltimore, 1997, Williams & Wilkins.
10. US Department of Health and Human Services, Centers for Disease Control and Prevention, National Center for Health Statistics: Stroke and cerebrovascular diseases, 2005. http://www.cdc.gov/nchs/.
11. US Department of Health and Human Services, Centers for Disease Control and Prevention, National Center for Health Statistics: Hypertension, 2005. http://www.cdc.gov/nchs/.
12. Abrams K et al: Management of trauma in the geriatric patient. *Curr Opin Anaesthesiol* 17(2):165, 2004.
13. Carey J: Brain facts: a primer on the brain and nervous system. *Society for Neuroscience,* Washington, DC, 2002. http://www.sfn.org/skins/main/pdf/brainfacts/2008/brain_facts.pdf. Accessed April 21, 2010.
14. US Department of Health and Human Services, National Institutes of Health, National Eye Institute: Cataract: what you should know, 2005. http://www.nei.nih.gov/health/cataract/cataract_facts.asp. Accessed April 21, 2010.
15. Alexander J, Shneiderman A: Vertebral fracture, 2004. http://www.emedicine.com/med/topic2895.htm. Accessed April 21, 2010.
16. Blackmore C: Cervical spine injury in patients 65 years old and older: Epidemiologic analysis regarding the effects of age and injury mechanism on distribution, type, and stability of injuries. *Am J Roentgenol* 178:573, 2002.
17. Tinetti M: Preventing falls in elderly persons. *N Engl J Med* 348:42, 2003.
18. US Department of Health and Human Services, Centers for Disease Control and Prevention, National Center for Health Statistics: Older adult drivers: fact sheet, 2005. http://www.cdc.gov/nchs/.
19. US Department of Health and Human Services, US Administration on Aging, National Center on Elder Abuse, 2005, http://www.elderabusecenter.org/.
20. US Department of Health and Human Services, US Administration on Aging: Elder rights and resources, 2005. http://www.aoa.gov/eldfam/Elder_Rights/Elder_Rights.asp.
21. Heffner J, Reynolds S: Airway management of the critically ill patient. *Chest* 127:1397, 2005.
22. American Geriatric Society: *Geriatric education for emergency medical services (GEMS),* Sudbury, MA, 2003, Jones & Bartlett.
23. Eastern Association for the Surgery of Trauma: Guidelines for geriatric trauma. In *Practice management guidelines,* www.east.org/tpg/geriatric.pdf. Accessed April 21, 2010.
24. Milzman DP, Boulander BR, Rodriguez A, et al: Pre-existing disease in trauma patients: A predictor of fate independent of age and injury severity score. *J Trauma* 32:236–243, 1992.

Suggested Reading

American College of Surgeons Committee on Trauma: Extremes of age: Geriatric trauma. In *Advanced trauma life support for doctors, student course manual*, ed 8, Chicago, Pages 247-258, 2008, ACS.

Callaway D, Wolfe R: Geriatric Trauma. *Emer Med Clin No Am* 25(3):837–860, 2007.

Lavoie A, Ratte S, Clas D, et al: Pre-injury warfarin use among elderly patients with closed head injuries in a trauma center. *J Trauma* 56:802, 2004.

Tepas JJ III, Veldenz HC, Lottenberg L, et al: Elderly trauma: A profile of trauma experience in the sunshine (retirement) state. *J Trauma* 48:581, 2000.

Victorino GP, Chong TJ, Pal JD: Trauma in the elderly patient. *Arch Surg* 138:1093–1097, 2003.

CHAPTER 17

Golden Principles of Prehospital Trauma Care

CHAPTER OBJECTIVES

At the completion of this chapter, the reader will be able to do the following:

✓ Understand the importance of the "golden period."

✓ Discuss why trauma patients die.

✓ Understand and discuss the 14 "Golden Principles" of prehospital trauma care.

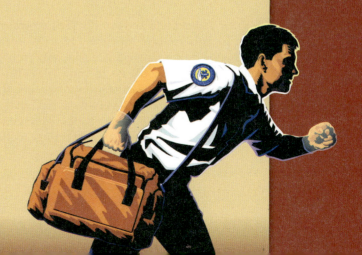

In the late 1960s, R Adams Cowley, MD, conceived the idea of a crucial time period during which it was important to begin definitive patient care for a critically injured trauma patient. In an interview he said, "There is a 'golden hour' between life and death. If you are critically injured, you have less than 60 minutes to survive. You might not die right then—it may be 3 days or 2 weeks later—but something has happened in your body that is irreparable."

Is there a basis for this concept? The answer is definitely "yes." However, an important realization is that a patient does not always have the luxury of a "Golden Hour." A patient with a penetrating wound of the heart may have only a few minutes to reach definitive care before the shock caused by the injury becomes irreversible. At the other end of the spectrum is a patient with slow, ongoing internal hemorrhage from an isolated femur fracture. Such a patient may have several hours to reach definitive care and resuscitation. Because the "Golden *Hour*" is not a strict 60-minute time frame and varies from patient to patient based on the injuries, the more appropriate term is the "Golden *Period*." If a critically injured patient is able to obtain definitive care—that is, hemorrhage control and resuscitation—within that particular patient's "Golden Period," the chance of survival is greatly improved.[1]

No call, scene, or patient is the same. Each requires flexibility of the health care team members to act and react to situations as they develop. The management of prehospital trauma must reflect these contingencies. The goals, however, have not changed: (1) gain access to the patient; (2) identify and treat life-threatening injuries; and (3) package and transport the patient to the closest appropriate facility in the least amount of time. The majority of the techniques and principles discussed are not new, and most are taught in an initial education program. This text is different in the following ways:

1. It provides current, evidence-based practices of management for the trauma patient.
2. It provides a systematic approach for establishing priorities of patient care for trauma patients who have sustained injury to multiple body systems.
3. It provides an organizational scheme for interventions.

The Prehospital Trauma Life Support (PHTLS) program teaches that the prehospital care provider can make correct judgments leading toward a good outcome only if the provider is supplied with a good base of knowledge. The foundation of the PHTLS program is that patient care should be *judgment* driven, not *protocol* driven—thus, the medical detail provided in this course. This chapter addresses the key aspects of prehospital trauma care and "brings it all together."

Why Trauma Patients Die

Studies that analyze the causes of death in trauma patients have several common themes. A study from Russia of more than 700 trauma deaths found that most patients who rapidly succumbed to their injuries fall into one of three categories: massive acute blood loss (36%), severe injury to vital organs such as the brain (30%), and airway obstruction and acute ventilatory failure (25%).[2] In an analysis of 753 trauma patients who died of their injuries at a Level I trauma center, Dr. Ronald Stewart and coworkers found that 51% of trauma patients died from severe trauma to the central nervous system (CNS) (e.g., traumatic brain injury), 21% from irreversible shock, 25% from both severe CNS trauma and irreversible shock, and 3% from multiple organ failure.[3]

But what is happening to these patients on a cellular level? As discussed in Chapter 8, the metabolic processes of the human body are driven by energy, similar to any other machine. As with machines, the human body generates its own energy but must have fuel to do this. Fuel for the body is oxygen and glucose. The body can store glucose as complex carbohydrates (glycogen) and fat to use at a later time. However, oxygen cannot be stored. It must be constantly supplied to the cells of the body. Atmospheric air, containing oxygen, is drawn into the lungs by the action of the diaphragm and intercostal muscles. Oxygen then diffuses across the alveolar and capillary walls, where it binds to the hemoglobin in the red blood cells (RBCs) and is transported to the body's tissues by the circulatory system. In the presence of oxygen, the cells of the tissues then "burn" glucose though a complex series of metabolic processes (glycolysis, Krebs cycle, and electron transport) to produce the energy needed for all body functions. This energy is stored as adenosine triphosphate (ATP). Without sufficient energy (ATP), essential metabolic activities cannot function normally, and organs begin to fail.

Shock is viewed as a failure of energy production in the body. The sensitivity of the cells to oxygen deprivation varies from organ to organ (Figure 17-1). The cells within an organ can be fatally damaged but can continue to function for a period of time (see Chapter 8 for complications of prolonged shock). This delayed death of cells, leading to organ failure, is what Dr. Cowley referred to in his statement quoted earlier. The condition he described, shock, resulted in death if a patient was not treated promptly. His definition included transporting the patient to the operating room for control of internal hemorrhage. The American College of Surgeons (ACS) Committee on Trauma has used this concept of a "Golden Hour" to emphasize the importance of transporting a patient to a facility where expert trauma care is immediately available.

The Golden Period represents a time interval during which shock is worsening, but this condition is almost always **reversible** if proper care is received. Failure to initiate

---

FIGURE 17-1   Shock

When the heart is deprived of oxygen, the myocardial cells cannot produce enough energy to pump blood to the other tissues. For example, a patient has lost a significant number of red blood cells and blood volume from a gunshot wound to the aorta. The heart continues to beat for several minutes before failing. Refilling the vascular system after the heart has been without oxygen for several minutes will not restore the function of the injured cells of the heart. This process is called irreversible shock. The specific condition in the heart is known as pulseless electrical activity (PEA). Cellular function is still present; however, it is not sufficient to pump blood to the body's cells. The patient has an ECG rhythm but not enough contractile power to force blood out of the heart to the rest of the body.

Another example of this same process but with a less severe outcome is congestive heart failure. Many of the cells of the heart

have been damaged by ischemia secondary to coronary artery disease, but some are not. The damage is not complete, so enough functioning cells are left for the pumping process to continue.

Although ischemia, as seen in severe shock, may damage virtually all tissues, the damage to the organs does not become apparent at the same time. In the lungs, acute respiratory distress syndrome (ARDS) often develops within 48 hours after an ischemic insult, whereas acute renal failure and hepatic failure typically occur several days later. Although all body tissues are affected by insufficient oxygen, some tissues are more sensitive to ischemia. For example, a patient who has sustained a traumatic brain injury may develop cerebral edema (swelling) that results in permanent brain damage. Although the brain cells cease to function and die, the rest of the body may survive for years.

---

appropriate interventions aimed at improving oxygenation and controlling hemorrhage allows shock to progress, becoming **irreversible.** For trauma patients to have the best chance of survival, interventions should start in the field with prehospital care providers and then continue in the emergency department (ED), the operating room (OR), and the intensive care unit (ICU). Trauma is a "team sport." The patient "wins" when all members of the trauma team—from those in the field to those in the trauma center—work together to care for the individual patient.

The Golden Principles of Prehospital Trauma Care

The preceding chapters discuss the assessment and management of patients who have sustained injury to specific body systems. Although this text presents the body systems individually, most severely injured patients have injury to more than one body system, thus the name *multisystem trauma patient* (also known as *polytrauma*). A prehospital care provider needs to recognize and prioritize the treatment of patients with multiple injuries, following the "Golden Principles of Prehospital Trauma Care" described next.

1. Ensure the Safety of the Prehospital Care Providers and the Patient.

Prehospital care providers need to ensure that scene safety remains their highest priority (Figure 17-2). This includes not only the safety of the patient, but their own safety as well.

Based on information provided by dispatch, potential threats can often be anticipated before arrival at the scene. For a motor vehicle crash (MVC), threats may include traffic, hazardous materials, fires, and downed power lines; for a shooting victim, providers need to be aware that the perpetrator may still be in the area. When a violent crime is involved, law enforcement personnel should first enter the scene and secure the area. A prehospital care provider who takes needless risk may also become a victim; in doing so, the provider is no longer of help to the original trauma patient. Except in the most unusual circumstances, only those with proper training should attempt rescues.

Another fundamental aspect of safety involves the use of standard precautions. Blood and other body fluids can transmit infections, such as human immunodeficiency virus (HIV)

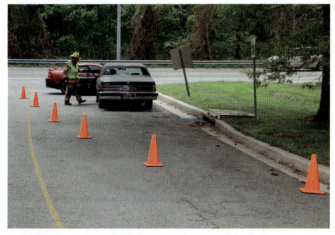

FIGURE 17-2 Ensure the safety of the prehospital care providers and the patient.

and hepatitis B virus (HBV). Protective gear should always be worn, especially when caring for trauma patients in the presence of blood.

The safety of the patient and possible hazardous situations should also be identified. Even if a patient involved in an MVC has no life-threatening conditions identified in the primary survey, rapid extrication is appropriate if threats to patient safety are noted, such as a significant potential for fire or a precarious vehicle position.

2. Assess the Scene Situation to Determine the Need for Additional Resources.

During the response to the scene and immediately on arrival, a quick assessment is performed to determine the need for additional or specialized resources. Examples include additional emergency medical services (EMS) units to accommodate the number of patients, fire suppression equipment, special rescue teams, power company personnel, medical helicopters, and physicians to aid in the triage of a large number of patients. The need for these resources should be anticipated and requested as soon as possible.

3. Recognize the Kinematics that Produced the Injuries.

Chapter 4 provides the reader with a foundation of how kinetic energy can translate into injury to the trauma patient. As the scene and the patient are approached, the kinematics of the situation are noted (Figure 17-3). Understanding the principles of kinematics leads to better patient assessment. Knowledge of specific injury patterns aids in predicting injuries and knowing where to examine. Consideration of the kinematics should not delay the initiation of patient assessment and care but can be included in the global scene assessment and in the questions directed to the patient and bystanders. The kinematics may also play a key role in determining the destination facility for a given trauma patient (mechanism of injury

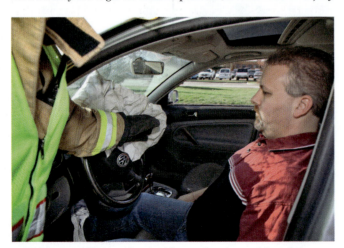

FIGURE 17-3   Recognize the kinematics that produced the injuries.

criteria for triage to trauma centers). The key aspects of the kinematics noted at the scene should also be relayed to the physicians at the receiving facility.

4. Use the Primary Survey Approach to Identify Life-Threatening Conditions.

The central concept in the PHTLS program is the emphasis on the primary survey adopted from the Advanced Trauma Life Support Program for Doctors, taught by the ACS Committee on Trauma. This brief survey allows vital functions to be rapidly assessed and life-threatening conditions to be identified through systematic evaluation of the ABCDEs: **a**irway, **b**reathing, **c**irculation, **d**isability, and **e**xpose/**e**nvironment (Figure 17-4). On initial approach to the scene and as field care is provided, the prehospital care provider receives input from several senses (sight, hearing, smell, touch) that must be sorted—placed in a priority scheme of life-threatening or limb-threatening injuries—and used to develop a plan for correct management.

FIGURE 17-4   **Critical or Potentially Critical Trauma Patient: Scene Time of 10 Minutes or Less**

Presence of any of the following life-threatening conditions:

1. Inadequate or threatened airway
2. Impaired ventilation as demonstrated by the following:
    - Abnormally fast or slow ventilatory rate
    - Hypoxia (SpO_2 <95% even with supplemental oxygen)
    - Dyspnea
    - Open pneumothorax or flail chest
    - Suspected pneumothorax
3. Significant external hemorrhage or suspected internal hemorrhage
4. Shock, even if compensated
5. Abnormal neurologic status
    - GCS score ≤ 13
    - Seizure activity
    - Sensory or motor deficit
6. Penetrating trauma to the head, neck, or torso, or proximal to the elbow and knee in the extremities
7. Amputation or near-amputation proximal to the fingers or toes
8. Any trauma in the presence of the following:
    - History of serious medical conditions (e.g., coronary artery disease, chronic obstructive pulmonary disease, bleeding disorder)
    - Age > 55 years
    - Hypothermia
    - Burns
    - Pregnancy

The primary survey involves a "treat as you go" philosophy. As life-threatening problems are identified, care is initiated at the earliest possible time. Although taught in a stepwise fashion, many aspects of the primary survey can be performed simultaneously. During transport, the primary survey should be reassessed at reasonable intervals so that the effectiveness of the interventions can be evaluated and new concerns addressed.

In children, pregnant patients, and elderly persons, injuries should be considered (1) to be more serious than their outward appearance, (2) to have a more profound systemic influence, and (3) to have a greater potential for producing rapid decompensation. In pregnant patients, there are at least two patients to care for—the mother and the fetus—both of whom may have sustained injury. Compensatory mechanisms differ from younger adults and may not reveal abnormalities until the patient is profoundly compromised.

The primary survey also provides a framework to establish management priorities when faced with numerous patients. At a multiple-casualty incident, for example, patients who have serious problems identified with their airway, ventilation, or perfusion are managed and transported before patients with only altered levels of consciousness.

5. Provide Appropriate Airway Management While Maintaining Cervical Spine Stabilization.

Management of the airway remains the highest priority in the treatment of critically injured patients. This should be accomplished while maintaining the head and neck in a neutral in-line position, if indicated by the mechanism of injury. All prehospital care providers must be able to perform the "essential skills" of airway management with ease: manual clearing of the airway, manual maneuvers to open the airway (trauma jaw thrust and trauma chin lift), suctioning, and the use of oropharyngeal and nasopharyngeal airways.

For many years, endotracheal intubation (ETI) has been the "gold standard" technique for controlling the airway of a critically injured trauma patient in the prehospital setting. This recommendation, based upon ATLS standards, has become increasingly controversial as more prehospital data on airway management has emerged (see Airway and Ventilation, Chapter 7). As previously discussed, concerns related to prehospital ETI include: unrecognized malpositioning, insufficient performance of the procedure to maintain proficiency, and conflicting data on outcome of patients who have received ETI.

Although performing intubation in the field seems to make sense, there is no conclusive evidence that endotracheal intubation results in lower morbidity or mortality rates in the trauma patient. The need for advanced airway management must be balanced with a number of factors, including training and skill of providers and distance from the receiving facil-

ity. *In some circumstances, such as the close proximity of an appropriate receiving facility, the most prudent decision may be to focus on the essential skills of airway management and rapidly transport the patient to that facility.*

If the prehospital care provider is properly trained, ETI should be considered for all trauma patients who are unable to protect their airway, including those who have a Glasgow Coma Scale (GCS) score of 8 or less, require high concentrations of oxygen to maintain oxygen saturation (SpO_2) greater than 95%, or require assisted ventilations because of a decreased ventilatory rate or decreased minute volume. Intubation may also be considered for those patients with potential threats to their airway, such as an expanding hematoma in the neck or findings consistent with airway or pulmonary burns. After performing endotracheal intubation, a combination of clinical assessments and adjunct devices should be used to confirm that the tube has been properly placed. After moving an intubated patient, tube placement should always be reconfirmed each time.

When intubation is indicated but cannot be performed, there are alternative options (see Airway Management Algorithm, p. 141). Ventilation can be attempted using the essential skills alone, or ventilation can be attempted with a dual-lumen airway or a laryngeal mask airway. If adequate ventilation can be achieved, additional attempts at intubation using retrograde or digital techniques may be considered. If ventilation cannot be accomplished, percutaneous transtracheal ventilation is an acceptable option.

6. Support Ventilation and Deliver Oxygen to Maintain an SpO_2 Greater than 95%.

Assessment and management of ventilation is another key aspect in the management of the critically injured patient. The normal ventilatory rate in the adult patient is 12 to 20 ventilations per minute. A rate slower than this often significantly interferes with the body's ability to oxygenate the RBCs passing through the pulmonary capillaries and to remove the carbon dioxide (CO_2) produced by the tissues. These patients with bradypnea require assisted or total ventilatory support with a bag-mask device connected to supplemental oxygen ($FiO_2 > 0.85$). When patients are tachypneic (adult rate >20 breaths/minute), their minute ventilation (tidal volume multiplied by their ventilatory rate) should be estimated. For a patient with a significant decrease in minute volume (rapid, shallow ventilations), ventilation should be assisted with a bag-mask device connected to supplemental oxygen ($FiO_2 > 0.85$). If available, end-tidal CO_2 monitoring ($ETCO_2$) can prove useful to ensure sufficient ventilatory support. A sudden decrease in the $ETCO_2$ may indicate dislodgment of the endotracheal tube or a sudden decrease in perfusion (profound hypotension or cardiopulmonary arrest).

Supplemental oxygen is administered to any trauma patient with obvious or suspected life-threatening conditions. If available, pulse oximetry can be used to titrate the oxygen administration to keep the SpO_2 greater than 95% (at sea level). If concern exists about the accuracy of a pulse oximetry reading or if this technology is not available, oxygen can be administered through a nonrebreathing mask to the spontaneously breathing patient or with a bag-mask connected to supplemental oxygen (FiO_2 >0.85) for those patients receiving assisted or total ventilatory support.

7. Control Any Significant External Hemorrhage.

In the trauma patient, significant external hemorrhage is a finding that requires immediate attention. Because blood is not available for administration in the prehospital setting, hemorrhage control becomes a paramount concern for prehospital care providers in order to maintain a sufficient number of circulating RBCs; *every RBC counts.* Extremity injuries and scalp wounds, such as lacerations and partial avulsions, may be associated with life-threatening blood loss.

Most external hemorrhage is readily controlled by the application of direct pressure at the bleeding site or, if resources are limited, by the use of a pressure dressing created with gauze 4 x 4 pads and an elastic bandage. If direct pressure or a pressure dressing fails to control external hemorrhage from an extremity, the prehospital care provider may consider applying a tourniquet. Although taught for many years in first aid and basic emergency care courses, evidence shows that elevation of an extremity or applying pressure over a pressure point adds little to direct pressure or a pressure dressing.[4] Tourniquets are routinely used in surgical procedures, with an excellent safety record, and may be lifesaving in the prehospital setting. When faced with a patient who has external hemorrhage that is difficult to control and not amenable to application of a tourniquet, the provider may consider application of a topical hemostatic agent.

For a patient in obvious shock from external hemorrhage, measures aimed at resuscitation (e.g., administration of IV fluids) should be avoided before adequately controlling the bleeding. *Attempted resuscitation will never be successful in the presence of ongoing external hemorrhage.*

Control of external hemorrhage and recognition of suspected internal hemorrhage, combined with prompt transport to the closest appropriate facility, represent opportunities in which prehospital care providers can make significant impact and save many lives.

8. Provide Basic Shock Therapy, Including Appropriately Splinting Musculoskeletal Injuries and Restoring and Maintaining Normal Body Temperature.

At the end of the primary survey, the patient's body is exposed so that the prehospital care provider can quickly scan for additional life-threatening injuries. Once this is completed, the patient should be covered again because hypothermia can be fatal to a critically injured trauma patient. The patient in shock is already handicapped by a marked decrease in energy production resulting from widespread inadequate tissue perfusion. Severe hypothermia can ensue if the patient's body temperature is not maintained. Hypothermia drastically impairs the ability of the body's blood clotting system to achieve hemostasis. Blood coagulates (clots) as the result of a complex series of enzymatic reactions leading to the formation of a fibrin matrix that traps RBCs and stems bleeding. These enzymes function in a very narrow temperature range. A drop in body temperature below 95° F (35° C) may significantly contribute to the development of a *coagulopathy* (decreased ability for blood clotting to occur). Therefore, it is important to maintain and restore body heat through the use of blankets and a warmed environment inside the ambulance.

When fracture of a long bone occurs, surrounding muscle and connective tissue are often torn. This tissue damage, along with bleeding from the ends of the broken bones, can result in significant internal hemorrhage. This blood loss can range from about 500 ml from a humerus fracture up to 1 to 2 liters from a single femur fracture. Rough handling of a fractured extremity can worsen the tissue damage and aggravate bleeding. Splinting assists in reducing the loss of additional blood into surrounding tissues, helping to preserve circulating RBCs for oxygen transport. For this reason, as well as for pain management, fractured extremities are splinted.

With a critically injured trauma patient, there is no time to splint each individual fracture. Instead, immobilizing the patient to a long backboard will splint virtually all fractures in an anatomic position and diminish internal hemorrhage. The one possible exception to this is a midshaft fracture of the femur. Because of the spasm of the very strong muscles in the thigh, the muscles contract, causing the bone ends to override one another, thereby damaging additional tissue. These types of fractures are best managed by use of a traction splint if time allows its application during transport. For the vast majority of trauma calls, when no life-threatening conditions are identified in the primary survey, each suspected extremity injury can be appropriately splinted. The pneumatic antishock garment (PASG), if available, can be used to splint and compress a suspected pelvic fracture when decompensated shock is present.

9. Maintain Manual Spinal Stabilization Until the Patient is Immobilized on a Long Backboard.

When contact with a trauma patient is made, manual stabilization of the cervical spine should be provided and maintained until the patient is either (a) immobilized on a long backboard or (b) deemed not to meet indications for spinal immobilization (Figure 17-5). Satisfactory spinal immobilization involves immobilization from the head to the pelvis. Immobilization

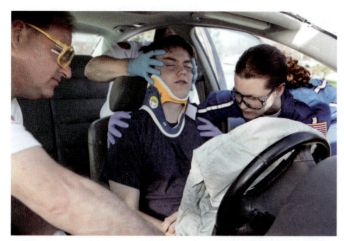

FIGURE 17-5 Maintain manual spinal immobilization until the patient is immobilized on a long backboard.

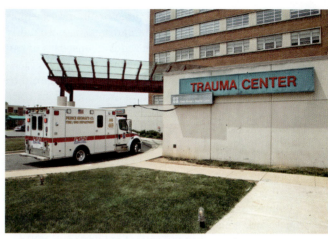

FIGURE 17-6 For critically injured trauma patients, initiate transport to the closest appropriate facility within 10 minutes of arrival on scene.

should not interfere with the patient's ability to open the mouth and should not impair ventilatory function.

For the victim of penetrating trauma, spinal immobilization is performed if the patient has spine-related neurologic complaints or if a motor or sensory deficit is noted on physical examination. In a patient with blunt trauma, spinal immobilization is indicated if the patient has an altered level of consciousness (GCS score <15) or a neurologic complaint, or if spinal tenderness, an anatomic abnormality, or a motor or sensory deficit is identified on physical examination. If the patient has sustained a mechanism of injury that causes concern, spinal immobilization is indicated if the patient has evidence of alcohol or drug intoxication, a significant distracting injury, or an inability to communicate because of an age or language barrier (see Indications for Spinal Immobilization Algorithm, p. 257).

10. For Critically Injured Trauma Patients, Initiate Transport to the Closest Appropriate Facility within 10 Minutes of Arrival on Scene.

Numerous studies have demonstrated that delays in transporting trauma patients to appropriate receiving facilities lead to increases in mortality rates (Figure 17-6). Although prehospital care providers have become proficient at endotracheal intubation, ventilatory support, and administration of intravenous (IV) fluid therapy, most critically injured trauma patients are in hemorrhagic shock and are in need of two things that cannot be provided in the prehospital setting: blood and control of internal hemorrhage. Because human blood is a perishable product, it is impractical for administration in the field in most circumstances. Crystalloid solution temporarily restores intravascular volume but does not replace the oxygen-carrying capacity of the lost RBCs. Although some blood substitutes have shown

promising results in early clinical trials, none are yet nearing approval for use in the field setting. Similarly, control of internal hemorrhage almost always requires emergent surgical intervention best performed in an OR. Resuscitation can never be achieved in the patient with ongoing internal hemorrhage. Therefore, the goal of the prehospital care provider is to spend as little time on scene as possible.

This concern for limiting scene time should not be construed as a "scoop-and-run" mentality in which no attempts are made to address key problems before initiating transport. Instead, the PHTLS program advocates a philosophy of "limited scene intervention," focusing on a rapid assessment aimed at identifying threats to life and performing interventions that are *believed* to improve outcome. Examples include airway and ventilatory management, control of external hemorrhage, and spinal immobilization. Precious time should not be wasted on procedures that can be instituted en route to the receiving facility. Patients who are critically injured (see Figure 17-4) should be transported within 10 minutes of the arrival of EMS on the scene whenever possible—the "Platinum 10 Minutes" of the Golden Period. Reasonable exceptions to the Platinum 10 Minutes include situations that require extensive extrication or time needed to secure an unsafe scene, such as law enforcement ensuring that a perpetrator is no longer present.

The *closest* hospital may not be the *most appropriate* receiving facility for many trauma patients. Those patients who meet certain physiologic, anatomic, or mechanism of injury criteria benefit from being taken to a trauma center—a facility that has special expertise and resources for managing trauma. Ideally, patients who meet physiologic, anatomic, or mechanism of injury criteria, and those with special circumstances, should be transported directly to a trauma center if one is within a reasonable distance (i.e., 30 minutes driving time). Air medical helicopters can also be utilized to transport patients from the scene directly to trauma centers, provided the delay in transport related to awaiting arrival of the helicopter does not exceed the time of ground transport to the closest hospital when a trauma center is not readily available. Thus, each community, through a consensus of surgeons, emergency physicians, and prehospital care providers, must decide where these types of trauma patients should be transported. These decisions should be incorporated into protocols that designate the best destination facility—the closest *appropriate* facility. In some situations, it is appropriate to bypass nontrauma centers to reach a trauma center. Even if this causes a moderate increase in the transport time, the overall time to definitive care will be shorter. Ideally, in the urban setting, a critically injured patient arrives at a trauma center within 25 to 30 minutes of being injured. The hospital also must work equally efficiently to continue resuscitation and, if necessary, transport the patient quickly to the OR (all within the Golden Period) to control hemorrhage.

11. Initiate Warmed Intravenous Fluid Replacement En Route to the Receiving Facility.

Initiation of transport of a critically injured trauma patient should never be delayed simply to insert IV catheters and administer fluid therapy. Although crystalloid solutions do restore lost blood volume and improve perfusion, they do not transport oxygen. Additionally, restoring normal blood pressure may result in additional hemorrhage from clot disruption in damaged blood vessels that initially clotted off.

While en route to the receiving facility, the prehospital care provider can insert two large-bore IV catheters and start an infusion of warmed (102° F [39° C]) crystalloid solution, preferably Lactated Ringer's. Warmed solution is given to aid in the prevention of hypothermia. Volume resuscitation is individualized to the clinical situation and involves balancing the need for perfusion of vital organs with the risk of rebleeding as the blood pressure increases (see Managing Volume Resuscitation Algorithm, p. 208). For adult patients with suspected uncontrolled hemorrhage in the chest, abdomen, or retroperitoneum, IV fluid therapy is titrated to maintain a mean arterial pressure of 60 to 65 mm Hg (SBP of 80 to 90 mm Hg) unless a CNS injury (TBI or spinal cord injury) is suspected, in which case a target systolic blood pressure of at least 90 mm Hg is appropriate. If hemorrhage has been controlled (i.e., application of a tourniquet to an amputated extremity), warmed IV fluid is provided in order to return vitals to normal levels unless the patient develops evidence of recurrent Class III or IV shock, in which case fluid is titrated to a MAP of 60 to 65 mm Hg. IV lines and fluid therapy may be initiated during extrication or while awaiting the arrival of an air medical helicopter. These situations do not result in a delay in transport to initiate volume resuscitation. Basic life support (BLS) providers should consider a rendezvous with an advanced life support (ALS) service (by air or ground units) when faced with prolonged transport time.

12. Ascertain the Patient's Medical History and Perform a Secondary Survey when Life-Threatening Problems Have Been Satisfactorily Managed or Have Been Ruled Out.

If life-threatening conditions are found in the primary survey, key interventions should be performed and the patient prepared for transport within the Platinum 10 Minutes. Conversely, if life-threatening conditions are not identified, a secondary survey is performed. The secondary survey is a systematic, head-to-toe physical examination that serves to identify all injuries. At this time a SAMPLE history (**s**ymptoms, **a**llergies, **m**edications, **p**ast medical history, **l**ast meal, **e**vents preceding the injury) is also obtained. For critically injured trauma patients, a secondary survey is performed only if time permits and once life-threatening conditions have been appropriately managed. In some situations in which the patient is located close to an appropriate receiving facility, a secondary survey may never be completed. This approach ensures that the prehospital care provider's attention is focused on the most serious problems—those that may result in death if not properly managed—and not on lower-priority injuries. The patient should be reassessed frequently because patients who initially present without life-threatening injuries may subsequently develop them.

13. Provide Thorough and Accurate Communication Regarding the Patient and the Circumstances of the Injury to the Receiving Facility.

Communication about a trauma patient involves three components: 1) pre-arrival warning; 2) verbal report upon arrival; and 3) written documentation of the encounter in the patient care report (PCR). Care of the trauma patient depends upon a team effort. The response to a critical patient begins with the prehospital provider and continues in the hospital. Thus, providing information from the prehospital setting to the receiving hospital allows for notification and mobilization of appropriate hospital resources to assure an optimal reception of the patient in the receiving institution. Then, upon arrival at the receiving facility, ideally a trauma center for the most critically injured, the prehospital care provider relates a verbal report to those who are assuming the care of the trauma patient. This report should be succinct and accurate and should serve to inform receiving personnel of the patient's presenting condition, kinematics of the injury, assessment findings, interventions, and response to interventions. Because of their ability to interview family members and bystanders and because a patient's mental status may deteriorate during transport, prehospital care providers may have key information essential to assessment and management of the patient that the in-hospital personnel may not be able to ascertain. Direct communication from provider to provider during patient hand-off ensures continuity of care.

Upon completion of patient care duties, the prehospital care provider carefully and accurately completes a patient care report (PCR). Like other medical records, this document serves as an organized record of the encounter with this patient. A PCR includes all important information from the patient and family or bystanders, as well as findings identified in the physical examination. Additionally, interventions performed are listed as well as any changes in the patient's condition noted during ongoing assessment. Although several different options exist for documentation, this record should "paint a picture" to the reader of the patient's appearance and provide chronology of interventions. PCRs should be accurate because they are a medicolegal document and they provide crucial information that is included in hospital trauma registries and may be utilized for research.

14. Above All, Do No Further Harm.

The medical principle that states "Above all, do no further harm" dates back to the ancient Greek physician Hippocrates. Applied to the prehospital care of the trauma patient, this principle can take many forms: developing a backup plan for airway management before initiating rapid sequence intubation, protecting a patient from flying debris during extrication from a damaged vehicle, or controlling significant external hemorrhage before initiating volume resuscitation. Recent experience has shown that prehospital care providers can safely perform many of the lifesaving skills that can be delivered in a trauma center. However, the issue in the prehospital setting is not, "What *can* providers do for critically injured trauma patients?" but rather, "What *should* providers do for critically injured trauma patients?"

When caring for a critically injured patient, prehospital care providers need to ask themselves if their actions at the scene and during transport will reasonably benefit the patient. If the answer to this question is either "no" or "uncertain," those actions should be withheld and emphasis placed on transporting the trauma patient to the closest appropriate facility. Interventions should be limited to those that prevent or treat physiologic deterioration. Trauma care must follow a given set of priorities that establish an efficient and effective plan of action, based on available time frames and any dangers present at the scene, if the patient is to survive (Figure 17-7). Appropriate intervention and stabilization should be integrated and coordinated between the field, the ED, and the OR. It is essential that every provider at every level of care and at every stage of treatment be in harmony with the rest of the team.

Another important component to the principle of "above all, do no further harm" relates to the issue of "secondary injury." It has become clear that injury occurs, not only from the initial traumatic event, but also from the physiologic consequences that result from the direct trauma. Specifically, hypoxia, hypotension, and hypothermia all produce addi-

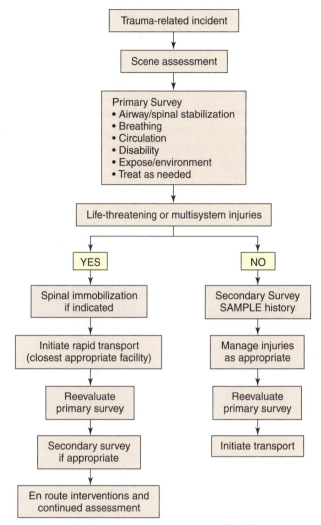

FIGURE 17-7 Trauma response algorithm.

tional injury, over and above the primary insult. Failure to recognize that these problems are present, allowing them to develop during the course of treatment, or failure to correct them in a timely fashion, offers an opportunity for added complications and greater morbidity and mortality.

In discussing the issue of "do no further harm," the concept of "financial" harm should be considered in addition to the common thought of "physical" harm. Specifically, on a regular basis, manufacturers introduce new medications and devices designed to replace or improve existing modalities of treatment. It is important to consider a number of issues prior to implementing new treatments including:

- What is the medical evidence supporting the efficacy of the new treatment?
- Is the new intervention as good as or better than existing interventions?
- How does the cost of providing the new intervention compare to the existing intervention?

As a general principle, there should be convincing medical evidence that demonstrates that a new intervention is at least as good as, and preferably better than, existing treatments before it is formally accepted and implemented. As the cost of a new intervention often exceeds that of an existing intervention, the absence of evidence indicating superiority of the new intervention leads to added charges to the patient resulting in "financial" harm.

As discussed in Chapter 1, critically injured trauma patients arriving at a trauma center can have a worse outcome when transported by EMS rather than private vehicle. A significant factor that probably accounts for the increased mortality rate is the actions of well-intentioned prehospital care providers who fail to understand that trauma is a *surgical* disease; most critically injured patients require immediate surgery to save their lives. Anything that delays surgical intervention translates into more hemorrhage, more shock, and ultimately death.

Even with the best-planned and executed resuscitation, not all trauma patients can be saved. However, with attention focused on the reasons for early traumatic death, a much larger percentage of patients may survive, with a lower residual morbidity rate than would otherwise result without the benefit of correct and expedient field management. *The fundamental principles taught in PHTLS—rapid assessment, key field interventions, and rapid transport to the closest appropriate facility—have been shown to improve outcomes in critically injured trauma patients.*

SUMMARY

The following are the Golden Principles of Prehospital Trauma Care:

1. Ensure the safety of the prehospital care providers and the patient.
2. Assess the scene situation to determine the need for additional resources.
3. Recognize the kinematics that produced the injuries.
4. Use the primary survey approach to identify life-threatening conditions.
5. Provide appropriate airway management while maintaining cervical spine stabilization.
6. Support ventilation and deliver oxygen to maintain an SpO_2 greater than 95%.
7. Control any significant external hemorrhage.
8. Provide basic shock therapy, including restoring and maintaining normal body temperature and appropriately splinting musculoskeletal injuries.
9. Maintain manual spinal stabilization until the patient is immobilized on a long backboard.
10. For critically injured trauma patients, initiate transport to the closest appropriate facility within 10 minutes of arrival on scene.
11. Initiate warmed intravenous fluid replacement en route to the receiving facility.
12. Ascertain the patient's medical history and perform a secondary survey when life-threatening conditions have been satisfactorily managed or have been ruled out.
13. Provide thorough and accurate communication regarding the patient and the circumstances of the injury to the receiving facility.
14. Above all, **do no further harm.**

References

1. Lerner EB, Moscati RM. The Golden Hour: Scientific fact of medical "urban legend?" *Acad Emerg Med* 8:758, 2001.
2. Tsybuliak GN, Pavlenko EP. Cause of death in the early post-traumatic period. *Vestn Khir Im I I Grek* 114(5):75, 1975.
3. Stewart RM, Myers JG, Dent DL, et al. 753 Consecutive deaths in a Level 1 trauma center: The argument for injury prevention. *J Trauma* 54:66, 2003.
4. 2005 International Consensus on Cardiopulmonary Resuscitation (CPR) and Emergency Cardiovascular Care (ECC) Science with Treatment Recommendations. Part 10. First aid. *Circulation* 112(suppl I):111–115, 2005.

Disaster Management

CHAPTER OBJECTIVES

At the completion of this chapter, the reader will be able to do the following:

✓ Describe the components of the disaster cycle.

✓ Discuss common pitfalls encountered during disaster response.

✓ Understand and discuss the components that comprise the medical response to a disaster.

✓ Recognize how disaster response may affect the psychological well-being of prehospital care providers.

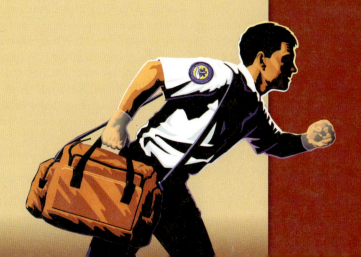

SCENARIO

You are dispatched to a report of an explosion at an apartment building. The dispatcher says that the local gas company was called for an odor of gas leaking at an apartment, but before anyone arrived, the explosion occurred. The force of the explosion was enormous. It heavily damaged the apartment building and left an enormous crater on one side with partial collapse of the structure. The blast was felt for several blocks around the area.

What safety and security concerns would first responders encounter? What triage system should be utilized? Who should be selected as incident commander? What level of personal protection should first responders utilize? What are important features of the casualty collection station?

Unlike the trauma patient who has a finite period of time for presentation, treatment, and recovery, the response to and recovery from a disaster are time consuming, encompass multiple agencies, and include not only medical and psychosocial issues, but also the rebuilding of public health, physical safety, and sociological resources and infrastructures.

The World Health Organization (WHO) has defined a disaster as a sudden ecologic phenomenon of sufficient magnitude to require external assistance. This broad definition does not provide specific reference to the medical response but is inclusive of the overall community response and sociopolitical response to any disaster of significant magnitude.

From a medical perspective, the definition can be more focused. A disaster is defined when the number of patients presenting for medical assistance within a given time is such that the medical providers cannot provide care for them with the usual resources at hand and require additional, and sometimes external, assistance.[1] This is commonly referred to as a "mass-casualty incident" or MCI. The acronym "MCI" has also been used to refer to "multiple-casualty incidents," which are events that involve more than one casualty, but which can be handled with the usual resources available to respond. In this text, MCI will be used to refer to mass casualty incidents that overwhelm the available resources.

In short, these definitions identify two key concepts: (1) a disaster is independent of a specific number of victims; and (2) the impact exceeds the available resources of the medical response. Simply stated, all mass casualty incidents are disasters, but not all disasters are mass casualty incidents.

Disasters are often thought to follow no rules because no one can predict the time, location, or complexity of the next disaster. Traditionally, medical providers have thought that all disasters are different, especially those involving terrorism. However, all disasters, regardless of etiology, have similar medical and public health consequences. Disasters differ in the degree to which these consequences occur and the degree to which they disrupt the medical and public health infrastructure of the disaster scene.

The key principle of disaster medical care is to do the greatest good for the greatest number of patients with the resources available, whereas the objective of "conventional" non-disaster-related medical care is to do the greatest good for the individual patient.

Natural disasters, man-made disasters, and terrorism encompass the spectrum of possible disaster threats. Weapons of mass destruction (WMD), creating huge numbers of casualties and "contaminated environments," may be the greatest challenge of all (see Chapter 19).

A consistent approach to disasters, based on an understanding of their common features and the response expertise required to deal with the incident, is becoming the accepted practice throughout the world. This strategy forms the framework for *mass-casualty incident* (MCI) *response.* The primary objective of the MCI response is to reduce the morbidity (injury, disease) and mortality (death) caused by the disaster. All medical responders need to incorporate the key principles of the MCI response in their training, given the complexity of current disasters (Figure 18-1).

The Disaster Cycle

Noji[1] and others have defined a theoretic framework by which the sequence of events in a disaster can be broken down and analyzed. This conceptual description not only provides an overview of the natural history of an event but also provides the basis for the development of the response process.[2,3] Five phases have been identified, as follows:

1. The *quiescence level,* or the interdisaster period, represents the time during which risk assessment and mitigation activities should be undertaken and when plans for the response to likely events are developed, tested, and implemented.
2. The next phase is the *prodrome phase,* or warning phase. At this point, a specific event has been identified as inevitably going to occur. This could reflect a natural weather condition (e.g., impending landfall of a hurricane) or the active unfolding of a hostile and potentially violent situation. During this period, specific steps may be taken to

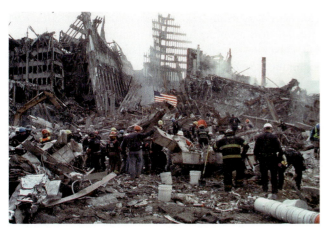

FIGURE 18-1 Mass-casualty management at Ground Zero, World Trade Center, New York, 2001.

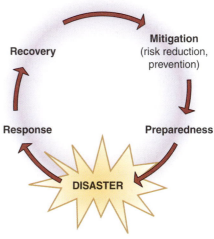

FIGURE 18-2 The life cycle of a disaster. The quiescence phase is represented by the mitigation and preparedness arrows. The warning phase comes just before the impact of the event. This is followed by the response and recovery periods.

mitigate the effects of the ensuing events. These defensive maneuvers may include such actions as fortifying physical structures, initiating evacuation plans, and mobilizing public health resources to mount a postevent response.

3. The third phase is the *impact phase,* or the occurrence of the actual event. During this period, there is often little that can be done to alter the actual impact or outcome of what is occurring.

4. The fourth phase is the *rescue phase,* which is the time period immediately following the impact during which response occurs and appropriate management and intervention can save lives. The skills of the first responders, rescue teams, and medical support services will be brought to bear to maximize survival from the event.

5. The fifth phase is the *recovery phase,* or reconstruction phase, which addresses the community's resources to endure and emerge from the effects of the disaster through the coordinated efforts of the medical, public health, and community infrastructure (physical and political). This period is by far the longest, lasting months, and perhaps years, before a community fully recovers.

Understanding the disaster cycle (Figure 18-2) allows prehospital care providers to evaluate the preparations that have been made in anticipation of the likely hazards and events that may be encountered in their community. After an incident has occurred, it allows for critical evaluation of the after-action report and assessment of the provider's individual area of responsibility and response, as well as the response of others, to determine the efficiency and efficacy of the response process and identify areas for future improvement. These concepts apply to all disasters, regardless of size.

The duration of each component of the disaster life cycle will vary depending upon the frequency with which incidents occur in a given community, the nature of the incident, and the degree to which the community is prepared. For example, the quiescent period in some locations can be extremely long (measured in years), whereas in other communities it may be measured in months. A specific example is that of hurricanes. The southeastern states of the United States prepare for hurricanes annually with a quiescent period between events of approximately 6–8 months. In contrast, although the New England states have been the victims of hurricanes, it is a rare event with a quiescent period of years in between hurricane strikes. The response and recovery phases from something like a refinery explosion will be measured in hours or at most a few days. The response and recovery from a major flood may take weeks to months or longer.

Comprehensive Emergency Management

Knowledge of the life cycle or natural history of disasters can be used to implement the steps needed to manage an incident. This is accomplished using a process referred to as "comprehensive emergency management." Comprehensive emergency management consists of four components: mitigation, preparation, response, and recovery.

Mitigation: This component of emergency management generally occurs during the "quiescence" phase. Potential hazards or likely etiologies of mass casualty incidents are identified and assessed. Steps are then taken to prevent these hazards from causing an incident or to minimize their effect should something untoward occur.

Preparedness: This step of comprehensive emergency management involves identification, in advance of the incident, of the specific supplies, equipment, and personnel that would be needed as well as the specific action plan that would be taken if an incident occurred.

Response: This phase involves the activation and deployment of the various resources identified in the Preparedness phase in order to manage an incident that has now occurred.

Recovery: This component of emergency management addresses the actions necessary to return the community back to its pre-incident status.

While this process is typically applied to the management of a disaster, these same steps may also be utilized for the emergency preparedness of each responder.

Responder Personal Preparedness

Just as it is vital that each community and each agency undertake a comprehensive planning process in order to be prepared to meet the challenges of dealing with a disaster, so too is it important that each responder be ready to face the many issues that a disaster may present.

The prehospital provider must have a complete understanding of the many potential hazards that may accompany a disaster response in advance of the actual incident and be prepared to take the necessary steps to protect himself or herself from these dangers. Gaps in knowledge about such issues as building collapse, hazardous materials and situations, weapons of mass destruction and their effects and treatment, and overall incident management should be identified in advance and addressed.

Many disasters will go on for a long period of time and the responder must have discussed their role, responsibilities, and potentially prolonged absence with their family. This includes preparing the family, in advance, for what they should do and where they should go during such an event to assure their safety as well. In similar fashion to the procurement of supplies and equipment that occurs for the medical response, the provider should assure that adequate supplies are available at home to meet family needs (Figure 18-3, 18-4, and 18-5).

All of these actions will help reassure the provider that their family is safely dealing with their needs during the incident, provide comfort to the family knowing that the provider is as prepared as possible for his or her role in disaster response, and allow the provider to continue to provide care to those requiring medical assistance.

Mass-Casualty Incident Management

Mass-casualty incidents (MCIs) are events that cause casualties in numbers large enough to overwhelm the available medical and public health services of the affected community. The severity and diversity of injuries and illness, in addition to the number of victims, will be major factors in determining whether an MCI requires resources and assistance from outside the impacted community.

Today's complex disasters, especially those involving terrorism and weapons of mass destruction (chemical, biological, or nuclear), may result in an austere environment. An *austere environment* is a setting in which resources, supplies, equipment, personnel, transportation, and other aspects of the physical, political, social, and economic environments are limited. As a result of these limitations, severe constraints on the availability and adequacy of immediate care for the population in need will be imposed. Prehospital providers must anticipate the reality that, in such situations, the level of care provided to the sick and injured will be altered and interventions normally offered to all patients may be provided only to those individuals who meet specific criteria and who are likely to survive.[4]

Medical concerns related to MCIs include the following four elements:

- Search and rescue—This involves the process of systematically looking for those individuals who have been impacted by an event and rescuing them from the hazardous situation. This often requires the use of specially trained teams, particularly when extrication issues are involved.
- Triage and initial stabilization—This is the process of systematically evaluating and categorizing each victim as to the seriousness of their injury or illness and providing initial medical care to address immediate life- or limb-threatening problems.
- Definitive medical care—This is the provision of the specific care needed to treat the patient's specific injuries. This care will usually be provided at hospitals; however, alternate care facilities may be used in major events when hospitals are overwhelmed with casualties or when hospitals have been directly impacted and damaged by the incident.
- Evacuation—This is the process of transporting disaster victims and injured patients away from the disaster site, either to a safe location or to a definitive care facility.

Public health concerns related to MCIs include the following:

- Water (ensuring a safe supply of potable water)
- Food (ideally nonperishable and needing no refrigeration or cooking)
- Shelter (a place for cover, protection, refuge)
- Sanitation (protection from contact with human and animal feces, solid waste, and wastewater)
- Security and safety
- Transportation
- Communication (includes information about communicable diseases)
- Endemic and epidemic diseases (endemic diseases are ones that are always present in a given area or population but which usually occur with low frequency, whereas an epidemic disease is one that develops and spreads rapidly to the population at risk)

FIGURE 18-3   Emergency Supply List

All Americans should have some basic supplies on hand in order to survive for at least three days if an emergency occurs. Following is a listing of some basic items that every emergency supply kit should include. However, it is important that individuals review this list and consider where they live and the unique needs of their family in order to create an emergency supply kit that will meet these needs. Individuals should also consider having at least two emergency supply kits, one full kit at home and smaller portable kits in their workplace, vehicle or other places they spend time.

- Water. Three gallons for each person who would use the kit and an additional four gallons per person or pet for use if you are confined to your home.
- Food. A three-day supply in the kit and at least an additional four-day supply per person or pet for use at home. (*You may want to consider stocking a two-week supply of food and water in your home. See Figure 18-4*)
- Battery-powered or hand-crank radio and a NOAA Weather Radio with tone alert and extra batteries for both.
- Flashlight and extra batteries.
- First aid kit (see Figure 18-5).
- Whistle to signal for help.
- Dust mask, to help filter contaminated air and plastic sheeting and duct tape to shelter-in-place.
- Moist towelettes, garbage bags and plastic ties for personal sanitation.
- Wrench or pliers to turn off utilities.
- Can opener for food (if kit contains canned food).
- Local maps.

   Additional items to consider adding to an emergency supply kit:

- **Items for infants**—including formula, diapers, bottles, pacifiers, powdered milk, and medications not requiring refrigeration.
- **Items for seniors, disabled persons or anyone with serious allergies**—including special foods, denture items, extra eyeglasses, hearing aid batteries, prescription and nonprescription medications that are regularly used, inhalers and other essential equipment.
- Prescription medications and glasses.
- Pet food and extra water for your pet.
- Important family documents such as copies of insurance policies, identification, and bank account records in a waterproof, portable container.
- Cash or traveler's checks and change.
- Emergency reference material such as a first aid book or information from www.ready.gov.
- Sleeping bag or warm blanket for each person. Consider additional bedding if you live in a cold-weather climate.
- Complete change of clothing including a long sleeved shirt, long pants and sturdy shoes. Consider additional clothing if you live in a cold-weather climate.

- Household chlorine bleach and medicine dropper. When diluted nine-parts water to one-part bleach, bleach can be used as a disinfectant. In an emergency, you can use it to treat water by using 16 drops of regular household liquid bleach per gallon of water. Do not use scented, color safe, or bleaches with added cleaners.
- Fire Extinguisher.
- Matches in a waterproof container.
- Feminine supplies and personal hygiene items.
- Mess kits, paper cups, plates and plastic utensils, paper towels.
- Paper and pencil.
- Entertainment—including games and books, favorite dolls, and stuffed animals for small children.
- Kitchen accessories—a manual can opener; mess kits or disposable cups, plates and utensils; utility knife; sugar and salt; aluminum foil and plastic wrap; re-sealable plastic bags.
- Sanitation and hygiene items—shampoo, deodorant, toothpaste, toothbrushes, comb and brush, lip balm, sunscreen, contact lenses and supplies, any medications regularly used, toilet paper, towelettes, soap, hand sanitizer, liquid detergent, feminine supplies, plastic garbage bags (heavy-duty) and ties (for personal sanitation uses), medium-sized plastic bucket with tight lid, disinfectant, household chlorine bleach.
- Other essential items—paper, pencil, needles, thread, small A-B-C-type fire extinguisher, medicine dropper, whistle, emergency preparedness manual.
- A map of the area marked with places you could go and their telephone numbers.
- An extra set of keys and IDs—including keys for cars and any properties owned and copies of driver's licenses, passports, and work identification badges.
- Cash and coins and copies of credit cards.
- Copies of medical prescriptions.
- A small tent, compass, and shovel.

   Pack the items in easy-to-carry containers, label the containers clearly, and store them where they would be easily accessible. Duffle bags, backpacks, and covered trash receptacles are good candidates for containers. In a disaster situation, you may need access to your disaster supplies kit quickly—whether you are sheltering at home or evacuating. Following a disaster, having the right supplies can help your household endure home confinement or evacuation.

   Make sure the needs of everyone who would use the kit are covered, including infants, seniors and pets. It is a good idea to involve whoever is going to use the kit, including children, in assembling it.

(Adapted from FEMA: Ready America (www.ready.gov) and the Centers for Disease Control and Prevention: Emergency Preparedness and Response (www.bt.cdc.gov/planning/).)

FIGURE 18-4 Food Kit

- Store *at least* a three-day supply of nonperishable food.
- Select foods that require no refrigeration, preparation or cooking and little or no water.
- Pack a manual can opener and eating utensils.
- Avoid salty foods, as they will make you thirsty.
- Choose foods your family will eat.
  - Ready-to-eat canned meats, fruits and vegetables
  - Protein or fruit bars
  - Dry cereal or granola
  - Peanut butter
  - Dried fruit
  - Nuts
  - Crackers
  - Canned juices
  - Nonperishable pasteurized milk
  - High energy foods
  - Vitamins
  - Food for infants
  - Comfort/stress foods

(Adapted from FEMA: Ready America (www.ready.gov) and the Centers for Disease Control and Prevention: Emergency Preparedness and Response (www.bt.cdc.gov/planning/).)

FIGURE 18-5 First Aid Kit

In any emergency a family member or you yourself may be cut, burned or suffer other injuries.
   Things you should have:

- Two pairs of Latex, or other sterile gloves (if you are allergic to Latex).
- Sterile dressings to stop bleeding.
- Cleansing agent/soap and antibiotic towelettes to disinfect.
- Antibiotic ointment to prevent infection.
- Burn ointment to prevent infection.
- Adhesive bandages in a variety of sizes.
- Eye wash solution to flush the eyes or as general decontaminant.
- Thermometer.
- Prescription medications you take every day such as insulin, heart medicine and asthma inhalers. You should periodically rotate medicines to account for expiration dates.
- Prescribed medical supplies such as glucose and blood pressure monitoring equipment and supplies.

Things it may be good to have:

- Cell phone
- Scissors
- Tweezers
- Tube of petroleum jelly or other lubricant

Nonprescription drugs:

- Aspirin or non-aspirin pain reliever
- Anti-diarrhea medication
- Antacid (for upset stomach)
- Laxative

(Adapted from FEMA: Ready America (www.ready.gov) and the Centers for Disease Control and Prevention: Emergency Preparedness and Response (www.bt.cdc.gov/planning/).)

Both medical and public health disaster-response activities are coordinated through one organizational structure: the incident command system.

Incident Command System

Many different organizations participate in the response to a disaster. The incident command system (ICS) was created to allow different types of agencies and multiple jurisdictions of similar agencies (fire, police, emergency medical services [EMS]) to work together effectively, using a common organizational structure and language in response to a disaster (Figure 18–6). (See Chapter 5.)

The incident command system recognizes that, regardless of the specific nature of the incident (police, fire, or medical), there are a number of functions that must always happen. The ICS is organized around these necessary functions. The components of the ICS are:

- Command
- Planning
- Logistics
- Operations
- Finance

These functions apply to all incidents and are now used in the medical setting to organize the response to a disaster.

From a medical perspective, several important ICS principles will help during an MCI response:

1. ICS must be started early, preferably upon arrival to the scene, before the incident management gets out of control.
2. Medical and public health responders, often used to working independently, need to implement the ICS management structure and coordinate their response assets to better respond to an MCI.
3. Using ICS will allow for the integration of the medical response into the overall response to the incident.

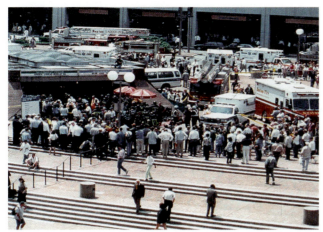

FIGURE 18-6 Incident command system (ICS) allows integration of fire, police, and EMS assets at a disaster scene.

Detailed information and training about the Incident Command System is available on the FEMA website, http://training.fema.gov/EMIWeb/IS/ICSResource/index.htm.

FIGURE 18-7 The Basic Steps in Medical Response to Disasters

The basic steps in Medical Response to Disasters
1) Initial response
2) Notification and activation of EMS
3) EMS response to the scene
4) Assess the situation
   a) Cause
   b) Number of casualties
   c) Additional resources
      i) Medical
      ii) Other
   d) Communicate the situation and needs
5) Activation of the medical community
   a) Notify receiving facilities
6) Search and rescue
7) Triage (treat airway and hemorrhage life-threats)
8) Casualty collection
9) Treatment
10) Transport
11) Re-triage

Medical Response to Disasters

The effective response to an MCI depends upon the initiation of a series of actions which, when combined, will help to minimize the mortality and morbidity of victims of the event. Although these actions will be discussed sequentially in this chapter, it is important to remember that during an actual disaster many of these will be occurring simultaneously (Figure 18-7).

Initial Response

The first step is notification and activation of the EMS response system. This is usually performed by witnesses to the event who then call the local emergency dispatch center seeking response by appropriate police, fire, and emergency medical agencies.

The first medical responders to arrive at the scene have a number of important functions to fulfill that will set the stage for the entire medical response to the incident. Most importantly, these actions do *not* include finding and treating the most critically injured patients, as would be the case in most non-MCI situations. This can be paraphrased as "Don't just do something, stand there." Before beginning the process of providing medical assistance, the first medical personnel should take the time to perform an overall scene assessment. The goals of this assessment are to evaluate any potential hazards, estimate the potential number of casual-

ties, determine what additional medical resources will be needed at the scene, and evaluate whether any specialized equipment or personnel, such as search-and-rescue teams, will be required.

Once this assessment is complete, the next step is to communicate the overall assessment to the dispatch center, where the process of acquiring and dispatching the needed resources can be performed. After this, the medical personnel should identify appropriate locations to perform triage, to collect casualties, and to stage incoming ambulances, personnel, and supplies so as not to impede rapid ingress and egress when necessary or expose responding assets to potential hazards from the event.

In addition to providing for the medical response to the disaster scene, it is essential that the responding EMS agency notify the likely receiving hospitals in the community so that they can activate their disaster plans to prepare to receive casualties. EMS agencies must remember that the field component of the disaster response is the first link in the overall chain of medical care for a disaster patient and that they are responsible for notifying and activating the other components of the health care system.

Search and Rescue

At this point, the on-scene process of initiating patient care can begin. Generally, this will start with a search-and-rescue effort to identify and evacuate casualties from the impacted site to a safer location. The local population near a disaster site as well as survivors themselves, if they are able, are often the immediate search-and-rescue resource and may have already begun to search for victims.[5] Experience has demonstrated that the local community will respond to a disaster site and begin the process of aiding victims. In addition, many countries and communities have developed formal, specialized search-and-rescue teams as an integral part of their national and local disaster-response plans. Members of these teams receive specialized training in "confined-space environments" and are activated as needed for a particular event. These search-and-rescue units generally include the following:

- A cadre of medical specialists
- Technical specialists knowledgeable in hazardous materials, structural engineering, heavy equipment operation, and technical search-and-rescue methods (e.g., listening equipment, remote cameras)
- Trained canines and their handlers

Local construction companies may provide valuable search-and-rescue assets by providing equipment, tools, and wooden planks that can be used at the disaster site to assist in moving heavy debris.

Triage

As patients are identified and evacuated, they are brought to the triage site, where they can be assessed and a triage category assigned (Figure 18-8). The term "triage" is a French word that means "to sort." From a medical perspective, triage means sorting casualties based on the severity of their injuries. This further serves to prioritize the patient's need for medical care and transportation to the hospital.

Triage is one of the most important missions of any disaster medical response. As noted previously, the objective of conventional triage in the nondisaster setting is to do the greatest good for the individual patient. This usually means finding and treating the sickest patient. The objective of mass-casualty triage is to do the greatest good for the greatest number of people. Mass-casualty triage in the field must be overseen by a trained triage officer. A *triage officer* should have a wide breadth of clinical experience in the assessment and management of field injuries as potentially difficult decisions may have to be made about patients who will be deemed critical versus those who will be classified as mortally wounded with little chance of survival. A paramedic with significant field experience usually meets this requirement. A trained physician with experience in the field may also function in this capacity.[6,7]

A number of different methodologies exist for evaluating and assigning the triage category.[8] One common method is to evaluate the anatomic injuries and assign the priority for medical care and transport based on the severity of the injury and the likelihood of need for surgical intervention. Another method involves a rapid physiological and mental status evaluation. This triage process is referred to as the "START" triage algorithm (**s**imple **t**riage **a**nd **r**apid **t**reatment). This system evaluates the respiratory status, perfusion status, and mental status of the patient in making a prioritization for initial transfer to definitive care facilities (see Chapter 5, pages 106–107).[7,9] In addition, other triage systems include M.A.S.S. (**M**ove, **A**ssess, **S**ort, **S**end) and the Sacco Triage Method.

In an effort to provide national guidance and bring uniformity to the triage process, the Centers for Disease Control in the United States convened a multi-disciplinary group of experts to develop a consensus-based triage system, now known as SALT (see Chapter 5, page 107).[8] This triage system involves **s**orting the patient based upon their ability to move, **a**ssessing the patient for the need for **l**ife-saving interventions, performing those interventions, and **t**reatment and **t**ransport.

Regardless of the exact triage method used, all these systems ultimately classify patients into one of (usually) four injury-severity categories. Highest priority patients are those who are identified as having critical, but likely survivable, injuries and are usually categorized as *immediate* and color-coded *red*. Patients with moderate injuries who can potentially tolerate a short delay in care are categorized as *delayed* patients and color-coded *yellow*. Patients with relatively minor injuries, often referred to as the "walking wounded," are classified as *minimal* victims and color-coded *green*. Patients who have expired on the scene or whose injuries are so severe that death is imminent or is likely are categorized as "dead" or "expectant," respectively, and color-coded *black*. Of note, some triage systems, particularly SALT, specifically separate those patients classified as mortally wounded from those who are dead and color code the expectant as *gray*. All these color codes refer to the use of "disaster tags," which are used at disaster scenes and attached to patients once they have been triaged. The "color code" provides an immediate visual reference to their triage category. Some triage systems also use a classification system in which critical, delayed, minimal, and the dead or expectant patients are referred to as Class I, Class II, Class III, and Class IV, respectively.

It is important that all triage personnel keep in mind that they must avoid the temptation to stop performing triage in

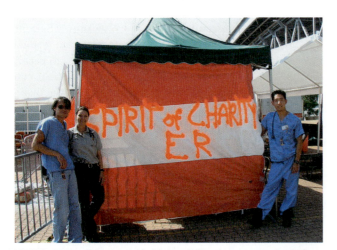

FIGURE 18-8 Triage and initial stabilization at a makeshift medical treatment facility, Hurricane Katrina, Louisiana, 2005.

favor of treating a critically injured patient that they encounter. As mentioned earlier, the primary principle involved in dealing with an MCI is to do the most good for the most people. During this initial triage phase, medical interventions are limited to those actions that are performed easily and rapidly and that are not labor intensive. Generally, this means performing only procedures such as manual airway opening and external hemorrhage control. Interventions such as bag-mask ventilation and closed chest compression involve the use of significant personnel and are not performed.

Once patients have been triaged, they are collected together at casualty collection points according to their triage priority. Specifically, all the "red" category or immediate patients are grouped, as are the delayed ("yellow") and minimal ("green") patients. Casualty collection sites should be located close enough to the disaster site to easily carry the victim to and offer rapid treatment, but far enough away from the impact site to be safe. Important features include the following:

- Proximity to the disaster site
- Safety from hazards and uphill and upwind from contaminated environments
- Protection from climatic conditions (when possible)
- Easy visibility for disaster victims and assigned personnel
- Convenient exit routes for air and land evacuation

As additional medical staff and resources arrive and become available on-scene, medical care and interventions are provided at the casualty collection points according to the triage priority. These are appropriate locations to which physicians responding to the scene may be assigned to further evaluate and treat injured patients.

Finally, as transportation resources become available, patients are then transported for definitive care according, once again, to their triage priority (Figure 18-9). Critical patients are not held on scene for the provision of further medical care if transport is available (Figure 18-10). Needed medical interventions should be conducted during transport to the definitive care facility.

Because of visible, critical injuries, emergency personnel often have a tendency to move individual patients forward for immediate treatment and transport and to bypass the triage process. This must be avoided so that all victims can be evaluated, the most life-threatening casualties can be treated first, and the best care can be provided for the majority of victims. However, bypassing the triage process is indicated in certain situations. These conditions include (1) risk, as in bad weather; (2) potential impending darkness without the capabilities of lighting resources; (3) the continued risk of injury as a result of natural or unnatural events; (4) no triage facility or triage officer immediately available; and (5) any tactical situation in a law enforcement scenario in which the victims are rapidly moved from the impact site to the collection point for transportation.[9,10]

Lastly, triage is not a static process, meaning that once a patient is evaluated and categorized, the patient carries that

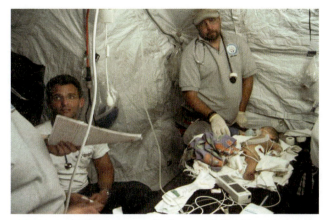

FIGURE 18-9 Definitive medical care, US field hospital, Bam, Iran earthquake, 2005.

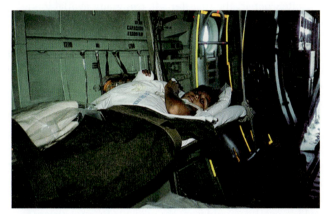

FIGURE 18-10 Interior of a military transport plane converted for medical evacuation with patient litters.

triage category for the remainder of their care. Instead, it is dynamic and ongoing. As a patient's condition changes, the triage category may change as well. For example, a patient with a major extremity wound and hemorrhage may initially be categorized as an "immediate" patient; however, after pressure is applied to the wound and the bleeding is controlled, the patient may be re-triaged as "delayed." Alternatively, a patient initially categorized as "immediate" could deteriorate and subsequently be re-triaged as "expectant."

Re-triage should occur on the scene while patients are waiting for transport resources. In addition, patients will undergo re-triage upon arrival at the receiving destination and again as they are prioritized for surgery.

Treatment

Since the number of casualties will initially exceed the available resources, treatment on the scene is generally limited to manually opening the airway, correction of tension pneumothorax, external hemorrhage control, and administration of chemical agent antidote. Only when adequate resources have arrived on scene or during transport to the hospital will additional interventions be provided.

Transport

The transport of patients from a mass-casualty incident to the receiving hospitals involves a coordinated effort using a variety of transport vehicles. Critically injured or ill patients will be taken to the hospital in ambulances or helicopters (if available and conditions permit). Those incidents that result in huge numbers of casualties, particularly casualties in the *minimal* category, may require the use of non-traditional transport vehicles such as buses and vans. It is important to remember, however, that when such alternate transport mechanisms are used, medical personnel with adequate supplies and equipment must be assigned to accompany the casualties in that vehicle.

Another important issue in effectively responding to an MCI relates to the decision-making process for patient destination once transport is initiated.[11] Recent events have demonstrated that casualties with non-life-threatening injuries will often depart the disaster site using any available means of transportation and make their own way to the hospital.[5] Often this results in large numbers of "walking wounded" arriving at the hospital closest to the disaster site. In fact, approximately 70% to 80% of casualties will get to a hospital without EMS ambulance transport.

Prehospital providers must, therefore, understand that the hospital closest to a disaster scene may be overwhelmed with casualties even before the arrival of the first transporting ambulance. Before taking a patient to the closest hospital, contact should be made to ascertain the status of the emergency department (ED) and the capability to accept and treat victims transported by ambulance. If the closest hospital is overwhelmed, the EMS system should transport patients to more distant facilities when possible. Although the transport time will be longer, the patient's care will not be complicated by the presence of numerous other casualties. Dispersal of casualties to multiple institutions will ultimately better preserve the ability of all the receiving hospitals to optimize the patient care they provide.

Even if the closest medical facility is not overwhelmed with self-transported patients, it is imperative that prehospital providers, themselves, not overwhelm the nearest hospital with patients transported by ambulance. Often, the natural desire is to transport a patient to the closest hospital so that the ambulance and its crew can quickly return to the disaster scene to pick up and transport another patient. Transferring the mass-casualty incident from the disaster site to the closest hospital will negatively impact the ability of medical facilities to provide the "most good for the most patients." However, in those communities that have limited numbers of hospitals, EMS will have no option other than to transport patients to the nearest hospital.

Medical Assistance Teams

If the disaster is of significant proportion that additional on-scene resources are needed, some hospitals have developed disaster-response teams to help augment the EMS field response and provide on-site care, thus allowing prehospital providers to be freed from the task of providing medical care at casualty collection points and, instead, perform patient transport. If outside resources are needed from the state or federal government, other medical response teams are available in many municipalities (Figure 18-11). As a result of the Metropolitan Medical Response System (MMRS) in the United States, MMRS task forces or strike teams have been created in many cities. These response assets comprise medical personnel from emergency medicine, trauma surgery, surgical subspecialties, and nursing. These teams can respond with resources that have been purchased through state and federal funds. These teams can be used to augment and backfill medical facilities or to staff mobile medical facilities that are established to provide surge capacity and medical care to victims.

On a larger-scale basis, the US government has capabilities through the National Disaster Medical System to mobilize Disaster Medical Assistance Teams (DMATs). These teams are able to provide field care as well as create mobile medical facilities, some of which have the capability to perform surgical interventions and meet the critical care needs of the victims. A request for these teams must come through the appropriate channels via the state emergency management authority and the governor's office through the federal government to the Department of Health and Human Services (DHHS), which houses the National Disaster Medical System's response program.

Threat of Terrorism and Weapons of Mass Destruction

Terrorism may present one of the most challenging MCIs for emergency responders. The spectrum of terrorist threats is limitless, ranging from suicide bombers, conventional explosives, and military weapons to weapons of mass destruction (nuclear, biologic, or chemical WMDs). Terrorist events have the greatest potential of all man-made disasters to generate large numbers of casualties and fatalities. (See

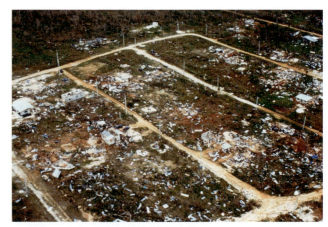

FIGURE 18-11 Aerial view of devastation caused by Super-Typhoon Pongsona, Guam, 2002.

Chapter 19: Explosions and Weapons of Mass Destruction, for detailed information about specific weapons.)

Terrorists have demonstrated their ingenuity and capacity to not be limited by conventional technology or weaponry. During the terrorist attacks on September 11, 2001, the terrorists used passenger jets full of fuel as "flying bombs," generating massive destruction of life and property.

One of the unique features of a terrorist threat, especially involving WMDs, is that psychologic casualties usually predominate. Terrorists do not need to kill a large number of people to achieve their goals; they only need to create a climate of fear and panic to overwhelm the medical infrastructure. In the March 1995 sarin attacks in Tokyo, 5000 casualties presented to hospitals. Of these, fewer than 1000 had physical effects from the sarin gas; the remaining presented with psychological stress. The anthrax incidents in the United States also dramatically increased the number of individuals presenting to EDs with nonspecific respiratory symptoms that ultimately did not result from actual anthrax infection.

Explosions and bombings continue to be the most frequent cause of mass casualties in disasters caused by terrorists. The majority of these bombings consist of relatively small explosives that produce low mortality rates. However, when strategically placed in buildings, pipelines, or moving vehicles, their impact can be much greater (Figure 18-12). The high morbidity and mortality is related not only to the intensity of the blast, but also to the subsequent structural damage that leads to collapse of the targeted buildings. A greater threat will be disasters caused by conventional explosives in combination with a chemical, biologic, or radiologic agent, such as a "dirty bomb" that combines a conventional explosive with radioactive material.

The WMDs that create "contaminated environments" may prove to be the greatest disaster challenge. Emergency responders will not be able to bring victims into hospitals because of the risk of further contaminating medical facilities. Medical responders must be prepared and equipped to perform triage, not only to determine the extent of the injuries, but also to assess the potential for contamination and need for decontamination and initial stabilization. At the same time, prehospital care providers need to take appropriate steps to protect themselves from potential contamination.

Decontamination

Decontamination is an important consideration for all disasters involving hazardous materials (hazmat) and WMDs (Figure 18-13). Terrorist events, with their larger number of patients, unknown substances, and large numbers of "worried well," significantly increase the possibility of contaminated or potentially contaminated casualties (see Chapter 19 for additional information).

Treatment Area

When responding to a disaster involving hazmat and WMDs, it is critical that the triage and treatment areas be at least 300 yards (275 meters) upwind and uphill of the contaminated area.

Psychological Response to Disasters

Psychological trauma and other adverse psychological sequelae are frequently the side effects of events such as natural disasters and unintentional disasters caused by humans.[12] In contrast, one of the objectives of terrorism is to inflict psychological pain, trauma, and disequilibrium.

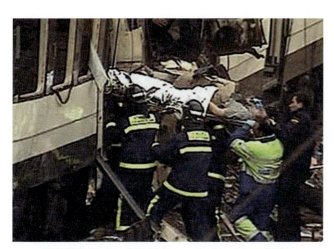

FIGURE 18-12 Madrid terrorist bombing, 2004.

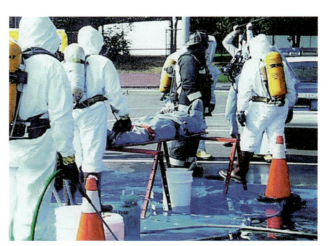

FIGURE 18-13 Decontamination of casualties in the "warm zone" by personnel in Level B personal protective equipment (PPE).

Characteristics of Disasters That Affect Mental Health

Not all disasters have the same level of psychological impact. Disaster characteristics that seem to have the most significant mental health impact include the following:

- Little or no warning
- Serious threat to personal safety
- Potential unknown health effects
- Uncertain duration of the event
- Human error or malicious intent
- Symbolism related to the terrorist target

Factors Impacting Psychological Response

Everyone who experiences a disaster, either as a victim or as a responder, is affected by it in some fashion. Fortunately, this does not mean that most individuals will develop a mental health disorder. It does mean, however, that all affected individuals will have some type of psychological or emotional response to the event.

Similarly, there are both individual and collective reactions that interact with each other as individuals and communities recover from these extraordinary events.

Factors affecting individual response to disasters include the following:

- Physical and psychological proximity to the event
- Exposure to gruesome or grotesque situations
- Diminished health status before or because of the disaster
- Magnitude of loss
- Trauma history

Factors impacting collective response to trauma are as follows:

- Degree of community disruption
- Pre-disaster family and community stability
- Community leadership
- Cultural sensitivity of recovery efforts

Psychological Sequelae of Disasters

Post-disaster psychological responses are wide ranging, from mild stress responses to full-blown *post-traumatic stress disorder* (PTSD), major depression, or acute stress disorder.[13] Although many people may exhibit signs of psychological stress, relatively few (typically 15%–25%) of those most directly impacted will subsequently develop a diagnosable mental disorder.

Interventions

A number of relatively simple actions can help individuals to minimize the psychologic effects of an event and assist them in returning to normal function. These include:

1. Return to normal activities as soon as possible.[13]
2. In persons with no diagnosed mental disorder, it is helpful to provide educational materials that help people understand what they and their families are experiencing.
3. Brief crisis counselling should be provided, followed by referral when treatment is indicated.
4. When a mental disorder is diagnosed, therapeutic interventions can be helpful, including cognitive-behavioral therapy and psychiatric medications.

Worker Stress

Disaster workers can also become secondary victims of stress and other psychological sequelae. This can adversely affect their functioning during and after an event. It can also adversely impact their personal well-being as well as their family and work relationships. Supervisory personnel and colleagues should be alert for the development or manifestations of stress and psychological distress in those individuals who were involved in the incident response.

A number of intervention strategies are often used in an effort to help prevent and manage stress after an incident. These include debriefing, defusing, and grief management sessions. Collectively, these processes have been referred to as Critical Incident Stress Management (CISM).

Signs of Stress in Workers

Some common signs of stress in workers include physiological, emotional, cognitive, and behavioral elements.

Physiological signs
- Fatigue, even after rest
- Nausea
- Fine motor tremors
- Tics
- Paresthesia
- Dizziness
- Gastrointestinal upset
- Heart palpitations
- Choking or smothering sensations

Emotional signs
- Anxiety
- Irritability
- Feeling overwhelmed
- Unrealistic anticipation of harm to self or others

Cognitive signs
- Memory loss
- Decision-making difficulties
- *Anomia* (inability to name common objects or familiar people)
- Concentration problems or distractibility
- Reduced attention span
- Calculation difficulties

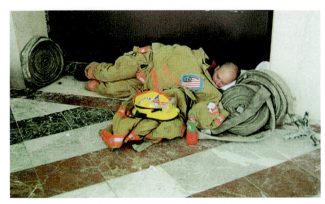

FIGURE 18-14 Fatigue contributes greatly to worker stress.

Behavioral signs
- Insomnia
- Hypervigilance
- Crying easily
- Inappropriate humor
- Ritualistic behavior

Managing Worker Stress On-Site

The following on-site interventions can assist in reducing worker stress:
- Limited exposure to traumatic stimuli
- Reasonable hours
- Adequate rest and sleep (Figure 18-14)
- Reasonable diet
- Regular exercise program
- Private time
- Talking to somebody who understands
- Monitoring signs of stress
- Identifiable endpoint for involvement

Disaster Education and Training

The development and implementation of a formal educational and training program will improve the prehospital care provider's ability to respond efficiently to an MCI. The prehospital provider may well fulfill a variety of roles in disaster and mass-casualty management, including mitigation and preparedness, search and rescue, triage, acute medical care, transport, and postevent recovery. Preparedness with regard to education and learning can be accomplished in various structured, as well as unstructured, learning environments. Each has its individual advantages and disadvantages, as measured by educational impact and comparative cost. For optimal learning from educational exercises, it is imperative that interdisciplinary training events be conducted often to include all the appropriate agencies and participants in a disaster response.

Independent learning is the foundation of disaster preparedness. A multitude of resources are available through printed literature as well as via the Internet. The Centers for Disease Control and Prevention (CDC), public health agencies, Federal Emergency Management Agency (FEMA), and the military forces all have internet-based learning opportunities and resources that are available to individuals. Courses can be completed on an independent basis on a time-flexible schedule. The limitation of this modality of learning is that it does not allow for an interactive learning experience.

Group training is directed at specific response teams with regard to disaster response. Training programs are broadly available and include understanding command structure and WMD preparedness. Numerous professional and paraprofessional organizations have developed training programs and modules specific to their scope of professional practice, including public health, emergency medicine, critical care, and surgical and medical specialties, as well as all levels of prehospital care providers.

Simulations provide a training opportunity that brings together many individuals from varied and different backgrounds who are essential to the implementation of a disaster response. As mentioned earlier, these exercises come in two specific forms: a tabletop exercise and a fully active, field-training exercise. *Tabletop exercises* are cost-effective and highly useful methods to test and evaluate a disaster response. A starting point with focused-incident goals and accomplishments and order for completion of the exercise are usually established in advance. Tabletop exercises can allow for real-time communications and interaction between multidisciplinary agencies. These activities require direction in the form of an experienced facilitator guiding the participants through the objective and critical evaluation of the results at the conclusion.

Field exercises are the most realistic training events, involving the actual execution and performance of the community disaster-response plan. The field exercise allows for a real-time assessment of the physical capacity to meet the objectives as defined in writing. Ideally, the exercises will involve moving victims from the point of impact and injury through the EMS response system and into definitive care at medical facilities. These events, however, are labor intensive and long in duration and have significant cost.

Common Pitfalls of Disaster Response

Numerous studies performed after significant MCIs have identified several consistent shortcomings in the medical response to these events. Identification of these deficiencies has resulted from subsequent evaluations of the response to these incidents as well as from communities that have performed risk, vulnerability, and needs assessments mandated by the US government in order to receive funding resources to enhance the disaster-response infrastructure.

Preparedness

As responders in a community, prehospital care providers prepare for the devastation that can occur in a mass-casualty event and plan for such events in a variety of ways. Although one method of preparing is the tabletop drill, it does not truly test the ability of the provider to perform the necessary duties or the ability of the EMS agency to bring resources and assets to the site in a timely and efficient manner. Realistic functional disaster drills—during which victims are triaged, evaluated, "treated," and transported through the medical response system to a hospital facility's doors in a realistic fashion—better test the emergency medical response that will be required. The ability to provide for "surge capacity" and for supplying the large number of staff, ambulances, and other equipment needed for victims must be appropriately addressed by the medical response community.

Unfortunately, few agencies have actually tested a surge-capacity response in real time and, instead, have relied on tabletop drills as a measure of their ability to respond. Only through community-wide drills that involve multiple EMS agencies and ambulance services can the true level of preparedness to respond to an MCI as a community be assessed.

Communications

Many events have demonstrated that the lack of a unified communication system significantly hinders the ability to mount a coordinated response to an MCI. Individual communication systems are effective, but relying on a single system for communication is doomed to failure. The use of cellular phones became impossible when the central communication center located in the World Trade Center was no longer in existence. Also, the failure of police, fire, and EMS agencies to be able to communicate with each other because of different radio technologies or frequencies is a serious deficiency that significantly reduces the ability to respond to MCIs effectively. Redundancy in the system is of paramount importance, regardless of the chosen source for primary communications. Landlines, hardwired phone systems, cellular phone systems, satellite phone systems, VHF radios, and 800–900 MHz frequency systems all have some degree of vulnerability. The following two principles are essential:

1. A unified communication system to which all pertinent responders in the community have access.
2. System redundancy such that if one modality of communication fails or is disabled, another source can be used efficiently and effectively as an appropriate backup.

Another common problem is the use of "codes" as a form of communication shorthand. Unfortunately, there is no single, agreed-upon set of codes for all agencies to use; thus, a response agency may find itself at a scene with other agencies, all of whom are using codes that have the same terminology but different meanings. It is for this reason that ICS and the National Incident Management System recommend the use of plain English during an incident to avoid any confusion in meaning.

Scene Security

Scene security has become an ever-increasing problem in MCIs. Scene security is important for the following reasons:

1. To protect the response teams from a second strike, resulting in further casualties.
2. To provide for the ingress and egress of rescue workers and victims unencumbered by onlookers at the disaster.
3. To protect and assist in securing the scene and physical evidence.

Scene security becomes a significant challenge during a disaster event because, by definition, all resources are stretched to the maximum of their capabilities and limits. Coordination with local law enforcement leaders is essential for the prehospital and medical community to ensure that security will be available.

Self-Dispatched Assistance

In many MCIs, public safety and EMS agencies (as well as medical responders of all other types) from adjacent and even distant communities have responded to the scene without any formal request for assistance from the impacted jurisdiction.[5] These self-dispatched responders, although well intentioned, often serve only to further complicate and confuse an already chaotic situation. Interagency communications issues are often made more difficult by incompatible radio systems. Coordinated rescue efforts are often impossible because of the lack of participation in the incident command structure. Ideally, public safety and EMS agencies should respond to a disaster site only if they have been specifically requested to do so by the responsible jurisdiction and incident commander.[14] In addition, it is extremely helpful if access to the scene is controlled and a staging area is established as soon as possible to which all responding units and volunteers can be directed to better incorporate them into the incident response.

Supply and Equipment Resources

Most municipalities have plans for the routine utilization of supplies and have purchased supplies based on this demand. Events of large magnitude will rapidly exhaust these resources. Having a seamless plan for the reconstitution of supplies is essential for the ongoing mission of treating victims. Supplies must be available in a timely fashion, and appropriate mechanisms must be in place for distribution, which cannot include the care providers in the field, who will already be utilized to their fullest availabilities. A plan for pharmaceutical replenishment must also be in place. In those communities that have been designated to receive Metropolitan Medical Response System (MMRS) funds, community stockpiles have been or are being purchased in preparation for such events.

Failure to Notify Hospitals

In the confusion of responding to and assessing a mass-casualty incident as well as performing the numerous tasks that must be accomplished in initiating the medical response to such an event, it is often easy for EMS providers to overlook the need to contact hospitals and have them activate their internal disaster plans. Numerous actual events have demonstrated that unless hospital notification and activation are integral parts of the EMS agency's MCI plan, hospitals may be left on their own to discover that an incident has occurred, either when patients self-transport and report the event or when the first ambulance arrives to an unprepared facility. It is essential that EMS agencies include hospital notification

as part of their plan so that a coordinated seamless transition from field care to hospital care can occur.

In addition, on-going communication from the field (or Emergency Operations Center) to the hospital and from the hospital to the field are important for monitoring the status of the event and the patient load at hospitals.

Media

The media are often seen as a detriment to the physical and operational process of disaster response. However, communities are encouraged to partner with the media because these outlets can be an asset during a disaster response. The media can provide for the dissemination of appropriate and accurate information to the general population, giving them directions as to how to respond to maintain personal safety and where to report to obtain information or to reunite with family members, as well as communicating other needed information. It is inevitable that the media will broadcast information to the public, and as responders, prehospital care providers have the responsibility to partner with the media to ensure that the information provided is accurate as well as helpful to the response process.

SUMMARY

- Disasters result from natural climactic or geologic events; however, they may also result from intentional or unintentional acts of man.
- Although disasters may be unpredictable, adequate preparation can turn an unthinkable event into a manageable situation.
- Appropriate disaster response involves much more than the medical component.
- Implementation of the Incident Command System allows multiple agencies to collaborate in the disaster response.

- Despite the fact that disasters occur in varying sizes and result from many different causes, common pitfalls have been identified that hinder management of such an event.
- Disaster response may take a heavy psychological toll on those involved, both victims and rescuers.
- The best outcomes in response to MCIs result from the creation of a well-devised disaster plan that has been rehearsed, tested, and critiqued to identify and improve problem areas.

SCENARIO SOLUTION

After the blast event, precautionary measures are taken to evaluate the risk potential for collapse of the damaged structure as well as ongoing gas leak, exposed electrical sources, and the potential for a second explosion. Appropriate personal protective equipment (PPE) and standard precautions must be used when treating patients.

Crowd control is of the utmost importance after such an event to prevent well-meaning bystanders from entering the building to search for victims and help with rescue. The ICS should be used to manage the resources required to deal with this event. A staging area for responding units should be designated. Patients will need to be triaged using whatever triage system the EMS provider has in place. Casualty collection points will be set up and located in strategic areas to allow for rapid loading and evacuation of victims.

In addition to patient care needs, remember that rescue workers will have hydration, nutrition, and sanitary needs throughout the rescue effort. ■

References

1. Noji EK. *The public health consequences of disasters,* New York, 1997, Oxford University Press.
2. Noji EK, Siverston KT. Injury prevention in natural disasters: A theoretical framework. *Disasters* 11:290, 1987.
3. Cuny SC. Introduction to disaster management. Lesson 5: Technologies of disaster management. *Prehosp Disaster Med* 6:372, 1993.
4. Mass Medical Care with Scarce Resources: A Community Planning Guide. AHRQ Publication No. 07–0001, February 2007. Agency for Healthcare Research and Quality, Rockville, MD. http://www.ahrq.gov/research/mce/. Accessed September 1, 2008.
5. Auf der Heide E: The importance of evidence-based disaster planning. *Ann Emerg Med* 47:34–49, 2006.
6. Burkle FM, editor: *Disaster medicine: Application for the immediate management and triage of civilian and military disaster victims,* New Hyde Park, NY, 1984, Medication Examination Publishing.
7. Burkle FM, Hogan DE, Burstein JL: *Disaster medicine,* Philadelphia, 2002, Lippincott, Williams & Wilkins.
8. Lerner EB, Schwartz RB, Coule PL, et al: Mass casualty triage: An evaluation of the data and development of a proposed national guideline. *Disaster Med Public Health Preparedness* 2 (Suppl 1): S25-S34, 2008.
9. Super G. START: A triage training module, Newport Beach, Calif, 1984, Hoag Memorial Hospital Presbyterian.
10. Burkle FM, Newland C, Orebaugh S, et al: Emergency medicine in the Persian Gulf. Part II. Triage methodology lessons learned. *Ann Emerg Med* 23:748, 1994.
11. Bloch YH, Schwartz D, Pinkert M, et al: Distribution of casualties in a mass-casualty incident with three local hospitals in the periphery of a densely populated area: Lessons learned from the medical management of a terrorist attack. *Prehosp Disast Med* 22:186–192, 2007.
12. Hick JL, Ho JD, Heegaard WG, et al: Emergency Medical Services Response to a Major Freeway Bridge Collapse. *Disaster Med Public Health Preparedness* 2 (Suppl 1): S17-S24, 2008.
13. West H: Addressing the Traumatic Impact of Disasters on Individuals, Families, and Communities (White Paper). http:// www.nh.gov/safety/divisions/bem/behavhealth/documents/atc_white_paper.Accessed September 1, 2008.
14. Asaeda G, Cherson A, Richmond N, Clair J, Guttenberg M: Unsolicited medical personnel volunteering at disaster scenes. A joint position paper from the National Association of EMS Physicians and the American College of Emergency Physicians. *Prehosp Emerg Care* 7:147–148, 2003.

Suggested Reading

Briggs SM, Brinsfield KH: *Advanced disaster medical response: manual for providers,* Boston, 2003, Harvard Medical International.

De Boer J, Dubouloz M: *Handbook of disaster medicine, emergency medicine in mass casualty situations,* National Society of Disaster Medicine, Netherlands, 2000, Van der Wees.

De Boer J, Rutherford WH: Definition and quantification of disaster: Introduction of a disaster severity scale. *J Emerg Med* 8:602, 1990.

Eachempati SR, Flomenbaum N, Barie PS: Biological warfare: Current concerns for the health care provider. *J Trauma* 52:179, 2002.

Emerg Med Clin North Am 14(2), 1996 (entire issue).

Feliciano DV, et al: Management of casualties from the bombing at the centennial Olympics. *Am J Surg* 176(6):538, 1998.

Hirshberg A, Holcomb JB, Mattox KL: Hospital trauma care in multiple-casualty incidents: A critical view. *Ann Emerg Med* 37(6):647, 2001.

Hogan DE, Burstein, JL, editors: *Disaster Medicine,* ed 2, Philadelphia, 2007, Lippincott, Williams & Wilkins.

Rutherford WH, De Boer J: The definition and quantification of disaster. *Injury* 15:1, 1983.

Slater MS, Trunkey DD: Terrorism in America: an evolving threat. *Arch Surg* 132(10):1059, 1997.

Stein M, Hirshberg A: Medical consequences of terrorism: the conventional weapon threat. *Surg Clin North Am* 79(6):1537, 1999.

Explosions and Weapons of Mass Destruction

CHAPTER OBJECTIVES

At the completion of this chapter, the reader will be able to do the following:

✓ Understand the essential considerations regarding mitigation of a weapon of mass destruction (WMD) event:

- Scene assessment
- Incident command
- Personal protective equipment
- Patient triage
- Principle of decontamination

✓ Understand the mechanisms of injury, evaluation and management, and transport considerations associated with specific categories of WMD agent:

- Explosive agents
- Incendiary agents
- Chemical agents
- Biologic agents
- Radiologic agents

✓ Know how to access and utilize resources for further study.

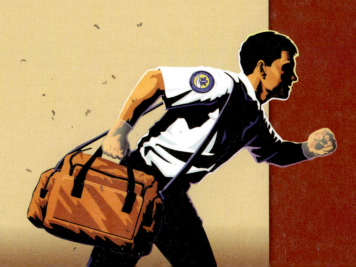

SCENARIO

You are dispatched to the scene of a reported explosion at an outdoor fair. The number of victims is unknown. Other public safety agencies have been dispatched to the location.

On arrival at the location, you note that you are the first EMS responder on scene. No incident command has yet been established. Dozens of people are running about the scene. Many are screaming for you to assist victims who are obviously bleeding. Other patients are laying on the ground; at least one of the victims is seizing.

What will you do first? What are your priorities as you determine your course of action? How will you care for so many people?

Preparing to manage a weapons of mass destruction (WMD) event challenges emergency medical services (EMS) systems every day. Recent history has demonstrated that these events can occur at any time and in any location. The 1993 World Trade Center bombing resulted in only six deaths, but yielded 548 casualties, with more than 1000 victims assisted by EMS. Responders became casualties as well, with 105 firefighters reporting injuries. The 1995 explosion at the Murrah Federal Building in Oklahoma City resulted in 168 deaths, with 700 injuries. One third of the patients brought to one Oklahoma City hospital came by EMS, and they were the sickest, with 64% requiring admission to the hospital, whereas only 6% of those who self-referred to the emergency department (ED) needed admission. The 2001 World Trade Center attacks resulted in over 1100 injured survivors, with almost a third of those patients arriving at the hospital by EMS. Rescue workers accounted for 29% of the injured victims.

Although conventional high explosives are the most commonly used and most likely form of WMD event, EMS systems have also been challenged by chemical and biohazard events. The 1994 sarin gas attack in Matsumoto, Japan, killed seven and injured more than 300. The more widely known 1995 sarin gas attack in the Tokyo subway system killed 12, but more than 5000 victims sought medical attention. The Tokyo Fire Department sent 1364 firefighters to the 16 affected subway sites; 135 responders (10%) were affected by direct or indirect exposure to the nerve agent.

No life-threatening bioterrorism assault in the United States has yielded a large number of casualties, but this does not mean that EMS systems have not been challenged to prepare for bioterrorism threats. During 1998 and 1999, almost 6000 persons across the United States were affected by a series of anthrax-related hoaxes in more than 200 incidents. The anthrax letters delivered in the fall of 2001 resulted in only 22 cases of clinical anthrax but generated countless calls for EMS to respond to suspicious packages and powders. Also, although not a bioterrorist event, a naturally occurring

biohazard, severe acute respiratory syndrome (SARS), seriously challenged the Toronto EMS system. During the epidemic, 526 of their paramedics had to be quarantined, the vast majority secondary to potential unprotected exposure to the virus, seriously straining that EMS system's ability to mitigate the crisis.

The threat that EMS may one day have to respond to a radiologic WMD event grows, with increasing speculation that terrorists may detonate a radiologic dispersal device ("dirty bomb") that will generate injuries and panic about radioactive contamination.

General Considerations

Scene Assessment and Incident Command System

The ability of the prehospital care provider to assess the scene properly is crucial to assuring the provider's safety and that of other responders and ensures the best delivery of service to the patient. WMD events pose significant threats to responding emergency services. In the case of a high-explosives detonation, there may be fire, spilled hazardous materials, power line hazards, and risk of falling debris or subsidence. One rescue worker was killed by falling debris in response to the Oklahoma City bombing.[1] Many more were killed in the 2001 World Trade Center attack. Chemical attacks potentially expose the emergency responder to the offending agent not only from the primary source—the weapon—but also from contamination of victims' skin, clothing, and personal belongings. Biohazards, depending on the form of their delivery, pose a risk of illness from the offending agent (e.g., aerosolized anthrax spores) or from transmission of a communicable disease (e.g., plague or smallpox). A further risk to emergency responders and patients alike is the possibility of a secondary device, for example, a second bomb placed at the scene of the incident, set to explode after arrival of emergency responders, with the intention of increasing not only injury, but also confusion and panic.

As many of the WMDs pose an inhalation risk, particularly the chemical and biologic agents, responding units from all involved agencies must take care to approach the scene from an upwind direction to minimize the potential for inadvertent exposure. In addition, any incident that involves the release of liquid chemical mandates that responders stage uphill from the spill.

Access to and egress from the potentially contaminated site must be controlled. Concerned bystanders and volunteers must not be allowed to enter the scene as they may contribute to the casualty count if they expose themselves to the agent. Victims of the incident must also be contained as they seek to evacuate the scene, since self-transport may only serve to further disseminate a dangerous chemical or substance to unsuspecting contacts. Just as would occur at a hazardous materials incident, scene control zones (hot, warm, cold) should be established with controlled access points and transit corridors to prevent spread of the contaminants, inadvertent exposure, and safe areas for patient evaluation and treatment (Figure 19-1). The zones are further described in the following section on Personal Protective Equipment.

All of these factors must be taken into consideration when evaluating a scene and their significance comprehended before taking action. In addition, a critical evaluation, from a safe distance, of how patients are presenting must be included as part of the scene assessment, with particular attention to the clues suggesting a possible chemical or biologic agent release. Prehospital providers also need to communicate their observations through the chain of command so that proper steps can be taken to mount an appropriate response, increasing the safety of the responders and the delivery of care to patients. The *incident command system* (ICS) defines the chain of command through which this communication takes place. The ICS is the model tool for command, control, and coordination. It was developed to mitigate the recurring failures of response to disasters, which include the following:

1. Nonstandard terminology used by responding agencies
2. Nonstandard and nonintegrated command structures of responding agencies
3. Lack of capability to expand and contract as required by the situation
4. Nonstandard and nonintegrated communications
5. Lack of consolidated incident action plans
6. Lack of designated facilities

ICS offers a management structure that coordinates all available resources to ensure an effective response. All incidents, regardless of size or complexity, will have a designated *incident commander,* who may be the first responding prehospital provider until relieved by some other competent

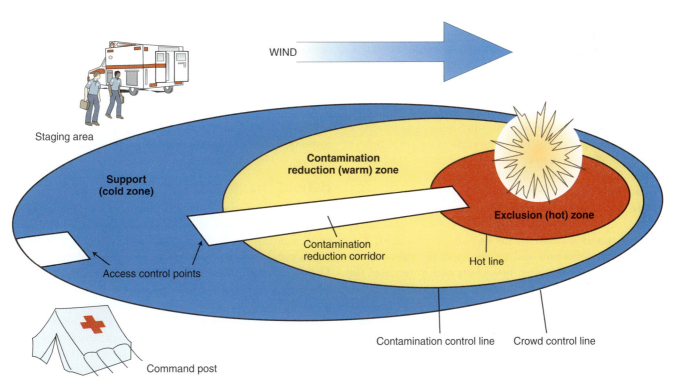

FIGURE 19-1 The scene of a WMD or hazmat incident is generally divided into hot, warm, and cold zones.
(Modified from Chapleau W: *Emergency first responder,* St. Louis, 2004, Mosby.)

authority (see Chapter 5). It is essential that prehospital providers are familiar with and have the opportunity to practice implementation of the ICS.

Personal Protective Equipment

When responding to WMD events, the wearing of proper personal protective equipment (PPE) needs to be considered. Requirements for PPE may range from the standard daily uniform to a fully encapsulated suit with *self-contained breathing apparatus* (SCBA) depending upon the specific agent involved and the specific role assigned to the responder. This equipment is designed to protect the prehospital provider from exposure to offending agents by providing defined levels of protection of the respiratory tract, skin, and other mucous membranes. Civilian PPE has generally been described in terms of the following levels (Figure 19-2):

- *Level A.* This level offers the highest respiratory and skin protection. The respiratory tract is protected by a SCBA or *supplied air respirator* (SAR) delivering air to the prehospital provider with positive pressure. A chemical-resistant barrier that completely encapsulates the wearer protects the skin and mucous membranes.
- *Level B.* The respiratory tract is protected in the same manner as in Level A protection, with positive-pressure-supplied air. Nonencapsulated chemical-resistant garments, including suit, gloves, and boots, which provide splash protection only, protect the skin and mucous membranes. The highest respiratory protection is afforded, with a lower level of skin protection.
- *Level C.* The respiratory tract is protected by an *air-purifying respirator* (APR). This may be a powered air-purifying respirator (PAPR), which draws ambient air through a filter canister and delivers it under positive pressure to a facemask or hood, or a nonpowered APR, which relies on the wearer to draw ambient air through a filter canister by breathing through a properly fitted mask. The skin protection is the same as for Level B.
- *Level D.* This represents standard work clothes (i.e., uniform for prehospital care provider) and may also include a gown, gloves, and surgical mask. This level provides minimal respiratory protection and minimal skin protection.

PPE is selected based on the known (or suspected) hazards of the environment and proximity to the threat. Proximity to the threat has often been described in terms of the following zones:

- The *hot zone* is the area where there is immediate threat to health and life. This includes an environment contaminated with a hazardous gas, vapor, aerosol, liquid, or powder. PPE adequate to protect the prehospital care provider is determined based on potential routes of exposure to the substance and the likely agent. Level A protection is most often used in the hot zone.

- The *warm zone* is characterized as an area where the concentration of the offending agent is limited. In the case of a WMD scene, this is the area to which victims are brought from the hot zone and where decontamination is taking place. The prehospital care provider is still at risk for hazmat exposure in this area as the agent is carried from the hot zone on victims, responders, and equipment. PPE is recommended based on potential routes of exposure to the substance.
- The *cold zone* is the area outside the hot and warm zones that is not contaminated, where there is no risk of hazmat exposure, and thus no specific level of PPE is required beyond standard universal precautions.

It is important to note that it is often difficult to define these hazard zones and that they may be dynamic and not static. Factors that contribute to the dynamics of the zones include the activity of the victims and responders and ambient conditions. Unless completely incapacitated, contaminated victims might walk toward prehospital care providers in the "cold zone" or leave the scene completely, either in panic or with the intention of seeking aid at a nearby medical treatment facility or their personal physician. By design, warm zones and cold zones are designated upwind of the hot zone, but if wind direction changes, prehospital care providers would be at risk of hazmat exposure if unable to don personal PPE or to retreat. These contingencies must be anticipated when planning for or responding to a WMD event.

It might be concluded that the best protective posture for a prehospital care provider is always to respond in the highest level of protection, Level A, regardless of the threat. This is, however, not a reasonable response. Level A protection is cumbersome, often making manual tasks difficult to perform. Significant training and experience are required when using an SCBA. Level A protection puts the wearer at risk for heat stress and physical exhaustion. It can make communication between responders and victims difficult. Appropriate PPE must be selected based on the threat and the operational responsibilities of the prehospital care provider.

Patient Triage

Prehospital care providers will potentially face a large and overwhelming number of victims who will require evaluation and treatment after a WMD event. Every EMS system should identify and rehearse a mechanism for rapidly triaging victims. The objective of patient triage in a WMD incident is to do the greatest good for the greatest number of victims. Field triage is typically based on easily measurable physiologic criteria that assign patients to severity categories in order to identify those victims who require treatment and transport to a medical treatment facility most urgently.[2] Several triage criteria are published.[3] The START (simple triage and rapid treatment) system is one such method that is commonly used. Patient severity is determined in an algorithmic fashion by first assessing ability to ambulate, then assessing airway, respirations, circulation,

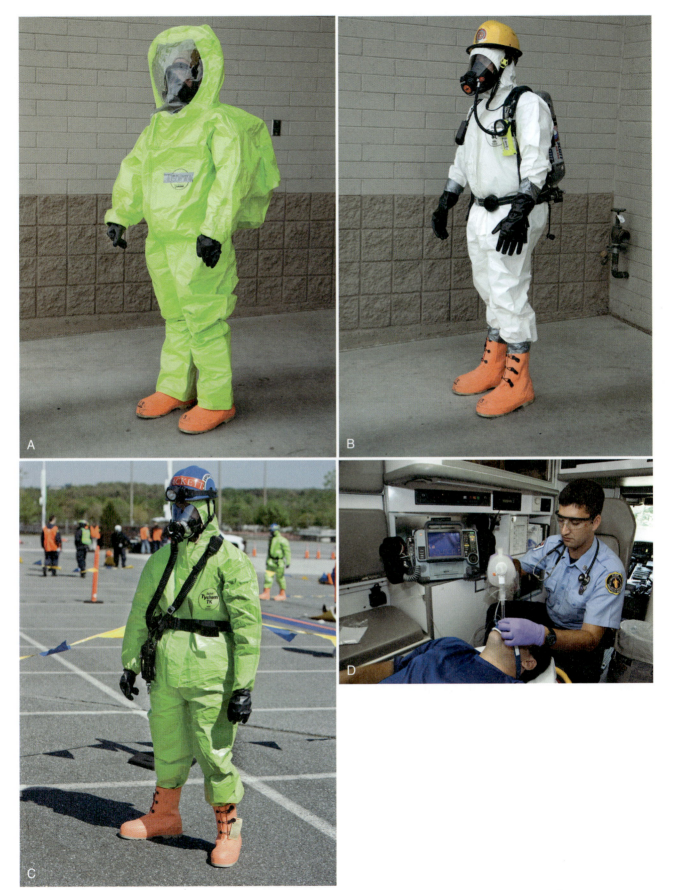

FIGURE 19-2 Personal protective equipment. **A.** Level A. **B.** Level B. **C.** Level C. **D.** Level D.

and mental status. Patients are usually assigned to one of four severity categories. *Minimal* ("green") patients do not have life-threatening injury and will likely do well even if care is withheld several hours or days. *Delayed* ("yellow") patients have a serious injury but will likely not deteriorate with a slight delay in care. *Emergent* ("red") patients are critical and will require immediate care. *Immediate* ("black") patients are dead or have injuries not compatible with life. A fifth category ("blue") has been used on occasion for patients requiring decontamination. Other triage systems include the M.A.S.S. method taught in the National Disaster Life Support courses and the S.A.L.T. system proposed by the CDC [4] (for more information please see Chapter 18: Disaster Management).

Whatever patient triage system is utilized, it must be employed in routine EMS operations to promote familiarity and to ensure recognition among emergency service providers at all levels of care, including the medical treatment facility.

Principles of Decontamination

Patients and prehospital care providers alike may require decontamination after exposure to adherent solids or liquids that may pose a risk to the patient or other health care personnel. These individuals should have decontamination procedures performed in the field in a designated decontamination area. Decontamination areas are typically upwind and uphill of the affected area when conditions allow. Known exposure to only vapor or gases does not require decontamination to prevent secondary contamination, although the victim's clothing should be removed.

Decontamination is a two-step process that first involves removal of all clothing, jewelry, and shoes, which are bagged and tagged for later identification. The simple act of removing clothing achieves removal of 70% to 90% of contamination. Any solid contaminant should be carefully brushed away from the patient, and any liquid contamination should be blotted off. The second step involves washing the skin surfaces with water or water and a mild detergent to ensure removal of all substances from the patient's skin. Avoid using harsh detergents or bleach solutions on skin as well as vigorous scrubbing. Chemically or physically aggravating the skin may contribute to increased absorption of the offending agent. When washing, skin folds, axillae, groin, buttocks, and feet must receive special attention because contaminants can collect in these areas and may be overlooked by patients in their cleansing efforts.

Decontamination should be performed in a systematic manner to avoid missing areas of contaminated skin. For the eyes, contact lenses should be removed and mucous membranes irrigated with copious amounts of water or saline, especially if the patient is symptomatic. Ambulatory patients should be able to perform their own decontamination under instruction from prehospital care providers. Nonambulatory patients will require the assistance of individuals properly outfitted with PPE to decontaminate litter patients. Expe-

ditious decontamination may be warranted in the effort to decrease exposure time to various life-threatening substances. All prehospital care providers need to be familiar with a hasty decontamination procedure that may be executed even before arrival of the formal hazmat/decontamination team, to minimize exposure time for both patients and responders.

Issues to consider include (1) offering privacy for males and females required to disrobe, (2) having warm water available for irrigation and showering, (3) providing a suitable substitute for clothing at the completion of decontamination, (4) assuring victims that their personal belongings will be secure until a final disposition is made regarding their return or necessary disposal, and (5) collection of effluent, if practical.

Specific Threats

Explosions and Explosives

Understanding injury from explosives is essential for all providers of emergency care in both civilian and military settings. Medical personnel need to understand the pathophysiology of injury resulting from unintentional, industrial, and the wide range of anti-personnel explosive devices such as letter bombs, shaped warheads from rocket-propelled grenades, antipersonnel land mines, aerial-delivered cluster bombs, enhanced blast weapons, and the improvised explosive devices (IEDs) so widely used by terrorists. A study of the 36,110 US bombing incidents reported by the Bureau of Alcohol, Tobacco, and Firearms (ATF) between 1983 and 2002 concluded, "...the US experience reveals that materials used for bombings are readily available [and] healthcare providers...need to be prepared."[5]

Explosions occur in homes (primarily due to gas leaks or fires) and are an occupational hazard of many industries, including mining and those involved in demolition, chemical manufacture, or handling fuel or dust-producing substances such as grain. Industrial explosions result from chemical spills, fires, faulty equipment maintenance, or electrical/machinery malfunctions and may produce toxic fumes, building collapse, secondary explosions, falling debris, and large numbers of casualties. Another common cause of explosion is the rupture of a pressurized containment vessel, such as boiler, when the internal pressure exceeds the capability of the container to withstand the elevated pressure.

As a whole, however, unintentional explosions are responsible for relatively few injuries and deaths (e.g., 150 in the United States in 2004[6]) compared with the large numbers of injuries and deaths produced by explosives used by terrorists and military adversaries.

Terrorists worldwide are increasingly using bombs, especially IEDs, against civilian targets. This is because these devices are inexpensive, made from easily obtained materials, and result in the devastating havoc that focuses international exposure on their cause. An emergency provider is thousands of times more likely to encounter injury from conventional explosives than from a chemical, biological, or nuclear attack. Because both civilian and military responders may be called upon during a bomb attack on civilian populations, all healthcare providers need to be familiar with their roles during these increasingly frequent occurrences.

Review of the US State Department's historical data on terrorist incidents worldwide between 1961 and 2003 reveals a significant increase beginning in 1996 and an exponential increase after the attacks of September 11, 2001.[7] In past decades, there has been a shift from bomb attacks occurring largely in certain "trouble spots," such as Northern Ireland (1970s) or Paris (1980s), to incidents occurring in all regions of the world, from Atlanta to Jerusalem to Nairobi. In recent years, however, a primary trouble spot has been Iraq, where 60% of the fatalities (a total of 13,606) caused by terrorist attacks occurred in 2007.[8]

At present, although the United States is not typically exposed to as many bomb attacks as other countries, bomb attacks reported in 2007 totalled 445 (more than one per day) and other explosive-related incidents occurred including theft/recovery of explosives, accidental explosions, etc. (Figure 19-3).[9]

Worldwide, a total of 14,499 terrorist attacks were reported in 2007, which resulted in 44,310 injuries and 22,685 deaths, a 20% to 30% increase over 2006.[10,11] A majority (~70%) were civilians.[12] Continuing the trend from the previous year of "the transition from expeditionary to guerilla terrorism," most attacks in 2007 were carried out by terrorists using bombs and small arms.[12] This large increase is in part attributed to the increase in suicide bomb attacks.[12] Also in 2007, terrorists continued to coordinate secondary attacks to target first responders and intensified their enhancement of IEDs with chlorine gas to create clouds of toxic fumes.[12] More recently, however, the number of terror attacks and their associated injuries and deaths declined, by 18%, 30%, and 23%, respectively (Figure 19-4).[13]

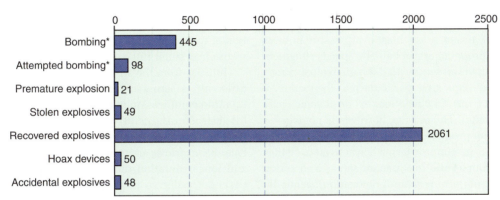

FIGURE 19-3 Explosion-related incidents, United States, 2007.

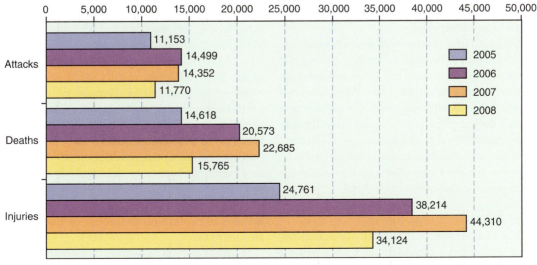

FIGURE 19-4 Terrorist attacks worldwide with associated injuries and deaths1: 2005−2008.

Categories of Explosives

Clinicians need to consider the type of explosive device and its location when evaluating casualties of terrorist blast incidents.[14] Explosives fall into one of two categories based on the velocity of detonation: high explosives and low explosives.

High explosives react almost instantaneously. Because they are designed to detonate and release their energy very quickly, HE are capable of producing a shock wave, or *overpressure phenomenon,* which can result in primary blast injury. The initial explosion creates an instantaneous rise in pressure, creating a shock wave that travels outward at supersonic speed (1400–9000 m/sec).[15] The *shock wave* is the leading front and an integral component of the *blast wave,* which is created on the rapid release of enormous amounts of energy, with subsequent propulsion of fragments, generation of environmental debris, and often intense thermal radiation.

Common examples of high explosives are 2,4,6-trinitrotoluene (TNT), nitroglycerin, dynamite, ammonium nitrate fuel oil, and the more recent polymer-bonded explosives that have 1.5 times the power of TNT, such as Gelignite and the ubiquitous plastic explosive, Semtex. High explosives have a sharp, shattering effect *(brisance)* that can pulverize bone and soft tissue, create blast overpressure injuries *(barotrauma),* and propel debris at ballistic speeds *(fragmentation).* It is also important to note that a high explosive may result in a low order explosion, particularly if the explosive has deteriorated as a result of age (Semtex) or in some cases become wet (dynamite). The reverse, however, is not true—a low explosive cannot produce a high-order explosion.

Low explosives (e.g., gunpowder), when activated, change relatively slowly from a solid to a gaseous state (in an action more characteristic of burning than of detonation), generally creating a blast wave that moves less than 2000 meters per second (m/second). Examples of LE include pipe bombs, gunpowder, and pure petroleum-based bombs such as Molotov cocktails.[16] Explosions resulting from container rupture and ignition of volatile compounds fall into this category as well. Because they release their energy much more slowly, LE are not capable of producing overpressure.

The type and amount of explosive will determine the size of the blast associated with detonation of the device. This fact makes the approach to the scene and the location for staging responders and equipment a critical decision. When responding to a scene that involves either a suspicious device or a potential secondary device, all responders must stage at a safe distance from the site in the event of a detonation. (See Chapter 5: Scene Assessment and Management for more information). Figure 19-5 provides guidelines for safe distances depending on the possible size of the explosion.

Mechanisms of Injury

Traumatic injury after explosions has generally been divided into three categories: primary, secondary, and tertiary blast injury.[17] In addition to the injuries that result directly from the blast, additional categories of injuries classified as quaternary and quinary have been described and result from complications or toxic effects that are related to the explosive or contaminants. Although these are described separately, they may occur in combination in victims of explosions. Figure 19-6 (page 456) shows the effects of explosions on the human body.

Primary blast injury (PBI) results from high-order explosive detonation and the interaction of the blast overpressure wave with the body or tissue to produce stress and shear waves. *Stress waves* are supersonic, longitudinal pressure waves that (1) create high local forces with small, rapid distortions; (2) produce microvascular injury; and (3) are reinforced and reflected at tissue interfaces, thereby enhancing injury potential, especially in gas-filled organs such as the lungs, ears, and intestines. This is not to be confused with wind generated by a blast; a *shock or blast wave* is significantly increased atmospheric pressure produced by the almost instantaneous combustion of HE. Overpressures from these detonations can exceed 4 million pounds per square inch (psi), compared with 14.7 psi ambient pressure. The shock wave or pressure wave then propagates from the point of origin, gradually dissipating as the distance from the point of combustion increases. Depending on the proximity of the victim to the blast, as well as shielding or augmentation of the wave secondary to detonations in a closed space, a victim may suffer PBI.

Injuries from the stress waves are caused by (1) pressure differentials across delicate structures such as the alveoli, (2) rapid compression of and subsequent re-expansion of gas-filled structures, and (3) reflection of the *tension wave* (a component of the compressive stress wave) at the tissue-gas interface. *Shear waves* are transverse waves with a lower velocity and longer duration that cause asynchronous movement of tissues. The degree of damage depends on the extent to which the asynchronous motions overcome inherent tissue elasticity, resulting in tearing of tissue and possible disruption of attachments. However, muscle, bone, and solid-organ injury are much more likely to result from the tertiary and quaternary effects of the blast than from the blast wave alone.[18,19]

Primary blast injury occurs in gas-filled organs such as the lung, bowel, and middle ear. The injury to the tissue occurs at the gas-fluid interface, presumably from a rapid compression of the gas in the organ, causing violent collapse of that organ, followed by an equally rapid and violent expansion, resulting in tissue injury. Damage to the lung manifests as pulmonary contusions, or possibly hemopneumothoraces, resulting in hypoxemia if the patient does not immediately succumb to the injuries (Figure 19-7, page 457). Alveoli can also become disrupted, resulting in arterial gas emboli, which may cause cerebral or cardiac embolic complications. Damage to the bowel may include petechiae or hematomas of the bowel wall or even perforation of the bowel. Tympanic membrane rupture or disruption of the middle ear ossicles also may occur.

Evidence of PBI to the lung is more often found in patients who die minutes after the explosion from associated injuries; however, pulmonary PBI has been noted more frequently among surviving victims of confined-space explosions.[20–22]

	Threat Description	Explosives Mass[1] (TNT equivalent)	Building Evacuation Distance[2]	Outdoor Evacuation Distance[3]
High Explosives (TNT Equivalent)	Pipe Bomb	5 lbs 2.3 kg	70 ft 21 m	850 ft 259 m
	Suicide Belt	10 lbs 4.5 kg	90 ft 27 m	1,080 ft 330 m
	Suicide Vest	20 lbs 9 kg	110 ft 34 m	1,360 ft 415 m
	Briefcase/Suitcase Bomb	50 lbs 23 kg	150 ft 46 m	1,850 ft 564 m
	Compact Sedan	500 lbs 227 kg	320 ft 98 m	1,500 ft 457 m
	Sedan	1,000 lbs 454 kg	400 ft 122 m	1,750 ft 534 m
	Passenger/Cargo Van	4,000 lbs 1,814 kg	640 ft 195 m	2,750 ft 838 m
	Small Moving Van/ Delivery Truck	10,000 lbs 4,536 kg	860 ft 263 m	3,750 ft 1,143 m
	Moving Van/Water Truck	30,000 lbs 13,608 kg	1,240 ft 375 m	6,500 ft 1,982 m
	Semitrailer	60,000 lbs 27,216 kg	1,570 ft 475 m	7,000 ft 2,134 m
	Threat Description	**LPG Mass/Volume[1]**	**Fireball Diameter[4]**	**Safe Distance[5]**
Liquefied Petroleum Gas (LPG - Butane or Propane)	Small LPG Tank	20 lbs/5 gal 9 kg/19 l	40 ft 12 m	160 ft 48 m
	Large LPG Tank	100 lbs/25 gal 45 kg/95 l	69 ft 21 m	276 ft 84 m
	Commercial/Residential LPG Tank	2,000 lbs/500 gal 907 kg/1,893 l	184 ft 56 m	736 ft 224 m
	Small LPG Truck	8,000 lbs/2,000 gal 3,630 kg/7,570 l	292 ft 89 m	1,168 ft 356 m
	Semitanker LPG	40,000 lbs/10,000 gal 18,144 kg/37,850 l	499 ft 152 m	1,996 ft 608 m

UNCLASSIFIED

FIGURE 19-5 Explosives Safe Distance Stand-off Chart (National Ground Intelligence Center, United States Army—unclassified).

---

[1] Based on the maximum amount of material that could reasonably fit into a container or vehicle. Variations possible.
[2] Governed by the ability of an unreinforced building to withstand severe damage or collapse.
[3] Governed by the greater of fragment throw distance or glass breakage/falling glass hazard distance. These distances can be reduced for personnel wearing ballistic protection. Note that the pipe bomb, suicide belt/vest, and briefcase/suitcase bomb are assumed to have a fragmentation characteristic that requires greater standoff distances than an equal amount of explosives in a vehicle.
[4] Assuming efficient mixing of the flammable gas with ambient air.
[5] Determined by U.S. firefighting practices wherein safe distances are approximately 4 times the flame height. Note that an LPG tank filled with high explosives would require a significantly greater standoff distance than if it were filled with LPG.

FIGURE 19-6   Blast Injury Categories

Effect	Impact	Mechanism of Injury	Typical Injuries
Primary	Direct blast effects (over- and under-pressurization)	■ Produced by contact of blast shockwave with body ■ Stress and shear waves occur in tissues ■ Waves reinforced/reflected at tissue density interfaces ■ Gas-filled organs (lungs, ears, etc.) at particular risk	■ Tympanic membrane rupture ■ Blast lung ■ Eye injuries ■ Concussion
Secondary	Projectiles propelled by explosion	Ballistic wounds produced by: ■ Primary fragments (pieces of exploding weapon) ■ Secondary fragments (environmental fragments, e.g., glass)	■ Penetrating injuries ■ Traumatic amputations ■ Lacerations ■ Concussion
Tertiary	Propulsion of body onto hard surface or object, or propulsion of objects onto individuals	■ Whole body translocation ■ Crush injuries caused by structural damage and building collapse	■ Blunt injuries ■ Crush syndrome ■ Compartment syndrome ■ Concussion
Quaternary	Heat and/or combustion fumes	■ Burns and toxidromes from fuel, metals ■ Septic syndromes from soil and environmental contamination	■ Burns ■ Inhalation injury ■ Asphyxiation
Quinary	Additives such as radiation or chemicals (e.g., dirty bombs)	Contamination of tissue from; ■ Bacteria, radiation, or chemical agents ■ Allogenic bone fragments	■ Variety of health effects, depending on agent

(Department of Defense Directive: Medical Research for Prevention, Mitigation, and Treatment of Blast Injuries. Number 6025.21E. http://www.dtic.mil/whs/directives/corres/html/602521.htm. Accessed November 21, 2008.)

It has also been associated with other severe injuries and is indicative of increased mortality in survivors. After an open-air explosion in Beirut, only 0.6% of survivors had evidence of PBI, and 11% of those died.[12] In a confined-space explosion in Jerusalem, 38% of survivors had evidence of PBI, with a similar mortality rate of approximately 9%.[23] Similarly, two of the three bombs that were detonated in the London subway system exploded in wide tunnels resulting in six and seven fatalities respectively. The third device detonated in the subway system was exploded in a narrow tunnel, causing 26 fatalities. This difference in mortality between open- and closed-space bombings results from the reflection of the blast wave back onto the victims rather than the dispersal of the blast wave into the surrounding area.

Secondary blast injury is caused by flying debris and bomb fragments. Fragment (fragmentation) injury, or secondary injury, is the most common category of injury in terrorist bombings and low-order explosions. These projectiles may be components of the bomb itself, as from military weapons designed to fragment, or from improvised bombs augmented with nails, screws, and bolts. Secondary blast injury is also caused by debris that is carried by the blast wind. Blast winds associated with the force required to create enough overpressure to rupture 50% of exposed tympanic membranes (approximately 5 psi) can briefly generate winds of 145 mph. Winds associated

with the force necessary to create an overpressure resulting in significant PBI may exceed 831 mph.[17] Although brief in duration, these winds can propel debris with great force and for great distances, causing both penetrating and blunt trauma.

Tertiary blast injury is caused by the blast wind throwing the body, resulting in tumbling and collision with stationary objects. This can result in the whole spectrum of injuries associated with blunt trauma and even penetrating trauma, such as impalement.

Following the blast itself, *quaternary effects* may be seen.[16] These injuries include burns and toxicities from fuel, metals, trauma from structural collapse, septic syndromes from soil, and environmental contamination (septic meliodosis). The increasing threat of radiation-enhanced explosives (i.e., "dirty bombs") has given rise to a fifth *(quinary)* category of effects, which includes injuries caused by radiation, chemicals, or biologic agents and material such as bone fragments of the bomber.[24,25]

Injury Patterns

The prehospital care provider will be confronted with a combination of familiar penetrating, blunt, and thermal injuries and possibly survivors with PBI.[26] The numbers and types of injury will depend on multiple factors, including explosion magnitude, composition, environment, and location and number of potential victims at risk.

FIGURE 19-7 Blast Lung Injury: What Prehospital Providers Need to Know

Current patterns in worldwide terrorist activity have increased the potential for casualties related to explosions, yet few civilian Emergency Medical Services (EMS) providers in the United States have experience treating patients with explosion-related injuries. Blast lung injury (BLI) presents unique triage, diagnostic, and management challenges and is a direct consequence of the blast wave from high-explosive detonations upon the body. Persons in enclosed space explosions or those in close proximity to the explosion are at a higher risk. BLI is a clinical diagnosis characterized by respiratory difficulty and hypoxia. BLI can occur, although rarely, without obvious external injury to the chest.

CLINICAL PRESENTATION

- Symptoms may include dyspnea, hemoptysis, cough, and chest pain.
- Signs may include tachypnea, hypoxia, cyanosis, apnea, wheezing, decreased breath sounds, and hemodynamic instability.
- Victims with greater than 10% BSA burns, skull fractures, and penetrating torso or head injuries may be more likely to have BLI.
- Hemothoraces or pneumothoraces may occur.
- Due to tearing of the pulmonary and vascular tree, air may enter the arterial circulation ("air emboli") and result in embolic events involving the central nervous system, retinal arteries, or coronary arteries.
- Clinical evidence of blast lung injury is typically present at the time of initial evaluation; however, it has been reported to occur over the course of 24 to 48 hours after an explosion.
- Other injuries are often present.

HOSPITAL MANAGEMENT CONSIDERATIONS

- Initial triage, trauma resuscitation, and transport of patients should follow standard protocols for multiple injured patients or mass casualties.
- Note the patient's location and the surrounding environment. Explosions in a confined space result in a higher incidence of primary blast injury, including lung injury.
- All patients with suspected or confirmed BLI should receive supplemental high-flow oxygen sufficient to prevent hypoxemia.
- Impending airway compromise requires immediate intervention.
- If ventilatory failure is imminent or occurs, patients should be intubated; however, prehospital providers must realize that mechanical ventilation and positive pressure may increase the risk of alveolar rupture, pneumothorax, and air embolism in BLI patients.
- High-flow oxygen should be administered if air embolism is suspected, and the patient should be placed in a prone, semi-left lateral, or left lateral position.
- Clinical evidence of or suspicion for a hemothorax or pneumothorax warrants close observation. Chest decompression should be performed for patients clinically presenting with a tension pneumothorax. Close observation is warranted for any patient with suspicion of BLI who is transported by air.
- Fluids should be administered judiciously, as overzealous fluid administration in the patient with BLI may result in volume overload and the worsening of pulmonary status.
- Patients with BLI should be transported rapidly to the nearest, appropriate facility, in accordance with community response plans for mass casualty events.

(From Centers for Disease Control and Prevention, Atlanta.)

Various mortality rates have been associated with different types of bombing. One study that examined 29 terrorist bombings showed that 1 of 4 victims died immediately after structural-collapse bombings, 1 of 12 died immediately in closed-space bombings, and 1 of 25 died immediately after open-space bombings.[14] Additional studies have documented the finding that mortality is higher when an explosion occurs in an enclosed space.[27,28] Soft tissue injuries, orthopedic trauma, and traumatic brain injury (TBI) are predominant among survivors (see Figure 19-8). For example, of 592 survivors of the Oklahoma City bombing, 85% had soft tissue injuries (lacerations, puncture wounds, abrasions, contusions), 25% had sprains, 14% had head injuries, 10% had fractures/dislocations, 10% had ocular injuries (nine with ruptured globes), and 2% had burns.[9] The most common location for soft tissue injury was the extremities (74%), followed by head and neck (48%), face (45%), and chest (35%). Eighteen survivors had severe soft tissue injuries, including carotid artery and jugular vein lacerations, facial and popliteal artery lacera-

FIGURE 19-8 Terrorist Bombings: Patterns of Injury

- Most wounds are noncritical soft tissue or skeletal injuries.
- Head injury predominates among casualties who die (50%–70%).
- Most head injury survivors (98.5%) have noncritical injuries.
- Head injuries are disproportionate to exposed total body surface area.
- Most casualties with blast lung die immediately.
- Survivors have a low incidence of abdominal and chest wounds, burns, traumatic amputations, and blast lung, although specific mortalities are high (10%–40%).

(Modified from Frykberg ER, Tepas JJ III: Terrorist bombings: lessons learned from Belfast to Beirut, *Ann Surg* 208:569, 1988.)

tions, and severed nerves, tendons, and ligaments. Seventeen survivors had serious internal organ injury, including partial bowel transection, lacerated kidney, spleen, and liver, pneumothorax, and pulmonary contusion. Of patients with fractures, 37% had multiple fractures. Of those diagnosed with a head injury, 44% required admission to the hospital.[29]

Evaluation and Management

The general evaluation and management of trauma victims (secondary and tertiary blast injury) are applicable to the WMD patient population and are addressed in other chapters. Unique to this patient population, however, is the possibility of PBI. Primary blast injuries might increase the likelihood that prehospital care providers will encounter patients with hemoptysis and pulmonary contusions, pneumothorax or tension pneumothorax, or even arterial gas embolism. Among survivors of primary blast injury, clinical manifestations may be present immediately[30,31] or may have a delayed onset of 24 to 48 hours.[32] Intrapulmonary hemorrhage and focal alveolar edema result in frothy bloody secretions and lead to ventilation/perfusion mismatch, increased intrapulmonary shunting, and decreased compliance. Hypoxia results, with increased work of breathing, pathophysiologically similar to pulmonary contusions induced by other mechanisms of nonpenetrating thoracic trauma.[33] The presence of rib fractures should increase suspicion of tertiary or quaternary injury to the thorax.

Primary blast injuries are not immediately apparent, and, therefore, care at the scene should include (1) monitoring for frothy secretions and respiratory distress, (2) sequential oxygen saturation (SpO_2) measurements, and (3) provision of oxygen. Decreased SpO_2 is a "red flag" for early blast lung even before symptoms begin. Fluid administration must be carefully managed, with care taken to avoid fluid overload.[1]

The likelihood of multisystem trauma is increased in bomb victims.[34] Management principles are similar to those for trauma from other mechanisms.

Transportation Considerations

Patients requiring transport must be brought to an appropriate medical treatment facility for further evaluation and management. These patients will often require the services of a designated trauma center. Prehospital providers should be aware of the epidemiology of patient transport after these events. Patient arrival at hospitals is usually bimodal, with ambulatory patients arriving first and more critically ill patients arriving later by ambulance. This was demonstrated in the Oklahoma City bombing. Patients began to arrive in the EDs 5 to 30 minutes after the bombing, with patients requiring admission taking longer to arrive. Also, the geographically closest hospitals in Oklahoma City received the majority of victims, as seen with other disasters. Nearby hospitals that are overwhelmed by the first wave of patients may experience some difficulty managing the critically ill patients that arrive in the second wave. In Oklahoma City, the aggregate peak arrival rate of patients to EDs was 220 per hour at 60 to 90 minutes; 64% of patients visited EDs within a 1.5-mile radius of the event. Prehospital

care providers should consider this latter fact when determining the destination of patients from the bomb scene.[1]

Incendiary Agents

Incendiary agents are typically encountered in the military and are used to burn equipment, vehicles, and structures. The three incendiaries recognized most often are thermite, magnesium, and white phosphorus. All three are highly flammable compounds that burn at extremely high temperatures.

Thermite is powdered aluminum and iron oxide that burns furiously at 3600° F (1982° C) and scatters molten iron.[35] Its primary mechanism of injury is partial-thickness or full-thickness burns. The primary and secondary assessment is performed with intervention directed at treating burns. Thermite wounds can be irrigated with copious amounts of water and any residual particles or material subsequently removed.

Magnesium is also a metal in powdered or solid form that burns furiously hot. In addition to its ability to cause second-degree and third-degree burns, magnesium can react with tissue fluid and cause alkali burns. The same chemical reaction produces hydrogen gas, which can cause the wound to bubble or can result in subcutaneous emphysema. Inhalation of magnesium dust can produce respiratory symptoms, including cough, tachypnea, hypoxia, wheeze, pneumonitis, and airway burns. Residual magnesium particles in a wound will react with water, so irrigation is discouraged until the wounds can be debrided and the particulates removed. If irrigation is required for other reasons, such as decontamination of another suspected material, care should be taken to ensure flushing or removal of magnesium particles from the wound.[35]

White phosphorus (WP) is a solid that spontaneously ignites when exposed to air, causing a yellow flame and white smoke. WP that comes in contact with skin can quickly result in second-degree and third-degree burns. WP can become embedded in the skin, propelled by the blast of WP munitions. The substance will continue to burn in the skin if exposed to air. Prehospital care providers can decrease the likelihood of combustion in the skin by immersing the affected areas in water or applying saline-soaked dressings to the area. Oily or greasy dressings are avoided in these patients because WP is lipid soluble, and application of these dressings may increase the likelihood of systemic toxicity. Copper sulfate has historically been used to neutralize WP and facilitate its removal because the reaction resulted in a black compound, which was easier to identify in the skin. Copper sulfate has fallen out of favor, however, because of complications from its use—specifically, intravascular hemolysis.[36]

Chemical Agents

Many scenarios could expose the prehospital care provider to chemical agents, including an industrial complex accident, a spilled tanker truck or railway car, unearthed military ordnance, or a terrorist attack. The 1984 Union Carbide industrial accident in Bhopal, India, and the sarin gas attack in Tokyo in 1995 are examples of such incidents.

Classification of Chemical Agents

Cyanides (blood agents or asphyxiants)
    Hydrogen cyanide, cyanogen chloride
Nerve Agents
    Tabun (GA), sarin (GB), Soman (GD), GF, VX
Lung toxicants (choking or pulmonary agents)
    Chlorine, phosgene, diphosgene, ammonia
Vesicants (blistering agents)
    Mustard, lewisite
Incapacitating agents
    BZ
Lacrimating agents (riot control agents)
    CN, CS
Vomiting agents
    Adamsite

Physical Properties of Hazardous Materials

The physical properties of a substance are affected by its chemical structure, the environmental temperature, and ambient pressure. These factors will determine whether a substance exists as a solid, liquid, or gas. Understanding the physical state of a material is important for the prehospital care provider because it gives clues as to the likely route of exposure and the potential for transmission and contamination.

A *solid* is in a state of matter that has a fixed volume and shape; a powder is an example of a solid. When heated to a melting point, solids become *liquids.* Liquids that are heated to their boiling point become a *gas.* Solid particles and liquid particles can become suspended in the air, similar to a dust particle or a liquid mist. This is considered an *aerosol.* A *vapor* is simply a solid or liquid that is in a gaseous state, but technically would be expected to be found as a solid or liquid at standard temperature and pressure, defined as 32 °F (0° C) and normal atmospheric pressure (1 ATA, 14.7 psi). Some solids and liquids can, therefore, emit vapors at room temperature. When solids emit vapors, bypassing the liquid state, this is called *sublimation.* The likelihood that solids or liquids vaporize into a gaseous form at room temperature is defined as the *volatility* of the substance. Highly volatile substances easily convert into a gas at room temperature.

These physical properties have implications for primary and secondary contamination and possible routes of exposure. *Primary contamination* is defined as exposure to the hazardous substance at its point of release. For example, primary contamination occurs, by definition, in the "hot zone." Gases (vapors), liquids, solids, and aerosols can all play a role in primary contamination. *Secondary contamination* is defined as exposure to the hazardous substance after it has been carried away from the point of origin by a victim, a responder, or a piece of equipment. Secondary contamination generally occurs in the "warm zone," although it may happen at more remote locations if the exposed victim is able to self-evacuate.

Solids and liquids (and sometimes aerosols) generally contribute to secondary contamination. Gases (vapors), which cause injury by inhalation of the substance, do not deposit on skin and, therefore, do not typically play a role in secondary contamination, although vapors can become trapped in clothing.

Volatility plays a significant role in risk of secondary contamination. More volatile substances are considered "less persistent," meaning that because they vaporize, the likelihood of long-lasting physical contamination is unlikely. These agents will readily disperse and be carried away by the wind. Less volatile substances are considered "more persistent." These substances do not vaporize, or do so at a very slow rate, thereby remaining on exposed surfaces for a long time, increasing the risk of secondary contamination. For example, the nerve agent sarin is a non-persistent agent, whereas the nerve agent VX is a persistent agent.[37]

Personal Protective Equipment

Personal protective equipment (PPE) is selected based on the threat of exposure to the hazardous substance. Level A provides respiratory and skin protection from gases (vapors), solids, liquids, and aerosols. This level of protection is appropriate for rescuers entering into the primary contaminated site. Because it also has supplied air, Level A PPE is suitable for oxygen-deprived environments. Level B provides the same respiratory protection as Level A, but only provides skin and splash protection suitable for solids and liquids. Level C provides respiratory protection from selected vapors and aerosols and skin and splash protection from solids and liquids. Level D provides no particular respiratory or skin protection from chemical hazards.

Evaluation and Management

After ensuring the safety of the scene, the prehospital provider will first confirm that victims are undergoing decontamination. Patients with likely skin exposure to the liquid form of a chemical will require decontamination with water. If available, soap may be used as well, but showering with copious amounts of water will generally suffice. Exposure to a gas only does not mandate decontamination, but does mandate removal from any ongoing exposure as well as removal of any clothing that may have trapped residual vapors.

Once the victim has been properly decontaminated, the prehospital care provider will likely encounter patients with signs and symptoms of exposure to a hazardous substance that has not yet been specifically identified. Victims of chemical agents can manifest signs and symptoms of exposure that affect (1) the respiratory system, affecting oxygenation and ventilation; (2) the mucous membranes, causing eye and upper airway injury; (3) the nervous system, resulting in seizures or coma; (4) the gastrointestinal (GI) tract, causing vomiting or diarrhea; and (5) the skin, causing burning and blistering. It is important to evaluate the presenting signs and symptoms and whether or not they are improving or progressing. Patients with worsening clinical findings likely had incomplete cleansing of the contaminant and should undergo repeat decontamination to assure complete removal.

Patients will require a primary survey to determine what lifesaving intervention may be immediately required. A secondary survey may then assist in the identification of symptom constellations that might indicate the nature of the hazardous substance and suggest a specific antidote. This constellation of signs and symptoms has been called a *toxidrome*. A toxidrome is a collection of clinical signs and symptoms that suggest exposure to a certain class of chemical or toxin.[38]

The *irritant gas toxidrome* will include mucous membrane burning and inflammation, coughing, and difficulty breathing. Agents responsible might include chlorine, phosgene, or ammonia.

The *asphyxiant toxidrome* is caused by cellular oxygen deprivation. This can result from inadequate oxygen availability, as in an oxygen-poor atmosphere; inadequate oxygen delivery to the cells, as in carbon monoxide poisoning; or inability to utilize oxygen at the cellular level, as in cyanide poisoning. Signs and symptoms include shortness of breath, chest pain, dysrhythmias, syncope, seizures, coma, and death.

The *cholinergic toxidrome* is characterized by rhinorrhea, respiratory secretions, difficulty breathing, nausea, vomiting, diarrhea, profuse sweating, pinpoint pupils and possible altered mental status, seizures, and coma. Pesticides and nerve agents can cause these cholinergic signs and symptoms.[40,41]

Most often, prehospital care providers will initiate supportive therapy without knowing the specific cause of the injury. If the offending agent is properly identified, or if its identity is suggested by the toxidrome or clinical presentation, therapy specific to the agent may be delivered. Cyanide and nerve-agent victims are examples of patients who can benefit from agent-specific antidote therapy.

Transportation Considerations

Patients must be brought to an appropriate medical treatment facility for further evaluation and management. Communities may identify preferred hospitals for the management of chemical casualties. These facilities may be more capable of managing these patients by virtue of specialized training or availability of critical care services and specific antidotes. Also, considerations similar to those previously noted for explosive incidents, regarding transport epidemiology, also apply to these patients. Nearby EDs may become overwhelmed by ambulatory, self-evacuated, self-transported patients. Of 640 patients presenting to one hospital in Tokyo after the sarin incident, 541 arrived without EMS assistance.[39] Hospitals closest to the event will likely receive the largest number of ambulatory patients. These factors should be considered in determining the destination of casualties transported via ambulance.

Selected Specific Agents

Cyanides. Most commonly, prehospital care providers might encounter cyanides when responding to a fire in which certain plastics are burning or in certain industrial complexes, where it is found in large quantities and used in chemical syntheses, electroplating, mineral extraction, dyeing, printing, photography, and agriculture, and in the manufacture of paper, textiles, and plastics. However, cyanide has been inventoried in military stockpiles and some terrorist websites have provided the instructions for making a cyanide dispersal device.

Hydrogen cyanide is a highly volatile liquid and, thus, will most often be encountered as a vapor or gas. Therefore, it has greater potential for mass casualties in a confined space with poor ventilation than if released outdoors. Although a smell of bitter almonds has been associated with this agent, this is not a reliable indicator of hydrogen cyanide exposure. It is estimated that as much as 40% to 50% of the general population is incapable of detecting the odor of cyanide.

Cyanide's mechanism of action is arrest of metabolism or respiration at the cellular level, quickly resulting in cell death. Cyanide binds in the mitochondria of cells, preventing oxygen usage in cellular metabolism. Victims of cyanide poisoning actually are able to inhale and absorb oxygen into the blood, but are unable to use it at the cellular level. Thus, patients who are ventilating will present with evidence of acyanotic hypoxia.

The organs most affected are the central nervous system (CNS) and the heart. Symptoms of mild cyanide poisoning include headache, dizziness, drowsiness, nausea, vomiting, and mucosal irritation. Severe cyanide poisoning includes alteration of consciousness, dysrhythmias, hypotension, seizures, and death. Death can occur within a few minutes after inhalation of high levels of cyanide gas.

Supportive therapy is important, including high-concentration oxygen delivery, correction of hypotension with fluids or vasopressors, and treatment of seizures. Cyanide antidote kits are available for patients with known or suspected cyanide poisoning. The traditional cyanide antidote treatment involved treatment with two medications, a nitrite followed by thiosulfate. The administration of inhaled amyl nitrite, or preferably intravenous (IV) sodium nitrite, creates methemoglobin (itself a poison which in high enough concentrations can kill), which binds cyanide in the bloodstream, making it less available to poison the victim's cellular respiration. This is followed by IV administration of sodium thiosulfate to assist the body in the conversion of cyanide to harmless thiocyanate, which is excreted by the kidneys. In late 2006, the United States Food and Drug Administration (FDA) approved the use of hydroxocobalamin for treatment of cyanide poisoning. This medication has been used in Europe for over a decade for cyanide therapy. Hydroxocobalamin given intravenously binds with cyanide to form cyanocobalamin (Vitamin B12), which is non-toxic.

Nerve Agents. Nerve agents were originally developed as insecticides, but once their effects on humans were recognized, numerous different types were developed in the early and mid-1900s. These deadly chemicals can be found in the military stockpiles of many nations. The most recent known use in a military conflict was in the Iraq-Iran war of the early 1990s. Nerve agents have also been produced by terrorist organizations, the most notorious releases occurring in Matsumoto (1994) and Tokyo (1995), Japan. Commonly available pesticides (e.g., malathion, Sevin®) and common therapeutic drugs (e.g., physostigmine, pyridostigmine) share properties with nerve agents, causing similar clinical effects.

Nerve agents are usually liquids at room temperature. *Sarin* is the most volatile of the group. *VX* is the least volatile and is found as an oily liquid. The main routes of intoxication are through inhalation of the vapor and absorption through the skin. Nerve agents can injure or kill at very low doses. A single, small drop of VX, the most potent nerve agent, if evenly distributed, could kill 1000 victims. Because nerve agents are liquids, they pose a risk for secondary contamination from contact with contaminated clothes, skin, and other objects.

The mechanism of action of nerve agents is inhibition of the enzyme acetylcholinesterase. This enzyme is necessary to inhibit the action of acetylcholine. *Acetylcholine* is a neurotransmitter that stimulates cholinergic receptors. These receptors are found in smooth muscles, skeletal muscles, the CNS, and most exocrine (secretory) glands. Some of these cholinergic receptors are termed *muscarinic* sites (because experimentally they are stimulated by muscarine), mostly found in smooth muscles and glands. Others are termed *nicotinic* sites (because experimentally they are stimulated by nicotine), mostly found in skeletal muscle. The mnemonic *DUMBELS* (**d**iarrhea, **u**rination, **m**iosis, **b**radycardia, bronchorrhea, bronchospasm, **e**mesis, **l**acrimation, **s**alivation, sweating) represents the constellation of symptoms associated with the muscarinic effects of nerve agent toxicity. The mnemonic *MTWHF* (**m**ydriasis [rarely seen], **t**achycardia, **w**eakness, **h**ypertension, hyperglycemia, **f**asciculations) represents the constellation of symptoms associated with stimulation of nicotinic receptors. The CNS effects, a result of both muscarinic and nicotinic receptors, include confusion, convulsions, and coma.

The clinical effects depend on the dose and route of nerve-agent exposure (inhalation or dermal) and whether the muscarinic or nicotinic effects predominate. Small amounts of vapor exposure primarily cause irritation to eyes, nose, and airways. Large amounts of vapor exposure can quickly lead to loss of consciousness, seizures, apnea, and muscular flaccidity. Miosis (constricted pupils) is the most sensitive marker of exposure to vapor. Symptoms of dermal exposure also vary according to dose and time of onset. Small doses may not result in symptoms for up to 18 hours. Underlying muscle fasciculations and local sweating at the site of the skin exposure may occur, followed by GI symptoms, nausea, vomiting, and diarrhea. Large dermal doses will result in onset of symptoms in minutes, with effects similar to a large vapor exposure.

Clinical symptoms of the nerve agents include rhinorrhea, chest tightness, miosis (pupil is pinpoint, and patient complains of blurry or dim vision), shortness of breath, excessive salivation and sweating, nausea, vomiting, abdominal cramps, involuntary urination and defecation, muscle fasciculations, confusion, seizures, flaccid paralysis, coma, respiratory failure, and death.

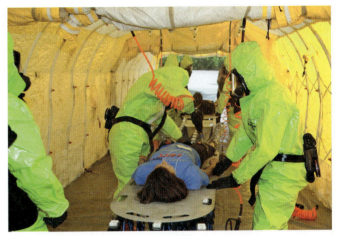

FIGURE 19-9 Decontamination from nerve agents.

Management of nerve-agent poisoning includes decontamination (Figure 19-9), a primary survey, administration of antidotes, and supportive therapy. Ventilation and oxygenation of the patient may be difficult because of bronchoconstriction and copious secretions. The patient will likely require frequent suctioning. These symptoms improve after the antidote is administered. The three therapeutic drugs for the management of nerve-agent poisoning are atropine, pralidoxime chloride, and diazepam.

Atropine is an anticholinergic drug that reverses most of the muscarinic effects of the nerve agent but has little effect on the nicotinic sites. Atropine is indicated for exposed victims with pulmonary complaints. Miosis alone is not an indication for atropine, and furthermore, atropine will not correct the ocular abnormalities. Atropine will be given according to system protocols. Atropine is titrated until the patient's ability to breathe or ventilate is improved or there is drying of pulmonary secretions. In moderate to severe exposures, it is not unusual to give 10 to 20 mg of atropine over a few hours.

Pralidoxime chloride (2-PAM chloride) is an oxime. Pralidoxime works by uncoupling the bond between the nerve agent and acetylcholinesterase, thereby reactivating the enzyme and helping to reduce the effects of the nerve agent, primarily on nicotinic receptors. The oxime therapy needs to be initiated within minutes to a few hours of the exposure to be effective, depending on the nerve agent released; otherwise, the bond between acetylcholinesterase and the nerve agent will become permanent ("aging"), delaying recovery of the patient.

Diazepam (Valium™) is a benzodiazepine and anticonvulsant. If patients develop seizures after significant exposure, benzodiazepine therapy is initiated to manage the seizures and help to reduce the brain injury and other life-threatening effects associated with status epilepticus. Diazepam given intramuscularly has erratic absorption; therefore, the preferred route for patients who are actively seizing is intravenous if access is available. In addition, diazepam administration is recommended for all patients with signs of severe nerve-agent poisoning, whether or not they have begun to

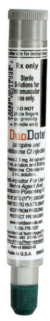

FIGURE 19-10 DuoDote™

seize. There are no data in either humans or animals for rectal administration of diazepam.[42] Lorazepam (Ativan™) has been studied in animal models and found to be less effective than diazepam.[42] Midazolam (Versed™), on the other hand, has been shown to be effective in animal models and, in the future, may become the first line medication for nerve-agent induced seizures.[43]

All three of these medications are available and packaged as autoinjectors. The Mark-1 kit supplies two autoinjectors, one filled with atropine (2 mg) and one filled with pralidoxime chloride (600 mg). These are intended for rapid intramuscular (IM) injection in the event of a nerve-agent exposure. Dosage is determined by protocol and titration of these drugs to effect. Diazepam is also available as an autoinjector. Recently, the manufacturer of the Mark-1 kit developed a single autoinjector that includes both the atropine and the pralidoxime in a single device (Figure 19-10, DuoDote™).

Lung Toxicants. Lung toxicants, including chlorine, phosgene, ammonia, sulfur dioxide, and nitrogen dioxide, are present in numerous industrial manufacturing applications. *Phosgene* has been stockpiled for military applications and was the most lethal chemical warfare agent used in World War I.

Chemical pulmonary agents may be gases (vapors) or aerosolized liquids or solids. The properties of the agent influence its ability to cause injury. For example, aerosolized particles of 2 microns (μm) or smaller readily access the alveoli of the lung, causing injury there, whereas larger particles are filtered out before reaching the alveoli. Water solubility of an agent also affects the injury pattern. Ammonia and sulfur dioxide, which are highly water soluble, cause irritation and injury to the eyes, mucous membranes, and upper airways. Phosgene and nitrogen oxides, which have low water solubility, tend to cause less immediate irritation and injury to the eyes, mucous membranes, and upper air-

ways, thus providing little warning to the victim and allowing for prolonged exposure to these agents. Prolonged exposure makes it more likely that the alveoli will be injured, resulting not only in upper-airway injury, but also in alveolar collapse and noncardiogenic pulmonary edema. Moderately water-soluble agents, such as chlorine, can cause both upper airway and alveolar irritation.

The mechanisms of injury vary among the lung toxicants. Ammonia, for example, combines with the water in the mucous membranes to form a strong base, ammonium hydroxide. Chlorine and phosgene, when combined with water, produce hydrochloric acid, causing injury to the tissues. Lung toxicants are not systemically absorbed but compromise the victim by damaging components of the pulmonary system, from the upper airway to the alveoli.

The agents with high water solubility cause burning of the eyes, nose, and mouth. Tearing, rhinorrhea, coughing, dyspnea, and respiratory distress secondary to glottic irritation or laryngospasm are possible. Bronchospasm can result in coughing, wheezing, and dyspnea. Agents with low water solubility, causing injury to the alveoli, can immediately injure the alveolar epithelium in the case of a large exposure, leading to death from acute respiratory failure or, with less massive exposure, can result in a delayed onset (24–48 hours) of respiratory distress, secondary to development of mild noncardiogenic pulmonary edema to fulminant acute respiratory distress syndrome (ARDS), depending on the dose.

Management of lung toxicants includes removal of the patient from the offending agent, decontamination with copious irrigation (if solid, liquid, or aerosol exposure, especially for ammonia), primary survey, and supportive therapy, which will likely require interventions to maximize ventilation and oxygenation. Eye irritation can be managed with copious irrigation using normal saline. Contact lenses should be removed. Expect to manage copious airway secretions, which will require suctioning. Bronchospasm may respond to inhaled β-adrenergic agonists. Hypoxia will require correction with high-flow oxygen and possibly intubation with positive-pressure ventilation. Prehospital care providers need to be prepared to encounter difficult airway management secondary to copious secretions, inflammation of glottic structures, and laryngeal spasm.

Vesicant Agents. The vesicants include sulfur mustard, nitrogen mustards, and lewisite. These agents have been stockpiled for military operations by many countries. Sulfur mustard was first introduced to the battlefield in World War I. It was reportedly used by Iraq against its Kurdish population and also in its conflict with Iran (1980). It is relatively easy and inexpensive to manufacture.

Sulfur mustard is an oily, clear to yellow-brown liquid that can be aerosolized by a bomb blast or a sprayer. Its volatility is low, allowing it to persist on surfaces for a week or more. This allows for easy secondary contamination. The agent is absorbed through the skin and mucous membranes, resulting in direct cellular damage within minutes of the exposure, although clinical symptoms make take 1 to 12 hours (usually 4–6 hours) after exposure to develop. The delayed onset of symptoms often makes it difficult for the victim to recognize that the exposure occurred and, therefore, increases the potential for secondary contamination. Warm, moist skin increases the likelihood of skin absorption, making the groin and axillary regions particularly susceptible. The eyes, skin, and upper airways can develop a range of findings, from erythema and edema to vesicle development and necrosis. Upper airway involvement can result in cough and bronchospasm. High-dose exposures can result in nausea and vomiting, as well as bone marrow suppression.

Treatment involves decontamination, primary survey, and supportive therapy; no antidote exists for the effects of mustard agents. Eyes and skin should be decontaminated with copious amounts of water as soon as exposure is recognized to minimize further absorption of the agent and prevent secondary contamination. Absorbed agent cannot be decontaminated and will result in cellular injury. The fluid in resulting vesicles and blisters is not a source of secondary contamination. Pulmonary bronchoconstriction may benefit from nebulized β-agonists. Skin wounds should be treated as burns, with regard to local wound care.

Lewisite has a similar constellation of symptoms, but the onset of action is much quicker than with sulfur mustard, resulting in immediate pain and irritation to the eyes, skin, and respiratory tract. Unlike mustard, Lewisite does not cause bone marrow suppression. Also unique to this agent is "Lewisite shock," the result of intravascular volume depletion secondary to capillary leak. As with mustard, prehospital treatment of these exposed patients involves decontamination, primary survey, and supportive care. British anti-lewisite (BAL) is an antidote available for the in-hospital treatment of lewisite-exposed patients. It is administered intravenously for patients with hypovolemic shock or pulmonary symptoms. Applied topically, BAL ointment has been reported to prevent mucous membrane and skin injury.

Biologic Agents

Biologic agents in the form of contagious disease represent a threat to prehospital care providers on a daily basis. Proper infection control procedures must be in place to prevent the contraction or transmission of tuberculosis, influenza, human immunodeficiency virus (HIV), methicillin-resistant staphylococci (MRSA), SARS, and a myriad of other organisms.

Preparing for bioterrorist events increases the complexity of EMS system preparation. An intentional terrorist act might include delivery of a hazardous agent with the potential to cause disease or illness, such as aerosolized spores, aerosolized live organisms, or an aerosolized biologic toxin. Patients with pathogens not typically seen by EMS personnel, such as plague, anthrax, and smallpox, might be encountered, requiring appropriate PPE and precautions. Familiar infection control procedures will be effective in the safe management of these potentially contagious patients. If the prehospital care provider is responding to an overt event, appropriate precautions regarding decontamination of victims and PPE are required, similar to other hazmat events.

Classification of Biologic Agents

Bacterial agents
    Anthrax
    Brucellosis
    Glanders
    Plague
    Q fever
    Tularemia
Viral agents
    Smallpox
    Venezuelan equine encephalitis
    Viral hemorrhagic fevers
Biologic toxins
    Botulinum
    Ricin
    Staphylococcal enterotoxin B
    T-2 mycotoxins

Concentrated Biohazard Agent versus Infected Patient

Prehospital care providers can experience bioterrorism in two forms. The first scenario involves the overt release of a material that is either identified as or thought to be a biologic agent. In this situation, the provider will encounter an environment or a patient contaminated with a suspicious substance. EMS services may be summoned to suspicious activity, such as a device delivering an unknown aerosol agent. The nature of the threat at these events is usually unknown, and precautions for personal safety should always be paramount. These events must be respected as hazmat events until characterized otherwise. If the suspicious substance is in fact a concentrated aerosol of an infectious organism or toxin, PPE appropriate for the hazard and decontamination are required. The anthrax hoaxes of 1998 and 1999 and the anthrax letters of 2001 are good examples. Prehospital providers responded on countless occasions to individuals covered in "white powder" or suspected anthrax.

In this situation, prehospital care providers will not be caring for patients with the clinical disease, but rather victims contaminated with suspected biologic agent on their skin or clothing. Any person coming in direct physical contact with a substance alleged to be a biologic should remove articles of clothing and perform a thorough washing of exposed skin with soap and water.[44] Clinically significant re-aerosolization of material from victims' skin or clothing is unlikely, and the risk to the provider is negligible.[45] As a matter of routine practice, however, clothing normally removed by pulling over the face and head should instead be cut off to minimize any risk of inadvertent inhalation of contaminant. Decontamination may then proceed using water or soap and water. Consultation with appropriate public health and law enforcement officials will then determine the need for antibiotic prophylaxis.

The second scenario involves a response to a patient who has been a victim of a remote, covert bioterrorist event. Perhaps an individual inhaled anthrax spores after a covert attack at work and now, several days later, is manifesting signs of pulmonary anthrax. Perhaps a terrorist has inoculated himself or herself with smallpox, and you are summoned to assist the victim with a suspicious rash. In these cases, personal and public safety can be assured by knowledge of proper infection control procedures and the proper donning and removal of PPE appropriate for the biohazard (Figure 19-11 and Figure 19-12). Decontamination of the patient in this scenario is not necessary because the exposure occurred several days in the past.

All prehospital care providers should be familiar with PPE for infection-control purposes. Different types of PPE are recommended, depending on the potential for transmission and the likely route of transmission. Transmission-based PPE is used in addition to the Standard Precautions, which are used in the care of all patients. These include contact, droplet, and aerosol precautions.

Contact Precautions. This level of protection is recommended to reduce the likelihood of transmission of microorganisms by direct or indirect contact. Contact precautions include the use of gloves and a gown. Commonly encountered organisms that require contact precautions include viral conjunctivitis, methicillin-resistant staphylococci, scabies, and herpes simplex or zoster virus. Organisms that might be encountered as a result of bioterrorism include bubonic plague or the viral hemorrhagic fevers, such as Marburg or Ebola, as long as the patient does not have pulmonary symptoms or profuse vomiting and diarrhea.

FIGURE 19-11 Sequence for Donning Personal Protective Equipment (PPE)

The type of PPE used will vary based on the level of precautions required (e.g., Standard Precautions and contact, droplet, or airborne infection isolation).

1. GOWN
   - Fully cover torso from neck to knees, arms to end of wrists, and wrap around the back
   - Fasten in back of neck and waist

2. MASK OR RESPIRATOR
   - Secure ties or elastic bands at middle of head and neck
   - Fit flexible band to nose bridge
   - Fit snug to face and below chin
   - Fit/check respirator

3. GOGGLES OR FACE SHIELD
   - Place over face and eyes and adjust to fit

4. GLOVES
   - Extend to cover wrist of isolation gown

   Use safe work practices to protect yourself and limit the spread of contamination:

   - Keep hands away from face
   - Limit surfaces touched
   - Change gloves when torn or heavily contaminated
   - Perform hand hygiene From Centers for Disease Control and Prevention, Atlanta.

(From Centers for Disease Control and Prevention, Atlanta.)

FIGURE 19-12 Sequence for Removing Personal Protective Equipment (PPE)

Except for the respirator, remove PPE at doorway or in an anteroom. Remove respirator after leaving patient room and closing door.

1. GLOVES
   - Outside of glove is contaminated!
   - Grasp outside of glove with opposite gloved hand; peel off
   - Hold removed glove in gloved hand
   - Slide fingers of ungloved hand under remaining glove at wrist
   - Peel glove off over first glove
   - Discard gloves in waste container

2. GOGGLES
   - Outside of goggles or face shield is contaminated!
   - To remove, handle by head band or ear pieces
   - Place in designated receptacle for reprocessing or in waste container

3. GOWN
   - Gown front and sleeves are contaminated!
   - Unfasten gown ties
   - Pull away from neck and shoulders, touching inside of gown only
   - Turn gown inside out
   - Fold or roll into a bundle and discard

4. MASK OR RESPIRATOR
   - Front of mask/respirator is contaminated—do not touch!
   - Grasp bottom, then top ties or elastics, and remove
   - Discard in waste container

(From Centers for Disease Control and Prevention, Atlanta.)

Droplet Precautions. This level of protection is recommended to reduce the likelihood of transmission of microorganisms that are known to be transmitted by large droplet nuclei (>5 μm) expelled by an infected person in the course of talking, sneezing, or coughing or during routine procedures, such as suctioning. These droplets infect the susceptible individual by landing on the exposed mucous membranes of the eye and mouth. Because the droplets are large, they do not remain suspended in air, and therefore, contact must be in close proximity, usually defined as 3 feet or less. Droplet precautions include the gloves and gown of contact precautions, but also add eye protection and a surgical mask. Because the droplets do not remain suspended in air, no additional respiratory protection or air filtration is required. Typically encountered organisms in this category include influenza, mycoplasma pneumonia, and invasive *Haemophilus influenzae* or *Neisseria meningitidis,* causing sepsis or meningitis. Pneumonic plague is an example of a possible agent encountered as a result of a bioterrorist event.

Aerosol Precautions. This level of protection is recommended to reduce the likelihood of transmission of microorganisms by the airborne route. Some organisms can become suspended in the air attached to small droplet nuclei (<5 μm) or attached to dust particles. In this case, microorganisms can become widely dispersed by air currents immediately around the source or far from the source, depending on conditions. These patients are kept in isolation rooms in which the exhaust ventilation can be filtered. Aerosol precautions include gloves, gown, eye protection, and a fit-tested high-efficiency particulate air (HEPA) filter mask, such as the N-95. Examples of illnesses typically encountered include tuberculosis, measles, chickenpox, and SARS. Smallpox and viral hemorrhagic fever with pulmonary symptoms are examples that could possibly be related to a bioterrorist event.

Note that many illnesses associated with bioterrorist events require no additional protection beyond Standard Precautions, provided there is no risk of exposure to a concentrated agent. Examples include patients with inhalational anthrax or a biologic toxin such as botulinum. However, in most cases, the specific biologic agent will likely not be identified for several days. Although some such as anthrax are not spread from person-to-person, providers must assume the worst—that the agent is contagious and, therefore, use all available precautions including standard and aerosol precautions.

Selected Agents

Anthrax. Anthrax is a disease caused by the bacterium *Bacillus anthracis. B. anthracis* is a spore-forming bacterium and, thus, can exist as a vegetative cell or as a spore. The vegetative cell lives well in a host organism but cannot survive long outside the body, unlike the spore, which can be viable in the environment for decades.

The disease is naturally occurring, contracted most often by persons in contact with infected animals or anthrax-contaminated animal products resulting in the cutaneous

form of the disease. The spores have been weaponized and are known to be inventoried in several nations' military stockpiles. The accidental release of aerosolized anthrax spores from a Soviet military facility at Sverdlovsk in 1979 resulted in approximately 79 cases of pulmonary anthrax with 68 reported deaths. Letters contaminated with anthrax spores were sent through the US mail in 2001 to prominent legislators and media outlets. Although only 22 cases (11 pulmonary, 11 cutaneous) and five deaths resulted, thousands required prophylaxis with antibiotics. An efficient release of 100 kg of anthrax spores over Washington, DC, is reported to be capable of causing 130,000 to 3 million deaths.[46]

Routes of exposure to anthrax include the respiratory tract, the GI tract, and breaks in the skin. Exposure to anthrax through the respiratory tract leads to inhalational or pulmonary anthrax. Exposure through the GI tract causes gastrointestinal anthrax, and skin exposure causes cutaneous anthrax.

Gastrointestinal anthrax is rare and would result from ingesting food substances contaminated with spores. Patients would have nonspecific symptoms of nausea, vomiting, malaise, bloody diarrhea, and acute abdomen; mortality is approximately 50%. Cutaneous anthrax follows deposition of spores or organisms into a break in the skin. This results in a papule, which subsequently ulcerates and causes a dry, black eschar with local edema. If not treated with antibiotics, mortality approaches 20%; with antibiotics, mortality is less than 1%.

For maximal effectiveness in a terrorist attack, anthrax would likely be disseminated in its spore form. Anthrax spores are approximately 1 to 5 μm in size, which allows the spores to be suspended in air as an aerosol. Aerosolized spores can be inhaled into the lungs and deposited in the alveoli. They are then consumed by macrophages and carried to the mediastinal lymph nodes, where they germinate, manufacture toxins, and cause acute hemorrhagic mediastinitis and often death. The onset of symptoms after inhalation of spores varies, with most victims developing symptoms within 1 to 7 days, although there may be a latency period as long as 60 days. Symptoms initially are nonspecific, including fever, chills, dyspnea, cough, chest pain, headache, and vomiting. After a few days, symptoms improve, followed by a rapidly deteriorating course of fever, dyspnea, diaphoresis, shock, and death.[44,47,48] Before the 2001 anthrax attacks, mortality from inhalational anthrax was thought to be 90%, but recent experience suggests that with early antibiotic therapy and critical care services, mortality may be less than 50%.[49]

Inhalational anthrax is not contagious and does not pose a risk to the prehospital care provider. Only exposure to aerosolized spores poses a risk of infectivity. Caring for patients known to be infected with inhalational anthrax requires only Standard Precautions; however, if the specific agent is unknown, standard and aerosol precautions are warranted. The prehospital care provider will provide supportive therapy and transport ill patients to facilities in which critical care services are available.

Prophylaxis with antibiotics is only required for individuals who have been exposed to spores. Local public health officials will determine the appropriate antibiotic and length of prophylactic treatment. The latest recommendations suggest 60 days of therapy with oral doxycycline or a quinolone antibiotic.

An anthrax vaccine does exist, and an immunization program for US military forces was instituted in 1998. The current regimen requires a series of six initial shots and annual boosters. It is currently recommended only for military personnel and for laboratory and industrial workers at high risk for exposure to spores.

Plague. Plague is a disease caused by the bacterium *Yersinia pestis.* It is naturally occurring, found in fleas and rodents. If an infected flea bites a human, the person can develop *bubonic plague.* If this local infection goes untreated, the patient can become systemically ill, resulting in septicemia and death. A number of patients may proceed to develop pulmonary symptoms *(pneumonic plague).* Plague was responsible for the "Black Death" of 1346, which killed 20 to 30 million people in Europe, approximately one third of its population at that time. *Y. pestis* has been weaponized for military stockpiles with techniques developed to aerosolize the organism directly, bypassing the animal vector. The World Health Organization (WHO) reports that in a worst-case scenario, 50 kg of *Y. pestis,* released as an aerosol over a city of 5 million, would result in 150,000 cases of pneumonic plague and 36,000 deaths.[50]

Naturally occurring plague, resulting from the bite of an infected flea, will cause symptoms in 2 to 8 days, with onset of fever, chills, weakness, and acutely swollen lymph nodes (buboes) in the neck, groin, or axilla. Untreated patients can deteriorate to systemic illness and death. Twelve percent have been described as developing pneumonic plague, with complaints of chest pain, dyspnea, cough, and hemoptysis, and these patients can also succumb from systemic illness.

Plague occurring from terrorist deployment of a weapon will likely result from aerosolized organisms, and thus, it will clinically present as the pneumonic form of the disease. Inhalation of *Y. pestis* aerosol will result in symptoms in 1 to 6 days. Patients will present with fever, cough, and dyspnea, with bloody or watery sputum. They may also develop nausea, vomiting, diarrhea, and abdominal pain. Buboes are not typically present. Without antibiotics, death occurs in 2 to 6 days after development of respiratory symptoms.[51]

Currently, no vaccine is available to protect from pneumonic plague. Treatment of the disease includes antimicrobial and supportive therapy, often requiring critical care services. Antibiotic regimens are also recommended for individuals with unprotected close exposure to patients with known pneumonic plague.

Patients with plague represent a communicable disease risk. If patients present with only cutaneous signs and symptoms (bubonic plague), contact precautions are adequate to protect the prehospital care provider. If patients present with pulmonary signs of plague (pneumonic plague), a more likely scenario after a terrorist attack, providers will be required to wear PPE suitable for respiratory droplet protection. Droplet precautions include a surgical mask, eye protection, gloves, and gown. Prehospital care providers responding to the scene of an overt *Y. pestis* aerosol delivery, which is unlikely to be a recognized event, would require PPE suitable for a hazmat environment if entering the hot zone or warm zone.

Plague victims are treated in the field with supportive therapy. Communication with the receiving facility is vital before arrival to ensure that the pneumonic plague patient can be properly isolated in the ED and that staff are prepared with the appropriate PPE. Asking the patient to wear a surgical mask, if tolerated, may also decrease the likelihood of secondary transmission.

Decontamination of the vehicle and equipment is similar to that required after transport of any patient with communicable disease. Contact surfaces should be wiped down with disinfectant approved by the Environmental Protection Agency (EPA) or 1:1000 diluted bleach solution. There is no evidence to suggest that *Y. pestis* poses a long-term environmental threat after dissolution of the primary aerosol.[51] The organism is sensitive to heat and sunlight and does not last long outside the living host. *Y. pestis* does not form spores.

Smallpox. Smallpox is also known as *variola major* and *variola minor.* This naturally occurring viral disease was eradicated in 1977 but still exists in at least two laboratories—Russia's Institute of Virus Preparations and the US Centers for Disease Control and Prevention (CDC). It has been alleged that the Soviet government began a program in 1980 to produce large quantities of smallpox virus for use in bombs and missiles, as well as to develop more virulent strains of the virus for military purposes. There is concern that smallpox virus may have changed hands after the dissolution of the Soviet Union.[52]

The smallpox virus infects its victim by entering the mucous membranes of the oropharynx or respiratory mucosa. After a 12- to 14-day incubation period, the patient develops fever, malaise, headache, and backache. The patient then develops a maculopapular rash that starts on the oral mucosa, but quickly progresses to a generalized skin rash with characteristic round, tense vesicles and pustules. The rash tends to affect the head and extremities more densely than the trunk (centrifugal), with the stage of the lesions appearing uniform (Figure 19-13). This distinguishes smallpox from *varicella,* or chickenpox (Figure 19-14), which begins on and is more dense on the trunk (centripetal) and has lesions at various stages of development (new lesions appear with older, crusted lesions) (Figure 19-15). Mortality from naturally occurring smallpox was approximately 30%. Little is known about the natural course of the disease in immunocompromised patients, such as those with HIV.

Smallpox is a contagious disease that is primarily spread by droplet nuclei projected from the oropharynx of infected patients and by direct contact. Contaminated clothing and bed linens can also spread the virus. Patients are contagious

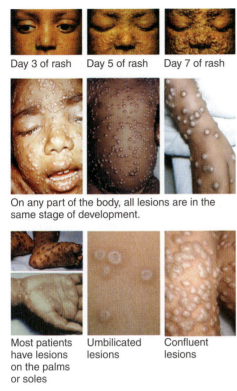

FIGURE 19-13 Smallpox.
(Courtesy Centers for Disease Control and Prevention, Atlanta.)

FIGURE 19-14 **Differentiating Chickenpox from Smallpox**

Chickenpox (varicella) is the most likely condition to be confused with smallpox.

In chickenpox:
- No prodrome or mild prodrome
- Lesions are superficial vesicles: "dewdrop on a rose petal"
- Lesions appear in crops; on any one part of the body, there are lesions in different stages (papules, vesicles, crusts)
- Centripetal distribution: greatest concentration of lesions on the trunk, fewest lesions on distal extremities. Lesions may involve the face/scalp; occasionally, entire body equally affected
- First lesions appear on the face or trunk
- Patients rarely toxic or moribund
- Rapid evolution: lesions evolve from macules→papules→vesicles→crusts quickly (<24 hours)
- Palms and soles rarely involved
- Patient lacks reliable history of varicella or varicella vaccination
- From 50% to 80% of patients recall an exposure to chickenpox or shingles 10 to 21 days before rash onset

(Courtesy Centers for Disease Control and Prevention, Atlanta.)

beginning slightly before the onset of the rash, although this might not always be obvious if the rash is subtle in the oropharynx. When managing a patient with smallpox, prehospital providers must wear PPE appropriate for contact, droplet, and aerosol precautions. This includes N-95 mask, eye protection, goggles, and gown. Ideally, persons managing patients with smallpox will have been immunized.[53]

The smallpox vaccination program in the United States was stopped in 1972. The residual immunity provided by this vaccination program is unknown, and it is suggested that individuals whose last immunization was 40 years ago will likely now be susceptible to contracting smallpox.[52] Vaccination for the smallpox virus is available to certain US Department of Defense and State Department members. It is also made available under a Department of Health and Human Services program to develop public health Smallpox Response Teams. It is currently only available to the general public for participants in clinical trials. In case of a public health emergency, the United States has stockpiles of vaccine that can be released for mass immunization of the public. Vaccination within 4 days of the exposure has been shown to offer some protection against contracting the illness and substantial protection against a fatal outcome.[52]

Prehospital care providers will provide supportive care to manage a patient with smallpox. The recommended PPE must be worn at all times, and it is imperative that there is no breach in infection-control procedures. Hospitals with

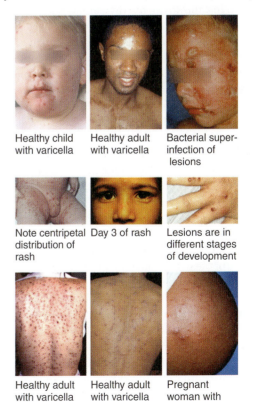

FIGURE 19-15 Chickenpox.
(Courtesy Centers for Disease Control and Prevention, Atlanta.)

the appropriate isolation facilities and properly trained staff should be identified in the community. The receiving facility must be contacted to inform the staff of the intention to transport the confirmed or suspected case of smallpox to their facility so that proper precautions can be taken to prevent transmission of the virus. The identification of a patient with smallpox will be considered a public health emergency of enormous significance.

Proper removal of PPE without breach in infection control procedures is important for the safety of the prehospital care provider. All contaminated disposable medical waste must be properly bagged, labelled, and disposed of as other regulated medical waste. Reusable medical equipment must be cleaned after use according to standard protocol, either autoclaved or subject to high-level disinfection. Environmental surfaces need to be cleaned only by an approved EPA-registered detergent-disinfectant. Air decontamination or fumigation of the emergency vehicle is not required.[54]

Botulinum Toxin. Botulinum toxin is produced by the bacterium *Clostridium botulinum* and is the most poisonous substance known. It is 15,000 times more toxic than the nerve agent VX and 100,000 times more toxic than sarin.[55] The Aum Shinrikyo cult, responsible for the Tokyo subway sarin attack, attempted to deliver an aerosol of botulinum toxin without success in 1995. Botulinum toxin has been weaponized for military use. Despite the reported difficulty of concentrating and stabilizing the toxin for dissemination, it is estimated that a terrorist point-source delivery of botulinum aerosol could incapacitate or kill 10% of persons downwind 0.5 km (0.3 mile). The toxin could also be introduced into the food supply in an attempt to poison large numbers of people.

Three forms of botulism exist naturally. *Wound botulism* occurs when toxins are absorbed from a dirty wound, often with devitalized tissue, in which *C. botulinum* is present. *Food-borne botulism* occurs when improperly canned foods allow the bacteria to grow and produce toxin, which is ingested by the victim. *Intestinal botulism* occurs when toxin is produced and absorbed within the GI tract. The fourth and man-made form of botulism is a result of aerosolized botulinum toxin, causing *inhalational botulism.*

Regardless of the route, botulinum toxin is carried to the neuromuscular junction where it binds irreversibly, preventing binding of the neurotransmitter acetylcholine and causing a descending flaccid paralysis. Onset of symptoms is several hours to a few days. All patients will present with diplopia (double vision) and multiple cranial nerve deficits, causing difficulty with sight, speech, and swallowing. The extent and rapidity of the descending paralysis depend on the dose of the toxin. Patients become fatigued, lose the ability to control the muscle from fallout of the head and neck, may lose their gag reflex, or may progress to paralysis of the muscles of respiration and develop respiratory failure, requiring intubation and months of mechanical ventilation. Untreated patients usually die of mechanical upper airway obstruction or inadequate ven-

tilation. The classic triad of botulinum toxicity is (1) descending symmetric flaccid paralysis with cranial nerve deficits, (2) afebrile, and (3) a clear sensorium. After weeks to months, patients may recover as new axon buds develop to innervate the denervated muscles.

Care for the patient with botulism is supportive, with administration of antitoxin. Early use of antitoxin will minimize further deterioration but cannot reverse existing paralysis. This antitoxin is available from the CDC.

Prehospital providers caring for victims of botulism need to be vigilant about airway compromise and inadequate ventilation. Patients may not be able to manage their secretions or maintain a patent airway. Because of diaphragm paralysis, patients may not be able to generate an adequate tidal volume. This may be exacerbated by having the patient in a supine or semi-recumbent position. Patients experiencing respiratory difficulty should be intubated and adequately ventilated.

Standard Precautions are adequate for the management of patients experiencing the effects of botulinum toxicity because it is not a contagious disease. Botulism aerosols degrade readily in the environment, and it is anticipated that after delivery in a terrorist incident, substantial inactivation will occur after 2 days. Prehospital care providers responding to an overt aerosol dissemination event will require PPE suitable for a hazmat environment if working in the hot zone or warm zone. Because the aerosol can persist for approximately 2 days under average weather conditions, victims who have been exposed to botulinum aerosol require decontamination by clothing removal and washing with soap and water. Equipment can be decontaminated using a 0.1% hypochlorite bleach solution.[56] Patients will not require isolation after arrival at the hospital, but critical care services may be needed for patients requiring mechanical ventilation.

Radiologic Disasters

Since the terrorist attacks of September 11, 2001, new consideration has been given to the likelihood of EMS systems needing to manage a radiologic emergency. Historically, planning has focused on civil-service preparation for a strategic exchange of military nuclear weapons or the rare occurrence of a nuclear power plant accident. Currently, however, there is increasing awareness of the possibility that terrorists could deploy an improvised nuclear detonation device, or perhaps more likely a radiologic dispersal device, that uses conventional explosives to disseminate radioactive material into the environment.

Although radiologic accidents are rare, there have been 243 radiation accidents since 1944 in the United States with 1342 casualties that met criteria for significant exposure. Worldwide, 403 accidents have occurred, with 133,617 victims, 2965 with significant exposure, and 120 fatalities. The Chernobyl disaster was responsible for 116,500 to 125,000 exposed casualties and close to 50 deaths as of 2005, although it is estimated that the total number of deaths could reach as many as 4,000 as additional cancer victims succumb.[57, 58,]

Radiation disasters have the potential to generate fear and confusion in both victims and responders. Familiarization with the hazard and management principles will help to ensure an appropriate response and help to reduce panic and disorder (Figure 19-16).

Exposure to ionizing radiation and radioactive contamination may result from several different scenarios: (1) detonation of a nuclear weapon, whether high grade or an improvised low-yield device; (2) detonation of a "dirty bomb" or radiation dispersion device (RDD), in which there is no nuclear detonation, but rather conventional explosives are detonated to disperse a radionuclide; (3) sabotage or accident at a nuclear reactor site; and (4) mishandled nuclear waste.

Medical Effects of Radiation Catastrophes

The injuries and risks associated with a radiologic catastrophe will be multifactorial. In the case of a nuclear detonation, casualties will be produced by the explosion, resulting in primary, secondary, and tertiary blast injuries, thermal injury, and structural collapse. Victims may be further subject to radiation injury from irradiation; from external radioactive contamination, which can be deposited on skin and clothing from fallout; or from internal radiation through radioactive particulate contamination, which victims may inhale, ingest, or have deposited in wounds.

Accidents at nuclear reactors can generate large doses of ionizing radiation, without a nuclear detonation, especially under circumstances in which the reactor reaches a point of "criticality." Explosions, fire, and gas release can also result in radioactive gas or particulate matter, which may expose responders to risk of exposure to contamination with radioactive particles.

Radiation dispersion devices (RDDs) typically would not deliver enough radiation to cause immediate injury. However, RDDs would complicate management for prehospital care responders by distributing radioactive particulates that could contaminate victims and responders and make it difficult to manage the injuries caused by the conventional explosive. RDDs could cause confusion and panic among responders concerned about radioactivity, hindering efforts to assist victims.

Ionizing radiation causes injury to cells by interacting with atoms and depositing energy. This interaction results in *ionization*, which can either damage the cell nucleus directly, causing cell death or malfunction, or indirectly, damaging cell components by interacting with water in the body and resulting in toxic molecules. Acute exposure to large doses of penetrating ionizing radiation (irradiation with gamma rays and neutrons) in a short time can result in acute radiation illness. Types of ionizing radiation include alpha particles, beta particles, gamma rays, and neutrons.

Alpha particles are relatively large and cannot penetrate even a few layers of skin. Intact skin or a uniform offers adequate protection from external contamination emitting alpha particles. Ionizing radiation from alpha particles is a concern only if it is internalized by inhaling or ingesting alpha-particle emitters. When internalized, alpha-particle radiation can cause significant local cellular injury to adjacent cells.

Beta particles are small charged particles that can penetrate more deeply than alpha particles and can affect deeper layers of the skin with the ability to injure the base of the skin, causing a "beta burn." Beta-particle radiation is found most frequently in nuclear fallout. Beta particles also result in local radiation injury.

Gamma rays are similar to x-rays and have the ability to easily penetrate tissue. Gamma rays are emitted with a

---

FIGURE 19-16	Principles of Management of a Radiologic Disaster

1. Assess the scene for safety.
2. All patients should be medically stabilized from their traumatic injuries before radiation injuries are considered. Patients are then evaluated for their external radiation exposure and contamination.
3. An external source of radiation, if great enough, can cause tissue injury, but it does not make the patient radioactive. Patients with even lethal exposures to external radiation are not a threat to medical staff.
4. Patients can become contaminated with radioactive material deposited on their skin or clothing. More than 90% of surface contamination can be removed by removal of clothing. The remainder can be washed off with soap and water.
5. Protect yourself from radioactive contamination by observing, at a minimum, Standard Precautions, including protective clothing, gloves, and a mask.
6. Patients who develop nausea, vomiting, or skin erythema within 4 hours of exposure have likely received a high external radiation exposure.
7. Radioactive contamination in wounds should be treated as dirt and irrigated as soon as possible. Avoid handling any metallic foreign body.
8. Potassium iodine (KI) is only of value if there has been a release of radioactive iodine. KI is not a general radiation antidote.
9. The concept of time/distance/shielding is key in the prevention of untoward effects from radiation exposure. Radiation exposure is minimized by *decreasing time* in the affected area, *increasing distance* from a radiation source, and using metal or concrete *shielding*.

(Modified from Department of Homeland Security Working Group on Radiological Dispersion Device Preparedness/Medical Preparedness and Response Subgroup, 2004, http://www1.va.gov/emshg/docs/Radiologic_Medical_Countermeasures_051403.pdf.)

nuclear detonation and with fallout. They can also be emitted from some radionuclides that might be present in an RDD. Gamma radiation can result in what is termed *whole-body exposure*. Whole-body exposure can result in acute radiation illness (Figures 19-17, 19-18, and 19-19).

Neutrons can penetrate tissue easily, with 20 times the destructive energy of gamma rays, disrupting the atomic structure of cells. Neutrons are released during a nuclear detonation but are not a fallout risk. Neutrons also contribute to whole-body radiation exposure and can result in acute radiation illness. Neutrons have the ability to convert stable metals into radioactive isotopes. This has significance in patients with metal hardware or those in possession of metal objects at the time of exposure.

FIGURE 19-17   Terrorism with Ionizing Radiation: General Guide

DIAGNOSIS

Be alert to the following:

1. The acute radiation syndrome follows a predictable pattern after substantial exposure or catastrophic events (Figure 19-18).
2. Individuals may become ill from contaminated sources in the community and may be identified over much longer periods based on specific syndromes (Figure 19-19).
3. Specific syndromes of concern, especially with a 2- to 3-week prior history of nausea and vomiting, are:
   - Thermal burn–like skin effects without documented thermal exposure
   - Immunologic dysfunction with secondary infections
   - Tendency to bleed (epistaxis, gingival bleeding, petecchiae)
   - Marrow suppression (neutropenia, lymphopenia, and thrombocytopenia)
   - Epilation (hair loss)

UNDERSTANDING EXPOSURE

Exposure may be known and recognized or clandestine through:

1. Large recognized exposures, such as a nuclear bomb or damage to a nuclear power station.
2. Small radiation source emitting continuous gamma radiation, producing group or individual chronic intermittent exposures (e.g., radiologic sources from medical treatment devices, environmental water or food pollution).
3. Internal radiation from absorbed, inhaled, or ingested radioactive material (internal contamination).

(Modified from Department of Veterans Affairs pocket guide produced by Employee Education System for Office of Public Health and Environmental Hazards. This information is not meant to be complete, but to be a quick guide; please consult other references and expert opinion.)

Whole-body exposure is measured in terms of the *gray* (Gy). The *rad* (radiation absorbed dose) was a familiar dose unit that was replaced by the gray; 1 Gy equals 100 rad. The *rem* (radiation equivalent–man) describes the dose in rad multiplied by a "quality factor," which takes into account the intrinsic special deposition pattern of different types of radiation. The rem has been replaced with the *sievert* (Sv); 1 Sv equals 100 rem.

Radiation affects rapidly dividing cells most readily, resulting in injury to the bone marrow and GI tract where high cell-turnover rates occur. Higher doses can affect the CNS directly. The dose of whole-body exposure determines the medical consequences of the exposure. Patients receiving up to 1 Gy of whole-body irradiation would typically not exhibit signs of injury. At 1 to 2 Gy, less than half of patients will develop nausea and vomiting, many will subsequently develop leukopenia (decreased white blood cell count), and deaths will be minimal. Most victims receiving greater than 2 Gy will become ill and require hospitalization; at greater than 6 Gy, mortality becomes high. At doses greater than 30 Gy, neurologic signs are manifest, and death is most likely.[18]

Acute radiation illness generally follows a defined progression that first manifests in a prodromal phase characterized by malaise, nausea, and vomiting. This is followed by a latent phase, in which the patient is essentially asymptomatic. The length of the latent phase depends on the total absorbed dose of radiation. The greater the dose of radiation, the shorter the latent phase. The latent phase is followed by the subsequent illness, as manifested by the organ system that has been injured. Damage to the bone marrow occurs with total doses of 0.7 to 4.0 Gy and results in decreasing levels of white blood cells and decreased immunity over several days to weeks. Decreased platelets can result in easy bruising and bleeding. Decreased red blood cells will result in anemia. At 6 to 8 Gy, the GI tract will also be affected, resulting in diarrhea, volume loss, and hematochezia (bloody stools). Above 30 Gy, the patient will manifest symptoms of the neurovascular syndrome, experiencing the prodromal phase of nausea and vomiting, a short latent phase lasting only a few hours, followed by a rapid deterioration of mental status, coma, and death, sometimes accompanied by hemodynamic instability. Doses this high can occur after a nuclear detonation, but the victim will most likely have been killed by injuries associated with the blast. Victims could also be exposed to these high doses at a nuclear power facility where no blast has occurred, but a reactor core has reached criticality.[18]

Not all radiation accidents or terrorist events will result in high-dose radiation exposure. Low-dose radiation exposure, as would most likely occur after an RDD detonation, probably would not produce acute injury secondary to radiation. Dependent on dose, the patient may have an increased future risk of developing cancer. The acute effects of RDD detonation, besides the effects of the detonation of the conventional explosive, will likely be psychological, including

FIGURE 19-18 **Acute Radiation Syndrome**

Feature	Efffects of whole-body irradiation or internal absorption, by dose range in rad (1 rad = 1 cGy; 100 rad = 1 Gy)					
	0–100	100–200	200–600	600–800	800–3000	>3000
PRODROMAL PHASE OF SYNDROME						
Nausea, vomiting	None	5%–50%	50%–100%	75%–100%	90%–100%	100%
Time of onset		3–6 hours	2–4 hours	1–2 hours	<1 hour	Minutes
Duration		<24 hours	<24 hours	<48 hours	48 hours	N/A
Lymphocyte count	Unaffected	Minimally decreased	<1000 at 24 hours	<500 at 24 hours	Decreases within hours	Decreases within hours
Central nervous system (CNS) function	No impairment	No impairment	Routine task performance Cognitive impairment for 6–20 hours	Simple, routine task performance Cognitive impairment for >24 hours	Rapid incapacitation May have a lucid interval of several hours	
LATENT PHASE OF SYNDROME						
No symptoms	>2 weeks	7–15 days	0–7 days	0–2 days	None	None
MANIFEST ILLNESS						
Signs/symptoms	None	Moderate leukopenia	Severe leukopenia, purpura, hemorrhage, pneumonia, hair loss after 300 rad		Diarrhea, fever, electrolyte disturbance	Convulsions, ataxia, tremor, lethargy
Time of onset		>2 weeks	2 days–4 weeks	2 days–4 weeks	1–3 days	1–3 days
Critical period		None	4–6 weeks; greatest potential for effective medical intervention		2–14 days	1–46 hours
Organ system	None		Hematopoietic; respiratory (mucosal) systems		GI tract Mucosal systems	CNS
Hospitalization duration	0%	<5% 45–60 days	90% 6 0–90 days	100% 100+ days	100% Weeks to months	100% Days to weeks
Mortality	None	Minimal	Low with aggressive therapy	High	Very high; significant neurologic symptoms indicate lethal dose	

(Modified from Armed Forces Radiobiology Institute: *Medical management of radiological casualties,* Bethesda, MD, 2003.)

FIGURE 19-19 **Symptom Clusters as Delayed Effects after Radiation**

1	2	3	4
Headache Fatigue Weakness	Anorexia Nausea Vomiting Diarrhea	Partial-thickness and full-thickness skin damage Epilation (hair loss) Ulceration	Lymphopenia Neutropenia Thrombocytopenia Purpura Opportunistic infections

(Modified from Armed Forces Radiobiology Institute: *Medical management of radiological casualties,* Bethesda, MD, 2003.)

stress reactions, fear, acute depression, and psychosomatic complaints, which will significantly strain the EMS agencies and medical infrastructure.

Patients can become contaminated with material that emits alpha, beta, and even gamma radiation, but the most common contaminants will emit alpha and beta radiation. Only gamma radiation contributes to whole-body irradiation, as previously described. Alpha and beta radiation have limited ability to penetrate, but still can cause local tissue injury. Patients can easily be decontaminated by clothing removal and washing with water or soap and water. It is impossible for a patient to be so contaminated as to be a radiologic hazard to health care providers caring for the individual, so management of traumatic life-threatening injury is an immediate priority and should not be delayed pending decontamination.[18]

As described, radioactive particles can be inhaled, ingested, or absorbed through the skin or contaminated wounds. This type of exposure to radiation will not result in acute effects of radiation exposure but can result in delayed effects. Any victims or responding personnel who operate in an area at risk for airborne radioactive particles without the benefit of respiratory protection will require subsequent evaluation to identify internal contamination, which may require medical intervention to dilute or block the effects of the radionuclide.

Personal Protective Equipment

Prehospital care providers will be operating in an environment with risk of exposure to ionizing radiation after a radiologic disaster. The radiation risk will depend greatly on the type of radiologic event.

The PPE available to prehospital care providers for use in chemical and biologic hazards will offer some protection from radioactive particulate contamination. However, it will not provide protection from high-energy radiation sources, such as a damaged reactor or nuclear blast at ground zero.

Radioactivity can be present in gases, aerosols, solids, or liquids. If radioactive gases are present, SCBA will offer the highest protection. If aerosols are present, an APR may be adequate to prevent internal contamination caused by inhalation of contaminated particles. An N-95 mask will offer some protection from inhaled particulates. A standard splash-resistant suit will protect against particulates that emit alpha radiation and will offer some protection from beta radiation, but will provide no protection from gamma radiation or neutrons. This type of barrier protection will assist in the decontamination of particulate matter from an individual, but it does not protect against the risks of acute radiation illness when the person is exposed to high-energy sources of external radiation. None of the typical PPE carried by prehospital providers protects from a high-energy point source of radiation. This type of radiation is encountered during the first minute of a nuclear detonation, in a critical reactor core, or with a high-energy radiation source

such as cesium-137, which may be dispersed in an RDD. The best protection from these sources is decreased time of exposure, increased distance from the source, and shielding. Some new materials that may offer some protection from low-level gamma radiation for first-responder PPE are under investigation.

Unlike insufficient PPE for a chemical hazmat, the inhalation, ingestion, or skin absorption of radiation-emitting gas or particulate will not immediately incapacitate a prehospital care provider or victim. All prehospital providers who have operated in an environment potentially contaminated with radioactive material will have to undergo a radiation survey to determine if internal contamination has occurred and undergo active management if warranted.

Dose rate meters or alarms should be worn if available. Standards exist for acceptable doses of ionizing radiation in the occupational environment under normal and emergency conditions.[19] Dose rates of ionizing radiation can be measured to prevent responders from putting themselves at risk for acute radiation illness or an unacceptably higher incidence of cancer. The incident commander should be approached for guidance on radiation-exposure readings and limits.

Evaluation and Treatment

Patients who have been injured in a radiologic catastrophe should receive primary and secondary surveys as dictated by the mechanism of injury. Prehospital care providers can expect to evaluate patients who have sustained blast injury and thermal injury in the case of a nuclear detonation, or from the conventional HE detonation of an RDD (Figure 19-20). Decontamination of the victim is recommended to eliminate radioactive particulate contamination but should not delay care of patients requiring immediate intervention for their injuries. If the patient does not show signs of serious injury requiring immediate intervention, the patient can be decontaminated first. If radioiodine is present in the environment, as might be encountered in a nuclear reactor or spent fuel rod accident or with detonation of a nuclear device, giving potassium iodide (KI) to responders and victims may help prevent accumulation of radioiodine in the thyroid, where it can increase the likelihood of cancer. Other blocking and decorporation therapy may be recommended by the hospital or federal assistance agencies when more information about the catastrophe is available.

Transportation Considerations

Patients should be transported to the nearest appropriate medical center that is capable of managing trauma and radiation injuries. All hospitals are required to have a plan for management of a radiologic emergency, but communities may have identified institutions that have decontamination facilities, are capable of managing trauma, and have staff trained to deal effectively with possible external or internal radioactive contamination, as well as the complications of whole-body exposure to ionizing radiation.

FIGURE 19-20   Treatment and Decontamination Considerations for Radiation Exposure

TREATMENT CONSIDERATIONS
- If trauma is present, treat
- If external radioactive contaminants are present, decontaminate (after treatment of life-threatening problems)
- If radioiodine (e.g., reactor accident) is present, consider giving prophylactic potassium iodide (Lugol's solution) within first 24 hours only (ineffective later)
- See http://www.afrri.usuhs.mil or http://www.orau.gov/reacts/guidance.htm

DECONTAMINATION CONSIDERATIONS
- Exposure without contamination requires no decontamination
- Exposure with contamination requires Standard (Universal) Precautions, removal of patient clothing, and decontamination with water

- Internal contamination will be determined at the hospital
- Treating contaminated patients before decontamination may contaminate the facility; plan for decontamination before arrival
- Patient with life-threatening condition: treat, then decontaminate
- Patient with non-life-threatening condition: decontaminate, then treat

(Modified from Armed Forces Radiobiology Institute, *Medical management of radiological casualties,* Bethesda, MD, 2003.)

SUMMARY

- Weapons of mass destruction manufactured by terrorist regimes pose a significant threat to civilized society.
- Prehospital care providers may also come in contact with explosions and with chemical and radiologic material as the result of industrial mishaps.
- The safety of providers is paramount, and they should possess a working knowledge of levels of personal protective equipment and the fundamentals of decontamination.
- Explosive agents have predominated in recent terrorist attacks. High-order explosives produce primary blast injuries in survivors who are in close proximity to the blast, and secondary injuries result from flying debris.

- Chemical agents may not only injure the skin and pulmonary system, but may also result in systemic illness, manifesting as a specific toxidrome that yields clues to the agent. Antidotes are used for some of these agents.
- Biologic agents can be highly virulent bacteria or viruses, or toxins produced by living organisms. The types of protective precautions used by providers vary with the specific agents.
- Several types of radiation exist. Exposure to these agents may result in acute radiation sickness, which is typically a function of the type of radiation and the length of exposure.

SCENARIO SOLUTION

The first priority is safety. Assess the scene. Look also for obvious evidence of a secondary device that may pose a threat to responders. Are there other hazards? Look for hanging debris, downed or exposed power lines, or hazmat spills. Briefly observe the crowd for evidence of a toxidrome. Is there an unusually high proportion of respiratory difficulty? Are victims vomiting and seizing? Is there evidence of agent dispersal in addition to the explosive blast? Don PPE appropriate for the scenario.

Communicate with your chain of command. As the first EMS responder, the communications center will be relying on you for information. Describe pertinent details of the scene, observed hazards, numbers of victims, and likely number of resources required to manage the scene and victims. Based on your observations, the communications center and the on-duty supervisor can apprise other units and agencies of your situation and dispatch the necessary resources. A predefined disaster response plan may be activated.

Once the personal safety of the team has been assured and information has been communicated to the chain of command, prepare to serve as the incident commander until relieved by another competent authority. As soon as is feasible, approach the victims with the intention of triaging them for treatment and transport using the START algorithm. Without engaging in the medical management of victims initially, sort the victims into immediate, urgent, delayed, and expectant categories. As other assistance arrives, direct personnel to assume roles of the incident command system until supervisory personnel arrive to assume command and control functions.

References

1. Hogan DE, Waeckerle JF, Dire DJ, et al: Emergency department impact of the Oklahoma City terrorist bombing. *Ann Emerg Med* 34:160, 1999.

2. Kennedy K, Aghababian R, Gans L, et al: Triage: Techniques and applications in decision making. *Ann Emerg Med* 28(2):136, 1996.

3. Garner A, Lee A, Harrison K: Comparative analysis of multiple-casualty incident triage algorithms. *Ann Emerg Med* 38:541, 2001.

4. Lerner EB, Schwartz RB, Coule PL, et al: Mass casualty triage: An evaluation of the data and development of a proposed national guideline. *Disaster Med Public Health Preparedness* 2 (Suppl 1): S25-S34, 2008.

5. Kapur GB, Hutson HR, Davis MA, Rice PL: The United States twenty-year experience with bombing incidents: Implications for terrorism preparedness and medical response. *J Trauma* 59:1436–1444, 2005.

6. Hall JR Jr: Deaths due to unintentional injury from explosions. Quincy, MA: National Fire Protection Association, Fire Analysis and Research Division. March 2008. http://www.arfireprevention.org/pdf/Deaths_Due_to_Unintentional_Injury_from_Explosions.pdf. Accessed December 17, 2008.

7. Significant terrorist incidents, 1961–2003: A brief chronology, Washington, DC, 2004, Office of the Historian, Bureau of Public Affairs, US Department of State. http://www.state.gov/r/pa/ho/pubs/fs/5902.htm. Accessed October, 2004.

8. National Counterterrorism Center: 2007 Report on Terrorism. 30 April 2008. http://www.terrorisminfo.mipt.org/GetDoc.asp?id=6051&type=d. Accessed December 15, 2008.

9. Explosive Incidents 2007. 2007 USBDC Explosives Statistics. United States Bomb Data Center. http://www.atf.gov/aexis2/statistics.htm. Accessed December 15, 2008.

10. United States Department of State: Country Reports on Terrorism 2007. http://www.state.gov/s/ct/rls/crt/2007/index.htm. Accessed December 15, 2008.

11. National Counterterrorism Center: Report on Terrorist Incidents—2006. 30 April 2007. http://www.wits.nctc.gov/reports/crot2006nctcannexfinal.pdf. Accessed December 15, 2008.

12. Frykberg ER, Tepas JJ, Alexander RH. The 1983 Beirut Airport terrorist bombing: Injury patterns and implications for disaster management. *Am Surg* 55:134, 1989.

13. National Counterterrorism Center: 2008 Report on Terrorism. 30 April 2009. http://wits.nctc.gov/ReportPDF.do?f=crt2008nctcannexfinal.pdf. Accessed May 25, 2009.

14. Arnold J, Halpern P, Tsai M: Mass casualty terrorist bombings: A comparison of outcomes by bombing type. *Ann Emerg Med* 43:263, 2004.

15. DePalma RG, Burris DG, Champion HR, et al: Blast injuries. *N Engl J Med* 352(13):1335–1342, 2005.

16. Explosions and blast injuries: A primer for clinicians. 2003. http://www.bt.cdc.gov/masstrauma/explosions.asp. Accessed August 2004.

17. Wightman JM, Gladish JL: Explosions and blast injuries. *Ann Emerg Med* 37:664, 2001.

18. Armed Forces Radiobiology Institute: *Medical management of radiological casualties,* Bethesda, MD, 2003, AFRI.

19. Department of Homeland Security Working Group on Radiological Dispersion Device Preparedness/Medical Preparedness and Response Subgroup. http://www1.va.gov/emshg/docs/Radiologic_Medical_Countermeasures_051403.pdf. Accessed September 2004.

20. Almogy G, Mintz Y, Zamir G, et al: Suicide bombing attacks: Can external signs predict internal injuries? *Ann Surg* 243(4):541–546, 2006.

21. Garner MJ, Brett SJ: Mechanisms of injury by explosive devices. *Anesthesiol Clin* 25(1):147–160, 2007.

22. Avidan V, Hersch M, Armon Y, et al: Blast lung injury: Clinical manifestations, treatment, and outcome. *Am J Surg* 190(6):927–931, 2005.

23. Katz E, Ofek B, Adler J, et al: Primary blast injury after a bomb explosion in a civilian bus. *Ann Surg* 209:484, 1989.

24. Kluger Y, Nimrod A, Biderman P, et al: Case report: The quinary pattern of blast injury. *J Emerg Mgmt* 4(1):51–55, 2006.

25. Sorkine P, Nimrod A, Biderman P, et al: The Quinary (Vth) Injury Pattern of Blast (Abstract). *J Trauma* 56[1]:232. 2007.

26. Nelson TJ, Wall DB, Stedje-Larsen ET, et al: Predictors of mortality in close proximity blast injuries during Operation Iraqi Freedom. *J Am Coll Surg* 202(3):418–422, 2006.

27. Arnold JL, Tsai MC, Halpern P, et al: Mass-casualty, terrorist bombings: Epidemiological outcomes, resource utilization, and time course of emergency needs (Part I). *Prehosp Disaster Med* 18(3):220–234, 2003.

28. Halpern P, Tsai MC, Arnold JL, et al: Mass-casualty, terrorist bombings: Implications for emergency department and hospital emergency response (Part II). *Prehosp Disaster Med* 18(3):235–241, 2003.

29. Mallonee S, Shariat S, Stennies G, et al. Physical injuries and fatalities resulting from the Oklahoma City bombing. *JAMA* 276:382, 1996.

30. Caseby NG, Porter MF: Blast injury to the lungs: clinical presentation, management and course. *Injury* 8:1, 1976.

31. Leibovici D, Gofrit ON, Shapira SC: Eardrum perforation in explosion survivors: Is it a marker of pulmonary blast injury? *Ann Emerg Med* 34:168, 1999.

32. Coppel DL: Blast injuries of the lungs. *Br J Surg* 63:735, 1976.

33. Cohn SM: Pulmonary contusion: review of the clinical entity. *J Trauma* 42:973, 1997.

34. Peleg K, Limor A, Stein M, et al: Gunshot and explosion injuries: Characteristics, outcomes, and implications for care of terror-related injuries in Israel. *Ann Surg* 239(3):311, 2004.

35. Burstein JL: CBRNE. Incendiary agents: Magnesium and thermite. http://www.emedicine.com/emerg/topic917.htm. Accessed October, 2004.

36. Irizarry L, Diaz-Acala J: CBRNE. Incendiary agents: White phosphorus. http://www.emedicine.com/emerg/topic918.htm. Accessed October 2004.

37. Sidell FR, Takafuji ET, Franz DR, editors: *Medical aspects of chemical and biological warfare, TMM series, Part 1, Warfare, weaponry and the casualty,* Washington, DC, 1997, Office of the Surgeon General, TMM Publications.

38. Walter FG, editor: *Advanced HAZMAT life support,* ed 2, Tucson, 2000, Arizona Board of Regents.

39. Okumura T, Takasu N, Ishimatsu S, et al: Report on 640 victims of the Tokyo subway sarin attack. *Ann Emerg Med* 28(2):129, 1996.

40. US Army, Medical Research Institute of Chemical Defense: *Medical management of chemical casualties handbook,* ed 3, Aberdeen Proving Ground, MD, 2000, US Army Research Institute.

41. Greenfield RA, Brown BR, Hutchins JB, et al: Microbiological, biological and chemical weapons of warfare and terrorism. *Am J Med Sci* 323(6):326, 2002.

42. Rotenberg JS, Newmark J: Nerve-agent attacks on Children: Diagnosis and management. *Pediatrics* 112:648, 2003.

43. McDonough JH, Capacio BR, Shih TM: Treatment of nerve-agent-induced status epilepticus in the nonhuman primate. In US Army Medical Defense—Bioscience Review, June 2–7, 2002, Hunt Valley, MD.

44. Ingelsby TV, Henderson DA, Bartlett JG, et al: Anthrax as a biological weapon: Medical and public health management. *JAMA* 281(18):1735, 1999.

45. Keim M, Kaufmann AF: Principles for emergency response to bioterrorism. *Ann Emerg Med* 34(2):177, 1999.

46. US Congress, Office of Technology Assessment: *Proliferation of weapons of mass destruction,* Pub No OTA-ISC-559, Washington, DC, US Government Printing Office.

47. Inglesby TV, O'Toole T, Henderson DA, et al: Anthrax as a Biological Weapon, 2002: Updated Recommendations for Management. *JAMA* 287:2236–2252, 2002.

48. Kman NE, Nelson RN: Infectious Agents of Bioterrorism: A Review for Emergency Physicians. *Emerg Med Clin North Amer* 26:517–547, 2008.

49. Bell DM, Kozarsky PE, Stephens DS: Conference summary: Clinical issues in the prophylaxis, diagnosis and treatment of anthrax. *Emerg Infect Dis* 8(2):222, 2002.

50. World Health Organization (WHO): *Health aspects of chemical and biological weapons,* Geneva, 1970, WHO.

51. Inglesby TV, Dennis DT, Henderson DA: Plague as a biological weapon: Medical and public health management. *JAMA* 283(17):2281, 2000.

52. Henderson DA, Inglesby TV, Bartlett, JG: Smallpox as a biological weapon: Medical and public health management. *JAMA* 281(22):2127, 1999.

53. Centers for Disease Control and Prevention (CDC): *Smallpox response plan and guidelines*, Version 3.0, Guide C, Part 1, Atlanta, 2002, CDC, pp 1–13.

54. Centers for Disease Control and Prevention (CDC): *Smallpox response plan and guidelines,* Version 3.0, Guide F, Atlanta, 2003, CDC, pp 1–10.

55. Franz DR, Jahrling PB, Friedlander AM, et al: Clinical recognition and management of patients exposed to biological warfare agents. *JAMA* 278(5):399, 1997.

56. Arnon SS, Schechter R, Inglesby TV, et al: Botulinum toxin as a biological weapon: Medical and public health management. *JAMA* 285(8):1059, 2001.

57. Hogan DE, Kellison T: Nuclear terrorism. *Am J Med Sci* 323(6):341, 2002.

58. World Health Organization, International Atomic Energy Agency, United Nations Development Programme. Chernobyl: The true scale of the event. Accessed August 27, 2010. http://www.who.int/mediacentre/news/releases/2005/pr38/en/index.html.

Suggested Reading

Centers for Disease Control and Prevention Emergency Preparedness and Response Site. http://www.bt.cdc.gov/

US Army Center for Health Promotion and Preventive Medicine. http://phc.amedd.army.mil/home/

US Army Medical Research Institute of Infectious Diseases. http://www.usamriid.army.mil/

US Army Soldier and Biological Chemical Command (SBCCOM). http://hld.sbccom.army.mil/

CHAPTER 20

Environmental Trauma I: Heat and Cold

CHAPTER OBJECTIVES

At the completion of this chapter, the reader will be able to do the following:

✓ Give the reason why heatstroke is considered a life-threatening condition.

✓ Differentiate between heatstroke and hyponatremia.

✓ List two effective cooling procedures for heat exhaustion and heatstroke.

✓ List the five factors that place prehospital care providers at risk for heat illness.

✓ Explain the fluid hydration guidelines and how they should be used to prevent dehydration in hot or cold environments.

✓ Differentiate the management of mild hypothermia from that of severe hypothermia.

✓ List the signs of mild frostbite, and discuss how to prevent its progression.

✓ Discuss the rationale for the statement, "patients are not dead until they are warm and dead."

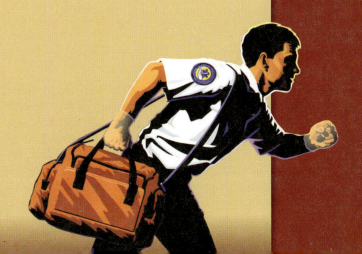

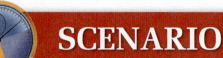

SCENARIO

At 2:00 a.m., your ambulance unit responds to a dispatch on a cold and windy evening (28° F [−2° C], 25 mph NE wind) following an 8-hour urban search for a 76 year-old female who wandered from an assisted-care retirement facility. She was recently moved closer to her daughter at this new location from her home in another state. She apparently was reported missing around 6:00 p.m. and was noted to be agitated most of the day. After a lengthy search, a volunteer search-and-rescue member found her disorientated and lightly dressed in a wind breaker and pants 400 yards from the facility. She was located on the ground, cold and wet, and stuck in some briars near an icy drainage ditch. The initial assessment shows that she is unresponsive, respirations are shallow, pulse is weak, and skin is cold.

What are possible causes for this patient to wander and her medical condition? How best to assess this patient for cold-related injuries and other potential medical conditions? Is this a life-threatening situation for the patient? How would you treat this patient? Should you attempt to rewarm the patient? If you transport the patient immediately, how do you treat the patient in route to the closest emergency room? What is the wind-chill index during this incident and how do you best protect the patient from ongoing cold injury?

This chapter focuses on recognizing and treating exposure to heat and to cold temperatures because the most significant morbidity and mortality in the United States from all environmental traumas are caused by thermal trauma.[1-4]

Thermal Trauma

Environmental extremes of heat and cold have a common outcome of injuries and potential death that can affect many individuals during the peak summer and winter months. Individuals who are especially susceptible to both highs and lows of temperature are very young persons, the elderly population, urban poor people, individuals who take specific medications, chronically ill patients, and alcoholic persons.[3-7] The majority of emergency medical services (EMS) responses in the United States for heat and cold injuries are for the *hyperthermic* and *hypothermic* patient in an urban setting. However, expanding interest in recreational and high-risk adventure activities in the wilderness backcountry during periods of environmental extremes places more individuals at risk for heat-related and cold-related injuries and fatalities.[8-11]

Epidemiology

Heat-Related Illness

During a 20-year period (1979–1999) in the United States, 8015 heat-related deaths from all causes were recorded.[2] More deaths were caused by heat stress than by hurricanes, lightning, tornadoes, floods, and earthquakes combined. Of these, 3829 (48%) deaths were related to high ambient temperatures. This averages to about 182 heat-related deaths per year during the four warmest months (May through August). The greatest percentage of deaths (1891, or 45%) occurred in

those who are 65 years of age and older. Furthermore, morbidity and mortality can be extremely high when periodic seasonal heat waves occur (≥3 consecutive days of air temperatures 90° F or higher [≥32.2° C]). The Centers for Disease Control and Prevention reported a total of 3,442 deaths (1999–2003) resulting from exposure to extreme heat (annual mean: 688). In 2239 (65%) of the deaths recorded, the underlying cause was exposure to excessive heat, whereas in the remaining 1203 (35%), hyperthermia was recorded as a contributing factor. Males accounted for 66% of deaths and outnumbered deaths among females in all age groups. Of the 3401 decedents for whom age information was available, 228 (7%) were aged less than 15 years; 1810 (53%) were aged 15 to 64 years; and 1363 (40%) were aged 65 years and older.[3]

In 1995, a record heat wave occurred during a 17-day period in Chicago, Illinois.[12,13] The Chicago Medical Examiner's office reported 1177 heat-related deaths during this short period. These cases included deaths in which heat was determined to be the underlying (primary) cause of death and in which cardiovascular disease was listed as the cause of death and heat as a contributing factor (secondary). Compared with the same period in 1994, this was an 84% increase in heat-related deaths. Of these 1177 cases, heat was the primary cause of death in 465 (39.5%).[13]

Cold-Related Illness

Mild to severe cold weather conditions caused 13,970 unintentional hypothermia-related deaths in the United States between 1978 and 1998 (an average of 699 deaths per year), and 6857 (49%) of these deaths occurred in persons 65 years of age and older.[4] When adjusted for age, death from hypothermia occurred approximately 2.5 times more often in men than women. The incidence of hypothermia related-deaths progressively increases with age and is three times higher in males than females after age 15 years. In 2003, 599 deaths were reported from exposure to cold weather in the United States, and 67% were males and 51% were older than 65 years of age.[7] Major contributing factors for accidental hypothermia are urban poverty, socioeconomic conditions, alcohol intake, malnutrition, and age (very young, senior citizens).[4,7]

Anatomy

The skin, the largest organ of the body, interfaces with the external environment and serves as a layer of protection. It prevents the invasion of microorganisms, maintains fluid balance, and regulates temperature. Skin is composed of three tissue layers—the epidermis, dermis, and subcutaneous tissue (Figure 20-1). The outermost layer, called the *epidermis,* or the stratum corneum, is made up entirely of epithelial cells, with no blood vessels. Underlying the epidermis is the thicker dermis. The *dermis,* or deeper layer of skin, is 20 to 30 times thicker than the epidermis. The dermis is made up of a framework of connective tissues that contain blood vessels, blood products, nerves, sebaceous glands, and sweat glands. The innermost layer, the *subcutaneous* layer, is a combination of elastic and fibrous tissue as well as fatty deposits; below this layer is skeletal muscle. The skin, nerves, blood vessels, and other underlying anatomic structures have major roles in regulating body temperature.

Physiology

Thermoregulation and Temperature Balance

Humans are considered *homeotherms,* or warm-blooded animals. A key feature of homeotherms is that they are able to regulate their own internal body temperature independent of varying environmental temperatures. The body is essentially divided into a warmer, inner *core* layer (including the brain and the thoracic and abdominal organs) and the skin and subcutaneous outer *shell* layer. *Core temperature* is regulated through a

balance of heat-production and heat-dissipation mechanisms. The temperatures on the skin surface and the thickness of the shell depend on the *environmental temperature,* so the shell becomes thicker in the colder temperatures and thinner in the warmer temperatures based on shunting blood away or to the skin, respectively. This shell or tissue insulation, as induced by vasoconstriction, has been estimated to be about the same outer protection as wearing a light business suit, compared with six to eight times the insulation created when wearing heavy, insulated clothing in cold temperatures.

Metabolic heat production will vary based on activity levels. Independent of the variation of external temperature, the body normally functions within a narrow temperature range, known as *steady-state metabolism,* of about 1° on either side of 98.6° F (37° C, ±0.6° C). Normal body temperature is maintained in a narrow range by homeostatic mechanisms regulated in the *hypothalamus,* which is located in the brain. The hypothalamus is known as the *thermoregulatory center* and functions as the body's thermostat to control neurologic and hormonal regulation of body temperature. As noted in preceding chapters, trauma to the brain can disrupt the hypothalamus, which in turn causes an imbalance in the regulation of the body temperature.

Humans have two systems to regulate body temperature: *behavioral regulation* and *physiologic thermoregulation.* Behavioral regulation is governed by the individual thermal sensation and comfort, and the distinguishing feature is the conscious effort to reduce thermal discomfort (e.g., adding additional clothing, seeking shelter in cold environments). The processing of sensory feedback to the brain of thermal information in behavioral thermoregulation is not well understood, but the feedback of thermal sensation and comfort responds more quickly than physiologic responses to changes in environmental temperature.[14]

Heat Production and Thermal Balance. *Basal metabolic rate* is the heat produced primarily as a by-product of metabolism, primarily from the large organs of the core and from skeletal muscle contraction. The heat generated is transferred throughout the body by blood in the circulatory system. Heat transfer and dissipation from the body by the cardiopulmonary system are important in the assessment and management of heat illness, as discussed later. Shivering increases the metabolic rate by increasing muscle tension, which leads to repeated bouts of muscular contraction and relaxation. There are some individual differences, but typically shivering starts when the core temperature drops to between 94° to 97° F (34.4°–36° C) and continues until the core temperature is 88° F [31° C].[15] With maximal shivering, heat production is increased by five to six times the resting level.[15,16]

The physiologic thermoregulation systems that control heat production and heat loss responses are well documented.[14,16,17] Two principles in thermoregulation are key to understanding how the body regulates core temperature: thermal gradient and thermal equilibrium. A *thermal gradient* is the difference in temperature (high vs. low temperature) between two objects. A *thermal equilibrium* is the transfer

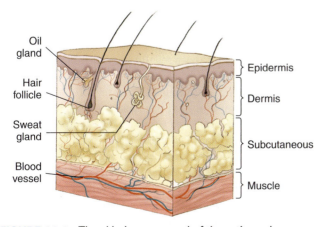

FIGURE 20-1 The skin is composed of three tissue layers—epidermis, dermis, and subcutaneous layer—and associated muscle. Some layers contain structures such as glands, hair follicles, blood vessels, and nerves. All these structures are interrelated to the maintenance, loss, and gain of body temperature.

of heat from a warmer object to a colder object in an effort to create the same temperature between them.

When body temperature rises, the normal physiologic response is to increase skin blood flow and to begin sweating. The majority of body heat is transferred to the environment at the skin surface by conduction, convection, radiation, and evaporation, as defined next. Because heat is transferred from greater temperature to lower temperature, the human body can gain heat by radiation and conduction during hot weather conditions. Methods to maintain and dissipate body heat are important concepts for prehospital care providers. They must understand how both heat and cold are transferred to and from the body so that they can effectively manage a patient who has hyperthermia or hypothermia (Figure 20-2).

■ *Radiation* is the loss or gain of heat in the form of electromagnetic energy; it is the transfer of energy from a warm object to a cooler one. Radiation does not use an intermediary source such as air or water. The sun warms the earth through space by this method of energy transfer. A patient with heat illness can acquire additional body heat from the hot ground or directly from the sun. These sources of heat will increase body temperature and impede interventions to cool the patient until the prehospital care provider eliminates these sources of radiant heat when assessing and treating the patient.

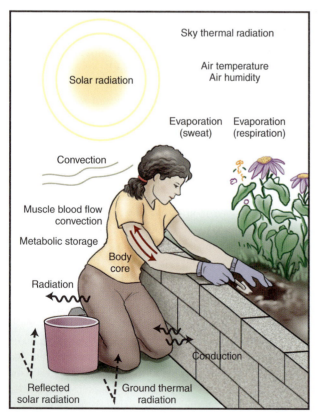

FIGURE 20-2   How humans exchange thermal energy with the environment.

■ *Conduction* is the transfer of heat between two objects in direct contact with each other, as with a patient lying on a frozen lawn after a fall. A patient will generally lose heat faster when lying on the cold ground than when exposed to cold air. Therefore, prehospital care providers need to lift the patient off the ground in cold temperatures rather than merely cover the patient with a blanket.

■ *Convection* is the transfer of heat from a solid object to a medium that moves across that solid object. Air or water currents are the two mediums generally considered in convective heat loss because they come into contact with the human body. The movement of cool air or water across the warmer skin provides for the continuous elimination of heat from the warmer skin. Furthermore, a patient will lose body heat 25 times faster in water than in air of the same temperature, so it is important to keep a patient dry and to remove wet clothing in mild to cold temperatures. A scuba diver's wetsuit helps to minimize the loss of body heat from convective heat loss when diving in water colder than skin temperature. When prehospital care providers are effectively managing a heat-illness patient, they use the principle of convective heat loss by moistening and fanning their patient to dissipate body heat quickly.

■ *Evaporation* of sweat from a liquid to a vapor is an extremely effective method of heat loss from the body, depending on the relative humidity or moisture in the air. A basal level of both water and accompanying heat loss from exhaled air, skin, and mucous membranes is called *insensible loss* and is caused by evaporation. This insensible loss is normally about 10% of basal heat production, but when the body temperature rises, this process becomes more active (sensible), and sweat is produced. Evaporative heat loss increases in cool, dry, and windy conditions (e.g., southwestern US deserts). Collectively, convection and evaporation are more important than other methods of heat transfer because they are regulated by the body to control core temperature.[5]

Increases (*hyperthermia*) and decreases (*hypothermia*) in body temperature beyond the steady-state range (98.6° F ±1.0° F [37° C, ±0.6° C]) can result from different internal and external causes and return to steady-state temperature without complications.[17] Hyperthermia occurs primarily in one of three ways: (1) as a normal response to sustained exercise, in which the heat produced elevates core temperature and is the stimulus for heat-dissipating responses (e.g., sweating, increased blood flow in skin); (2) when the sum of heat production and heat gained from the environment is greater than the body's heat dissipation capability; and (3) from a fever. Unlike the first two ways, fever usually occurs in response to inflammation because of a change in the thermoregulatory set point, and the body responds by elevating body temperature to a higher value (100°–106° F [38°–41° C]). Heat production increases only temporarily to achieve a new set point temperature in an attempt to make the environment less hospitable for the invading infection.[17]

FIGURE 20-3   Heat Illness Risk Factors

CONDITIONS
- Cardiovascular disease
- Dehydration
- Autonomic neuropathies
- Parkinsonism
- Dystonias
- Skin disorders: psoriasis, sunburn, burns
- Endocrine disorders
- Fever
- Delirium tremens
- Psychosis
- Neonates, elderly persons
- History of heatstroke
- Obesity
- Low fitness

TOXINS/DRUGS
- **Increase Heat Production**
  - Thyroid hormone
  - Cyclic antidepressants
  - Hallucinogens (e.g., LSD)
  - Cocaine
  - Amphetamines

Decrease Thirst
- Haloperidol
- Angiotensin-converting enzyme (ACE) inhibitors

Decrease Sweating
- Antihistamines
- Anticholinergics
- Phenothiazines
- Glutethimide
- Beta blockers

Increase Water Loss
- Diuretics
- Ethanol
- Nicotine

BEHAVIOR
- Injudicious exertion
- Inappropriate clothing
- Poor acclimatization
- Poor fluid intake
- Poor supervision
- High motivation
- Athletic profile
- Military recruit profile

(Modified from Tek D, Olshaker JS: Heat illness. *Emerg Med Clin North Am* 10(2):299, 1992.)

Homeostasis

All of these anatomic structures and physiologic systems are interacting so that the body functions properly when exposed to temperature changes. The body is in a constant state of neurologic feedback from peripheral and internal regions to the thermoregulatory center and other regions in the brain—all in an effort to maintain constant, stable internal conditions, or *homeostasis,* in the body. However, at times, this does not occur. For example, when an imbalance occurs in the cardiovascular and thermoregulatory adjustments to eliminate excessive body heat, one outcome is the loss of excessive body fluid through sweating, which causes acute dehydration and may lead to signs and symptoms of heat illness.

Injuries Produced by Heat

Risk Factors in Heat Illness

Many studies on humans have demonstrated large individual differences in their tolerance to hot environments.[18] These differences can be partially explained by both physical characteristics and medical conditions that are associated with an increased risk for heat illness (Figure 20-3). It is important to realize that any situation in which heat production exceeds the body's ability to dissipate heat may result in heat injury. Key risk factors that contribute to the onset of heat illness are alcohol consumption, medications, dehydration, higher body mass index, obesity, inadequate diet, improper clothing, low fitness, sleep loss, extremes of age, cardiovascular disease, skin injuries, previous heat-related illness, sickle cell trait, sunburn, viral illness, and exercise during the hottest hours of day.[19,29] Transient conditions include those affecting individuals who travel from cooler climates and are not heat-acclimatized to warmer climates on arrival. Other transient factors that place individuals at risk for heat illness are common illnesses, including colds and other conditions that cause fever, vomiting, and diarrhea, along with poor dietary and fluid intake.[20,21]

Factors considered to be *chronic* conditions that place individuals at greater risk for heat illness are fitness, body size, age, medical condition, and medications.

Fitness and Body Mass Index

Low levels of physical fitness caused by genetic factors or a sedentary lifestyle with inadequate daily physical activity will reduce tolerance to heat exposure. Physical fitness provides a cardiovascular reserve to maintain cardiac output as needed to sustain thermoregulation. Overweight individuals have a normal response to heat exposure of vasodilation of skin blood vessels and increased sweating, but the combination of low fitness, lack of heat acclimatization, and excessive body weight (higher body mass index) increases the energy cost of movement, placing them at greater risk for heat illness.

Age

Thermoregulatory capacity and tolerance to heat diminish with age. However, this state can be improved by maintaining a low body weight and a high level of physical fitness.

Gender

A long-held belief was that women were less tolerant of heat compared to men. Although wide variation was reported previously, these differences resulted from women who were less physically fit and had less exposure to heat compared with men in conditions that would induce full *heat acclimatization*. More recent studies have controlled for differences in physical fitness and heat acclimatization between men and women and indicate that women demonstrate equal work tolerance in heat and, in some studies, are more tolerant of heat than men.

Medical Conditions

Medical conditions that can increase the risk for heat intolerance and heat illness are diabetes mellitus, thyroid disorders, and renal disease. Cardiovascular disease and circulatory problems that increase cutaneous blood flow and circulatory demand are aggravated by heat exposure. A mild form of heat illness seen in individuals is "prickly heat rash," which has been shown to cause reduced heat tolerance.

Medications

The use of specific prescription or over-the-counter medications can place individuals at a greater risk for heat illness (see Figure 20-3). Certain medications can increase metabolic heat production, suppress body cooling, reduce cardiac reserve, and alter renal electrolyte and fluid balance. Sedative and narcotic drugs will affect mental status and can affect logical reasoning and judgment, suppressing decision-making ability, when the individual is exposed to heat.

Dehydration

Body water is the largest component of the human body, representing 45% to 70% of body weight; for example, a 165-pound (75-kg) man contains approximately 45 liters of water, representing 60% of body weight. Excessive changes in the normal body water balance *(euhydration)* resulting from either overconsumption of water *(hyperhydration;* see section on hyponatremia) or fluid loss (causing acute dehydration) alter homeostasis, producing specific signs and symptoms. Acute dehydration can be a serious outcome of both heat and cold exposure, but it is also seen as a dangerous side effect of diarrhea, vomiting, and fever.

Dehydration is a common finding in many cases of heat illness occurring over many days as seen in senior citizens or during physical activity as seen with profuse sweating in athletes. Generally, these individuals consume no fluid or low volumes of fluid during daily activities, not replacing the depleted body water. Children and persons over age 60 are particularly susceptible to dehydration. Body water is lost daily through sweat, tears, urine, and stool. Normally, drink-

ing fluids and eating foods that contain water replace body water. When a person becomes sick with fever, diarrhea, or vomiting, or an individual is exposed to heat, dehydration occurs. Occasionally, drugs that deplete body fluids and electrolytes, such as diuretics, can cause dehydration.

During heat exposure, body water is primarily lost as sweat. Individuals can sweat 0.8 to 1.4 liters per hour (liter/hour), and it has been reported that some elite athletes who are heat-acclimatized can sweat up to 3.7 liter/hour during competition in hot environments.[22] The keys to avoiding the onset of heat illness are to maintain a body fluid balance and to minimize dehydration during daily activities, particularly during any physical activity in moderate to high heat exposure. Individuals normally do not perceive thirst until a deficit of approximately 2% of body weight has resulted from sweating.[23] Thus, thirst provides a poor indicator of body water needs during rest or physical activity.

With mild to moderate levels of acute dehydration (2%–6% body weight), individuals experience fatigue, headache, decreased heat tolerance, and cognitive deterioration, along with reductions in strength and aerobic physical capacity.[24,25] People will consistently under consume fluids and remain dehydrated at approximately 1% to 2% of body weight without some form of fluid hydration guidelines (see Prevention of Heat-Related Illness later in this chapter) to direct them regarding the amount of fluids to consume per hour when exposed to mild or high heat exposure. The under consumption of fluid to restore normal water balance is currently known as "voluntary" dehydration.[21]

When individuals are encouraged to drink fluids frequently during heat exposure, the rate at which fluids can be replaced by mouth is limited by the rate of gastric emptying and the rate of fluid absorption in the small intestine.[26] Fluids empty from the stomach to the small intestine, where absorption occurs into the bloodstream, at a maximal rate of approximately 1 to 1.2 liter/hour.[26] Furthermore, gastric emptying rates are decreased approximately 20% to 25% when sweat-induced weight loss causes dehydration of 5% of total body weight (e.g., 5% of 200-pound male = 10-pound weight loss).[27] The important message is that once dehydration occurs, it becomes more challenging to rehydrate the individual adequately with oral fluids. In addition, rapid oral administration of fluids may lead to nausea and vomiting, thus further exacerbating the dehydration problem. The key to minimizing the amount of dehydration during heat exposure is to begin consuming oral fluids before heat exposure and to maintain fluid intake frequently during and after heat exposure. The goal of oral hydration throughout physical activity is to prevent excessive dehydration (>2% body-weight loss) and excessive changes in electrolytes (e.g., sodium, potassium, and chloride).[29]

The following are the most common signs and symptoms of dehydration in infants, children, and adults, although each individual may experience symptoms differently:

- Less frequent urination and dark color urine
- Thirst
- Dry skin

- Fatigue
- Light headedness
- Headache
- Dizziness
- Confusion
- Dry mouth and mucous membranes
- Increased heart rate and breathing

In infants and children, additional symptoms may include the following:

- Dry mouth and tongue
- No tears when crying
- No wet diapers for more than 3 hours
- Sunken abdomen, eyes, or cheeks
- High fever
- Listlessness
- Irritability
- Skin that does not flatten when pinched and released

Heat-Related Disorders

Heat-related disorders can range from minor to severe in patients with heat illness.[9,29,30] It is important to note that prehospital care providers may or may not see a progression of signs and symptoms, starting with minor syndromes (e.g., heat cramps) and then advancing to major heat-related illness (e.g., classic heatstroke). In the majority of heat exposures, the patient is able to dissipate core body heat adequately and maintain core temperature within the normal range. However, when heat-related conditions do result in a call for EMS assistance, the minor heat-related conditions may be apparent to the prehospital care provider during patient assessment, along with signs and symptoms of a major heat illness (Figure 20-4).

Minor Heat-Related Disorders

The minor heat-related disorders include heat rash, heat edema, heat tetany, muscle (heat) cramps, and heat syncope.

Heat Rash. Heat rash, also known as "prickly heat" and *miliaria rubra,* is a red, pruritic, papular rash normally seen on the skin in areas of restrictive clothing and heavy sweating. This condition is caused by inflammation of the sweat glands that blocks the sweat ducts. As a result, affected areas cannot sweat, putting individuals at increased risk of heat illness, depending on the amount of skin surface involved.

Management. Treatment is by cooling and drying the affected area and by preventing further conditions that cause sweat in these areas.

Heat Edema. Heat edema is a mild, dependent edema in the hands, feet, and ankles seen during early stages of heat acclimatization when plasma volume is expanding to compensate for the increased need for thermoregulatory blood flow.

This form of edema does not indicate excessive fluid intake or cardiac, renal, or hepatic disease. In the absence of other diseases, this condition is of no clinical significance and is self-limited. Heat edema is observed more often in females.

Management. Treatment consists of loosening any constricting clothes and elevating the legs. Diuretics are not indicated and may increase risk of heat illness.

Heat Tetany. Heat tetany is a rare and self-limited condition that may occur in patients acutely exposed to short, intense heat conditions. The hyperventilation that results from these conditions is considered to be the principle cause. Respiratory alkalosis, paresthesia, carpopedal spasm, and tetany may develop.

Management. Treatment consists of removal from the source of heat and controlling hyperventilation. Dehydration is not a common occurrence with these short heat exposures. Heat tetany may be seen along with signs and symptoms of heat exhaustion and heatstroke.

Muscle (Heat) Cramps. Heat cramps are manifested by short-term, painful muscle contractions frequently seen in the calf (gastrocnemius) muscles, but also in the voluntary muscles of the abdomen and extremities, and are commonly observed following prolonged physical activity often in warm to hot temperatures. These occur in individuals during exercise that produces profuse sweating or during the exercise-recovery period. Smooth muscle, cardiac, diaphragm, and bulbar muscles are not involved. Muscle (heat) cramps can occur alone or in association with heat exhaustion. The cause is unknown, but it is believed to be caused by muscle fatigue, body water loss, and large sodium loss. Salt supplementation in the diet has been shown to reduce the incidence of heat cramps.

Management. Treatment consists of rest in a cool environment, prolonged stretching of the affected muscle, and consuming oral fluids and food containing sodium chloride (i.e., ⅛–¼ teaspoon of table salt added to 300–500 ml of fluids or sport drinks, 1–2 salt tablets with 300–500 ml of fluid, bullion broth, or salty snacks). Intravenous (IV) fluids are rarely needed, but prolonged and severe muscle cramps can be resolved rapidly with IV normal saline. Avoid the use of salt tablets by themselves because these can cause gastrointestinal (GI) distress.

Heat Syncope. Heat syncope is seen with prolonged standing in warm environments and is caused by low blood pressure that results in fainting or feeling faint or lightheaded. Heat causes vasodilation, and venous blood pools in the legs, causing low blood pressure.

Management. After removal to a cool environment, patients rest in a recumbent position and are provided oral or IV rehydration. If a fall occurred, patients should be thoroughly evaluated for any injury. Patients with a significant history of car-

FIGURE 20-4 **Common Heat-Related Disorders**

Disorder	Cause/problem	Signs/symptoms	Treatment
Muscle (heat) cramps	Failure to replace NaCl lost through sweating; electrolyte and muscle problems	Painful muscle cramps, usually in legs or abdomen	Move to cool place; massage/stretch muscle; drink athletic drinks or drinks with NaCl (e.g., tomato juice); transport those with signs or symptoms listed below.
Dehydration	Failure to replace sweat loss with fluids	Thirst, nausea, excessive fatigue, headache, hypovolemia, decreased ermoregulation; reduces physical and mental capacity	Replace sweat loss with lightly salted fluids; rest in cool place until body weight and water losses are restored. In some patients, IV rehydration is necessary.
Heat exhaustion	Excessive heat strain with inadequate water intake; cardiovascular problems with venous pooling, decreased cardiac filling time, reduced cardiac output; untreated, may progress to heatstroke	Low urine output, tachycardia, weakness, unstable gait, extreme fatigue, wet clammy skin, headache, dizziness, nausea, collapse	Remove from heat source and place in cooler location; cool body with water and fanning; drink lightly salty fluids (e.g., athletic drinks); IV 0.9 % NaCl or Lactated Ringer's solution.
Heatstroke	High core temperatures >105° F (40.6° C); cellular disruption; dysfunction of multiple organ systems common; neurologic disorder with thermoregulatory center failure	Mental status changes; irrational behavior or delirium; possible shivering; tachycardia initially, then bradycardia late; hypotension; rapid and shallow breathing; dry or wet, hot skin; loss of consciousness; seizures and coma	*Emergency:* Rapid, immediate cooling by water immersion, or wet patient or wrap in cool wet sheets and fan vigorously. Continue until core temperature is <102° F (39° C). Treat for shock if necessary once core temperature is lowered. Immediately transport to emergency department.
Exertional (dilutional) hyponatremia (also referred to as water intoxication)	Low plasma sodium concentration; typically seen in individuals during prolonged activity in hot environments; drinking water (>4 liters/hour) that exceeds sweat rate; failure to replace sodium loss in sweat.	Nausea, vomiting, malaise, dizziness, ataxia, headache, altered mental status, polyuria, signs of intracranial pressure, seizures, and coma; core temperature <102° F; mimics signs of heat illness	Restrict water intake; eat salty foods; unresponsive patients receive "ABC" standard care, 15 liters/minute O_2 NRM; IV 0.9 % NaCl at TKO rate; immediate transport alert; patient in sitting position or left-lateral position if unresponsive.

diac or neurologic disorders need further evaluation for the cause of their syncopal episode. Monitoring of vital signs and the electrocardiogram (ECG) during transport is essential.

Major Heat-Related Disorders

The major heat-related disorders include exertion-associated collapse, heat exhaustion, and heatstroke (classic and exertional forms).

Exertion-Associated Collapse. This disorder occurs when an individual collapses after strenuous exercise.[31,32] During exercise, contraction of the muscles of the lower extremities assists in augmenting venous blood return to the heart. When exercise stops, such as at the end of a jog, the muscle contraction that assisted blood return to the heart slows significantly. This in turn causes venous blood return to the heart to decrease, resulting in a decreased cardiac output to the brain.

Assessment. Signs and symptoms include nausea, light-headedness, collapse, or syncope. Patients may feel better when lying down but become lightheaded when they attempt to stand or sit *(orthostatic hypotension).* Profuse sweating is not unusual. Ventilations and pulse rates may be rapid. The patient's core body temperature may be normal or slightly elevated. It is difficult to rule out dehydration, but this type of post-exercise collapse is not from hypovolemia. In contrast, collapse that occurs during exercise needs immediate evaluation for other causes (e.g., cardiovascular).

Management. The patient is removed to a cool environment and rests in a recumbent position. Oral or IV rehydration is provided as needed. Since many of these patients experienced collapse because of the decreased venous return at the end of exercise and not from dehydration, it is highly recommended to withhold IV therapy until further assessment is completed following recumbent rest with elevated legs and "cool down." As with any form of collapse, further evaluation is necessary to rule out other disorders (e.g., exercise-associated hyponatremia, cardiac or neurologic causes). Monitoring of vital signs and ECG during transport is essential to detect cardiac arrhythmias.

Heat Exhaustion. Heat exhaustion is the most common heat-related disorder seen by prehospital care providers. This condition can develop over days of exposure, as in elderly persons living in poorly ventilated spaces, or acutely, as in athletes. This condition results from cardiac output that is insufficient to support the increased circulatory load caused by competing demands of thermoregulatory heat dissipation, increased skin blood flow, reduced plasma volume, reduced venous return to the heart from vasodilation, and sweat-induced depletion of salt and water.[21] Patients with heat exhaustion normally present with a rectal temperature less than 104° F (<40° C), but this is a guide and not always a reliable finding.[32]

Another form of heat exhaustion is known as exertional heat exhaustion. This occurs with physical exercise or heavy exertion in all temperatures. It is defined as the inability to continue the exercise or exertion and may or may not be associated with physical collapse.[29] The key predisposing factors are dehydration and high body mass index that place one at greater risk for exertional heat exhaustion.

Distinguishing severe heat exhaustion from *heatstroke* often may be difficult, but a quick mental status assessment will determine the level of neurologic involvement. If heat exhaustion is not effectively treated, it may lead to heatstroke, a life-threatening form of heat illness. Heat exhaustion is a *diagnosis of exclusion* when there is no evidence of heatstroke. These patients will need further physical and laboratory evaluation in the emergency department.

Assessment. Signs and symptoms of heat exhaustion are neither specific nor sensitive. They include low fluid intake, decreased urine output, frontal headache, drowsiness, eupho-ria, nausea, vomiting, light-headedness, anxiety, fatigue, irritability, decreased coordination, heat sensation on head and neck, chills, and apathy. Patients may feel better when lying down but may become lightheaded when they attempt to stand or sit (orthostatic hypotension). During the acute stage of heat exhaustion the blood pressure is low, the pulse and respiratory rates are rapid. The radial pulse may feel thready. The patient generally appears sweaty, pale, and ashen. The patient's core body temperature may be either normal or slightly elevated, but generally below 104° F (40° C). It is important to obtain a good history of prior heat illness and the current heat exposure incident because these patients may display signs and symptoms of other conditions of fluid and sodium loss (e.g., hyponatremia; see later discussion). Ongoing assessment is critical. Continuously look for any changes in mentation and personality (i.e., confusion, disorientation, irrational or unusual behavior). Any such change should be taken as a progressive sign of hyperthermia indicating heatstroke—*a life-threatening condition!*

Management. Immediately remove the patient from the hot environment to a cooler location either in the shade or air conditioned space (i.e., ambulance). Place the patient in a supine resting position. Remove clothing and anything restricting heat dissipation, such as a hat. Assess the patient's heart rate, blood pressure, respiratory rate, rectal temperature (if a thermometer is available and conditions permit), and particularly for central nervous system status changes as an early indicator of life threatening heatstroke. Oral rehydration should be considered for any patient who can take fluids by mouth and who is not at risk of aspirating, using sport electrolyte fluids diluted to half-strength. Large amounts of oral fluids may increase bloating, nausea, and vomiting. Normally IV fluids are not needed as long as blood pressure, pulse, and rectal temperature are normal. However, in patients who are not able to consume fluids by mouth, IV fluids provide rapid recovery from heat exhaustion.[29] If IV fluids are needed, Lactated Ringer's (LR) solution or normal saline (NS) should be used. IV solutions produce more rapid fluid recovery than fluids by mouth due to delays in gastric emptying and absorption in the small intestine caused by dehydration.

In exertional heat exhaustion, most exercising patients recover with recumbent rest and oral fluids. Before any decision in made for IV therapy in these patients, there needs to be a thorough assessment for signs and symptoms of dehydration, orthostatic pulse, blood-pressure changes, and the ability to ingest oral fluids. Ongoing mental status changes should prompt further evaluation for hyponatremia, hypoglycemia, and other medical problems. In the exertional heat exhaustion patient, the recommended IV fluids are NS or 5% dextrose in NS for patients who are mildly hypoglycemic. However, caution should be used to ensure that large amounts of IV fluids are not administered to a patient who has been participating in prolonged exercise (>4 hours), especially individuals who do not have obvious clinical signs of dehydration, or in a collapsed athlete with suspected heat exhaustion who has been drinking a large amount of water. This type of patient may have exertional hyponatremia, and providing oral and/or IV fluids will cause further dilutional hyponatremia, potentially causing a life-threatening condition. See discussion on exertional hyponatremia about how best to correctly assess the patient for heat-related illness or hyponatremia.

Because heat exhaustion may be difficult to distinguish from heatstroke and because heatstroke patients should be cooled rapidly, the best course of action is to provide some active cooling procedures to all heat exhaustion patients. Active cooling can be done simply and quickly by wetting the head and upper torso with water and fanning the patient to increase *convective* body-heat dissipation. Body-cooling procedures will also improve mental status. Transport all patients who are unconscious, who do not recover rapidly, or who have a significant medical history. Proper environmental temperature control and monitoring of vital signs and mental status are essential during transport.

Heatstroke. Heatstroke is considered the most emergent and life-threatening form of heat illness. Heatstroke is a form of hyperthermia resulting in failure of the thermoregulatory system—a failure of the body's physiologic systems to dissipate heat and cool down. Heatstroke is characterized by an elevated core temperature of 104° F or greater (40° C) and central nervous system (CNS) dysfunction, resulting in delirium, convulsions, or coma.[30,33]

The most significant difference in heatstroke compared with heat exhaustion is *neurologic disability,* which presents to the prehospital care provider as mental status changes. Pathophysiologic changes often result in multiple organ failure.[30,34] These pathophysiologic changes occur when organ tissue temperature rise above a critical level: cell membranes are damaged, leading to disruption in cell volume, metabolism, acid-base balance, and membrane permeability that causes cellular and a whole organ dysfunction with ultimate cell death and organ failure.[29] The degree of complications in patients with heatstroke is not entirely related to the magnitude of core temperature elevation. This pathophysiologic dysfunction is the underlying reason for early heatstroke recognition by prehospital care providers who can quickly provide aggressive whole-body cooling in effort to rapidly reduce core temperature and decrease the associated heatstroke morbidity and mortality too frequently seen in the emergency departments.

Morbidity and mortality are directly associated with the duration of elevated core temperature. Even with aggressive prehospital intervention and in-hospital management, heatstroke can be fatal, and many patients who survive have permanent neurologic disability.

Heatstroke has two different clinical presentations: classic heatstroke and exertional heatstroke (Figure 20-5).

Classic heatstroke is a disorder of infants, febrile children, poor people, the elderly population, alcoholic persons, and sick patients, which may be compounded by the risk factors listed in Figure 20–3 (e.g., medications). A classic presentation is a patient who is exposed to elevated humidity and high room temperatures over several days without air conditioning, leading to dehydration and high core temperature. Often their sweating mechanism has stopped, known as *anhidrosis*. This is especially common in large cities during summer heat waves, when effective home ventilation is either not possible or not used.[12] Scene assessment will provide information helpful in the identification of classic heatstroke.

Exertional heatstroke (EHS) is a preventable disorder often seen in those individuals with poor physical fitness or lack of heat acclimatization who are involved in short-term, strenuous physical activity (e.g., industrial workers, athletes, military recruits, firefighters, and other public safety personnel) during a hot, humid environment. These conditions can rapidly elevate internal heat production and limit the body's ability to dissipate heat. Almost all EHS patients exhibit sweat-soaked and pale skin at time of collapse as compared to dry, hot, and flushed skin in the classic heatstroke patient.[29] Even though drinking fluids can slow the rate of dehydration during strenuous activity and reduce the rate at which core temperature rises, hyperthermia and EHS may still occur in the absence of significant dehydration.

Assessment. The appearance of signs and symptoms depends on the degree and duration of hyperthermia.[27] Heatstroke patients typically present with hot, flushed skin. They may or may not be sweating, depending on where they are found and whether they have classic or exertional heatstroke. Blood pressure may be elevated or diminished, and the radial pulse is usually tachycardic and thready; 25% of these patients are hypotensive. The patient's level of consciousness (LOC) can range from confused to unconscious, and seizure activity may also be present, particularly during cooling.[33] As confirmed in hospitals, rectal temperature may range from 104° to 116° F (40°–47° C).[30,33]

The keys to distinguishing heatstroke from one of the other heat-related conditions are the elevation in body temperature and altered mental status. Any patient who is warm to the touch with an altered mental status (confused, disoriented, combative, or unconscious) should be suspected of having heatstroke and managed immediately and aggressively.

Management. Heatstroke is a true emergency—immediately remove the patient from the source of heat. Cooling the patient should begin immediately in the field by one prehospital care provider as another provider assesses and stabilizes the patient's airway, breathing, and circulation (ABCs). Cooling of the patient begins immediately with whatever means are available (e.g., garden hose, fire hose, bottled water), even before removing clothing. Ideally, ice water immersion is the fastest method of cooling, but this is generally limited in the prehospital setting.[35–37] The next most effective method is application of ice water towels/sheets combined with ice packs on head, trunk, and extremities.[29] If cold water and ice are not immediately available, remove excess clothing, wet down the

FIGURE 20-5 **Classic Versus Exertional Heat Stroke**

	Classic	Exertional
Patient characteristics	Elderly	Men (15–45 years)
Health status	Chronically ill	Healthy
Concurrent activity	Sedentary	Strenuous exercise
Drug use	Diuretics, antidepressants, antihypertensives, anticholinergics, antipsychotics	Usually none
Sweating	May be absent	Usually present
Lactic acidosis	Usually absent; poor prognosis if present	Common
Hyperkalemia	Usually absent	Often present
Hypocalcemia	Uncommon	Frequent
Hypoglycemia	Uncommon	Common
Creatine	Mildly elevated	Greatly elevated
Rhabdomyolysis	Mild	Frequently severe

(Modified from Knochel JP, Reed G: Disorders of heat regulation. In Kleeman CR, Maxwell MH, Narin RG, editors: *Clinical disorders of fluid and electrolyte metabolism*, New York, 1987, McGraw-Hill.)

patient head to toe and provide fanning of the skin. This is the next most effective technique causing evaporation and convective heat loss when humidity is low.[35] Since the late 1950s, it has been thought that cold- or ice-water immersion will cause vasoconstriction sufficient to decrease heat loss from the body and cause the onset of shivering so that internal heat is produced. However, recent research has shown that this does not interfere with the critical lowering of the elevated core temperature.[35,37] Individuals who rapidly become lucid during whole-body cooling usually have the best prognosis. *The most important intervention prehospital care providers can deliver to a heatstroke patient (along with ABCs) is immediate and rapid whole-body cooling to reduce core temperature.*

During transport, the patient should be placed in a prepared, air-conditioned ambulance. It is an error to place a heatstroke patient in a hot internal cabin of the ambulance even if it is a short transfer time to the hospital. Remove any additional clothing, cover the patient with a sheet, and wet down the sheet with irrigation fluids along with continuous fanning. Ice packs, if available, should be placed in the groin area, in the axillae, and around the anterior lateral neck because blood vessels are closest to the skin surface in these areas. However, ice packs alone are insufficient to lower core body temperature rapidly and should be considered only as an extra cooling method.[4,35] If able, rectal temperature should be measured every 5 to 10 minutes during transport to ensure effective cooling and prevent hypothermia. Other means to assess the patient's temperature (e.g., oral, skin, axillary) should not be used for treatment decisions since they do not adequately reflect core temperature.[29] Active cooling should

stop when the rectal temperature reaches 102.2° F (39° C).[4,37] Provide high-flow oxygen, support ventilations with a bag-mask device as needed, and monitor the cardiac rhythm.

Heatstroke patients generally do not require extensive fluid resuscitation and typically are initially given IV fluids consisting of 1.0 to 1.5 liter of NS. Provide a 500-ml fluid challenge and assess vital signs. Fluid volume should not exceed 1 to 2 liters in the first hour, or follow local medical protocol. Monitor blood glucose because these patients are frequently hypoglycemic and may require a bolus of 50% dextrose IV. Seizures can be managed with 5 to 10 mg of diazepam or other benzodiazepines as per local protocol. Transport the patient in a right or left lateral recumbent position to maintain an open airway and to avoid aspiration.

Exercise-Associated Hyponatremia. Exercise-associated hyponatremia (EAH), also known as exertional hyponatremia or water intoxication, is a life-threatening condition that has been increasingly described after prolonged physical exertion in recreational hikers, marathoners, ultra-marathoners, triathletes, adventure racers, and military infantry personnel.[38–40] With the increasing popularity of these outdoor activities, the incidence rate of mild to severe EAH has steadily increased since it was first reported in the mid 1980s.[41] It is now known to be one of the most common medical complications of long-distance running and is an important cause of race-related fatalities. Also, EAH is commonly associated with consumption of excessive water intake during prolonged activities.[42] It can take two forms depending on presenting symptoms. Low plasma sodium concentration disturbs the osmotic balance across the blood-brain barrier, resulting in rapid influx of water into the brain, which in turn causes cerebral edema.[41] In similar fashion to the signs and symptoms of increased intracranial pressure (ICP) in head trauma (see Chapter 9), a progression of neurologic symptoms from hyponatremia will occur, including headache, malaise, confusion, and seizures to coma, permanent brain damage, brainstem herniation, and death.[41] These individuals are said to have exercise-associated hyponatremic encephalopathy (EAHE).[42] Symptomatic EAHE patients generally have a serum sodium concentration below 126 mEq/liter (normal range, 135–145 mEq/liter) with rapidly developing (<48 hours) hyponatremia, as seen frequently in prolonged endurance events.[38,42] Alternatively, the milder form generally presents with isolated serum sodium levels 135 to 128 mEq/liter, without easily discernable symptoms (i.e., weakness, nausea/vomiting, headache, or no symptoms).

Studies have reported that 18% to 23% of ultra-marathoners and 29% of the Hawaiian Ironman Triathlete finishers had EAH.[32–46] In 2003, 32 cases of EAH were reported in hikers in the Grand Canyon National Park, requiring an extensive rescue efforts by park rangers and paramedics in many cases.[47]

Exertional-associated hyponatremia can occur in the following situations:

1. Excessive sodium and water loss in sweat throughout an endurance event, resulting in dehydration and sodium depletion.
2. Athletes overhydrate solely with water while maintaining plasma sodium, creating a dilution of sodium concentration.
3. Combination of excessive sodium and fluid loss in sweat and an excessive overhydration only with water.

The evidence indicates that exertion-induced hyponatremia is a result of fluid retention in the extracellular space (dilutional) rather than fluid remaining unabsorbed in the intestine.[38] Typically, these patients have not consumed sport electrolyte drinks, have consumed energy food supplements containing no salt, or consumed them in quantities insufficient to balance the loss of sodium in sweat or the dilution from excessive water intake.

A few key risk factors that have been linked to the development of EAH:

1. exercise duration (>4 hours) or slow running/exercise pace at these events, allowing for greater water drinking
2. female gender (maybe explained by lower body weight)
3. low body weight
4. excessive drinking (>1.5 liter/hour) during an event
5. overhydration from abundant availability of drinking fluids at the event
6. nonsteroidal anti-inflammatory drugs (NSAID), which decrease renal filtration
7. extreme hot or cold environments[42]

Exercise-associated hyponatremia has been described as the "other heat-related illness" because the symptoms are nonspecific and are similar to those exhibited in minor and major heat-related disorders.[47] Many endurance events and multi-day adventure activities are conducted in warm to hot environments; therefore, it is assumed that the signs and symptoms of EAH are some form of heat illness, and patients are managed with standard protocols that address the presumed hypovolemia and excessive body heat. Standard protocols that provide body cooling and IV fluid challenge to correct hyperthermia, sweat-induced dehydration, and mental status changes can complicate the dilutional hyponatremia and place the patient at further risk for seizure and coma. Treating an EAH patient with fluids and rest will worsen their condition, unlike the heat exhaustion patient.

This "other heat-related disorder" is becoming more widely recognized and correctly treated today by EMS and ED personnel, largely because of an increased effort to educate medical personnel and the public in its prevention, early recognition, and management. Prehospital care providers directly supporting or responding to calls at these athletic endurance events in the cities or in the wilderness settings need to be aware that EAH is more frequently reported today. It is important to remember that, in general, dehydration is more common in prolonged exertional activities and that it can lead to impaired performance during exercise or work-related tasks and to serious heat illness, but that overdrinking with symptomatic hyponatremia is more dangerous and potentially a life-threatening illness.[56]

Assessment. A wide range of signs and symptoms may be found in the endurance-athlete population with hyponatremia (see Figure 20-4). Core temperature is usually normal but can be low or slightly elevated, depending on the ambient temperature, body-heat dissipation, and recent exercise intensity at assessment. Heart rate and blood pressure can be low, normal, or elevated, depending on core temperature, exercise intensity, hypovolemia, or shock. Respiratory rate ranges from within normal limits to slightly elevated. Hyperventilation observed with exertional hyponatremia can account for vision disturbances, dizziness, tingling in hands, and paresthesias in the extremities. The hallmark assessment and findings are mental-status changes, fatigue, malaise, headache, and nausea. Other forms of neurologic changes include slowed speech, ataxia, and cognitive changes, including irrational behavior, combativeness, and fear. These patients also often report that they have a sense of "impending doom."

Management. The first step in treatment is recognizing the disorder and determining the severity. Management is based on the severity of exertional hyponatremia. Figure 20-6 provides an algorithm for assessing patients to determine whether hyponatremia or a heat illness is present. Mild symptoms should be managed conservatively by observing the patient and waiting for normal diuresis of excessive fluid. Symptomatic patients should be placed in an upright position to maintain their airway and to minimize any positional effect on ICP. These patients are known to have projectile vomiting when transported. Place unconscious patients in the left lateral recumbent position, anticipate vomiting, and consider active airway management. Provide high-flow oxygen, establish IV access at the keep vein open (KVO) rate, and monitor for seizures. As needed, administer anticonvulsant therapy (e.g., titrate benzodiazepine intravenously, per medical protocol). Check with your medical control for volume of NS fluid, if any, to be administered, depending on patient severity and transport time to hospital. Because these patients are already fluid-overloaded, infusion of intravenous hypotonic fluids is contraindicated, as this can worsen the degree of hyponatremia and fluid overload.[48,] Patients with extensive signs and symptoms of EAHE (i.e., cerebral edema and pulmonary edema) need to have their plasma sodium concentration increased. The current consensus for management in the prehospital setting is to provide a bolus infusion of 3% NaCl over ten minutes to acutely reduce brain edema and to raise sodium (Na^+) 2–3 mEq/L, if this solution is available. With no clinical improvement, up to two additional 100 ml—3% bolus infusions can be given per medical protocol.[48] These severe cases of EAHE have a poor outcome if they do not receive hypertonic saline.[51] Keep the patient calm while en route to the ED, and continue to monitor for mental status changes or seizures.

Prevention of Heat-Related Illness

Because heat stress is a significant public health factor in the United States, methods for preventing heat illness are vital to any community, particularly for those individuals who must work in high-heat occupational settings. For example, in 2006, there were a total of 106 firefighter deaths in the United States from all causes and, of these deaths, 54 (50.9%) occurred at the scene due to stress/overexertion, which included heat illness as a cause of death in this category.[52] Prehospital care providers and

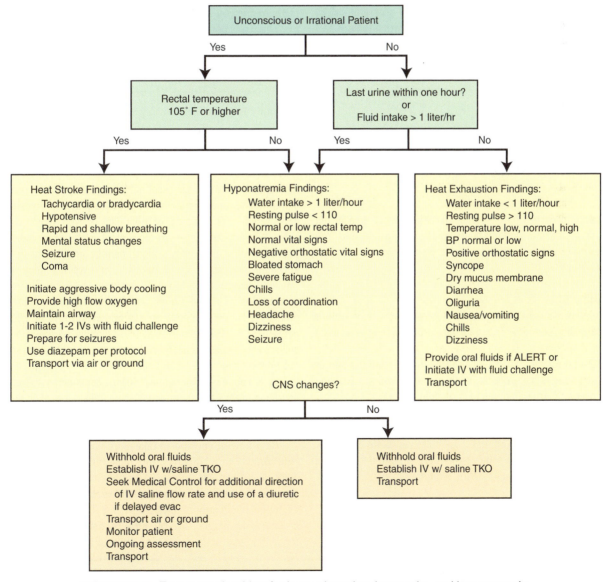

FIGURE 20-6   Treatment algorithm for heat exhaustion, heatstroke, and hyponatremia.

their EMS agencies are a good resource as partners for community education on heat stress prevention strategies in many different formats, including educational handouts, agency Web site or newsletter, community presentations, and local newspaper.

As with the general public, it may not be possible to prevent all forms of heat-related illness in prehospital care providers; therefore, EMS and other public safety personnel need to use prevention strategies and prepare for exposure to high ambient temperature and high occupational exposures. These strategies, which include administrative policies, procedures, engineering controls, use of equipment, and medical surveillance programs, are designed to help minimize the overall impact from acute or chronic heat exposure. The implementation of simple preventive procedures can have a dramatic impact on lowering the incidence of heat illness, but individuals in an organization often do not consider these strategies. Figure 20-7 provides an overview of heat stress prevention strategies for EMS providers, firefighters, and other public safety personnel.[53]

FIGURE 20-7 Prevention of Heat-Related Disorders in Prehospital Care Providers

You can prevent the serious consequences of heat disorders by improving your level of fitness and becoming acclimated to the heat.

Maintaining a high level of aerobic fitness is one of the best ways to protect yourself against heat stress. The fit worker has a well-developed circulatory system and increased blood volume. Both are important to regulate body temperature. Fit workers start to sweat sooner, so they work with a lower heart rate and body temperature. They adjust to the heat twice as fast as the unfit worker. They lose acclimatization more slowly and regain it quickly.

Heat acclimatization occurs in 5 to 10 days of heat exposure as the body:

- Increases sweat production
- Improves blood distribution
- Decreases the heart rate, and lowers the skin and body temperatures

You can acclimatize by gradually increasing work time in the heat, taking care to replace fluids, and resting as needed. You maintain acclimatization with periodic work or exercise in a hot environment.

ON THE JOB
The heat stress index (Figure 20-8) illustrates how temperature and humidity combine to create moderate-heat or high-heat stress conditions.

Be alert for heat stress when radiant heat from the sun or nearby flames is high, the air is still, or when you are working hard, creating large amounts of metabolic heat.

Some organizations use the WBGT heat stress index (Figure 20-9). The index, which is often available locally from the National Weather Service, uses dry bulb, wet bulb, and black globe temperatures. The temperatures are weighted to indicate the impact of each measure on the worker:

- *Wet bulb* (humidity) accounts for 70%
- *Black globe* (radiant heat and air movement) accounts for 20%
- *Dry bulb* (air temperature) accounts for 10%

Heat stress indexes do not take into account the effects of long hours of hard work, dehydration, or the impact of personal protective clothing and equipment.

When heat stress conditions exist, you must modify the way you work or exercise. Pace yourself. There are individual differences in fitness, acclimatization, and heat tolerance. Push too hard and you will be a candidate for a heat disorder.

When possible:

- Avoid working close to heat sources
- Do harder work during cooler morning and evening hours
- Change tools or tasks to minimize fatigue
- Take frequent rest breaks

Most important, maintain hydration by replacing lost fluids.

HYDRATION
Maintaining body fluids is essential for sweating and the removal of internal heat generated during physical activities. To minimize dehydration and the risk of heat illness, you must hydrate before, during, and after exercise or physical work. Individual characteristics (e.g., body weight, genetic predisposition, heat acclimatization state, and metabolic state) will influence sweat rate for a given activity. These factors will result in large individual sweat rates and total sweat loss. For example, long distance running is known to cause an average sweat rate of 1.8 liters per hour (1.0–2.6 liter/hour) in summer months, whereas football players (large body mass and wearing protective gear) are known to sweat on average 2.1 liters per hour (1.1–3.2 liter/hour) and up to 8.8 liters per day.[48] There needs to be a commitment to frequent hydration breaks to ensure dehydration does not exceed greater than 2% of body weight (based on pre-activity nude body weight) throughout the duration of physical activity.

Before work, you should take extra fluids to prepare for the heat. Drink 1 to 2 cups of water, juice, or a sport drink before work. Avoid excess caffeine; it hastens fluid loss in the urine. There is no physiologic advantage to excessively consume large amounts of fluid prior to physical activity. The American College of Sports Medicine (ACSM) now recommends prehydrating slowly for several hours before a physical activity and consume

---

(Modified from US Department of Agriculture, US Forest Service: Heat stress brochure, http://www.fs.usda.gov/fire/safety/fitness/heat_stress/hs_pg1.html. See also: American College of Sports Medicine Position Stand: Exercise and Fluid Replacement. *Med Sci Sports Exerc* 39(2):377, 2007.)

FIGURE 20-7—cont'd

~5–7 ml per kg of body weight. The goal is to produce urine output that is clear to straw color in appearance and prevent starting an activity in a dehydrated state.

While working, take several fluid breaks every hour, drinking approximately 1 quart of fluid per hour. Individual sweat rates will vary as will the amount of water needed to consume per hour. Caution should be used to prevent consumption of excessive fluids greater than 1.5 liters/hour for prolonged periods unless you have determined your individualized sweat loss rate per hour. ACSM now recommends a starting point of 0.4 to 0.8 liters on average per hour for exercise activities (e.g., marathon running) and adjusting the amount consumed based on individual lower or higher sweat rates for activities in cool or warm temperature conditions, lighter or heavier individuals.[48] Water is your greatest need during work in the heat. Studies show that workers drink more when lightly flavored beverages are available. Providing a portion of fluid replacement with a carbohydrate/electrolyte sport beverage will help you retain fluids and maintain energy and electrolyte levels. Unfortunately, many sports drinks contain large amounts of sugar which can actually slow absorption of ingested fluid.

After work, you need to continue drinking to replace fluid losses. To achieve rapid and complete recovery for activities resulting is large sweat loss (i.e., firefighting) you should drink ~1.5 liters of fluids for each kilogram of body weight loss.[48] *Thirst always underestimates fluid needs,* so you should drink more than you think you need. Rehydration is enhanced when fluids contain sodium and potassium or when foods with these electrolytes are consumed along with the fluid.

Sodium lost in sweat is easily replaced at meals with liberal use of the salt shaker. Unacclimatized workers lose more salt in the heat, so they need to pay particular attention to salt replacement. Do not overdo salt intake; too much salt impairs temperature regulation. Excessive salt can cause stomach distress, fatigue, and other problems.

Make potassium-rich foods like bananas and citrus fruits a regular part of your diet, and drink lots of lemonade, orange juice, or tomato juice. Limit the amount of caffeine drinks such as coffee and colas because caffeine increases fluid loss in the urine. Avoid alcoholic drinks. They also cause dehydration. Avoid sharing water bottles except in emergencies.

You can reassess your hydration by observing the volume, color, and concentration of your urine; low volumes of dark, concentrated urine and painful urination indicate a serious need for rehydration. Other signs of dehydration include a rapid heart rate, weakness, excessive fatigue, and dizziness. Rapid loss of several pounds of body weight is a certain sign of dehydration. Rehydrate before returning to work. Continuing to work in a dehydrated state can lead to serious consequences, including heatstroke, muscle breakdown, and kidney failure.

CLOTHING

Personal protective clothing strikes a balance between protection and worker comfort. Australian researchers have concluded that *the task for personnel wearing personal protection equipment is not to keep heat out, but to let it out.* About 70% of the heat load comes from within, from metabolic heat generated during hard work. Only 30% comes from the environment and the fire. Wear loose-fitting garments to enhance air movement. Wear cotton T-shirts and underwear to help sweat evaporate. Avoid extra layers of clothing that insulate, restrict air movement, and contribute to heat stress.

INDIVIDUAL DIFFERENCES

Individuals differ in their response to heat. Some workers are at greater risk for heat disorders. The reasons include inherited differences in heat tolerance and sweat rate; excess body weight, which raises metabolic heat production; illness, drugs, and medications, which can also influence your body's response to work in a hot environment. Check with your physician or pharmacist if you are using prescription or over-the-counter medications, or if you have a medical condition.

You should always train and work with a partner who can help in the event of a problem. Remind each other to drink lots of fluids, and watch each other. If your partner develops a heat disorder, start treatment immediately.

SUMMARY
Prevention
- Improve or maintain aerobic fitness
- Acclimate to the heat

On the Job
- Be aware of conditions (temperature, humidity, air movement)
- Take frequent rest breaks
- Avoid extra layers of clothing
- Pace yourself

Hydrate
- The hydration goal is to prevent dehydration (sweat loss) of greater than 2% of nude body weight
- Before work, drink several cups of water, juice, or a sport drink
- During work, take frequent fluid breaks
- After work, keep drinking to ensure rehydration
- Remember, only you can prevent dehydration

Partners
- Always work or train with a partner

FIGURE 20-7—cont'd

Drinks

■ Sport drinks with carbohydrates (no more than 6–8%; ~30–60 grams/hour) and electrolytes (e.g., sodium 20–50 mEq per liter) encourage fluid intake, provide energy, and diminish urinary water loss. The carbohydrates also help maintain immune function and mental performance during prolonged, arduous work. Drinks with caffeine and alcohol interfere with rehydration by increasing urine production.

(Modified from US Department of Agriculture, US Forest Service: Heat stress brochure, http://www.fs.usda.gov/fire/safety/fitness/heat_stress/hs_pg1.html. See also: American College of Sports Medicine Position Stand: Exercise and Fluid Replacement. *Med Sci Sports Exerc* 39(2):377, 2007.)

A complex interaction of factors that combine to exceed the tolerance limits for individual heat exposure can eventually lead to the onset of signs and symptoms of heat illness. The capacity of humans to work in moderate to hot environments can be maximized through advanced preparation of physical fitness, heat acclimatization, living and working conditions, personal hygiene, and use of food and beverages to maintain and replace electrolytes and water in the body. Environment, fluid hydration, physical fitness, and heat acclimatization are essential factors to understand.

Environment

Prehospital care providers and other public safety personnel are subjected to high heat environments as part of their occupational requirements. During training or an emergency response, many personnel will encounter high levels of heat stress while working in *personal protection equipment* (PPE) (impermeable clothing), such as turnout gear, hazardous material (hazmat) suit, or chemical/biologic protective garment. This heat stress is further compounded by the need to enter poorly ventilated or confined spaces or to work on a multivehicle crash in the sun on a hot, humid day. PPE compromises the body's ability to dissipate body heat and prevents the evaporation of sweat during a heavy workload. With high sweat rates from internal heat production during physically demanding tasks and the external heat exposure, personnel are at a high risk of dehydration and heat illness. Thus, the use of PPE diminishes the physiologic advantage gained through heat acclimatization and physical fitness.

These risks can be minimized by measuring the environmental heat conditions and, when applicable, following the recommended work/rest and hydration guidelines for work in highly thermal environments.[18,54]

One traditional method for measuring the thermal load is by use of the *heat stress index* (Figure 20-8). This index uses the combination of ambient temperature (read on a thermometer) and relative humidity. This is a better method of predicting potential systemic heat injury than the ambient temperature alone. If working in direct sunlight, near surfaces that radiate large amounts of heat, or in heavy protective clothing, 10° F should be added to the value in the table.

A more widely used method for measurement of environmental heat strain used in many industrial and military settings is the *wet-bulb globe temperature* (WBGT) *index*[5,18,55] (Figure 20-9). This index uses the combination of a dry bulb for ambient temperature, wet bulb for humidity measurement, black globe for radiant heat, and air movement to provide a

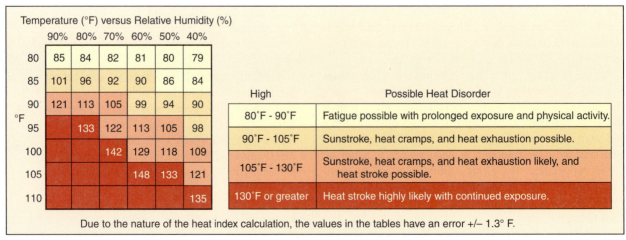

Temperature (°F) versus Relative Humidity (%)

°F	90%	80%	70%	60%	50%	40%
80	85	84	82	81	80	79
85	101	96	92	90	86	84
90	121	113	105	99	94	90
95		133	122	113	105	98
100			142	129	118	109
105				148	133	121
110						135

High	Possible Heat Disorder
80°F - 90°F	Fatigue possible with prolonged exposure and physical activity.
90°F - 105°F	Sunstroke, heat cramps, and heat exhaustion possible.
105°F - 130°F	Sunstroke, heat cramps, and heat exhaustion likely, and heat stroke possible.
130°F or greater	Heat stroke highly likely with continued exposure.

Due to the nature of the heat index calculation, the values in the tables have an error +/– 1.3° F.

FIGURE 20-8 Heat stress index.
(Courtesy National Weather Service, Pueblo, Colo, www.crh.noaa.gov/pub/heat.htm.)

FIGURE 20-9 Fluid Replacement Guidelines for Warm-Weather Training

Heat category	WBGT Index (°F)	Easy work Work/rest (minutes)	Easy work Water intake (qt/hour)	Moderate work Work/rest (minutes)	Moderate work Water intake (qt/hour)	Hard work Work/rest (minutes)	Hard work Water intake (qt/hour)
1	78–81.9	NL	$1/2$	NL	$3/4$	40/20	$3/4$
2	82–84.9	NL	$1/2$	50/10	$3/4$	30/30	1
3	85–87.9	NL	$3/4$	40/20	$3/4$	30/30	1
4	88–89.9	NL	$3/4$	30/30	$3/4$	20/40	1
5	>90	50/10	1	20/40	1	10/50	1

The work/rest times and fluid replacement volumes will sustain performance and hydration for at least 4 hours of work in the specified heat category. Individual water needs will vary ±qt/hr. *NL*, No limit to work time per hour. *Rest* means minimal physical activity (sitting or standing), accomplished in shade if possible.
Caution: Hourly fluid intake should not exceed 1.5 quarts. Daily fluid intake should not exceed 12 quarts.
Wearing body armor: Add 5° F to WBGT index in humid climates. Wearing personal protective equipment (PPE) over garment: add 10° F to WBGT index for easy work and 20° F for moderate and hard work.

Easy work	Moderate work	Hard work
Walking on hard surface at 2.5 mph, <31-lb load.	Walking on hard surface at 3.5 mph, <41-lb load. Walking in loose sand at 2.5 mph, no load. Calisthenics.	Walking on hard surface at 3.5 mph, >40-lb load. Walking in loose sand at 2.5 mph with load.

(Current version of WBGT, hydration, and work/rest guidelines as updated by US Army Research Institute for Environmental Medicine (USARIEM) and published by Montain SJ, Latzka WA, Sawka MN: *Mil Med* 164:502, 1999.)

more accurate impact of the environmental conditions. Integrated in the five-level WBGT index range of temperatures are hourly work/rest (minutes) and hydration (quarts) guidelines. A color flag (no flag, green, yellow, red, or black) represent each of the five WBGT ranges of temperatures. The WBGT can be monitored hourly and the corresponding color flag placed on a flagpole outdoors for all personnel to see throughout the day. When applicable, the appropriate adjustments of clothing, physical activity, work/rest cycles, and fluid intake can then be made based on these WBGT conditions. This integrated WBGT system and related policies can easily be developed at various public safety locations and training sites to ensure that effective heat illness prevention programs are in use to reduce fatigue, injuries, and heat illness.

Hydration

If the WBGT flag system is not used to provide guidelines for hydration, another excellent resource is published by the American College of Sports Medicine (ACSM), based on years of research.[56] These guidelines are easily applied to any individual engaged in physical activity. Hydration guidelines should be established within an agency in an effort to prevent excessive dehydration (>2% body weight loss) by creating easy access to water and sport electrolyte drinks, particularly

during activity in warm environments (Figures 20-10 and 20-11). Studies show that the average individual does not drink sufficient quantities of fluids before, during, and after work or exercise to recover body fluids lost from sweating, even though they believe they are consuming enough fluids.[56] Even though overconsumption of fluids can lead to hyponatremia (see Exertional Hyponatremia section), a potential life-threatening condition of clinical to low sodium concentration in the blood, it is more common for individuals to become dehydrated (>2% of body weight) during a given physical activity. Ideally, fluid-replacement programs should be customized based on individualized sweat rate loss as determined from a pre/post physical activity nude body weight loss measurement.

Fitness

To increase heat tolerance effectively in high-heat conditions, individuals should increase their aerobic fitness (e.g., walk, jog, bike, swim, stair stepping, elliptical exercise machines) through individualized programs.[57] These programs will provide the cardiac reserve to sustain the cardiac output required to meet the competing demands of physical (muscular) work and heat dissipation mechanisms (thermoregulation) in a high-temperature environment.[57,58]

FIGURE 20-10 Hydration Guidelines to Minimize Dehydration

1. Start exercise well hydrated.
Drink 2 to 3 cups (16–24 ounces) of fluid 2 to 3 hours before physical activity to allow excess fluid to be lost as urine. About 30 minutes before physical activity, drink 5 to 10 ounces. There is no benefit to overconsumption of fluids (hyperhydration), so do not drink excessively.

2. Weigh yourself.
The best way to determine if you have replaced sweat loss during heavy work or exercise is to check to see how much weight you have lost. Determine your body weight before and after physical activity. Minimal weight loss means that you have done a good job staying hydrated. Remember that weight loss during exercise or work is water loss, not fat loss, and must be replaced.

3. Drink during physical activity.
Drink 5 to 10 ounces of water or sport electrolyte drink every 10 to 20 minutes during a workout. Heavy sweaters can benefit from drinking more often (e.g., every 10 minutes) and light sweaters should drink less often (every 20+ minutes).

4. Ingest sodium during physical activity.
The best time to begin replacing the sodium lost in sweat is during exercise. That is one reason why a good sports electrolyte drink is better than plain water.

5. Follow your own plan.
Everybody sweats differently, so everybody needs a drinking plan tailored to his or her individual needs.

6. Drink plenty during meals.
If you were not able to drink enough during heavy work or exercise to keep from losing weight, be sure to drink enough before the next practice or returning to work. Mealtime is the best time to do that because of the ease of drinking and the sodium that comes along with food.

7. Do not rely solely on water.
Drinking only water keeps you from replacing the electrolytes lost in sweat and from ingesting carbohydrates that help you work or exercise longer and stronger. Excessive water drinking can lead to dangerous electrolyte disturbances (hyponatremia).

8. Do not overdrink.
Water is definitely a good thing, but you can get too much of a good thing. Drinking large amounts of fluid not only is unnecessary, but can be dangerous (hyponatremia). Bloated stomach, puffy fingers and ankles, a bad headache, and confusion are warning signs of hyponatremia.

9. Do not gain weight during exercise.
A sure sign of drinking too much is weight gain during heavy work or exercise. If you weigh more after work or exercise than you did before, it means that you drank more than you needed. Be sure to cut back the next time so that you do not gain weight.

10. Do not restrict salt in your diet.
Ample salt (sodium chloride) in the diet is essential to replace the salt lost in sweat. Because athletes sweat a lot, their need for salt is much greater than for nonathletes. (This principle holds true for those who work and sweat heavily each day in occupations conducted in moderate to hot environments.)

11. Do not use dehydration to lose weight.
Restricting fluid intake during work or exercise impairs physical performance and increases the risk of heat-related problems. Dehydration should be kept to a minimum by following a wise fluid replacement plan.

12. Do not delay drinking during exercise or work.
Stick to a drinking schedule so that you avoid dehydration early in exercise or work. Once dehydrated, it is almost impossible to catch up to what your body needs, because dehydration actually slows the speed at which fluid exits the stomach.

(Modified from: Murray B, Eichner ER, Stofan J: Hyponatremia in athletes. *Sports Sci Exchange* 16(1):88, 2003, http://www.gssiweb.com/.)

The American College of Sports Medicine, American Heart Association, and Health and Human Services have collaborated recently to establish an updated nationwide physical activity recommendations to maintain health and well-being.[58] Figure 20-12 shows the most recent physical activity guidelines.

Heat Acclimatization

A policy and protocol for heat acclimatization should be provided within a public safety organization.[60] Heat acclimatiza-tion can be achieved with 60 to 90 minutes of exercise a day in hot conditions for approximately 7 to 14 days.[9,61] The benefits of heat acclimatization are increased work performance, heat tolerance, and reduced physiologic strain. These adjustments include increased blood volume, increased stroke volume, decreased heart rate at a given activity level, reduced sodium concentration in sweat, sodium conserved in the body, earlier onset of sweating, and *increased* sweat volume rate (Figure 20-13). These changes improve the transfer of body heat from the core to the skin in an effort to increase the heat transfer

FIGURE 20-11   Simple Test to Determine if You are Dehydrated

There are three simple questions you can ask yourself to determine if you are dehydrated:

- Am I thirsty?
- Is my morning urine dark yellow?
- Is my bodyweight this morning noticeably lower when compared to yesterday morning?

If the answer to any one of these questions is "Yes," you may be dehydrated. If the answer to any two of these questions is "Yes," it is likely that you are dehydrated. If the answer to all three of these questions is "Yes," it is <u>very</u> likely that you are dehydrated.

Drinking too little or too much during physical activity can be dangerous to your health and can worsen your performance. Here are some tips to help you stay in fluid balance.

- To determine how much fluid you lose or gain during physical activity, exercise or hard work, use a chart like the one below to record your nude body weight to the nearest pound before and after your workouts.
- If you lost more than 1% of your body weight, you drank too little during exercise; if you gained weight, you drank too much.
- If you regularly lose more than 1% of your body weight, try to drink more during and after physical activity to keep your body weight stable.
- Remember, it can be dangerous to gain weight during physical activity by drinking too much.

RECORD OF BODY WEIGHT, THIRST, AND URINE COLOR
Loss of >1% body weight or persistent thirst or dark urine indicates possible dehydration.
If any two of these indicators occurs, dehydration is likely.
If all three occur, dehydration is <u>very</u> likely.

Date	Nude Weight Yesterday Morning (lb)	Nude Weight this Morning (lb)	Weight Change (lb)	Thirsty? (Yes/No)	Dark Yellow Urine in Morning? (Yes/No)	Your Comments
Example 1/1/2006	146	142	−4	Yes	Yes	- Very likely dehydrated - Need to drink more during and after exercise

(Modified from: Cheuvront SN and Sawka MN: Hydration Assessment of Athletes. *Sports Science Exchange 97,* Vol 18(2), 2005. http://www.gssiweb.com)

from the skin to the environment. Although heat tolerance is improved in these individuals (e.g., endurance athletes, military infantry personnel) and is considered desirable, the greater sweat-volume production (1–2 liter/hour) results in large fluid losses, leading to dehydration. Consequently, the greater volume of sweat loss in heat-acclimatized individuals increases the hydration requirements during heat exposure, particularly when the person does not adhere to a rigorous oral hydration schedule. Figure 20-14 provides an overview of heat acclimatization guidelines.

Emergency Incident Rehabilitation

A standard for fire rehabilitation that complements other standards (e.g., Occupational Safety Health Administration [OSHA], US Fire Administration [USFA]) in the areas of safety, health, and fitness provides guidance about incident rehabilitation. The 2008 edition of *NFPA 1584: Standard on the Rehabilitation Process for Members During Emergency Operations and Training Exercises* reflects current science and knowledge on rehabilitation of fire service members and upgrades the previous document from a recommended practice to a standard.[62–65] The introduction of NFPA 1584 as a standard means every department must have standardized procedure outlining how they provide rehabilitation at incidents and training exercises.

The nine key components of rehab required by NFPA 1584 are:

1. **Relief from climactic conditions**—An area free of smoke and sheltered from extreme heat or cold is provided. This might be a nonfire floor in a high-rise building, a shaded area upwind from a brush fire, or the heated fire-

FIGURE 20-12   Physical Activity Guidelines for Americans

The following guidelines are from the Department of Health and Human Services (HHS) with support from the American College of Sports Medicine (ACSM) and the American Heart Association (AHA).[58] Physical activity is one of the most important steps that Americans of all ages can take to improve their health. The *2008 Physical Activity Guidelines for Americans* provides science-based guidance to help Americans aged 6 and older improve their health through appropriate physical activity.

Key Guidelines for Adults
- All adults should avoid inactivity. Some physical activity is better than none, and adults who participate in any amount of physical activity gain some health benefits.
- For substantial health benefits, adults should do at least 150 minutes (2 hours and 30 minutes) a week of moderate-intensity, or 75 minutes (1 hour and 15 minutes) a week of vigorous-intensity aerobic physical activity, or an equivalent combination of moderate- and vigorous intensity aerobic activity. Aerobic activity should be performed in episodes of at least 10 minutes, and preferably, it should be spread throughout the week.
- For additional and more extensive health benefits, adults should increase their aerobic physical activity to 300 minutes (5 hours) a week of moderate intensity, or 150 minutes a week of vigorous intensity aerobic physical activity, or an equivalent combination of moderate- and vigorous-intensity activity. Additional health benefits are gained by engaging in physical activity beyond this amount.
- Adults should also do muscle-strengthening activities that are moderate or high intensity and involve all major muscle groups on 2 or more days a week, as these activities provide additional health benefits.

Ways to get the equivalent of 150 minutes (2 hours and 30 minutes) of moderate-intensity aerobic physical activity a week plus muscle-strengthening activities:

- Thirty minutes of brisk walking (moderate intensity) on 5 days, exercising with resistance bands (muscle strengthening) on 2 days
- Twenty-five minutes of running (vigorous intensity) on 3 days, lifting weights on 2 days (muscle strengthening)
- Thirty minutes of brisk walking on 2 days, 60 minutes (1 hour) of social dancing (moderate intensity) on 1 evening, 30 minutes of mowing the lawn (moderate intensity) on 1 afternoon, heavy gardening (muscle strengthening) on 2 days
- Thirty minutes of an aerobic dance class on 1 morning (vigorous intensity), 30 minutes of running on 1 day (vigorous intensity), 30 minutes of brisk walking on 1 day (moderate intensity), calisthenics (such as sit-ups, push-ups) on 3 days (muscle strengthening)
- Thirty minutes of biking to and from work on 3 days (moderate intensity), playing softball for 60 minutes on 1 day (moderate intensity), using weight machines on 2 days (muscle-strengthening on 2 days)
- Forty-five minutes of doubles tennis on 2 days (moderate intensity), lifting weights after work on 1 day (muscle strengthening), hiking vigorously for 30 minutes and rock climbing (muscle strengthening) on 1 day

For adults who are already doing at least 150 minutes of moderate-intensity physical activity, here are a few ways to do even more. Physical activity at this level has even greater health benefits.

- Forty-five minutes of brisk walking every day, exercising with resistance bands on 2 or 3 days;
- Forty-five minutes of running on 3 or 4 days, circuit weight training in a gym on 2 or 3 days;
- Thirty minutes of running on 2 days, 45 minutes of brisk walking on 1 day, 45 minutes of an aerobics and weights class on 1 day, 90 minutes (1 hour and 30 minutes) of social dancing on 1 evening, 30 minutes of mowing the lawn, plus some heavy garden work on 1 day;
- Ninety minutes of playing soccer on 1 day, brisk walking for 15 minutes on 3 days, lifting weights on 2 days; and
- Forty-five minutes of stationary bicycling on 2 days, 60 minutes of basketball on 2 days, calisthenics on 3 days.

For more information or additional details on the physical activity guidelines, visit:

http:/www.americanheart.org/fitness
http:/www.acsm.org/physicalactivity
http:/www.health.gov/PAGuidelines

(Source: Haskell, WL, Lee, IM, Pate, RR, Powell, KE, Blair, SN, Franklin, BA, Macera, CA, Heath, GW, Thompson, PD and Bauman, A: Physical activity and public health: Updated recommendation for adults from the American College of Sports Medicine and the American Heart Association. *Medicine & Science in Sports & Exercise* 39(8), 1423, 2007.)

FIGURE 20-13   Benefits of heat acclimatization

1. Thermal comfort: improved
2. Core temperature: reduced
3. Skin blood flow: earlier
4. Heart rate: lowered
5. Salt losses (sweat and urine): reduced
6. Exercise performance: improved
7. Sweating: earlier and greater
8. Body heat production: lower
9. Thirst: improved
10. Organ protection: improved

(From the Heat Acclimatization Guide, Ranger and Airborne School Students, 2003, www.usariem.army.mil/download/heatacclimatization guide.pdf.)

apparatus cab during cold winter months. The theme is providing shelter from environmental extremes.

2. **Rest and recovery**—Members are afforded the ability to rest for at least 10 minutes or as long as needed to recover work capacity.

3. **Cooling or rewarming**—Members who feel hot should be able to remove their PPE, drink water, and have the means to cool off. Members who are cold should be able to add clothing, wrap in blankets, and have the means to warm themselves.

4. **Rehydration**—Fluid replacement. Fluid volume requirements were eliminated from the standard with the exception of prehydration with 500 ml (16 ounces) of fluids consumed two hours prior to scheduled events. On scene, potable fluids must be provided so members can satisfy thirst. Fluids should also be provided to encourage continued hydration after the incident.

5. **Calorie and electrolyte replacement**—When appropriate for longer duration events, such as incidents exceeding three hours duration or situations in which members are likely to work for more than one hour. Of note, whenever food is available, means for members to wash their hands and faces must also be provided.

6. **Medical monitoring**—Specifies a minimum of six conditions that EMS must assess in each member during rehabilitation:
   a. Presence of chest pain, dizziness, shortness of breath, weakness, nausea, or headache.
   b. General complaints such as cramps or aches and pains.
   c. Symptoms of heat- or cold-related stress.
   d. Changes in gait, speech, or behavior.
   e. Alertness and orientation to person, place, and time.

FIGURE 20-14   Heat acclimatization guidelines

The following is a modified version of the heat acclimatization guidelines designed for healthy and physically fit infantry personnel in preparation for physical activity in hot environments.

SHOULD YOU BE CONCERNED ABOUT HOT WEATHER?

If you are used to working in cool or temperate climates, exposure to hot weather will make it much more difficult to complete your advanced training course. Hot weather will make you feel fatigued, make it more difficult to recover, and increase your risk of becoming a heat casualty. Individuals with the same abilities but who are used to training in hot weather will have a greater heat tolerance and physical ability during heat exposure.

WHAT IS HEAT ACCLIMATIZATION?

Heat acclimatization refers to biologic adaptations that reduce physiologic strain (e.g., heart rate, body temperature), improve physical work capabilities, improve comfort and protect vital organs (brain, liver, kidneys, muscles) from heat injury. The most important biologic adaptation from heat acclimatization is an earlier and greater sweating response, and for this response to improve, it needs to be invoked.

Heat acclimatization is specific to the climate (desert) and physical activity level. However, acclimatization to desert climates greatly improves the ability to work in other climates. Individuals who only perform light or brief physical work will achieve the level of heat acclimatization needed to perform that task. If they attempt a more strenuous or prolonged task, additional acclimatization and improved physical fitness will be needed to perform that task successfully in the heat.

HOW DO YOU BECOME HEAT ACCLIMATIZED?

Heat acclimatization occurs when repeated heat exposures are sufficiently stressful to elevate body temperature and provoke profuse sweating. Resting in the heat, with limited physical activity to that required for existence, results in only partial acclimatization. Physical exercise in the heat is required to achieve optimal heat acclimatization for that exercise intensity in a given hot environment.

Generally, about 2 weeks of daily heat exposure is needed to induce heat acclimatization. Heat acclimatization requires a minimum daily heat exposure of about 2 hours (can be broken into two 1-hour exposures) combined with physical exercise that requires cardiovascular endurance (e.g., jogging) rather than strength training. Gradually increase the exercise intensity or duration each day. Work up to an appropriate physical training schedule adapted to the required physical activity.

(For complete report: http://www.usariem.army.mil/download/heatacclimatizationguide.pdf.)

FIGURE 20-15—cont'd

The benefits of heat acclimatization will be retained for about 1 week and then decay, with about 75% lost by about 3 weeks, once heat exposure ends. One or 2 days of intervening cool weather will not interfere with acclimatization to hot weather.

HOW FAST CAN YOU BECOME HEAT ACCLIMATIZED?
For the average individual, heat acclimatization requires about 2 weeks of heat exposure and progressive increases in physical work. By the second day of acclimatization, significant reductions in physiologic strain are observed. By the end of the first week and second week, >60% and >80% of the physiologic adaptations are complete, respectively. Less fit individuals or those unusually susceptible to heat exposure may require several days or weeks more to fully acclimatize.

Physically fit individuals should be able to achieve heat acclimatization in about 1 week. However, several weeks of living and working in the heat (seasoning) may be required to maximize tolerance to high body temperatures.

WHAT ARE THE BEST HEAT ACCLIMATIZATION STRATEGIES?
1. Maximize physical fitness and heat acclimatization before hot weather exposure. Maintain physical fitness with maintenance programs tailored to the environment, such as physical training in the cooler morning or evening hours.
2. Integrate training and heat acclimatization. Train in the coolest part of the day and acclimatize in the heat of the day. Start slowly by reducing your usual training intensity and duration (compared to what you could achieve in temperate climates). Increase training and heat exposure volume as your heat tolerance permits. Use interval training to modify your activity level.
3. If the new climate is much hotter than what you are accustomed to, recreational activities may be appropriate for the first 2 days with periods of run/walk. By the third day, you should be able to integrate training runs (20–40 minutes) at a reduced pace.
4. Consume sufficient water to replace sweat losses. Sweat rates of more than 1 quart per hour are common. Heat acclimatization increases the sweating rate, and, therefore, increases water requirements. As a result, heat-acclimatized individuals will dehydrate faster if they do not consume fluids. Dehydration negates many of the thermoregulatory advantages conferred by heat acclimatization and high physical fitness.

f. Any vital signs considered abnormal in local protocol. The specific vital signs and what defines normal is entirely up to local medical control and department medical authorities. Vital signs listed in the NFPA 1584 annex include temperature, pulse, respirations, blood pressure, pulse oximetry, and carbon monoxide assessment, using either an exhaled breath CO monitor or a pulse CO-oximeter (i.e., a pulse oximeter designed to measure carboxyhemoglobin).

7. **EMS treatment in accordance with local protocol**—Available on scene for members who require treatment or transport. Note that medical monitoring is documented in the fire department data collection system. When EMS treatment or transport is provided, a medical report must be generated and included in the member's employee medical record.

8. **Member accountability**—A personnel accountability system must track members assigned to rehabilitation by Incident Command as they enter and leave.

9. **Release**—Prior to leaving rehabilitation, EMS must confirm that members are able to safely perform full duty. [63]

The NFPA 1584 new standards for fire rehabilitation compliments the United States Fire Administration (USFA) standardized approach for evaluating and rehabilitating firefighters and emergency personnel during environmental extremes (Figure 20-15). In 1992 the USFA stated the following:

The physical and mental demands of EMS, firefighting and emergency operations that are associated with extreme heat and humidity create conditions that can have an adverse impact upon the safety and health of the individual emergency responder. Members who are not provided adequate rest and rehydration during emergency operations and training exercises are at increased risk for illness, and may jeopardize the safety of others on the incident scene. When emergency responders become fatigued, their ability to operate safely is impaired. As a result, their reaction time is reduced, and their ability to make critical decisions diminishes. Rehabilitation is an essential element on the incident scene to prevent more serious conditions such as heat exhaustion or heatstroke from occurring.[62]

EMS Drug Storage in Thermal Extremes

Prehospital care providers work in regions within the United States and elsewhere where annual extremes range from below freezing to high heat and humidity. Their vehicles, including mobile intensive care units, paramedic units, and medical helicopters, and the medications stored in those vehicles, are also subjected to the environmental extremes unless a temperature-controlled storage device is on board. Medications used by prehospital care providers are intended for storage at controlled room tem-

FIGURE 20-15 **US Fire Administration (USFA) Standard Operating Procedure (SOP) on Emergency Incident Rehabilitation**

PURPOSE

To ensure that the physical and mental conditions of members operating at the scene of an emergency or a training exercise do not deteriorate to a point that affects the safety of each member or that jeopardizes the safety and integrity of the operation.

SCOPE

This procedure will apply to all emergency operations and training exercises in which strenuous physical activity or exposure to heat or cold exists.

RESPONSIBILITIES

The Incident Commander will consider the circumstances of each incident and make adequate provisions early in the incident for the rest and rehabilitation for all members operating at the scene. These provisions will include medical evaluation, treatment, and monitoring; food and fluid replenishment; mental rest; and relief from extreme climatic conditions and the other environmental parameters of the incident. The rehabilitation will include the provision of emergency medical services (EMS) at the basic life support (BLS) level or higher. The Incident Commander will establish a rehabilitation sector or group when conditions indicate rest and rehabilitation is needed for persons operating at the incident scene or training evaluation.

GUIDELINES

Climatic or environmental conditions of the emergency scene should not be the sole justification for establishing a rehabilitation area. Any activity or incident that is large in size, long in duration, or labor intensive will rapidly deplete the energy and strength of personnel and, therefore, merits consideration for rehabilitation. Climatic or environmental conditions that indicate the need to establish a rehabilitation area are a heat stress index above 90° F (32° C) (see Figure 20-8) or windchill index below 10° F (-12° C) (see Figure 20-23).

HYDRATION

During heat stress, the member should consume at least 1 quart per hour and not to exceed 1.5 quarts per hour. The rehydration should be a 50/50 mixture of water and a commercially prepared activity beverage (sport electrolyte beverage) and administered at about 40° F (4.4° C). Alcohol and caffeine beverages should be avoided before and during heat stress because both interfere with the body's water conservation mechanisms. Carbonated beverages should also be avoided.

NOURISHMENT

The department will provide food at the scene of an extended incident when units are engaged for 3 or more hours. A cup of soup, broth, or stew is highly recommended because it is digested much faster than sandwiches and fast-food products.

REST

The "two-bottle rule," or 45 minutes of work time, is recommended as an acceptable level before mandatory rehabilitation. Members will rehydrate (at least 8 ounces) while SCBA cylinders are charged. Firefighters having worked for two full 30-minute-rated bottles, or 45 minutes, will be immediately placed in the rehabilitation area for rest and evaluation. Rest will not be less than 10 minutes and may exceed an hour, as determined by the Rehabilitation Officer.

RECOVERY

Members in the rehabilitation area should maintain a high level of hydration. Certain drugs impair the body's ability to sweat, and extreme caution must be exercised if the member has taken antihistamines, such as Actifed™ or Benadryl™ or has taken diuretics or stimulants.

MEDICAL EVALUATION

EMS should be provided and staffed by the most highly trained and qualified prehospital care providers on the scene (at a minimum of BLS level). They will evaluate vital signs, examine members, and make proper disposition (return to duty, continued rehabilitation, or medical treatment and transport to medical facility). Continued rehabilitation should consist of additional monitoring of vital signs, providing rest, and providing fluids for rehydration. Prehospital care providers will be assertive in an effort to find potential medical problems early. If a member's heart rate exceeds 110 beats/minute, an oral temperature should be taken. If the member's temperature exceeds 100.6° F (38° C), he or she should not be permitted to wear protective equipment. If it is below 100.6° F and heart rate remains above 110 beats/minute, rehabilitation time should be increased. If the heart rate is less than 110 beats/minute, the chance of heat stress is negligible. Document all medical evaluations.

(Modified from SOP for USFA Emergency Incident Rehabilitation, www.smemsc.org/EmergencyIncidentRehabilitation.pdf.)

perature according to recommendations of the drug manufacturers. The *United States Pharmacopeia (USP)* has oversight responsibilities in the United States for establishing drug standards intended to ensure the quality of medications, and *USP* defines controlled room temperature as follows:

A temperature maintained thermostatically that encompasses the usual and customary working environment of 68° to 77° F (20° to 25° C); that results in a mean kinetic temperature calculated to be not more than 77° F (25° C); and allows for excursions between 59° to 86° F (15° to 30° C) that are experienced in pharmacies, hospitals and warehouses. Provided the mean kinetic temperature remains in the allowed range, transient spikes up to 104° F (40° C) may be permitted if the manufacturer so instructs.[66]

Manufacturers will guarantee a medication's stability, quality, and potency only when the drugs are stored within the recommended temperature range. In many cases across the country, EMS vehicles have been shown periodically to have stored medications at temperatures outside the *USP*-recommended range.[67–70] These studies have examined thermal exposure of drugs in both field and laboratory settings for short (1–4 weeks) and long (12–26 weeks) durations.[67] What remains unclear is the effect of these thermal fluctuations on the bioavailability of many common prehospital drugs. Laboratory assessment shows that the majority of these drugs remain stable, except for epinephrine, which significantly degrades in extreme cold and heat.[67,71,72]

To improve compliance with the *USP* standards and manufacturers' recommendations, some states have implemented specific rules regarding storage of medication. For example, the New Jersey Office of Emergency Medical Services (Department of Health and Senior Services) passed regulations requiring the following:

Each vehicle and cabinet or other storage place for medications shall be sufficiently climate controlled so that the medications and solutions are kept within temperature range recommended by the manufacturer. Each vehicle shall have a temperature recording device which shall, at least, record the highest and lowest temperature during a specified time period.[73]

EMS agencies need to consider how they will deal with this concern for the efficacy of the medications used in their vehicles to assure that these drugs always work as intended when used by the EMS personnel. The cost for implementing environmentally controlled storage for all advanced life support (ALS) units, as recommended by each drug manufacturer and the *USP*, is certainly not insignificant, but to take no action based on these studies is unacceptable as well. It is suggested that each EMS agency develop a policy to investigate the thermal conditions in the vehicle medication storage area and consider a medication rotation system during periods of extreme cold and heat, or some other system to minimize the exposure of medications to thermal extremes in their region.[67]

Injuries Produced by Cold

Dehydration

Dehydration occurs very easily in the cold, particularly with increased physical activity. This occurs for three primary reasons: (1) evaporation of sweat, (2) increased respiratory heat and fluid losses caused by the dryness of cold air, and (3) cold-induced diuresis.

Cold-induced diuresis is a normal physiologic response resulting from skin vasoconstriction from prolonged cold exposure. This is the body's response to reduce body heat loss by shunting blood away from the colder periphery to deeper veins of the body. This response causes a central blood volume expansion, which results in a rise in the mean arterial pressure (MAP), stroke volume, and cardiac output.[74] The expanded blood volume can produce a diuresis, manifested by frequent urination. Cold-induced diuresis can reduce plasma volume by 7% to 15%, resulting in hemoconcentration and acute dehydration from almost a twofold fluid loss over normal.

As with exposure to heat, adherence to fluid hydration guidelines (see Figure 20-10) while working in cold environments is necessary to minimize dehydration along with the associated fatigue, and physical and cognitive changes. Because thirst is suppressed in cold environments, dehydration is a significant risk.

Cold-Related Disorders
Minor Cold-Related Disorders

Contact Freeze Injury. When cold material comes into contact with unprotected skin, it can produce local frostbite immediately. Do not touch any metal surface, alcohol, gasoline, antifreeze, ice, or snow with the hands. (See the frostbite section for assessment and management.)

Frostnip. Frostnip is a precursor to *frostbite* and produces reversible signs of skin blanching and numbness in localized tissue. It is typically seen on the face, nose, and ears.[10] Frostnip is a self-limited tissue injury as long as cold exposure does not continue; it does not require prehospital care provider intervention and transport.

Cold Urticaria. Cold urticaria ("hives") is a disorder characterized by the rapid onset (within minutes) of itchiness, redness, and swelling of the skin after exposure to cold. The sensation of burning may be a prominent feature. This condition, caused by a local release of histamine, is sometimes observed when ice is applied directly to the skin during cold therapy for sprains and strains. Individuals with a history of cold urticaria are advised to avoid cold-water immersion, which could potentially cause death from systemic anaphylaxis. Treatment includes avoiding the cold and possibly taking antihistamines.

Chilblains (Pernio). Chilblains are small skin lesions that are itchy, tender, and appear as red or purple bumps that occur on the extensor skin surface of the finger or any skin surface (e.g., ears, face) from chronic cold exposure. Chilblains occur several hours after exposure to the cold in temperate humid climates. They are sometimes aggravated by sun exposure. Cold causes constriction of the small arteries and veins in the skin, and rewarming results in leakage of blood into the tissues and swelling of the skin.

Chilblains are more likely to develop in those with poor peripheral circulation. Some contributing factors are a familial tendency, peripheral vascular disease caused by diabetes, smoking, hyperlipidemia, poor nutrition (e.g., anorexia nervosa), connective tissue disease, and bone marrow disorders. Each chilblain comes up over a few hours as an itchy, red swelling and subsides over the next 7 to 14 days. In severe cases, blistering, pustules, scabs, and ulceration can occur. Occasionally the lesions may be ring shaped. They may become thickened and persist for months.

Symptoms will subside with removal of the individual from the cold. Management involves protection from cold with appropriate gloves and clothing.

Solar Keratitis (Snow Blindness). Without protection from dry air and from exposure to bright reflections on snow, the risk of ultraviolet burns to skin and eyes increases. This risk is greatly enhanced at higher altitudes. Solar keratitis is insidious during the exposure phase, with corneal burns occurring within 1 hour, but not becoming apparent until 6 to 12 hours after exposure.

Management of snow blindness is based on symptoms, which include excessive tearing, pain, redness, swollen eyelids, pain when looking at light, headache, a gritty sensation in the eyes, and decreased (hazy) vision. Prehospital care providers need to consider patching affected eyes if there is no other method to prevent further ultraviolet exposure (e.g., sunglasses), then transport the patient. Topical ophthalmic anesthetic drops, if available, may be used to provide symptomatic relief. Medical attention is required to determine the level of severity and the need for antibiotics and analgesics.

Major Cold-Related Disorders

Localized Cutaneous Cold Injury. Cold injuries occur at peripheral sites on the body and are classified as either freezing (e.g., frostbite) or nonfreezing (e.g., immersion foot) injuries. Localized cold injuries are preventable with proper preparation for cold exposure, early recognition of cold injury, and effective medical care. However, frostbite, potentially the most serious form of freezing injury because of the risk of limb loss, is the primary injury of interest in this section.

It is imperative to recognize, manage, and prevent further tissue freezing in mild to severe forms of freezing injury. Nicotine, alcohol intoxication, homelessness, and major psychiatric disorders remain important predisposing factors.[75]

When comparing cold weather injuries by ethnicity, African Americans are reported to be at greater risk for cold weather injuries, including frostbite. This relationship is related to the greater susceptibility of pigmented cells to freeze compared with nonpigmented cells.[76,77] Tight or constricting clothes, too many socks, and tight-fitting footwear are predicable factors in the onset of frostbite. With an increase in adventure sports and other recreational activities conducted in the winter season, localized cold injuries are now seen more often. Prehospital care providers need to prevent body heat loss and protect exposed skin from frostbite in patients during prolonged exposure to cold conditions. For example, in patients needing vehicular extrication, in scenarios resulting in the inability to move the patient, and in patients in cold environments with soft tissue swelling, impaired circulation can lead to an increased incidence of localized cold injury.

Nonfreezing Cold Injury. Nonfreezing cold injury (NFCI), a syndrome also called immersion foot and trench foot, results from damage to peripheral tissues caused by prolonged (hours to days) wet/cold exposure.[78-80] NFCI does not involve freezing of tissue but may coexist with freezing injury such as frostbite. This syndrome involves primarily the feet and is reflected in two types of NFCI. *Trench foot* occurs primarily in military personnel during infantry operations and is related to the combined effects of prolonged cold exposure and restricted circulation in the feet without immersion in water.[78] *Immersion foot* is caused by prolonged immersion of extremities to wet and cool to cold temperatures. Prehospital care providers may see immersion foot in homeless, alcoholic, or elderly persons; in hikers and hunters; in multiday adventure sport athletes; and in ocean survivors.[78,81,82] Frequently, this syndrome goes unrecognized during assessment of individuals who have been exposed to cold or wet conditions because of the lack of formal medical training in NFCI.[78]

This syndrome occurs as a result of many hours of cooling of the lower extremities in temperatures ranging from 32° to 65° F (0°–18° C). Soft tissue injury occurs to the skin of the feet, known as *maceration*. The breakdown of the skin will predispose individuals to infection as well. The greatest injury is seen to the peripheral nerves and blood vessels, caused by secondary ischemic injury. Mild NFCI is self-limited initially, but with continued prolonged cold exposure, it becomes irreversible. When the feet are wet and cold, this increases the risk and accelerates the injury because wet socks insulate poorly, and water cools more effectively than air at the same temperature. Any factors that reduce circulation to the extremities also contribute to the injury, such as constrictive clothing, boots, prolonged immobility, hypothermia, and crouched posture.

NFCI is classified in four degrees of severity, as follows:

- *Minimal.* Hyperemia or engorgement caused by an increase in blood flow to the feet and slight sensory change will remain 2 to 3 days after injury. Condition is self-limited, and no signs of injury remain after 7 days. Occasionally, cold sensitivity will remain.

- *Mild.* Edema, hyperemia, and slight sensory change remain 2 to 3 days after injury. Seven days after injury, anesthesia is found on the plantar surface of the foot and tips of the toes and lasts 4 to 9 weeks. Blisters and skin loss are not observed. Ambulation is possible when walking does not cause pain.
- *Moderate.* Edema, hyperemia, blisters, and mottling are present 2 to 3 days after injury. At 7 days, anesthesia to touch is present to both dorsal and plantar surface and toes. Edema persists 2 to 3 weeks, and pain and hyperemia last up to 14 weeks. Some blister sloughing occurs, but no loss of deep tissue. Some patients will have permanent injury.
- *Severe.* Severe edema, blood forced into surrounding tissues *(extravasation)*, and gangrene are present 2 to 3 days after injury. Complete anesthesia of the entire foot remains at 7 days, with paralysis and muscle wasting in the affected extremities. The injury goes beyond the foot into the lower leg. This severe injury produces significant tissue loss, resulting in autoamputation. Gangrene is a constant risk until tissue loss is complete. The patient is expected to have prolonged convalescence and a permanent disability. [78]

Assessment. Because the patient has experienced mild or moderate cold exposure, it is essential to rule out hypothermia and assess for dehydration. Even though this is not a freezing injury, NCFI still is an insidious and potentially disabling injury; the common finding with these two localized cold injuries is that the extremity is cooled to the point of anesthesia or numbness while the injury is occurring.

The key to management of NCFI is detection and recognition during assessment. During the initial assessment, injured tissue appears macerated, edematous, pale, anesthetized, pulseless, and immobile, but not frozen. Patients complain of clumsiness and stumbling when attempting to walk. After removal from cold, and during or after rewarming, peripheral blood flow increases as reperfusion of ischemic tissue begins. Extremities change color from white to mottled pale blue while remaining cold and numb. The diagnosis of trench foot or immersion foot is generally made when these signs have not changed after passive rewarming of the feet. From 24 to 36 hours after rewarming, a marked hyperemia develops, along with severe burning pain and reappearance of sensation proximally, but not distally. This is caused by venous vasodilation. Edema and blisters develop in the injured areas as perfusion increases. Skin will remain poorly perfused after hyperemia appears, and the skin is likely to slough as the injury evolves. Any pulselessness after 48 hours in the injured extremity suggests severe, deep injury and a greater chance of substantial tissue loss.

Management. Once a possible NFCI is detected, the priorities are to eliminate any further cooling, prevent further trauma to the extremity, and transport the patient. Do not allow the patient to walk on an injured extremity. Carefully remove the footwear and socks. Cover the injured part or extremity with a loose, dry, sterile dressing; protect it from the cold; and begin passive rewarming of injured tissue during transport. The affected area may be aggravated by the weight of a blanket. No active rewarming is necessary. Do not massage the affected area because this may cause further tissue damage. As needed, treat the patient for dehydration with a bolus of IV fluids, and reassess. Depending on length of transport, severe pain may develop during passive rewarming as tissues begin to reperfuse, and it may be necessary to manage with adequate opiate analgesia (e.g., begin initially with 5 mg morphine IV as needed).

Freezing Cold Injury. On the continuum of further peripheral cold tissue exposure beginning with frostnip, *frostbite* ranges from mild to severe tissue destruction and possibly the loss of tissue. [6,10] The most susceptible body parts for frostbite are those tissues with large surface-to-mass ratios, such as the ears and nose or areas farthest from the body's core, such as the hands, fingers, feet, toes, and male genitalia. These structures are most susceptible to cold injury because they contain many arteriovenous capillary *anastomoses* that easily shunt blood away during vasoconstriction. The body's normal response to lower-than-desirable temperatures is to reduce blood flow to the skin surface to reduce heat exchange with the environment. The body accomplishes this by vasoconstriction of peripheral blood vessels in an attempt to shunt warm blood to the body's core to maintain a normal body temperature. Reduction of this blood flow greatly reduces the amount of heat delivered to the distal extremities.

The longer the period of exposure to the cold, the more the blood flow is reduced to the periphery. The body conserves core temperature at the expense of extremity and skin temperature. The heat loss from the tissue becomes greater than the heat supplied to that area.

When an extremity is cooled to 59° F (15° C), maximal vasoconstriction and minimal blood flow occur. If cooling continues to 50° F (10° C), vasoconstriction is interrupted by periods of *cold-induced vasodilation* (CIVD), known as the "hunting response," and an associated increase in tissue temperature caused by an increase in blood flow. CIVD recurs in 5- to 10-minute cycles to provide some protection from the cold. Individuals show differences in susceptibility to frostbite when exposed to the same cold conditions, which may be explained by the amount of CIVD. [10]

Tissue does not freeze at 32° F (0° C) because cells contain electrolytes and other solutes that prevent tissue from freezing until skin temperature reaches approximately 28° F (−2° C). In cases of below-freezing temperatures, when the extremities are left unprotected, the intracellular and extracellular fluids can freeze. This results in the formation of ice crystals. As the ice crystals form, they expand and cause damage to local tissues. Blood clots may also form, further impairing circulation to the injured area.

The type and duration of cold exposure are the two most important factors in determining the extent of freezing injury. Frostbite is classified by depth of injury and clinical presentation.[10] The degree of injury in many cases will not be known for at least 24 to 72 hours after thawing, except in very minor or severe exposures. Skin exposure to cold that is short in duration but very intense will create a superficial injury, whereas severe frostbite to a whole extremity can occur during prolonged exposures. Direct cold injury is usually reversible, but permanent tissue damage occurs during rewarming. In more severe cases, even with appropriate rewarming of tissue, microvascular thrombosis can develop, leading to early signs of gangrene and necrosis. If the injured site freezes, thaws, and then refreezes, the second freezing causes a greater amount of severe thrombosis and vascular damage and tissue loss. For this reason, prehospital care providers need to prevent any frozen tissue that thaws during initial field treatment from refreezing.

Traditional methods of frostbite classification present four degrees of injury (similar to burns) based on initial physical findings after freezing and rewarming (Figures 20-16 and 20-17), as follows:

- *First-degree frostbite.* An epidermal injury; limited to skin that has brief contact with cold air or metal; skin appears white or as yellowish plaque at site of injury; no blister or tissue loss; skin thaws quickly, feels numb, and appears red with surrounding edema; healing occurs in 7 to 10 days.
- *Second-degree frostbite.* Involves all the epidermis and superficial dermis; initially appears similar to first-degree injury, however, frozen tissues are deeper; tis-

sue feels stiff to the touch, but tissue beneath gives way to pressure; thawing is rapid; after thawing, results in superficial skin blister or vesiculation that has clear or milky fluid after several hours; surrounded by erythema and edema; no permanent loss of tissue; healing occurs in 3 to 4 weeks.
- *Third-degree frostbite.* Involves the epidermis and dermis layers; frozen skin is stiff with restricted mobility; after tissue thaws, skin swells along with blood-filled blister (hemorrhagic bulla), indicating vascular trauma to deep tissues; swelling restricts mobility; skin loss occurs slowly, leading to mummification and sloughing; healing is slow.
- *Fourth-degree frostbite.* Frozen tissue involves full thickness completely through the dermis, with muscle and bone involvement; no mobility when frozen and passive movement when thawed, with no intrinsic muscle function; poor skin perfusion; blisters and edema do not develop; early signs of necrotic tissue; slow mummification process will occur along with sloughing of tissue and autoamputation of nonviable tissue. [9]

Although traditional classification of frostbite is by the four degrees of injury, it is easiest for EMS providers in the prehospital setting to classify as either superficial or deep.[83–85] *Superficial frostbite* (first and second degree) affects the skin and subcutaneous tissues, resulting in clear blisters when rewarmed. *Deep frostbite* (third and fourth degree) affects skin, muscle, and bone, and the skin has hemorrhagic blisters when rewarmed.

In special situations, frostbite may occur rapidly, and prehospital care providers may respond to the following:

- Hydrocarbon fluid spills on skin; for example, gasoline will cause rapid evaporation and conduction in below-freezing temperatures
- Touching extremely cold metal with warm skin
- Intense windchill on exposed skin caused by rotary wind from a medical helicopter

Assessment. On arrival, assess scene safety and then the patient for ABCs. Remove the patient from the cold, and place

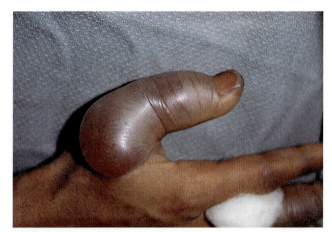

FIGURE 20-16   Edema and blister formation 24 hours after frostbite injury.
(From McCauley RL, Killyon GW, Smith DJ, Robson MC, Heggers JP: Frostbite. In Auerbach PS: *Wilderness medicine,* ed 5, St. Louis, 2007, Mosby Elsevier. Photograph courtesy Cameron Bangs, MD.)

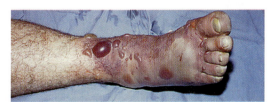

FIGURE 20-17   Deep second-degree and third-degree frostbite with hemorrhagic blebs, 1 day after thawing.
(From McCauley RL, Killyon GW, Smith DJ, Robson MC, Heggers JP: Frostbite. In Auerbach PS: *Wilderness medicine,* ed 5, St. Louis, 2007, Mosby Elsevier. Photograph courtesy Murray P. Hamlet, DVM.)

in an area protected from moisture, cold, and wind. Many frostbite victims may have additional associated medical conditions, such as dehydration, hypovolemia, hypothermia, hypoglycemia, and traumatic injury. Remove any wet clothing to minimize further body heat loss. When in doubt, treat hypothermia first. Superficial frostbite is usually assessed through a combination of recognizing the environmental conditions, locating the patient's chief complaint of pain or numbness, and observing discolored skin in the same area. The environmental conditions during exposure must be below freezing.

Frostbite injuries are insidious because the patient may have no pain at the injury site when skin is frozen and covered by a glove or footwear. Detection of the affected area requires direct visual inspection of highly suspect body regions, as previously listed. Gentle palpation of the area can determine if the underlying tissue is compliant or hard. Ensure that the patient or prehospital care provider does not rub or massage the affected skin, because this will cause further cellular damage to frozen tissues. The patient with superficial freezing will usually complain of discomfort during the manipulation of the frostbitten area. In patients with deep frostbite, the frozen tissue will be hard and usually is not painful when touched. After inspection of the affected area, a decision is necessary about the method of rewarming, which is usually based on transport time to the emergency department. The State of Alaska EMS protocol for frostbite rewarming in the prehospital phase states:

1. If transport time is short (1–2 hours at most), then the risks posed by improper rewarming or refreezing in the prehospital phase outweigh the risks for delaying treatment for deep frostbite.
2. If transport time will be prolonged (more than 1–2 hours), frostbite will often thaw spontaneously. It is more important to prevent hypothermia than to rewarm frostbite rapidly in warm water. This does not mean that a frostbitten extremity should be kept in the cold to prevent spontaneous rewarming. Anticipate that frostbitten areas will rewarm as a consequence of keeping the patient warm and protect them from refreezing at all costs.[87]

Management

Patients with superficial frostnip or frostbite should be placed with the affected area against a warm body surface, such as covering the patient's ears with warm hands or placing affected fingers into armpits, axillae, or groin regions. Superficial frostbite only needs to be warmed at normal body temperatures. Management of deep frostbite in the prehospital setting includes the following:

1. Assess and treat the patient for hypothermia, if present.
2. Provide supportive care and appropriate shelter for the patient and the affected part to minimize heat loss.

3. Assess frostbite area; remove any clothing and jewelry from affected area and check for loss of sensation.
4. If there is frostbite distal to a fracture, attempt to align the limb unless there is resistance. Splint the fracture in a manner which does not compromise distal circulation.
5. Cover with a loose, dry, sterile dressing that is noncompressive and nonadherent.
6. Do not allow the patient to walk on affected feet.
7. Fingers and toes should be separated by and protected with sterile cotton gauze.
8. Do not drain blisters.
9. Hands and feet should be splinted and elevated to reduce edema.
10. Intravenous opiate analgesics are usually required for pain relief and should be initiated before tissues have thawed.
11. Initiate normal saline IV with a 250-ml bolus to treat dehydration and reduce blood viscosity and capillary sludging.
12. Protect fragile tissues from further trauma during patient movement.
13. *Attempts to begin rewarming of deep frostbite patients in the field can be hazardous to the patient's eventual recovery and are not recommended unless prolonged transport times are involved.* If prolonged transport is involved, thaw in a warm water bath at a temperature no greater than 102° F (>39° C) on the affected area; if refreezing is a concern, do not thaw.
14. Do not allow the thawed part to thaw and refreeze.
15. Ensure early transport to an appropriate facility.

The patient can drink something warm (and nonalcoholic) if it is available, depending on the patient's LOC and other injuries. Tobacco use (smoking, chewing, using nicotine patches) should be discouraged because nicotine causes further vasoconstriction.

Accidental Hypothermia. Hypothermia is defined as the condition in which the core body temperature is below 95° F (35° C), as measured by a rectal thermometer probe placed at least 6 inches (15 cm) into the rectum.[11] Hypothermia can be viewed as a decrease in core temperature that renders a victim unable to generate sufficient heat production to return to homeostasis or normal bodily functions. Hypothermia can occur in many different situations, resulting from cold ambient air, cold-water immersion, or cold-water submersion (cold-water near-drowning), and can be intentionally induced during surgery.[11,87,88] Immersion ("head out") hypothermia typically occurs when an individual is accidentally placed into a cold environment without preparation or planning. For example, a person who has fallen into ice water is immediately in danger of becoming a submersion casualty, resulting from "cold shock" gasp reflex, loss of motor skills, hypothermia, and drowning. These unique aspects of submersion incidents can lead to hypoxia and hypothermia (see later discussion and Chapter 21).

The progression of hypothermia in cold air or cold water can be delayed as long as the metabolic heat production can match heat loss. Surviving an overwhelming cold exposure is possible, with many reported cases of survival at sea and in other extreme situations.[74,89] Many factors are known to increase survival after cold exposure, including age, gender, body composition (e.g., body surface area to body mass ratio), onset and intensity of shivering, level of physical fitness, nutritional state, and alcohol consumption. Hypoglycemia can occur during progressive phases of hypothermia and may be more common in immersion hypothermia. This occurs due to depletion of blood glucose and muscle glycogen as sources of fuel for contracting muscles during shivering. Also, the hypothalamus as the thermoregulatory center in the brain needs optimal blood glucose concentration since it is the primary fuel for best brain function. Consequently, an alcoholic is at greater risk for hypothermia since alcohol blocks the production of glucose in the body and inhibits maximal shivering for heat production.[11] Thus, rapid assessment and effective management of low blood glucose in the hypothermic patient is essential to achieve effective increase in metabolism and shivering during rewarming.

Unlike frostbite, hypothermia can occur in environments with temperatures well above freezing. *Primary hypothermia* generally occurs when healthy individuals are in adverse weather conditions unprepared for overwhelming acute or chronic cold exposure. Deaths by primary hypothermia are a direct result of cold exposure and are documented by the medical examiner as accidental, homicides, or suicides.[11]

Secondary hypothermia is considered a normal consequence of a patient's systemic disorders, including hypothyroidism, hypoadrenalism, trauma, carcinoma, and sepsis. If unrecognized or improperly treated, hypothermia can be fatal, in some cases within 2 hours. Mortality is greater than 50% in cases of secondary hypothermia caused by complications of other injuries and in severe cases in which the core body temperature is below 89.6° F (32° C).[11]

Rapid attention to preventing further body heat loss in the traumatic patient is needed by the prehospital care provider since mild hypothermia is very common following injury in all weather conditions. Therefore, the trauma patient should be moved off of cold ground as soon as possible and placed in a warm ambulance. The temperature in the ambulance should be adjusted to minimize heat loss from the patient and not for the comfort of the provider. Warmed IV fluids will also help to maintain the patient's body temperature.

It is all too common to receive hypothermic patients arriving at a trauma center and to have further body heat loss during the initial patient assessment.[90,91] The development of hypothermia that begins in the prehospital setting is related to the effect of trauma on thermoregulation and the inhibition of shivering as a primary mechanism for heat production.[92] In many patients, further heat loss continues after arrival at the hospital due to a multitude of reasons: an exposed patient in a cold emergency department or trauma center, administration of cool resuscitation fluids, open abdominal or thoracic cavities, the use of anesthetic and neuromuscular blocking agents that prevent heat-producing shivering, and further cold exposure in an operating room environment.[97,98]

One cause of higher mortality in hypothermic trauma patients is related to the lethal combination of *hypothermia, acidosis,* and *coagulopath*y (inability of blood to clot normally). This is known as the "lethal triad" in trauma patients.[93] It is essential to assess and treat patients both for trauma and hypothermia because the coagulopathy is reversible with patient rewarming.[91] In one study, 57% of the trauma patients admitted to a level I trauma center were hypothermic at some point in the continuum of care. The mortality rate approaches 100% when core temperature falls below 32° C in a trauma patient. This is in contrast to a mortality of 20% in a primary hypothermic (nontraumatic) patient at moderate levels (28–32° C).[98] Consequently, the mortality rate associated with hypothermia in the trauma victim is so high that the definition of mild, moderate, and severe hypothermia in the trauma patient has resulted in a special classification[93,94] (Figure 20-18).

It is well established that the detrimental "lethal triad" in trauma victims increases mortality. However, there is mounting evidence showing that intentionally induced hypothermia has a beneficial role in shock, organ transplantation, cardiac arrest, and controlling intracranial pressure from traumatic brain injury.[94,95] The fastest growing application of therapeutic hypothermia treatment in the prehospital setting is for victims of sudden nontraumatic cardiac arrest.[94,96] It is well

FIGURE 20-18 **Ranges of Severity of Hypothermia: Trauma Versus Accidental Hypothermia**

Classification	Traditional	Trauma
Mild hypothermia	95.0–89.6° F (35.0–32.0° C)	96.8–93.2° F (36.0–34.0° C)
Moderate hypothermia	89.6–82.4° F (32.0–28.0° C)	93.2–89.6° F (34.0–32.0° C)
Severe hypothermia	82.4–68.0° F (28.0–20.0° C)	<89.6° F (32° C)
Profound hypothermia	68.0–57.2° F (20.0–14.0° C)	
Deep hypothermia	<57.2° F (14.0° C)	

(Source: Gentilello LM: *Surg Clin North Am*, 1995.)

known that the outcome following cardiac arrest is very poor with only 3% to 27% of all cardiac arrest patients surviving to discharge. However, based on the growing amount of evidence for increased survival rate with therapeutic hypothermia in the past decade, the International Liaison Committee on Resuscitation (ILCOR) published an advisory statement in 2003 on the role of hypothermia following nontraumatic cardiac arrest, which recommended intentional cooling of the patient to 32° C to 34° C for 12 to 24 hours in unconscious adults with spontaneous circulation after an out-of-hospital cardiac arrest.[95]

Immersion Hypothermia. During immersion, if there is no heat gain or heat loss by the body, water temperature is considered *thermoneutral.* Thermoneutral water temperature is 91° to 95° F (33°–35° C), at which temperatures a naked individual passively standing in neck-level water can maintain a nearly constant core temperature for at least 1 hour.[98,99] Individuals in thermoneutral water are at almost no risk for the initial immersion "cold shock" and hypothermia experienced in sudden cold-water exposure.[100]

When immersion occurs in water temperature colder than the lower thermoneutral limit, the immediate physiologic changes are a rapid decline in skin temperature, peripheral vasoconstriction resulting in shivering, and increased metabolism, ventilation, heart rate, cardiac output, and MAP. To offset any heat loss in water, heat production must occur by increasing physical activity, shivering, or both. If not, core temperature continues to fall and shivering ceases, and these physiologic responses decrease proportionally with the fall in core temperature.[88]

The greatest risk of immersion hypothermia usually begins in water temperature less than 77° F (25° C).[101] Because the heat dissipation capacity of water is 24 times greater than that of air, individuals are at risk for more rapid hypothermia in water. However, continued physical activity (i.e., swimming to keep warm) in cold water will eventually become a detriment by increasing convective heat loss to the colder water surrounding the body, resulting in a faster onset of hypothermia. This understanding has lead to the recommendation for individuals to minimize heat loss during cold-water immersion by using the *heat escape lessening posture* (HELP) or the *huddle position* when multiple immersion victims are together[101] (Figure 20-19).

The lowest recorded core temperature for an infant with an intact neurologic recovery from accidental hypothermia is 59° F (15° C).[103] In an adult, 56.8° F (13.7° C) is the lowest recorded core temperature for a survivor of accidental hypothermia. This occurred in a 29-year-old female who struggled to self-rescue for more than 40 minutes before symptoms of severe hypothermia affected muscular contraction.[89] She was immersed for more than 80 minutes before a rescue team arrived and cardiopulmonary resuscitation (CPR) was initiated during transport to a local hospital. After 3 hours of continuous rewarming, her core temperature returned to normal, and she survived with normal physiologic function.

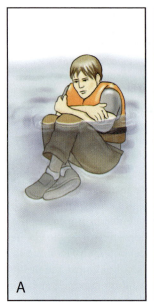 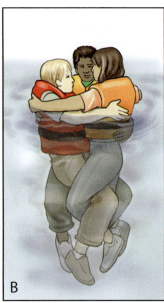

FIGURE 20-19 Techniques for decreasing cooling rates of survivors in cold water. **A.** Heat escape lessening posture (HELP). **B.** Huddle technique.

This case of accidental hypothermia illustrates why all prehospital care providers managing hypothermic patients should not stop treatment interventions and declare the patient deceased until they have been rewarmed to over 95° F (>35° C) and still have no evidence of cardiorespiratory and neurologic function. This is one of many hypothermic survivor scenarios in which patients are discharged from the hospital with full neurologic function after prolonged CPR in the field. The lessons from this case and others with a similar outcome are that the initial impression of these patients as likely dead is not sufficient justification to withhold basic or advanced life support. This is the reason the following phrase was created:

"Patients are not dead until they are warm and dead."

Whether intentional or unintentional, cold-water immersion (head out) occurs throughout the year in the United States as a result of recreational and industrial activities, as well as from accidents. If the individual survives the initial submersion incident without drowning, he or she is at risk for hypothermia, depending on the water temperature. The body's responses to cold-water immersion can be divided into the following three phases:

■ *First phase.* This phase begins with a cardiovascular reflex known as "cold shock" response that occurs quickly (within 2–4 minutes) after immersion and begins with rapid skin cooling, peripheral vasoconstriction, a gasp reflex and the inability to breath-hold, hyperventilation, and tachycardia.[75,87] The gasp response may lead to aspiration and drowning, depending on the individual's head location above or below water. These responses can lead to immediate sudden death or death within minutes following immersion because of several conditions in this setting, including syncope or convulsions resulting in drowning, vagal arrest, and ventricular fibrillation.[88,104–106]

■ *Second phase.* If a victim survives the cold shock phase, significant cooling of peripheral tissues occurs over the first 30 minutes of immersion. This cooling has a deleterious effect on gross and fine motor skills of the extremities, causing finger stiffness, poor coordination, and loss of muscle power, making it nearly impossible to swim, grasp a rescue line, or perform other survival motor skills.[88,101]

■ *Third phase.* Surviving the first two phases without drowning places an individual at risk of hypothermia from continued heat loss and core temperature reduction from immersion longer than 30 minutes. If the victim is not able to remain above the water surface because of fatigue and hypothermia, the individual is at risk to become a submersion casualty, leading to aspiration and drowning.[75,90] How long an individual can survive in cold water depends on many factors. It has been estimated that a submersion victim cannot survive for more than 1 hour at a water temperature of 32° F (0° C), and at a water temperature of 59° F (15° C), survival is uncommon after 6 hours.[108]

The US Coast Guard and other search-and-rescue organizations use guidelines to assist in estimating how long individuals can survive in the cold water. These guidelines are mathematical models that estimate core temperature cooling rate based on the influence of the following variables: (1) water temperature and sea state; (2) clothing insulation; (3) body composition (amount of fat, muscle, and bone); (4) amount of the body immersed in water; (5) behavior (e.g., excessive movement) and posture (e.g., HELP, huddle) of the body in the water; and (6) shivering thermogenesis.[109–111]

Early studies in the 1960s–70s suggested that during accidental immersion in cold water, it was a better option not to self-rescue by attempting to distance-swim to safety, but stay in place, float still in lifejackets, or hang on to wreckage and not swim around to keep warm. More recent research has suggested that self-rescue swimming during accidental immersion in cold water (10–14° C) is a viable option based on the following conditions:

a. Initially survive the cold-shock phase within the first few minutes of cold water exposure.

b. Make a decision early to attempt self-rescue or wait for rescue since decision-making ability will become impaired as hypothermia progresses.

b. Low probability for rescue by first responders in the area.

c. The victim can reach shore within 45 minutes of swimming based on his or her fitness level and swimming ability.

d. On average, a cold-water immersion victim wearing a PFD should be able to swim approximately 800 meters in 50° F (10° C) water before incapacitation due to muscle cooling and fatigue of the arms rather than general hypothermia.

e. Cold water swim distance is about ⅓ of the distance covered in warmer water.[112]

Pathophysiologic Effects of Hypothermia on the Body. Whether from exposure to a cold environment or immersion, the influence of hypothermia on the body affects all major organ systems, particularly the cardiac, renal, and central nervous systems. As the body's core temperature decreases to 95° F (35° C), maximal rate of vasoconstriction, shivering, and metabolic rate occurs, with increases in heart rate, respiration, and blood pressure. Cerebral metabolism oxygen demand decreases by 6% to 10% per 1° C drop in core temperature, and cerebral metabolism is preserved. When core temperature falls to between 86° F (30° C) and 95° F (35° C), cognitive function, cardiac function, metabolic rate, respiratory rate, and shivering rate are all significantly decreased or completely inhibited. At this point, the limited physiologic defensive mechanisms to prevent heat loss from the body are overwhelmed and core temperature falls rapidly. At a core temperature of 85° F (29.5° C), cardiac output and metabolic rate are reduced approximately 50%. Ventilation and perfusion are inadequate and do not keep up with the metabolic demand, causing cellular hypoxia, increased lactic acid, and an eventual metabolic and respiratory acidosis. Oxygenation and blood flow are maintained in the core and brain.

Bradycardia occurs in a large percentage of patients as a direct effect of cold on the depolarization of pacemaker cells and their slower propagation through the conduction system. It is important to note that the use of atropine, as well as other cardiac medications, is often ineffective to increase the heart rate when the myocardium is cold.[6] When core temperature falls below 86° F (30° C), the myocardium becomes irritable. The PR, QRS, and QTC intervals are prolonged. ST-segment and T-wave changes and J (or Osborne) waves may be present and may mimic other ECG abnormalities, such as an acute myocardial infarction (AMI). The J waves are a striking ECG feature in hypothermic patients and are seen in approximately one third of moderately to severely hypothermic patients (<90° F [<32° C]). The J wave is described as a "humplike" deflection between the QRS complex and the early part of the ST segment.[113] The J wave is best viewed in the aVL, aVF, and left lateral leads (Figure 20-20).

Atrial fibrillation and extreme bradycardia develop and may continue between 83° and 90° F (28° and 32° C). When the core temperature reaches 80° to 82° F (26.7°–28° C), any physical stimulation of the heart can cause ventricular fibrillation (VF). CPR or rough handling (patient assessment and movement) of the patient could be sufficient to cause VF. At these extremely low core temperatures, pulse and blood pressure are not detectable, and the joints are stiff. The pupils become fixed and dilated at extremely low core temperatures. Again, a patient should not be assumed to be dead until he or she is rewarmed and still has no signs of life (ECG, pulse, ventilation, and CNS function).

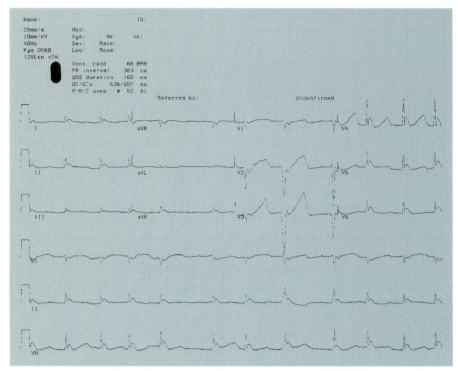

FIGURE 20-20 Osborne or J-wave in hypothermia patient.

With acute cold exposure, renal blood flow increases because of the shunting of blood during vasoconstriction. This may result in a phenomenon known as cold diuresis in which patients produce more urine and may, as a result, become dehydrated. At 81° to 86° F (27°–30° C), renal blood flow is depressed by 50%. At this moderate to severe hypothermic level, the decrease in cardiac output causes a fall in renal blood flow and glomerular filtration rate, which in turn results in acute renal failure (ARF).

Assessment. It is imperative to assess scene safety on arrival. All responders need to ensure their safety and protection from cold exposure while working in this environment. There should be a high suspicion for hypothermia even when the environmental conditions are not highly suggestive (e.g., wind, moisture, temperature). Some patients may present with vague complaints of fatigue, lethargy, nausea, vomiting, and dizziness. With trauma and critically ill patients, it is important to begin assessment and assume hypothermia by protecting the patient from the cold environment; assessment starts with the ABCs. Neurologic function is assessed and monitored frequently. Severely hypothermic patients generally present with bradypnea, stupor, and coma. Rectal temperatures are not usually assessed in the field or widely used as a vital sign in most prehospital systems. Ambulances that do have access to a thermometer usually carry a standard-range oral or rectal (for infants) thermometer with a lower limit of 96° F (35.5° C). Electronic thermometers are not useful in hypothermic situations for accurate readings. Tympanic membrane (TM) infrared temperature measurement is generally accurate if careful technique is used to assure aiming the probe at the TM and not the ear canal which can affect the reading. In addition the ear must be clear of cerumen (ear wax) and blood. To accurately measure hypothermic temperatures, a low-range rectal thermometer is often necessary. Figure 20-21 provides the anticipated physiologic responses with decreasing core temperature.

Signs of shivering and mental status change are important in the assessment of suspected hypothermia. Mildly hypothermic patients (core temperature >90° F, or 32° C) will be shivering and usually show signs of altered LOC (e.g., confusion, slurred speech, altered gait, clumsiness). They will be slow in their actions and are usually found in a nonambulatory state, sitting or lying. Law enforcement personnel and prehospital care providers may misinterpret this condition as drug or alcohol intoxication or as cerebrovascular accident (CVA, stroke) in elderly patients. However, a patient's LOC is not a reliable indicator of the degree of hypothermia; some patients have remained conscious at core temperature below 80° F (27° C).

When the patient's core temperature falls below 90° F (32° C), moderate hypothermia is present, and the patient will probably not complain of feeling cold. Shivering will be absent, and the patient's LOC will be greatly decreased, possibly to the point of unconsciousness and coma. The patient's pupils

FIGURE 20-21 **Physiologic Characteristics of Hypothermia**

°C	°F	Characteristics
37.6	99.6 ±1	Normal rectal temperature
37.0	98.6 ±1	Normal oral temperature
36.0	96.8	Increase in metabolic rate and blood pressure and pre-shivering muscle tone
35.0	95.0	Urine temperature 34.8° C; maximum shivering thermogenesis
34.0	93.2	Amnesia, dysarthria, and poor judgment develop; maladaptive behavior; normal blood pressure; maximum respiratory stimulation; tachycardia, then progressive bradycardia
33.3	91.4	Ataxia and apathy develop; linear depression of cerebral metabolism; tachypnea, then progressive decrease in respiratory minute volume; cold diuresis
32.0	89.6	Stupor; 25% decrease in oxygen consumption
31.0	87.8	Extinguished shivering thermogenesis
30.0	86.0	Atrial fibrillation and other dysrhythmias develop; poikilothermia; pupils and cardiac output two thirds of normal; insulin ineffective
29.0	84.2	Progressive decrease in level of consciousness, pulse, and respiration; pupils dilated; paradoxical undressing
28.0	82.4	Decreased ventricular fibrillation threshold; 50% decrease in oxygen consumption and pulse; hypoventilation
27.0	80.6	Loss of reflexes and voluntary motion
26.0	78.8	Major acid-base disturbances; no reflexes or response to pain
25.0	77.0	Cerebral blood flow one third of normal; loss of cerebrovascular autoregulation; cardiac output 45% of normal; pulmonary edema may develop
24.0	75.2	Significant hypotension and bradycardia
23.0	73.4	No corneal or oculocephalic reflexes; areflexia
22.0	71.6	Maximum risk of ventricular fibrillation; 75% decrease in oxygen consumption
20.0	68.0	Lowest resumption of cardiac electromechanical activity; pulse 20% of normal
19.0	66.2	Electroencephalographic silencing
18.0	64.4	Asystole
15.0	59.0	Lowest infant accidental hypothermia survival
13.7	56.8	Lowest adult accidental hypothermia survival
10.0	50.0	92% decrease in oxygen consumption
9.0	48.2	Lowest therapeutic hypothermia survival

(Modified from Danzl DF: Accidental hypothermia. In Auerbach PS: *Wilderness medicine,* ed 5, St. Louis, 2007, Mosby Elsevier.)

will react slowly or may be dilated and fixed. The patient's palpable pulses may be diminished or absent, and SBP may be low or indeterminate. The patient's ventilations may have slowed to as few as 2 breaths/minute. An ECG may show atrial fibrillation, the most common dysrhythmia. As the myocardium becomes progressively colder and more irritable at about 82° F (28° C), VF is observed more often. Because of the changes in cerebral metabolism, evidence of "paradoxical undressing" may be observed before the patient loses consciousness. This is an attempt by the patient to remove the clothing while in the cold environment, and it is thought to represent a response to an impending thermoregulatory failure.

The clinical management of hypothermia is based on the following three ranges of rectal body temperature as presented by the American Heart Association for the use of advanced cardiac life support:

- *Mild hypothermia* is above 93° to below 97° F (>34° to <36° C)
- *Moderate hypothermia* is 86° to 93° F (30° to 34° C)
- *Severe hypothermia* is below 86° F (<30° C) [114]

Management

Prehospital care of the hypothermic patient consists of preventing further heat loss, gentle handling, initiating rapid transport, and rewarming. This includes moving the patient away from any cold source to a warm ambulance or to a warm shelter if transportation is not immediately available (see Prolonged Transport section). Wet clothing should be removed by cutting with trauma shears to avoid unnecessary movement and agitation of the patient. Concern for initiating ventricular dysrhythmia based on the handling of the patient should not delay any critical interventions. This concern becomes more realistic in severe hypothermic patients (<86° F, or 30° C). The patient's head and body should be covered with warm blankets or sleeping bags, followed by an outer windproof layer to prevent convective and evaporative heat loss.

If the patient is conscious and alert, the patient should avoid alcohol and caffeine drinks. Anticipate hypoglycemia and assess blood glucose level. For the mildly hypothermic patient with normal glucose levels, provide warm, high-caloric or glucose fluids. For moderate hypothermic victims with low blood glucose concentration, establish IV fluids and administer 50% dextrose (D50) IV per medical protocol and repeat glucose determination every 5 minutes to determine the need for an additional D50 bolus. Hypothermic patients need high-flow oxygen because they have decreased oxygen delivery to the tissues; the oxyhemoglobin dissociation curve shifts to the left with a decrease in core temperature. High-flow oxygen should be delivered using a nonrebreather mask or BVM. Ideally, the patient may benefit more if the oxygen can be warmed and humidified (108°–115° F [42°–46° C]). If possible, warmed oxygen administered before movement may prevent VF during transport.

In unresponsive hypothermic patients, passive rewarming will be insufficient to increase core temperature. These patients will need an airway adjunct to protect the airway, and this should be initiated depending on jaw rigidity. If endotracheal intubation cannot be successfully achieved without rough handling, continue ventilation with a bag-mask device and consider another advanced airway device (e.g., Combitube, laryngeal mask airway, nasal intubation). At a minimum, use an oral or nasal pharyngeal airway with bag-mask ventilation.

Intravenous NS, ideally with 5% dextrose, should be warmed to 109° F (43° C) and administered without agitating the patient. *The hypothermic patient should not be given "cold" (room-temperature) fluids* because this could make the patient colder or could delay rewarming. When NS and dextrose solutions are unavailable, any warm crystalloid solution is satisfactory. Provide a fluid challenge of 500 to 1000 ml, and prevent the solution from freezing or becoming colder by placing the IV bag under the patient to infuse warm fluids under pressure. The rewarming effect of warmed IV fluids is minimal at best, and the prehospital care provider should use good judgment to decide whether fluids (orally or IV) are worth the risks of aspiration, coughing, and painful stimuli to the patient. Hot packs or massaging of the patient's extremities are not recommended. Typically, active external rewarming occurs only to the thoracic region, with no active rewarming of the extremities. This will prevent increased peripheral circulation, causing an increased amount of colder blood returning from the extremities to the thorax before central core rewarming. Increased return of peripheral blood can increase acidosis and hyperkalemia and can actually decrease the core temperature ("afterdrop"). This complicates resuscitation and may precipitate VF.

National Guidelines for Treatment of Cold-Related Disorders

Emergency Cardiovascular Care: Basic and Advanced Lifesaving Guidelines for Management of Hypothermia

Guidelines for resuscitation of the hypothermic patient have evolved over many decades. The most recent revision of the Emergency Cardiovascular Care (ECC) guidelines by the American Heart Association in collaboration with the International Liaison Committee on Resuscitation represents the latest findings in cardiovascular care research. The current ECC guidelines were published by the American Heart Association in the journal *Circulation* in December 2005.[115]

The hypothermic victim can present many challenges to the EMS provider, particularly the unconscious, moderately to severely hypothermic patient. Because severe hypothermia is a core temperature less than 86° F (<30° C), the patient can present with no detectable pulse or respiration because of the reduced cardiac output and decreased arterial pressure. Historically, the challenge has been to determine whether to initiate basic (BLS) or advanced (ALS) life support interventions on these patients based on the viability of the patient. Furthermore, it may be difficult to determine from any bystanders whether these patients had a primary hypothermic exposure or, for example, a cardiac arrest or stroke, that preceded the hypothermia. Other concerns for a prehospital care provider are protecting the hypothermic patient with a potential irritable myocardium from any rough handling and initiating chest compression for the patient with nondetectable pulse, in whom both these interventions may initiate VF.[114]

Independent of any scenario that created the primary or secondary hypothermia, lifesaving procedures should generally not be withheld on the basis of clinical presentation, whether in an urban setting with short transport distances or in the backcountry environment with potentially significant delays in transport, in which extended patient care may be necessary (see later discussion).

Basic Life Support Guidelines for Treatment of Mild to Severe Hypothermia

Hypothermic patients should be kept in a horizontal position at all times to avoid aggravating hypotension because these patients are often volume-depleted from cold diuresis. It may be difficult to feel or detect respiration and a pulse in the hypothermic patient. Therefore, it is recommended initially to assess for breathing and then a pulse for 60 seconds to confirm one of the following:

- Respiratory arrest
- Pulseless cardiac arrest (asystole, ventricular tachycardia, VF)
- Bradycardia (requiring CPR)

If the patient is not breathing, start rescue breathing immediately. Start chest compressions immediately in any hypothermic patient who is pulseless and has no detectable signs of circulation.[114] If there is a doubt about detecting a pulse, begin compressions. Never withhold BLS interventions until the patient is rewarmed. If the patient is determined to be in cardiac arrest, use the current BLS guidelines, as outlined elsewhere.[115]

An automated external defibrillator (AED) should be used if pulseless ventricular tachycardia or VF is present. The current ECC guidelines (see ACLS hypothermia algorithm) recommend that these patients should be treated by providing up to 5 cycles (2 minutes) of CPR (one cycle is 30 compressions to 2 breaths) before checking the ECG rhythm and attempting to shock when an AED arrives.[115] If a shockable rhythm is determined, give one shock, then continue 5 cycles of CPR. If the hypothermic patient does not respond to one shock with a detectable pulse, further attempts to defibrillate the patient should be deferred and efforts directed toward effective CPR with an emphasis on rewarming the patient to above 86° F (>30° C) before attempting further defibrillation.[115] When performing chest compression in a hypothermic patient, a greater force is required because chest wall elasticity is decreased when cold.[116] If core temperature is below 86° F (30° C), the conversion to normal sinus rhythm does not normally occur until rewarming above this core temperature is accomplished.[117]

The importance of not declaring a patient dead until they have been rewarmed and remain unresponsive is even greater today, with new evidence from studies of hypothermic victims indicating that cold exerts a protective effect on the vital organs.[117,118]

ACLS Guidelines for Treatment of Hypothermia

The treatment of severe hypothermia in the field remains controversial.[114] However, the guidelines for administering advanced cardiac life support (ACLS) procedures are different than with a normothermic patient. Unconscious hypothermic patients need a protected airway and should be intubated. Do not delay airway management based on concern for initiating VF. As noted earlier, if a shockable rhythm is detected, defibrillate once at 120–200 biphasic joules or 360 monophasic joules, resume CPR, and then defer cardiac drugs and subsequent defibrillation attempts until core temperature is above 86° F (30° C). If possible, initiate active rewarming procedures with warm, humid oxygen and warm IV solutions, and package the patient for transport by preventing further heat loss.

The challenge with ACLS procedures in a hypothermic patient is that the heart may be unresponsive to ACLS drugs, pacing, and defibrillation.[119] Furthermore, ACLS drugs, (e.g., epinephrine, amiodarone, lidocaine, procainamide) can accumulate to toxic levels in the circulation with repeated administration in the severely hypothermic patient, particularly when the patient rewarms.[114] Consequently, it is recommended to withhold IV medications in patients with a core temperature below 86° F (30° C). If a hypothermic patient initially presents with a core temperature above 86° F, or if a severely hypothermic patient has been rewarmed above this temperature, IV medications may be administered. However, longer intervals between drug administration are recommended than with standard drug intervals in ACLS.[114] The use of repeated defibrillation is indicated if the core temperature continues to rise above 86° F (30° C), consistent with the current ACLS guidelines.[115]

Finally, BLS/ACLS procedures performed in the field should be withheld only in patients with injuries incompatible with life or if the body is frozen such that chest compressions are impossible, or if the mouth and nose are blocked with ice.[11,114] Figure 20-22 provides an algorithm of mild, moderate, and severe hypothermia guidelines for both pulse and pulseless patients.[114]

Prevention of Cold-Related Injuries

The prevention of cold injuries in patients, yourself, and other prehospital care providers is vital when on the scene. Recommendations to prevent cold-related injuries include the following:

1. Note the risk factors generally accepted for cold injury:
   - Fatigue
   - Dehydration
   - Undernutrition
   - Lack of cold weather experience
   - Black race
   - Tobacco use
   - Windchill
2. When you cannot stay dry under conditions of cold, wet, and wind, end your session outdoors and seek shelter as soon as possible.
3. Remember that individuals with a history of cold injury are at a greater risk of a subsequent cold injury.
4. Avoid dehydration.
5. Avoid alcohol in cold environments.
6. Use the huddle technique with others if accidental water immersion in cold water occurs. You are more likely to survive if you remain still in cold water less than 68° F (20° C) and do not attempt to swim to shore unless it is nearby.

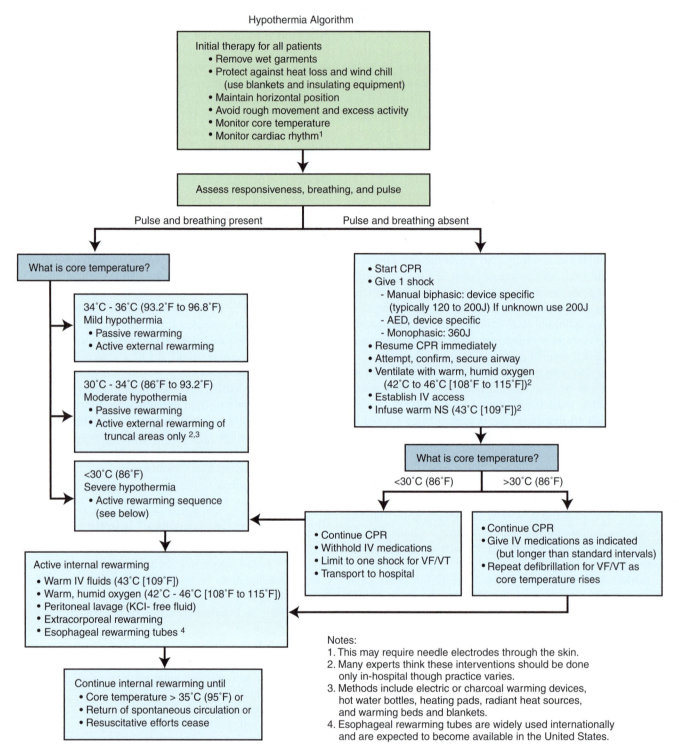

FIGURE 20-22 American Heart Association (AHA) hypothermia algorithm from the 2005 Cardiopulmonary Resuscitation and Emergency Cardiovascular Care guidelines. *Note:* Peritoneal lavage, extracorporeal rewarming, and esophageal rewarming tubes are usually hospital-only procedures.

(American Heart Association: *Handbook of emergency cardiovascular care for healthcare providers,* Chicago, 2006, AHA.)

7. Increase your likelihood of survival in cold environments by:
   - Maintaining a will to survive
   - Adaptability and improvisation
   - Optimism and belief that event is only a temporary situation
   - Maintaining a calm rationality to bizarre experiences and a sense of humor
8. Cold or nearly frozen extremities may be warmed with body heat by placing fingers in the armpits or groin area. Toes and feet can be placed on another person's stomach.
9. Keep protective cold weather clothing (e.g., boots, socks, gloves, winter hat, insulated pants and jacket, windproof outer shell) in your car for unexpected car emergencies during cold weather months. Avoid clothing that absorbs moisture as wet clothing will exacerbate heat loss (use wool or fleece).
10. Frostbite can occur rapidly when touching metal objects in the cold with your bare hands; always wear gloves.
11. Understand that the windchill index (Figure 20-23) is composed of wind speed and air temperature, and dress for extreme cold with insulated clothing and a windproof garment.
12. Keep feet dry with socks that transfer moisture from your feet to the footwear.
13. Do not walk through snow with low-cut shoes; if you lack appropriate shoes and protective clothes,

attempt to stay in a protected area; do not lie or rest directly on snow. Lie on tree boughs, a sleeping pad, or a poncho.
14. Use a sleeping bag outdoors, and do not wear clothing that will absorb and retain sweat; any sweat retained in your clothes will increase heat loss and cause shivering.
15. Water-based lotions on face, hands, and ears will increase the risk for frostnip and frostbite. Use an oil-based lotion (e.g., Chapstick®, Vaseline®).
16. Mittens are more effective at trapping warm air around all fingers than a five-finger glove.
17. When protecting the lower extremities from cold weather, it is common not to consider protecting the genital region. Use of sweat pants, long underwear, Lycra® tights, Gore-Tex® pants, and any combination of these garments work well.
18. To prevent frostbite:
    - Do not wear tight clothing, gloves, or boots that restrict circulation.
    - Exercise fingers, toes, and face periodically to keep them warm and to detect numb areas.
    - Work or exercise with a partner, who watches for warning signs of cold injury and hypothermia.
    - Wear properly insulated clothing, and keep it dry; carry extra undergarments, socks, and shoes at all times.
    - Watch for numbness and tingling.[120]

Wind Chill Chart

	Temperature (°F)																	
Calm	40	35	30	25	20	15	10	5	0	-5	-10	-15	-20	-25	-30	-35	-40	-45
5	36	31	25	19	13	7	1	-5	-11	-16	-22	-28	-34	-40	-46	-52	-57	-63
10	34	27	21	15	9	3	-4	-10	-16	-22	28	-35	-41	-47	-53	-59	-66	-72
15	32	25	19	13	6	0	-7	-13	-19	-26	-32	-39	-45	-51	-58	-64	-71	-77
20	30	24	17	11	4	-2	-9	-15	-22	-29	-35	-42	-48	-55	-61	-68	-74	-81
25	29	23	16	9	3	-4	-11	-17	-24	-31	-37	-44	-51	-58	-64	-71	-78	-84
30	28	22	15	8	1	-5	-12	-19	-26	-33	-39	-46	-53	-60	-67	-73	-80	-87
35	28	21	14	7	0	-7	-14	-21	-27	34	-41	-48	-55	-62	-69	-76	-82	-89
40	27	20	13	6	-1	-8	-15	-22	-29	-36	-43	-50	-57	-64	-71	-78	-84	-91
45	26	19	12	5	-2	-9	-16	-23	-30	-37	-44	-51	-58	-65	-72	-79	-86	-93
50	26	19	12	4	-3	-10	-17	-24	-31	-38	-45	-52	-60	-67	-74	-81	-88	-95
55	25	18	11	4	-3	-11	-18	-25	-32	-39	-46	-54	-61	-68	-75	-82	-89	-97
60	25	17	10	3	-4	-11	-19	-26	-33	-40	-48	-55	-62	-69	-76	-84	-91	-98

Wind (MPH) — [left axis label]

Frostbite Times: ▢ 30 minutes ▢ 10 minutes ▢ 5 minutes

$$\text{Wind Chill } (°F) = 35.74 + 0.6215T - 35.75(V^{0.16}) + 0.4275T(V^{0.16})$$
Where, T = Air temperature (°F) V = Wind speed (mph)

FIGURE 20-23 Wind chill index.
(Courtesy National Weather Service.)

Prolonged Transport

At times, the location of a patient will result in a delay in transport or a prolonged transport to an appropriate facility, necessitating extended prehospital care. Consequently, EMS providers may need to consider management options beyond what would be used with a rapid transport. How the patient is managed will depend on the time to definitive care, approved medical protocols, equipment and supplies on hand, additional personnel and resources, and location of the patient and severity of the injuries.

Some extended care considerations for moderately to severely injured patients from each of the environments discussed in this chapter are provided here. As with all patient care, it is understood that the first priorities are scene safety, ABCDEs, and the use of standard assessment and management procedures appropriate to these environments. If medical control is available, always obtain a consult early, and communicate routinely throughout the extended care period. Any of the procedures listed that fall outside the scope of practice are to be used by other, credentialed medical providers.

Also, it is important to know that all agencies have established guidelines for discontinuation of CPR. (See a discussion by the American Heart Association on the ethical issues arising from withholding or withdrawing BLS or ALS resuscitation efforts.[115]) The Wilderness Medical Society recommends that once CPR is initiated, it should be continued until resuscitation is successful with an awake patient, until rescuers are exhausted, until rescuers are placed in danger, until the patient is turned over to more definitive care, or until the patient does not respond to prolonged (30 minutes) resuscitative efforts.[121] The National Association of EMS Physicians also provides guidelines for the termination of CPR in the prehospital environment (see discussion in Patient Assessment chapter, p. 129.[122] If medical control is available, begin patient consult early, if possible, for consideration of CPR termination after a total time of 20 minutes, depending on special patient circumstances (see Chapter 21 for further situations—e.g., cold-water submersion, lightning strike—in which CPR may be extended longer than 20 to 30 minutes).[121]

Heat-Related Illness

Heatstroke

- Provide whole-body cooling as quickly as possible. Think about using any available access to water. Immerse the body to neck level in cool water (maintain body control and protect the airway), or spray the whole body with water (e.g., IV fluids, saline, water bottles, water from hydration backpacks), and provide a source of continuous wind current (e.g., natural wind current, fanning with towel, fire ventilation fans).
- When possible, keep medical control informed of patient status and to receive further medical directions.

- Stop body cooling when rectal temperature reaches 102° F (39° C). Then, protect the patient from shivering and hypothermia.
- As you are cooling the patient, manage the airway in unresponsive patients and initiate good ventilation with bag-mask device with high-flow oxygen. Insert an IV line, provide a 500-ml NS fluid challenge, and assess vital signs. Patient should have vital signs assessed after every 500 ml. Total fluid volume should not exceed 1 to 2 liters in the first hour. An additional liter can be considered during the second hour if prehospital care is extended.[9]
- The next priorities are to manage any seizure activity and hypoglycemia per medical protocol with diazepam and dextrose, respectively.
- Place the patient in recovery position, and continue assessment to include level of consciousness, vital signs, rectal temperature, and blood glucose. Provide supportive care and basic bodily needs throughout the remaining extended care period.

Hyponatremia

- Correct the presumed low blood sodium concentration. If the patient can take food by mouth and if available, provide potato chips, pretzels, or other salty food, a sport electrolyte or other sodium-containing beverage, or give 2 teaspoons of salt mixed in 16 ounces of water. Salt tablets given alone are not recommended; additional fluid must accompany the tablets and there is the risk of increasing sodium levels too much.
- Establish an IV line. Start NS with a flow rate of TKO. Check with medical control to consider a flow rate of 250 to 500 ml/hour based on the estimated delay in transporting the patient to the hospital. Do not use hypotonic IV fluids because this will exacerbate cerebral edema.
- In a patient with severe signs or symptoms (seizure or coma), consider administration of furosemide (a diuretic, if available) to reduce extracellular body water content while providing some sodium by infusing NS, 250 to 500 ml/hour IV.
- Assess cerebral edema and increased ICP. Establish a baseline Glasgow Coma Scale (GCS) score, and reassess every 10 minutes as an indicator of progressive cerebral edema and increased ICP (manage per recommendation for cerebral edema; see Chapter 9).
- Be prepared to manage nausea and projectile vomiting. Take one side of a large trash bag and make a hole for the patient's head about 12 inches (30 cm) below the rim of the bag. Place the patient's head through the hole so that the patient can look down into the center of the bag.
- Be prepared to manage urine when diuresis begins. Use a large trash bag as a diaper or use a bucket or other container.
- Give supplemental oxygen to lethargic or obtunded patients. Manage the airway of unresponsive patients, and initiate good ventilation with a bag-mask device

(no hyperventilation; see Chapter 9), with oxygen at 10 breaths/minute.

- Measure blood sugar, and provide IV dextrose per protocol to hypoglycemic patients.
- Monitor for seizures, and administer an anticonvulsant (e.g., diazepam, initially 2–5 mg IV/IM, and titrate per medical protocol).
- Place unconscious patients in left lateral recumbent position. Continue ongoing assessment of patient.

Cold-Related Illness

Frostbite

- Start IV fluids KVO before initiation of rewarming procedures. If a vein cannot be accessed, the IO route is an alternative.
- In a situation of significant transport delay, active rewarming should be considered. Rapid, active rewarming can reverse the direct injury of ice crystals in tissues, but it may not change the injury severity.[10] It is critical to keep the thawed tissue from refreezing because this significantly worsens the outcome compared with passive thawing. Thus, when and where to begin active rewarming becomes critical in the decision making, if it is to be done at all.
- A standard rewarming procedure is to immerse the affected extremity in circulating water warmed to between 99° and 102° F (37° and 39° C) in a large enough container to accommodate the frostbitten tissues without them touching the sides or bottom of the container.[86] Water should feel warm, but not hot, to the normal hand. (Note that this new temperature range is lower than previously recommended since this temperature range decreases pain for the patient while only slightly slowing the rewarming phase). If available, an oral or rectal thermometer should be used to measure water temperature. A temperature below that recommended will thaw tissue but is less beneficial for rapid thawing and for tissue survival. Any greater temperature will cause greater pain and may cause a burn injury.[10] Avoid active rewarming with intense sources of dry heat (e.g., placing near campfire). Continue immersion until tissue is soft and pliable, which may take up to 30 minutes. Active motion of the extremity during immersion is beneficial, without directed rubbing or massaging of the affected part.
- Extreme pain is experienced during rapid thawing. Treat with morphine, 5 to 10 mg IV, and titrate as needed. Provide ibuprofen, 400 mg orally every 12 hours, alone or in combination with morphine. Aspirin may be given if ibuprofen is not available although the optimal dosage regimen has not been determined (aspirin is contraindicated in pediatric patients because of the risk of Reye's syndrome).
- The return of normal skin color, warmth, and sensation in the affected part are all favorable signs. Dry all affected parts with warm air (do not towel dry affected parts), and ideally, apply topical aloe vera on skin, place sterile gauze between toes or fingers, bandage, splint, and elevate extremity. Cover any extremity with insulating material, and wrap a windproof and waterproof material (e.g., trash bag) as the outer layer, particularly if continuing patient extraction outdoors to a transport location.

Hypothermia

- Start active rewarming procedures. The key point is to prevent further heat loss.
- Heated IV fluids (104°–108° F [40°–42° C]).
- Shivering is the single best way for rewarming mildly hypothermic patients in the prehospital setting compared with external methods for rewarming. Hypothermic patients who are able to shiver maximally can increase core temperature by up to 6° to 8° F (~3°–4° C) per hour. However, external heat sources are often used but may provide only minimal benefit.[88] For the moderately to severely hypothermic patient, these remain important considerations in the extended-care situation when used in combination with the hypothermia insulation wrap.
- Some external heat sources are as follows:

  1. Warmed, (maximum 108° F [42° C]) humidified oxygen by mask can prevent heat loss during ventilation and provide some heat transfer to the chest from the respiratory tract.
  2. Body-to-body contact has merit for heat transfer, but many studies fail to show any advantage except in mildly hypothermic patients.
  3. Electric and portable heating pads provide no additional advantage.
  4. Forced-air warming has some benefit in minimizing postcooling core temperature ("afterdrop"); it provides effective warming rate comparable to shivering for mildly hypothermic patients.

- Insulate all hypothermic patients in the remote setting to minimize heat loss. Prepare a multilayer hypothermia wrap. Place a large, waterproof plastic sheet on the floor or ground. Add an insulation layer of blankets or a sleeping bag on top of the waterproof layer. Lay the patient on top of the insulation layer along with any external heat sources. Add a second insulating layer on top of the patient. The left side of the hypothermia wrap is folded over the patient first, then the right side. The patient's head is covered to prevent heat loss, keeping an opening at the face to allow patient assessment.
- Assess for hypoglycemia. Providing dextrose will ensure that adequate fuel (sugar) is available for muscular metabolism during shivering and will prevent further hypoglycemia. Alert patients can consume warm sugar fluids by mouth.

SCENARIO SOLUTION

This 76 year-old female victim has mild to moderate Alzheimer's disease. Individuals with this disease are subject to wandering and may experience bouts of hallucination and psychosis. These victims have a high mortality if not found within 24 hours, caused by dehydration and hypothermia, or drowning. There is a greater rate of fatality when these victims are exposed to high temperature or in cold and rainy climates. These patients can have narrowing of their vision resulting in poor peripheral field of view that corresponds with a trademark behavior of moving straight forward until they reach some form of barrier (e.g., fence, bushes, briars, drainage or sources of water). It is not uncommon for these patients who have been recently relocated to attempt to return to their previous residence even though they are not sure of the direction. Approach these victims from the front with good eye contact and move slowly to their side. Speak to them in slow and simple terms. Use of forceful directions and arguing will be not beneficial and may lead to an undesirable patient reaction. After initial rapid ABCs and assessing for all primary and secondary illness or injury, think about "E" or environment early since this victim has been exposed for many hours in approximately 16° F (−9° C) wind-chill temperature that accelerates convective body-heat loss along with conductive heat loss when lying or sitting on cold surface (e.g., bench, rock, or ground). A quick decision is necessary to get some protective material under and on top of the patient to slow down body heat transfer if there are any delays getting the victim onto a stretcher and into a heated ambulance. Do not delay transport waiting for a paramedic unit to arrive on scene since you can rendezvous en route to the hospital unless it is a very short transport time. Furthermore, do not delay patient transport to the hospital in the attempt to provide any means of active rewarming, or IV fluids, since these attempts will have limited benefit to rewarm the patient. In regions with prolonged transport, consider assessing rectal temperature with a hypothermic temperature probe (reads low body temperature) if available, provide warm humidified oxygen (maximum 108° F [42° C]), heated (104–108° F [40–42° C]) IV fluids and thoroughly surround the victim in a hypothermia wrap (i.e., multiple blankets surrounding the patient with a vapor barrier tarp [wind-water proof outer layer] from head to toe). Gently handle all hypothermic victims since aggressive movement can trigger ventricular tachycardia or ventricular fibrillation because the myocardium is irritable when cold. Provide supportive care with high-flow oxygen and monitor both oxygen saturation with pulse oximetry and cardiac rhythm. Remember that all hypothermic victims are not considered dead until they have been rewarmed and declared dead at the hospital. ■

SUMMARY

- Prehospital care providers will inevitably be faced with environmental encounters, such as those described in this chapter.
- Basic knowledge of common environmental emergencies is necessary to provide rapid assessment and treatment in the prehospital setting.
- It is not easy to remember this type of information because these problems are infrequently encountered, so remember the general principles involved.
- For heat-related illness, treat heat-stroke patients with effective, rapid, whole-body cooling to reduce core temperature quickly.

- For cold-related illness, manage all moderately to severely hypothermic patients gently, taking the time to remove them from the cold environment and begin passive rewarming while monitoring core temperature—the key is to prevent further body-heat loss.
- Remember, drugs and defibrillation are generally ineffective when core temperature is less than 86° F (<30° C).
- Patients are not dead until they are warm and dead.
- Remember that you must maintain your own safety. There are too many cases in which prehospital care providers have lost their lives as a result of attempting a rescue.

References

1. National Center for Health Statistics: *Compressed mortality file,* Hyattsville, MD, 2002, US Department of Health and Human Services, Centers for Disease Control and Prevention.
2. Center for Disease Control and Prevention: Heat-related deaths—Chicago, Illinois, 1996–2001, and United States, 1979–1999. *MMWR* 52(26):610, 2003.
3. Centers for Disease Control and Prevention: Heat-related deaths—United States, 1999–2003, *MMWR* 55(29):796, 2006.
4. Center for Disease Control and Prevention: Hypothermia-related deaths—Utah, 2000, and United States, 1979–1998. *MMWR* 51(4):76, 2002.
5. Lugo-Amador NM, Rothenhaus T, Moyer P: Heat-related illness. *Emerg Med Clin North Am* 22:315, 2004.
6. Ulrich AS, Rathlev NK: Hypothermia and localized injuries. *Emerg Med Clin North Am* 22:281, 2004.
7. Center for Disease Control and Prevention: Hypothermia-related deaths—United States, 2003. *MMWR* 53(8):172, 2004.
8. Speedy DB, Noakes TD: Exercise-associated hyponatremia: A review. *Emerg Med* 13:17, 2001.
9. Moran DS, Gaffen SL: Clinical management of heat-related illnesses. In Auerbach PS: *Wilderness medicine.* ed 5, St. Louis, 2007, Mosby Elsevier.
10. McCauley RL, Killyon GW, Smith DJ, Robson MC, Heggers JP: Frostbite. In Auerbach PS: *Wilderness medicine,* ed 5, St. Louis, 2007, Mosby Elsevier.
11. Danzl, DF: Accidental hypothermia. In Auerbach PS: *Wilderness medicine,* ed 5, St. Louis, 2007, Mosby Elsevier.
12. Semenza JC, Rubin CH, Flater KH, et al: Heat-related deaths during the July 1995 heat wave in Chicago. *N Engl J Med* 335(2):84, 1996.
13. Center for Disease Control and Prevention: Heat related mortality—Chicago, July 1995. *MMWR* 44 (21):577, 1995.
14. Hardy JD: Thermal comfort: Skin temperature and physiological thermoregulation. In Hardy JD, Gagge AP, Stolwijk JAJ, editors: *Physiological and Behavioral Temperature Regulation,* Springfield, IL, 1970, Charles C Thomas.
15. Pozos RS, Danzl DF: Human physiological responses to cold stress and hypothermia. In: Pandolf KB, Burr RE, editors: *Medical aspects of harsh environments,* Vol 1, Washington, DC, 2001, Office of The Surgeon General, Borden Institute/TMM Publications, pp 351–382.
16. Stocks JM, Taylor NAS, Tipton MJ, Greenleaf JE: Human physiological responses to cold exposure. *Aviat Space Environ Med* 75:444, 2004.
17. Wenger CB: The regulation of body temperature. In Rhoades RA, Tanner GA, editors: *Medical physiology,* Boston, 1995, Little, Brown.
18. Nunnelely SA, Reardon MJ: Prevention of heat illness. In Pandolf KB, Burr RE, editors: *Medical aspects of harsh environments,* Vol 1, Washington, DC, 2001, Office of The Surgeon General, Borden Institute/TMM Publications, pp 209–230.
19. Yeo T: Heat Stroke: A comprehensive review. *AACN Clin Issues* 15:280, 2004.
20. Sonna LA: Practical medical aspects of military operations in the heat. In Pandolf KB, Burr RE, editors: *Medical aspects of harsh environments,* Vol 1, Washington, DC, 2001, Office of The Surgeon General, Borden Institute/TMM Publications, pp 293–309.
21. Tek D, Olshaker JS: Heat illness. *Emerg Med Clin North Am* 10(2):299, 1992.
22. Armstrong LE, Hubbard RW, Jones BH, Daniels JT: Preparing Alberto Salazar for the heat of the 1984 Olympic marathon. *Phys Sportsmed* 14:73, 1986.
23. Hubbard RW, Sandick BL, Matthew WT: Voluntary dehydration and alliesthesia for water. *J Appl Physiol* 57:868, 1984.
24. Johnson RF, Kobrick JL: Psychological aspects of military performance in hot environments. In Pandolf KB, Burr RE, editors: *Medical aspects of harsh environments,* Vol 1, Washington, DC, 2001, Office of The Surgeon General, Borden Institute/TMM Publications.
25. Sawka MN, Pandolf KB: Physical exercise in hot climates: Physiology, performance, and biomedical issues. In Pandolf KB, Burr RE, editors: *Medical aspects of harsh environments,* Vol 1, Washington, DC, 2001, Office of The Surgeon General, Borden Institute/TMM Publications.
26. Dutchman SM, Ryan AJ, Schedl HP, et al: Upper limits of intestinal absorption of dilute glucose solution in men at rest. *Med Sci Sport Exerc* 29:482, 1997.
27. Neufer PD, Young AJ, Sawka MN: Gastric emptying during exercise: Effects of heat stress and hypohydration. *Eur J Appl Physiol* 58:433, 1989.
28. American College of Sports Medicine: Position stand: Exertional heat illness during training and competition. *Med Sci Sports Exerc* 39(3):556, 2007.
29. Wenger CB: Section I: Human adaption to hot environments. In Pandolf KB, Burr RE, editors: *Medical aspects of harsh environments,* Vol 1, Washington, DC, 2001, Office of The Surgeon General, Borden Institute/TMM Publications, pp 51–86.
30. Bouchama A, Knochel JP: Medical progress: Heatstroke. *N Engl J Med* 346(25):1978-1988; 2002.
31. Holtzhausen LM, Noakes TD: Collapsed ultra-endurance athlete: Proposed mechanisms and an approach to management. *Clin J Sport Med* 7(4):292, 1997.
32. Gardner JW, Kark, JA: Clinical diagnosis, management and surveillance of exertional heat illness. In Pandolf KB, Burr RE, editors: *Medical aspects of harsh environments,* Vol 1, Washington, DC, 2001, Office of The Surgeon General, Borden Institute/TMM Publications, pp 231–279.
33. Knochel JP, Reed G: Disorders of heat regulation. In Narins RE, editor: *Maxwell & Kleenman's clinical disorders of fluid and electrolyte metabolism,* ed 5, New York, 1994, McGraw-Hill.
34. Gaffin SL, Hubbard RW: Pathophysiology of heatstroke. In Pandolf KB, Burr RE, editors: *Medical aspects of harsh environments,* Vol 1, Washington, DC, 2001, Office of The Surgeon General, Borden Institute/TMM Publications, pp 161–208.
35. Armstrong LE, Crago AE, Adams R, et al: Whole-body cooling of hyperthermic runners: Comparison of two field therapies. *Am J Emerg Med* 14:335, 1996.
36. Costrini A: Emergency treatment of exertional heatstroke and comparison of whole-body cooling techniques. *Med Sci Sports Exerc* 22:15, 1984.
37. Gaffin SL, Gardner J, Flinn S: Current cooling method for exertional heatstroke. *Ann Intern Med* 132:678, 2000.
38. Speedy DB, Noakes TD: Exercise-associated hyponatremia: A review. *Emerg Med* 13:17, 2001.
39. Backer HD, Shopes E, Collins SL, Barkan H: Exertional heat illness and hyponatremia in hikers. *Am J Emerg Med* 17(6):532, 1999.
40. Gardner JW: Death by water intoxication. *Mil Med* 164(3):432, 2002.

41. Noakes TD, Goodwin N, Rayner BL et al: Water intoxication: A possible complication during endurance exercise. *Med Sci Sports Exerc* 17:370, 1985.

42. Rosner MH and Kirven J: Exercise-associated hyponatremia. *Clin J Am Soc Nephrol* 2:151, 2007.

43. Adrogue HJ, Madias NE: Hyponatremia. *N Engl J Med* 342(21):1581, 2000.

44. Hiller WDB: Dehydration and hyponatremia during triathlons. *Med Sci Sports Exerc* 21:S219, 1989.

45. Speedy DB, Noakes TD, Rodgers IR: Hyponatremia in ultra-distance triathletes. *Med Sci Sports Exerc* 31:809, 1999.

46. Laird RH: Medical care at ultra-endurance triathlons. *Med Sci Sports Exerc* 21:S222, 1989.

47. Collins S, Reynolds, B: The other heat-related emergency. *JEMS*, July 2004.

48. Hew-Butler T, Ayus JC, Kipps C, Maughan RJ, Mettler S, et al: Statement of Second International Exercise-Associated Hyponatremia Concensus Development Conference, New Zealand, 2007. *Clin J Sport Med* 18:111, 2008.

49. Irving RA, Noakes TD, Buck R: Evaluation of renal function and fluid homeostasis during recovery from exercise-induced hyponatremia. *J Appl Physiol* 70:342, 1991.

50. Eichner ER: Exertional hyponatremia: Why so many women? *Sports Med Digest* 24:54, 2002.

51. Ayus JC, Arieff A, Moritz ML: Hyponatremia in marathon runners. *N Engl J Med* 353:427, 2005.

52. US Fire Administration: Firefighter fatalities in the United States in 2006. FEMA, July 2007, http://www.usfa.dhs.gov/downloads/pdf/publications/ff_fat06.pdf.

53. US Department of Agriculture, US Forest Service: Heat stress brochure. http://www.fs.fed.us/t-d/pubs/pdfpubs/pdf98512841/pdf98512841dpi300.pdf. Accessed Sep 3, 2010.

54. Montain SJ, Latzka WA, Sawka MN: Fluid replacement recommendations for training in hot weather. *Mil Med* 164(7):502, 1999.

55. Parson KC: International standards for the assessment of the risk of thermal strain on clothed workers in hot environments. *Ann Occup Hyg* 43(5):297, 1999.

56. American College of Sports Medicine: Position stand on exercise and fluid replacement. *Med Sci Sports Exerc* 39(2):377, 2007.

57. American College of Sports Medicine: Position stand on the recommended quantity and quality of exercise for developing and maintaining cardiorespiratory and muscular fitness, and flexibility in adults. *Med Sci Sports Exerc* 30(6):975, 1998.

58. Haskell WL, Lee IM, Pate RR, et al: Physical activity and public health: Updated recommendation for adults from the American College of Sports Medicine and the American Heart Association. *Med Sci Sports Exerc* 39(8):1423, 2007.

59. Pate RR, Pratt M, Blair SB, et al: Physical activity and public health: A recommendation from the Centers for Disease Control and Prevention and the American College of Sports Medicine. *JAMA* 273(5):402, 1995.

60. Heat acclimatization guide, Ranger and Airborne school students, 2003, www.usariem.army.mil/pages/download/heatacclimatizationguide.pdf. Accessed Sep 3, 2010.

61. Eichna LW, Park CR, Nelson N, et al: Thermal regulation during acclimatization in a hot, dry (desert type) environment. *J Appl Physiol* 163:585, 1950.

62. NFPA 1584: Standard on the rehabilitation process for members during emergency operations and training exercises, 2008 edition. http://www.nfpa.org/catalog/product.asp?pid=158408&src=nfpa&order_src=A292.

63. McEnvy, Mike: Making a rehab a requirement: NFPA 1584. *FireRescue1* December, 2007. http://www.firerescue1.com/firerehab/articles/327047-Making-Rehab-a-Requirement-NFPA-1584/.

64. Hostler D: First responder rehab: Good, better, best. *JEMS*, 32(12): 2007. http://www.jems.com/article/mobile-treatment-facilities/first-responder-rehab-good44-b. Accessed Sep 3, 2010.

65. Federal Emergency Management System, United States Fire Administration: Emergency incident rehabilitation, Report #FA-114, July 1992. http://www.usfa.dhs.gov/downloads/pdf/publications/fa-114.pdf. Accessed Sep 3, 2010.

66. US Pharmacopeia, National Formulary, USP-25/NF-20, Rockville, MD, US Pharmacopeia Convention, 2000.

67. Brown LH, Krumperman K, Fullagar CJ: Out of hospital medical storage temperature. *Prehosp Emerg Care* 8:200, 2004.

68. Mehta SH, Doran JV, Lavery RF, Allegra JR: Improvements in prehospital medication storage practices in response to research. *Prehosp Emerg Care* 6:319, 2002.

69. Allegra JR, Brennan J, Lanier V: Storage temperatures of out-of-hospital medications. *Acad Emerg Med* 6:1098, 1999.

70. Palmer RG, Zimmerman J, Clawson JJ: Altered states: The influence of temperature on prehospital drugs. *J Emerg Med Serv* 10(12):29, 1985.

71. Johansen RB, Schafer NC, Brown PI: Effects of extreme temperature on drugs for prehospital ACLS. *Am J Emerg Med* 11:450, 1993.

72. Church WH, Hu SS, Henry AJ: Thermal degradation of injectable drugs. *Am J Emerg Med* 12:306, 1994.

73. New Jersey Department of Health and Senior Services, Suppl Section 8:41-43.12, paragraph (f), August 17, 1998.

74. Stocks JM, Taylor NAS, Tipton MJ, Greenleaf JE: Human physiological responses to cold exposure. *Aviat Space Environ Med* 75:444, 2004.

75. Ulrich AS, Rathlev NK: Hypothermia and localized injuries. *Emerg Med Clin North Am* 22:281, 2004.

76. Chandler W, Ivey H: Cold weather injuries among US soldiers in Alaska: A five-year review. *Mil Med* 162:788, 1997.

77. DeGroot DW, Castellani JW, Williams JO, Amoroso PJ: Epidemiology of US Army cold-weather injuries, 1980–1999. *Mil Med* 74:564, 2003.

78. Thomas JR, Oakley EHN: Nonfreezing cold injury. In Pandolf KB, Burr RE, editors: *Medical aspects of harsh environments*, Vol 1, Washington, DC, 2001, Office of The Surgeon General, Borden Institute/TMM Publications, pp 467–490.

79. Montgomery H: Experimental immersion foot: Review of the physiopathology. *Physiol Rev* 34:127, 1954.

80. Francis TJR: Nonfreezing cold injury: A historical review. *J R Nav Med Serv* 70:134, 1984.

81. Wrenn K: Immersion foot: A problem of the homeless in the 1990s. *Arch Intern Med* 151:785, 1991.

82. Ramstead KD, Hughes RB, Webb AJ: Recent cases of trench foot. *Postgrad Med J* 56:879, 1980.

83. Biem J, Koehncke N, Classen D, Dosman J: Out of cold: Management of hypothermia and frostbite. *Can Med Assoc J* 168(3):305, 2003.

84. Vogel JE, Dellon AL: Frostbite injuries of the hand. *Clin Plast Surg* 16:565, 1989.

85. Mills WJ: Clinical aspects of freezing injury. In Pandolf KB, Burr RE, editors: *Medical aspects of harsh environments*, Vol 1,

Washington, DC, 2001, Office of The Surgeon General, Borden Institute/TMM Publications.

86. Gilbertson J, Mandsager R: State of Alaska cold injuries guidelines. Department of Health and Social Services, Juneau, Alaska, 2005 (revision). http://www.ems.alaska.gov/EMS/documents/AKColdInj2005.pdf. Accessed Sep 3, 2010.

87. Sessler DI: Mild preoperative hypothermia. *N Engl J Med* 336:1730, 1997.

88. Giesbrecht GG: Cold stress, near drowning and accidental hypothermia: A review. *Aviat Space Environ Med* 71:733, 2000.

89. Gilbert M, Busund R, Skagseth A, et al: Resuscitation from accidental hypothermia of 13.7° C with circulatory arrest. *Lancet* 355:375, 2000.

90. Danzl DF, Pozos RS, Auerbach PS: Multicenter hypothermia survey. *Ann Emerg Med* 16:1042, 1987.

91. Tsuei BJ, Kearney PA: Hypothermia in the trauma patient. *Injury Int J Care Injured* 35:7, 2004.

92. Stoner HB: Effects of injury on the responses to thermal stimulation of the hypothalamus. *J Appl Physiol* 33:665, 1972.

93. Jurkovich G: Hypothermia in the trauma patient. *Adv Trauma* 4:111, 1989.

94. Jurkovich, GJ: Environmental cold-induced injury. *Surg Clin N Am* 87:247, 2007.

95. Nolan JP, Morley PT, Vanden Hoek TL, et al: Therapeutic hypothermia after cardiac arrest. An advisory statement by the Advance Life Support Task Force of the international liaison committee on resuscitation, *Circulation* 108:118, 2003.

96. Alzaga AG, Cerdan M, Varon J: Therapeutic hypothermia. *Resuscitation* 70:369, 2006.

97. Ferrara A, MacArthur J, Wright H: Hypothermia and acidosis worsen coagulopathy in the patient requiring massive transfusion. *Am J Surg* 160:515, 1990.

98. Epstein M: Renal effects of head-out immersion in man: Implications for understanding volume homeostasis. *Physiol Rev* 58:529, 1978.

99. Carlson LD: Immersion in cold water and body tissue insulation. *Aerospace Med* 29:145, 1958.

100. Wittmers LE, Savage M: Cold water immersion. In Pandolf KB, Burr RE, editors: *Medical aspects of harsh environments*, Vol 1, Washington, DC, 2001, pp 531–552, Office of The Surgeon General, Borden Institute/TMM Publications.

101. Giesbrecht GG, Steinman AM: Immersion into cold water. In Auerbach PS: *Wilderness medicine,* ed 5, St. Louis, 2007, Mosby Elsevier.

102. Hayward JS, Eckerson JD, Collis ML: Effect of behavioral variables on cooling rate of man in cold water. *J Appl Physiol* 38:1073, 1975.

103. Nozaki R, Ishibashi K, Adachi N, et al: Accidental profound hypothermia. *N Eng J Med* 315:1680, 1986 (letter).

104. Tipton MJ: The initial responses to cold-water immersion in man. *Clin Sci* 77:581, 1989.

105. Keatinge WR, McIlroy MB, Goldfien A: Cardiovascular responses to ice-cold showers. *J Appl Physiol* 19:1145, 1964.

106. Mekjavic IB et al: Respiratory drive during sudden cold water immersion. *Respir Physiol* 70:21, 1987.

107. Golden FSC, Tipton MJ, Scott RC: Immersion, near-drowning and drowning. *Br J Anaesth* 79:214, 1997.

108. Schoene RB, Nachat A, Gravatt AR, Newman AB: Submersion incidents. In Auerbach PS: *Wilderness medicine,* ed 5, St. Louis, 2007, Mosby Elsevier.

109. Wissler EH: Probability of surviving during accidental immersion in cold water. *Aviat Space Environ Med* 74:47, 2003.

110. Tikuisis P: Predicting survival time at sea based on observed body cooling rates. *Aviat Space Environ Med* 68:441, 1997.

111. Hayward JS, Errickson JD, Collis ML: Thermal balance and survival time prediction of man in cold water. *Can J Physiol Pharmacol* 53:21, 1975.

112. Ducharme MB, Lounsbury DS: Self-rescue swimming in cold water: The latest advice. *Appl Physiol Nutr Metab* 32:799, 2007.

113. Van Mieghem C, Sabbe M, Knockaert D: The clinical vales of the ECG in noncardiac conditions. *Chest* 125:1561, 2004.

114. American Heart Association, International Liaison Committee on Resuscitation: Guidelines 2005 for cardiopulmonary resuscitation and emergency cardiovascular care. *Circulation*; 112; IV-136–IV-138, 2005.

115. International Liaison Committee on Resuscitation: 2005 International consensus on cardiopulmonary resuscitation and emergency cardiovascular care science with treatment recommendations. *Circulation* 112(suppl 1):IV–1, 2005.

116. Danzl DF, Lloyd EL: Treatment of accidental hypothermia. In Pandolf KB, Burr RE, editors: *Medical aspects of harsh environments*, Vol 1, Washington, DC, 2001, pp 491–529, Office of The Surgeon General, Borden Institute/TMM Publications.

117. Southwick FS, Dalglish PH: Recovery after prolonged asystolic cardiac arrest in profound hypothermia: A case report and literature review. *JAMA* 243:1250, 1980.

118. Bernard MB, Gray TW, Buist MD, et al: Treatment of comatose survivors of out-of-hospital cardiac arrest with induced hypothermia. *N Engl J Med* 346(8):557, 2002.

119. Reuler JB: Hypothermia: Pathophysiology, clinical setting, and management. *Ann Intern Med* 89:519, 1978.

120. Armstrong LE: Cold, windchill, and water immersion. In *Performing in extremes environments*, Champaign, IL, 2000, Human Kinetics.

121. Wilderness Medical Society: Myocardial Infarction, Acute Coronary Syndromes, and CPR. In Forgey WW, editor: *Practice guidelines for wilderness emergency care*, ed 5, Guilford, 2006, Globe Pequot Press.

122. Bailey DE, Wydro GC, Cone DC: Position paper of the National Association of EMS Physicians: Termination of resuscitation in the prehospital setting for adult patients suffering nontraumatic cardiac arrest. *Prehosp Emerg Care* 4:190, 2000.

Suggested Reading

Auerbach PS, editor: *Wilderness medicine,* ed 5, St. Louis, 2007, Mosby.

Fregly MJ, Blatteis CM: *Environmental physiology,* Vols I & II, American Physiological Society, New York, 1996, Oxford University Press.

Pandolf KB, Burr RE, editors: *Medical aspects of harsh environments,* Vol 1, Washington, DC, 2001, Office of the Surgeon General, Borden Institute/TMM Publications.

CHAPTER 21

Environmental Trauma II: Drowning, Lightning, Diving, and Altitude

CHAPTER OBJECTIVES

At the completion of this chapter, the reader will be able to do the following:

✓ List five risk factors for a near-drowning incident.

✓ List three signs or symptoms that can occur in a patient after a near-drowning incident.

✓ List five methods for preventing a drowning incident.

✓ Explain the "30–30" rule in lightning injury prevention.

✓ Differentiate the use of "reverse" triage for multiple lightning casualties from its use for other multiple-casualty scenarios.

✓ Differentiate signs and symptoms of Type I and Type II decompression sickness.

✓ Explain two primary treatment interventions for Type II decompression sickness and arterial gas embolism.

✓ List two key risk factors for high-altitude illness.

✓ Discuss the similarities and differences between acute mountain sickness and high-altitude cerebral edema.

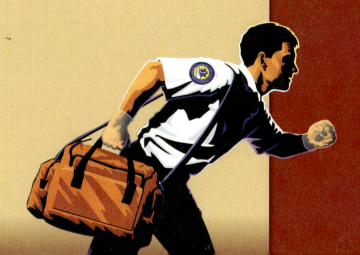

SCENARIO

At 4:15 p.m. on a hot and humid summer afternoon, Medic 10 with two paramedics and an EMT intern was returning to station when they received a dispatch for an unconscious male on the 18th hole at the city country club. En route to the scene, the duty chief provided an update that a fast moving thunderstorm passed through the country club less than 15 minutes ago with rain, hail, and lightning, and stressed scene safety due to additional lightning nearby. As you arrive on the 18th hole, you observe one golfer lying on the fairway and another golfer sitting against a nearby tree along with a number of bystanders in the area. The scene now appears safe with one downed large tree branch and dark thunderclouds moving fast eastward. As you prepare to assess the victims, the other paramedic and EMT student bring out the medic bags and are gathering bystander information. An uninjured golfer from the foursome stated that a thunderstorm approached the area rapidly with high winds, heavy rain with severe lightning, and thunder. The two injured golfers ran for cover at the base of a large tree and two others ran to the clubhouse nearby. Apparently, lightning struck the tree and traveled down the trunk and hit the ground near the two huddled golfers. He initially thought they both were hit by lightning—one looked dead, another look injured and dazed.

Is the scene safe? How would you begin to immediately assess these two victims? What are your priorities for triage? How would you assess and manage lightning injuries? What is the underlying medical concern for lightning-strike victims? Are there other primary or secondary injuries to consider in this scenario?

Each year in the United States, significant morbidity and mortality are caused by a variety of environmental conditions, including drowning or near-drowning, lightning, recreational scuba diving, and high altitude (see Chapter 20 for heat and cold conditions). Thus, it is important for prehospital care providers to know the major and minor disorders associated with each type of environment; understand the anatomy, physiology, and pathophysiology involved; and perform patient assessment and management. At the same time, they must prevent injury to themselves and other public safety personnel.

Drowning or Near-Drowning

Submersion incidents in water that lead to injury are all too common in the United States and the world. Drowning remains a leading cause of preventable death across all age groups,[1] but is an epidemic in children.[2] The World Health Organization estimates that there are over 400,000 deaths annually from unintentional submersion incidents, not including deaths from drowning resulting from floods, suicide or homicide.[3] Submersion injuries have a substantial cost to society; an estimated $450 million to $650 million or more is spent on these patients each year in the United States alone.[4] The terminology describing these patients continues to evolve. Thirty-five years ago, "drowning" was defined as

the process by which air-breathing animals succumb on submersion in a liquid, and "near-drowning" was defined as submersion with at least temporary survival.[5] The term "secondary drowning" was used to describe patients who recovered initially from a submersion injury, but then died from respiratory failure secondary to submersion.[6,7] However, this latter term has come under question lately, and some suggest that it should not be used.[6]

The more accepted definitions for drowning and near-drowning are as follows:

- **Drowning:** death within 24 hours of the submersion incident.
- **Near-drowning:** survival for at least 24 hours after the submersion.[5,6,8,9]

Because resuscitative care at the scene is initiated for all water-related casualties, it may be more practical to avoid using these two terms and instead use the term *submersion incident*, which encompasses drowning *and* near-drowning. Furthermore, the term submersion incident implies no particular outcome of the patient at the scene, en route to the hospital, or later at the hospital. This should help prevent providers of all types from making any judgment about withholding resuscitative efforts based on the mechanism of injury, length of submersion, water temperature, or the patient who presents without vital signs.[10] This last point is critical because there are numerous reports of those who have survived prolonged periods (>30 minutes) of cold-water submersion.[11–13] Immediate and effective delivery of cardiopulmonary resuscitation (CPR) and the activation of emergency medical services (EMS) by bystanders are two important factors that influence the survival of a submersion patient.[14]

Prevention strategies are vital in the effort to lower the rates of submersion incidents in the United States. Many education programs are emphasizing the reduction of *unintentional* water entry of infants and children by encouraging the installation of various types of barriers around pools (e.g., isolation fences, pool covers, alarms, etc.) and the use of personal flotation devices such as life vests. Furthermore, CPR initiated by a bystander before the arrival of prehospital care personnel is associated with improved patient prognosis.[15]

Epidemiology

Death by unintentional drowning is the seventh leading cause of death for all ages, the second leading cause of death for ages 1 to 14 years, and the fifth leading cause of death of infants (<1 year of age).[1] Infants are at risk from drowning in bathtubs, buckets, and toilets.[14] The incidence of near-drowning may be 500 to 600 times the rate of drowning.[15] In 2000, there were 3281 cases of unintentional drowning in the United States, and for every child who drowned, three others survived and required emergency care for their submersion incident. Each week, approximately 40 children die from drowning, 115 are hospitalized, and 12 have irreversible brain injury.[2]

The Centers for Disease Control and Prevention (CDC) reported a total of 7546 submersion casualties (fatal and nonfatal) in 2001 and 2002[1] (Figure 21-1). Of these, 3372 persons experienced unintentional drowning in various recreational settings, such as pools, oceans, and rivers. In comparison, 4174 unintentional nonfatal submersion incidents were treated in emergency departments (EDs) in the United States. The nonfatal and fatal injury rates were the highest for children age 4 years or younger and for males of all ages. The nonfatal rate for males was almost twice that of females, whereas the fatal rate for males was almost five times that of females. Nonfatal submersion injuries in pools accounted for 75%, whereas 70% of the fatal submersions occurred in natural settings, such as oceans, lakes, and rivers.

Submersion Factors

Specific factors place individuals at an increased risk for submersion incidents.[5,6,14,16] Recognizing these factors will increase awareness and assist in the creation of preventive strategies and policies to minimize these occurrences. For infants and young children, the major risk factor is inadequate supervision, and for adolescents and adults, it is risky behavior and use of drugs or alcohol.[14]

Ability to Swim

Swimming ability is not consistently related to drowning. White males have a higher incidence of drowning than

FIGURE 21-1   **Unintentional Drowning/Near-Drowning— United States, 2001–2002**

Characteristic	Nonfatal*	Fatal*
AGE (yr)		
0–4	2168	442
5–14	1058	333
≥15	948	2563
Unknown	—	34
GENDER		
Male	2721	2789
Female	1452	583
LOCATION		
Pool	2571	596
Natural water (ocean, lakes, rivers)	909	1467
Other	513	1309
DISPOSITION		
Treated/released	1925	—
Hospitalized	2233	—
Other	16	—
Total	**4174**	**3372**

(Data from Centers for Disease Control and Prevention: Nonfatal and fatal drownings in recreational water settings—United States, 2001–2002. *MMWR* 53(21):447, 2004.)
*Estimated number.

white females, even though they are reported to have better swimming ability.[5] Although black females have poor swimming skills, they have a very low drowning rate.[17] One study reported that nonswimmers or beginners accounted for 73% of drownings in home swimming pools and 82% of incidents in canals, lakes, and ponds.[18]

Shallow-Water Blackout

Some swimmers, in an effort to increase their swim distance, will intentionally hyperventilate immediately before underwater swimming in effort to lower the partial pressure of arterial carbon dioxide ($PaCO_2$) since CO_2 level provides the stimulus to breath in non-COPD patients.[19] This decrease in $PaCO_2$ will decrease the feedback to the respiratory center in the hypothalamus to take a breath during breath holding. These individuals are at risk of a submersion incident because the partial pressure of arterial oxygen (PaO_2) does not change significantly with hyperventilation. As the individual continues to swim underwater, PaO_2 will decrease significantly and cause a possible loss of consciousness and cerebral hypoxia.

Accidental Cold-Water Immersion

Another situation that places individuals at greater risk of drowning or near-drowning is cold-water immersion ("head out"). The physiologic changes that occur with cold-water immersion can have either a disastrous outcome or a protective effect of cold on the body, depending on many circumstances. Adverse outcomes are more common, resulting from both cardiovascular collapse and sudden death within minutes of cold-water immersion.

Age

Drowning is recognized as a young person's accident, with toddlers as the largest group, based on their inquisitive nature and a lack of parental supervision. Children under 1 year of age have the highest drowning rate.[1,20]

Gender

Males account for more than half of submersion victims with two age-related peak incidences. The first peak incidence occurs in males at age 2 years, decreases until age 10 years, and then rises rapidly to peak again at age 18 years. Older males may be more at risk for drowning because of higher exposure rates to aquatic activities, higher alcohol consumption while at the waterfront, and more risk-taking behavior.[5,21]

Race

Black children experience more submersion incidents than white children. Black children tend to drown in ponds, lakes, and other natural sources of water.[1] The drowning rate of black male children has been estimated to be as high as three times that of white males.[22]

Location

Submersion incidents typically occur in backyard swimming pools and in the ocean, but also occur in buckets.[6] Houses in rural areas with open wells increase the risk of a young child drowning by sevenfold.[5] Other hazardous locations are water barrels, fountains, and underground cisterns.

Alcohol and Drugs

Alcohol is the primary drug associated with submersion incidents,[23] most likely because it causes a loss of judgment.[24] As many as 20% to 30% of adult boating fatalities and submersion incidents involve alcohol use in which occupants used poor judgment, were speeding, failed to wear life jackets, or handled the craft recklessly.[5,25,26]

Underlying Disease or Trauma

The onset of illness from underlying disease can account for submersion victims. Hypoglycemia, myocardial infarction, cardiac arrhythmia, depression and suicidal thoughts, and syncope predispose to drowning incidents.[14] A recent study reported that the risk of drowning in people with epilepsy is raised 15- to19-fold compared to people in the general population.[24] Cervical spine injuries and head trauma should be suspected in all unwitnessed incidents and injuries involving body surfers, board surfers, and victims diving in shallow water or water with submerged objects such as rocks or trees (Figures 21-2 and 21-3).

Child Abuse

A high incidence of child abuse from submersion incidents is reported, particularly in bathtubs. A study of children sustaining bathtub submersion between 1982 and 1992 found that 67% had historical or physical findings compatible with a diagnosis of abuse or neglect.[16] Consequently, it is highly recommended that any suspicious child-submersion bathtub incident be reported to local social services for appropriate investigation.

Hypothermia

Drowning may result directly from prolonged immersion leading to hypothermia. (See Cold-Related Disorders in Chapter 20 for further discussion of accidental hypothermia.)

Mechanism of Injury

A common scenario of *head-out immersion* in water or a whole-body submersion incident begins with a situation that creates a panic response, leading to breath-holding, air hunger, and increased physical activity in effort to stay or get above the

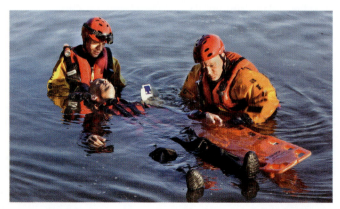

FIGURE 21-2 Spine board immobilization in water.

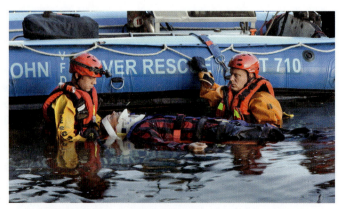

FIGURE 21-3 Spine board immobilization in water.

water surface. According to most bystander reports, *submersion victims are rarely seen screaming and waving for assistance while struggling to stay above the surface of the water.* Rather, they are seen either floating on the surface or in a motionless position, or they dive underwater and fail to come up. As the submersion incident continues, a reflex inspiratory effort draws water into the pharynx and larynx, causing a choking response and laryngospasm. The onset of laryngospasm represents the first step in suffocation, which in turn causes the victim to lose consciousness and submerge underwater even further.

Over the years, controversies have surrounded the pathophysiology of drowning and near-drowning, mostly about the differences between drowning in freshwater versus salt water and whether water entered or did not enter the lungs.[6,10,14] Approximately 15% of drownings are termed "dry drowning" because the severe laryngospasm prevents the aspiration of fluid into the lungs. The remaining 85% of submersion incidents are considered "wet drownings," in which the laryngospasm relaxes, the glottis opens, and the victim aspirates water into the lungs.[27] Theoretically, there are different effects on the pulmonary system when freshwater (hypotonic) versus salt water (hypertonic) enters in the lung. In freshwater drowning, the hypotonic fluid enters the lung and then moves across the alveolus into the intravascular space, causing a volume overload and dilutional effect on serum electrolytes and other serum components. Conversely, in saltwater aspiration, the hypertonic fluid enters the lung, which in turn causes additional fluid from the intravascular space to enter the lung across the alveolus, causing pulmonary edema and hypertonicity of serum electrolytes.

It has since been shown that no real differences exist between wet and dry drowning and freshwater and saltwater aspiration.[14,28,29] For prehospital care providers, the common denominator in any of these four submersion scenarios is hypoxia caused by either laryngospasm or water aspiration. Management at the scene should be aimed at reversing any hypoxia in these patients, thereby preventing cardiac arrest.

Surviving Cold-Water Submersion

In numerous cases of prolonged submersion—in one case for as long as 66 minutes—patients have presented to the hospital with severe hypothermia and recovered with either partial or full neurologic function.[12] In these submersion incidents, the lowest recorded core temperature of a survivor is 56.6° F (13.7° C) in an adult female.[11] In another case, a child survived fully intact after submersion in ice water for 40 minutes, with a core temperature of 75° F (24° C). After 1 hour of resuscitation, spontaneous circulation returned.[30]

No explanation exists for such cases, but hypothermia is thought to be protective. Immersion in cold water may lead quickly to hypothermia because of surface heat loss and core cooling. In addition, swallowing or aspiration of cold water may contribute to rapid cooling. Rapid onset of hypothermia during freshwater drowning may result from core cooling caused by pulmonary aspiration and rapid absorption of cold water and subsequent brain cooling.

Another factor that may explain why some young children survive is the mammalian diving reflex. The *mammalian diving reflex* slows heart rate, shunts blood to the brain, and closes the airway. However, recent evidence suggests that the diving reflex present in various mammals is active in only 15% to 30% of human subjects, although this still may explain in part why some children survive.[5]

Every submersion patient should have full resuscitation efforts made, regardless of the presence or absence of any of these factors. The factors described next appear to influence the outcome of a cold-water submersion patient.

Age. Many successful infant and child resuscitations have been well documented in the United States and Europe. The smaller mass of a child's body cools faster than an adult's body, thus permitting fewer harmful by-products of anaerobic metabolism to form and causing less irreversible damage.

Submersion Time. The shorter the duration of submersion, the lower is the risk for cellular damage caused by hypoxia. Accurate information concerning submersion time needs to be obtained. Submersion longer than 66 minutes is probably fatal. Therefore, a reasonable approach to resuscitation of a submersion victim is that efforts should be initiated if the duration of submersion is less than one hour.

Water Temperature. Water temperatures of 70° F (21° C) and below are capable of inducing hypothermia. The colder the water, the better is the chance of survival, probably because of the rapid decrease in brain temperature and metabolism when the body is quickly chilled.

Struggle. Submersion victims who struggle less have a better chance of resuscitation (unless their struggling efforts are successful enough to avoid drowning). Less struggling means less hormonal release (e.g., epinephrine) and less muscle activity; this translates to less heat (energy) production and less vasodilatation. These in turn cause decreased muscular oxygen demand, which results in smaller muscle oxygen deficit and less CO_2 and lactic acid production. Thus, the rate of cooling of the patient is increased which may improve resuscitation chances.

Cleanliness of Water. Patients generally do better after resuscitation if they were submerged in clean water rather than muddy or contaminated water.

Quality of CPR and Resuscitative Efforts. Patients receiving adequate and effective CPR, combined with proper rewarming and advanced life support (ALS) measures, generally do better than patients receiving one or more substandard measures. Immediate initiation of CPR is a key factor for submersion-hypothermia patients. Past and current studies reveal that poor CPR technique is directly related to poor resuscitation outcome.[31,32] See the current basic life support (BLS) guidelines as outlined elsewhere.[33]

Associated Injuries or Illness. Patients with an existing injury or illness, or who become ill or injured in combination with the submersion, do not fare as well as otherwise healthy individuals.

Assessment

The initial priorities for any submersion patient include:

1. Prevent injuries to the patient and emergency responders.
2. Initiate plans early for water extraction and rapid transport to ED.
3. Conduct a safe water rescue (consider a possible diving-related cause and the need for spine immobilization).
4. Assess for ABCs (airway, breathing, circulation).
5. Reverse hypoxia and acidosis.
6. Restore or maintain cardiovascular stability.
7. Prevent further loss of body heat and initiate rewarming efforts in hypothermic patients.

Initially, it is safest to presume the submersion patient is hypoxic and hypothermic until proved otherwise. Consequently, all efforts should be made to establish effective respirations during water rescue and to remove the patient from water and other sources of cold to minimize further body heat loss. Quickly assess the patient for any life threats, and assess for head trauma and cervical spine injuries, particularly if there is suspicion of trauma associated with the submersion incident (e.g., falls, boat accidents, diving into water with underwater hazards). However, it has been shown that the typical submersion casualty has a low chance of traumatic injury, unless the victim dove into the water.[34] Acquire vital signs, and assess all lung fields of submersion patients because they present with a wide range of pulmonary distress, including shortness of breath, rales, rhonchi, and wheezing. These patients can present without symptoms initially and then deteriorate rapidly with signs of pulmonary edema.

Assess oxygen saturation with pulse oximetry. Assess for cardiac rhythm disturbances; submersion patients often have dysrhythmias secondary to hypoxia and hypothermia. Assess for altered mental status and neurologic function of all extremities because many submersion victims develop sustained neurologic damage. Determine the patient's blood glucose level as hypoglycemia may have been the cause for the submersion incident. Acquire a baseline Glasgow Coma Scale (GCS) score and continue to assess for trends. Remove all wet clothing and assess rectal temperature (if appropriate thermometers are available and the situation permits) to determine the level of hypothermia, and initiate steps to minimize further heat loss (see Chapter 20 for management of hypothermia).

The following variables are predictive of a more favorable outcome in near-drowning patients:

- Children age 3 years and older
- Female

- Water temperature less than 50° F (10° C)
- Duration of submersion less than 10 minutes
- No aspiration
- Time to effective BLS less than 10 minutes
- Rapid return of spontaneous cardiac output
- Spontaneous cardiac output on arrival in ED
- Core temperature less than 95° F (35° C)
- No coma on arrival and GCS score greater than 6
- Pupillary responses present

Management

A patient who has experienced some form of submersion incident, but who is not presenting with any signs or symptoms at the time of the initial assessment, still needs follow-up care in a hospital after assessment at the scene due to the potential for delayed onset of symptoms. Many asymptomatic patients are released in 6 to 8 hours, depending on clinical findings in the hospital. In one study of 52 swimmers who experienced a submersion incident and were all initially asymptomatic immediately after the incident, 21 (40%) went on to develop shortness of breath and respiratory distress due to hypoxemia within 4 hours.[35] In general, all symptomatic patients are admitted to the hospital for at least 24 hours for supportive care and observation because the initial clinical assessment can be misleading. It is critical to obtain a good history of the incident detailing the estimate of submersion time and any past medical history.

All suspected submersion patients should receive high-flow oxygen (12–15 liters/minute) independent of their initial breathing status or oxygen saturation, based on the concern for delayed pulmonary distress, particularly if the patient develops shortness of breath. Monitor electrocardiogram (ECG) for dysrhythmias. Obtain intravenous (IV) access and provide normal saline (NS) or Lactated Ringer's (LR) solution at keep-vein-open (KVO) rate. Transport to the ED for evaluation. Because many near-drowning patients are asymptomatic, some may refuse transport because they have no immediate chief complaint. If so, take the time necessary to provide good patient education about the delayed signs and symptoms in a near-drowning incident and that many victims develop secondary complications from pulmonary injury. Firm and persistent persuasion is needed for them to agree to be transported or for them to report to the closest ED for further evaluation and observation. If the patient is adamant about refusing care, the patient must be informed of the potential ramifications of refusing care and a signed refusal of care against medical advice obtained.

A symptomatic patient with a history of submersion who presents with signs of distress (e.g., anxiety, rapid respirations, difficulty breathing, coughing) is considered to have a submersion pulmonary injury until hospital evaluation has proved otherwise. Emphasis should be placed on correcting hypoxia, acidosis, and hypothermia. Provide cervical spine immobilization in all patients with suspicion of trauma. In unresponsive patients, use suction to clear the airway and keep the airway open with an airway adjunct. Hypoxia and acidosis can be corrected with effective ventilation support. Apneic patients should be supported with bag-mask ventilation. Intubation should be considered early to protect the airway in patients who are apneic or cyanotic or who have decreased mental status, since submersion victims swallow large amounts of water and are at risk of vomiting and aspirating stomach contents. The Sellick maneuver (cricoid pressure) should be applied during manual ventilation with a bag-mask and intubation to prevent regurgitation and aspiration. Monitor the ECG for rate and rhythm disturbances and investigate for evidence of a cardiac event that might have preceded or followed the submersion incident. Provide 100% oxygen (12–15 liters/minute) with a nonrebreather mask. Obtain IV access and provide NS or LR solution at KVO rate. Provide transport to local ED.

Patient Resuscitation

Rapid initiation of effective CPR and standard ALS procedures for submersion patients in cardiopulmonary arrest is associated with the best chance of survival.[6] Victims may present in asystole, pulseless electrical activity, or pulseless ventricular tachycardia/ventricular fibrillation. Follow the current version of the American Heart Association (AHA) guidelines for pediatric and adult ALS and advanced cardiac life support (ACLS) for managing these rhythms.[33] As briefly presented in Chapter 20, it is currently recommended to use therapeutic hypothermia in patients who remain in a coma from cardiac arrest caused by ventricular fibrillation and that it might be equally effective for other causes of cardiac arrest, but it has not been proven beneficial to induce hypothermia for drowning victims.[8]

Routine stabilization of the cervical spine during in-water rescue is not necessary unless the reasons leading to the submersion indicate that trauma is likely (e.g., diving, use of water slide, signs of injury, alcohol use).[8] When these indicators are not present, spinal injury is unlikely. Cervical stabilization and other means to immobilize the spine during a water rescue can cause delays in opening the airway so that rescue breathing can begin.

The use of CPR during in-water rescue is not recommended because the depth of chest compressions is ineffective in water. Besides delaying effective CPR out of water, attempting to provide CPR in water puts rescuers at risk from fatigue, cold water, wave, surge, and current dangers. Place a greater emphasis on establishing an open airway and providing rescue breathing for apneic patients as soon as possible, depending on the patient's in-water position, number of rescuers, and rescue equipment (e.g., in-water backboard).

When a beach rescue (or any location) involves sloping terrain, it is no longer recommended to place a patient in a head-down (or head-up) position in an effort to drain the airway. Resuscitation efforts are shown to be more successful when the patient is placed supine on the ground, parallel to the water, with effective ventilation and chest compressions. Maintaining a level position on the ground will prevent a decrease in forward blood flow during chest compressions in the head-up position or an increase in intracranial pressure in the head-down position. Furthermore, no evidence suggests that lung drainage is effective with any particular maneuver.

The Heimlich maneuver has been previously suggested for use in drowning victims. However, the Heimlich maneuver is designed for airway obstruction and does not remove water from the airway or lungs. Rather, it may induce vomiting in drowning victims and place them at greater risk for aspiration. Currently, the AHA and the Institute of Medicine advise against the Heimlich maneuver except when the airway is blocked with foreign material.[36] If the patient recovers with spontaneous breathing, the patient should be placed in a lateral recumbent position with head slightly lower than the trunk to reduce the risk of aspiration if the patient vomits. (Chapter 20 outlines ALS procedures regarding resuscitation of a hypothermic patient. See Figure 20-6 for the hypothermia algorithm. These guidelines are the same for all hypothermic patients regardless of the source of cold exposure.)

Use the regional EMS medical protocol for established guidelines that determine the criteria for an obviously dead individual. Acceptable guidelines for an obviously dead victim are a normal rectal temperature in a patient who presents with asystole, apnea, postmortem lividity, rigor mortis, or other injuries incompatible with life. A patient who has been recovered from warm water without vital signs or unsuccessful resuscitative efforts lasting 30 minutes may be considered dead on the scene.[5,9] Consult local medical control early for any individual recovered from cold-water submersion. As stated previously, many individuals have fully recovered from more than 60 minutes of cold-water submersion. These patients should be managed as a hypothermic patient, based on the rectal temperature.

Figure 21-4 summarizes assessment and management of a submersion patient.

Prevention

Prehospital care providers have great opportunities to be advocates of water safety and education in their respective communities, with an emphasis on communication of the risk factor areas previously identified. Furthermore, prevention should be emphasized to EMS providers and other public safety personnel who arrive on the scene so that they do not become additional submersion victims. A panicked and struggling near-drowning victim can be a danger to an unprepared in-water rescuer, potentially resulting in a double drowning. EMS providers need to assess the problem quickly, control the scene to prevent bystanders from entering the water, and ensure their own safety.

Many water safety organizations recommend the use of highly skilled professionals who regularly train for water

FIGURE 21-4 **Submersion Patient: Summary of Assessment and Management**

History	Examination	Intervention
ASYMPTOMATIC PATIENT		
Time submerged	Appearance	Administer oxygen by facemask at 8–10 liters/minute
Description of incident	Vital signs	Initiate IV line at KVO rate
Complaints	Head and neck trauma	Re-examine patient as needed
	Chest examination: lung fields	
Past medical history	ECG monitor	Transport patient to ED
SYMPTOMATIC PATIENT		
Description of incident	General appearance	Administer oxygen by nonrebreather mask at 12–15 liters/minute
Time submerged, water temperature, water contamination, vomiting, type of rescue	Level of consciousness (AVPU)	Initiate IV line at KVO rate; intubate early as needed
Symptoms	Vital signs; monitor ECG	Transport patient to ED
On-scene field resuscitation	Assess ABCDEs; vital signs; AED or ECG monitor	Initiate CPR early; intubate; 100% oxygen at 12–15 liters/minute via bag-valve mask; consider NG tube for gastric distension; use ACLS procedures for VF and asystole; use ACLS hypothermia algorithm

(Modified from Schoene RB, Nachat A, Gravatt AR, Newman AB: Submersion incidents. In Auerbach PS: *Wilderness medicine*, ed 5, St. Louis, 2007, Mosby Elsevier.)

IV, Intravenous; *KVO,* keep vein open; *ECG,* electrocardiogram; *ED,* emergency department; *AED,* automatic external defibrillator; *CPR,* cardiopulmonary resuscitation; *ACLS,* advanced cardiac life support; *NG,* nasogastric; *VF,* ventricular fibrillation.
AVPU, **A**lert; responds to **v**erbal stimulus; responds to **p**ainful stimulus; **u**nresponsive.
ABCDEs, Airway, breathing, circulation, disability, expose.

rescue, retrieval, and resuscitation. If no professional water rescue teams are available, however, first responders must consider their own safety and the safety of all responders before attempting an in-water rescue. The following guidelines are recommended to safely rescue a victim out of the water:

REACH—Attempt to perform the water rescue by reaching out with a pole, stick, paddle or anything so that the rescuer stays on land or on a boat. Use caution to avoid being inadvertently pulled into the water.
THROW—When reaching is not possible, throw something to a victim, such as a life preserver or rope so that it floats to the victim.
TOW—Once the victim has a rescue line, tow them to safety.
ROW—If a water entry is necessary, it is preferable to use a boat or paddleboard to reach the victim and wear a personal floatation device (PFD) if entering the water in a boat or to swim.[5]

Swimming rescues are not recommended unless the responder has been trained appropriately to manage a victim who can rapidly turn violent from panic, creating a potential double drowning. Too many well-intentioned first responders have become additional victims because their own safety was not the priority. See Figure 21-5A–C for a few options for in-water rescue systems, equipment for a submersion and/or trauma victim (C-spine precaution), and movement when in deep water.

Community education regarding submersion incidents should include the following recommendations:

Beaches

- Always swim near a lifeguard
- Ask a lifeguard about a safe place to swim
- Do not overestimate your swimming capability
- Always look out for your children
- Swim away from piers, rocks, and stakes

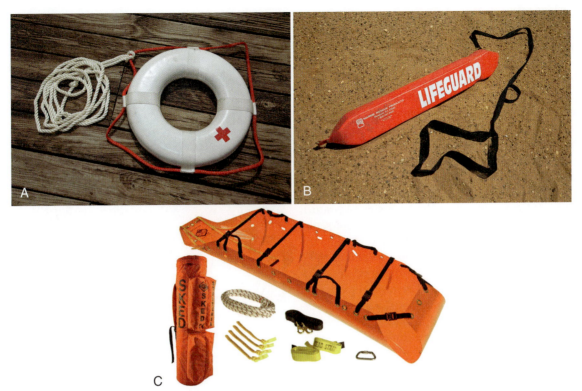

FIGURE 21-5 Options for in-water rescue equipment and patient packaging. **A.** Rescue throw lines. **B.** Tow device. **C.** In-water patient packing equipment.

- Avoid drinking alcohol and having a heavy meal before swimming
- Take lost children to the nearest lifeguard tower
- Be aware that more than 80% of ocean drownings occur in rip currents
- Never try to rescue someone without knowing what you are doing; many people have died in such attempts
- If you are fishing on rocks, be cautious with waves that may sweep you into the ocean
- Do not dive in shallow water; cervical injury could result
- Keep away from marine animals
- Read and heed signs posted on the beach

Residential

- Adult supervision is necessary, closely observing all children
- Never leave a child alone near a pool or a source of water, such as a bathtub or bucket
- Install a four-side (4-foot) fence around the pool with a self-closing and self-latching gate
- Do not allow children to use arm buoys or other air-filled swim aids
- Avoid toys that will attract children around pools
- Turn off pump filters when using pools
- Use cordless or cell phones near pool to prevent leaving the poolside to answer the phone elsewhere
- Keep rescue equipment (e.g., shepherd's hook, life preserver) and a telephone by the pool

- Do not try or allow hyperventilation to increase underwater swim time
- Do not dive in shallow water
- Provide swimming lessons for all children by age 2 years
- After the children have finished swimming, secure the pool so they cannot return (locks or audible alarms on gates are recommended)
- All family members and others watching children should learn CPR[10]

Recreational Scuba-Related Injuries

Recreational diving using *self-contained underwater breathing apparatus* (scuba) is a common activity enjoyed by many age groups. The popularity of this activity continues to grow, with more than 400,000 new certified divers each year, now totalling over 5 million scuba divers in the United States.[37,38] Relative to the increasing number of new divers each year, the injury rate is low, but the concern for medical fitness to dive has increased because of the diversity of divers, increasing age, low physical fitness, and underlying medical conditions. Water is an unforgiving environment when problems occur. Currently, there are medical guidelines that indicate relative and temporary health risks and absolute contraindications for scuba diving.[38]

Injuries to divers occur from many underwater hazards (e.g., shipwrecks, coral reefs) or from handling hazardous marine life. More often, however, prehospital care providers respond to scuba-related injuries and fatalities caused by *dysbarism,* or altered environmental pressure, which accounts for the majority of the serious diving medical disorders. The mechanism of injury is based on the principles of gas laws when breathing compressed gases (e.g., oxygen, carbon dioxide, nitrogen) at varying underwater depths and pressures.

Most scuba-related injuries caused by dysbarism present with immediate signs and symptoms or within 60 minutes after surfacing, but some symptoms are delayed up to 48 hours after individuals depart the dive site and return home. Consequently, with the increasing number of scuba divers today flying to and from popular dive sites in the United States, Caribbean, and other remote locations, there is a greater possibility of responding to diving-related injuries at locations distant from the actual dive site. Prehospital care providers need to recognize these scuba-related disorders, provide initial treatment, and initiate plans early for transportation to the local ED or for treatment at the closest recompression chamber.[39]

Epidemiology

Divers Alert Network (DAN) compiles an extensive morbidity and mortality database based on casualty data provided from participating recompression chambers in North America. In 2000, they published a report summarizing 11 years (1987 to 1997) of data.[40] The majority of the scuba-related diving injuries occur in the Northwest (38%) and Southeast (32%) regions of the United States during the months of May to September, with August as the peak month. Eighty-seven percent of the injuries occur in the ocean and 9% in freshwater areas (lake and quarry). Three to four times more male divers are injured than female divers. The primary cause of diving-related injury is decompression sickness. From 1970 to 1998, the number of diving-related deaths ranged from 66 to 147 per year.[41] Eighty percent of the fatalities occurred in males with a mean age between 38 and 42 years. The causes of death were drowning (50%–70%), cardiovascular factors (6%–14%), arterial gas embolism (5%–14%), and decompression sickness (0%–2%). Even though drowning was the leading cause of fatalities, it is unclear what led to the drowning, such as equipment issues, panic, disorientation, hypothermia, heart attack, or arterial gas embolism. Many drowning deaths during scuba diving are actually arterial gas embolism leading to secondary drowning.[42] Figure 21-6 summarizes the 2000 DAN report on scuba injuries and fatalities. See Figures 21-7 and 21-8 for summary of annual diving injuries and fatalities for DAN 2006 annual report.[43]

Panic or near-panic may explain many recreational diving accidents and be the reason for many diving fatalities (Figure 21-9).[40,44] In a recent national survey, more than half of divers reported experiencing at least one panic or near-panic

episode. The primary cause of diving fatalities is listed as drowning; 60% of all deaths are usually caused by specific problems such as lack of air, entanglement (in fishing nets, rope, or kelp), air embolism, narcosis, and panic. Panic was significantly higher in women (64%) than in men (50%), but more men (48%) perceived the events as life-threatening than women (35%).[43]

FIGURE 21-6   **Eleven-Year (1987–1997) Profile of SCUBA Diving Injuries**

INJURIES	1987–1997
Age (range of average age each year)	33–37
Percentage divers >50 years	7% (1997)
Male/female ratio	3–4:1
DIVE PROFILES	
Mean number of days diving	1
Median number of days diving	2–4
Number of dives	1–7
Mean maximum depth	75–95 feet saltwater
SYMPTOMS	
Pain and numbness	50%–65%
Paralysis	3%–10%
Unconsciousness	4%–7%
Bladder dysfunction	0.5%–2%
DECOMPRESSION SICKNESS	
Type II	65%–70%
Type I	20%–30%
Arterial gas embolism	10%–20%
FATALITIES (RANGE = 66–147)	**1970–1998**
Average age	38–42
Male gender	80%
CAUSES OF DEATH	
Drowning	50%–70%
Cardiovascular	6%–14%
Arterial gas emboli	5%–14%
Decompression sickness	0%–2%

(From Divers Alert Network: Eleven-year trends (1987–1997) in diving activity: The DAN annual review of recreational SCUBA diving injuries and fatalities based on 2000 data. In *Report on decompression illness, diving fatalities and Project Dive exploration,* Durham, NC, 2000, Divers Alert Network.)

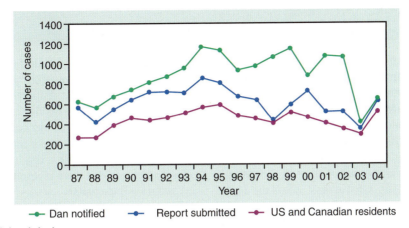

FIGURE 21-7   Annual diving injuries.
(From DAN Report on Decompression Illness, Diving Fatalities and Project Dive Exploration: 2006 Edition [Based on 2004 Data] © 2006 Divers Alert Network.)

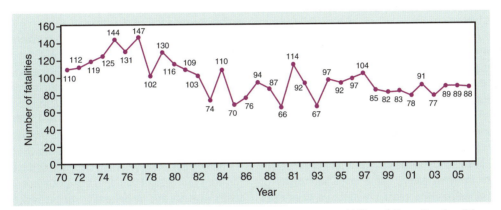

FIGURE 21-8   Annual number of US and Canadian diving fatalities. The number of US and Canadian fatalities recorded annually has varied substantially from year to year. The annual count has been fairly stable in recent years, lower than the overall mean ± standard deviation of 98±21 (range 66–147).
(From Annual Record of US and Canadian Diving Fatalities from the DAN Report on Decompression Illness, Diving Fatalities and Project Dive Exploration: 2006 Edition [Based on 2004 Data] © 2006 Divers Alert Network. [The annual record of US and Canadian diving fatalities that was started in 1970 by Mr. John McAniff of the University of Rhode Island and transitioned to DAN in 1989.])

Mechanical Effects of Pressure

Scuba-related diving injuries incurred by the changing atmospheric pressure, or dysbarism, can be separated into two types: (1) the conditions when a change in pressure from the underwater environment results in tissue trauma or *barotrauma* in closed air spaces in the body (e.g., ears, sinuses, intestines, lungs); and (2) the problems that occur from breathing compressed gases at elevated partial pressure, such as decompression sickness.

Barotrauma associated with scuba diving relates directly to the pressure effects of air and water on the diver. When standing at sea level, the atmospheric pressure is 760 Torr, which is essentially the same as millimeters of mercury [mm Hg]) or 14.7 pounds per square inch (PSI) on the body. This is also known as one atmosphere (1 atm). As a diver descends deeper in water, the absolute pressure increases 1 atm for every 33 feet of seawater. Consequently, a depth of 33 feet

of seawater is equivalent to 2 atm (air [1 atm] and 33 feet of water [1 atm]) of pressure on the body. Figure 21-10 lists common units of pressure in the underwater environment.

When a diver descends under the increasing pressure of seawater, the effect of the forces exerted on the body differs depending on the tissue compartments. The force applied to solid tissue acts in similar fashion to a fluid medium, and the diver is generally unaware of compressive force. The air in air-containing spaces of the body is compressed as the diver descends. Conversely, these gases expand as the diver ascends toward the surface. Boyle's law and Henry's law explain the effects of pressure on the body when underwater.

Boyle's Law

Boyle's law states that the volume of a given mass of gas is inversely proportional to the absolute pressure found in that environment. Stated another way, as a diver descends

FIGURE 21-9 Diver Panic

In *Diving Medicine for Scuba Divers,** the authors reviewed over 2,500 recreational diving fatalities over a 20-year period. These involved cases from the United States, Australia, and New Zealand. The average age of the divers was 33, but 10% were over 50. It is pertinent that 90% of these divers died with their weight belt still on. Fifty percent of these divers did not inflate their buoyancy compensator. Furthermore, 25% had trouble first develop on the surface, and 50% of these divers actually died on the surface.

Most important, however, is that at least 39% of the deaths were associated with panic, and this figure could, as reported by other authors, be as high as 80%. This probably accounts for so many deaths occurring on the surface. In a panic situation, the over-stressed diver usually has only one thought in mind: to get to the surface as rapidly as possible. Under such a situation, the diver is very likely to forget to breathe normally, which can result in a gas embolism.

Today in our fast-moving world, anxiety, stress, and even panic attacks are increasingly common. The reasons for diving panic are similar: excessive anxiety causes loss of self-control. Divers may feel they are losing control of a situation and are unable to extricate themselves. This generates the beginning of the panic cycle—rising apprehension and fear can add to stress, causing even more apprehension and fear. This can produce the irrational decision to flee upward regardless of the costs.

Individuals whose personalities include a tendency toward anxiety are more likely to panic. Some immediate signs of stress in an individual include rapid breathing, a wide-eyed appearance, agitation, frequent jerky movements, or appearing "frozen with fear."

A number of stressors can act to provoke the panic cycle. They include poor physical condition, when fatigue sets in at the end of a dive or when fighting a strong current. Panic can occur when the out-of-condition diver cannot find the boat and is low on air. In general, equipment failure is not a cause, although there are factors that are relevant: poor maintenance, resulting in a free-flowing regulator; or, all too common, too much weight, causing fatigue and poor buoyancy control. Loss of equipment—a fin, face mask, or computer—can initiate stress. Poor monitoring of air, depth, and time can lead to a sudden realization that there is insufficient air to return to the boat when still underwater.

The environment can add its share of stresses, with rough seas, swift currents, and poor visibility. It may be a diver's first night dive or first deep dive. From a psychological standpoint, there are a number of factors which may be involved, including use of alcohol and/or drugs; limited time frames of depth and time; required to go beyond your own performance limits; and a strong dependence on a buddy.

How, then, can the panic cycle be prevented? First, be well trained, physically fit, and informed about the dive environment and conditions you are about to make. Dive within the limits of your training, experience, and fitness. If you do feel panic rising, STOP, REST, and THINK, what is happening, why it's occurring, and decide the best remedy. Only then should you ACT. If that is to go to the surface, do so slowly—in a controlled manner, not in a hurry. If you do think you are ascending too fast, slow down and breathe out.

Remember when you're back on the surface, inflate your BC and drop your weight belt. If this is an emergency, you will have good buoyancy and be better able to get back to the boat.

If you feel you have a tendency to panic, try to avoid any diving in which stress may occur, and dive with buddies who know you well and who can help you manage in an anxious situation.

Whatever happens, don't panic.

(Modified from Bennett, PB: Don't Panic—Whatever happens, try to keep a cool head in a hot situation. *Alert Diver*, January/February, 1998.)
* Edmonds C, McKenzie B, Thomas R, Pennefather J. *Diving Medicine for Scuba Divers*. 3rd Edition, Carl Edmonds-Publisher, Manly, Australia, 2010.

FIGURE 21-10 Common Units of Pressure in Underwater Environment

Depth (FSW)	PSIA	ATA	Torr or mm Hg (absolute)
Sea level	14.7	1	760
33	29.4	2	1520
66	44.1	3	2280
99	58.8	4	3040
132	73.5	5	3800
165	88.2	6	4560
198	102.9	7	5320

FSW, Feet seawater; *PSIA*, pounds per square inch absolute; *ATA*, atmosphere absolute; *mm Hg*, millimeters of mercury.

in water to a lower depth, pressure increases and the volume of the gas (e.g., the volume in the lung or ear) decreases; the reverse is also true, the volume increases in size when the diver returns toward the surface. This is the principle behind the effects of barotrauma and arterial gas embolism in the body. Figure 21-11 shows the effects of pressure on the volume and diameter of a gas bubble.

Henry's Law

At a constant temperature, the amount of gas that will dissolve in a liquid is directly proportional to the partial pressure of that gas outside the liquid. Henry's law is fundamental in the understanding of how gas from a compressed air cylinder (scuba tank) behaves in the body as the diver descends. For example, the increasing partial pressure of nitrogen will cause it to dissolve in tissue fluid as the pressure increases during descent, and on return toward the surface, nitrogen will bubble

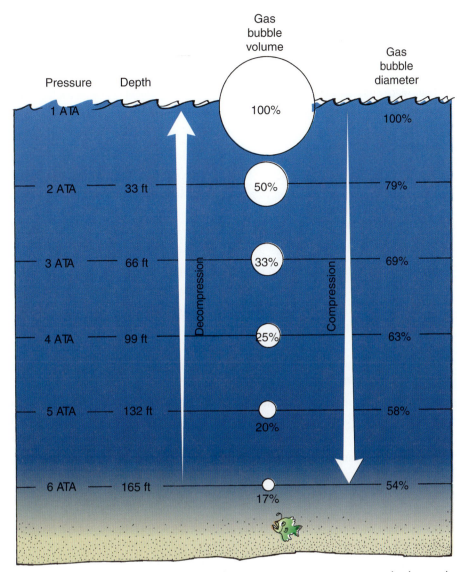

FIGURE 21-11   Boyle's law. The volume of a given quantity of gas at constant temperature varies inversely with pressure. (From Kizer KW, Van Hoesen KB: Diving medicine. In Auerbach PS: *Wilderness medicine*, ed 5, St. Louis, 2007, Mosby Elsevier.)

out of solution in the tissues. This law describes the principle that explains why decompression sickness occurs.

Diving-Related Injuries

Barotrauma

Barotrauma, also known as "squeeze," is the most common form of scuba-related diving injury.[45] Although many forms of barotraumas cause pain, most resolve spontaneously and do not require EMS involvement or recompression chamber therapy. However, some pulmonary overpressurization injuries are very serious. During scuba diving, barotrauma occurs within noncompressible, gas-filled body cavities (e.g., sinuses). If the pressure in these spaces cannot equalize during a dive as ambient pressure increases, vascular engorgement, hemorrhage, and mucosal edema result from decreasing air volume when the diver descends, and tissue disruption results from

increasing air volume when the diver ascends. Figure 21-12 summarizes signs and symptoms of barotrauma and its treatment. The various forms of barotraumas are described next.

Barotrauma of Descent

Mask Squeeze. This generally occurs in inexperienced or inattentive divers who fail to equalize pressure in their facemask with increasing external water pressure during descent.

Assessment. Examine the soft tissue around the eyes and conjunctival tissues for capillary rupture. Signs and symptoms include skin ecchymoses and conjunctival hemorrhage.

Management. Mask barotrauma is self-limited; no diving until tissue damage clears. Provide cold compresses over eyes; rest and pain medication as needed.

FIGURE 21-12 **Barotrauma: Common Signs, Symptoms, and Treatment**

Type	Signs/symptoms	Treatment*
Mask squeeze	Corneal injection, conjunctival hemorrhage	Self-limited; rest, cold compresses, pain medication
Sinus squeeze	Pain, bloody nasal discharge	Pain medication, decongestants, antihistamines
Middle-ear squeeze	Pain, vertigo, tympanic membrane rupture, hearing loss, vomiting	Decongestants, antihistamines, pain medication; may need antibiotics; avoid diving and flying
Internal-ear barotrauma	Tinnitus, vertigo, ataxia, hearing loss	Bed rest; elevate head; avoid loud noises; stool softeners; avoid strenuous activity; no diving or flying for months
External-ear barotrauma	Difficulty with Valsalva maneuver, earache, bloody discharge, possible tympanic membrane rupture	Maintain dry ear canal; antibiotics may be needed for infection
Tooth squeeze	Tooth pain while diving	Self-limited; pain medication
Alternobaric vertigo	Pressure, pain in affected ear, vertigo, tinnitus	Usually short lived; decongestants; prohibit diving until resolution with normal hearing
Pulmonary barotrauma	Substernal pain; voice change; dyspnea; subcutaneous emphysema	Assess ABCs, neurologic functions; 100% oxygen 12–15 liters/minute nonrebreather mask; transport patient lying supine; need to rule out AGE
Subcutaneous emphysema	Substernal pain and crepitus, brassy voice, neck swelling, dyspnea, bloody sputum	Rest; avoid diving and flying; oxygen and recompression therapy only in severe cases
Pneumothorax	Sharp chest pain, dyspnea, diminished breath sounds	100% oxygen 12–15 liters/minute nonrebreather mask; monitor pulse oximetry; transport in position of comfort; assess for tension pneumothorax
Tension pneumothorax	Cyanosis, distended neck veins, tracheal deviation	14-gauge needle thoracentesis; 100% oxygen 12–15 liters/minute nonrebreather mask; monitor pulse oximetry
Arterial gas embolism (AGE)	Unresponsive, confusion, headache, visual disturbances, seizure	Assess ABCs, neurologic functions; initiate BLS/ALS; control seizures; 100% oxygen 12–15 liters/minute nonrebreather mask; transport patient lying supine; glucose-free IV fluid therapy (1–2 ml/kg /hr); monitor ECG; Consult *DAN* (919–684–8111) for closest recompression chamber (primary treatment)

(From Clenney TL, Lassen LF: Recreational scuba diving injuries. *Am Fam Physician* 53(5):1761, 1996; and Kizer KW, Van Hoesen KB: Diving medicine. In Auerbach PS: *Wilderness medicine*, ed 5, St. Louis, 2007, Mosby Elsevier.)
*Good patient education on scene for minor barotrauma injuries because some of these injuries are self-limiting and others need physician evaluation; others need patient referral to family physician or emergency department and will not necessitate EMS transport.

Tooth Squeeze. A very infrequent finding, this form of barotrauma occurs to divers when gas is trapped in the interior portion of a tooth after dental fillings, recent extractions, or a root canal, or with defective restorations. During descent, the tooth can fill with blood or can implode with increasing external pressure. During ascent, any air forced into the tooth will expand, causing either pain or explosion of the tooth. To prevent tooth squeeze, it is recommended not to dive for 24 hours after any dental treatment.

Assessment
Examine the affected tooth to see if it is intact. Signs and symptoms include pain and fractured tooth.

Management
Refer for dental evaluation; give pain medication as needed.

Middle-Ear Squeeze. This squeeze occurs in 40% of scuba divers and is considered the most common diving injury.[46] Ear squeeze occurs near the surface, when the greatest changes in pressure occur as the diver descends. Divers need to begin equalizing their middle ear early as they start to descend so a pressure differential across the tympanic membrane (TM) leading to rupture of the eardrum does not occur. Divers need to equalize the pressure by forcing air into the middle ear through the Eustachian tube by either a Valsalva or Frenzel maneuver.[42] The diver will experience pain and vertigo if the

TM ruptures, allowing water to enter the middle ear. Divers with upper respiratory infection or allergies may have difficulty equalizing their middle ear during a dive and should determine if they can perform a Valsalva maneuver before the dive.

Assessment. Examine the ear canal for blood caused by ruptured TM. Signs and symptoms include pain, vertigo, conductive hearing losses with TM rupture, and vomiting.

Management. No pressure changes are permitted (diving or flying). Patients may need decongestants if the TM has not ruptured; antibiotics may be needed with ruptured TM; and antiemetics may be necessary for vertigo and vomiting. The patient should be referred for audiometric evaluation. Transport in upright position or position of comfort.

Sinus Squeeze. Normally, pressure in the sinuses equalizes easily as the diver is descending and ascending. Pressure develops by the same mechanism as middle ear squeeze, but sinus squeeze is not as common. As a diver descends, there is an inability to maintain pressure in the sinuses, and a vacuum develops in the sinus cavity, causing intense pain, mucosal wall trauma, and bleeding in the sinus cavity. This squeeze may be caused by congestion, sinusitis, mucosal hypertrophy, rhinitis, or nasal poyps.[45] A reverse sinus squeeze during ascent can occur as well (see later discussion on Sinus Barotrauma).

Assessment. Examine the nose for discharge; signs and symptoms include severe pain over the affected sinus or bloody discharge, usually from frontal sinuses.

Management. No specific management is needed at the scene unless extensive bleeding is observed, in which case, treat for epistaxis by pinching firmly on the fleshy part of the patient's nostrils just below the nasal bones. Transport in a position of comfort.

Internal-Ear Barotrauma. Although much less common than middle-ear squeeze, this is the most serious form of ear barotrauma because it may lead to permanent deafness.[47] Internal-ear barotrauma occurs when a diver descends and has failed attempts to equalize the middle ear. Further forceful attempts can result in a large rise in middle-ear pressure and can rupture the round window structure.

Assessment. Examine the ear canal for any discharge. Signs and symptoms include roaring tinnitus, vertigo, hearing loss, a feeling of fullness or "blockage" in the affected ear, nausea, vomiting, pallor, diaphoresis, disorientation, and ataxia.

Management. The patient should avoid strenuous activities and loud noises, with no pressure changes (diving or flying). Transport in upright position. Early medical consultation

with DAN or an ED is recommended because it may be difficult to determine if this is inner-ear decompression sickness and if there is an immediate need for recompression chamber therapy.

Barotrauma of Ascent (Reverse Squeeze)

Alternobaric Vertigo. This is an unusual form of barotrauma in that it occurs as expanding gas moves through the Eustachian tube and unequal pressure develops in the middle ear, which can cause vertigo. Although the symptoms are brief, vertigo can trigger panic in divers, leading to other forms of injury caused by a rapid ascent to the surface (e.g., air embolism, near-drowning, drowning).

Assessment. Examine the ear canal for any discharge; assess any hearing loss. Signs and symptoms are short in duration, resulting in transient vertigo, pressure in the affected ear, tinnitus, and hearing loss.

Management. No specific intervention is required; diving is not recommended until any hearing loss returns. Provide decongestants as needed. No transport is needed if symptoms resolve quickly; arrange physician referral as needed.

Sinus Barotrauma. This form of sinus squeeze can occur on ascent when some form of blockage in the sinus openings prevents expanding gas from escaping. The expanding gas puts pressure on the mucosal lining of the sinus, causing pain with hemorrhage. Sinus barotrauma occurs in divers with upper respiratory infections or allergies. It is common for divers to take a decongestant before a dive as a preventive measure to help equalize the middle ear when diving. However, the vasoconstrictive benefits can wear off at depth, causing mucosal tissue expansion and forming a sinus blockage of expanding gas during the return to the surface.

Assessment. Examine the nose for discharge. Signs and symptoms include severe pain over the affected sinus and bloody discharge, usually from the frontal sinuses.

Management. No specific management is needed at the scene unless extensive bleeding is observed, in which case treat for epistaxis by pinching firmly on the fleshy part of the patient's nostrils, just below the nasal bones. Transport in a position of comfort.

Gastrointestinal Squeeze. This occurs when expanding gas in the gut becomes trapped as the diver surfaces. Gastrointestinal (GI) barotrauma occurs in novice divers who frequently perform Valsalva maneuvers in the head-down position, which forces air into the stomach. It can also occur in divers who chew gum when diving or who have consumed carbonated beverages or other gas-producing foods before diving.

Assessment. Examine the abdominal quadrants. Signs and symptoms include abdominal fullness, belching, and flatulence.

Management. GI squeeze normally resolves on its own and rarely needs medical attention; arrange physician referral if pain and fullness do not resolve. Only in severe cases is recompression chamber therapy needed.

Pulmonary Overinflation Barotrauma.

Pulmonary overinflation is a serious form of barotrauma resulting from the expansion of gas in the lungs during ascent. Normally the diver eliminates expanding gas with normal exhalations when returning to the surface. If the expanding gas does not escape, there is a rupture of the alveoli, which in turn causes one of many forms of injury, depending on the amount of air that escapes outside the lung and its final location. A common scenario is a diver who has a rapid and uncontrollable ascent to the surface caused by running out of air, panic, or a dropped weight belt. These types of injuries are collectively called *pulmonary overpressurization syndrome* (POPS), or "burst lung."

The five forms of POPS are: (1) overdistension with local injury, (2) mediastinal emphysema, (3) subcutaneous emphysema, (4) pneumothorax, and (5) arterial gas embolism.

Overdistension with Local Injury.

This is the mildest form of POPS, with only a small, isolated lung barotrauma.

Assessment. Auscultate the lung fields for diminished breath sounds. Chest pain may or may not be present. Blood is often seen in the sputum (*hemoptysis).*

Management. Ensure rest, and treat symptoms as needed. Monitor vital signs and oxygen saturation with pulse oximetry; provide oxygen at 2 to 4 liters/minute with nasal cannula. Transport the patient in position of comfort. The patient needs further medical evaluation to rule out a more severe form of POPS and should avoid further pressure exposure (diving or commercial flying).

Mediastinal Emphysema.

This is the most common form of POPS, caused by escaping gas from ruptured alveoli entering the interstitial space to the mediastinum.

Assessment. This condition is usually benign; examine the lung fields for diminished breath sounds. Signs and symptoms include hoarseness, neck fullness, and minor substernal chest pain; often a dull ache or tightness worsens with breathing and coughing. Examine chest and neck for subcutaneous emphysema. In severe cases, the diver presents with chest pain, dyspnea, and difficulty swallowing.

Management. Ensure rest. Monitor vital signs and oxygen saturation with pulse oximetry; provide oxygen at 2 to 4 liters/minute with nasal cannula. Usually, mediastinal emphysema requires no specific treatment or recompression therapy. Rare cases need to be medically evaluated to rule out other causes of chest pain and severe forms of POPS. Transport the patient in a supine position; avoid further pressure exposure (diving or commercial flying).

Subcutaneous Emphysema.

Air escaping from ruptured alveoli continues to move superiorly into the neck and clavicle regions of the chest.

Assessment. Examine the lung fields for diminished breath sounds. Signs and symptoms include swelling, crepitus, hoarseness, sore throat, and difficulty swallowing.

Management. No specific treatment is required besides rest. Monitor vital signs and oxygen saturation with pulse oximetry; provide oxygen by nasal cannula at 2 to 4 liters/minute. The patient needs further medical evaluation to rule out more severe forms of POPS. Transport in supine position. The patient should avoid further pressure exposure (diving or commercial flying).

Pneumothorax.

Pneumothorax is seen in less than 10% of POPS cases because air must escape through the visceral pleura around the lung, which presents greater resistance than air escaping through the interstitial space between the lung and visceral pleura. If the diver is at depth when the pulmonary rupture occurs, a tension pneumothorax can result as the volume of escaping gas expands as the diver continues toward the surface.

Assessment. Examine the lung fields for diminished breath sounds. Signs and symptoms will vary based on the size of the pneumothorax and include sharp chest pain, diminished breath sounds, breathlessness, subcutaneous emphysema, and dyspnea. Provide ongoing assessment for conversion from simple to tension pneumothorax.

Management. Ensure rest. Monitor vital signs and oxygen saturation with pulse oximetry; provide oxygen by nasal cannula at 2 to 4 liters/minute. Provide standard ALS management of tension pneumothorax with 14-gauge needle thoracostomy as necessary. Transport the patient in a position of comfort. The patient needs further medical evaluation to rule out more severe forms of POPS and should avoid further pressure exposure (diving or commercial flying). Recompression therapy is generally not necessary.

Arterial Gas Embolism (AGE).

This is the most feared complication of POPS and, after drowning, is a leading cause of death in divers, accounting for about 30% of fatalities.[48] AGE can occur from any of the four POPS conditions previously presented as a result of air escaping and forming an air embolism. AGE typically occurs in divers who have an uncontrolled ascent to the surface without appropriate exhalation, causing an overinflation pulmonary injury. However, AGE can occur in divers who surface slowly without underlying lung pathology. During ascent, once the pulmonary overinflation bursts alveoli, air enters the pulmonary venous capillary circulation; the gas bubbles enter the left atrium and left ventricle, then exit the heart through the aorta, and are distributed to the cerebral, coronary, and other systemic vasculature. Gas bubbles can enter the coronary circulation, causing an occlusion resulting in cardiac dysrhythmia, cardiac arrest, or myocardial infarction.[49] If gas bubbles enter the cerebral circulation, the diver presents with signs and symptoms similar to an acute stroke.

Unlike decompression sickness, which can present with delayed symptoms hours after diving, symptoms of AGE appear either immediately at the water surface or typically within 2 minutes. Any loss of consciousness once a diver surfaces must be presumed to be AGE until proved otherwise.[35] The primary treatment for AGE is recompression chamber (hyperbaric) therapy.

Historically, it was recommended that patients with AGE be placed in the Trendelenburg position for transport, based on the belief that this would help keep bubbles from circulating in the systemic vasculature. However, recent evidence has shown that the head-down position does not prevent systemic circulation of nitrogen bubbles, makes it more difficult to oxygenate the patient, and may worsen cerebral edema.[50] It is currently recommended that all AGE patients be placed in a supine position in the field and during transport. The supine position also provides a greater rate of nitrogen bubble washout.[51,52]

Decompression Sickness

Decompression sickness (DCS) is directly related to Henry's law. When scuba divers breathe compressed air containing oxygen (21%), carbon dioxide (0.03%), and nitrogen (79%), the amount of gas that will be dissolved in liquid is directly proportional to the partial pressure of gas in contact with liquid. Oxygen is used in the body for tissue metabolism when in solution and does not form gas bubbles during ascent from depth.

Nitrogen, an inert gas not used for metabolism, is the primary source of concern in DCS. Nitrogen is five times more soluble in fat than in water and becomes dissolved in tissue proportionately to the increasing ambient pressure. Consequently, the deeper underwater the diver goes and the longer the diver stays at depth, the greater the amount of nitrogen that dissolves into tissue. As the diver ascends toward the surface, the absorbed nitrogen must be eliminated. If there is inadequate time to eliminate nitrogen during ascent, nitrogen comes out of solution in the tissues in the form of intravascular gas bubbles, causing obstruction of the vascular and lymphatic systems and tissue distension, and activating inflammatory responses.[53]

Most divers experience DCS within the first hour after surfacing, although some will present with symptoms up to 6 hours after surfacing. Only 2% of divers will have delayed symptoms between 24 to 48 hours after surfacing. Traditionally, symptoms of DCS are categorized as *Type I,* a mild form involving cutaneous, lymphatic, and musculoskeletal systems, or *Type II,* a severe form involving neurologic and cardiopulmonary systems. The term *decompression illness* (DCI) has been proposed to encompass Type I and Type II DCS and AGE.[54,55] Mild symptoms of DCS include fatigue and malaise. However, mild symptoms

can be precursors to more severe signs and symptoms, such as numbness, weakness, and paralysis. Studies now suggest that it is more important clinically to describe DCS by the region of the body affected and not as Type I or Type II.[38] This suggestion is applicable for prehospital care providers to ensure that even patients with mild DCS symptoms are treated aggressively with 100% oxygen and an early consult for recompression therapy. Many divers with the mild form of DCS will not have a medical evaluation. Divers may delay up to 32 hours before seeking medical care for DCS because denial of DCS is a common finding in the scuba-diving population.[56]

Several factors predispose a diver to DCS.[57,58] Some risk factors are known to enhance the uptake of nitrogen in tissues during descent and slow the release of nitrogen during ascent. Certain host and environmental factors, as well as equipment failures and improper technique, increase the risk for DCS (Figure 21-13).

FIGURE 21-13   Factors Related to Decompression Sickness (DCS)

HOST FACTORS
Lack of fitness
Advancing age
Female sex
Hypothermia
Alcohol or drug use
Patent foramen ovale
Obesity
Sleep deprivation
Dehydration
Inadequate nutrition
Heavy exertion at depth or fatigue
Underlying medical illness (e.g., asthma)
Prior history of DCS

ENVIRONMENTAL FACTORS
Extremes of temperature
Rough seas
Flying after diving
Heavy exercise at depth
Nitrogen narcosis
Elevated arterial carbon-dioxide tension
Low water temperature

EQUIPMENT FAILURES AND IMPROPER TECHNIQUE
Violating the decompression tables
Difficulty with buoyancy
Rapid ascent
Running out of air
Regulator malfunction
Unfamiliar or improper equipment

(From Barratt DM, Harch PG, Van Meter K: Decompression illness in divers: A review of the literature. *Neurologist* 8:186, 2002.)

Limb Pain (Type I DCS). This form of DCS results from bubble formation in the musculoskeletal system, typically occurring in one or more joints. The most common joints involved are the shoulder and elbow, followed by the knee, hip, wrist, hand, and ankle.[37] This pain is described as a severe tendonitis, joint pain with a grating sensation on movement. The pain starts gradually, presenting as a deep, dull ache of mild to severe intensity. Victims often attempt to relieve their pain by flexion of their joints, hence the common name for this condition—the "bends." Although this form of DCS is not life threatening, it indicates that bubbles are present in the venous circulation. It can lead to more severe forms if left untreated.

Cutaneous and Lymphatic (Type I DCS). This form of DCS is uncommon. It represents inadequate elimination of bubbles forming in the skin or lymphatic systems. Cutaneous "skin bends" are uncommon and usually not serious, but signs of mottling and marbling are considered precursors of delayed neurologic problems.[38] Symptoms include an intense rash that progresses to a red patchy or bluish discoloration of the skin.[59] Lymphatic obstruction can result in swelling and an orange-peel appearance (peau d'orange).

Cardiopulmonary (Type II DCS). This severe form of DCS is referred to as the "chokes" and results when venous bubbles overwhelm the pulmonary capillary system. Hypotension can occur from a massive venous air embolism in the lung. Symptoms include nonproductive cough, substernal chest pain, cyanosis, dyspnea, shock, and cardiopulmonary arrest. This disorder resembles acute respiratory distress syndrome (ARDS).[60]

Spinal Cord (Type II DCS). The white matter of the spinal cord is vulnerable to bubble formation, and nitrogen is highly soluble in spinal cord tissue (myelin). The most common site for this form of DCS is the lower thoracic spine, followed by the lumbar/sacral and cervical regions.[56] Common signs and symptoms include low back pain and "heaviness" in the legs. With this form of DCS, the patient often gives a vague statement in an effort to describe "strange sensations," or *paresthesia*, which can progress to weakness, numbness, and paralysis. Bowel and bladder dysfunction, leading to urinary retention, also has been reported.[61]

Figure 21-14 summarizes signs and symptoms of decompression sickness and its treatment.

FIGURE 21-14   Decompression Sickness (DCS): Common Signs, Symptoms, and Treatment

Condition	Signs/symptoms	Treatment
DCS TYPE I		
Skin bends	Intense itching (pruritus); red rash patches over shoulders and upper chest; skin marbling may precede burning sensation and itching over shoulders and torso; localized cyanosis and pitting edema.	Self-limiting; resolves on its own; observe for delayed signs of limb-pain DCS.
Limb-pain DCS	Large joint tenderness; mild to severe joint or extremity pain; pain is usually steady but may throb and present in 75% of cases; grating sensation on joint motion; worse with movement. DCS Type I may progress to DCS Type II.	Mild pain only often resolves on its own; observe 24 hours; moderate to severe pain. Start with 100% oxygen, 12–15 liters/minute nonrebreather mask; transport all patients in supine position; glucose-free IV fluid therapy (1–2 ml/kg/hr); early consult *DAN* (919–684–8111) for closest recompression chamber for definitive treatment.
DCS TYPE II		
Cardiopulmonary "Chokes"	Substernal pain, mild cough, dyspnea, nonproductive cough, cyanosis, tachypnea, tachycardia, shock and cardiac arrest	ABCs; 100% oxygen, 12–15 liters/minute nonrebreather mask; BLS or ALS as needed; glucose-free IV fluid therapy (1–2 ml/kg/hr); transport all patients in supine position; early consult *DAN* (919–684–8111) for closest recompression chamber for definitive treatment.
Neurologic		
Brain	Many visual changes, headache, confusion, disorientation, nausea and vomiting	
Spinal cord	Back pain, heaviness or weakness, numbness, paralysis, urine retention, fecal incontinence	
Inner ear	Vertigo, ataxia	

(From Barratt DM, Harch PG, Van Meter K: Decompression illness in divers: A review of the literature. *Neurologist* 8:186, 2002; and Kizer KW Van Hoesen KB: Diving medicine. In Auerbach PS: *Wilderness medicine*, ed 5, St. Louis, 2007, Mosby Elsevier.)

Assessment

A standardized approach for patients with AGE and DCS is provided to ensure that consistent care is given. It is recommended that all patients with scuba-related diving injuries be examined for signs and symptoms of AGE and DCS because the primary and essential lifesaving treatment is recompression chamber therapy.

Arterial Gas Embolism

About 5% of all AGE patients present with immediate apnea, unconsciousness, and cardiac arrest. Others present with signs and symptoms similar to acute stroke, with loss of consciousness, stupor, confusion, hemiparesis, seizure, vertigo, visual changes, sensory changes, and headache.

Decompression Sickness

Type I DCS is characterized by deep pain in a joint, including minor forms of cutaneous pruritus (severe itching) and obstruction of lymph vessels (lymphedema). Type II DCS is characterized by symptoms involving the central nervous system, ranging from weakness and numbness to paralysis. Obtain a dive profile and medical history of the events that led to the diving-related injury from a fellow diver, including: (1) time of onset of signs and symptoms; (2) source of breathing medium (e.g., air or mixed gases; Heliox); (3) dive profile (dive activity, depth, duration, dive frequency, surface interval, interval between dives); (4) dive location and water conditions; (5) dive risk factors; (6) underwater medical and equipment problems on ascent and descent; (7) whether a no-decompression dive or a decompression dive; (8) rate of ascent; (9) decompression stop(s); (9) postdive activity level; (10) postdive aircraft travel, with type and duration; (11) past and present medical history (DCI); (12) medication use; and (13) current use of alcohol or illicit drugs.[62]

Management

Assure the ABCs, protect the airway, and initiate BLS or ALS procedures as required. Initiate 100% oxygen at 12 to 15 liters/minute, and give NS or LR (no dextrose) IV fluid therapy (1–2 ml/kg/hour). Monitor vital signs, pulse oximetry, and ECG; check and treat blood glucose as required; control seizures. Protect the patient from hypothermia, and consult early with local medical control or DAN for the closest recompression chamber (primary treatment) (see Figure 21-15 for DAN contact information). Standard recompression therapy with 100% hyperbaric oxygen is given according to the US Navy treatment tables.[63] Transport the patient in a supine position. For any scuba-related diving injury, if air evacuation is provided by helicopter or other nonpressurized aircraft, it is recommended to fly as low as possible (e.g., 500 feet), but not to exceed 1000 feet to minimize further expansion of air bubbles (Boyle's law) and further dysbarism trauma.[38,52]

Definitive treatment for specific barotraumas, including AGE and DCS, is to administer 100% oxygen by mask at two to three times the atmospheric pressure at sea level in a recompression chamber.[64] (For further discussion of recompression chamber treatment methods for scuba-related diving injuries, see the US Navy Diving Manual or other sources.[38,63]) The patient immediately benefits, based on the principles of Boyle's law, by increasing the ambient pressure and decreasing the size of bubbles formed and increasing the oxygen concentration in tissues. Figure 21-16 describes recompression and hyperbaric oxygen therapy (HBO).

Prevention of Scuba-Related Diving Injuries

Millions of certified scuba divers need frequent skill refresher training to prevent and recognize scuba-related dive injuries. This includes many professional scuba dive teams in the United States, such as lifeguards, fire and law enforcement personnel, search and rescue, Coast Guard, and Department of Defense, who depend on local EMS providers to provide initial and follow-up medical care and transport to local hospitals or recompression chambers. Collaboration among dive teams and local EMS agencies to develop medical scenarios during dive training is strongly encouraged. This should include frequent scuba

---

FIGURE 21-15 Divers Alert Network (DAN) Contact Information for Emergency and Nonemergency Consult

Diving Emergencies (Remember: Call local EMS first, then DAN!)
1–919–684–9111
1–919–684–9111 (collect)

Travel Assistance
1–929–684–9111
If outside the USA, Canada, Puerto Rico, Bahamas, British Virgin Islands or U.S. Virgin Islands, call +1–919–684–9111 (collect).

Nonemergency Medical Questions
1–800–446–2671 or 1–919–684–2948
Monday–Friday, 8:30 AM–5:00 PM (EST)

All Other Inquiries
1–800–446–2671 or 1–919–684–2948
1–919–490–6630 (fax)
1–919–493–3040 (fax–Medical Department)

Contact Information to Send a Letter
Divers Alert Network
The Peter B. Bennett Center
6 West Colony Place
Durham, NC 27705 USA

(From http://www.diversalertnetwork.org/contact/index.asp. Accessed Sept 4, 2010.)

FIGURE 21-16 Recompression Therapy for Scuba-Related Diving Injuries

The goals of recompression therapy for scuba-related diving injuries caused by pulmonary overinflation barotrauma and decompression sickness (DCS) are to compress the bubbles and increase oxygen delivery to tissues. Recompression therapy includes the following mechanisms:

- Reduces volume of the bubbles where they are circulated to the pulmonary capillaries and filtered out
- Promotes reabsorption of bubbles in solution
- Increases oxygen delivery to the tissues
- Corrects hypoxia
- Provides an increased diffusion gradient for nitrogen
- Reduces edema
- Reduces blood vessel permeability

All divers with arterial gas embolism (AGE) and DCS must be considered early for recompression in a hyperbaric treatment facility because the treatment is more successful if started within 6 hours after the onset of symptoms. Divers are not always near a recompression chamber when symptoms occur, and there can be considerable delays getting to a chamber by ground or by arranging for air transport. Contact Diver's Alert Network (DAN) to consult for diving medical assistance and to determine the closest recompression chamber (see Figure 21-15).

In the meantime, place the patient in a supine position. Nitrogen washout can be increased by providing 100% oxygen by mask and by starting an IV fluid line with normal saline or Lactated Ringer's solution at 1 to 2 ml/kg/hr to ensure adequate intravascular volume and capillary perfusion. During recompression treatment, patients with AGE or DCS normally will receive recompression treatment at 2.5 to 3.0 atm for 2 to 4 hours while breathing 100% oxygen. Longer and repeated treatment will be necessary if the patient has no clinical improvement of symptoms. Recompression treatment principles include the following:

- Any painful or neurologic signs or symptoms occurring within 24 hours of a dive are caused by decompression sickness (DCS) until proved otherwise.
- Any painful or neurologic signs or symptoms occurring within 48 hours of flying after diving are caused by DCS until proved otherwise.
- Contact the Diver's Alert Network 24-hour emergency hotline for consultation at 919–684–9111.
- Every diver with signs or symptoms of DCI should receive recompression treatment.
- Never fail to treat doubtful cases.
- Early treatment improves outcomes, whereas delayed treatment worsens outcomes.
- Long delays should never preclude treatment because divers respond to recompression therapy days to weeks after injury.
- Monitor patient closely for signs of relief or progression of symptoms.
- Inadequate treatment can lead to a recurrence.
- Continue to treat until clinical plateau.

(Modified from: Tibbles PM, Edelsberg JS: Hyperbaric oxygen therapy. *N Engl J Med* 334(25):1642, 1996; from Barratt DM, Harch PG, Van Meter K: Decompression illness in divers: A review of the literature. *Neurologist* 8:186, 2002; and from Kizer KW, Van Hoesen KB: Diving medicine. In Auerbach PS: *Wilderness medicine*, ed 5, St. Louis, 2007, Mosby Elsevier.)

training in varying underwater conditions and locations, along with in-water rescue scenarios and initial medical care, which are paramount to responding safely and effectively for in-water swimmer/diver rescues and recoveries. Scuba-training coordination among medical dive team members and local EMS providers will ensure effective communication and appropriate field-care continuity. This should be included with scenario-based consults with local medical control and with DAN.

Medical Fitness to Dive

Prehospital care providers responding to diving-related incidence not only must assess divers, in all ages groups, for primary diving disorder related to a submersion incident, DCS or AGE, but also for underlying medical conditions (e.g., cardiac, pulmonary, neurologic, endocrine, psychiatric, or a combination of both medical and dysbaric disorders). Ideally, all new divers should be cleared medically before the start of scuba training. Five general medical screening recommendations for identifying individuals who are at an increased risk for a diving-related problem are listed below. These recommendations are based on consensus of medical diving specialists.[38,65] Also refer to Figure 21-17 for the absolute contraindications and specific conditions of concern for scuba diving. Recommendations include:

- Inability to equalize pressure in one or more of the body's air spaces increases the risk for barotrauma.
- Medical or psychiatric conditions may manifest underwater or at a remote diving site and can endanger the diver's life because of the condition itself, because it occurs in the water, or because inadequate medical help is available.
- Impaired tissue perfusion or diffusion of inert gases increases the risk of DCS.

FIGURE 21-17 Fitness to Dive: Disqualifying and Specific Conditions of Concern for Scuba Diving

ABSOLUTE CONTRAINDICATION FOR DIVING
Epilepsy or other seizure disorder
Pregnancy
Symptomatic coronary artery disease
Sickle cell disease
Ménière's disease
Chronic inability to equalize sinus and/or middle ear
Acute asthma with abnormal pulmonary function
Cystic or cavitary disease of the lungs
Obstructive or restrictive lung disease
Atrial septal defect (ASD)
Spontaneous pneumothorax
Chronic perforated tympanic membrane
Intraorbital gas

SPECIFIC CONDITIONS OF CONCERN WITH REGARDS TO DIVING
Seizures
Head injury
Unexplained syncope
Pneumothorax
Asthma
Bullous lung disease
Atrial septal defect
Patent foramen ovale
Coronary artery disease
Dysrhythmia
Hypertension
Ear, nose, throat disorders
Diabetes
Pregnancy
Migraine headaches
Sickle-Cell disease or trait
Panic disorders

(From Kizer KW, Van Hoesen KB: Diving medicine. In Auerbach PS: *Wilderness medicine*, ed 5, St. Louis, 2007, Mosby Elsevier.)

■ Poor physical condition increases the risk of DCS or exertion-related medical problems. The factors compromising physical condition may be physiologic or pharmacologic.
■ In women who are pregnant, the fetus may be at increased risk of dysbaric injury.

For many years, diabetics have questioned the diving medical experts about scuba-diving waivers for individuals who have control of their blood sugar. In June 2005, an international workshop was held in the United States that was jointly sponsored by the Undersea and Hyperbaric Medical Society (UHMS) and Divers Alert Network (DAN). They brought together over 50 medical and research experts from around the world to develop guidelines for recreational divers with diabetes.[66] The panel indicated that dive candidates who use medication (oral hypoglycemic agents [OHAs] or insulin) to treat diabetes, but who are otherwise qualified to dive may undertake recreational scuba diving. However, they stated that strict criteria need to be met before diving. The panel agreed that those diabetics using dietary control will easily meet the new guidelines. The consensus guidelines (Figure 21-18) consist of 19 points, under the categories of selection and surveillance, scope of diving, and glucose management on the day of diving.

Flying after Diving

Because diving is conducted at many popular dive locations in the United States and at remote locations outside the United States, persons may dive the day before flying. Because of Boyle's principle, flying too soon after a dive can increase the risk of decompression sickness during flight or after arriving at the destination because of the reduced atmospheric pressure in either a pressurized or a nonpressurized commercial aircraft. Figure 21-19 lists the current guidelines recommended by DAN for flying safely after diving.[38]

Lightning

Lightning is the most widespread threat to people and property during the thunderstorm season and has been second only to floods in causing storm-related death in the United States since 1959.[67] The National Weather Service estimates that 100,000 thunderstorms occur each year in the United States and that lightning is present in all storms. Lightning is reported to start approximately 75,000 forest fires annually and starts 40% of all fires.[68] The most destructive form of lightning is the cloud-to-ground strike (Figure 21-20). Based on real-time lightning-detection systems, it is estimated that cloud-to-ground lightning strikes occur approximately 20 million times per year, with as many as 50,000 flashes per hour during a summer afternoon.[69,70] Central Florida is the region with the highest number of lightning ground strikes each year (see Figure 21-21 for distribution of lightning flashes in the United States). Lightning occurs most frequently from June through August, but occurs in Florida and along the southeastern coast of the Gulf of Mexico throughout the year.[71]

Since the 1950s, the number of deaths from lightning in the United States has been decreasing, possibly because of fewer people working outdoors in rural areas, improved warning systems for approaching storms, increased public education on lightning safety, and improved medical care.[72] Latest reports indicate that lightning kills 50 to 300 individuals each year and injures about 1000.[68,73] The greatest life threats from lightning strikes are neurologic and cardiopulmonary injuries.

FIGURE 21-18   **Guidelines for Recreational Diving with Diabetes**

SELECTION AND SURVEILLANCE

- Age ≥18 years (≥16 years if in special training program)
- Delay diving after start/change in medication
  - 3 months with oral hypoglycemic agents (OHA)
  - 1 year after initiation of insulin therapy
- No episodes of hypoglycemia or hyperglycemia requiring intervention from a third party for at least one year
- No history of hypoglycemia unawareness
- HbA1c ≤9% no more than one month prior to initial assessment and at each annual review
  - values >9% indicate the need for further evaluation and possible modification of therapy
- No significant secondary complications from diabetes
- Physician/Diabetologist should carry out annual review and determine that the diver has a good understanding of the disease and the effect of exercise in consultation with an expert in diving medicine, as required
- Evaluation for silent ischemia for candidates >40 years of age
  - after initial evaluation, periodic surveillance for silent ischemia can be in accordance with accepted local/national guidelines for the evaluation of diabetics
- Candidate documents intent to follow protocol for divers with diabetes and to cease diving and seek medical review for any adverse events during diving possibly related to diabetes

SCOPE OF DIVING

- Diving should be planned to avoid
  - depths >100 fsw (30 msw)
  - durations >60 minutes

- compulsory decompression stops
- overhead environments (e.g., cave, wreck penetration)
- situations that may exacerbate hypoglycemia (e.g., prolonged cold and arduous dives)
- Dive buddy/leader informed of diver's condition and steps to follow in case of problem
- Dive buddy should not have diabetes

GLUCOSE MANAGEMENT ON THE DAY OF DIVING

- General self-assessment of fitness to dive
- Blood glucose (BG) ≥150 mg·dL-1 (8.3 mmol·L-1), stable or rising, before entering the water
  - complete a minimum of three pre-dive BG tests to evaluate trends at 60 minutes, 30 minutes and immediately prior to diving
  - alterations in dosage of OHA or insulin on evening prior or day of diving may help
- Delay dive if BG
  - <150 mg·dL-1 (8.3 mmol·L-1)
  - >300 mg·dL-1 (16.7 mmol·L-1)
- Rescue medications
  - carry readily accessible oral glucose during all dives
  - have parenteral glucagon available at the surface
- If hypoglycemia noticed underwater, the diver should surface (with buddy), establish positive buoyancy, ingest glucose and leave the water
- Check blood sugar frequently for 12–15 hours after diving
- Ensure adequate hydration on days of diving
- Log all dives (include BG test results and all information pertinent to diabetes management)

(From Pollock NW, Uguccioni DM, Dear GdeL, editors: Diabetes and recreational diving: Guidelines for the future. Proceedings of the UHMS/DAN 2005 June 19 Workshop. Durham, NC: Divers Alert Network; 2005.)

Epidemiology

Based on the National Oceanic and Atmospheric Administration (NOAA) publication called *Storm Data,* 3529 deaths (average 98 deaths per year), 9818 injuries, and 19,814 property-damage reports occurred during the 36-year period from 1959 to 1994 due to lightning.[67] This report showed that the top four states for casualties (death and injuries) from lightning are Florida (523), Michigan (732), Pennsylvania (644), and North Carolina (629). The highest number of deaths occurred in Florida (345), North Carolina (165), Texas (164), and New York (128). Figure 21-22 shows the ranking of lightning injuries and deaths by state from 1959 to 1994.

There were 1318 lightning deaths between 1980 and 1995 in the United States, on review of medical examiners' death certificates listing lightning as the cause of death.[74] Of those who died during this 16-year period, 1125 (85%) were male and 896 (68%) were age 15 to 44 years. The highest death rate from lightning occurred among those age 15 to 19 years (6

deaths per 10,000,000). Analysis shows that about 30% die and 74% of the survivors have permanent disabilities. Furthermore, victims with cranial or leg burns are at a greater risk for death.[75] Of the individuals who died from a lightning strike, 52% were outside (25% of whom were at work). Death occurred within 1 hour in 63% of the lightning victims.[72]

Mechanism of Injury

Injury from lightning can result from the following five mechanisms:

- *Direct strike* occurs when a person is in the open environment unable to find shelter.
- *Side flash* or *splash contact* occurs when lightning hits an object (e.g., ground, building, tree) and splashes onto a victim or multiple victims. The current will jump from the primary strike object and can splash over to a person.

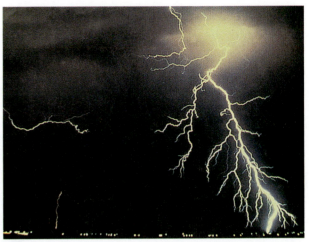

FIGURE 21-20   A cloud-to-ground lightning strike, with streak lightning pattern.
(From Cooper MA, Andrews CJ, Holle RL, Lopez RE: Lightning injuries. In Auerbach PS: *Wilderness medicine*, ed 5, St. Louis, 2007, Mosby Elsevier.)

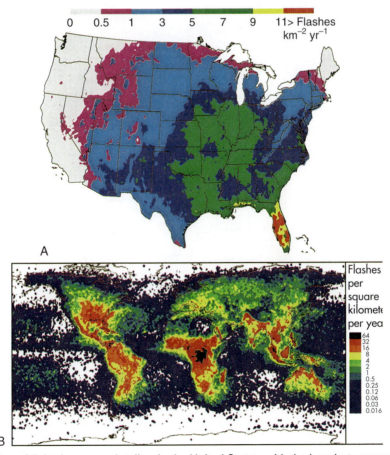

FIGURE 21-21   **A.** Distribution of lightning ground strikes in the United States, with the heaviest concentration in the southeast region. **B.** Distribution of lightning ground strikes worldwide.
(From Huffines GR, Orville RE: Lightning ground flash density and thunderstorm duration in the continental United States, 1989–1996. *J Appl Meteorol* 38:1013, 1999.)

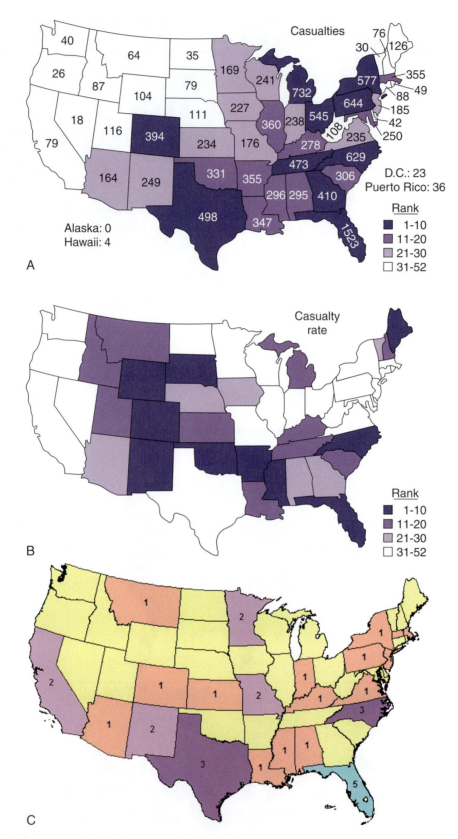

FIGURE 21-22 Rank of each state in lightning casualties (deaths and injuries combined) from 1959 to 1994. **A**. Casualties per state. **B**. Casualties weighted by state population. **C**. 2009 lightning fatalities.
(Data [A & B] from Curran EB, Holle RL, Lopez RE: Lightning fatalities, injuries, and damage reports in the United States from 1959–1994. *NOAA Tech Memo NWS SW-193*, 1997. Part C from http://www.weather.gov/om/lightning/fatalities09.htm. Accessed Sept 5, 2010.)

Splashes occur from person to person, tree to person, and even indoors from telephone wire to a person talking on the phone.

- *Contact* occurs when a person is in direct contact with an object that is struck directly or by a splash.
- *Step voltage,* also known as *stride voltage* or *ground current,* occurs when lightning hits the ground or a nearby object. The current will spread outward radially. Human tissue provides less resistance than the ground, and the current will travel, for example, up one leg and down the other in the path of least resistance.
- *Indirectly.* Blunt trauma can occur from a shock wave produced by lightning, which can move a person up to 10 yards. Injuries can result from lightning that causes forest fires, building fires, and explosions.[68,76,77]

There are six known factors that determine the injury severity from electrical and lightning current: type of circuit, duration of exposure, voltage, amperage, resistance of tissue, and the pathway of current. Once contacted by lightning or other high-voltage electrical source, the heat generated within the body is directly proportional to the amount of current, tissue resistance, and the duration of contact. As resistance of various tissues increases (e.g., from nerve to muscle and bone), so does the heat generated by the passage of current.

It is easy to assume that lightning injuries are similar to high-voltage electrical injuries. However, significant differences exist between the two mechanisms of injury.

A lightning strike is direct current (DC) as opposed to alternating current (AC) that is responsible for industrial and household electrical injuries. Lightning produces millions of volts of current, 30,000 to 50,000 amps and the duration of exposure to the body is instantaneous (10–100 milliseconds). The temperature of lightning varies with the diameter, but the average temperature is approximately 14,430° F (8000° C).[73] In comparison, high-voltage electrical exposure tends to be a much lower voltage than lightning. However, the key factor that distinguishes lightning from high-voltage electrical injury and the different patterns of injury is the duration of current exposure within the body.[76] Figure 21-23 lists differences between lightning and generator-produced, high-voltage electrical injuries.

At times, lightning can show injury patterns similar to those seen with high-voltage electricity because of a rare lightning pattern that produces a prolonged strike lasting up to 0.5 second. This type of lightning, called "hot lightning," is capable of causing deep burns, exploding trees, and setting fires. Lightning can show entry and exit wounds on the body, but a more common pathway of lightning once it strikes a victim is to pass over the body. This is referred to as a "flashover" current. A flashover current can also enter the eyes, ears, nose, and mouth. It is theorized that the flashover current flow is the reason why many survive lightning strikes. It is also known that a flashover current may vaporize moisture on skin or blast a part of clothing or shoes off a victim. The immense flashover current generates large magnetic fields, which in turn can induce secondary electric currents within the body and are thought to cause cardiac arrest and other internal injuries.[78,79]

Injuries from Lightning

Lightning injuries range from minor superficial wounds to major multisystem trauma and death. Figure 21-24 lists common signs and symptoms of lightning injury. As a tool to determine the likely recovery or prognosis from lightning strikes, victims can be placed in one of three injury categories: minor, moderate, and severe.[42]

Minor Injury

Patients with minor injury are awake and report an unpleasant and abnormal sensation (dysesthesia) in the affected extremity. In a more serious lightning strike, victims report they have been hit in the head or state that an explosion hit

FIGURE 21-23   **Comparison of Lightning and High-Voltage Electrical Injuries**

Factor	Lightning	High voltage
Energy level	30 million volts; 50,000 amperes	Usually much lower
Time of exposure	Brief, instantaneous	Prolonged
Pathway	Flashover, orifice	Deep, internal
Burns	Superficial, minor	Deep, internal
Cardiac	Primary and secondary arrest, asystole	Ventricular fibrillation
Renal	Rare myoglobinuria or hemoglobinuria	Myoglobinuric renal failure common
Fasciotomy	Rarely if ever necessary	Common, early, and extensive
Blunt injury	Explosive thunder effect	Falls, being thrown

(Modified table from Cooper MA, Andrews CJ, Holle RL, Lopez RE: Lightning injuries. In Auerbach PS: *Wilderness medicine*, ed 5, St. Louis, 2007, Mosby Elsevier.)

FIGURE 21-24 **Lightning Injury: Common Signs, Symptoms, and Treatment**

Injuries	Signs/symptoms	Treatment
Minor	Feeling of strange sensation in extremity; confusion; amnesia; temporary unconsciousness, deafness, or blindness; tympanic membrane rupture	Scene safety; ABCDEs; medical history and secondary exam; monitor ECG; give oxygen and transport all patients with mild injuries.
Moderate	Disoriented, combative, paralysis, fractures, blunt trauma, absent pulses in lower extremities, spinal shock, seizures, temporary cardiorespiratory arrest, comatose	Scene safety; ABCDEs; medical history and secondary exam; monitor ECG; CPR early when needed; give oxygen and transport all patients.
Severe	Any from above, otorrhea in ear canal, cardiac fibrillation or cardiac asystole	CPR and advanced lifesaving procedures; use "reverse" triage with multiple patients.

(Data from O'Keefe GM, Zane RD: Lightning injuries. *Emerg Med Clin North Am* 22:369, 2004; and Cooper MA, Andrews CJ, Holle RL, Lopez RE: Lightning injuries. In Auerbach PS: *Wilderness medicine*, ed 5, St. Louis, 2007, Mosby Elsevier.)

them, because they are unsure of the source. A patient may present at the scene with the following:

- Confusion (short term or hours to days)
- Amnesia (short term or hours to days)
- Tympanic membrane rupture
- Temporary deafness
- Blindness
- Temporary unconsciousness
- Temporary paresthesia
- Muscular pain
- Cutaneous burns (rare)
- Transient paralysis

Victims present with normal vital signs or with mild, transient hypertension, and recovery is usually gradual and complete.[73]

Moderate Injury

Victims with moderate injury have progressive, single or multisystem injuries, some of which are life threatening. Some patients in this category also have a permanent disability. Patients may present at the scene with the following:

Immediate effects
- Neurological signs
- Seizures
- Cardiac arrest
- Confusion, amnesia
- Blindness
- Dizziness
- Contusion from shockwave
- Blunt trauma (e.g., fractures)
- Chest pain, muscle aches

- Tympanic membrane rupture
- Headache, nausea, post-concussion syndrome
- Tympanic membrane rupture (common)

Delayed effects
- Memory deficits
- Neuropsychological changes
- Coding and retrieval problems
- Distractibility
- Personality changes
- Irritability
- Chronic pain
- Seizures[73]

Depending on the location of the lightning strike, a strike affecting the respiratory center of the brain can result in prolonged respiratory arrest that may lead to secondary cardiac arrest as a result of hypoxia.[73] Victims in this category may experience immediate cardiopulmonary arrest, although the inherent automaticity of the heart may produce a spontaneous return to normal sinus rhythm.[75] Because immediate cardiopulmonary arrest is the greatest threat, prehospital care providers need to assess the ABCs quickly in all lightning-strike victims and continuously monitor the ECG for secondary cardiac events.

Severe Injury

Victims with severe injury from a direct lightning strike (cardiovascular or neurologic injuries) or delays in CPR have a poor prognosis. On arrival at the scene, the prehospital care provider may find the patient in cardiac arrest with asystole or ventricular fibrillation (VF). Lightning causes a massive DC countershock, which simultaneously depolarizes the entire myocardium.[78] The American Heart Association recommends vigorous resuscitation measures for those who appear dead on initial evaluation. This is based on many reports of excellent recovery after lightning-induced cardiac arrest and on the fact that victims in this category are mostly young and without heart disease.[77]

It is not uncommon to observe the initial cardiac arrest with spontaneous recovery of electrical activity following the lightning strike, but any ongoing respiratory arrest may cause secondary hypoxic cardiac arrest.[77,78] If prolonged cardiac and neurologic ischemia has occurred, it may be very difficult to resuscitate these patients.[73] Other common findings are tympanic membrane rupture with cerebrospinal fluid (CSF) and blood in the ear canal, ocular injuries, and various forms of blunt trauma from falls, including soft tissue contusions and fractures of the skull, ribs, extremities, and spine. Many patients in this category have no evidence of burns. In those patients presenting with cutaneous burns caused by lightning, it is generally reported to be less than 20% total body surface area.[77]

Injury to the central nervous system (CNS) is common in a lightning victim and has been classified into four groups of CNS injuries:

Group 1 CNS Effects (Immediate and Transient): Loss of consciousness (75%), paresthesia (80%); weakness (80%); confusion, amnesia and headaches.

Group 2 CNS Effects (Immediate and Prolonged): hypoxic ischemic neuropathy; intracranial hemorrhage; post-arrest cerebral infarction.

Group 3 CNS Effects (Possible Delayed Neurological Syndromes): motor neuron diseases and movement disorders.

Group 4 CNS Effects (Trauma from Fall or Blast): subdural and epidural hematomas and subarachnoid hemorrhage.

Assessment

On arrival at the scene, as with any other call, the priority is the safety of the prehospital care providers and other public safety personnel. Know whether or not there is still the chance of lightning in the area. As a storm approaches or has passed, there still is a source of danger that is not always apparent since lightning remains a very real threat as far as 10 miles away.[75] The mechanism of injury may be unclear without a witness because lightning can strike during a sunny day. When in doubt about the mechanism of injury, immediately assess for ABCDEs and any life-threatening conditions, as for any emergency. These patients do not carry an electrical charge and touching them poses no risk in providing patient care. Assess the victim's heart rhythm with the ECG. It is common to see nonspecific ST-segment and T-wave changes, but more specific evidence of myocardial infarction with Q-wave or ST-segment elevation is rarely seen.[80]

Once the patient is stable, a detailed head-to-toe assessment is necessary to identify the wide range of injuries that can occur with this type of trauma. Assess the patient's situational awareness and the neurologic function of all extremities because the upper and lower extremities may experience transient paralysis (known as keraunoparalysis). Lightning victims are known to have an autonomic dysfunction causing dilated pupils, which will mimic head trauma.[81] Assess the eyes because 55% of victims have some form of ocular injury. Look for blood and cerebrospinal fluid in the ear canals—50% of these victims will have one or two ruptured tympanic membranes. All victims of lightning injury have a high probability of blunt trauma from being thrown against a solid object or from objects falling on the patient. Cervical spine precautions are needed during the assessment to minimize further injury. Assess the skin for signs of any burns, ranging from first degree to full thickness. It is common to see a feathering appearance in the skin, known as "Lichtenberg's figures," but these patterns are not burns and resolve in 24 hours. It is more common to see burns secondary to igniting of clothes and heating of jewelry or other objects.

Management

The priorities for managing a lightning victim are to ensure scene safety for yourself and your crew, stabilize airway, breathing, and circulation. If spontaneous respiration or circulation is absent, initiate effective CPR up to 5 cycles (2 minutes), and evaluate the heart rhythm with an automatic external defibrillator (AED) based on current guidelines.[30] Use ALS measures to manage lightning-induced cardiopulmonary arrest based on current AHA guidelines for ACLS and PALS, as discussed elsewhere.[33] Evaluate and treat for shock and hypothermia. Apply high-flow oxygen for all moderately and severely injured patients. Intravenous fluids should be started KVO, since lightning-injured patients, unlike conventional high-voltage electrical-injured patients, do not have massive tissue destruction and burns requiring a larger amount of fluids. Stabilize any fractures, and package the blunt trauma patient for cervical spine immobilization. Lightning-strike victims with minor to severe injuries need to be transported to an ED for further evaluation and observation. Transport the patient by either ground or air based on availability, distance, and time to the hospital and overall risk to the flight crew and benefit to patient.

As mentioned previously, lightning victims have a higher probability of a positive outcome from early and effective resuscitation. However, there is little evidence to suggest that these patients can regain a pulse from prolonged BLS or ALS procedures lasting longer than 20 to 30 minutes.[68] Before terminating resuscitation, all efforts should be made to stabilize the patient by establishing an airway, along with high-flow oxygen and supported ventilation, and to correct any hypovolemia, hypothermia, and acidosis.

If the incident involves multiple victims, principles of triage should be implemented immediately. The normal rules of triage are to focus limited personnel and resources on patients with moderate and severe injuries and quickly bypass those patients without respiration and circulation. However, with multiple lightning-strike patients, the rule changes to use "reverse" triage and "resuscitate the dead," because these patients are either in respiratory arrest or cardiac arrest and have a high probability of recovery if managed expeditiously.[75,82] In contrast, other patients who have survived a lightning strike have little likelihood of deteriorating, unless there is associated trauma and occult hemorrhage.

Prevention

With numerous thunderstorms throughout the year, lightning ground strikes are common. The public and prehospital care providers must be educated about prevention and the many lightning myths and misconceptions (Figure 21-25). Numerous lightning-prevention resources are provided by such agencies as the National Weather Service/NOAA, National Lightning Safety Institute, American Red Cross, and Federal Emergency Management Agency (FEMA).[47]

Official guidelines are published for lightning-injury prevention and treatment by both national and international mountain medicine commissions.[83] Prehospital care providers servicing areas in mountainous regions are at greater risk for lightning strike, especially those who serve as Park Rangers, Search and Rescue, and other public safety personnel in high altitude and in remote areas. It is difficult to find protected areas in the wilderness when a lightning storm occurs. It is always recommended to take note of the weather forecast since thunder and lightning in the mountains occur mainly during summer months in the late afternoons and night. Thus, the saying, "up by noon and down by 2:00 p.m.," to remind individuals to return to lower elevations by the middle to late afternoon to decrease the risk for lightning strike. The best place to get out of a lightning storm in the mountains is a hut or mountain refuge. Stay away from open doors and windows. Tents do not provide any protection from lightning strike and tent poles may act as lightning rods. Larger caves and valleys are protective, but small caves provide little protection if the person is near the opening and side walls. Wet stream beds are more dangerous than open areas. Stay off mountain ridges and summits, power lines, and ski lifts. Stay clear of the base of taller trees since lightning will travel down the trunk to the base. In a forest, it is best to get into a cluster of smaller trees. If caught in the open, do not sit or lie flat. It is best to crouch down with feet or knees together and keep contact with as small an area of the ground as possible to minimize injury from ground current. Try to use some insulation between yourself and the ground, such as a dry pack on which to kneel or sit. If in a group, stay apart from each other, but within sight, to reduce the number of people injured by ground current or side flashes between persons. Consider the use of small, portable lightning detectors so that advance warning is received and prevention steps can be implemented before the storm arrives.

FIGURE 21-25 Myths and Misconceptions about Lightning

GENERAL MYTHS
- Lightning strikes are invariably fatal
- Major cause of death is from burns
- A victim struck by lightning bursts into flames or is reduced to ashes
- Victims remain charged or electrified after they are struck
- Individuals are only at risk for being struck when there are storm clouds overhead
- Occupying a building during the storm affords 100% protection from lightning
- The belief that lightning never strikes the same place twice is false
- Wearing rubber-soled shoes and raincoat will protect a person
- Rubber tires in a vehicle are what protect a person from injury
- Wearing metal jewelry increases the risk of attracting lightning
- Lightning always hits the highest object
- There is no danger from lightning unless it is raining
- Lightning can occur without thunder

MISCONCEPTIONS
Some myths and misconceptions held by prehospital care providers can adversely affect the care and outcome of their patients.

- If you are not killed by lightning, you will be OK
- If the victim has no outward signs of injury, the damage cannot be that serious
- Lightning injuries should be treated similar to other high-voltage electrical injuries
- Lightning victims who have resuscitation for several hours might still recover successfully

(Modified from O'Keefe GM, Zane RD: Lightning injuries. *Emerg Med Clin North Am* 22:369, 2004; and Cooper MA, Andrews CJ, Holle RL, Lopez RE: Lightning injuries. In Auerbach PS: *Wilderness medicine*, ed 5, St. Louis, 2007, Mosby Elsevier.)

Prehospital care providers and other public safety personnel should establish procedures for a severe weather watch that provides storm warnings updated through the day as one method of safety prevention.

One public education motto used for children and adults is, "If you see it, flee it; if you hear it, clear it." Another useful rule is the "30–30 rule." When the time between seeing lightning and hearing thunder is 30 seconds or less, individuals are in danger and need to seek appropriate shelter. Furthermore, it is recommended to resume outdoor activity only after 30 minutes following the last lightning or thunder, because a passing thunderstorm still is a threat and lightning can strike up to 10 miles after the storm passes.[84,85] Another measure of lightning proximity is the "flash-to-bang" rule, 5 seconds = 1 mile: following lightning, for every 5 seconds until the sound of thunder equals 1 mile.

The following are safety guidelines for lightning prevention as a storm develops:

Indoors

1. Seek a building and stay away from windows, open doors, fireplaces, bath and shower, and metal objects such as sinks and appliances.
2. Turn off the radio and computer and avoid hard-wired telephones; use a telephone only in emergency.
3. Turn off all faucets, electrical appliances, and devices *before* a storm arrives.

Outdoors

1. Avoid metal objects such as bikes, tractors, and fences.
2. Avoid tall objects such as trees, and make yourself small.
3. Avoid areas near pipelines, power lines, and ski lifts.
4. Avoid open fields.
5. Avoid open shelters (e.g., carport, bus shelter), depending on overall size, because side flashes or ground strikes can occur.
6. Drop ski poles and golf clubs, which may attract lightning.
7. In large public outdoors events, seek out nearby buses or minivans.
8. Seek the inside of a hardtop vehicle, and avoid convertibles; keep windows up and avoid metal items in the vehicle.
9. Tents offer little if any protection, and avoid metal tent poles and wet objects.
10. When no immediate shelter is available, all persons should spread out 30 to 50 feet apart to avoid splash contact and ground current.
11. Seek to make the smallest contact with ground, if possible, to minimize ground contact.
12. Lightning position requires squatting, feet together, ears covered with hands; squat on a ground pad, backpack, or some insulation material. An alternative position of comfort is to kneel or sit cross-legged.
13. Do not stand, hug, squat, or huddle near tall trees; seek out a low area of lower trees or saplings.
14. Seek out large caves, and stay away from the opening and side walls.
15. If on high ground or side of a mountain, seek out lower terrain in area.
16. Seek out ditches unless there is contact with water.
17. If on water, seek shore immediately and move inland, away from the water: avoid swimming, boating, or tallest object on water.[67,73]

Support for survivors of lightning injury can contact Lightning Strike & Electric Shock Survivors International, Inc. LS&ESSI, Inc. is a nonprofit support group by and for survivors, their families, and other interested parties. There are members throughout the United States and in more than 13 other countries (http://www.lightning-strike.org/).

High Altitude

In the United States, more than 40 million people each year travel above 8000 feet (about 2400 m) to participate in activities that include snowboarding, alpine skiing, hiking, camping, concerts, and festivals. Thus, many people are at risk for altitude-related illness, which can develop within hours to days after they arrive at altitude. Prehospital care providers, therefore, need to become familiar with the predisposing factors, signs and symptoms, medical management, and prevention techniques to reduce the morbidity and mortality of high-altitude illness. This section presents three medical conditions directly caused by the high-altitude environment and highlights specific underlying medical conditions that worsen as a result of high-altitude-induced hypoxia, also known as *altitude-exacerbated* medical conditions.[86]

Epidemiology

High-altitude illness is a term that encompasses two cerebral and one pulmonary syndrome: (1) acute mountain sickness (AMS); (2) high-altitude cerebral edema (HACE); and (3) high-altitude pulmonary edema (HAPE). Even though the risks of acquiring high-altitude illness are low, once it develops, progression can be fatal.[87]

Acute mountain sickness is a mild form of high-altitude illness, rarely experienced at altitudes below 6540 feet (2000 m), but the incidence increases to 1.4% to 25% with increasing altitudes of 6754 to 8000 feet (2060–2440 m).[88,89] AMS develops in 20% to 25% of cases above 8200 feet (2500 m) and in 40% to 50% of cases at 14,000 feet (3123 m).[81] The incidence of AMS is greater than 90% when the rate of ascent to approximately 14,000 feet (3123 m) occurs over hours versus days.[90] Furthermore, a small number of AMS cases (5%–10%) progress from mild symptoms to become HACE, a severe form of AMS.[91] HACE is a severe neurologic form of high-altitude illness and has a low incidence rate of 0.01% in the general population at an altitude above 8200 feet (2500 m); this rate increases to 1% to 2% in more physically active individuals.[86]

HAPE is rare but accounts for the most deaths from high-altitude illness.[91] The incidence rate for HAPE is 0.01% to 0.1% at 8200 feet (2500 m) in the general population and increases to 2% to 6% in climbers at an altitude of 13,120 feet (4000 m). The overall mortality for HAPE is 11% and increases to 44% when no treatment interventions are made.[92] Forty-seven cases of HAPE were reported in Vail, Colorado, from 1975 to 1982. These were young, healthy males who skied at an average altitude of 7644 feet (2330 m).[92]

Hypobaric Hypoxia

There are three defined levels of altitude. *High-altitude* is defined as an elevation above 5000 to 11,480 feet (1500–3500 m). This is a common altitude in the western mountain ranges of the United States, where high-altitude illness is reported with greater frequency than in other regions.[93] *Very high altitude* is defined as an elevation between 11,480 to 18,045 feet (3500–5500 m) and is the more common altitude for serious forms of high-altitude illness.[94] *Extreme altitude* is defined as elevations higher than 18,045 feet (5500 m).[91] With a progressive increase in altitude, the environment becomes very hostile to an individual not acclimatized to the decreased availability of oxygen, also known as *hypobaric hypoxia.*

High altitude is a unique environment because there is a decreased availability of oxygen for respiration, which results in cellular *hypoxia.* Boyle's law states that the volume of gas is inversely proportional to external pressure applied to it; thus, air is less dense in higher altitudes (see section on scuba-related diving injuries for gas laws). Compared to sea level, or 1 atm, atmospheric pressure at 18,045 feet (5500 m) is reduced by approximately 50% (0.5 atm).[91,95] This relationship relates to Henry's law, which states that the concentration of gas in solution is proportional to the partial pressure of that gas.

Even though the concentration of oxygen remains at 21% at all altitudes, decreased atmospheric pressure at higher altitude results in a decreased partial pressure of oxygen (PO_2). For example, PO_2 is 160 mm Hg at sea level (1 atm) and 80 mm Hg at 18,045 feet (0.5 atm at 5500 m), resulting in less oxygen available during respiration. Figure 21-26 shows that as altitude increases from sea level to extreme altitude, there is a proportional decrease in barometric pressure, arterial blood gases, and arterial oxygen saturation (SaO_2). It is worth noting that SaO_2 remains, on average, above 91% in a healthy, acclimatizing adults until reaching an altitude above 9200 feet (2810 m). *Prehospital care providers are trained to provide aggressive ventilatory support with 100% oxygen for all patients who are symptomatic with a pulse oximetry reading of 91% SaO_2, because this is indicative of moderate hypoxia (86%–91%).*

This relationship between increasing altitude and progressive hypoxia forms the basis for the acute physiologic adjustments in respiratory rate and cardiac output and biochemical changes.[96] Consequently, it is the hypobaric hypoxia and hypoxemia that set up nonacclimatized individuals for high-altitude illness.[87]

High-Altitude Illness

Factors Related to High-Altitude Illness

The development of high-altitude illness depends on many factors specific to each high-altitude exposure.

Increased Altitude and Ascent Rate. The incident and severity of high-altitude illness are primarily related to the speed of ascent, altitude reached, and the length of stay because these three factors increase the hypoxic stress in the body.[87,96]

Previous History of High-Altitude Illness. A documented past history of high-altitude illness is a valuable predicator of who is susceptible for subsequent high-altitude illness when returning to the same altitude at the same ascent rate.[97] Incidence rates for HAPE increase from 10% to 60% for those with a previous history of HAPE who abruptly ascend to an altitude of 14,960 feet (4560 m).[98]

Preacclimatization. Having a permanent residence above 2950 feet (900 m) provides some preacclimatization and is associated with a lower rate of and severity of high-altitude illness

FIGURE 21-26   **Relationship of Altitude, Barometric Pressure (P_B), Arterial Blood Gases, and Oxygen Saturation***

Altitude (meters)	Altitude (feet)	Pb (mm Hg)	PaO$_2$ (mm Hg)	SaO$_2$ (%)	PaCO$_2$ (mm Hg)
Sea level	Sea level	760	100	98.0	40.0
1,646	5,400	630	73.0	95.1	35.6
2,810	9,200	543	60.0	91.0	33.9
3,660	12,020	489	47.6	84.5	29.5
4,700	15,440	429	44.6	78.0	27.1
5,340	17,500	401	43.1	76.2	25.7
6,140	20,140	356	35.0	65.6	22.0

(Modified from Hackett PH, Roach RC: High-altitude medicine. In Auerbach PS: *Wilderness medicine*, ed 5, St. Louis, 2007, Mosby Elsevier.)
*Data are mean values for subjects age 20 to 40 years.
Pao$_2$, Arterial oxygen partial pressure; *Sao$_2$*, arterial oxygen saturation; *Paco$_2$*, arterial carbon dioxide partial pressure.

when ascending to higher altitudes. However, this protection is limited if the ascent rate is rapid or reaches an extreme altitude.[96,97]

Age and Gender. Age, but not gender, is a factor in developing AMS; the incidence is lower in those older than 50 years. HAPE occurs more frequently and with greater severity in children and young adults and is reported in equal proportions of males and females in these age groups.[87,99]

Physical Fitness and Exertion. The onset and severity of high-altitude illness is independent of physical fitness; fitness does not accelerate altitude acclimatization. A high level of fitness does allow individuals to exert themselves more, but vigorous exertion on arrival at high altitude further exacerbates hypoxemia and hastens the onset of high-altitude illness.[93,100]

Medications and Intoxicants. Any substance that depresses ventilation and disrupts sleep patterns at altitude should be avoided because this will further exacerbate altitude-induced hypoxemia. These substances include alcohol, barbiturates, and opiates.[91,101]

Pre-existing Medical Conditions. It is important to note that when clinical studies are used to determine effective dose of medication for altitude illness, they generally include only healthy individuals without underlying medical problems. However, today many more high-altitude travelers and those who move their residence to altitude do, in fact, have underlying disease such as diabetes, hypertension, heart disease, or depression. The current medication recommendations for managing altitude illness may not be appropriate for these patients due to potential for drug interactions and for those patients with renal and/or hepatic insufficiencies. A recent review article discusses the medications for the prevention and treatment of altitude illness (i.e., AMS, HAPE, and HACE) for healthy individuals and the drug selection and dosing for patients with underlying medical conditions.[102] Figure 21-27 lists underlying medical conditions that are aggravated by high altitude (low risk, caution, and contraindicated). Additionally, specific medical conditions known to increase susceptibility to high-altitude illness include the following:

- Cardiopulmonary congenital abnormalities: absent pulmonary artery, primary pulmonary hypertension, congenital heart defects
- Carotid artery surgery: irradiation or abolishing carotid bodies

Cold. Exposure to cold ambient temperatures increases the risk for HAPE because cold increases the pulmonary arterial pressure.[102]

Acute Mountain Sickness

AMS is a self-limited, nonspecific syndrome that is easily mistaken for a number of other conditions because of common symptoms, including influenza, hangover, exhaustion, and dehydration. A consensus panel defined AMS as the presence of headache in an unacclimatized person who has recently arrived at an altitude above 8202 feet (2500 m) and has one or more symptoms of AMS.[103] However, AMS can occur at levels as low as 6562 feet (2000 m). AMS is now viewed as a mild form of cerebral edema, often preceding both HACE and HAPE (at the other end of the spectrum, HACE is a severe form of AMS).[104,105] The majority of AMS cases do not progress to more severe forms of high-altitude illness unless there is continued exposure to higher altitude.

FIGURE 21-27   **Common Medical Conditions that Worsen at High Altitude without Supplemental Oxygen**

PROBABLY NO EXTRA RISK	CAUTION	CONTRAINDICATED
Young and old	Moderate COPD	Sickle cell anemia (with history of crises)
Fit and unfit	Compensated congestive heart failure (CHF)	Severe COPD
Obesity	Sleep apnea syndromes	Pulmonary hypertension
Diabetes	Troublesome arrhythmias	Uncompensated CHF
After coronary artery bypass grafting (without angina)	Stable angina/coronary artery disease	
Mild chronic obstructive pulmonary disease (COPD)	High-risk pregnancy	
Asthma	Sickle cell trait	
Low-risk pregnancy	Cerebrovascular diseases	
Controlled hypertension	Any cause for restricted pulmonary circulation	
Controlled seizure disorder	Seizure disorder (not receiving medication)	
Psychiatric disorders	Radial keratotomy	
Neoplastic diseases		
Inflammatory conditions		

(From Hackett PH, Roach RC: High-altitude medicine. In Auerbach PS: *Wilderness medicine*, ed 5, St. Louis, 2007, Mosby Elsevier.)

The hallmark symptom of AMS is a mild to severe, protracted headache believed to be caused by the hypoxia-induced cerebral vasodilation.[106] Patients describe their headache as throbbing, as located in the occipital or temporal regions, and as worsening at night or on awakening. Other symptoms include nausea, vomiting, insomnia, dizziness, lassitude, fatigue, and difficulty sleeping. Malaise and lack of appetite may be present along with a decrease in urine output. It is important to recognize early symptoms of AMS so that continued ascent does not cause a preventable condition to progress into a severe form of HACE.

The onset of symptoms in AMS can occur as early as 1 hour after arriving at high altitude but typically develop after 6 to 10 hours of exposure. Symptoms usually peak in 24 to 72 hours and subside in 3 to 7 days. If the onset of symptoms occurs beyond 3 days after arriving at altitude and does not include headache, and if oxygen therapy provides no benefit, the condition is probably not AMS.[87]

Assessment. If patients are alert, the key is to obtain a good medical history, including the onset and severity of symptoms, rate of ascent, duration of exposure, use of medications which may cause dehydration, use of alcohol, and level of physical exertion. Obtain vital signs, including pulse oximetry. Also, assess the status of any underlying medical condition, as determined by the medical history.

Because a headache is the most common finding with AMS, assess for location and quality. Cheyne-Stokes respirations are a common finding in individuals who have ascended above 10,000 feet (3000 meters). Findings of a dry cough and dyspnea on exertion are common at altitude and may not always be specific for AMS. Auscultate all lung fields because crackles are common with AMS. Assess neurologic function, and assess specifically for ataxia and excessive lethargy; these symptoms are indicative of HACE.

Management. Descending 1640 to 3280 feet (500–1000 m) will provide the quickest resolution of symptoms. Mild AMS will resolve on its own, but patients should avoid further ascent and any exertion until symptoms resolve. Provide analgesics for headache and antiemetics for nausea. For moderate symptoms, descend to lower altitude and provide oxygen at 2 to 4 liters/minute by nasal cannula initially. Assess pulse oximetry for SaO_2 greater than 90%. If lower than 90%, titrate oxygen by 1 to 2 liters/minute and reassess. For patients with neurologic symptoms, see management of HACE. Patients with underlying medical problems exacerbated by altitude should be transported on oxygen for medical evaluation of their primary illness and the secondary development of high-altitude illness.

Figure 21-28 summarizes the signs and symptoms, management, and prevention of AMS.

In 2001, the International Society for Mountain Medicine published a consensus statement that recommends that adult treatment algorithms (for AMS, HACE and HAPE) be followed with adjustments for pediatric drug dosages (Figure 21-29).[107]

High-Altitude Cerebral Edema

HACE is a very serious neurologic syndrome that can develop in individuals with AMS or HAPE. At altitudes above 8000 feet (2438 m), cerebral blood flow increases as a result of hypoxia-induced vasodilation. The mechanism of injury appears to be related to a combination of sustained cerebral vasodilation, increased capillary permeability across the blood-brain barrier, and the inability to compensate sufficiently for the excess cerebral edema.[107]

HACE can occur within 3 to 5 days after arrival at 9022 feet (2750 m), but generally it occurs at altitudes above 12,000 feet (3600 m), with an onset of symptoms within hours. Some mild to moderate symptoms of AMS may be present, but the hallmark features of HACE are altered level of consciousness (LOC) and ataxia, along with drowsiness, stupor, and irrational behavior progressing to coma. Death results from brain herniation.[108]

Assessment. If patients are alert, as with AMS, the key in HACE patients is to obtain a good medical history, including the onset and severity of symptoms, rate of ascent, duration of exposure, and level of physical exertion. Obtain vital signs, including pulse oximetry. Also, assess the status of any underlying medical condition, as determined by the medical history. It is important to assess lung sounds because a strong association exists between HACE and HAPE.

Management. Do not delay planning for treatment and evacuation at the first signs or symptoms of HACE. The highest priority for any patient with HACE is immediate descent, along with initiation of high-flow oxygen (15 liters/minute) by nonrebreather mask and monitoring of SaO_2 until 90% or greater. Unconscious patients should be managed as a patient with head injury (see Chapter 8), including intubation and other ALS procedures.[94]

See Figure 21-28 for a summary of the signs and symptoms, management, and prevention of HACE.

High-Altitude Pulmonary Edema

The onset of HAPE follows a pattern similar to that seen with AMS and HACE, occurring in unacclimatized individuals after a rapid ascent to high altitude. This high-altitude illness has a different mechanism of injury than AMS and HACE, however, because HAPE is induced by hypobaric hypoxia. HAPE is a form of noncardiogenic pulmonary edema associated with pulmonary hypertension and elevated capillary pressure.[97] More than 50% of patients with HAPE have AMS, and 14% have HACE.[109] The signs and symptoms generally appear during the second night (1–3 days onset) and rarely occur 4 days after arriving at a given altitude.[110] The development of HAPE and the rate of progression are hastened by cold exposure,

FIGURE 21-28   **High-Altitude Illness (AMS, HACE, HAPE): Signs, Symptoms, Treatment, and Prevention**

Signs/symptoms	Treatment	Prevention
ACUTE MOUNTAIN SICKNESS (AMS)		
Mild: Headache, nausea, dizziness, and fatigue in first 12 hours	Oxygen 1–2 liters/minute by nasal cannula, and/or descend 1700–3300 feet (500–1000 m); avoid further ascent until symptoms resolve; consider acetazolamide (125–250 mg PO BID) to speed acclimatization; give analgesics and antiemetics as needed	Ascend at slow rate; spend night at intermediate altitude; avoid overexertion; avoid direct transport to 9000 feet (2750 m) Consider acetazolamide 125–250 mg PO BID, starting day before ascent and continued for 2 days at maximum altitude Treat AMS early
Moderate: Moderate to severe headache, marked nausea, vomiting, decreased appetite, dizziness, insomnia, fluid retention for ≥12 hours	Descend, consider dexamethasone (4 mg PO/IM every 6 hours); and/or acetazolamide (125–250 mg PO BID); if unable to descend, vigilant observation for deterioration; oxygen (1–2 liters/minute) and/or portable hyperbaric therapy (2–4 psi) for a few hours if available	Same as listed above. Dexamethasone 2 mg q 6 hours, or 4 mg q 12 hours PO, starting day of ascent and discontinued cautiously after 2 days at maximum altitude; consider Ginkgo biloba 120–180 mg/day in divided doses, begin 1–5 days before ascent
HIGH-ALTITUDE CEREBRAL EDEMA (HACE)		
AMS for ≥24 hours, ataxia, confusion, bizarre behavior, severe lassitude	Immediately descend or evacuate ≥3300 foot (1000 m); give oxygen 2–4 liters/minute; titrate to maintain SaO_2 ≥90% with pulse oximetry; dexamethasone (8 mg IV/IM/PO initially, then 4 mg q 6 hours); hyperbaric therapy if cannot descend	As listed above for AMS
HIGH-ALTITUDE PULMONARY EDEMA (HAPE)		
Dyspnea at rest, moist cough, rales, severe exercise limitation, cyanosis, drowsiness, tachycardia, tachypnea, desaturation	Start oxygen 4–6 liters/minute, then titrate to maintain SaO_2 ≥90% with pulse oximetry Minimize exertion; keep warm; descend or evacuate 1700–3300 feet (500–1000 m); consider nifedipine (10 mg PO, then 30 mg extended-release PO q 12–24 hours) if no HACE; consider inhaled beta-agonists (salmeterol, 125 mcg inhaled q 12 hours, or albuterol); consider EPAP mask; dexamethasone only if HACE develops	Ascend at a slow rate; avoid overexertion; consider nifedipine (20–30 mg extended-release dose every 12 hours BID PO) in person with repeated episodes of HAPE; start 1 day prior to ascent and continue for 2 days at maximum altitude

(Modified from Gallagher SA, Hackett PH: High-altitude illness. *Emerg Med Clin North Am* 22:329, 2004; and Hackett PH, Roach RC: High-altitude illness. *N Engl J Med* 345(2):107, 2001.)

FIGURE 21-29   **Drug Dosing for Children with Altitude Illness**

AMS	Acetazolamide 2.5 mg/kg/dose p.o. 8 to 12 hourly (maximum 250 mg per dose) Dexamethasone 0.15 mg/kg/dose p.o. 6 hourly
HACE	Nifedipine 0.5 mg/kg/dose p.o. 8 hourly (maximum 20 mg for capsules and 40 mg for tabs, slow release preparation is preferred). Nifedipine is necessary only in the rare case when response to oxygen and/or descent is unsatisfactory.
HAPE	Dexamethasone 0.15 mg/kg/dose p.o. 6 hourly

(From Pollard AJ, Niermeyer S, Barry PB, Bartsch P, Berghold F, Bishop RA, et al: Children at high altitude: An international consensus statement by an ad hoc committee of the International Society for Mountain Medicine. *High Alt Med Biol* 2001:2:389–401.)

vigorous exertion, and continued ascent. Compared with the other two high-altitude illnesses, HAPE accounts for the greatest number of fatalities.

Assessment. Patient assessment, including vital signs, lung sounds, and medical history, are vital in the determination of HAPE, which is defined by at least two or more symptoms (e.g., dyspnea at rest, cough, weakness, or decreased exertion performance; chest tightness or congestion) and at least two signs (e.g., crackles or wheezing, central cyanosis, tachypnea, or tachycardia).[111] Rales are generally present in lung fields, starting in the right axilla and eventually becoming bilateral. Assess for fever, which is a common sign with HAPE. Late findings as HAPE progresses are resting tachycardia, tachypnea, and blood-tinged sputum. If treatment interventions are not provided, symptoms will progress over hours to days to include audible gurgling, respiratory distress, and eventually death.

Management. Descending to a lower altitude by at least 1640 to 3280 feet (500–1000 m) provides the fastest recovery, but initially patients show good improvement with rest and oxygen. Keep patients warm, and prevent any exertion. These patients need to improve their arterial oxygenation; start oxygen at 4 to 6 liters/minute or titrate oxygen flow until SaO_2 is 90% or greater. Reassess vital signs after starting oxygen because improved arterial oxygenation decreases the tachycardia and tachypnea. As HAPE is a form of noncardiogenic pulmonary edema, diuretics have not been shown to be helpful. Anecdotal case reports have suggested favorable results with the use of CPAP for serious cases of HAPE; however, specific research is lacking and such equipment is often not available in the environment most likely to be associated with HAPE.[112,113]

See Figure 21-28 for a summary of the signs and symptoms, management, and prevention of HAPE.

Prevention

Acute high-altitude illness in unacclimatized individuals is preventable. The common factor for the onset of AMS, HACE, and HAPE is the rate of ascent to higher altitude. Altitude illness may be experienced by skiers who travel by commercial airlines and start in the early morning from cities at sea level, arrive at high altitude, and begin skiing by early afternoon at about 7000 to 14,000 feet (2100–4500 m). Another scenario with risk of high-altitude illness is a call for mutual aid to various public safety personnel living below 3300 feet (1000 m). They quickly assemble and then arrive at 9000 feet (2750 m) or higher to assist local volunteer search-and-rescue teams trekking to higher altitudes in search of a missing backcountry hiker. Therefore, prehospital care personnel, whether ground crew or flight crew, who have responsibilities at high altitude for patient transfer to another hospital or for medical evacuation from the backcountry need to possess the knowledge to minimize the risk of high-altitude illness for their own safety and the safety of coworkers.

General guidelines for prevention of high-altitude illness in those who fly to altitudes above 8200 feet (2500 m) include the following:

- Perform minimal activity during the first 24 hours at altitude
- A layover at 4900 to 5900 feet (1500–1800 m) for 24 to 36 hours is more beneficial
- Conduct graded ascent with no more than 1900 feet (600 m)/day
- Take a rest day every 1900 to 3950 feet (600–1200 m)
- Avoid heavy exertion for the first 3 days
- Keep well hydrated with water
- Avoid alcohol, sleeping pills, and other sedatives
- Eat a high-carbohydrate diet
- Avoid overexertion
- Avoid smoking
- Physical training is not preventive for high-altitude illness[94]

The "golden rules" of high-altitude illness are as follows:

1. If you are ill at altitude, your symptoms are caused by the altitude until proved otherwise.
2. If you have altitude symptoms, do not go any higher.
3. If you are feeling ill or are getting worse, or if you cannot walk heel-to-toe in a straight line, descend immediately.
4. A person ill with altitude illness must always be accompanied by a responsible companion who can accomplish or arrange for descent should it become necessary.[94]

Medications as Prophylaxis for High-Altitude Illness

For the prevention of AMS and HACE, individuals traveling from sea level to over 9850 feet (3000 m) as their sleeping altitude in 1 day or individuals who have a history of AMS should consider prophylactic treatment. The drug of choice is oral acetazolamide (Diamox™), 125 to 250 mg twice daily, beginning 1 day before ascent and continuing for 2 days at maximum altitude. The alternative drug is dexamethasone (Decadron™), 2 mg orally or intramuscularly (IM) every 6 hours and continuing for 2 days at maximum altitude. The combination of both drugs has been shown to be more effective than either drug alone.[101,102] Other studies have shown the benefit of *Ginkgo biloba* to prevent AMS during gradual ascent to 16,400 feet (5000 m) or reduce AMS symptoms by 50% during rapid ascent to 13,450 feet (4100 m).[103,114] Aspirin (325 mg) taken every 4 hours for three doses reduced the incidence of headache from 50% to 7%.[104] For the prevention of HAPE in individuals with a history of repeated episodes, prophylaxis with oral nifedipine, 20 to 30 mg (extended-release formulation) every 12 hours, is recommended. Currently, prophylactic treatment should be avoided as a method to prevent altitude illness in children because of insufficient clinical studies.[115]

PROLONGED TRANSPORT

Near-drowning

- Asymptomatic patients can become symptomatic in an extended-care situation with a delay of 4 hours before pulmonary symptoms.
- Obtain a pulse oximetry reading before and after administration of oxygen. Provide high-flow oxygen via a nonrebreather mask at 12 to 15 liters/minute.
- Any patient with pulse oximetry values less than 90%, altered mental status, apnea, or coma may require early active airway management to protect from aspiration. Any patient who continues to be hypoxic with pulse oximetry readings less than 85% after administration of high-flow oxygen is a candidate for CPAP or rapid-sequence intubation (RSI) protocol.
- Liberal use of suction through the endotracheal tube is necessary to remove pulmonary secretions and water aspirated during submersion.
- Consult with medical control, if available, to sedate and paralyze the patient to ensure successful intubation, oxygenation, and effective ventilation.
- Another effective method to ensure effective oxygenation and ventilation is the use of positive end-expiratory pressure (PEEP) in apneic submersion patients.[5,14] PEEP increases the diameter of small and large airways and improves the ventilatory/perfusion ratio and arterial oxygenation.
- Determine the GCS score and assess routinely for trends because it is predictive of patient outcome.
- Monitor for hypothermia and hypoglycemia. Any comatose patient should have blood glucose measured or, if unable, receive IV dextrose.
- The placement of a nasogastric tube may be needed to reduce gastric content and water swallowed during submersion.

Lightning Injury

- Initiate CPR very quickly.
- When in the extended-care situation with multiple victims, use "reverse triage" and first resuscitate those who appear dead. However, prolonged (multiple hours) CPR on these victims has a poor patient outcome, and there is little benefit from CPR or ACLS procedures lasting longer than 20 to 30 minutes. All measures to stabilize the patient to correct for hypoxia, hypovolemia, hypothermia, and acidosis should be attempted before terminating resuscitative efforts.[68]
- Assess cerebral edema and increased intracranial pressure (ICP). Establish a baseline GCS score, and reassess every 10 minutes as an indicator of progressive cerebral edema and increased ICP (manage per recommendation for cerebral edema; see Chapter 9).

Recreational Scuba-Related Diving Injuries

- The standard treatment protocol for scuba-related injuries causing pulmonary overpressurization syndrome (e.g., AGE, DCS) is to provide high-flow oxygen (12–15 liters/minute via nonrebreather mask) at the scene and continue oxygen therapy during transport of the patient to the closest recompression chamber for hyperbaric oxygen (HBO) therapy.
- Conduct an extensive neurologic evaluation, and reassess frequently for progression of signs and symptoms.
- Use analgesics for pain control. Also consider giving aspirin (325 or 650 mg) for its antiplatelet activity.[38] Anecdotal data suggest benefits for DCS and AGE patients with cerebral edema, shock, and other conditions after treatment with HBO and high-dose parenteral corticosteroids.[38,116] The standard regimen used has been to administer hydrocortisone hemisuccinate (1000 mg) or methylprednisolone sodium succinate (125 mg), followed by dexamethasone, 4 to 6 mg every 6 hours, with continuation of the dexamethasone for 72 hours. However, this therapeutic approach lacks acceptance because there are no published clinical trials demonstrating the efficacy of these drugs in these patients.[38]
- Use Divers Alert Network (DAN, telephone 919–684–9111) and local medical control for the closest location of a functional recompression chamber. Before transporting a patient for HBO therapy, contact the chamber directly because the status of chamber readiness can change without notification. DAN is the primary medical source for diving consultation and for recommending recompression chamber location and availability worldwide. When transporting by air, use aircraft that can preferably maintain sea-level atmosphere during flight. Any nonpressurized aircraft should maintain an altitude below 1000 feet en route to the chamber site.

High-Altitude Illness

- Mild to moderate acute mountain sickness (AMS) can be managed with low-volume oxygen at 2 to 4 liters/minute by nasal cannula, titrated to 1 to 2 liters/minute ($>$90% SaO_2), with a combination of analgesics (e.g., aspirin, 650 mg; acetaminophen, 650–1000 mg; ibuprofen, 400–600 mg) for headache and prochlorperazine (5–10 mg IM) for nausea. Other medications used for treating mild to moderate AMS include oral acetazolamide (125–250 mg twice daily) and dexamethasone (4 mg PO or IM every 6 hours) until symptoms resolve. Treat HACE with oxygen at 2 to 4 liters/minute by nasal cannula, to maintain greater than 90% SaO_2, and with dexamethasone (8 mg PO, IV, or IM initially, then 4 mg every 6 hours); consider using oral acetazolamide (125–250 mg twice daily) with prolonged delays to descent.

- If a severe form of HACE develops and the patient is comatose, manage according to recommendations for cerebral edema (see Chapter 9).
- Prolonged management of HAPE primarily consists of administering oxygen at 4 to 6 liters/minute by nasal cannula (>90% SaO_2) until improvement of symptoms, then 2 to 4 liters/minute for conserving oxygen. If oxygen is not available, give oral nifedipine (10 mg initially, then 30 mg extended-release dose every 12 to 24 hours). If the patient acquires HACE, add dexamethasone (8 mg PO or IM every 6 hours).

- Use of portable hyperbaric chambers, such as the Gamow bag (Altitude Technologies), has been successful for treating high-altitude illness.[91] These lightweight, fabric pressure bags simulate descending to a lower altitude with or without the use of supplemental oxygen or medication (e.g., acetazolamide, dexamethasone, nifedipine). They inflate with manual pumps up to 2 psi, which is equivalent to descending 5250 feet (1600 m), depending on the initial altitude. The use of these chambers for 2 to 3 hours can effectively improve symptoms. This is an ideal use of technology while waiting for transportation to definitive care.

SUMMARY

Prehospital care providers will inevitably be faced with unpredictable environmental encounters, such as those described in this chapter. Basic knowledge of common environmental emergencies is necessary so that rapid assessment and treatment in the prehospital setting can be provided. It is not easy to remember this type of information because these problems are not frequently encountered. Therefore, remember the general principles involved, as follows:

- *Drowning or near-drowning.* Assume all near-drowning patients have pulmonary distress until proven otherwise; correct hypoxia, acidosis, and hypothermia as indicated.
- *Lightning.* Patients with severe lightning injury need rapid assessment of cardiopulmonary status. Use the "reverse triage" principle for multiple victims. Initiating CPR early is the key to survival.

- *Recreational scuba-related diving injuries.* Patients with severe decompression sickness and arterial gas embolism need high-flow oxygen and rapid treatment in a recompression chamber for the best outcome. Consult early with medical control and Divers Alert Network (919–684–9111).
- *High-altitude illness.* Key interventions for acute mountain sickness and high-altitude cerebral or pulmonary edema are to descend at least 1640 to 3280 feet in altitude (500–1000 m) and provide rest and oxygen.

In every case, remember that personal safety must be maintained. There are too many cases in which EMS and other prehospital care providers have lost their lives as a result of attempting a rescue.

SCENARIO SOLUTION

As you respond into the country club you are anticipating a single, unconscious male on the 18th fairway, but you should be thinking about additional injured players since golfers normally play in a group of four. It has been frequently reported that when a lightning ground strike occurs the electrical energy splashes in many directions hitting multiple golfers standing near each other. Therefore, it is important to conduct a remote assessment and look for multiple victims, note where they are located, whether or not they are moving around or unconscious, and if there are any potential threats to the victims, bystanders or your medic team. Even though you do not hear thunder or see lightning, the lead paramedic should communicate that there is still a environmental threat and to be continually aware for lightning since there are dark thunder clouds in the area. It is known that lightning can strike in the same area more than once and that lightning has struck people outdoors even when the storm has passed and is up to 10 miles away. Note that the victims are not electrically charged and pose no electrical threat to the medical personnel or other first responder personnel, so treatment should not be withheld based on this unfounded belief.

With multiple lightning-strike casualties, rapid assessment of the ABCs is paramount, but use reverse triage on the victims. Resuscitate the "dead" first because these victims are usually in respiratory or cardiac arrest and have a high probability of recovery if rescue breathing, CPR, and/or cardiac defibrillation are performed soonest after a lightning strike. Then, conduct a thorough head-to-toe assessment with specific emphasis on a looking at eyes, ear canals, and signs of blunt trauma. Perform a rapid neurological exam since many victims experience transient paralysis in the upper or lower extremities. Your exam should also identify any lightning entry or exit wounds on the body. Direct contact burns from lightning are rare, but can occur from burning clothes, shoes, or hot metal objects (e.g., belt buckles) touching the skin, which should be removed from the body. Once all victims have been assessed, provide all severely injured victims with high-flow oxygen and an IV with KVO fluids, monitor the ECG for heart rhythm abnormalities, splint any fractures, and backboard all victims with blunt trauma. Think early on about the onset of hypothermia if the patient is wet from rain and lying on a cool surface. All victims, both minor and severely injured, need to be transported to the emergency department for evaluation and treatment for any neurological, cardiopulmonary, or metabolic complications from lightning strike. ■

References

1. Centers for Disease Control and Prevention. Nonfatal and fatal drowning in recreational water settings—United States, 2001–2002. *MMWR* 53(21):447, 2004.
2. Zuckerman GB, Conway EE Jr. Drowning and near-drowning. *Pediatr Ann* 29:6, 2000.
3. Facts about Injuries: Drowning. http://www.who.int/violence_injury_prevention/publications/other_injury/en/drowning_factsheet.pdf. Accessed November 25, 2009.
4. Zamula WW. In *Social costs of drowning and near-drowning from submersion accidents occurring to children under five in residential swimming pools,* Washington, DC, 1987, US Consumer Product Safety Commission.
5. Schoene RB, Nachat A, Gravatt AR, Newman AB. Submersion incidents. In Auerbach PS: *Wilderness medicine,* ed 5, St. Louis, 2007, Mosby.
6. DeNicola LK, Falk JL, Swanson ME, Kissoon N. Submersion injuries in children and adults. *Crit Care Clin* 13(3):477, 1997.
7. Olshaker JS. Near-drowning. *Emerg Med Clin North Am* 10(2):339, 1992.
8. Anonymous. 2005 American Heart Association guidelines for cardiopulmonary resuscitation and emergency cardiovascular care: Part 10.3: Drowning. *Circulation* 112:IV-126–132, 2005.
9. Wilderness Medical Society. Submersion Injuries. In Forgey WW: *Practice guidelines for wilderness emergency care,* ed 5, Helena, 2006, Globe Pequot Press.
10. Orlowski JP, Szppilman D. Drowning. *Pediatr Clin North Am* 48(3):627, 2001.
11. Gilbert M, Busund R, Skagseth A. Resuscitation from accidental hypothermia of 13.7° C with circulatory arrest. *Lancet* 355:375, 2000.
12. Bolte RG, Black PG, Bowers RS: The use of extracorporeal rewarming in a child submerged for 66 minutes. *JAMA* 260:377, 1988.
13. Lloyd EL. Accidental hypothermia. *Resuscitation* 32:111, 1996.
14. Olshaker JS. Submersion, *Emerg Med Clin North Am* 22:357, 2004.
15. Kyriacou DN, Arcinue EL, Peek C, Kraus JF. Effect of immediate resuscitation on children with submersion injury. *Pediatrics* 94:137, 1994.
16. Lavelle JM. Ten-year review of pediatric bathtub near-drownings: Evaluation for child abuse and neglect. *Ann Emerg Med* 25:344, 1995.
17. Karkal MB, Rasch DK, Gilbert J. Optimizing salvage in drowning and near-drowning victims. *Emerg Med Rep* 10(16), 1989.

18. Rowe MI, Arango A, Allington G. Profile of pediatric drowning victims in a water-oriented society. *J Trauma* 17:587, 1977.

19. Craig AB Jr. Underwater swimming and loss of consciousness. *JAMA* 176:255, 1961.

20. Jensen LR, et al. Submersion injuries in children younger than 5 years in urban Utah. *West J Med* 157:641, 1992.

21. Howland J, Smith GS, Mangione TW, et al. Why are most drowning victims men? Sex differences, aquatic skills and behaviors. *Am J Public Health* 86:93, 1996.

22. Schuman SH, et al. The iceberg phenomenon of near-drowning. *Crit Care Med* 4:127, 1976.

23. Howland J, Smith GS, Mangione T, et al. Missing the boat on drinking and boating. *JAMA* 270:91, 1993.

24. Bell GS, Gaitatzis A, Bell CL, Johnson AL, Sander JW. Drowning in people with epilepsy. *Neurology* 71:578, 2008.

25. Howland J, Mangione T, Hingson R, et al. Alcohol as a risk factor for drowning and other aquatic injuries. In: Watson RR, editor. *Alcohol and accidents: Drug and alcohol abuse reviews.* Vol 7. Totowa, NJ, 1995, Humana Press, Inc.

26. Howland J, Hingson R. Alcohol as a risk factor for drownings: A review of the literature (1950–1985). *Accid Anal Prev* 20(1):19–25, 1988.

27. Karch KB. Pathology of the lung in near-drowning. *Am J Emerg Med* 4(1):4, 1986.

28. Orlowski JP, Drowning, near-drowning, and ice water submersion. *Pediatr Clin North Am* 34(1):75, 1987.

29. Modell JH, Moya F. Effects of volume of aspirated fluid during chlorinated fresh-water drowning. *Anesthesiology* 27:663, 1966.

30. Siebke H, et al. Survival after 40 minutes submersion without cerebral sequelae. *Lancet* 1:1275, 1975.

31. Abella BS, Alvarado JP, Myklebust H, et al. Quality of cardiopulmonary resuscitation during in-hospital cardiac arrest. *JAMA* 293(3):305, 2005.

32. Wik L, Kramer-Johansen J, Myklebust H, et al. Quality of cardiopulmonary resuscitation during out-of-hospital cardiac arrest. *JAMA* 293(3):299, 2005.

33. International Liaison Committee on Resuscitation. 2005 International consensus on cardiopulmonary resuscitation and emergency cardiovascular care science with treatment recommendations. *Circulation* 112(suppl 1):IV-58–66, 2005.

34. V. Hwang, S. Frances, D. Durbin, et al: Prevalence of traumatic injuries in drowning and near-drowning in children and adolescents. *Arch Pediatr Adolesc Med* 157(1):50–53, 2003.

35. Pratt FD, Haynes BE. Incidence of "secondary drowning" after saltwater submersion. *Ann Emerg Med* 15(9):1084, 1986.

36. Rosen P, Stoto M, Harley J. The use of the Heimlich maneuver in near-drowning: Institute of Medicine report. *J Emerg Med* 13:397, 1995.

37. Melamed Y, Shupak A, Bitterman H. Medical problems associated with underwater diving. *N Engl J Med* 326:30, 1992.

38. Kizer, KW, Van Hoesen KB. Diving medicine. In Auerbach PS: *Wilderness medicine*, ed 5, St. Louis, 2007, Mosby Elsevier.

39. Strauss MB, Borer RC Jr. Diving medicine: Contemporary topics and their controversies. *Am J Emerg Med* 19:232, 2001.

40. Morgan WP. Anxiety and panic in recreational scuba divers. *Sports Med* 20(6):398, 1995.

41. Divers Alert Network. Eleven-year trends (1987–1997) in diving activity: The DAN annual review of recreational SCUBA diving injuries and fatalities based on 2000 data. In *Report on decompression illness, diving fatalities and Project Dive exploration*, Durham, NC, 2000, Divers Alert Network, pp 17–29.

42. Cooper MA. Electrical and lightning injuries. *Emerg Med Clin North Am* 2:489, 1984.

43. DAN Report on Decompression Illness, Diving Fatalities and Project Dive Exploration. 2006 Edition (Based on 2004 Data). Durham, NC, 2006, Divers Alert Network. http://www.diversalertnetwork.org/medical/report/2006DANDivingReport.pdf.

44. Morgan WP, Raglin JS, O'Connor PJ. Trait anxiety predicts panic behavior in beginning scuba students. *Int J Sports Med* 25(4):2004.

45. Hardy KR. Diving-related emergencies. *Emerg Med Clin North Am* 15(1):223, 1997.

46. Green SM. Incidence and severity of middle-ear barotraumas in recreational scuba diving. *J Wilderness Med* 4:270, 1993.

47. Zimmerman C, Cooper MA, Holle RL. Lightning safety guidelines, *Ann Emerg Med* 39:660, 2002.

48. Kizer KW. Dysbaric cerebral air embolism in Hawaii. *Ann Emerg Med* 16:535, 1987.

49. Cales RH, Humphreys N, Pilmanis AA, Heilig RW. Cardiac arrest from gas embolism in scuba diving. *Ann Emerg Med* 10(11):589, 1981.

50. Butler BD, Laine GA, Leiman BC, et al. Effect of Trendelenburg position on the distribution of arterial air emboli in dogs. *Ann Thorac Surg* 45(2):198, 1988.

51. Moon RE. Treatment of diving emergencies. *Crit Care Clin* 15:429, 1999.

52. Van Meter K. Medical field management of the injured diver. *Respir Care Clin North Am* 5(1):137, 1997.

53. Francis TJ, Dutka AJ, Hallenbeck JM. Pathophysiology of decompression sickness. In Bove AA, Davis JC, editors: *Diving medicine*, ed 2, Philadelphia, 1990, Saunders.

54. Neuman TS. DCI/DCS: Does it matter whether the emperor wears clothes? *Undersea Hyperb Med* 24:2, 1997.

55. Bove AA. Nomenclature of pressure disorders. *Undersea Hyperb Med* 24:1, 1997.

56. Spira A. Diving and marine medicine review. Part II. Diving diseases. *J Travel Med* 6:180, 1999.

57. Clenney TL, Lassen LF. Recreational scuba diving injuries. *Am Fam Physician* 53(5):1761, 1996.

58. Kizer KW. Women and diving. *Physician Sportsmed* 9(2):84, 1981.

59. Baratt DM, Harch PG, Van Meter K. Decompression illness in divers: A review of the literature. *Neurologist* 8:186, 2002.

60. Francis TJ, Dutka AJ, Hallenbeck JM. Pathophysiology of decompression sickness. In Bove AA, Davis JC, editors: *Diving medicine*, ed 2, Philadelphia, 1990, Saunders.

61. Greer HD, Massey EW. Neurologic injury from undersea diving. *Neurol Clin* 10(4):1031, 1992.

62. Kizer KW. Management of dysbaric diving casualties. *Emerg Med Clin North Am* 1:659, 1983.

63. Department of the Navy. *US Navy diving manual,* Vol 1, Rev 4, Washington, DC, 1999, US Government Printing Office.

64. Tibbles PM, Edelsberg JS. Hyperbaric-oxygen therapy. *N Engl J Med* 334(25):1642, 1996.

65. Davis JC. Hyperbaric medicine: Critical care aspects. In Shoemaker WC, editor: *Critical care: State of the art,* Aliso Viejo, CA, 1984, Society of Critical Care Medicine.

66. Pollock NW, Uguccioni DM, Dear Gde L, editors: Diabetes and recreational diving: Guidelines for the future. Proceedings of the Undersea and Hyperbaric Medical Society/Divers Alert Network 2005 June 19 Workshop. Durham, NC: Divers Alert Network; 2005.

67. Curran EB, Holle RL, Lopez RE: Lightning fatalities, injuries and damage reports in the United States, 1959–1994. *NOAA Tech Memo NWS SR-193*, 1997, http://www.nssl.noaa.gov/papers/techmemos/NWS-SR-193/techmemo-sr193.html.

68. Gatewood MO, Zane RD: Lightning Injuries. *Emerg Med Clin North Am* 22:369, 2004.

69. Huffins GR, Orville RE: Lightning ground flash density and thunderstorm duration in the contiguous United States. *J Appl Meteorol* 38:1013, 1999.

70. Cummins KL, Krider EP, Malone MD: A combined TOA/MDF technology upgrade of the US National Lightning Detection Network. *J Geophys Res* 103:9035, 1998.

71. MacGorman, DR, Rust WD: *Lightning strike density for the contiguous United States from thunderstorm duration records,* Pub No NUREG/CR03759, Washington, DC, 1984, Office of Nuclear Regulatory Research.

72. Dulcos PJ, Sanderson LM, Klontz KC. Lightning-related mortality and morbidity in Florida. *Pub Health Rep* 105:276, 1990.

73. Cooper MA, Andrews CJ, Holle RL, Lopez RE. Lightning injuries. In Auerbach PS: *Wilderness medicine*, ed 5, St. Louis, 2007, Mosby Elsevier.

74. Centers for Disease Control and Prevention. Lightning associated deaths: 1980–1995. *MMWR* 47(19):391, 1998.

75. Cooper MA. Lightning injuries: Prognostic signs of death. *Ann Emerg Med* 9:134, 1980.

76. Andrews CJ, Darveniza M, Mackerras D. Lightning injury: A review of the clinical aspects, pathophysiology and treatment. *Adv Trauma* 4:241, 1989.

77. Anonymous. 2005 American Heart Association guidelines for cardiopulmonary resuscitation and emergency cardiovascular care: Part 10.9: Electric shock and lightning strike. *Circulation* 112:IV-154, 2005.

78. Ritenour AE, Morton MJ, McManus JG, Barillo DJ, Cancio LC. Lightning injury: A review. *Burns* 34:585, 2008.

79. Beir M, Chen W, Bodnar E, Lee RC. Biophysical injury mechanisms associated with lightning injury. *Neurorehabilitation* 20(1):53, 2005.

80. Kleiner JP, Wilkin JH. Cardiac effects of lightning stroke. *JAMA* 240:2757, 1978.

81. Casten JA, Kytilla J. Eye symptoms caused by lightning. *Acta Ophthalmol* 41:139, 1963.

82. Taussig HB. Death from lightning and the possibility of living again. *Ann Intern Med* 68:1345, 1968.

83. Zafren K, Durrer B, Henry JP, Brugger H. Lightning injuries: prevention and on-site treatment in mountains and remote areas—Official guidelines of the international commission for mountain emergency medicine and medical commission of the international mountaineering and climbing federation (ICAR and UIAA MEDCOM). *Resuscitation* 65:369, 2005.

84. Lightning safety myths and truths. http.//www.lightningsafety.noaa.gov/resources/LightningMyths-1.pdf. Accessed November 28, 2009.

85. Lightning risk reduction outdoors. http.//www.lightningsafety.noaa.gov/outdoors.htm. Accessed November 28, 2009.

86. Gallagher SA, Hackett PH: High-altitude illness. *Emerg Med Clin North Am* 22:329, 2004.

87. Hackett PH, Roach RC: High-altitude illness. *N Engl J Med* 345(2):107, 2001.

88. Houston CS: High-altitude illness disease with protean manifestations. *JAMA* 236:2193, 1976.

89. Montgomery AB, Mills J, Luce JM: Incidence of acute mountain sickness at intermediate altitude. *JAMA* 261:732, 1989.

90. Gertsch JH, Seto TB, Mor J, Onopa J: Ginkgo biloba for the prevention of severe acute mountain sickness (AMS) starting day one before rapid ascent. *High Alt Med Biol* 3(1):29, 2002.

91. Hackett PH, Roach RC: High-altitude medicine. In Auerbach PS: *Wilderness medicine*, ed 5, St. Louis, 2007, Mosby Elsevier.

92. Tso E: High-altitude illness. *Emerg Clin North Am* 10(2):231, 1992.

93. Honigman B, Theis MK, Koziol-McLain J, et al: Acute mountain sickness in a general tourist population at moderate altitudes. *Ann Intern Med* 118(8):587, 1993.

94. Zaphren K, Honigman B: High-altitude medicine. *Emerg Clin North Am* 15(1):191, 1997.

95. Sutton JR, Reeves JT, Wagner PD, et al: Operation Everest II: Oxygen transport during exercise at extreme stimulated altitude. *J Appl Physiol* 64(4):1309, 1988.

96. Hultgren HN: *High-altitude medicine,* Stanford, CA, 1997, Hultgren Publications.

97. Schneider M, Bernasch D, Weymann J, et al: Acute mountain sickness: Influence of susceptibility, pre-exposure, and ascent rate. *Med Sci Sports Exerc* 34(12):1886, 2002.

98. Bartsch P: High-altitude pulmonary edema. *Med Sci Sports Exerc* 31(suppl 1):S23, 1999.

99. Roach RC, Houston CS, Honigman B: How well do older persons tolerate moderate altitude? *West J Med* 162 (1):32, 1995.

100. Roach RC, Maes D, Sandoval D, et al: Exercise exacerbates acute mountain sickness at simulated high altitude. *J Appl Physiol* 88(2):581, 2000.

101. Roeggla G, Roeggla H, Roeggla M, et al: Effect of alcohol on acute ventilation adaptation to mild hypoxia at moderate altitude. *Ann Intern Med* 122:925, 1995.

102. Luks AM, Swenson ER: Medication and dosage considerations in the prophylaxis and treatment of high-altitude illness. *Chest* 133:744, 2008.

103. Roach RC, Bartcsh P, Oelz O, Hackett PH, Lake Louise Scoring Committee: The Lake Louise Acute Mountain Sickness Scoring System. In Sutton JR, Houston CS, Coates G, editors: *Hypoxia and molecular medicine*, Burlington, 1993, Charles S Houston.

104. Muza SR, Lyons TP, Rock PB: Effect of altitude on exposure on brain volume and development of acute mountain sickness (AMS). In Roach RC, Wagner PD, Hackett PH, editors: *Hypoxia: Into the next millennium,* Vol 474, Advances in experimental medicine and biology, New York, 1999, Kluwer Academic/Plenum.

105. Hacket PH: High-altitude cerebral edema and acute mountain sickness: A pathological update. In Roach RC, Wagner PD, Hackett PH, editors: *Hypoxia: Into the next millennium,* Vol 474, Advances in experimental medicine and biology, New York, 1999, Kluwer Academic/Plenum.

106. Sanchez del Rio M, Moskkowitz MA: High-altitude headache: Lessons from aches at sea level. In Roach RC, Wagner PD, Hackett PH, editors: *Hypoxia: Into the next millennium,* Vol 474, Advances in experimental medicine and biology, New York, 1999, Kluwer Academic/Plenum.

107. Hackett PH: The cerebral etiology of high-altitude cerebral edema and acute mountain sickness. *Wilderness Environ Med* 10(2):97, 1999.

108. Yarnell PR, Heit J, Hackett PH: High-altitude cerebral edema (HACE): The Denver/Front Range experience. *Semin Neurol* 20(2):209, 2000.

109. Hultgren HN, Honigman B, Theis K, Nicholas D: High-altitude pulmonary edema at ski resort. *West J Med* 164:222, 1996.

110. Stenmark KR, Frid M, Nemenoff R, et al: Hypoxia induces cell-specific changes in gene expression in vascular wall cells: Implications for pulmonary hypertension. In Roach RC, Wagner PD, Hackett PH, editors: *Hypoxia: Into the next millennium*, Vol 474, Advances in experimental medicine and biology, New York, 1999, Kluwer Academic/Plenum.

111. The Lake Louise Consensus on the Definition and Quantification of Altitude Illness. In Sutton JR, Coates G, Houston C, editors: *Hypoxia and mountain medicine*, Burlington, 1992, Queen City Press.

112. Luks AM: Do we have a "best practice" for treating high-altitude pulmonary edema? *High Alt Med Biol* 9:111–114, 2008.

113. Koch RO, Burtscher M: Do we have a "best practice" for treating high-altitude pulmonary edema? Letter to the Editor. *High Alt Med Biol* 9:343–344, 2008.

114. Roach RC, Wagner J, Zafren K, et al: Seasonal variation in barometric pressure and temperature in Summit County: Effect on altitude illness. In Sutton JR, Houston CS, Coates G, editors: *Hypoxia and molecular medicine*, Burlington, 1993, Charles S Houston.

115. Pollard AJ, Niermeyer S, Barry PB, Bartsch P, Berghold F, Bishop RA, et al: Children at high altitude: An international consensus statement by an ad hoc committee of the International Society for Mountain Medicine. *High Alt Med Biol*, 2:389, 2001.

116. Kizer KW: Corticosteroids in the treatment of serious decompression sickness. *Ann Emerg Med* 10:485, 1981.

Suggested Reading

Auerbach PS: *Wilderness medicine*, ed 5, St. Louis, 2007, Mosby Elsevier.

Bennett P, Elliott D: *The physiology and medicine of diving*, ed 4, Philadelphia, 1993, Saunders.

Bove AA: *Bove and Davis' diving medicine,* ed 5, Philadelphia, 2003, Saunders.

Sutton JR, Coates G, Remmers JE, editors: *Hypoxia: The adaptations,* Philadelphia, 1990, BC Dekker.

CHAPTER 22

Wilderness Trauma Care

CHAPTER OBJECTIVES

At the completion of this chapter, the reader will be able to do the following:

✓ List four factors that distinguish the "wilderness" and "street" EMS contexts.

✓ Given a particular patient situation and location, list four factors that affect the decision whether "wilderness" or "street" care is more appropriate.

✓ Describe methods used for improvised wilderness evacuation.

✓ Describe methods for dealing with elimination needs during evacuations, as well as potential medical consequences if this is not addressed.

✓ Explain the reasons for the dictum that "every wilderness patient is hypothermic, hypoglycemic, and hypovolemic until proven otherwise."

✓ Explain the meaning of the term "SPF" (sun protection factor).

✓ Describe standard ways to manage bleeding wounds in the backcountry.

✓ Describe the reasons, specific indications, and technique for wound irrigation.

✓ Explain when, in the wilderness context, an attempt at CPR is appropriate, and when it is not appropriate.

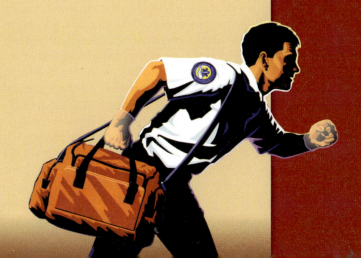

SCENARIO

It is 9 a.m. in the morning and you are working as a member of the local search-and-rescue team that has been looking for a lost hunter since 6 p.m. last night. The hunter is found a short distance from your location by a K9 team. On your arrival you find that the hunter, although cold, is alert and oriented and is complaining of a fractured right lower leg and a 5 cm laceration to the occipital area of his head. The temperature overnight dropped to 38° F (3° C). He explains that late yesterday afternoon he was trying to make his way back to the road and slipped on a wet rock, catching his leg between two rocks. He has fashioned a splint of sorts using some sticks and torn cloth from his shirt. He is approximately 2 miles from the nearest access point over rocky terrain. On examination, you find an alert and oriented 40-year-old male with a GCS of 15. Secondary examination reveals only an angulated, open, right-lower leg fracture with no active bleeding and the scalp laceration that is clotted over.

How would you manage this patient in the field?

Proper Care Depends on Context

Although our medical knowledge, understanding, and technology change from month to month, the *principles* of medical care change little over the years. "[T]he critically injured patient must be transported as quickly as possible, without detailed examination and treatment of noncritical conditions."[1] However, *proper* care is still somewhat context dependent, and the definition of "detailed examination" and "noncritical conditions" may be different on an urban street than deep in the backcountry (Figure 22-1). This concept was introduced in Chapter 3 (Art and Science), showing how situation, knowledge level, skill, scene conditions, and equipment available may alter management of the trauma patient.

Consider a patient with a complex fracture-dislocation of the shoulder. What is the proper care in the operating room (OR)? In many cases it involves an open reduction and internal fixation (ORIF). However, proper care in the OR may not be proper care in the emergency department (ED). It would *not* be proper care to attempt an open reduction in the ED. In the ED, the patient will have x-ray films taken to evaluate the fracture-dislocation, a short-acting pain medication, and a *closed* reduction of the dislocation to reduce pain and swelling, to realign the bones grossly, and to decrease pressure on nerves and blood vessels. However, the definitive ORIF will occur later, in the OR.

Furthermore, proper care in the ED may not be proper care on the street. The ambulance crew may not have the advantage of a large, warm, dry area. They may be working in the rain or snow, where the patient is hanging upside down inside a crushed vehicle, or where a rescue crew is using

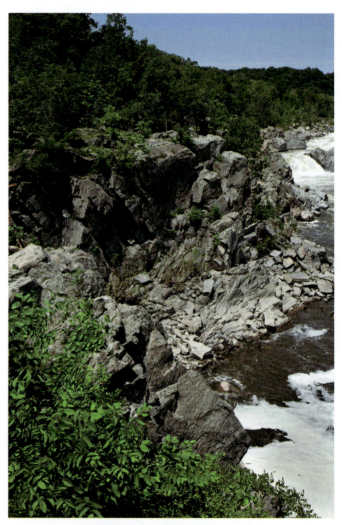

FIGURE 22-1 Wilderness terrain.

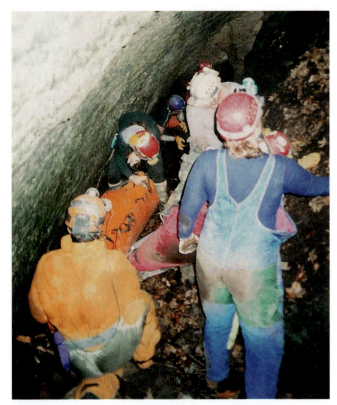

FIGURE 22-2 Trauma care in the wilderness is often hampered by adverse environmental conditions, mud, underbrush, and confined spaces.

power tools to cut and crush metal all around them. On the street, the provider will assess for scene safety, rescue the victim from immediate dangers, assess the patient for other injuries, check distal neurovascular status in the arm, immobilize the shoulder, provide some pain medication, and transport rapidly to the ED. On the street, it would *not* be proper care to attempt an open reduction to reduce the fracture-dislocation.

Finally, proper care on the street may not be proper care in the backcountry (Figure 22-2). What if, instead of in a crushed vehicle, the patient had fallen off a rope while a half-mile into a limestone cave in the mountains, facing a multihour evacuation through the cave passages, followed by a several-hour drive to the nearest hospital? For most conditions, proper care is proper care whether it is done in the OR, in the ED, on the street, or in the backcountry, limited only by equipment and training.

For a small but significant number of situations, however, great differences exist between proper "street" emergency medical services (EMS) care and proper backcountry EMS care. This brings up the following important questions, as discussed later in this chapter:

- Is "street" EMS care always optimal in the backcountry?
- If "street" EMS care is not optimal, how do you know *what* the optimal care is? Is this written down?
- How do you deal with situations in the field when you are not sure precisely what the injury might be? For

example, in the previous case, how do you determine a fracture-dislocation is present when you are examining the patient while you are hanging upside down, whether in a crushed vehicle or from a rope dangling down a pit deep within a cave?
- How do you decide, for a particular patient in a particular situation, which is *more* proper, street or backcountry care?
- What makes a situation "backcountry" or "street?" What about all the "in-between" cases?

Keep the patient with the fracture-dislocation of the shoulder and these questions in mind as you read further. Definitive answers to all the questions cannot be provided—often the answer is "it depends"—but at least good background information can be provided so that providers may, as needed in a particular patient care situation, answer the question. The prehospital trauma life support (PHTLS) philosophy has always been that, given a good fund of knowledge and key principles, prehospital care providers such as emergency medical technicians (EMTs) are capable of making reasoned decisions regarding patient care.

This chapter considers several "backcountry" issues, chosen either because they are critical for optimal backcountry patient care or because they are common backcountry problems for which management is different than on the "street."

Most importantly, this chapter provides an overview of the many issues involved in wilderness-related medical emergencies. Prehospital care providers who will be functioning in a formal capacity in the wilderness setting should obtain specific training in managing these patients. In addition, medical direction by a knowledgeable physician should be an integral component of wilderness medicine activities.

The "Wilderness EMS" Context

Many terms are used for areas far from civilization: backcountry, remote, wilderness, isolated. EMS personnel tend to lump these together under the rubric "wilderness" and to speak of "wilderness EMS." The dictionary definition of "wilderness" follows:

1. a: a tract or region uncultivated and uninhabited by human beings;
   b: an area essentially undisturbed by human activity together with its naturally developed life community;
   c: an empty or pathless area or region;
   d: a part of a garden devoted to wild growth;
2. wild or uncultivated state;
3. a: a confusing multitude or mass: an indefinitely great number or quantity;
   b: a bewildering situation.[2]

Our use of "wilderness" differs from the dictionary definition, however, because we are thinking about *patient care*. Our definition is really the answer to a question: "When should we think about wilderness EMS?" That is, "When should we think and work differently from what we do on the street?"

The answer to this question goes beyond simple geography and involves the following considerations:

- Access to the scene
- Weather
- Daylight
- Terrain
- Special transport and handling needs
- Access and transport times
- Available personnel
- Communications
- Hazards present
- Medical and rescue equipment available
- Injury patters for the specific environment

Numerous potential examples exist besides the traditional view of wilderness:

1. In a city after an earthquake, it may be very difficult to access those who are injured or trapped, there may be no road for transport, and local EMS systems may be out of action. In this situation, patients are likely to remain in their location for considerable time. They will have the same care requirements as a hiker who has fallen in the mountains and is hours—or days—away from a hospital.
2. A person who has fallen into a suburban landfill site, late in the evening, during an ice storm, is at risk from the same factors as in the wilderness. The patient may need a rescue team with ropes, ice axes, and crampons, and medics who can anticipate and cope with issues such as hypothermia, toileting needs, prevention of pressure sores, wound management, and food and fluid requirements.

We often talk of "wilderness EMS," but in reality, *all* EMS lies on a spectrum. At one extreme is a scene half a block from a Level I trauma center, and at the other extreme are scenes such as the summit of Mount Everest or the deepest part of the Mammoth–Flint Ridge cave system in Kentucky. Therefore, in the final analysis, where does "the street" end and "the wilderness" begin? The answer is, "It depends." It depends on the distance from the ambulance (and the ED). It depends on the weather. It depends on the terrain. Even more importantly, it depends on the nature of the injury or illness and the capabilities of the EMS and rescue personnel on-scene. We will return to this topic at the end of the chapter.

Backcountry Injury Patterns

As mentioned in Chapter 1, death from trauma has a trimodal (three-peaked) distribution. The *first peak of death* is within seconds to minutes of injury. Deaths occurring during this period are usually caused by lacerations of the brain, brainstem, high spinal cord, heart, aorta, or other large vessels and can best be managed by preventive measures such as helmets and seat belts. Only a few of the patients can be saved, and then only in large urban areas where rapid emergency transport is available. The *second death peak* occurs within minutes to a few hours after injury. **Rapid assessment and resuscitation are carried out to reduce this second peak of trauma deaths.** Deaths occurring during this period are usually caused by subdural and epidural hematomas, hemopneumothoraces, a ruptured spleen, lacerations of the liver, pelvic fractures, or multiple injuries associated with significant blood loss. The fundamental principles of trauma care learned in this course can best be applied to these patients. The *third death peak* occurs several days or weeks after the initial injury and is almost always caused by sepsis and organ failure.

The PHTLS course focuses mostly on saving patients from the second "peak" of the trimodal death distribution. In the backcountry, most of those who survive to be rescued have already weathered the first, and usually most of the second, "peak" of the trimodal death graph; however, the presence of medically-trained individuals on the rescue team may also prevent deaths related to this second peak. More often, backcountry care focuses on "what can we do *now* that will keep the patient from dying or having major complications later?" We need to make sure the patient does not develop problems such as kidney failure from dehydration, overwhelming infection from poor resistance due to starvation, pulmonary embolism from deep venous thrombosis (blood clots in the legs breaking off and going to the lungs), and infections from decubiti (bedsores).

Safety

In the backcountry, even more so than on the street, scene safety is paramount. An injured or dead rescuer never does anyone any good. "Street" scene safety considerations still apply—even in the backcountry, a civilian aircraft crash can offer problems similar to an automobile crash—but there are other considerations as well. In the backcountry, scene dangers are usually much less obvious than on the street; they tend to slowly "sneak up" on unwary rescuers.

The provider and patient will be exposed to the weather, and changes in weather, such as an incoming cold front with freezing rain, may complicate the operation or even injure or kill the provider and patient. If a rescue lasts for hours, the lack of food and water may cause debilitation. The terrain is often rugged, and poisonous plants and wildlife may complicate patient care (Figure 22-3). Providers need to be aware of dangers specific to the environment, such as rockfall, avalanche risk, rising water, bad air or altitude exposure, and recirculating eddies at the base of waterfalls.

Thus, it is essential that appropriate preparations and precautions are taken to assure the safety, health, and well-being of the medical team. All members of the team must be educated about the hazards and dangers of the specific environment in which they will be working. Each member of the team must know their limitations and not exceed their capabilities trying to rescue an injured individual. Each member of the team must be appropriately prepared with the necessary clothing and equipment for the rescue at hand. Lastly, assuring that the medical needs of the response team are met must be an integral component of the response effort.

The Wilderness Is Everywhere

In the rest of this chapter, we talk about "wilderness EMS" and "in the wilderness" and "wilderness patients." Remember, however, that "the wilderness" might be a short distance from the road, if it is dark and the weather is bad, or even

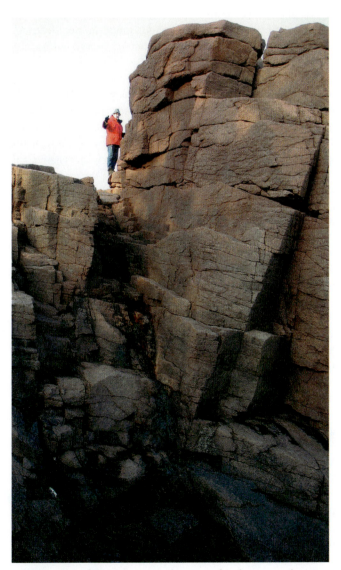

FIGURE 22-3   Steep slopes and uneven footing are a danger in wilderness rescue.

on the road if a disaster has made roads impassable or made nearby hospitals unable to accept patients.

EMS Decision Making: Balancing Risks and Benefits

Experienced EMTs and paramedics (and even doctors and nurses) know that procedures such as airway management and wound management are the easy part of medicine. The difficult part is in knowing *when* to do *what*: critical thinking. Even more often than on the street, in the wilderness, one risk needs to be weighed carefully against another and against the potential benefits.

For *this* particular patient, in *this* particular setting, and with *these* particular resources, and with *this* particular likelihood of *this* particular help arriving at *this* particular time in the future, what are the potential risks? What are the potential benefits? Wilderness EMS is largely the art of compromise: balancing the particular risks and benefits for each patient.

To illustrate wilderness EMS decision making, we continue the discussion on management of potential spinal injury presented in Chapter 10.

"Clearing" the Cervical Spine in the Wilderness

A healthy 22-year-old woman was rock climbing along a river gorge when she fell 65 feet. All her chocks (anchors placed in cracks in the cliff) came out one by one, so she fell all the way to the ground, but was slowed by each anchor as it failed. She was wearing a helmet but hit her head and had a brief loss of consciousness. When you and your partner arrive, after an hour-long hike up the river gorge from where you parked the ambulance at the end of the road, she is conscious and alert, complaining of only a mild headache, with a normal neurologic examination and a normal physical examination. It is late fall, it is getting dark, the nearest helicopter landing zone is back at the road an hour away, and the forecast is for a blizzard to start tonight. Does she need to be immobilized? Do you have to call for a team with a Stokes litter and a long backboard? Or can you walk her out?

"Street" Cervical Spine Management History

Spinal immobilization for severely injured trauma patients became the standard of care decades ago. Even if unstable cervical spine fractures were rare in alert trauma patients, and even if no evidence indicated that spinal immobilization was effective at preventing paralysis in alert patients, strapping a patient to a board seemed unlikely to hurt anyone. Therefore, over the intervening years, prehospital care providers used spinal immobilization for more and more patients. It has since been recognized that patients experience gradually increasing pain from the long backboard. Studies show moderate pain at 30 minutes and severe pain after about 45 minutes.[3]

As EMT training became more and more widely used by backcountry search-and-rescue teams, the practice of strapping everyone to a board after an accident did not seem to make sense, especially if the patient was on the side of a mountain in a snowstorm, and the nearest board was 10 miles away and 10,000 feet down. So search-and-rescue teams and the physicians working with them developed guidelines, based on the available literature, for when *not* to immobilize trauma patients in the backcountry.[4]

A large and important multicenter study called "NEXUS" showed that, in the hospital, many trauma patients can have their spinal column "cleared" without the need for x-ray films, if the following selection criteria are used:

- Absence of tenderness at the posterior midline of the cervical spine
- Absence of a focal neurologic deficit
- Normal level of alertness
- No evidence of intoxication
- Absence of clinically apparent pain that might distract the patient from the pain of a cervical spine injury

Variants of these criteria have been used by many EMS systems. A few studies suggest some problems with using these criteria in the field. The wording of some EMS "selective spinal-immobilization protocols" deviates significantly from the previous wording, raising concerns about whether they really reflect the NEXUS criteria. However, it is generally accepted that the NEXUS criteria, properly applied, are a reasonable guide for the selection of patients who do not need to be strapped to a board, whether on the street or in the backcountry. Although NEXUS may be useful for inference in the EMS setting, one should remember that the study was not designed as a prehospital spinal-immobilization trial, but rather an evaluation of the need for cervical spine x-rays in-hospital.

The problem in the backcountry, however, is not as simple. What if a patient doesn't quite meet these criteria? Does that mean that the patient *has* to be immobilized?

As discussed earlier, wilderness EMS is the art of compromise, and nowhere is this more apparent than in making decisions about spinal immobilization.

What if the patient has a potential spine injury and it is a 2-hour walk from the nearest road, and no spinal-immobilization equipment is at hand? Is it necessary to send someone on the 4-hour round-trip hike back to the ambulance for it?

What if the patient is in a cave, with the water level rising? Could the patient and rescuers be cut off from an escape route and drown if the team delays?

What if the patient is in the mountains, far from the ambulance, and a storm is moving in? What are the risks to the patient and rescuers if they are forced to spend the night on the mountain?

In each of these situations, prehospital care providers at the scene are faced with the following two options:

- Stay and wait for the spinal-immobilization equipment to arrive.
- Start an improvised evacuation without spinal immobilization.

Neither option is ideal; however, prehospital care providers need to choose. To make this choice intelligently, the following questions must be asked and answered:

- What are the risks of an improvised evacuation without spinal immobilization, and what are the risks of waiting for spinal-immobilization equipment to arrive, *for this particular patient in this particular situation*?
- What are the benefits of moving without waiting for spinal immobilization versus waiting for spinal-immobilization equipment to arrive, *for this particular patient in this particular situation*?

The benefits of spinal immobilization depend on the likelihood that this particular patient has an unstable spinal injury.

In the NEXUS study, even those who did *not* meet the NEXUS criteria, and who could not be "cleared," still had a very low risk of unstable spinal fracture, as follows:

- Only 2% of those who *failed* the NEXUS "clearing" protocol had "clinically significant" fractures.
- Of that 2%, only a small fraction likely required specific treatment.
- Of *that* small fraction, only a small fraction likely had injuries that might endanger the spinal cord if not immobilized, and most of those were in patients with multiple major fractures and multiple life-threatening injuries.

Therefore, it seems likely that, for backcountry trauma patients who have survived long enough to be rescued, the incidence of unstable spine injury will be less than 1%.

Prehospital care providers at the scene need to assess these potential risks and benefits to make an informed decision.

Improvised Evacuations

When discussing spinal injury in the wilderness context, we mentioned the idea of starting an improvised evacuation rather than waiting for a litter and spinal-immobilization equipment.

Carrying patients in the backcountry is an extremely difficult, time-consuming, and potentially dangerous activity for both the patient and those doing the carrying. Those with no search-and-rescue (SAR) experience generally underestimate the time and difficulty of a backcountry evacuation by at least

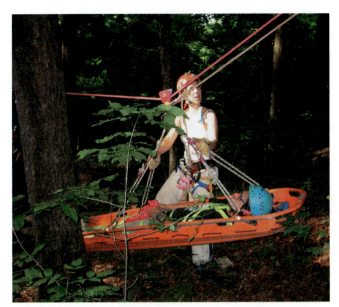

FIGURE 22-4 Because of uneven terrain, creativity and technical rescue skills may be needed to evacuate patients safely out of the backcountry.

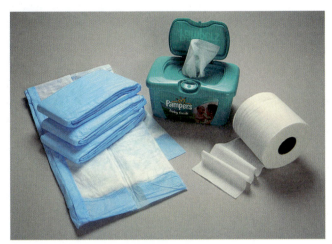

FIGURE 22-5 Elimination supplies.

half, or sometimes up to a factor of five for more difficult evacuations, especially cave rescues.

If someone without SAR experience says, "It'll take us about 2 hours to get the patient out of here," triple the time, and expect it to take 6 hours, or longer if the patient is in a cave, if the team is short on people, if the terrain is particularly difficult, or if the weather is bad. This is especially important to remember if darkness is approaching or the weather is deteriorating.

Walking a patient out, even with a couple of people helping, is almost always *much* faster. If the patient is able to and starts moving *now*, rather than waiting for a litter or spinal immobilization, the evacuation will be much, much faster and completed much earlier. If the patient cannot walk (e.g., because of an ankle fracture), it may be possible to do a piggyback carry or to make an improvised stretcher out of sticks and rope (Figure 22-4).

Patient Care in the Wilderness

Elimination Needs

The truth described in a popular children's book called *Everyone Poops*[5] applies to backcountry patients as well. Given the relatively short transport times in an urban setting, most patients do not have an elimination need. Trauma patients almost never defecate during their prehospital and ED care. However, if you are caring for a patient who has been in the backcountry for a day or more and it takes you several hours

to get to the patient, it is *much* more likely that the patient will need to urinate or defecate.

Having patient care supplies that include "blue pads (chux)" for placing under the patient, having some toilet paper, or even stopping to let the patient urinate or defecate are all reasonable measures (Figure 22-5).

It is possible for men and women to urinate even while immobilized in a Stokes litter (Figure 22-6) with a full body vacuum splint, if packaging is planned carefully and the litter is tipped up on the foot end. For women, a small funnel device often carried by women when backpacking will be needed.

However, people who are lying on their backs for a long time tend to develop decubiti (bedsores). These may end up requiring surgery, resulting in a longer hospital admission. Some patients even die from infection and other complications from bedsores.

Lying in one's own urine and feces for a long time (just hours, not even days) may make bedsores more likely. If patient care occurs for only for a few minutes during a short transport, urine and feces are not a major issue. However, if a provider has been taking care of a patient for several hours and then delivers the patient to the ED lying in his own feces, the nurses might (legitimately) complain about the level of care.

Food and Water Needs

Every backcountry patient should be considered to be cold, hungry, and thirsty; that is, hypothermic, starved, and dehydrated, or if you prefer a good mnemonic at a slight expense of accuracy—*hypothermic, hypoglycemic,* and *hypovolemic.*

Starvation is much more than just hypoglycemia (low blood sugar), and not all starving patients are significantly

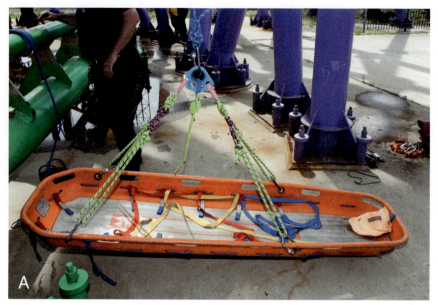

FIGURE 22-6 Stokes litter.

hypoglycemic. Dehydration is more than just hypovolemia, which refers only to intravascular volume within the blood vascular system. Patients who are dehydrated have also lost water out of their cells and the interstitial spaces between the cells.

On the street, water or food are *not* generally given to patients. There are good reasons not to feed patients on the street. A patient will not starve or dehydrate in a few minutes. If the patient might need to go to the OR, having food or fluid in the stomach is harmful; it increases the likelihood of vomiting or, more likely, passive regurgitation leading to possible aspiration when under anesthesia.

However, the stomach only needs to be empty for a few hours before anesthesia. If a patient rescued from the backcountry needs to go the OR, it will almost always take a few hours for the patient to get prepared for the OR in any event.

As noted earlier, with wilderness patients, the focus is to ensure that the patient does not die sometime after hospital admission. Starving people is seldom good for them. Feeding the patient today will make the patient better tomorrow. Therefore, provide food and water to any reasonably alert backcountry patient.

Vomiting and aspiration are always a danger, and careful attention to the patient's airway is always important (e.g., positioning on the side for long transports, even if the patient needs spinal immobilization). However, rescuers should still attempt to provide food and water for backcountry patients, even though they have vomited once or twice, as long as their airway is protected.

Backboard Use

Other important preventive measures for backcountry patients, especially those who face prolonged evacuation, include prevention of decubiti (bedsores), as follows:

- Allow (and assist) the patient to turn from side to side in the litter.
  - Keep the patient's sacrum (buttocks) clean and dry.
  - Provide adequate padding.

If the patient truly needs spinal immobilization, prevention of decubiti is even more important, although correspondingly more difficult. Techniques to avoid decubiti during spinal immobilization include the following:

- Put the patient in a full-body vacuum splint rather than on a long backboard. Vacuum mattresses provide excellent spinal immobilization and are much less likely to cause decubiti.[6–9]
- If no full-body vacuum splint is available, pad the long backboard well and add support under the lumbar spine, knees, and neck. Studies show that immobilization on an unpadded long backboard causes even uninjured people to experience excruciating pain in about 45 minutes and skin necrosis (cell death) in about 90 minutes.[3,10–13]
- Carry the litter first on one side, then the other, so that pressure alternates between the two hips rather than always on the sacrum.

To prevent deep venous thrombosis and pulmonary embolism, do the following:

- Package patients so that they can move their legs; do not tie them down tight.
- Consider rest stops to allow patients to get out of the litter to stretch their legs.
- Consider administering a dose of aspirin if there are no contraindications.

If there is mild suspicion of a cervical spine injury but not a lumbar spine injury, it might even be appropriate to allow an alert patient to get out of the litter, still wearing a cervical collar, and, with many trained hands to help, allow the patient to stretch their legs and take care of any elimination needs. Speaking with a physician knowledgeable with wilderness EMS might be reassuring if this is contemplated.

Sun Protection

Other backcountry hazards to consider include rockfalls, avalanches, and cave-stream flooding. However, one hazard worth discussing in more detail here is sun protection.

The ultraviolet (UV) rays of the sun can damage the skin—acutely, sometimes severely, and in a delayed fashion. Acute injury can include second-degree and third-degree sunburns seen in some victims of exposure, and such severe sunburn can cause shock or death. Delayed injury is manifested as increased risk for skin cancer.

Ultraviolet light comes in two frequencies, A and B (UVA and UVB). UVA was once thought to be harmless, but now we know that it works synergistically with UVB to cause sunburn. Thus, sun-blocking materials or creams must block both UVA and UVB to be effective.

Sun protection is measured by the *sun protection factor* (SPF) (Figure 22-7). The SPF is a numeric measure of how much the clothing or cream increases the minimum dose of UV light to make the skin red. For example, a sunscreen lotion with a rating of SPF 45 provides protection from sunburn for about 45 times longer than without the sunscreen.

To check clothing for SPF, hold a piece of clothing up against a light bulb. If an image of the light bulb is seen through it, the SPF is slightly below 15. If light is seen through it but not the image of the light bulb, the SPF is in the range of 15 to 60 SPF.

Protective lotions with a minimum SPF of 15 should be applied to exposed skin to minimize the potential injury from sun exposure. For prolonged evacuations, lotion with a SPF value of 30 should be used. With profuse sweating, lotion should be reapplied frequently. Some patients may have an acute allergic reaction if the lotion contains para-amino benzoic acid (PABA), therefore PABA-free products are recommended to avoid this complication.

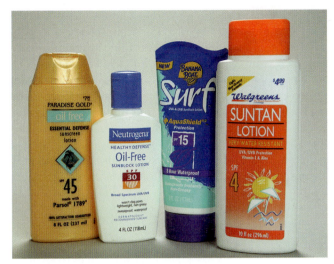

FIGURE 22-7 Sunscreen.

Sunburn is treated as any other burn, and the care is essentially the same in the wilderness as on the street. The only major difference is that in the backcountry, the prehospital care provider needs to be aware of and treat the potential fluid loss, dehydration, or sometimes even shock, and to recognize that patients with sunburn are at higher risk for hypothermia.

Specifics of Wilderness EMS

This section reviews a few of the most important situations in which proper backcountry trauma care differs from that on the street.

Wound Management

Wound management encompasses the following:

- Hemostasis (stopping bleeding)
- Antisepsis (prevention of infection)
- Restoration of function (returning the skin to its protective function, and restoring a limb or other body part to normal function)
- Cosmesis (pleasant appearance)

In the backcountry, prevention of infection and restoration of function assume great importance.

Hemostasis

Control of bleeding is part of the primary survey. On the street, arterial bleeding can kill. In the backcountry, however, even venous bleeding can kill, if it continues for a sufficient amount of time; every RBC counts. Therefore, bleeding control, using standard measures such as direct pressure, are as important or more important in the wilderness. Unless medical personnel are part of the actual injured party's group, severe bleeding that is not stopped will probably result in the patient's demise prior to the rescue party's arrival. Educational programs for those venturing into wilderness situations should address these lifesaving skills:

- Direct digital pressure should be applied for 10 to 15 minutes on the bleeding site followed by a pressure bandage.
- Topical hemostatic agents may have a useful purpose in wilderness care in the control of severe bleeding. Wilderness responders may encounter injured patients that have had such agents already applied by others in their group. Some of these agents are available for sale to the general public. It is important to remember, however, that even if these agents are used, direct pressure on the wound remains part of the treatment process (see Chapter 8, Shock Assessment and Management).
- Tourniquets may be used when all other methods to control the hemorrhage have failed and the priority is life preservation over limb preservation. The tourniquet should be applied above the wound as close to the wound as possible. The tourniquet should be released every 10 to 15 minutes to allow for reassessment of the need for continued application of the tourniquet and to permit blood flow into the extremity in an effort to prolong the viability of the extremity.

Prevention of Infection

After injury in the backcountry, it may be a long time before the wound receives definitive treatment in an ED. Routine wound care in the ED includes appropriate cleaning to prevent infection. Wounds contaminated by dirt or caused by penetration from a dirty object are cleaned with high-pressure irrigation. Uncontaminated wounds are cleaned with low-pressure irrigation.

High-pressure irrigation may cause swelling of wounds, but in the case of contaminated wounds full of dirt and bacteria, the benefit of removing bacteria outweighs the risks from wound swelling.[14,15] Infection may set in quickly. After a wound has been open for about 8 hours, bacteria have spread from the skin deep into the wound, and sewing up a wound is likely to create a deep wound infection. Deep wound infections develop pressure, which keeps out white blood cells, the body's normal defense mechanism against infection.

Routine wound care on the "street" does *not* include cleansing the wound because it makes sense to delay cleansing for a few minutes until the patient reaches the ED, which is better suited for wound cleansing and evaluating the patient. The ED can determine if the patient has a tendon or nerve laceration, an associated fracture, a spleen laceration, or a subdural hematoma in the head.

Delaying wound care does *not* make sense in the backcountry. If it will take hours to get to the ED, the wound should be cleaned. In extremely remote areas, the wound could even become infected before the patient arrives at the ED several days later.

Studies have shown that early irrigation is essential to removing bacteria and reducing wound infections.[16–18] It is not necessary or practical to carry sterile solutions for wound irrigation. There is no need to add an antiseptic to the water.[19] Water that is good enough to drink is good enough to irrigate a wound. Water from streams or melted snow can be treated with any standard backcountry drinking water treatment.[14,20–24]

When cleaning an uncontaminated wound, such as a laceration sustained from banging the forehead against a teammate's helmet, it is only necessary to wash it out with water poured through the wound." A bulb syringe, usually available in the ED, is commonly used but squirting some clean available water from a drinking-water bottle, for example, will do as well.

If the wound is contaminated, it must be irrigated with enough pressure to clean out bacteria. The original studies showed that a 35-ml syringe with an 18-gauge needle provided an appropriate amount of pressure (5–15 psi).[25–27] Squirt the water, at high pressure, throughout the wound. However, this is a major blood-borne pathogen risk; protection from the spray of blood when irrigating is necessary. Eye protection and gloves are essential.

Sometimes it is necessary to use a gauze pad or clean cloth with gloved fingers to clean out some gross dirt or foreign material. The patient's pain may need to be treated before the wound can be cleaned. Once the irrigation is done, dress and bandage the wound. Reapply a clean dressing at least daily.

If the wound is gaping open, a wet dressing will prevent tissue damage as a result of drying out; change or at least rewet the dressing with clean water several times a day. In most cases, however, because the wound will be mostly closed by bandaging, a dry dressing can be used.

Early antibiotic administration is commonly used upon arrival at the Emergency Department for patients with significant trauma. Antibiotics are not given in most civilian prehospital emergency medical systems because of the very short transport times encountered in the urban environment. Definitive care may, however, be significantly delayed in wilderness settings due to the longer distances to be covered and tactical rescue considerations in rugged terrain.

Antibiotics must be given as soon as possible after injury to maximize their ability to prevent wound infections. Intramuscular benzyl penicillin begun within 1 hour of wounding was found to be effective in preventing streptococcal infections in a swine model of wound infection. If administration was delayed until 6 hours after wounding, however, the medication was not effective.[28] A recent military review of antibiotic use on the battlefield recommended that antibiotics be used if arrival at a medical treatment facility was anticipated to be 3 hours or longer.[29] There was no evidence cited in this review, however, to document the efficacy of antibiotics administered beyond the one-hour period in preventing wound infections.

Restoration of Function and Cosmesis: Closing Backcountry Wounds

Because of the lack of good lighting, x-ray films, and a warm dry place to work, it does not make sense to perform definitive wound closure in the backcountry. However, it is possible simply to cleanse the wound, dress and bandage, do good wound care for 4 days, and then do a *delayed primary closure.* Four days later, as long as the wound is not infected, it is safe to close the wound as if it had just occurred. Although bacteria move into the wound soon after injury, eventually enough of the body's defenses (e.g., white blood cells) have entered the wound and make it safe to close. This occurs about 4 days after the initial injury.

Because delayed primary closure is available, there is no pressing reason to close wounds in the backcountry. If a surgeon or someone else experienced at wound closure is present, the wound may be closed at the scene. However, it is still reasonable to only cleanse, dress, and bandage the wound and allow closure to occur later.

Closing a backcountry wound may be important in one situation: when bleeding cannot be controlled in any other way. These situations are uncommon and usually involve a scalp laceration. For this reason, some wilderness EMS personnel are trained to use disposable surgical staplers to repair scalp wounds. However, wound repair is complex and should not be attempted without sufficient training and experience.

Dislocations

A healthy 20-year-old man was kayaking along a white-water stream when the top of his kayak paddle hit a low-hanging tree branch. Now his right shoulder is swollen and deformed and painful. He cannot bring his right arm across his chest. Distal pulses, capillary refill, sensation, and movement are intact. From the ambulance, you and your partner EMT hiked a mile through the woods to get to the stream. Should you "splint it as it lies" or try to reduce what looks like an anterior shoulder dislocation?

The common practice for fractures and dislocations on the street is to "splint it as it lies" and transport for definitive treatment. The only exception is the patient whose pulse is not palpable; in which case the extremity is realigned anatomically.

Although "splint it as it lies" is a good general rule for the street, "make it look normal" is a better general rule for the wilderness context. It is certainly appropriate for both fractures and dislocations when transport is delayed.

There are many types of dislocations—finger, toe, shoulder, patella, knee, elbow, hip, ankle, and jaw—and all have been successfully reduced in the backcountry, some more easily than others. It is usually very easy to reduce dislocations of the ankle (which are almost always fracture-dislocations), patella, toe, or finger, except the proximal interphalangeal joint of the index finger in some cases. Elbow, knee, and hip dislocations are usually quite difficult. All are much easier with training and practice, and, in particular, it takes training or experience to know, without a radiograph, *when* a joint is likely dislocated and to attempt reduction.

EMT and paramedic courses seldom provide training in dislocation reduction. Because backcountry dislocations are so common, however, dislocation reduction is covered in almost all wilderness first-aid, wilderness first-responder, and wilderness EMT training. Those who might provide EMS in the backcountry or who regularly travel in the backcountry are advised to take one of these courses.

Cardiopulmonary Resuscitation in the Wilderness

Wilderness Traumatic Arrest

A few signs can be uniformly equated with nonsurvivability, as follows:

- Decapitation
- Transection of the torso
- Patient is frozen so hard that the chest cannot be compressed
- Patient's rectal temperature is very cold and the same as the environment
- Well-progressed decomposition (see later discussion)

The following presumptive signs of death may be of use to prehospital care providers, although no one sign by itself is reliable:

- *Rigor mortis.* Postmortem rigidity is well known but not always present, and similar rigidity is often observed in hypothermic, but semiconscious, patients.
- *Dependent lividity.* This is common in corpses but also is found along with pressure necrosis and frostbite in some patients exposed to the elements for a long time.
- *Decomposition.* This is usually self-evident.
- *Lack of presumptive signs of life.* Hypothermia can mimic death, in that pulses may not be palpable and

respirations may be undetectable, with dilated unreactive pupils and no signs of consciousness. However, such severely hypothermic patients have occasionally been resuscitated, with full neurologic recovery.

We know that traumatic cardiac arrest "on the street" has a poor prognosis, even if the scene is within minutes of a Level I trauma center. No person survives more than a few minutes of cardiopulmonary resuscitation (CPR) after traumatic arrest.[30–33] This reality is recognized in many EMS protocols, as follows:

For traumatic cardiac arrest, initiate CPR with cervical spine stabilization if:

1. Cardiac arrest occurs in the presence of EMS personnel.
2. Victim of penetrating trauma had signs of life within 15 minutes before the arrival of EMS personnel.

Therefore, in the wilderness context, CPR is inappropriate for traumatic arrest. It is appropriate for prehospital care providers and the mountain rescue team members to examine the patient, then gently but firmly tell the companions that the victim is dead and there is no reason to initiate resuscitation. Although it is oftentimes difficult to use the word "dead," euphemisms often lead to misunderstanding and misinterpretation of what is actually being said. The prehospital care providers and mountain rescue team members should then deal appropriately with the expected denial and grief reactions, with a check of scene safety, especially if oncoming darkness may make exiting the area hazardous to the victim's mentally and physically exhausted companions.

Wilderness Medical Arrest

A medical arrest applies to a patient who has chest pain and then sustains a cardiac arrest. Again, in the wilderness context, the chances of survival are poor or nonexistent when the patient is more than a few minutes from CPR or defibrillation.[34–39] It is possible that a rescue team might be carrying out a patient with chest pain when the patient sustains a cardiac arrest. Although some lightweight defibrillators are now being manufactured, the weight-to-need-for-use ratio of defibrillators is so poor that they are seldom carried by wilderness rescue teams.

There are a variety of other causes of cardiac arrest in the backcountry, and in the previous example, ventricular fibrillation (VF) cardiac arrest secondary to hypothermia or cardiac arrest secondary to pulmonary embolism is likely. For such cardiac arrests, however, survival is even less likely than with a cardiac arrest secondary to a myocardial infarction.

However, "nontraumatic" backcountry cardiac arrest might be survivable in the following situations:

- Hypothermia[40]
- Cold-water submersion[41–44]
- Lightning strike[45]

- Electrocution
- Drug overdose
- Avalanche burial[46]

In all these cases, a patient may appear to be in cardiac arrest but still might be resuscitated by basic CPR. For hypothermia in particular, there is a saying that "nobody's dead until they're warm and dead" (see Chapter 20). A significant minority of those who appear dead from the mechanisms listed can be resuscitated. There are special considerations for each of these situations; for example, scene safety for those who have been electrocuted and are still attached to a backcountry power line, or knowing that external cardiac compression can actually induce a VF cardiac arrest in a hypothermic patient whose heart is beating just enough to keep the patient alive.[47–50] Although appropriate in a wilderness EMT course, detailed discussion of these topics is beyond the scope of this chapter.

However, two standard wilderness CPR rules are as follows:

- If the patient appears to be in cardiac arrest from causes other than trauma, attempt CPR for 15 to 30 minutes; if this does not resuscitate the patient, stop CPR and consider the patient dead.
- However, do *not* start CPR if it will put rescuers at risk and decrease their chances of retreating from the scene safely, given concerns about daylight, terrain, weather, and available nearby shelter. [36]

Bites and Stings

Bites and stings are common backcountry problems. The exact type of bite or sting likely in a backcountry area depends on the specific locale.

Bee Stings

The most widespread, common, and deadly sting is that of the common honeybee, at least to those who are allergic. Most reactions to bee stings are severe (although brief) local pain and in some cases local swelling and redness persist for 1 or 2 days; these latter reactions are likely directly related to injected toxins, and not an indication of allergy.

Some individuals who are stung will progress within a few minutes to a generalized allergic reaction. This may range from urticaria to a full-blown anaphylactic reaction. Although the exact spectrum of generalized allergic reaction depends on the contents of the injected toxin (which varies among the many species of bees and wasps) and the allergic history of the patient, one or more of the following are usually seen:

- Urticaria (hives) (Figure 22-8)
- Lip swelling
- Hoarseness or stridor

- Wheezing and/or shortness of breath
- Abdominal cramping, vomiting, or diarrhea
- Tachycardia *or* bradycardia
- Hypotension
- Syncope
- Shock

Those with a history of a generalized allergic reaction to a sting are more likely to have another generalized reaction to the next sting. However, venom among different species varies enough that, despite a history of generalized allergy in the past, a patient might have no generalized reaction to the next sting.

A patient with mild urticaria after a sting probably will do well. If a patient with hives after a sting progresses to "real" anaphylaxis, however, the best early sign is hoarseness. The major cause of death after bee sting allergy is airway obstruction from hives in the airway, and hoarseness is usually the first sign of airway swelling. Any patient with a generalized reaction to a bee sting needs treatment immediately.

Basic life support (BLS) interventions generally involve keeping the patient flat or in a position of comfort, performing standard airway management, and providing oxygen.

One simple but useful intervention is to remove an embedded stinger properly. Although only a small fraction of bee stings still have an embedded stinger, it often requires good eyes and bright light or a magnifying glass to see the stinger, and improper removal could be deadly. Squeezing an embedded stinger with a pair of forceps, clamps, or tweezers can squeeze more venom into the skin. Instead, *carefully* scraping with a credit card or knife blade can remove the stinger without squeezing additional venom into the skin.

It is important to remove embedded stingers as soon as possible; the venom sac continues to squeeze in venom even after the bee has flown away.

The main medications to treat bee stings include the following:

1. Epinephrine (adrenalin). Although epinephrine only acts for a few minutes, it can be lifesaving.
2. Antihistamines (e.g., diphenhydramine [Benadryl®]). Anyone who requires epinephrine for a bee sting allergy should receive an antihistamine.
3. Steroids (e.g., prednisone). Most people who require epinephrine also require steroids.

Some wilderness SAR teams carry drugs for bee-sting allergy in their medical kits; the team's wilderness EMTs have special training in their use. Also, some people with a history of bee-sting allergy will carry these medications in their personal first-aid kits.

The most important drug is epinephrine. Epinephrine is available as a pen-sized autoinjector (e.g., EpiPen®), which is often prescribed to any patient who has had a generalized allergy to bee stings. These autoinjectors are found in many wilderness first-aid kits.

Snakebite

There are many species of poisonous snakes. Few are found in northern latitudes. Most occur in tropical areas, and many are deadly. Although many snakes have venom glands, there are only two types of snakes in North America with venom strong enough to cause more than minor irritation to humans.

Coral snakes are small snakes found in the southern parts of North America that have venom that is neurotoxic and causes paralysis (Figure 22-9). However, the snakes are small, have small fangs, cannot open their mouths very far compared to larger snakes, and have to chew to allow the venom to penetrate; therefore, serious envenomations are not common.

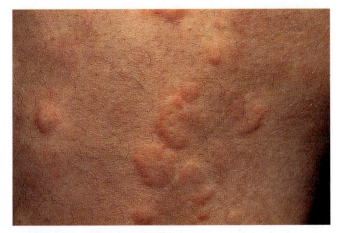

FIGURE 22-8 Allergic urticaria.
(From Forbes CD, Jackson WF: *World atlas and text of clinical medicine*, ed 3, London, 1993, Mosby–Year Book Europe Limited.)

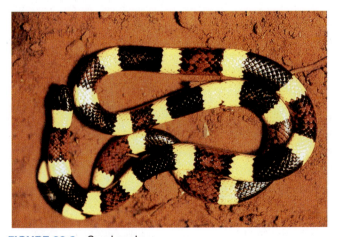

FIGURE 22-9 Coral snake.
(From Sanders M: *Mosby's paramedic textbook*, ed 3, St. Louis, 2006, Mosby.)

Pit vipers (Figure 22-10) are found throughout large portions of North America and include *rattlesnakes* of various types, *copperheads* (Figure 22-11), and *water moccasins,* or *cottonmouths* (Figure 22-12). The majority of pit viper bites do not occur in the backcountry, but rather occur in rural, suburban, or even urban areas. A classic example is the intoxicated man who was kissing his pet rattlesnake when he was bitten on the lips or tongue.

Snakebites are not as rare as one might think. This is further complicated by the variety of prehospital treatments attempted by patients, bystanders, or sometimes EMS personnel. The only treatment shown to be effective for envenomated pit viper bites is antivenin (antivenom), which is very expensive (thousands of dollars for a single treatment) and, thus, not routinely carried in first-aid kits. Indeed, the only "street" care proven to be helpful is transportation to the hospital.

The first thing to do to treat snakebite is to *watch for signs of envenomation* (venom was injected). Only a fraction of

bites by pit vipers actually result in envenomation and the signs of envenomation are fairly distinct. Although signs and symptoms of envenomation usually develop in a few minutes, sometimes they are delayed by 6 to 8 hours or perhaps even longer, so starting to the hospital after a suspected poisonous snakebite is appropriate. Signs of envenomation include the following:

a. Severe local swelling, bruising, and pain
b. Continued bleeding from the bite
c. Paresthesias in the fingers and toes (paresthesia is unusual sensation, usually caused by damage to nerves or biochemical abnormalities; a feeling of "pins and needles" is a common paresthesia)
d. Metallic taste in the mouth
e. Feeling of severe anxiety ("impending doom")
f. Nausea, vomiting, and abdominal pain

The following are treatments that have been recommended over the years but are **not** supported by the literature and **should not be performed:**

1. *Rest.* Some recommendations insist that those who have been bitten should always avoid exertion. Deaths from North American snakebite are very rare,[51] and it is very unlikely that the exertion of hiking out from a backcountry area will make a snakebite victim significantly more ill. If the victim can be carried out, that is ideal. However, if waiting for a carryout will delay the victim's arrival at a hospital, the victim should walk out with whatever assistance can be given.

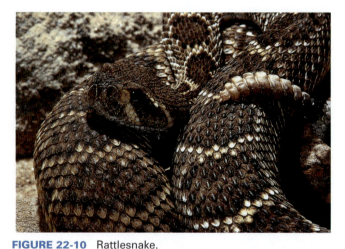

FIGURE 22-10 Rattlesnake.
(From Sanders M: *Mosby's paramedic textbook,* ed 3, St Louis, 2006, Mosby.)

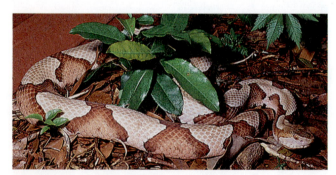

FIGURE 22-11 Copperhead snake.
(From Auerbach PS: Wilderness medicine: *Management of wilderness and environmental emergencies,* ed 4, St. Louis, 2001, Mosby.)

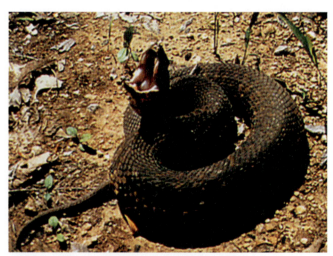

FIGURE 22-12 Water moccasin (cottonmouth) snake.
(From Auerbach PS: *Wilderness medicine: Management of wilderness and environmental emergencies,* ed 4, St. Louis, 2001, Mosby.)

2. *Catch the snake and bring it to the hospital.* There are numerous reports of bystanders who tried to catch a suspected poisonous snake and were bitten during the attempt. A single antivenin is used for all domestic pit-viper venoms, and treatment is based on clinical degree of envenomation, relying on the previous signs and symptoms. Therefore, identifying a domestic snake is of minor importance compared with the dangers of attempting to catch the snake. A digital photograph of the snake might be useful, but identification is not worth the risk of an additional bite.

3. *Suction.* Suction, with or without cutting, has been shown to be useless for poisonous snakebite. Snakebite kits consisting of suction devices should be left out of all first-aid kits and should never be used.[52,53]

4. *Electric shock.* Electric shock, whether applied to the snake or to the snakebite, has been shown to be totally ineffective and should never be used.[54,55]

5. *Cold packs.* Cold packs have been shown to increase tissue damage from North American pit-viper bites and should not be used.[56]

6. *Splinting, arterial or venous tourniquets, lymph constrictors, or elastic bandages.* Although widely recommended, none of these treatments has been shown to be effective and may worsen local damage to the bite area.[57,58]

The "Wilderness EMS" Context Revisited

At the beginning of this chapter, we asked *when* EMS is "wilderness EMS:" "When should we think about wilderness EMS; that is, when should we think and work differently from what we do on the street?"

Based on this chapter, the reader can probably provide the short answer: "It depends."

Time, distance, weather, and terrain all enter into the decision. The decision that a particular patient, in a particular situation, with a particular set of injuries, needs "wilderness" care rather than "street" care is a medical decision—one best made by the prehospital care provider directly attending the patient. If the provider at the scene can contact a knowledgeable EMS physician, especially one with wilderness EMS experience or training, the advice is definitely worth seeking. Ultimately, the decision is up to the prehospital care provider at the scene.

PHTLS has always held that, given a good fund of knowledge and key principles, prehospital care providers, other EMS personnel, and EMTs are capable of making reasoned decisions regarding patient care.

SUMMARY

- While many of the principles of wilderness EMS are the same as "street" EMS, preferences and practice may change because of the unique circumstances.
- Wilderness patients seldom need more or different invasive procedures; they do usually need prehospital care providers with keen critical thinking skills.
- Clinical situations in which wilderness care is different include clearing the cervical spine, irrigating wounds, reducing dislocations, and terminating CPR.

- Managing patients in the wilderness setting requires that the medical care providers have a good understanding of environmental medical issues (see Chapters 20 and 21).
- When managing patients in the wilderness, the prehospital care providers have to also consider food and water requirements and elimination needs.
- A basic principle of wilderness care is that all patients are hypothermic, hypoglycemic, and hypovolemic.

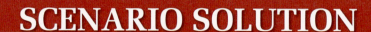

SCENARIO SOLUTION

You, as the team's wilderness EMT, briefly examine the patient and find an open fracture of the tibia and fibula. While the fall also caused a laceration to the scalp, a cervical spinal exam does not reveal any necessity for spinal immobilization. You are also concerned that the patient has been in low temperatures overnight, but are somewhat relieved as the patient's level of consciousness is normal suggesting only mild hyperthermia at worst. You decide to treat the hypothermia using passive rewarming techniques. You radio for the incoming extraction team to bring a lower leg splint along with a Stokes basket. While waiting for the extrication crew to arrive, you realign the fracture and dress the lower leg wound. You also begin to rehydrate the hunter as he did not have any water with him overnight. You provide him some high carbohydrate energy bars since he has not eaten since noon yesterday. You then examine the head wound and find that it is contaminated with dirt and debris. You irrigate the wound

and dress it. It takes the extraction team 90 minutes to reach your location. You splint the lower leg with the commercial splint. Since you have determined by examination that no cervical immobilization is needed, you place the patient directly into the Stokes basket for transport. At this point, you have 12 rescuers available and begin to transport the patient toward the extraction point. After an hour, you have only made it a half mile from the site. Additional rescuers are called to help with the extraction. As the team medic, besides providing care for the patient, you are also responsible for the team's health and safety. You make sure team members have sunscreen available as it is reaching the middle of the day. You monitor the hydration status of not only the patient, but also the team members, reminding them to take breaks and drink plenty of fluid. Finally, after two and a half hours you reach the waiting ambulance and turn the patient over to the crew for transport to the local hospital 17 miles away. ■

References

1. Demarest JH. *Prehospital trauma life support,* Akron, OH, 1986, Emergency Training.
2. *Merriam-Webster's collegiate dictionary,* ed 10, Springfield, MA, 1996, Merriam-Webster, Inc.
3. Chan D, Goldberg R, Tascone A, et al. The effect of spinal immobilization on healthy volunteers. *Ann Emerg Med* 23(1):48, 1994.
4. Conover K. EMTs should be able to clear the cervical spine in the wilderness (editorial). *J Wild Med* 3(4):339, 1992.
5. Gomi T. *Everyone poops,* Brooklyn, NY, 1993, Kane/Miller Book Publishers.
6. Goldberg R, Chan D, Mason J, Chan L. Backboard versus mattress splint immobilization: A comparison of symptoms generated. *J Emerg Med,* 14(3):293, 1996.
7. Hamilton RS, Pons PT. The efficacy and comfort of full-body vacuum splints for cervical-spine immobilization. *J Emerg Med* 14(5):553, 1996.
8. Johnson DR, Hauswald M, Stockhoff C. Comparison of a vacuum splint device to a rigid backboard for spinal immobilization. *Am J Emerg Med* 14(4):369, 1996.
9. Lovell ME, Evans JH. A comparison of the spinal board and the vacuum stretcher, spinal stability and interface pressure. *Injury* 25(3):179, 1994.
10. Cordell WH, Hollingsworth JC, Olinger ML, et al: Pain and tissue-interface pressures during spine-board immobilization. *Ann Emerg Med* 26(1):31, 1995.
11. Delbridge TR, Auble TE, Garrison HG, Menengazzi JJ: Discomfort in healthy volunteers immobilized on wooden backboards and

vacuum mattress splints. *Prehosp Disaster Med* 8(suppl 2), 1993.
12. Linares HA, Mawson AR, Suarez E: Association between pressure sores and immobilization in the immediate postinjury period. *Orthopedics* 10:571, 1987.
13. Mawson AR, Bundo JJ, Neville P: Risk factors for early occurring pressure ulcers following spinal cord injury. *Am J Phys Med Rehab* 67:123, 1988.
14. Edlich RF, Rodeheaver GT, Morgan RF, et al: Principles of emergency wound management. *Ann Emerg Med* 17(12):1284, 1988.
15. Edlich RF, Thacker JG, Buchanan L, Rodeheaver GT: Modern concepts of treatment of traumatic wounds. *Adv Surg* 13:169, 1979.
16. Bhandari M, Thompson K, Adili A, Shaughnessy SG: High and low pressure irrigation in contaminated wounds with exposed bone. *Int J Surg Invest* 2(3):179, 2000.
17. Bhandari M, Adili A, Lachowski RJ: High pressure pulsatile lavage of contaminated human tibiae: An in vitro study. *J Orthop Trauma* 12(7):479, 1998.
18. Bhandari M, Schemitsch EH, Adili A, et al: High and low pressure pulsatile lavage of contaminated tibial fractures: An in vitro study of bacterial adherence and bone damage. *J Orthop Trauma* 13(8):526, 1999.
19. Anglen JO: Wound irrigation in musculoskeletal injury. *J Am Acad Orthop Surg* 9(4):219, 2001.
20. Valente JH, Forti RJ, Freundlich LF, et al: Wound irrigation in children: Saline solution or tap water? *Ann Emerg Med* 41(5):609, 2003.

21. Backer HD: Field water disinfection. In Auerbach PS, Geehr EC, editors: *Wilderness medicine: Management of wilderness and environmental emergencies,* ed 2, St. Louis, 1989, Mosby.

22. Griffiths RD, Fernandez RS, Ussia CA: Is tap water a safe alternative to normal saline for wound irrigation in the community setting? *J Wound Care* 10(10):407, 2001.

23. Moscati R, Mayrose J, Fincher L, Jehle D: Comparison of normal saline with tap water for wound irrigation. *Am J Emerg Med* 16(4):379, 1998.

24. Moscati RM, Reardon RF, Lerner EB, Mayrose J: Wound irrigation with tap water. *Acad Emerg Med* 5(11):1076, 1998.

25. Rodeheaver GT, Pettry D, Thacker JG, et al: Wound cleansing by high pressure irrigation. *Surg Gynecol Obstet* 141(3):357, 1975.

26. Edlich RF, Reddy VR: Revolutionary advances in wound repair in emergency medicine during the last three decades: A view toward the new millennium. 5th Annual David R. Boyd, MD, Lecture. *J Emerg Med* 20(2):167, 2001.

27. Singer AJ, Hollander JE, Subramanian S, et al: Pressure dynamics of various irrigation techniques commonly used in the emergency department. *Ann Emerg Med* 24(1):36, 1994.

28. Mellor SG, Cooper GJ, Bowyer GW: Efficacy of delayed administration of benzylpenicillin in the control of infection in penetrating soft tissue injuries in war. *J Trauma* 40(3 Suppl):S128–134, 1996.

29. Hospenthal DR, Murray CK, Andersen RC, et al: Guidelines for the prevention of infection after combat-related injuries. *J Trauma* 64(3 Suppl):S211–220, 2008.

30. Fulton RL, Voigt WJ, Hilakos AS: Confusion surrounding the treatment of traumatic cardiac arrest. *J Am Coll Surg* 181:209, 1995.

31. Pasquale MD, Rhodes M, Cipolle MD, et al: Defining "dead on arrival:" Impact on a Level I trauma center. *J Trauma* 41:726, 1996.

32. Mattox KL, Feliciano DV: Role of external cardiac compression in truncal trauma. *J Trauma* 22:934, 1982.

33. Shimazu S, Shatney CH: Outcomes of trauma patients with no vital signs on admission. *J Trauma* 23(3):213, 1983.

34. Forgey WW, Wilderness Medical Society: *Practice guidelines for wilderness emergency care,* ed 2, Guilford, Conn, 2001, Globe Pequot Press.

35. Goth P, Garnett G, Rural Affairs Committee, National Association of EMS Physicians: Clinical guidelines for delayed/prolonged transport. I. Cardiorespiratory arrest. *Prehosp Disaster Med* 6(3):335, 1991.

36. Bowman WD: CPR and wilderness rescue: When and when not to use it. *Response,* 1987.

37. Eisenberg MS, Bergner L, Hallstrom AP: Cardiac resuscitation in the community: Importance of rapid provision and implications of program planning. *JAMA* 241:1905, 1979.

38. Kellermann AL, Hackman BB, Somes G: Predicting the outcome of unsuccessful prehospital advanced cardiac life support. *JAMA* 270(12):1433, 1993.

39. Bonnin MJ, Pepe PE, Kimball KT, Clark PS: Distinct criteria for termination of resuscitation in the out-of-hospital setting. *JAMA* 270(12):1457, 1993.

40. Leavitt M, Podgorny G: Prehospital CPR and the pulseless hypothermic patient. *Ann Emerg Med* 13:492, 1984.

41. Keatinge WR: Accidental immersion hypothermia and drowning. *Practitioner* 219:183, 1977.

42. Olshaker JS: Near drowning. *Emerg Med Clin North Am* 10(2):339, 1992.

43. Bolte RG, Black PG, Bowers RS, et al: The use of extracorporeal rewarming in a child submerged for 66 minutes. *JAMA* 260(3):377, 1988.

44. Orlowski JP: Drowning, near-drowning, and ice-water drowning. *JAMA* 260(3):390, 1988.

45. Cooper MA: Lightning injuries. In Auerbach PS, Geehr EC, editors: *Wilderness medicine: Management of wilderness and environmental emergencies,* ed 2, St. Louis, 1989, Mosby.

46. Durrer B, Brugger H: Recent advances in avalanche survival. Presented at the Second World Congress on Wilderness Medicine, Aspen, CO, 1995.

47. Steinman AM: Cardiopulmonary resuscitation and hypothermia. *Circulation* 74(6, pt 2):29, 1986.

48. Zell SC: Epidemiology of wilderness-acquired diarrhea: Implications for prevention and treatment. *J Wild Med* 3(3):241, 1992.

49. Lloyd EL: *Hypothermia and cold stress,* Rockville, MD, 1986, Aspen Systems.

50. Maningas PA, DeGuzman LR, Hollenbach SJ, et al: Regional blood flow during hypothermic arrest. *Ann Emerg Med* 15(4):390, 1986.

51. Curry SC, Kunkel DB: Death from a rattlesnake bite. *Am J Emerg Med* 3(3):227, 1985.

52. Bush SP: Snakebite suction devices don't remove venom: They just suck. *Ann Emerg Med* 43(2):187, 2004.

53. Alberts MB, Shalit M, LoGalbo F: Suction for venomous snakebite: A study of "mock venom" extraction in a human model. *Ann Emerg Med* 43(2):181, 2004.

54. Davis D, Branch K, Egen NB, et al: The effect of an electrical current on snake venom toxicity. *J Wild Med* 3(1):48, 1992.

55. Howe NR, Meisenheimer JL Jr: Electric shock does not save snakebitten rats. *Ann Emerg Med* 17(3):254, 1988.

56. Gill KA Jr: The evaluation of cryotherapy in the treatment of snake envenomation. *South Med J* 63:552, 1968.

57. Norris RL: A call for snakebite research. *Wilderness Environ Med* 11(3):149, 2000.

58. Stewart ME, Greenland S, Hoffman JR: First-aid treatment of poisonous snakebite: Are currently recommended procedures justified? *Ann Emerg Med* 10(6):331, 1981.

Suggested Reading

Auerbach PS, editor: Wilderness medicine: Management of wilderness and environmental emergencies, ed 5, St. Louis, 2007, Mosby Elsevier.

Goth P, Garnett G: Clinical guidelines for delayed or prolonged transport: II. Dislocations. Rural Affairs Committee, National Association of Emergency Medical Services Physicians. Prehosp Disaster Med 8(1):77, 1993.

Goth P, Garnett G: Clinical guidelines for delayed or prolonged transport: IV. Wounds. Rural Affairs Committee, Nation Association of Emergency Medical Services Physicians. Prehosp Disaster Med 8(3):253, 1993.

CHAPTER 23

Civilian Tactical Emergency Medical Support (TEMS)

CHAPTER OBJECTIVES

At the completion of this chapter, the reader will be able to do the following:

✓ Describe the components of tactical emergency medical support.

✓ Understand the operational and support functions of TEMS.

✓ Explain the benefits of a TEMS program.

✓ Discuss how emergency medical care differs in each of the three zones of care.

✓ Relate how remote assessment methodogology may be used on a tactical mission.

✓ Describe the role of medical support for counterterrorism operations.

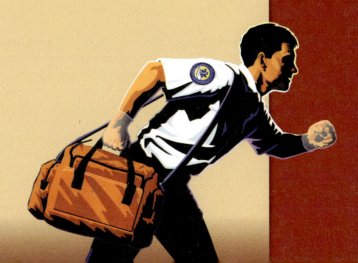

SCENARIO

Your ambulance service provides coverage for the local SWAT team and has a rigorous, integrated training program with local law enforcement. Your team receives a call regarding a domestic disturbance. When you arrive, two officers cross the suspect's yard and approach the house. Shots ring out from the front window, wounding the officers. One officer falls in the door way of the suspect's house. The second falls near a low dividing wall. A patrol officer standing next to you yells, "We need to go get them. Come on!" You grab the officer by the arm and look to the SWAT Commander.

What should your actions be? How will you assess and treat the fallen officers given the danger of the scene?

HISTORY AND EVOLUTION OF TEMS

Tactical Emergency Medical Support (TEMS) is an out-of-hospital system of care dedicated to enhancing the probability of special operations law enforcement mission success and promoting public safety.[1] TEMS builds upon the principles of military medicine, wilderness medicine, disaster response, urban search and rescue, and conventional EMS to create a system of care that supports law enforcement missions *and* maximizes the clinical outcome for casualties in what is often a resource-poor, prolonged-transport environment while minimizing the threat to the provider. This chapter provides a brief overview of TEMS roles and responsibilities. Participation in TEMS requires specific training and expertise that is beyond the scope of this chapter.

The first SWAT team was developed in Los Angeles in 1968. Shortly thereafter, the thought of having a "medic" attached to the team was pushed forward. TEMS encompasses a broad spectrum of medical services modified in structure and function to operate within the high-risk, high-paced tactical environment. Since its origin in the 1960s to support SWAT operations, TEMS has evolved into an area of special expertise. Professional support for TEMS began within the law enforcement community and expanded into the medical arena following the military model of having a "medic" available during high-risk operations. Broad support for TEMS now exists within both communities. Over 20 years ago, the Counter Narcotics and Terrorism Operational Medical Support (CONTOMS) course was developed. This program developed an evidence-based TEMS curriculum that took seasoned field providers and, in 56 hours, immersed them in providing medical care in the tactical environment. Through CONTOMS, an injury database was developed providing the research base needed to support the efficacy of tactical medicine. The National Tactical Officers Association (NTOA) endorsed TEMS as "an important element of tactical law enforcement" and began to promote training of

tactical medics.[2] After the September 11, 2001 attacks, both the National Association of Emergency Medical Service Physicians (NAEMSP) and the American College of Emergency Physician (ACEP) formally endorsed integrating EMS capabilities into law enforcement special operations.[3,4]

The Tactical Combat Casualty Care (TCCC) guidelines are currently considered to be the standard of care for military tactical medicine. Both the American College of Surgeons Committee on Trauma (ACS-COT) and the National Association of Emergency Medical Technicians (NAEMT), through its PHTLS program, endorse the TCCC guidelines.[5] Though military and law enforcement special operations are unique, similarities exist in the operational medical care aspects. The TCCC guidelines represent a strong starting point for standardization of TEMS protocols and are endorsed by the NTOA.

TEMS COMPONENTS

Basic Concepts and Considerations

In the United States, most federal and many state and local law enforcement agencies have tactical medical support programs. In law enforcement, "special operations" denotes those activities that are too dangerous, complex, or technical to assign to uniformed patrol units. Special teams carry out these missions and emphasize training, coordination and speed, stealth, and violence of action to ensure success. They often use advanced technology, such as less lethal weapons systems, encrypted communications, armour, remote imaging, acoustic capture devices, and similar equipment. Special operations teams are generally comprised of the fittest, fastest, brightest, and most motivated personnel. The units carry a wide variety of names, including Special Weapons and Tactics (SWAT), Special Response Team (SRT), Hostage Rescue Team (HRT), Counter Assault Team (CAT), Emergency Response Team (ERT), and Special Operations Unit (SOU).

SCENARIO SOLUTION

The SWAT commander orders you to utilize your Rapid Assess Methodology (RAM) to determine the utility of a rescue effort. You use your binoculars and the SWAT team acoustic device to examine the two fallen officers. The first officer, lying in the doorway of the gunman's house shows no chest wall movement or signs of condensation near his mouth. Despite calls from his fellow officers, you are unable to detect a response on the acoustic device. The second officer has moved behind a low brick wall. You can visualize bleeding from his lower thigh. Fortunately, you have conducted extensive tactical medical training for your officers. You communicate with him via the secure team radio and instruct him to apply a tourniquet two finger breadths above his wound. He secures the device and communicates that he has no further injuries.

Based upon your recommendation and the threat assessment, the SWAT Commander chooses not to undertake a high-risk rescue of the officer showing no signs of life. You remain in contact with the second injured officer while the negotiators work to convince the suspect to surrender. You contact the local Trauma Center and inform them of a potential incoming casualty. Thirty minutes later, the suspect surrenders and is taken into custody. Your team evacuates the casualty to the local hospital where he undergoes a vascular repair saving both his leg and his life. ■

References

1. Rinnert KJ, Hall WL: Tactical emergency medical support. *Emerg Med Clin N Am* 20:929–952, 2002.
2. National Tactical Officers Association: Position statement on the inclusion of physicians in tactical law enforcement operations in the USA. *The Tactical Edge* 86, Spring 1994.
3. Heck JJ, Pierluisi G: Law enforcement special operations and medical support. *Prehosp Emerg Care* 5:403–406, 2001.
4. American College of Emergency Physicians: Policy statement on tactical emergency medical support. *Ann Emerg Med* 45:108, 2005.
5. McSwain NE, Frame S, Paturas JL, editors: *Prehospital trauma life support manual*. ed 6, Akron, 2005, Mosby.
6. Kolman JA: *A guide to the development of special weapons and tactics teams*, Springfield, IL, 1982, Charles C Thomas.
7. Gildea JR, Janssen AR: Tactical emergency medical support: Physician involvement and injury patterns in tactical teams. *J Emerg Med* 35(4):411–414, 2008.
8. Sztajnkrycer MD, Callaway DW, Baez AA: Police officer response to the injured officer: A survey- based analysis of medical care decisions. *Prehosp Disaster Med* 22(4):335–341; discussion 342, 2007.
9. *Sams v Oelrich*, 717 So2d 1044 (1998), Court of Appeal of Florida, First District.
10. *Shepherd v Washington County*, AR, 962 SW2d 779 (1998), Supreme Court of Arkansas.
11. State of Massachusetts Statewide Treatment Protocols (7.02) Appendix U. April 2, 2009.
12. Campbell JP, Gratton MC, Salomone JA III, et al: Ambulance arrival to patient contact: The hidden component of prehospital response time intervals. *Ann Emerg Med* 22:1254, 1993.
13. Kanable R: Peak performance: well-trained tactical medics can help the team perform at its best. *Law Enforcement Technology*, August 1999.
14. Jagoda A, Pietrzek M, Hazen S, et al: Prehospital care and the military, *Mil Med* 157:11, 1992.
15. Bellamy RF: The causes of death in conventional land warfare: implications for combat casualty care research, *Mil Med* 149:55, 1984.
16. Callaway, DW: *Tactical emergency services. Disaster*, ed 2, Burstein & Hogan. Philadelphia, PA, 2007, Lippincott, Williams and Williams.
17. Delorenzo, TA, Porter RS: *Tactical emergency care*, Upper Saddle River, NY, 1999, Prentice- Hall.
18. Holcomb, J and Butler F. Personal Communication, 2009.
19. Kragh JF, Walters TJ, Baer DG, et al: Survival with emergency tourniquet use to stop bleeding in major limb trauma. *Ann Surg* 249 (1):1–7, 2009.
20. Butler FK, Hagmann JH, Butler EG: Tactical combat casualty care in special operations. *Mil Med* 161:3–16, 1996.
21. Ciccone TJ, Anderson PD, Chon AD, et al: Successful development and implementation of a tactical emergency medical technician training program for United States federal agents. *Prehosp Disaster Med* 20(1):36–39, 2005.
22. Sohn VY, Eckert MJ, Martin MJ, et al: Efficacy of three topical hemostatic agents applied by medics in a lethal groin injury model. *J Surg Res* 154(2):258–261, 2009.
23. Kheirabadi BS, Edens JW, Terrazas IB, et al: Comparison of new hemostatic granules/powders with currently deployed hemostatic products in a lethal model of extremity arterial hemorrhage in swine. *J Trauma* 66(2):316–326; discussion 327–328, 2009.
24. Butler FK Jr, Hagmann J, Butler EG: Tactical combat casualty care in special operations. *Mil Med* 161 (Suppl):3–16, 1996.
25. Tien HC, Jung V, Rizoli SB, et al: An evaluation of tactical combat casualty care interventions in a combat environment. *J Am Coll Surg* 207(2):174–178, 2008.
26. Rasumoff D, Carmona R: Suggested guidelines for TEMS policy and SOP. *Tactical Edge J* 95–96, Summer 1999.
27. Arishita GI, Vayer JS, Bellamy RF: Cervical spine immobilization of penetrating neck wounds in a hostile environment. *J Trauma* 29:332–337, 1989.
28. Rosemary AS, Norris PA, Olson SM, et al: Prehospital traumatic cardiac arrest: The cost of futility. *J Trauma* 38:468–474, 1998.
29. Revell M, Greaves I, Porter K: Endpoints for fluid resuscitation in hemorrhagic shock. *J Trauma* 54 (5 Suppl):S63–67, 2003.

30. Lavergne GM: *A sniper in the tower,* New York, 1997, Bantam Books.

31. Trainer key #412: *Transportation of prisoners II,* Arlington, VA: International Association of Chiefs of Police, 1992.

32. Casualty Care Research Center: *Counter narcotics and terrorism operational medical support medical director's course handbook,* ed 2, Bethesda, MD, Casualty Care Research Center.

33. *Emergency medical technician: tactical course manual,* ed 15, Bethesda, MD, 2000, Uniformed Services University of the Health Sciences.

34. Cloonan C: In *Proceedings of the Third International Conference on Tactical Emergency Medical Support,* Bethesda, MD, 1999, Uniformed Services University of the Health Sciences.

35. US Department of Health and Human Services, Centers for Disease Control and Prevention: Bioterrorism alleging use of anthrax and interim guidelines for management—United States, 1998. *MMWR* 48(4):69, 1999.

36. Okumura T, Takasu N, Ishimatsu S, et al: Report on 640 victims of the Tokyo subway sarin attack. *Ann Emerg Med* 28:129, 1996.

37. Downey R: Terrorism and the fire service: Preparing for today's threats. *Fire Engineering,* August 1996, 109–,111.

38. Stein M, Hirshberg A: Trauma care in the new millennium: Medical consequences of terrorism. *Surg Clin North Am* 79:1538, 1999.

39. MacIntyre AG, Christopher GW, Eitzen E, et al: Weapons of mass destruction events with contaminated casualties. *JAMA* 283:242, 2000.

40. Federal Response Plan, Terrorism Incident Annex, 2003, Federal Emergency Management Agency, http://www.fema.gov/rrr/frp/frpterr.shtm. Accessed Jun 2005.

41. Tang N, Kelen GD: Role of tactical EMS in support of public safety and the public health response to a hostile mass casualty incident. *Disaster Med Public Health Prep* 1(1 Suppl):S55–56, 2007.

Glossary

accelerated motion A sudden surge or increase in motion, e.g., from the transferring of energy in a rear-impact collision; occurs as a slower moving or stationary object is struck from behind.

acetabulum The cup-shaped hip socket on the lateral surface of the pelvis that holds the head of the femur.

acidosis Accumulation of acids and decreased pH of the blood.

acute radiation syndrome The physiologic consequences of whole-body radiation.

acute respiratory distress syndrome (ARDS) Respiratory insufficiency as a result of damage to the lining of the capillaries and alveoli in the lung, leading to the leakage of fluid into the interstitial spaces and alveoli.

acute tubular necrosis (ATN) Acute damage to the renal tubules, usually due to ischemia associated with shock.

adolescent A child with the body size and physical development normally found in children between 13 and 16 years of age.

adult A person (generally 16 years of age or older) whose body has reached maturity and has finished its progression through the phases of pediatric growth and development.

aerobic metabolism Oxygen-based metabolism that is the body's principal combustion process; most efficient process for the production of cellular energy.

aerosol Solid particles and liquid particles that are suspended in air.

afterload The pressure against which the left ventricle must pump out (eject) blood with each beat.

air bags Bags that automatically inflate in front of the driver or passenger upon collision to cushion the impact. The bags absorb the energy slowly by increasing the body's stopping distance. These bags are only designed to cushion forward motion on the initial impact.

alveoli The terminal air sacs of the respiratory tract where the respiratory system meets the circulatory system and gas exchange occurs.

Alzheimer's disease A form of brain disease commonly associated with premature senile dementia.

amnesia A loss of memory.

amputation A severed part or a part that is surgically totally separated (removed) from the rest of the body.

anaerobic metabolism Metabolism not using oxygen, an inefficient process for the production of cellular energy.

analgesia The relief of pain.

anatomical splinting "Splinting" the body on a long backboard, in a supine position and securing the patient to the board.

angina (angina pectoris) A cramping, crushing midsternal chest pain caused by myocardial anoxia. It often radiates to either arm, most commonly the left, or the jaw and is associated with a feeling of suffocation and impending death.

anhidrosis The absence of sweating.

anisocoria Inequality of pupil size.

anterior cord syndrome Damage to the anterior portion of the spinal cord, usually as a result of bony fragments or pressure on spinal arteries.

anterocaudad Forward and toward the feet.

anterograde amnesia Amnesia for events occurring after the precipitating trauma; inability to form new memories.

anticoagulant A substance or drug that prevents or delays coagulation or the forming of blood clots.

antihypertensive A drug that reduces high blood pressure (hypertension).

aortic tear Complete or partial tear of one or more layers of tissue of the aorta.

apnea An absence of spontaneous breathing.

arachnoid mater (arachnoid membrane) Spiderweb-like transparent membrane between the dura mater and the pia mater; the middle of the three meningeal membranes surrounding the brain.

ARDS See *acute respiratory distress syndrome.*

ascending nerve tracts Nerve pathways in the spinal cord that carry sensory impulses from body parts up to the brain.

ataxic breathing Erratic breathing with no rhythm. Commonly associated with head injury and increased intracranial pressure.

atelectasis Collapse of alveoli or part of the lung.

atherosclerosis A narrowing of the blood vessels; a condition in which the inner layer of the artery wall thickens while fatty deposits build up within the artery.

atlas First cervical vertebra (C1); the skull perches upon it.

austere environment A setting in which resources, supplies, equipment, personnel, transportation, and other aspects of the physical, political, social, and economic environments are extremely limited.

autonomic nervous system The part of the central nervous system that directs and controls the involuntary functions of the body.

avulsion The ripping or tearing away of a part; a flap or partially separated tissue or part.

axial unloading Taking the weight of the head off the cervical spine.

axis Second cervical vertebra (C2); its shape allows for the wide possible range of rotation of the head. Also, an imaginary line that passes through the center of the body.

bag-mask device Mechanical ventilation device consisting of a self-inflating bag made of plastic or rubber and several one-way valves; squeezing the bag results in positive-pressure ventilation through a mask or endotracheal tube. May be used with or without supplementary oxygen.

baroreceptor A sensory nerve ending that is stimulated by changes in blood pressure. Baroreceptors are found in the walls of the atria of the heart, vena cava, aortic arch, and carotid sinus.

basal metabolic rate The number of calories the body burns while at rest, resulting in heat production as a byproduct of metabolism.

basilar skull fracture Fracture of the floor of the cranium.

Battle's sign Discoloration posterior and slightly inferior to the outer ears due to bleeding into the subcutaneous tissue caused by an occipital basilar skull fracture.

birdshot Small metal pellets loaded into shotgun shells.

blunt trauma Nonpenetrating trauma caused by a rapidly moving object that impacts the body.

body surface area (BSA) Outer surface of the body covered by the skin; percentage of the body's total surface area represented by any body part. Used as one factor in determining size of a burn.

bradycardia Heart rate less than 60 beats per minute.

brain stem The stem-like part of the brain that connects the cerebral hemispheres with the spinal cord.

bronchioles The smaller divisions of the bronchial tubes.

Broselow Resuscitation Tape A commercially available system for estimating pediatric medication dosing and equipment sizing based on patient length.

Brown-Séquard syndrome Caused by penetrating injury and involves hemitransection of the spinal cord involving only one side of the cord.

buckshot Large metal pellets loaded into shotgun shells.

capillaries The smallest blood vessels. Minute blood vessels that are only one cell wide, allowing for diffusion and osmosis of oxygen and nutrients through the capillary walls.

capnography (end-tidal carbon dioxide) The method of monitoring the partial pressure of carbon dioxide in a sample of gas. It can correlate very closely to the arterial partial pressure of carbon dioxide ($PaCO_2$).

cardiac output The volume of blood pumped by the heart at each contraction (reported in liters per minute).

cardioaccelerator center The brain center that activates the sympathetic response that increases the rate of the heart.

cardiogenic shock Shock that results from failure of the heart's pumping activity; causes can be categorized as either intrinsic, a result of direct damage to the heart itself, or extrinsic, related to a problem outside the heart.

cardioinhibitory center A part of the medulla that slows or inhibits the heart's activity.

cardiovascular Referring to the combination of the heart and blood vessels.

cataract Milky lens that blocks and distorts light entering the eye and blurs vision.

catecholamines Group of chemicals produced by the body that work as important nerve transmitters. The main catecholamines made by the body are dopamine, epinephrine (also called adrenalin), and norepinephrine. They are part of the body's sympathetic defense mechanism used in preparing the body to act.

caudad Toward the tail (coccyx).

cavitation Forcing tissues of the body out of their normal position; to cause a temporary or permanent cavity (e.g., when the body is struck by a bullet, the acceleration of particles of tissue away from the missile produces an area of injury in which a large temporary cavity occurs).

cellular respiration The use of oxygen by the cells to produce energy.

central cord syndrome Damage to the central portion of the spinal cord that usually occurs with hyperextension of the cervical area.

central neurogenic hyperventilation Pathologic rapid and shallow ventilatory pattern associated with head injury and increased intracranial pressure.

cephalad Toward the head.

cerebellum A portion of the brain that lies beneath the cerebrum and behind the medulla oblongata and is concerned with coordination of movement.

cerebral perfusion pressure The amount of pressure needed to maintain cerebral blood flow; calculated as the difference between the mean arterial pressure (MAP) and the intracranial pressure (ICP).

cerebrospinal fluid (CSF) A fluid found in the subarachnoid space and dural sheath; acts as a shock absorber, protecting the brain and spinal cord from jarring impact.

cerebrum The largest part of the brain; responsible for the control of specific intellectual, sensory, and motor functions.

cervical flexion Bending the head forward or downward, causing bending of the neck.

cervical spine The neck area of the spinal column containing seven vertebrae (C1–C7).

chemical burn Burn that occurs when skin comes into contact with various caustic agents.

chemical energy The energy, usually in the form of heat, that results from the interaction of a chemical with other chemicals or human tissue.

chemoreceptor cells Cells that stimulate nerve impulses by reacting to chemical stimuli. Certain chemoreceptor cells control the ventilatory rate.

chemoreceptor A sensory nerve ending that is stimulated by and reacts to certain chemical stimuli; located outside of the central nervous system. Chemoreceptors are found in the large arteries of the thorax and neck, the taste buds, and the olfactory cells of the nose.

Cheyne-Stokes breathing Pathologic ventilatory pattern with periods of shallow, slow breathing increasing to rapid, deep breathing and then returning to shallow, slow breathing followed by a short apneic period. Commonly associated with traumatic brain injury and increased intracranial pressure.

chin lift A way to open the airway of a patient with suspected cervical spine injury; adaptation of chin lift airway maneuver that includes manual immobilization of the head in a neutral in-line position.

cilia Hair-like processes of cells that propel foreign particles and mucus from the bronchi.

cingulate herniation The cingulate gyrus along the medial surface of the cerebral hemispheres is forced under the falx, usually as a result of hemorrhage or edema, causing injury to the medial cerebral hemispheres and the midbrain.

closed fracture A fracture of a bone in which the skin is not interrupted.

coagulopathy Impairment in the normal blood-clotting capabilities.

coagulative necrosis The type of tissue damage that results from acid exposure; the damaged tissue forms a barrier that prevents deeper penetration of the acid.

coccygeal spine The most caudad part of the spinal column; contains the three to five vertebrae that form the coccyx.

cold zone A geographic area that is free from contamination from a hazardous material.

Colles' fracture Fracture of the wrist. If the victim falls forward onto outstretched hands to break a fall, this may result in a silver fork deformity.

compartment syndrome The clinical findings noted from ischemia and compromised circulation that can occur from vascular injury causing hypoxia of muscles in an extremity compartment. The cellular edema produces increased pressure in a closed facial or bony compartment.

compensated shock Inadequate peripheral perfusion as evidenced by signs of decreased organ perfusion but with normal blood pressure.

complacency A feeling of safety or security in the unacknowledged face of potential danger.

complete cord transection Complete damage and severing of the spinal cord; all spinal tracts are interrupted, and all cord functions distal the site are lost.

complication An added difficulty that occurs secondary to an injury, disease, or treatment. Also, disease or incident superimposed upon another without being specifically related yet affecting or modifying the prognosis of the original disease.

compressibility Ability to be deformed by the transfer of energy.

compression injuries Injuries caused by severe crushing and squeezing forces; may occur to the external structure of the body or to the internal organs.

compression Type of force involved in impacts resulting in a tissue, organ, or other body part being squeezed between two or more objects or body parts.

concussion A temporary alteration in neurologic function, most commonly a loss of consciousness, and no intracranial abnormality is identified by computed tomography (CT) scan.

conduction The transfer of heat between two objects in direct contact with each other.

consensual reflex The reflexive constriction of one pupil when a strong light is introduced into the other eye. A lack of consensual reflex is considered a positive sign of brain injury or eye injury.

contact wounds The type of wound that occurs when the muzzle of a gun touches the patient at the time of discharge, resulting in a circular entrance wound, often associated with visible burns, soot, or the imprint of the muzzle.

contraindication Any sign, symptom, clinical impression, condition, or circumstance indicating that a given treatment or course of treatment is inappropriate. Relative contraindication is usually considered as a contraindication but under special circumstances may be overruled by a physician as an accepted medical practice on a case-by-case basis.

contralateral On the opposite side.

contrecoup injury An injury to parts of the brain located on the side opposite that of the primary injury.

contusion A bruise or bruising.

convection The transfer of heat from the movement or circulation of a gas or liquid, such as the heating of water or air in contact with a body, removing that air (such as wind) or water, and then having to heat the new air or water that replaces what left.

cord compression Pressure on the spinal cord caused by swelling, which may result in tissue ischemia and, in some cases, may require decompression to prevent a permanent loss of function.

cord concussion The temporary disruption of the spinal cord functions distal to the site of a spinal cord injury.

cord contusion Bruising or bleeding into the tissue of the spinal cord, which may also result in a temporary loss of cord functions distal to the injury.

cord laceration Occurs when spinal cord tissue is torn or cut.

coup injury An injury to the brain located on the same side as the point of impact.

cranial vault The space within the skull or cranium.

crash Energy is exchanged between a moving object and the tissue of the human body or between the moving human body and a stationary object.

crepitus Crackling sound made by bone ends grating together.

cricothyroid membrane The thin, tough layer of tissue that is located between the thyroid and the cricoid cartilages, the site where a surgical opening is created during a cricothyrotomy.

crush syndrome The physiologic consequences that occur from severe muscle trauma after part of the body is crushed under a heavy weight, manifested by renal failure and death.

Cullen's sign Ecchymosis around the umbilicus.

Cushing's phenomenon The combination of increased arterial blood pressure and the resultant bradycardia that can occur with increased ICP.

cyanosis Blue coloring of skin, mucous membranes, or nail beds indicating unoxygenated hemoglobin and a lack of adequate oxygen levels in the blood; usually secondary to inadequate ventilation or decreased perfusion.

dead space The amount of space that contains air that never reaches the alveoli to participate in the critical gas exchange process.

decerebrate posturing Characteristic posture that occurs when a painful stimulus is introduced, the extremities are stiff and extended and the head is retracted. One of the forms of pathologic posturing (response) commonly associated with increased intracranial pressure.

decontamination Reduction or removal of hazardous chemical, biologic, or radiologic agents.

decorticate posturing A characteristic pathologic posture of a patient with increased intracranial pressure; when a painful stimulus is introduced, the patient is rigidly still with the back and lower extremities extended while the arms are flexed and fists clenched.

definitive care Care that resolves the patient's illness or injury after a definitive diagnosis has been established. Clear and final care that is without question what the particular patient needs for his or her individual problem.

density The number of particles in each given area of tissue.

dermatome The sensory area on the body for which a nerve root is responsible. Collectively, they allow the body areas to be mapped out for each spinal level and to help locate a spinal cord injury.

dermis Layer of skin just under the epidermis made up of a framework of connective tissues containing blood vessels, nerve endings, sebaceous glands, and sweat glands.

diaphragm The dome-shaped muscle that divides the chest and abdomen and which functions as part of the breathing process.

diaphragmatic rupture (diaphragmatic herniation) A tearing or cutting of the diaphragm so that the abdominal and thoracic cavities are no longer separated, allowing abdominal contents to enter the thoracic cavity. Usually a result of increased intra-abdominal pressure producing a tear in the diaphragm.

diaphyseal Part of or affecting the shaft of a long bone.

diastole Ventricular relaxation (ventricular filling).

diastolic blood pressure The resting pressure between ventricular contractions, measured in millimeters of mercury (mm Hg).

diffusion The movement of solutes (substances dissolved in water) across a membrane.

distraction The pulling apart of two structures; i.e., pulling apart the fractured components of a bone or part of the spine.

distributive shock Shock that occurs when the vascular container enlarges without a proportional increase in fluid volume.

Don Juan syndrome The pattern of injury that often occurs when victims fall or jump from a height and land on their feet. Bilateral calcaneus (heel bone) fractures are often associated with this syndrome. After the feet land and stop moving, the body is forced into flexion as the weight of the still-moving head, torso, and pelvis come to bear. This can cause compression fractures of the spinal column in the thoracic and lumbar areas.

dorsal root The spinal nerve root responsible for sensory impulses.

down-and-under pathway When a vehicle ceases its forward motion, the occupant usually continues to travel downward into the seat and forward into the dashboard or steering column.

dura mater The outer membrane covering the spinal cord and brain; the outer of the three meningeal layers. Literally means "tough mother."

dural sheath A fibrous membrane that covers the brain and continues down to the second sacral vertebra.

dysarthria Difficulty speaking.

dysbarism The changes that result physiologically as a result of changes in ambient environmental pressure.

dysrhythmia (cardiac) Abnormal, disordered, or disturbed rhythm of the heart.

ecchymosis A bluish or purple irregularly formed spot or area resulting from a hemorrhagic area below the skin.

eclampsia A syndrome in pregnant women that includes hypertension, peripheral edema and seizures; also called Toxemia of pregnancy.

edema A local or generalized condition in which some of the body tissues contain an excessive amount of fluid; generally includes swelling of the tissue.

edentulism The absence of teeth.

electrical energy The result of movement of electrons between two points.

electrolytes Substances that separate into charged ions when dissolved in solution.

empyema Collection of pus in the pleural space.

endotracheal intubation Insertion of a large tube into the trachea for direct ventilation from outside of the body.

epidermis The outermost layer of the skin, which is made up entirely of dead epithelial cells with no blood vessels.

epidural hematoma Arterial bleeding that collects between the skull and dura mater.

epidural space Potential space between the dura mater surrounding the brain and the cranium. Contains the meningeal arteries.

epiglottis Leaf-shaped structure that acts as a gate or flapper valve and directs air into the trachea and solids and liquids into the esophagus.

epinephrine Chemical released from the adrenal glands, it stimulates the heart to increase cardiac output by increasing the strength and rate of contractions.

epiphyseal The end of the long bone.

escharotomy Incision made to allow the tissues underlying the tough, leathery damaged skin created by severe burns to expand as they swell.

eucapnia Normal blood carbon dioxide level.

euhydration The physiologic state of normal body water balance.

euvolemia Normal circulating blood volume.

evaporation Change from liquid to vapor.

event phase The moment of the actual trauma.

evisceration When a portion of the intestine or other abdominal organ is displaced through an open wound and protrudes externally outside the abdominal cavity.

expiration The forcing of air out of the lungs from the relaxation of the intercostal muscles and diaphragm, resulting in the return of the ribs and diaphragm to their resting positions.

explosion Physical, chemical, or nuclear reactions that result in the almost instantaneous release of large amounts of energy in the form of heat and rapidly expanding, highly compressed gas, capable of projecting fragments at extremely high velocity.

exsanguination Total loss of blood volume, producing death.

external respiration The transfer of oxygen molecules from the atmosphere to the blood.

extraluminal pressure Pressure in the tissue surrounding the vessel.

extreme altitude Elevations higher than 18,045 feet.

fight-or-flight response A defense response that the sympathetic nervous system produces that simultaneously causes the heart to beat faster and stronger, constricts the arteries to raise blood pressure, and increases the ventilatory rate.

FiO$_2$ Fraction of oxygen in inspired air stated as a decimal. An FiO$_2$ of 0.85 means that 85 hundredths or 85% of the inspired air is oxygen.

flail chest A chest with an unstable segment produced by multiple ribs fractured in two or more places or including a fractured sternum.

flat bones Thin, flat, and compact bones, such as the sternum, ribs, and scapulae.

flexion A bending movement around a joint that decreases the angle between the bones at the joint. In the cervical region, it is a forward bending motion of the head, bringing the chin nearer to the sternum.

foot-pounds of force A measure of mechanical force brought to bear. Force = Mass × Deceleration or Acceleration.

foramen magnum The opening at the base of the skull through which the medulla oblongata passes.

foramina Small opening.

fourth-degree burn Burn injury that involves all layers of the skin, as well as the underlying fat, muscles, bone, or internal organs.

fracture A broken bone. A simple fracture is closed without a tear or opening in the skin. An open fracture is one in which the initial injury or bone end has produced an open wound at or near the fracture site. A comminuted fracture has one or more free-floating segments of disconnected bone.

fragmentation When an object breaks up to produce multiple parts or rubble, and, therefore, creates more drag and more energy exchange.

frostbite The actual freezing of body tissue as a result of exposure to freezing or below-freezing temperatures.

full-thickness (third-degree) burns Burn to the epidermis, dermis, and subcutaneous tissue (possibly deeper). Skin may look charred or leathery and may be bleeding.

G-force (gravitational force) Measured force of acceleration or deceleration or of centrifugal force.

gastric ventilation Air undesirably forced down the esophagus and into the stomach rather than into the lungs.

geriatric Dealing with aging and the diagnosis and treatment of injuries and diseases affecting the elderly.

Glasgow Coma Scale A scale for evaluating and quantifying level of consciousness or unconsciousness by determining the best responses of which the patient is capable to standardized stimuli, including eye-opening, verbal, and motor responses.

global overview The simultaneous 15- to 30-second overview of the patient's condition. The global overview focuses on the patient's immediate ventilatory, circulatory, and neurologic status.

glycogen Glucose molecules strung together, used for carbohydrate storage purposes.

Golden Period The period of time a patient has to reach definitive care to achieve the best possible outcome.

Grey Turner's sign Ecchymosis involving the flanks.

heat cramps Acute painful spasms of the voluntary muscles after hard physical work in a hot environment, especially when not acclimated to the temperature.

heat exhaustion Results from excessive fluid and electrolyte loss through sweating and lack of adequate fluid replacement when the patient is exposed to high environmental temperatures for a sustained period of time, usually several days.

heat stress index The combination of ambient temperature and relative humidity.

heat stroke An acute and dangerous reaction to heat exposure characterized by high body temperature and altered mental status.

hematocrit A measure of the packed cell volume of red blood cells in the total blood volume.

hemianesthesia Loss of sensation on one side of the body.

hemiparesis Weakness limited to one side of the body.

hemiplegia Paralysis on one side of the body.

hemoglobin The molecule found in red blood cells that carry oxygen.

hemopericardium Blood accumulation inside the pericardial space that can lead to pericardial tamponade.

hemoptysis Coughing up blood.

hemorrhage Bleeding. Also, a loss of a large amount of blood in a short period of time, either outside or inside the body.

hemorrhagic shock Hypovolemic shock resulting from blood loss.

hemothorax Blood in the pleural space.

high altitude An elevation above 5000–11.480 feet.

homeostasis A constant, stable internal environment. Balance necessary for healthy life processes.

homeotherm Warm-blooded animal.

hot zone The geographic area of highest contamination from a hazardous material; only specially trained and equipped workers may enter this area.

hypercarbia Increased level of carbon dioxide in the body.

hyperchloremia Increase in the blood chloride level.

hyperextension Extreme or abnormal extension of a joint; a position of maximum extension. Hyperextension of the neck is produced when the head is extended posterior to a neutral position and can result in a fracture or dislocation of the vertebrae or in spinal cord damage in a patient with an unstable spine.

hyperflexion Extreme or abnormal flexion of a joint. A position of maximum flexion. Increased flexion of the neck can result in a fracture or dislocation of the vertebrae or in spinal cord damage in a patient with an unstable spine.

hyperglycemia Elevated blood glucose.

hyperhydration Over-consumption of water.

hyperkalemia Increased blood potassium.

hyperrotation Excessive rotation.

hypertension Having a blood pressure greater than the upper limits of the normal range; generally considered to exist if the patient's systolic pressure is greater than 140 mm Hg.

hypertensive crisis A sudden severe increase in blood pressure with signs of organ damage, such as renal failure or cardiac compromise.

hyperthermia Body temperature much higher than normal range.

hypertonic Osmotic pressure greater than serum or plasma.

hypochlorite solutions Solutions used in the production of household bleaches and industrial cleaners.

hypoglycemia Decreased blood glucose.

hypoperfusion Inadequate blood flow to cells with properly oxygenated blood.

hypopharynx The lower portion of the pharynx that opens into the larynx anteriorly and the esophagus posteriorly.

hypotension Blood pressure below normal acceptable range.

hypothalamus The area of the brain that functions as the thermoregulatory center and the body's thermostat to control neurologic and hormonal regulation of body temperature.

hypothenar eminence Fleshy part of the palm along the ulnar margin.

hypothermia Subnormal core body temperature below normal range, usually between 78° and 90° F (26° and 32° C).

hypotonic A solution of lower osmotic pressure than another. Also, having a lower osmotic pressure than normal serum or plasma.

hypoventilation Inadequate ventilation when minute volume falls below normal.

hypovolemia Inadequate (below normal range) fluid or blood volume.

hypovolemic shock Shock caused by loss of blood or fluid.

hypoxia (hypoxemia) Deficiency of oxygen; inadequate available oxygen. Lack of adequate oxygenation of the lungs due to inadequate minute volume (air exchange in the lungs) or a decreased concentration of oxygen in the inspired air. Cellular hypoxia is inadequate oxygen available to the cells.

immune system A related group of responses by various body organs and cells that protects the body from disease organisms, other foreign bodies, and cancers. The main components of the immune response system are the bone marrow, thymus, lymphoid tissues, spleen, and liver.

incident command system A system that defines the chain of command and organization of the various resources that respond during a disaster.

incisura (tentorial incisura) Opening in the tentorium cerebelli at the junction of the midbrain and the cerebrum. The brain stem is inferior to the incisura.

incomplete cord transection Partial transection of the spinal cord in which some tracts and motor/sensory functions remain intact.

infant A child between 7 weeks and 1 year of age.

inhalation The process of drawing air into the lungs.

injury A harmful event that arises from the release of specific forms of physical energy or barriers to normal flow of energy.

intentional injury Injury associated with an act of interpersonal or self-directed violence.

intercostal muscles The muscles located between and that connect the ribs to one another.

internal respiration The movement or diffusion of oxygen molecules from the red blood cells into the tissue cells.

interstitial fluid The extracellular fluid located between the cell wall and the capillary wall.

intervertebral disc Cartilage-like discs that lie between the body of each vertebra and act as shock absorbers.

intervertebral foramina A notch through which nerves pass in the inferior lateral side of the vertebra.

intracellular fluid Fluid within the cells.

intracranial hypertension Increased intracranial pressure.

intraosseous Within the bone substance.

intubation Passing a tube into a body aperture. Endotracheal intubation is the insertion of a breathing tube through the mouth or nose into the trachea to provide an airway for oxygen or an anesthetic gas.

involuntary guarding Rigidity or spasm of the abdominal wall muscles in response to peritonitis.

ipsilateral On the same side.

ischemia Local deficiency of blood supply due to obstruction of circulation to a body part or tissue.

ischemic sensitivity The sensitivity of the cells of a tissue to the lack of oxygen before cell death occurs.

jaw thrust A maneuver that enables the airway of a trauma patient to be opened while the head and cervical spine are manually maintained in a neutral in-line position.

jugular vein distention (JVD) Backup of pressure on the right side of the heart resulting in venous pooling and neck vein distention (engorgement) due to decreased filling of the left heart and reduced left heart output.

keraunoparalysis Transient paralysis that results from a lightning strike.

kinematics The process of looking at the mechanism of injury of an incident to determine what injuries are likely to have resulted from the forces and motion and changes in motion involved; the science of motion.

kinetic energy (KE) Energy available from movement. Function of the weight of an item and its speed. KE = ½ of the mass × the velocity squared.

kyphosis A forward, humplike curvature of the spine commonly associated with the aging process. Kyphosis may be caused by aging, rickets, or tuberculosis of the spine.

larynx The structure located just above the trachea that contains the vocal cords and the muscles that make them work.

laws of motion Scientific laws relating to motion. Newton's first law of motion: A body at rest will remain at rest and a body in motion will remain in motion unless acted upon by some outside force.

ligament A band of tough, fibrous tissue connecting bone to bone.

ligamentum arteriosum A remnant of fetal circulation and point of fixation at the arch of the aorta.

limbus Junction of the cornea and the sclera.

liquefaction necrosis The type of tissue injury that occurs when alkali damages human tissue; the base liquefies the tissue which allows for deeper penetration of the chemical.

logroll A way to turn a person with a possible spine injury from one side to the other or completely over while manually protecting the spine from excessive, dangerous movement. Used to place patients with a suspected unstable spine injury onto a longboard.

long bones Femur, humerus, ulna, radious, tibia, and fibula.

lumbar vertebrae The five spine vertebrae located below the thoracic vertebrae, these are the most massive, and allow for movement in several directions.

lucid interval Period of normal mental functioning between periods of disorientation, unconsciousness, or mental illness.

lumbar spine Part of the spinal column found at the lower back inferior to the thoracic spine, containing the five lumbar vertebrae (L1–L5).

lymphedema Obstruction of lymph channels, leading to edema.

mass (multiple) casualty incident (MCI) An incident (such as a plane crash, building collapse, or fire) that produces a large number of victims from one mechanism, at one place, and at the same time.

mass The victim's weight.

mean arterial pressure The average pressure in the vascular system, estimated by adding one third of the pulse pressure to the diastolic pressure.

mechanical energy The energy that an object contains when it is in motion.

mediastinum The middle of the thoracic cavity containing the heart, great vessels, trachea, mainstem bronchi, and esophagus.

medulla (medulla oblongata) Part of the brain stem. The medulla is the primary regulatory center of autonomic control of the cardiovascular system.

meninges Three membranes that cover the brain tissue and the spinal cord.

metabolic acidosis Acidosis resulting from increase in acids produced by impaired or abnormal metabolic processes.

metabolism The sum of all physical and chemical changes that take place within an organism; all energy and material transformations that occur within living cells.

minute volume The amount of air exchanged each minute; calculated by multiplying the volume of each breath (tidal volume) by the number of breaths per minute (rate).

miosis Constricted pupil, the patient often complains of blurry or dim vision.

multisystem trauma patient Having injury to more than one body system.

myocardial contusion A bruising of the heart or the heart muscle.

myocardial hypertrophy An increase in the heart's muscle mass and size.

myocardium The middle and thickest layer of the heart wall; composed of cardiac muscle, often used as a general term to refer to all muscle in the heart.

myoglobin A protein found in muscle that is responsible for giving muscle its characteristic red color.

myoglobinuria The release of myoglobin into the bloodstream in considerable amounts, causing a reddish or tea-colored urine, toxicity to the kidneys, and kidney failure.

nares (singular naris) The openings in the nose that allow passage of the air from the outside to the throat. The anterior nares are the nostrils. The posterior nares are a pair of openings in the back of the nasal cavity where it connects with the upper throat.

nasopharyngeal airway An airway that is placed in the nostril and follows the floor of the nasal cavity directly posterior to the nasopharynx. This airway is commonly tolerated by patients with a gag reflex.

nasopharynx The upper portion of the airway, situated above the soft palate.

neural arches Two curved sides of the vertebrae.

neurogenic shock Shock that occurs when a cervical spine injury damages the spinal cord above where the nerves of the sympathetic nervous system exit, thus interfering with the normal vasoconstriction and leading to decreased blood pressure.

newborn A child from birth to 6 weeks of age.

Newton's first law of motion A body at rest will remain at rest and a body in motion will remain in motion unless acted on by an outside force.

norepinephrine Chemical released by the sympathetic nervous system, it triggers constriction of the blood vessels to reduce the size of the container and bring it more into proportion with the volume of the remaining fluid.

nonpatent airway An obstructed airway.

nonrebreather reservoir mask (NRB) An oxygen mask with a reservoir bag and nonrebreather valves that allow the exiting of exhaled air. It delivers high oxygen concentrations of between 85% and 100% to the patient when attached to a high-liter-flow oxygen source.

obtundation Diminished mental capacity, usually as a result of trauma or disease.

occipital condyles The two rounded knuckle-like bumps on either side of the occipital bone at the back of the head.

oculomotor nerve The third cranial nerve; controls pupillary constriction and certain eye movements.

odontoid process The toothlike protrusion on the upper surface of the second vertebra (axis) around which the first cervical vertebra (atlas) turns, allowing the head to rotate through approximately 180 degrees.

off-line medical direction Written protocols that can direct most prehospital care.

oncotic pressure Pressure that determines the amount of fluid within the vascular space.

online medical direction Medical direction that allows the prehospital care provider to discuss patient care over the radio or phone while in the field.

open fracture A fracture of a bone in which the skin is broken.

open pneumothorax (sucking chest wound) A penetrating wound to the chest causes the chest wall to be opened, producing a preferential pathway for air moving from the outside environment into the thorax.

oropharyngeal airway An airway that, when placed in the oropharynx superior to the tongue, holds the tongue forward to assist in maintaining an open airway. It is only used in patients with no gag reflex.

oropharynx The central portion of the pharynx lying between the soft palate and the upper portion of the epiglottis.

orthostatic hypotension Decrease in blood pressure when attempting to stand or sit after lying down, often manifested by lightheadedness, dizziness, or syncope.

osmosis The movement of water (or other solvent) across a membrane from an area that is hypotonic to an area that is hypertonic.

osteomyelitis Bone infection.

osteophysis Calcification of bone.

osteoporosis A loss of normal bone density with thinning of bone tissue and the growth of small holes in the bone. The disorder may cause pain (especially in the lower back), frequent broken bones, loss of body height, and various poorly formed parts of the body. Commonly a part of the normal aging process.

overtriage The problem of minimally or noninjured patients being taken to trauma centers.

oxygen consumption The volume of oxygen consumed by the body in 1 minute.

oxygen delivery The process of oxygen transfer from the atmosphere to the RBC during ventilation and the transportation of these RBCs to the tissues via the cardiovascular system.

palpation Process of physically examining a patient by application of the hands or fingers to the external surface of the body to detect evidence of disease, abnormalities, or underlying injury.

paradoxical motion The motion caused by the combination of the lower pressure in the chest and the higher atmospheric pressure outside the chest that causes a flail segment to move inward, rather than outward, during inspiration.

paradoxical pulse Condition in which the patient's systolic blood pressure drops more than 10 to 15 mm Hg during each inspiration, usually due to the effect of increased intrathoracic pressure such as would occur with tension pneumothorax or from pericardial tamponade.

para-anesthesia Loss of sensation in the lower extremities.

paraplegia Paralysis of the lower extremities.

parasympathetic acute stress reaction Slows bodily functions and may result in syncope.

parasympathetic nervous system The division of the nervous system that maintains normal body functions.

paresis Localized weakness or partial (less than total) paralysis related in some cases to nerve inflammation or injury.

parietal pleura A thin membrane that lines the inner side of the thoracic cavity.

Parkland formula Formula for fluid replacement in the burned patient.

partial-thickness (second-degree) burns Burns that involve both the epidermis and dermis. Skin presents with reddened areas; blisters; or open, weeping wounds.

patent airway An open unobstructed airway of sufficient size to allow for normal volumes of air exchange.

pathophysiology The study of how normal physiologic processes are altered by disease or injury.

PEARRL Pupils equal and round, reactive to light; the term used when checking the patient's eyes to determine if they are round, appear normal, and appropriately react to light by constricting, or whether they are abnormal and unresponsive. Generally the presence of consensual reflex is included in this examination term.

pediatric trauma score (PTS) A clinical scoring system based on clinical information that is predictive of severity of injury and can be used for triage decision making.

pediatric Dealing with children; dealing with injuries and diseases affecting children (birth to 16 years of age).

penetrating trauma Trauma that results when an object penetrates the skin and injuries underlying structures. Generally produces both permanent and temporary cavities.

percutaneous transtracheal ventilation (PTV) A procedure in which a 16-gauge or larger needle through which the patient is ventilated is inserted directly into the lumen of the trachea through the cricothyroid membrane, or directly through the tracheal wall.

perfusion Blood passing through an organ or a part of the body.

pericardial space The space existing between the heart muscle (myocardium) and the pericardium.

pericardial tamponade Compression of the heart by blood collecting in the pericardial sac, which surrounds the heart muscle (myocardium); also sometimes called cardiac tamponade.

pericardiocentesis A procedure to remove accumulated blood or fluid inside the pericardial space.

pericardium A tough, fibrous, flexible but inelastic membrane that surrounds the heart.

peristalsis The propulsive, muscular movements of the intestines.

peritoneal space Space in the anterior abdominal cavity that contains the bowel, spleen, liver, stomach, and gallbladder. The peritoneal space is lined with the peritoneum.

peritoneum Lining of the abdominal cavity.

peritonitis Inflammation of the peritoneum.

phantom pain The experience of sensation in the missing part or limb after amputation.

pharynx The throat; a tubelike structure that is a passage for both the breathing and digestive tracts. Oropharynx area of the pharynx posterior to the mouth; nasopharynx area of the pharynx beyond the posterior nares of the nose.

photophobia Light sensitivity.

pia mater A thin vascular membrane closely adhering to the brain and spinal cord and proximal portions of the nerves; the innermost of the three meningeal membranes that cover the brain.

pleura A thin membrane that lines the inner side of the thoracic cavity and the lungs. The part that lines the thoracic cavity is called the parietal pleura; the fold covering the lung is called the visceral pleura.

pleural fluid Fluid that creates surface tension between the two pleural membranes and causes them to cling together.

pneumatic antishock garment (PASG) A garment designed to put pressure on the lower portion of the body and prevent pooling of blood in the abdomen and pelvis. Also called military or medical antishock trousers (MAST).

pneumothorax Injury that results in air in the pleural space; commonly producing a collapsed lung. A pneumothorax can be open with an opening through the chest wall to the outside or closed resulting from blunt trauma or a spontaneous collapse.

polytrauma See *multisystem trauma patient.*

postevent phase This phase begins as soon as the energy from the crash is absorbed and the patient is traumatized; the phase of prehospital care that includes response time, "golden period," and critique of a call.

pre-event/precrash phase This phase includes all of the events that precede an incident (e.g., ingestion of drugs and alcohol) and conditions that predate the incident (e.g., acute or pre-existing medical conditions). This phase includes injury prevention and preparedness.

preload The volume and pressure of the blood coming into the heart from the systemic circulatory system (venous return).

premature ventricular contraction A premature, irregular, extra contraction of the ventricles due to an ectopic stimulus, causing a contraction rather than the normal stimuli from the normal pacing node. Second most common abnormal rhythm of the heart.

presbycusis Gradual decline in hearing.

presbyopia Farsightedness.

preschooler A child with the body size and physical development normally found between 2 and 6 years of age.

priapism Prolonged erection. It may be caused by a urinary stone, sickle cell disease, or an injury to the lower spinal column.

primary brain injury Direct trauma to the brain and associated vascular injuries.

primary contamination Exposure to a hazardous substance at its point of release.

primary hypothermia Decrease in body temperature that occurs when healthy individuals are unprepared for overwhelming acute or chronic cold exposure.

primary injuries of blasts Injuries that are caused by the pressure wave of the blast (e.g., pulmonary bleeding, pneumothorax, perforation of the gastrointestinal tract).

primary survey The initial assessment of airway, breathing, circulation, disability, and environment/exposure to identify and manage any life-threatening injuries.

pruritus Severe itching.

psychogenic shock A temporary neurogenic shock as a result of psychological stress (fainting).

pulmonary contusion A bruising of the lungs. This can be secondary to blunt or penetrating trauma.

pulmonary diffusion Movement of oxygen from the alveoli across the alveolar capillary membrane and into the red blood cells or the plasma.

pulmonary function Controlled patent airway, ventilation, diffusion, and perfusion, resulting in arterial blood that contains adequate oxygen for aerobic metabolism and a proper level of carbon dioxide to maintain tissue acid-base balance.

pulse oximeter A machine that provides measurement of arterial oxyhemoglobin saturation. It is determined by measuring the absorption ratio of red and infrared light passed through the tissue.

pulse pressure The increase in pressure (surge) that is created as each new bolus of blood leaves the left ventricle with each contraction. Also, the difference between the systolic and diastolic blood pressures (systolic pressure minus diastolic pressure equals pulse pressure).

quadriplegia Paralysis of all four extremities.

quaternary effects Injuries from a blast or explosion that include burns and toxicities from fuel, metals, trauma from structural collapse, septic syndromes from soil, and environmental contamination.

raccoon eyes (periorbital ecchymosis) Ecchymotic area around each eye, limited by the orbital margins.

radiation The direct transfer of energy from a warm object to a cooler one by infrared radiation.

radiation energy Any electromagnetic wave that travels in rays and has no physical mass to it.

rapid sequence intubation A method of patient intubation that includes pharmacologic adjuncts for sedation and muscle relaxation.

rebound tenderness A physical examination finding that occurs by pressing deeply on the abdomen and then quickly releasing the pressure causing more severe pain when the abdominal pressure is suddenly released.

residual volume Air that remains trapped in the alveoli and bronchi that cannot be forcibly exhaled.

respiration The total ventilatory and circulatory processes involved in the exchange of oxygen and carbon dioxide between the outside atmosphere and the cells of the body. Sometimes in medicine limited to meaning breathing and the steps in ventilation.

respiratory tract The pathway for air movement between the outside air and the alveoli; includes the nasal cavity, oral cavity, pharynx, larynx, trachea, bronchi, and lungs.

response time The time interval from the time an incident occurs until arrival of emergency medical services on scene.

retrograde amnesia Loss of memory for events and situations just preceding the time (immediate preinsult period) of the patient's injury or illness. Also, loss of memory for past events.

retroperitoneal space Space in the posterior abdominal cavity that contains the kidneys, ureters, bladder, reproductive organs, inferior vena cava, abdominal aorta, pancreas, a portion of the duodenum, colon, and rectum.

revised trauma score A method for scoring and quantifying the severity of trauma in patients.

rotational impact When one vehicle strikes the front or rear side of another, causing it to rotate away from the point of impact. Also, when one corner of the vehicle strikes an immovable object or one moving slower or in the opposite direction of the vehicle, resulting in it rotating.

rule of nines A topographic breakdown (mostly of 9% and 18% portions) of the body in order to estimate the amount of body surface covered by burns.

sacral spine (sacrum) Part of the spinal column below the lumbar spine containing the five sacral vertebrae (S1–S5), which are connected by immovable joints to form the sacrum. The sacrum is the weight-bearing base of the spinal column and is also a part of the pelvic girdle.

safety Evaluation of all possible dangers and ensuring that no unreasonable threats or risks still exist.

SAMPLE History A mnemonic to remember the components of the history of symptoms, allergies, medication, past medical and surgical history, last meal, and events leading up to the injury.

SAR Search and rescue.

scalp The outermost covering of the head.

scene Environment to be evaluated in which an injury occurred. In a motor vehicle crash, this includes evaluation of the number of vehicles, the forces that acted upon each, and the degree and type of damage to each.

school-age child A child with the body size and physical development normally found between about 6 and 12 years of age.

seat-belt sign Ecchymosis or abrasion across the chest or abdomen resulting from compression of the trunk against the shoulder harness or lap belt.

secondary brain injury An extension of the magnitude of the primary brain injury by factors such as hypoxia and hypertension that result in a larger, more permanent neurologic deficit.

secondary contamination Exposure to a hazardous substance after it has been carried away from the point of origin by a victim, a responder, or a piece of equipment.

secondary hypothermia Decrease in body temperature as a consequence of a patient's systemic disorder, including hypothyroidism, hypoadrenalism, trauma, carcinoma, and sepsis.

secondary injuries of blasts Injuries that occur when the victim is struck by flying glass, falling mortar, or other debris from the blast.

secondary survey Head-to-toe evaluation of the trauma patient. This assessment is only done after the primary survey is complete and there are no immediate life-threatening problems; usually done en route in urgent patients.

semipermeable membrane Membrane that will allow fluids (solvents) but not the dissolved substance to pass through it.

senescence The process of aging.

sensory examination A gross examination of sensory capability and response to determine the presence or absence of loss of sensation in each of the four extremities.

sepsis Infection that has spread to involve the entire body.

septic shock Shock resulting from locally active hormones due to widespread systemic infection, causing damage to the walls of blood vessels, producing both peripheral vasodilation and a leakage of fluid from the capillaries into the interstitial space.

sesamoid bones Bones, usually small and round, located within tendons.

shear Change-of-speed force resulting in a cutting or tearing of body parts.

shock A widespread lack of tissue perfusion with oxygenated red blood cells that leads to anaerobic metabolism and decreased energy production.

short bones Metacarpals, metatarsals, phalanges.

simple pneumothorax The presence of air within the pleural space.

sinoatrial node Node at junction of superior vena cava with right cardiac atrium; regarded as the pacing or starting point of the heartbeat. In healthy patients, pacing from this node causes atrial contraction and then results in contraction of the ventricles.

situation Events, relationships, and roles of those parties who, with the patient, were involved in a call. The situation (e.g., domestic dispute, single vehicle crash without an apparent reason, elderly person living alone, a shooting) is important in scene assessment.

skull (cranium) Several bones that fuse into a single structure during childhood to house and protect the brain.

slugs A single metallic missile; bullet.

sniffing position A slightly superior anterior position of the head and neck to optimize ventilation as well as the view during endotracheal intubation.

spinal shock A term that refers to an injury to the spinal cord that results in a temporary loss of sensory and motor function.

spinal stenosis Narrowing of the spinal canal.

spinous process Tail-like structure on the posterior region of the vertebrae.

sprain An injury in which ligaments are stretched or even partially torn.

stellate wound Star-shaped wound.

strain A soft tissue injury that occurs around a joint when the muscles or tendons are stretched or torn anywhere in the musculature.

stroke volume The volume of blood pumped out by each contraction (stroke) of the left ventricle.

subarachnoid hemorrhage Bleeding into the cerebrospinal fluid-filled space beneath the arachnoid membrane.

subarachnoid space Space between the pia mater proper and arachnoid membrane; contains cerebrospinal fluid and meningeal veins. The subarachnoid space is a common site of subdural hematomas.

subcutaneous layer Layer of skin just under the dermis that is a combination of elastic and fibrous tissue as well as fat deposits.

subdural hematoma A collection of blood between the dura mater and the arachnoid membrane.

sublimation When solids emit vapors, bypassing the liquid state.

superficial (first-degree) burns Burns to the epidermis only; red, inflamed, and painful skin.

supine hypotension syndrome Decrease in blood pressure caused by compression of the vena cava by the pregnant uterus.

surgical cricothyrotomy A procedure to open a patient's airway that is accomplished by cutting a slit into the cricothyroid membrane in the neck to open the airway into the trachea.

surveillance The process of collecting data within a community, usually for infectious diseases.

sutural bones The flat bones that make up the skull.

sympathetic acute stress reaction The "fight-or-flight" response in which bodily functions increase and pain masking occurs from a release of epinephrine and norepinephrine.

sympathetic nervous system Division of the nervous system that produces the fight-or-flight response.

syncope Fainting.

synovial fluid Fluid found inside joints.

systemic vascular resistance The amount of resistance to the flow of blood through the vessels. It increases as the vessel constricts. Any change in lumen diameter or vessel elasticity can influence the amount of resistance.

systole Ventricular contraction.

systolic blood pressure Peak blood pressure produced by the force of the contraction (systole) of the ventricles of the heart.

tachycardia Abnormally fast rate of heartbeats; defined as a rate over 100 beats per minute in an adult.

tachypnea Increased breathing rate.

tendon A band of tough, inelastic, fibrous tissue that connects a muscle to bone.

tension pneumothorax Condition when the air pressure in the pleural space exceeds the outside atmospheric pressure and cannot escape. The affected side becomes hyperinflated, compressing the lung on the involved side and shifting the mediastinum to partially collapse the other lung. A tension pneumothorax is usually progressive and is an imminently life-threatening condition.

tentorial herniation The process by which part of the brain is pushed down through the incisura as a result of increased intracranial pressure, tentorial herniation occurs.

tentorium cerebelli (tentorium) An infolding of the dura that forms a covering over the cerebellum. The tentorium is a part of the floor of the upper skull just below the brain (cerebrum).

tertiary injuries of blasts The injuries that occur from an explosion when the victim becomes a missile and is thrown against some object. These injuries are similar to those sustained in ejections from vehicles, in falls from significant heights, or when the victim is thrown against an object by the force wave resulting from an explosion. Tertiary injuries are usually blunt injuries.

tetany Muscle contraction or spasms that are sustained in duration.

thermal energy Energy associated with increased temperature and heat.

thoracic spine The part of the spinal column between the cervical spine (superiorly) and the lumbar spine (inferiorly) containing the 12 thoracic vertebrae (T1–T12). The 12 pairs of ribs connect to the thoracic vertebrae.

thorax (thoracic cavity) Hollow cylinder supported by 12 pairs of ribs that articulate posteriorly with the thoracic spine and 10 pairs that articulate anteriorly with the sternum. The 2 lowest pairs are only fastened posteriorly (to the vertebrae) and are called floating ribs. The thoracic cavity is defined and separated inferiorly by the diaphragm.

tidal volume Normal volume of air exchanged with each ventilation. About 500 ml of air is exchanged between the lungs and the atmosphere with each breath in a healthy adult at rest.

toddler A child with the body size and physical development normally found between about 1 and 2 years of age.

tonsil-tip catheter Rigid suction catheter designed for rapid removal of large amounts of fluid, vomitus, blood, and debris from the mouth and pharynx to avoid aspiration.

tonsillar herniation The process by which the brain is pushed down toward the foramen magnum and pushes the cerebellum and medulla ahead of it, causing damage and, ultimately, death.

total lung capacity The total volume of air in the lungs after a forced inhalation.

transmural pressure Difference between the pressure inside a blood vessel and the pressure outside the vessel.

transverse process Protuberances at each side of a vertebra near the lateral margins.

trauma chin lift This maneuver is used to relieve a variety of anatomic airway obstructions in patients who are breathing spontaneously. It is accomplished by grasping the chin and lower incisors and then lifting to pull the mandible forward.

trauma jaw thrust This maneuver allows an open airway with little or no movement of the head and cervical spine. The mandible is thrust forward by placing the thumbs on each zygomatic arch and placing the index and long fingers under the mandible and at the same angle, thrusting the mandible forward.

traumatic aneurysm An abnormal dilation, bursting, or tearing of a major blood vessel (usually an artery) caused by or related to an injury.

traumatic asphyxia Blunt and crushing injuries to the chest and abdomen with marked increase of intravascular pressure, producing rupture of the capillaries.

traumatic rhabdomyolysis See *crush syndrome*.

Trendelenburg position Simultaneous lowering of the patient's head while elevating the patient's legs. Usually done by raising the foot end of a flat bed or longboard higher than the head end. In this position (with the abdomen higher than the thorax), the weight of the abdominal contents presses on the diaphragm, producing some ventilatory difficulty. A modified Trendelenburg position with the head and torso horizontal and only the legs elevated will minimize ventilatory problems.

triage French word meaning "to sort;" a process in which a group of patients is sorted according to their priority of need for care. When only several patients are involved, triage involves assessing each patient, meeting all of the patients' highest priority needs first, and then moving to lower priority items. In a mass casualty incident with a large number of patients involved, triage is done by determining both urgency and potential for survival.

tumble End-over-end motion. Bullets commonly tumble when resistance is met by the leading edge of the missile.

uncal herniation The process by which an expanding mass (usually hemorrhage or swelling) along the convexity of the brain pushes the medial portion of the temporal lobe downward through the tentorium that supports the cerebrum, causing damage to the brainstem.

uncus The medial portion of the temporal lobe.

undertriage The problem that arises when seriously injured patients are not recognized as such and are mistakenly taken to nontrauma centers.

unified command The process by which the incident commanders of all of the various agencies responding to an event work together to manage the incident.

up-and-over pathway The pathway in a motor vehicle crash in which the body's forward motion carries it up-and-over the steering wheel; the chest or abdomen commonly impacts the steering wheel and the head strikes the windshield. In the semisitting position common in passenger vehicles, once the down-and-under motion has ended as the knees are stopped by the dashboard, the body then continues in an up-and-over movement. In some trucks, in which the driver is sitting fully upright with his feet stopped by the pedals, the up-and-over movement may occur initially.

vagal Dealing with stimulation of the vagus (tenth cranial) nerve; the parasympathetic system's response that slows the heart rate and reduces the force of contractions, keeping the body within workable limits. This response can normally override the sympathetic nervous system's chemical release, keeping the heart rate in an acceptable range. Accidental vagal stimulation, however, can result in producing an undesirable bradycardia, further reducing the patient's cardiac output and circulation.

vagus nerve The tenth cranial nerve; when stimulated, slows the heart rate regardless of levels of catecholamines. It contains motor and sensory functions and a wider distribution than any of the other cranial nerves.

vapor A solid or liquid in a gaseous state, usually visible as a fine cloud or mist.

velocity Speed, as in the speed of a moving mass, and the direction of movement.

ventilation Movement of air into and out of the lungs through the normal breathing process; the mechanical process by which air moves from the atmosphere outside the body through the mouth, nose, pharynx, trachea, bronchi, and bronchioles, and into and out of the alveoli. To ventilate a patient is to provide positive-pressure inspirations with a ventilating device, such as a bag-mask device, and then alternately allowing time for passive exhalation to occur; used in patients who are apneic or who cannot provide adequate ventilation for themselves.

ventral root The spinal nerve root responsible for motor impulses.

vertebra Any of the 33 bony segments of the spinal column.

vertebral body The part of the vertebrae that bears most of the weight of the spine.

vertebral foramen Holes in the bony structure of the vertebrae through which blood vessels and nerves pass.

vertebral foramina Openings in the vertebral body.

very high altitude Elevation levels between 11,480–18,045 ft.

vestibular folds The false vocal cords that direct airflow through the vocal cords.

visceral pleura A thin membrane that covers the outer surface of each lung.

volatility The likelihood that solids or liquids vaporizes into a gaseous form at room temperature.

voluntary guarding When palpating a tender area of the abdomen, the patient tenses up the abdominal muscles in that area.

warm zone A geographic area of diminished contamination from a hazardous material and the location for the contamination reduction corridor where exposed patients are decontaminated by the hazmat team.

whistle-stop catheter (whistle-tip catheter) A soft catheter used for suctioning the nasal passage, deep oropharynx, or endotracheal tube; allows for controlled intermittent suction. Its name is derived from the opening (whistle-stop) found in the side of the proximal end of the catheter. Suction is not produced at the distal tip until this hole or port is covered with one of the operator's fingers, producing a closed system to the opening at the distal tip.

white phosphorus An incendiary agent used in the production of munitions.

zygomatic arches The bones that form the superior area of the cheeks of the face. Laterally, superior to the molars, these extend more anteriorly than the maxilla, giving the individual some of his or her unique facial structure; commonly called the cheekbones.

Index

A

ABCDE assessment
  burns, 360–361
  geriatric trauma, 411–412
  head trauma, 228–229
  pediatric trauma, 382–387
  primary survey, 112–117
  shock, 193–197
ABCDE priority, 39
Abdomen, 122–123
Abdominal aorta, 320
Abdominal evisceration, 327
Abdominal trauma, 317–331
  anatomy, 318–319
  assessment, 321–326
  blunt trauma, 322–323
  children, 394
  evisceration, 327
  FAST, 324–326
  genitourinary injuries, 330
  impaled objects, 326–327
  kinematics, 321–322
  management, 326
  obstetrical patient, 327–330
  pathophysiology, 319–321
  penetrating trauma, 321–322
  primary survey, 323
  secondary survey, 323–324
  special examinations/key indicators, 324–326
Abducens nerve, 221f
Abuse, 130
A/C ventilation, 153
Accessory nerve, 221f
Accident, 3, 23
Accidental cold-water immersion, 524
Accidental Death and Disability: the Neglected Disease of Modern Society, 16
Accidental hypothermia. *See* Hypothermia
Acetabular fractures, 344
Achilles tendon, 336f
Acids, 370
Acticoat dressing, 364f
Active fragmentation, 70
Active strategies, 25
Acute injuries, process of caring, 40
Acute mountain sickness (AMS), 551–552, 553f
Acute radiation syndrome (ARS), 370, 470, 471f
Acute renal failure, 191
Acute respiratory distress syndrome (ARDS), 191
Acute tubular necrosis (ATN), 191
Adductor longus muscle, 336f
Adductor magnus muscle, 336f
Adequate exposure, 79
Aerobic metabolism, 181

Aerosol, 459
Aerosol precautions, 465
Afghanistan, 80
Afterload, 184
Age
  children. *See* Pediatric trauma
  drowning, 524, 525
  elderly persons. *See* Geriatric trauma
  heat-related illness, 482
  shock, 197
Aging, 405–410. *See also* Geriatric trauma
Air bags, 60, 380f
Air density, 48
Airway (ABCDE approach). *See also* Airway and ventilation
  burns, 360
  geriatric trauma, 411, 414
  head trauma, 228, 236
  pediatric trauma, 382–384, 389
  primary survey, 112
  shock, 198
Airway and ventilation, 133–177. *See also* Airway (ABCDE approach); Specific skills (airway and ventilation)
  algorithm, 140f
  anatomy, 134–136
  capnography, 155
  CQI, 152
  decreased neurologic function, 138
  digital intubation, 151
  endotracheal intubation, 144–151
  face-to-face intubation, 147–148
  LEMON assessment, 145, 146–147f
  LMA, 151, 170–171
  manual maneuvers, 141
  mechanical obstruction, 138–139
  nasotracheal intubation, 146–147
  NPA, 143, 162–163
  OPA, 143, 159–161
  orotracheal intubation, 145–146, 172–175
  oxygenation process, 138
  pharmacologically-assisted intubation, 148, 150f
  physiology, 136–138
  prolonged transport, 155–156
  PTV, 152, 176–177
  pulse oximetry, 154–155
  suctioning, 141–142
  supraglottic airway, 143–144, 166–169
  surgical cricothyrotomy, 152, 176–177
  ventilatory devices, 152–154
Airway management algorithm, 140f
Albumin, 205
Allergic urticaria, 573f
Alpha-particle radiation, 469
Alternate trauma jaw thrust, 158
Alternobaric vertigo, 535
Altitude-related illness. *See* High-altitude illness
Alveolar duct, 135f
Alveolar epithelium, 293f

Alveolar sacs, 135f
Alveolus, 136, 293, 293f
Ammonia, 462
AMPLE history, 229
Amputation, 347–348
AMS. *See* Acute mountain sickness (AMS)
Anaerobic metabolism, 181
Anal canal, 319f
Anaphylactic shock, 190
Anastomoses, 502
Ancient period, 6
Anemia, 227
Angular-impact collision, 61
Anhidrosis, 486
Anisocoria, 124
Anterior artery, 184f
Anterior clinoid process, 219f
Anterior cord syndrome, 253, 254f
Anterior-posterior compression fractures, 344
Anthrax, 465–466
Anticoagulants, 414
Anxiolysis, 347
Aorta artery, 184f
Aortic arch, 308f
Aortic tear, 68
Apoptosis, 223
Arachnoid membrane, 219f, 220
Arch of aorta, 184f
Arcuate artery, 184f
ARDS. *See* Acute respiratory distress syndrome (ARDS)
ARS. *See* Acute radiation syndrome (ARS)
Arterial bleeding, 114
Arterial gas embolism (AGE), 536–537, 539
Arterial oxyhemoglobin saturation (Spo_2), 154–155
Arteries, 184f
Arytenoid cartilage, 136f
Ascending colon, 319f, 320
Ascending nerve tracts, 250
Asphyxiant toxidrome, 460
Asphyxiants, 367–368
Aspirin, 554
Assessment. *See* Patient assessment and management
Assessment algorithm, 120–121f
Assessment terminology, 111f
Ataxic breathing, 225
Atherosclerosis, 408
Athletic equipment removal, 261f, 288–289
Ativan, 462
ATN. *See* Acute tubular necrosis (ATN)
Atropine, 150f, 461
Austere environment, 434
Autonomic nervous system, 186
Available equipment, 37
AVPU, 116–117, 386
Axial loading, 253
Axial unloading, 259
Axillary artery, 184f

Page numbers followed by f indicate figures.

B

Backcountry EMS. *See* Wilderness trauma care
Bag-mask, 153
Bag-mask ventilation, 164–165
BAL. *See* British anti-lewisite (BAL)
Banks, Sam, 7
Baroreceptors, 295
Barotrauma, 533–536
Basal metabolic rate, 479
Bases, 370
Basic principles. *See* Golden principles of prehospital care
Basilar skull fractures, 230
Battle of Bull Run, 7
Battle's sign, 230
Beck's triad, 306
Bee sting, 572–573
Behavioral regulation, 479
Bellows effect, 69
Bends, 538
Benzodiazepines, 347
Beta blockers, 414
Beta-particle radiation, 469
Biceps brachii muscle, 336f
Biceps femoris muscle, 336f
BIG. *See* Bone Injection Gun (BIG)
Bile duct, 320
Biologic agents, 463–468
Birdshot, 77, 78f
Black Death, 466
Blast injuries, 79–82
    blast waves and body, 80
    categorization, 81f
    explosion-related injuries, 80
    injury from fragments, 81
    multi-etiology injury, 81–82
    physics of blast, 79–80
Blast injury categories, 81f, 456f
Blast lung injury, 457f
Blast overpressure, 79
Blast wave, 454
Blind nasotracheal intubation (BNTI), 146–147
Blister agents, 372
Blisters, 358f
Blood, 185–186
Blood-borne pathogens, 92–94
Blood pressure
    aortic disruption, 308f
    pediatric patients, 386f
    shock, 196
Blood substitutes, 206
Blood vessels, 184–185
Blown pupil, 225
Blue Star of Life, 8
Blunt cardiac injury, 304–305
Blunt trauma, 51–69
    abdomen, 68–70
    abdominal trauma, 322–323
    defined, 49
    falls, 64–65
    head, 66
    mechanical principles, 51–52
    MVCs. *See* Motor vehicle crashes (MVCs)
    neck, 66

Blunt trauma *(Continued)*
    spinal trauma, 255–256
    sports injuries, 65–66
    thoracic trauma, 296
    thorax, 66–68
BNTI. *See* Blind nasotracheal intubation (BNTI)
Board splint, 343f
Body exposure. *See* Expose/environment
Bomb threats (safe evacuation distances), 98f
Bone Injection Gun (BIG), 204
Botulinum toxin, 468
Botulism, 468
Boyd, David, 8
Boyle's law, 531–532, 533f, 550
Brachial artery, 184f
Brachial plexus, 251f
Brachialis muscle, 336f
Brachiocephalic artery, 184f
Brachioradialis muscle, 336f
Bradyasystole, 129
Bradypnea, 113
Brain death, 239
Brain injuries, 233–235
Brainstem, 220f, 221
Breathing
    burns, 360
    geriatric trauma, 411–412, 416
    head trauma, 228, 236–237
    pediatric trauma, 384–385, 389–391
    primary survey, 113–114
    shock, 193–194, 198
    thoracic trauma, 293–295
British anti-lewisite (BAL), 463
Bronchioles, 136
Brown-Séquard syndrome, 254, 254f
Bubonic plague, 466
Buccinator muscle, 336f
Buckshot, 77, 78f
Bullet vehicle, 54
Burn cooling, 363
Burn depth, 357–359
Burn injuries, 355–375
    ABCDE assessment, 360–361
    anatomy of skin, 356–357
    burn cooling, 363
    burn depth, 357–359
    burn size estimation, 361–362
    chemical burns, 370–372
    children, 361, 365, 369–370
    circumferential burns, 366
    contact burns, 369
    dressings, 362
    elderly persons, 411
    electrical burns, 366
    fluid resuscitation, 364–365
    initial burn care, 363–364
    Lund-Browder chart, 361–362, 362f
    radiation burns, 370
    rule of nines, 361, 361f
    rule of palms, 362
    smoke inhalation injuries, 367–368
    toxin-induced/lung injury, 368
    transportation, 362
    zones of burn injury, 357, 357f
Burn size estimation, 361–362

Burst lung, 536
Bush, George W., 100

C

C-A-T. *See* Combat Application Tourniquet (C-A-T)
Calcaneal tendon, 336f
Calcium channel blockers, 414
Cancer patient, 2
Capillary, 293, 293f
Capillary bleeding, 114
Capillary endothelium, 293f
Capillary refilling time, 115, 195
Capnography, 155, 297
Carbon monoxide toxicity, 368, 369
Cardiac contusion, 304
Cardiac output (CO), 184
Cardiac tamponade, 191, 305–306
Cardiogenic shock, 190–191
Cardiopulmonary arrest, 128–129
Cardiopulmonary resuscitation (CPR), 5, 585
Care under fire, 37, 583
Care under fire evacuation, 585
Caroline, Nancy, 8
Carpals, 335f
Carroll, Robert, 39
Casualty evacuation (CASEVAC), 37
Cataract, 409
Cavitation, 49–50, 73
CBF. *See* Cerebral blood flow (CBF)
Cecum, 319f
Cefazolin, 352
Celiac artery, 184f
Cellular respiration, 293
Cement, 372
Central cord syndrome, 253, 254f
Central neurogenic hyperventilation, 225
Central sulcus, 220f
Cerebellum, 220f, 221, 221f
Cerebral blood flow (CBF), 221–222
Cerebral concussion, 233
Cerebral contusions, 235
Cerebral edema, 225
Cerebral hypoxia, 226–227
Cerebral perfusion pressure (CPP), 222
Cerebrospinal fluid (CSF), 220
Cerebrum, 220–221, 220f, 221f
Cervical collar, 259, 267–268
Cervical spine, 335f
Cervical spine stabilization, 112–113
Cervical vertebrae, 249
Cervical vessels, injuries to, 232
Champion, Howard, 8, 125
Chemical agents, 458–463
Chemical burns, 370–372
Chemical energy, 20
Chemoreceptors, 293
Chernobyl nuclear disaster, 468–469
Chest, 122, 292
Chest injury. *See* Thoracic trauma
Chest tube, 303
Cheyne-Stokes ventilation, 225
Chickenpox, 466, 467f
Chilblains, 501
Child abuse, 369–370, 396–398, 524

Child immobilization device, 286–287
Child safety seats, 4
Children. *See also* Pediatric trauma
  abuse, 369–370, 396–398
  altitude illness, 553f
  burns, 361, 365, 369–370
  seriousness of injuries, 425
  skull, 218
  spinal trauma, 261–262, 284–287
Chokes, 77, 538
Cholinergic toxidrome, 460
Cigarette burns, 396
Cilia, 407
Cingulate herniation, 224
Circulation
  burns, 360–361
  geriatric trauma, 412, 416
  head trauma, 228, 237
  pediatric trauma, 385–386, 391
  primary survey, 114–115
  shock, 194–195, 198–201
  thoracic trauma, 295
Circumferential burns, 366
CISM. *See* Critical Incident Stress Management (CISM)
CIVD. *See* Cold-induced vasodilation (CIVD)
Civilian tactical emergency medical support (TEMS), 579–590
  advantages of TEMS programs, 581–582
  barriers to traditional EMS access, 582–583
  historical overview, 580
  mass casualty events, 588
  medical counterterrorism operations, 587
  medical intelligence, 586–587
  operational components, 581
  patient advocacy, 587
  practice guidelines, 582, 583f
  RAM, 586
  screening for incarceration, 587
  support functions, 581
  zones of care/zones of operation, 583–586
Class I evidence, 9
Class I hemorrhage, 187–188
Class II evidence, 9
Class II hemorrhage, 187f, 188
Class III evidence, 9
Class III hemorrhage, 187f, 188
Class IV hemorrhage, 187f, 188
Classic heatstroke, 486, 487f
Clavicle, 335f
Clinical herniation syndromes, 225
Close range wounds, 78, 79f
Closed fracture, 340–342
CO. *See* Cardiac output (CO)
CO monitor, 367f
Coagulative necrosis, 370–371
Coccygeal vertebrae, 249
Coccyx, 249
Cold-induced diuresis, 500
Cold-induced vasodilation (CIVD), 502
Cold-related illness, 500
  dehydration, 500
  epidemiology, 478–479

Cold-related illness *(Continued)*
  frostbite, 502–504, 515
  hypothermia. *See* Hypothermia
  major disorders, 501–510
  minor disorders, 500–501
  prevention, 511–513
  prolonged transport, 515
Cold shock, 506f
Cold urticaria, 500
Cold zone, 96, 97, 98f, 372, 449f, 450, 585
Combat Application Tourniquet (C-A-T), 200
Combat Gauze, 201
Combitube, 166–167
Command structure, 99–101
Common iliac artery, 184f
Commotio cordis, 306–307
Community-wide intervention, 28–29
Compartment syndrome, 349–350
Complacency, 29
Complete cord transection, 253
Compression, 51
  abdomen, 68–69
  head, 66
  neck, 66
  thorax, 68–70
Computerized literature search, 10f
Condition of the patient, 36
Conduction, 480
Coning, 225
Consensus statement, 11
Contact area, 48–49
Contact burns, 369, 396
Contact freeze injury, 500
Contact precautions, 464
Contact wounds, 78, 79f
Continuous quality improvement (CQI), 152
CONTOMS. *See* Counter Narcotics and Terrorism Operational Medical Support (CONTOMS)
Contributory negligence, 56
Convection, 480
Copperhead snake, 574f
Coral snake, 573
Cord compression, 253
Cord concussion, 253
Cord contusion, 253
Cord laceration, 253
Core temperature, 479
Corneal abrasion, 230
Cost of care, 2
Cottonmouths, 574f
Counter Narcotics and Terrorism Operational Medical Support (CONTOMS), 580, 586
Courts, 26
Cowley, R. Adams, 5, 110, 181, 422
CPP. *See* Cerebral perfusion pressure (CPP)
CPR. *See* Cardiopulmonary resuscitation (CPR)
CQI. *See* Continuous quality improvement (CQI)
Cranial nerve, 221, 221f, 251f
Cranium, 122f
Crash, 45

Crash phase, 45
Crepitus, 337
Cribriform plate, 219f
Cricothyroid membrane, 152
Crime scene, 96–97
Critical Incident Stress Management (CISM), 442
Critical thinking, 37–40
Critical trauma patient, 118f
Crush syndrome, 350–351
CSF. *See* Cerebrospinal fluid (CSF)
Cue ball, 49
Cullen's sign, 324
Curry, George J., 7
Cushing's phenomenon, 225
Cutaneous anthrax, 465
Cutaneous skin bends, 538
Cyanide, 460
Cyanide antidote kit, 368
Cyanide poisoning, 367–368
Cyanokit, 368
Cyanosis, 296, 301f

D

DCS. *See* Decompression sickness (DCS)
Dead space, 136, 295f
"Death in a Ditch" (Farrington), 7
Decerebrate posturing, 116, 225
Decompression sickness (DCS), 537–539
Decontamination, 97–99, 441, 452
Decorticate posturing, 116, 225
Deep frostbite, 503
Deep second-degree burn, 358
Definitive medical care, 434
Dehydration, 482–483, 484f, 500
Deltoid muscle, 336f
Denaturation, 357
Density, 48
Dependent lividity, 571
Depressed skull fracture, 230
Dermatome, 251
Dermatome map, 252f
Dermis, 357, 357f, 479
Descending aorta, 308f
Descending colon, 319f, 320
Descending nerve tracts, 250
Dextran, 205
Diamox, 554
Diaphragm, 68, 123f, 292, 293f, 319f, 320
Diaphragmatic rupture, 309–310
Diaster education and training, 443
Diastole, 183, 184
Diazepam, 461
Dicobalt edetate, 368
Digital artery, 184f
Digital intubation, 151
Dilutional hyponatremia, 484f, 487–489
Direct pressure, 114
Dirty bomb, 441
Disability
  burns, 361
  geriatric trauma, 412
  head trauma, 228–229, 237–238
  pediatric trauma, 386–387
  primary survey, 115–117
  shock, 195, 201

Disaster, 432
Disaster cycle, 432–433
Disaster management, 431–446
   communications, 444
   comprehensive emergency management, 433–434
   decontamination, 441
   disaster cycle, 432–433
   education and training, 443
   emergency supply list, 435f
   failure to notify hospitals, 445
   first aid kit, 436f
   food kit, 436f
   ICS, 436
   initial response, 437
   media, 445
   medical assistance teams, 440
   medical concerns, 434
   pitfalls, 443–445
   preparedness, 434, 444
   psychological response, 441–443
   public health concerns, 434
   scene security, 444
   search and rescue, 437–438
   self-dispatched assistance, 444
   steps in process, 437f
   supply and equipment resources, 444–445
   terrorism/WMDs, 440–441
   transport, 440
   treatment, 439
   treatment area, 441
   triage, 438–439
   worker stress, 442–443
Disaster Medical Assistance Teams (DMATs), 440
Disease process, 20
Dislocation, 345–346, 571
Distended neck veins, 301f
Distributive shock, 189
Diver panic, 532f
Diverters, 77
Diving. *See* Scuba-related diving injuries
DMATs. *See* Disaster Medical Assistance Teams (DMATs)
Don Juan syndrome, 64–65
Dorsal metatarsal artery, 184f
Dorsal pedis artery, 184f
Double blinding, 9
Down-and-under path, 53–54
Droplet precautions, 465
Drowning, 522. *See also* Submersion incidents
Drug storage in thermal extremes, 498–500
Drunk driving, 4
DUMBELS, 461
Duodenum, 320
Dura mater, 218, 219f
Dying declaration, 97
Dysrhythmia, 190

E

EAH. *See* Exercise-associated hyponatremia (EAH)
Eclampsia, 329
Economics of injury, 18

Education, 25–26
EHS. *See* Exertional heatstroke (EHS)
Elasticity, 50
Elder abuse, 411, 417–418, 419f
Elderly persons. *See* Geriatric trauma
Electrical burns, 366
Electrical energy, 20
Elimination supplies, 567f
Emergency Care and Transportation of the Sick and Injured, 8
Emergency incident rehabilitation, 495–498, 499f
Emergency Medical Services Agenda for the Future, 28
Emergency Military Tourniquet (EMT), 200
Emergency Response Guidebook (ERG), 95
Emergency supply list, 435f
EMS Agenda for the Future, 16
EMS drug storage in thermal extremes, 498–500
EMS literature, 9–11
EMT. *See* Emergency Military Tourniquet (EMT)
EMT-Basic, 8
End-tidal carbon dioxide (ETCO$_2$), 155
Endophthalmitis, 231
Endotracheal intubation, 144–151, 390f
Endotracheal tube, 144f
Energy, 19–20, 45–50
Enforcement, 26
Engineering, 26
Entrance and exit wounds, 74–75
Environmental trauma, 477–560
   altitude. *See* High-altitude illness
   cold-related illness. *See* Cold-related illness
   diving. *See* Scuba-related diving injuries
   drowning. *See* Submersion incidents
   EMS drug storage in thermal extremes, 498–500
   heat-related illness. *See* Heat-related illness
   lightning. *See* Lightning injuries
   prolonged transport, 514–515, 555–556
EOD. *See* Explosive ordnance disposal (EOD)
Epidemiological triad, 20f
Epidermis, 357, 357f, 479
Epidural hematoma, 233–234
Epidural space, 218, 219f
Epiglottis, 134, 136f
Equipment available, 37
ERG. See Emergency Response Guidebook (ERG)
Escharotomies, 366, 367f
Esophagus, 123f, 136f, 320
ET tube, 144f
ETCO$_2$. *See* End-tidal carbon dioxide (ETCO$_2$)
Etomidate, 150f
Euhydration, 482
Eupnea, 114
Evacuation, 434
Evaporation, 480
Event phase, 4–5
Event-phase intervention, 23

Evidence, 9
Evisceration, 327
Executive protection medicine, 581
Exercise-associated hyponatremia (EAH), 484f, 487–489
Exercise-associated hyponatremia encephalopathy (EAHE), 488, 489
Exertion-associated collapse, 484–485
Exertional heat exhaustion, 485
Exertional heatstroke (EHS), 486, 487f
Exertional hyponatremia, 484f, 487–489
Exhalation, 293
Exit wound, 74–75
Expanding bullets, 70f
Expiration, 293
Explosion and weapons of mass destruction, 440–441, 447–475
   biologic agents, 463–468
   chemical agents, 458–463
   decontamination, 452
   evaluation and management, 458, 459–460, 472
   explosions and explosives, 452–458
   incendiary agents, 458
   injury pattern, 456–458
   mechanisms of injury, 454–456
   PPE, 450, 451f, 459, 464f, 472
   radiologic disasters, 468–473
   scene assessment/ICS, 448–450
   transport, 458, 460, 472
   triage, 450–452
Explosion-related injuries, 80
Explosions and explosives, 452–458
Explosive ordnance disposal (EOD), 581
Explosives Safe Distance Stand-off Chart, 455f
Expose/environment
   burns, 361
   geriatric trauma, 412
   head trauma, 229
   pediatric trauma, 387
   primary survey, 117
   shock, 195, 201–203
Exposure protocol, 95f
External carotid artery, 184f
External hemorrhage, 114
External iliac artery, 184f, 320
External iliac vein, 320
External nares, 136f
External oblique muscle, 336f
External respiration, 138
Extracellular fluid, 185
Extreme altitude, 550
Extremity trauma, 394–395
Eye, 124
Eye injuries, 230–231
Eye protection, 93–94
Eyelid laceration, 230
EZ IO device, 204, 204f

F

Face, 122f
Face shields, 93
Face-to-face intubation, 147–148
Face-to-face orotracheal intubation, 174–175

Facial artery, 184f
Facial injuries, 230–231
Facial nerve, 221f
Falling domino effect, 49
Falls, 64–65, 411
Farrington, J. D. "Deke," 7
Farrington era, 7
Fascia, 349
FAST. *See* Focused assessment sonography in trauma (FAST)
F.A.S.T.1, 204
Femoral artery, 184f
Femur, 335f
Femur fractures, 342–344
Fentanyl, 150f, 347
FGC. *See* Fire Ground Command System (FGC)
Fibula, 335f
Fick principle, 182
Field amputation, 348, 350f
Field amputation set, 350f
Field exercises, 443
Field management and care period, 8
Field triage scheme, 126
Fight-or-flight response, 186
Fildes, Sir Luke, 34
File of life, 414, 415f
Fire Ground Command System (FGC), 100
Firefighting Resources of California Organized for Potential Emergencies (FIRESCOPE), 99–100
First aid kit, 436f
First Battle of Bull Run, 7
First-degree burns, 358, 358f
First-degree frostbite, 503
First Geneva Convention, 7
First peak of death, 564
Fitness, 493–494, 496f
Flail chest, 67f, 297–298
Flares, 90
Flat bones, 335
Floating ribs, 292
Fluid resuscitation, 364–365
Fluid therapy, 118–119, 392
Focused assessment sonography in trauma (FAST), 324–326
Fontanelles, 218
Food-borne botulism, 468
Food kit, 436f
Foramen lacerum, 219f
Foramen magnum, 218, 219f
Foramen ovale, 219f
Forensic evidence, 117f
Formable splints, 343f
Fourth-degree burns, 359, 359f
Fourth-degree frostbite, 503
Fracpac, 343f
Fractured cervical spine, 2
Fractures, 340–345
Fragmental injury, 81
Fragmentation, 71
    active/passive, 71
    blast injuries, 81
    high-energy weapons, 73–74
Freezing cold injury, 502
Frontal bone, 122f, 219f

Frontal-impact collisions, 52–54
Frontal lobe, 220f
Frontalis muscle, 336f
Frostbite, 502–504, 503, 515
Frostnip, 500
Full-thickness burns, 359
Fund of knowledge of the provider, 36–37
Fundal height, 328f

G

Gallbladder, 320
Gamma radiation, 469–470
Gas, 459
Gastric distension, 385
Gastrointestinal anthrax, 465–466
Gastrointestinal (GI) squeeze, 535–536
GCS. *See* Glasgow Coma Scale (GCS)
Gelignite, 454
Gelofusine, 205
General impression, 112
General principles. *See* Golden principles of prehospital care
Genitourinary injuries, 330
Gentran, 205
Geriatric trauma, 403–420
    ABCDE assessment, 411–412
    airway, 411, 414
    assessment, 410–414
    breathing, 411–412, 414
    burns, 411
    cardiovascular system, 407–408
    chronic medical problems, 405–406
    circulation, 412, 416
    communication challenges, 413
    disability, 412
    disposition, 418
    ears, nose, and throat, 406
    elder abuse, 411, 417–418, 419f
    environmental factors, 413
    expose/environment, 412
    falls, 411
    file of life, 414, 415f
    immobilization, 416
    legal considerations, 417
    management, 414–416
    medications, 414
    musculoskeletal system, 409–410
    nervous system, 408
    nutrition and immune system, 410
    pain perception, 409
    physiologic changes, 413
    pre-existing disease, 406f, 407f
    prolonged transport, 418–419
    renal system, 409
    respiratory system, 406–407
    secondary survey, 412–414
    seriousness of injuries, 425
    skin, 410
    TBI, 411
    temperature control, 416
    transport, 418–419
    vehicular trauma, 411
    vision and hearing, 408–409
GI squeeze. *See* Gastrointestinal (GI) squeeze
Ginkgo biloba, 554

Glasgow Coma Scale (GCS), 8, 116, 116f, 228
Glossopharyngeal nerve, 221f
Gloves, 93
Gluteus maximus muscle, 336f
Gluteus medius muscle, 336f
Glycogen, 396
Golden Hour, 5, 110, 422
Golden Period, 110, 422
Golden principles of prehospital care, 421–430
    airway management, 425
    algorithm, 429f
    body temperature, 426
    communication with receiving facility, 428–429
    death, why it happens, 422–423
    hemorrhage, 426
    intravenous fluid, 428
    kinematics, 424
    medical history, 428
    no harm principle, 429–430
    primary survey approach, 424–425
    safety, 423–424
    scene situation, 424
    shock therapy, 426
    spinal immobilization, 426–427
    splinting, 426
    transport, 427–428
    ventilation/oxygen, 425–426
Gowns, 94
Grab and run period, 8
Gracilis muscle, 336f
Grades of Recommendation, Assessment, Development and Evaluation (GRADE), 9
Grey-Turner's sign, 324
Gross, Samuel, 180
Ground current, 545
Group training, 443
Gunpowder, 77
Guns, 73f

H

HACE. *See* High-altitude cerebral edema (HACE)
Haddon, William J., Jr., 21, 25
Haddon matrix, 21, 22f
Hague Convention of 1899, 74
Hampton, Oscar, 7
Hamstring, 336f
Hand washing, 94
Handguns, 77
Handheld end-tidal carbon dioxide detector, 155f
HAPE. *See* High-altitude pulmonary edema (HAPE)
Hard palate, 136f
Harris, Jeffrey, 8
Hazardous materials, 94–96, 97–99
Hazardous materials (HAZMAT) emergency medicine, 581
Hazardous materials training, 94
Hazmat scene control zones, 372
HBIG. *See* Hepatitis B immune globulin (HBIG)

HBOCs. *See* Hemoglobin-based oxygen carriers (HBOCs)
HBsAg. *See* Hepatitis B surface antigen (HBsAg)
HBV. *See* Hepatitis B (HBV)
HCV. *See* Hepatitis C (HCV)
Head, 121, 122f
Head-on collision, 61
Head trauma, 217–243
  airway, 228, 236
  algorithm, 240f
  anatomy, 218–221
  brain death, 239
  brain injuries, 233–235
  breathing, 228, 236–237
  cervical vessels, injuries to, 232
  children, 392–393
  circulation, 228, 237
  disability, 228–229, 237–238
  elderly persons, 411
  expose/environment, 229
  facial injuries, 230–231
  kinematics, 227
  laryngeal injuries, 232
  management, 235–239
  mandibular fractures, 232
  midface fractures, 231–232
  nasal fractures, 231
  physiology, 221–223
  primary brain injury, 223
  primary survey, 228–229
  scalp injuries, 229–230
  secondary assessment, 229
  secondary brain injury, 223–227
  skull fractures, 230
  transportation, 238–239
Headrest, 56, 56f
Heart, 182–183
Heart muscle damage, 190
Heat acclimatization, 494–495, 497–498f, 497f
Heat cramps, 483, 484f
Heat edema, 483
Heat escape lessening posture (HELP), 506, 506f
Heat exhaustion, 484f, 485–486
Heat rash, 483
Heat-related illness, 481–498
  dehydration, 482–483
  emergency incident rehabilitation, 495–498, 499f
  epidemiology, 478
  heat acclimatization, 494–495, 497–498f, 497f
  heat exhaustion, 484f, 485–486
  heat stress index, 492f
  heatstroke, 484f, 486–487, 514
  hyponatremia, 484f, 487–489, 514–515
  major disorders, 484–489
  minor disorders, 483–484
  prevention, 489–499
  prolonged transport, 514–515
  risk factors, 481–482, 481f
  treatment algorithm, 489f
  WGBT index, 492–493
Heat syncope, 483–484
Heat tetany, 483

Heatstroke, 484f, 486–487, 514
Helmet removal, 288–289
Helmets, 4
Hematologic failure, 191
Hemoglobin-based oxygen carriers (HBOCs), 206
Hemorrhage
  control of, 114–115
  external, 114
  golden principles, 426
  musculoskeletal trauma, 339–340
  pediatric trauma, 381–382
  shock, 194, 198–201, 207
  subarachnoid, 235
  subconjunctival, 230–231
  TEMS, 584
Hemorrhagic shock, 187–188
Hemostasis, 570
Hemostatic agents, 201
Hemothorax, 296, 304
Henry's law, 532–533, 550
Hepatic failure, 191
Hepatic flexure, 319f, 320
Hepatitis, 92–93
Hepatitis B (HBV), 92–93, 92f
Hepatitis B immune globulin (HBIG), 92
Hepatitis B surface antigen (HBsAg), 92
Hepatitis C (HCV), 92–93, 92f
Hepatocellular carcinoma, 92f
Herniation, 223–225
Hespan, 205
Hetastarch, 205
High-altitude, 550
High-altitude cerebral edema (HACE), 552, 553f
High-altitude illness, 549–556
  AMS, 551–552, 553f
  children, 553f
  epidemiology, 549–550
  factors to consider, 550–551
  HACE, 552, 553f
  HAPE, 552–554
  hypobaric hypoxia, 550
  medications, 553f, 554
  pre-existing medical conditions, 551, 551f
  prevention, 553f, 554
  prolonged transport, 555–556
  scientific data, 550f
  signs/symptoms, 553f
  treatment, 553f
High-altitude pulmonary edema (HAPE), 552–554
High-energy weapons, 72–74
High explosives, 454
High-quality overview, 11
High spinal cord injuries, 254
High-voltage electrical injuries, 545f
Highway design, 90
Historical overview
  ancient period, 6
  Farrington era, 7
  hospitals, military, and mortuaries, 7
  Larrey period, 6–7
  modern era, 8–9
HIV. *See* Human immunodeficiency virus (HIV)

HIV-1, 93f
HIV-2, 93f
Hives, 500
Holcomb, John, 8
Homeostasis, 481
Homeotherms, 479
Host, agent, and environment change, 20–22
Hot zone, 95, 97, 98f, 372, 449f, 450, 583
How to. *See* "Specific skills" entries
Hoyt, Walter, 8
Huddle technique, 506f
Human immunodeficiency virus (HIV), 93, 93f
Human skeleton, 335f
Humerus, 335f
Hunting response, 502
Hydration, 490–491, 493, 494f, 495f
Hydrofluoric acid, 372
Hydrogen cyanide, 460
Hydroxocobalamin, 368
Hypercapnia, 227
Hyperglycemia, 227
Hyperhydration, 482
Hyperoxygenation, 142
Hypertension, 408
Hypertonic crystalloid solutions, 205, 382
Hypertonic saline, 205
Hyperventilation, 222–223
Hyphema, 231
Hypobaric hypoxia, 550
Hypocapnia, 227
Hypochlorite solutions, 372
Hypoglossal canal, 219f
Hypoglossal nerve, 221f
Hypoglycemia, 227
Hypoglycemic agents, 414
Hyponatremia, 484f, 487–489, 514–515
Hypopharynx, 134, 136f
Hypophyseal fossa, 219f
Hypotension, 226
Hypothalamus, 479
Hypothermia, 117, 410, 504–512
  algorithm, 512f
  assessment, 508–510
  drowning, 524
  immersion, 506–507
  J-wave, 507, 508f
  management, 510
  national guidelines, 510–511
  pathophysiologic effects, 507–508
  physiologic characteristic, 509f
  prolonged transport, 515
  ranges of severity, 505f
Hypotonic crystalloid solutions, 382
Hypoventilation, 137, 138
Hypovolemic shock, 187
Hypoxemia, 138
Hypoxia, 138, 226–227, 380–381
Hypoxia hypoperfusion, 181
Hypoxic encephalopathy, 149

I

IAPs. *See* Incident action plans (IAPs)
ICS. *See* Incident command system (ICS)
Ileum, 319f

Iliopsoas muscle, 336f
Illustration. *See* "Specific skills" entries
Immersion foot, 501
Immersion hypothermia, 506–507
Immobilization of torso to board device, 260, 269–276
Immobilizing the patient, principles, 258
Impact phase, 433
Impaled objects, 326–327
IMS. *See* National Fire Incident Management System (IMS)
IMV. *See* Intermittent mandatory ventilation (IMV)
In-water patient packing equipment, 529f
Incendiary agents, 458
Incident action plans (IAPs), 101
Incident command system (ICS), 99–110, 102–103f, 436, 449
Incident command training resources, 103f
Incident commander (IC), 100, 449
Incomplete cord transection, 253
Independent learning, 443
Infant child seat, 284–285
Inferior vena cava, 320
Inhalation, 293
Inhalational anthrax, 465
Inhalational botulism, 468
Injury, 19
Injury prevention, 15–31
　classification of injury, 22–23
　community-wide intervention, 28–29
　education, 25–26
　EMS personnel, 19, 29
　energy out of control, 20
　enforcement, 26
　engineering, 26
　goal, 23
　Haddon matrix, 21, 22f
　injury, defined, 19
　injury as disease, 20–21
　one-on-one intervention, 28
　opportunities for intervention, 23, 25
　prevention as solution, 23
　public health approach, 26–27
　risk factor identification, 27
　role of EMS, 27–29
　scope of problem, 17–19
　strategies, 24–25f, 25
　surveillance, 27
　Swiss cheese model, 21, 23f
Injury prevention strategies, 24–25f, 25
Injury process, 20
Injury-related causes of mortality, 17
Injury triangle, 19
Insensible loss, 480
Intelligence, 101
Intentional injury, 22
Intercostal muscles, 292
Interior mesenteric artery, 184f
Intermediate-range wounds, 78, 79f
Intermittent mandatory ventilation (IMV), 153
Internal acoustic meatus, 219f
Internal carotid artery, 184f

Internal-ear barotrauma, 535
Internal iliac artery, 184f
Internal oblique muscle, 336f
Internal (cellular) respiration, 138
Interstitial fluid, 186
Intervertebral disk, 248f, 251
Intervertebral foramina, 248f, 250
Intestinal botulism, 468
Intracellular fluid, 185
Intracerebral hematoma, 226, 235
Intracranial hematoma, 233
Intracranial hypertension, 226
Intraosseous vascular access, 203–204, 213–214
Intravascular fluid, 186
Intravenous access, 203
Intravenous fluid, 428
Involuntary guarding, 324
Ionization, 469
Ionizing radiation, 469
Iraq, 80
Irritant gas toxidrome, 459
Ischemia, 181, 181f, 225
Isotonic crystalloid solutions, 205, 382
Israeli trauma bandage, 215

J

J-wave, 507, 508f
Jaslow, David, 29
Jaundice, 92f
Jejunum, 319f
Jennett, Bryan, 8
Joint dislocation deformities, 338f

K

KED. *See* Kendrick extrication device (KED)
Kelvin, Lord, 193
Kendrick extrication device (KED), 277
Kennedy, Robert, 7
Ketamine, 347
Kinematics, 45
Kinematics of trauma, 43–85
　assessment, 82
　blast injuries, 79–82
　blunt trauma. *See* Blunt trauma
　cavitation, 49–50
　contact area, 48–49
　density, 48
　energy, 45–50
　general principles, 45
　penetrating trauma. *See* Penetrating trauma
Kinetic energy, 47
King airway, 168–169
KING LT, 168–169
Kinnane, J. M., 29
Kocher, Emil Theodor, 73
Krebs cycle, 181
Kyphosis, 409, 409f

L

Lactated Ringer's, 118, 205
Larrey, Dominick Jean, 6–7
Larrey period, 6–7
Laryngeal injuries, 232

Laryngeal mask airway (LMA), 151, 151f, 170–171
Larynx, 123f, 134, 135f, 136f
Late age, 404
Lateral compression fractures, 344
Lateral-impact collisions, 56–57
Lateral sulcus, 220f
Latissimus dorsi muscle, 336f
Law of conservation of energy, 46
Laying the bike down, 61
Le Fort I fracture, 231, 232f
Le Fort II fracture, 231, 232f
Le Fort III fracture, 231, 232f
Left common carotid artery, 184f
Left coronary artery, 184f
Left heart, 183
Left subclavian artery, 184f
LEMON assessment, 145, 146–147f
Lethal triad, 505
Letterman, Jonathan, 7
Level A personal protective equipment, 450, 451f, 459
Level B personal protective equipment, 450, 451f, 459
Level B protection, 99
Level C personal protective equipment, 450, 451f, 459
Level D personal protective equipment, 450, 451f, 459
Level of consciousness (LOC), 115, 116, 138, 194
Lewis, Frank, 8
Lewisite, 463
Lidocaine, 150f
Life-threatening conditions, 424f
Ligament, 335
Lightning injuries, 541–549
　assessment, 547
　epidemiology, 542
　high-voltage electrical injuries, compared, 545f
　management, 546f, 547–548
　mechanism of injury, 542, 545
　minor injury, 545–546
　moderate injury, 546
　myths/misconceptions, 548f
　prevention, 548–549
　prolonged transport, 555
　safety guidelines, 549
　severe injury, 546–547
　signs/symptoms, 546f
Lilly kit, 368
Limited scene intervention, 117–118
Linea alba muscle, 336f
Linear fractures, 230
Liquefaction necrosis, 371
Liquids, 459
Literature, 9–11
Liver, 319f
Liver failure, 191
LMA. *See* Laryngeal mask airway (LMA)
LOC. *See* Level of consciousness (LOC)
Localized cutaneous cold injury, 501
Logroll, 269–272
Long bones, 334
Long-range wounds, 79, 79f

Lorazepam, 462
Low-energy weapons, 71–72
Low explosives, 454
Low-light intubation training, 584
Lower airway, 134–136
Lower respiratory tract, 135f
Lucid interval, 234
Lumbar spine, 335f
Lumbar vertebrae, 249
Lund-Browder chart, 361–362, 362f
Lung toxicants, 462

M

Maceration, 501
MADD. *See* Mothers Against Drunk Drivers (MADD)
Madrid terrorist bombing (2004), 441f
Magnesium, 458
Mainstem bronchus, 135f, 136
Mainstream technique, 155
Mallampati classifications, 147f
Mandible, 122f, 335f
Mandibular fractures, 232
Mangled extremity, 351, 352
Manual in-line stabilization of head, 259
MAP. *See* Mean arterial pressure (MAP)
Maritime medicine, 581
Mark-1 kit, 462
Masimo prehospital CO2 monitor, 367f
Mask squeeze, 533
Masks, 93
M.A.S.S., 438
Mass-casualty incident (MCI). *See* Disaster management
Mass-casualty incident (MCI) response, 432
Mass effect, 223
Masseter muscle, 336f
Mattox, Ken, 8
Maxilla, 122f
MCI. *See* Disaster management
MCI response. *See* Mass-casualty incident (MCI) response
McSwain, N. E., 6
Mean arterial pressure (MAP), 184, 221–222
Mechanical energy, 19
Mechanical obstruction, 138–139
Media, 445
Median nerve, 251f
Mediastinal emphysema, 536
Mediastinum, 293, 293f
Medical consultation, 581
Medical counterterrorism operations, 587
Medical evacuation (MEDEVAC), 37
Medical evidence, 9
Medical history, 428
Medical intelligence, 586–587
Medical intelligence and mission planning, 581
Medical literature, 9–11
Medium-energy weapons, 72
Medline, 10f
Medulla, 220f
Medulla oblongata, 221f
Meninges, 219f
Metabolic heat production, 479
Metabolism, 181

Metacarpals, 335f
Metatarsals, 335f
Metropolitan Medical Response System (MMRS), 440
Midazolam, 150f, 462
Middle age, 404
Middle-ear squeeze, 534–535
Midface fractures, 231–232
Miles, A. B ., 7
Miliaria rubra, 483
Minute ventilation (V_E), 295f
Minute volume, 137
Mitigation, 433
MMRS. *See* Metropolitan Medical Response System (MMRS)
Moist skin, 115
Mongolian blue spots, 397f
Monitoring and reassessment, 126–128
Monro-Kellie doctrine, 223, 224, 224f
Morando, Rocco, 8
Morphine, 347
Mothers Against Drunk Drivers (MADD), 4
Motor vehicle crashes (MVCs), 52–63
air bags, 60
frontal impact, 52–54
lateral impact, 56–57
motorcycle crashes, 61
pedestrian injuries, 62–63
rear impact, 54–56
rollover, 57–58
rotational impact, 57
seat belts, 59–60
three collisions, 52
vehicle incompatibility, 58–59
Motor vehicle injury prevention, 396
Motorcycle crashes, 61
Motorcycle deaths, 4
Motorcycle-helmet-usage laws, 4
MTWHF, 461
Mucocutaneous exposures, 92
Multisystem trauma patient, 111f, 423
Muscle (heat) cramps, 483, 484f
Muscle fascia, 349
Muscles, 336f
Musculoskeletal trauma, 333–353
algorithm, 349f
amputation, 347–348
anatomy/physiology, 334, 335
assessment, 336–338
associated injuries, 338, 339f
compartment syndrome, 349–350
critical multisystem trauma patient, 346
crush syndrome, 350–351
dislocation, 345–346
extremities, 338f, 339f, 351, 352
femur fractures, 342–344
fractures, 340–345
hemorrhage, 339–340
kinematics, 336–337
lower extremities, 339f
mangled extremity, 351, 352
pain management, 346–347
pelvic fractures, 341–342, 344–345
primary survey, 337
prolonged transport, 352
relief of anxiety, 347

Musculoskeletal trauma *(Continued)*
secondary survey, 337–338
sprain, 352
transport, 352
upper extremities, 338f
Myocardial hypertrophy, 408

N

Nasal bone, 122f
Nasal cavity, 135f
Nasal fractures, 231
Nasopharyngeal airway (NPA), 143, 143f, 162–163
Nasopharynx, 134, 136f
Nasotracheal intubation, 146–147
National Fire Incident Management System (IMS), 100
National Incident Management System (NIMS), 100, 103f
National Registry of EMTs (NREMT), 8
Near-drowning, 522. *See also* Submersion incidents
Neck, 122, 123f
Needle cricothyrotomy, 176–177
Needle decompression of thoracic cavity, 302–303, 314–316
Nerve agents, 460–462
Nervous system, 186
Neural arches, 247
Neurogenic shock, 189–190
Neurologic examination, 124
Neutral in-line position of head, 260–262
Neutrons, 470
Newton's first law of motion, 45, 47, 70
Newton's second law of motion, 46
NEXUS, 566
NFCI. *See* Nonfreezing cold injury (NFCI)
NFPA Standard 1561, 100
NFPA Standard 1584, 495–498
NIMS. *See* National Incident Management System (NIMS)
Nipple level, 251
Nitrogen, 537
No harm principle, 429–430
Nonfreezing cold injury (NFCI), 501–502
Nonsteroidal anti-inflammatory agents, 414
Norcuron, 150f
Normal saline (NS), 205
Nose, 123f
NPA. *See* Nasopharyngeal airway (NPA)
NREMT. *See* National Registry of EMTs (NREMT)
NS. *See* Normal saline (NS)

O

Occipital bone, 122f, 219f
Occipital lobe, 220f
Occupational health, 581
Oculomotor nerve, 221f
Older age, 404
Olfactory bulb, 221f
Olfactory tract, 221f
On-scene prevention counselling, 28
One-on-one intervention, 28
OPA. *See* Oropharyngeal airway (OPA)
Open fracture, 340–342

Open globe, 231
Open pneumothorax, 299–300
Open skull fracture, 230
Optic canal, 219f
Optic chiasma, 221f
Optic nerve, 221f
Oral cavity, 136f
Orbicularis oculi muscle, 336f
Orbicularis oris muscle, 336f
Orbit, 122f
Organ donation, 239
Oropharyngeal airway (OPA), 143, 143f,
    159–161
Oropharynx, 134, 136f
Orotracheal intubation, 145–146, 172–175
Orthostatic hypotension, 485
Osborne wave, 507, 508f
Osmosis, 186
Osteomyelitis, 340
Osteophytosis, 410
Osteoporosis, 409, 410
Over the counter (OTC) medications, 414
Overtriage, 126
Oxygen, 150f
Oxygen consumption, 138
Oxygen delivery, 138
Oxygenation, 293
Oxygenation process, 138

P

Packaging, 125
PaCO$_2$, 155
Pain management, 129–130, 346–347, 392
    musculoskeletal trauma, 346–347
    patient assessment and management,
        129–130
    pediatric trauma, 392
Pancreas, 320
Pancuronium, 150f
Paper bag effect, 67–68, 68f
Paradoxical pulse, 306f
Paranasal sinuses, 123f
Parasympathetic system, 186
Parietal bone, 122f, 219f
Parietal lobe, 220f
Parietal pleura, 293, 293f
Parkland formula, 364–365
Partial-thickness burns, 358
Pasadena kit, 368
PASG. *See* Pneumatic antishock garment
    (PASG)
Passive fragmentation, 70
Passive strategies, 25
Patella, 335f
Patient advocacy, 587
Patient assessment and management, 109–132
    ABCDE approach, 112–117
    abdomen, 122–123
    abuse, 130
    airway, 112–113
    assessment algorithm, 120–121f
    breathing (ventilation), 113–114
    cervical spine stabilization, 112–113
    chest, 122
    communication, 128
    disability, 115–117

Patient assessment and management
    (Continued)
    expose/environment, 117
    extremities, 124
    field triage scheme, 126
    fluid therapy, 118–119
    GCS, 116
    general impression, 112
    golden period, 110
    head, 121, 122f
    hemorrhage control, 114–115
    limited scene intervention, 117–118
    monitoring and reassessment, 126–128
    neck, 122, 123f
    neurologic examination, 124
    packaging, 125
    pain management, 129–130
    pelvis, 124
    perfusion, 115
    primary survey (initial assessment),
        111–117
    priorities, 111
    prolonged transport, 130–131
    resuscitation, 117–119
    RTS, 125–126
    SAMPLE history, 121
    secondary survey, 119–124
    see, hear, feel, 119
    terminology, 111f
    transport, 118, 125, 126, 130–131
    traumatic cardiopulmonary arrest, 128–129
    vital signs, 119–121
Patient care report (PCR), 429
Pavulon, 150f
PCO$_2$, 155
PCR. *See* Prehospital care report (PCR)
PEA. *See* Pulseless electrical activity (PEA)
PEARRL, 116
Pectoralis major muscle, 336f
Pedestrian injuries, 62–63
Pediatric endotracheal intubation, 390f
Pediatric intraosseous infusion, 391f
Pediatric trauma, 377–401
    ABCDE assessment, 382–387
    abdominal injuries, 394
    abuse, 369–370, 396–398
    airway, 382–384, 389
    breathing, 384–385, 389–391
    circulation, 385–386, 391
    CNS injury, 382
    common patterns of injury, 379, 379f
    disability, 386–387
    expose/environment, 387
    extremity trauma, 394–395
    fluid therapy, 392
    hemorrhage, 381–382
    hypoxia, 380–381
    kinematics, 379
    management, 389–392
    motor vehicle injury prevention, 396
    pain management, 392
    pediatric trauma score, 387–388, 387f
    prolonged transport, 398–399
    psychosocial issues, 379–380
    seat belts/air bags, 380f
    secondary survey, 388–389

Pediatric trauma *(Continued)*
    spinal trauma, 393–394
    TBI, 392–393
    thermal homeostasis, 379
    thermal injuries, 395–396
    thoracic injuries, 394
    transport, 392, 398–399
    vascular access, 391–392
    vital signs, 388f
Pediatric Trauma Score (PTS), 387–388
PEEP. *See* Positive end-expiratory pressure
    (PEEP)
Pelvic binders, 345f
Pelvic fractures, 341–342, 344–345
Pelvic ring fractures, 344
Pelvis, 124, 335f
Penetrating trauma, 70–79
    abdomen, 76–77
    abdominal trauma, 321–322
    defined, 49
    entrance and exit wounds, 74–75
    extremities, 77
    fragmentation, 71
    head, 75–76
    high-energy weapons, 72–74
    low-energy weapons, 71–72
    medium-energy weapons, 72
    profile, 70
    shotgun wounds, 77
    spinal trauma, 256
    thoracic trauma, 295–296
    thorax, 76
    tumble, 70–71
Percussion, 297
Percutaneous exposures, 92
Percutaneous transtracheal ventilation
    (PTV), 152, 176–177
Perfluorocarbons (PFCs), 206
Perfusion, 115
Periorbital ecchymosis, 230
Periosteum, 219f
Peritoneal cavity, 318
Peritonitis, 319, 323f
Permanent cavity, 50
Pernio, 501
Peroneal artery, 184f
Peroneus longus muscle, 336f
Personal protective equipment (PPE), 93–
    94, 97
    donning/removing, 464f
    levels, 450, 451f, 459
    radiologic disaster, 472
    WMD events, 450, 459
PFCs. *See* Perfluorocarbons (PFCs)
Phalanges, 335f
Phantom pain, 348f
Pharmacologically-assisted intubation, 148,
    150f
Pharyngeal tonsil, 123f
Pharynx, 123f, 134, 135f
Phosgene, 462
PHTLS. *See* Pre-hospital trauma life sup-
    port (PHTLS)
Physical activity guidelines, 496f
Physiologic thermoregulation, 479
Physiological PEEP, 154

Pia mater, 219f, 220
Pit vipers, 574
Pituitary gland, 221f
Placenta previa, 328f
Plague, 466
Plaque, 408
Platinum 10 Minutes, 427, 428
Pleural space, 293f
Pneumatic antishock garment (PASG), 201, 202f
Pneumonic plague, 466
Pneumothorax, 298–302, 536
Pocket masks, 153
Polytrauma, 423
Pons, 220f, 221f
Popliteal artery, 184f
Portable Pulse CO-Oximeters, 367
Positive end-expiratory pressure (PEEP), 153–154
Positive-pressure ventilators, 153–154
Postcrash phase, 45
Posterior tibial artery, 184f
Postevent intervention, 23
Postevent phase, 5–6
PPE. See Personal protective equipment (PPE)
Pralidoxime chloride, 461
Pre-eclampsia, 329
Pre-event interventions, 23
Pre-event phase, 3–4
Pre-hospital trauma life support (PHTLS)
    assessment terminology, 111f
    foundation, 37
    goal, 9
    golden principles. See Golden principles of prehospital care
    philosophy, 2, 35
    preferences, 35
    principles, 35
    science and art, 33–41
Precrash phase, 45
Pregnancy
    abdominal trauma, 327–330
    seriousness of injuries, 425
    shock, 197
Prehospital care report (PCR), 128
Prehospital pediatric intubation, 390f
Preoxygenation, 141
Preparedness, 433
Presbycusis, 409
Presbyopia, 409
Pressure phenomenon, 454
Prickly heat, 483
Primary blast injuries, 80, 81f, 454, 456, 456f
Primary brain injury, 223
Primary contamination, 459
Primary hypothermia, 505
Primary intervention, 23
Primary prevention, 21
Primary survey (initial assessment), 111–117
Primary survey algorithm, 349f
Procedure. See "Specific skills" entries
Prodrome phase, 432
Profile, 70

Prolonged transport, 130–131
    airway management, 155–156
    cold-related illness, 515
    crew, 131
    equipment, 131
    geriatric trauma, 418–419
    head trauma, 238–239
    heat-related illness, 514–515
    high-altitude illness, 555–556
    lightning injury, 555
    musculoskeletal trauma, 352
    near-drowning, 555
    patient issues, 130
    pediatric trauma, 398–399
    scuba-related diving injuries, 555
    shock, 207–210
    spinal trauma, 264
    thoracic trauma, 310–311
Protocols, 2
Psychogenic shock, 190
PTS. See Pediatric Trauma Score (PTS)
PTV. See Percutaneous transtracheal ventilation (PTV)
Public health approach to injury prevention, 26–27
Public health impact of injury, 18
Pulmonary artery, 184f
Pulmonary contusion, 296, 298
Pulmonary overpressurization syndrome (POPS), 536
Pulmonary volumes/relationships, 295f
Pulse
    circulatory status, 115
    pediatric patients, 386f
    shock, 194, 198
Pulse oximetry, 154–155, 297
Pulse pressure, 184
Pulseless electrical activity (PEA), 129, 305
Pulseless ventricular tachycardia, 129
Pulselessness, 350f
Pulsus paradoxus, 306f
Pupil, 124f
Pupil constriction, 124f
Pupil dilation, 124f
Pyramidal fracture, 231

Q

Quadriceps femoris muscle, 336f
Quaternary blast injuries, 81f, 456, 456f
Quiescence level, 432
Quinary blast injuries, 80, 81f, 456, 456f

R

Raccoon eyes, 230, 397f
Radial artery, 184f
Radial nerve, 251f
Radiation, 480
Radiation burns, 370
Radiation dispersion devices (RDDs), 469
Radiation energy, 20
Radiologic disasters, 468–473
Radius, 335f
RAM. See Rapid and Remote Assessment Methodology (RAM)
Rami fractures, 344
Randomization, 9

Rapid and Remote Assessment Methodology (RAM), 586
Rapid extrication, 280–283
Rapid-sequence intubation (RSI), 148, 149f
RAS. See Reticular activating system (RAS)
Rattlesnake, 574f
RDDs. See Radiation dispersion devices (RDDs)
Rear-impact collisions, 54–56
Reason, James, 21
Rebound tenderness, 324
Recompression therapy, 540f
Recovery, 434
Recovery phase, 433
Recreational scuba-related injuries. See Scuba-related diving injuries
Rectum, 319f
Rectus abdominis muscle, 336f
Rectus femoris muscle, 336f
Reflective clothing, 90
Reflective cones, 90, 91f
Relative hypovolemia, 189
Relief of anxiety, 347
Renal artery, 184f
Rescue phase, 433
Rescue throw lines, 529f
Respiration, 293
Respiratory rate, 113. See also Ventilatory rate
Respiratory system, 135f
Response, 434
Response time, 5
Resuscitation, 117–119
Reticular activating system (RAS), 221
Retroperitoneal space, 318
Revised Trauma Score (RTS), 125–126, 387
Rib fractures, 297
Ribs, 335f
Rifles, 77
Rifling, 77
Right common carotid artery, 184f
Right coronary artery, 184f
Right heart, 183
Rigid cervical collars, 259, 267–268
Rigid splints, 343f
Rigor mortis, 571
Risk factor identification, 27
Road traffic deaths, 3f
Road traffic injuries, 3
Rollover, 57–58
Rotational-impact collisions, 57
RSI. See Rapid-sequence intubation (RSI)
RTS. See Revised Trauma Score (RTS)
Rubber necking, 90
Rule of nines, 361, 361f, 395
Rule of palms, 362
Ruptured globe, 231
Ruptured uterus, 328f
Rural roads, 90

S

Sacral vertebrae, 249
Sacrum, 249, 250, 320, 335f
SALT triage, 107f, 438
SALT triage algorithm, 107f
SAMPLE history, 121

Sarin, 460
Sartorius muscle, 336f
SBP. *See* Systolic blood pressure (SBP)
Scalp injuries, 229–230
Scapula, 335f
Scene, 87–108
  blood-borne pathogens, 92–94
  command structure, 99–101
  crime, 96–97
  decontamination, 97–99
  hazardous materials, 94–96, 97–99
  highway design, 90
  IAPs, 101
  reflective clothing, 90
  scene control zones, 97, 98f
  secondary devices, 99
  standard precautions, 93–94
  traffic safety, 89
  triage, 101–107
  vehicle positioning and warning devices,
    90–91
  violence, 91–92
  weather/light conditions, 89
  WMD, 97
Scene assessment, 88–89
Scene control zones, 97, 98f
Schwartz, Lew, 8
Scuba-related diving injuries, 529–541
  barotrauma, 533–536
  Boyle's law, 531–532, 533f
  DAN contact information, 539f
  DCS, 537–539
  diabetes, 542f
  epidemiology, 530, 531f
  fitness to dive, 540–541
  flying after diving, 541, 543f
  Henry's law, 532–533
  management, 539
  mechanical effects of pressure, 531
  panic, 532f
  prevention, 539–541
  prolonged transport, 555
  recompression therapy, 540f
  units of pressure, 532f
Search and rescue, 434, 437–438
Seat belt sign, 324f, 394f
Seat belts, 59–60, 380f
Second Battle of Bull Run, 7
Second death peak, 564
Second-degree burns, 358, 358f
Second-degree frostbite, 503
Secondary blast injuries, 81f, 456, 456f
Secondary bombs, 99
Secondary brain injury, 223–227
Secondary contamination, 459
Secondary drowning, 522
Secondary hypothermia, 505
Secondary prevention, 21
Secondary survey, 119–124
See, hear, feel, 119
Seizures, 227
Self-dispatched assistance, 444
Semimembranosus muscle, 336f
Semitendinosus muscle, 336f
Semtex, 454
Senescence, 405

Sepsis, 319
Septic shock, 190
Serratus anterior muscle, 336f
Sesamoid bones, 335
Severe tachypnea, 114
Shallow-water blackout, 523
Sharps injury, 94, 94f
Shear, 51
  abdomen, 69–70
  head, 66
  neck, 66
  thorax, 68
Shear wave, 454
Shivering, 479
Shock, 179–216, 423f
  ABCDE assessment, 193–197
  airway, 198
  algorithm, 208f, 209f
  assessment, 192–197
  blood, 185–186
  blood vessels, 184–185
  body exposure and environment, 198,
    201–203
  breathing, 193–194, 198
  circulation, 194–195, 198–201
  complications, 191–192
  confounding factors, 196–197
  definition of, 180
  disability, 195, 201
  Fick principle, 182
  heart, 182–183
  hemorrhage, 194, 198–201, 207
  management, 197–207
  musculoskeletal injuries, 196
  nervous system, 186
  physiology, 181–182
  primary survey, 193–197
  prolonged transport, 207–210
  questions to ask, 198
  secondary survey, 195–196
  signs/symptoms, 189f
  specific skills (illustrations), 213–216
  tourniquet, 209–211, 211f, 215–216
  transport, 203, 207–210
  types, 187–191
  vascular access, 203–204, 213–214
  vital signs, 195–196
  volume resuscitation, 205–207, 208f
Shock management algorithm, 209f
Shock wave, 454
Short bones, 334
Side flash, 542
Sigmoid colon, 319f
Simple pneumothorax, 298, 299
Simulations, 443
Simultaneous evaluation, 118f
Single-system trauma patient, 111f
Sinus barotrauma, 535
Sinus squeeze, 535
Sitting immobilization, 277–279
Situation, 36
Skeleton, 335f
Skin, 115, 356–357, 410, 479
Skin color, 115, 194–195
Skin temperature, 115, 195
Skull, 122f, 335f

Skull fractures, 230
Slugs, 77
Smallpox, 466–468
Smoke inhalation injuries, 367–368
Snakebite, 573–575
Sniffing position, 382, 383f
Snow blindness, 501
Soft palate, 136f
Soft tissue injuries, 337
SOFTT. *See* Special Operations Force Tac-
  tical Tourniquet (SOFTT)
Solar keratitis, 501
Soleus muscle, 336f
Solid, 459
Solid density, 48
Spaite, Dan, 10
Special Operations Force Tactical Tourni-
  quet (SOFTT), 200
Special Operations Law Enforcement Mis-
  sions, 581
Specific skills (airway and ventilation),
  158–177
  alternate trauma jaw thrust, 158
  bag-mask ventilation, 164–165
  face-to-face orotracheal intubation,
    174–175
  LMA, 170–171
  needle cricothyrotomy, 176–177
  NPA, 162–163
  OPA, 159–161
  PTV, 176–177
  supraglottic airway, 166–169
  tongue blade insertion method, 161
  tongue jaw lift insertion method, 160
  trauma chin lift, 159
  trauma jaw thrust, 158
  visualized orotracheal intubation,
    172–173
Specific skills (spinal trauma), 267–289
  cervical collar, 267–268
  child immobilization device, 286–287
  helmet removal, 288–289
  infant child seat, 284–285
  logroll, 269–272
  rapid extrication, 280–283
  sitting immobilization, 277–279
  standing long backboard application,
    273–276
SPF. *See* Sun protection factor (SPF)
Sphenoid bone, 219f
Spinal cord, 221f, 250, 251f
Spinal cord injuries, 253–254
Spinal cord tracks, 250f
Spinal cord transection, 253
Spinal nerve, 251f
Spinal shock, 253
Spinal stenosis, 410
Spinal trauma, 245–289. *See also* Specific
  skills (spinal trauma)
  anatomy and physiology, 247–251
  assessment, 254–257
  athletic equipment removal, 261f,
    288–289
  blunt trauma, 255–256
  cervical collar, 259, 267–268
  children, 261–262, 284–287, 393–394

Spinal trauma *(Continued)*
  common mistakes, 263
  completing the immobilization, 262–263
  evaluating immobilization skills, 263f
  how caused, 246–247
  immobilization of torso to board device,
       260, 269–276
  immobilizing the patient, principles, 258
  indications for spinal immobilization,
       256, 257f
  management, 258–263
  manual in-line stabilization of head, 259
  mechanisms of injury, 253, 255
  neurologic examination, 254–255
  neutral in-line position of head, 260–262
  obese patients, 263–264
  pathophysiology, 251–254
  penetrating trauma, 256
  prolonged transport, 264
  scientific concepts, 246
  signs/symptoms, 258f
  skeletal injuries, 252–253
  spinal cord injuries, 253–254
  steroids, 264
  transport, 264
Spinous process, 247, 248f
Splash contact, 542
Spleen, 319f
Splenic artery, 184f
Splenic flexure, 319f
Splinting, 342, 343f
Spo$_2$. *See* Arterial oxyhemoglobin satura-
       tion (Spo$_2$)
Sport drinks, 492f
Sports injuries, 65–66
Sprain, 352
Squeeze, 533
St. Petersburg Declaration of 1868, 74
*Standard on Emergency Services Incident
       Management,* 100
Standard precautions, 93–94
Standing long backboard application,
       273–276
Starling's law, 184
START triage, 105f
START triage algorithm, 107f
START triage mnemonic, 106f
Statutory commands, 26
Stay and play period, 8
Steady-state metabolism, 479
Stellate (starburst) wound, 75
Step-by-step procedure. *See* "Specific
       skills" entries
Step voltage, 545
Stepped breaths, 164
Sternocleidomastoid muscle, 336f
Sternum, 123f, 335f
Stewart, Ronald, 422
Stomach, 319f
Stopping distance, 47
Stress waves, 454
Stride voltage, 545
Stroke volume, 184
Subarachnoid hemorrhage, 235
Subarachnoid space, 219f

Subconjunctival hemorrhage, 230–231
Subcutaneous emphysema, 536
Subdural hematoma, 234–235
Subdural space, 219f, 220
Sublimation, 459
Sublimaze, 150f
Submersion incidents, 522–529
  assessment, 526, 528f
  beaches, 528–529
  epidemiology, 523
  factors to consider, 523–524
  management, 526–527, 528f
  mechanism of injury, 524–525
  patient resuscitation, 527
  prevention, 527–529
  prolonged transport, 555
  surviving cold-water submersion, 525–526
Suboptimal restraint, 396
Succinylcholine, 150f
Sucking chest wound, 299
Suctioning, 141–142
Sulfur and nitrogen mustards, 372
Sulfur mustard, 462
Sun protection factor (SPF), 569
Sunburn, 569
Sunscreen, 569f
Superficial burns, 358
Superficial frostbite, 503
Superficial second-degree burns, 358
Superior mesenteric artery, 184f, 320
Superior vena cava, 320
Supraglottic airways, 143–144, 143f, 166–169
Surgical cricothyrotomy, 152, 176–177
Surveillance, 27
Sutural bones, 335
SVR. *See* Systemic vascular resistance (SVR)
Swiss cheese model, 21, 23f
Sympathetic nervous system, 186
Synthetic colloid solutions, 205–206
Systemic vascular resistance (SVR), 184
Systole, 183
Systolic blood pressure (SBP), 222

T

Tabletop exercises, 443
Tachypnea, 114
Tactical Combat Casualty Care Committee
       (TCCC), 37
Tactical emergency medical support
       (TEMS). *See* Civilian tactical emer-
       gency medical support (TEMS)
Tactical field care, 37, 584–585
Tactical field evacuation, 585
Tactile intubation, 151
Target vehicle, 54
Tarsals, 335f
TBI. *See* Head trauma
TCCC. *See* Tactical Combat Casualty Care
       Committee (TCCC)
Teachable moment, 28
Tear gas, 372
Teasdale, Graham, 8
Temperature balance, 479
Temporal bone, 122f, 219f
Temporal lobe, 220f

Temporalis muscle, 336f
Temporary cavity, 49
TEMS. *See* Civilian tactical emergency
       medical support (TEMS)
Tendon, 335
Tension pneumothorax, 191, 300–302, 385
Tension wave, 454
Terrorism, 440–441. *See also* Explosion
       and weapons of mass destruction
Tertiary blast injuries, 81f, 456, 456f
Tertiary prevention, 21
Thermal energy, 20
Thermal equilibrium, 479
Thermal gradient, 479
Thermal homeostasis, 379
Thermal injuries, 395–396
Thermal trauma, 478–481
Thermite, 458
Thermoregulation, 479–480
Thermoregulatory center, 479
Third death peak, 564
Third-degree burns, 358–359
Third-degree frostbite, 503
Thoracic spine, 335f
Thoracic trauma, 291–316
  anatomy, 292–293
  assessment, 296–297
  blunt cardiac injury, 304–305
  blunt force injury, 296
  cardiac tamponade, 305–306
  children, 394
  circulation, 295
  commotio cordis, 306–307
  diaphragmatic rupture, 309–310
  flail chest, 297–298
  hemothorax, 304
  needle decompression, 302–303,
       314–316
  penetrating injury, 295–296
  physiology, 293–295
  pneumothorax, 298–302
  prolonged transport, 310–311
  pulmonary contusion, 298
  rib fractures, 297
  specific skills (illustration), 314–316
  tracheobronchial disruption, 307–309
  transport, 310–311
  traumatic aortic disruption, 307
  traumatic asphyxia, 309, 310f
  tube thoracostomy, 303
  ventilation, 293–295
Thoracic vertebrae, 249
3-3-2 rule, 146f
Thyroid gland, 123f
Tibia, 335f
Tibialis anterior muscle, 336f
Tidal volume (V$_T$), 137, 295f
Tissue densities, 48
TLC. *See* Total lung capacity (TLC)
Tongue, 123f, 136f
Tongue blade insertion method, 161
Tongue jaw lift insertion method, 160
Tonsil, 136f
Tonsillar herniation, 224
Tooth squeeze, 534

Topical hemostatic agents, 201
Total lung capacity (TLC), 295f
Tourniquet, 115
   shock, 199–201
   specific skills (Israeli trauma bandage),
     215–26
Tow device, 529f
Toxemia of pregnancy, 329
Toxidrome, 460
Toxin-induced/lung injury, 368
Trachea, 123f, 134, 135f, 136f, 293f
Tracheal deviation, 301f
Tracheal or bronchial rupture, 309f
Tracheobronchial disruption, 307–309
Traction splints, 343f, 344
Traffic delineation devices, 91f
Traffic safety, 89
Transport, 125
   burns, 360
   disaster management, 440
   duration of, 126
   environmental trauma, 514–515,
     555–556
   explosions/WMDs, 458, 460, 472
   geriatric trauma, 418–419
   golden principles, 427–428
   head trauma, 238–239
   musculoskeletal trauma, 352
   pediatric trauma, 392, 398–399
   primary survey, 118
   prolonged. *See* Prolonged transport
   shock, 203, 207–210
   spinal trauma, 264
   thoracic trauma, 310–311
Transverse process, 247, 248f
Transversus abdominis muscle, 336f
Trapezius muscle, 336f
Trauma
   abdominal. *See* Abdominal trauma
   blunt. *See* Blunt trauma
   cause of death, as, 2
   cost of care, 2
   environmental. *See* Environmental trauma
   event phase, 4–5
   geriatric. *See* Geriatric trauma
   golden hour, 5
   head. *See* Head trauma
   kinematics. *See* Kinematics of trauma
   musculoskeletal. *See* Musculoskeletal
     trauma
   pediatric. *See* Pediatric trauma
   penetrating. *See* Penetrating trauma
   phases, 45
   postevent phase, 5–6
   pre-event phase, 3–4
   preparation, 4
   spine. *See* Spinal trauma
   thermal, 478–481
   thoracic. *See* Thoracic trauma
Trauma chin lift, 141, 141f, 159
Trauma jaw thrust, 141, 141f, 158
Trauma response algorithm, 429f
Trauma Score (TS), 125
Traumatic aortic disruption, 307
Traumatic asphyxia, 309, 310f

Traumatic brain injury (TBI). *See* Head
   trauma
Traumatic cardiopulmonary arrest, 128–129
Traumatic rhabdomyolysis, 350f
Traumatic subarachnoid hemorrhage
   (tSAH), 235
Treatment area, 441
Trench foot, 501
Triage
   disaster management, 438–439
   explosions and WMD, 450–452
   field triage scheme, 126
   scene, 101–107
Triage and initial stabilization, 434
Triage Decision Scheme, 126
Triage officer, 438
Triage tag, 104f
Triceps brachii muscle, 336f
Trigeminal nerve, 221f
Trochlear nerve, 221f
Trunkey, Donald, 5, 8
TS. *See* Trauma Score (TS)
tSAH. *See* Traumatic subarachnoid hemor-
   rhage (tSAH)
Tube thoracostomy, 303
Tumble, 70–71
Turbinates, 123f, 136f
Two-provider method (bag-mask ventila-
   tion), 165
2-PAM chloride, 461
Tympanic membrane rupture, 80
Type I DCS, 538, 538f, 539
Type II DCS, 538, 538f, 539

U

Ulna, 335f
Ulnar artery, 184f
Ulnar nerve, 251f
Ultraviolet light, 569
Umbilicus level, 251
Uncal herniation, 224
Uncontrolled release of energy, 20
Undertriage, 126
Unequal pupils, 124f
Unified command system, 100
Unintentional injuries, 22–23
Up-and-over path, 52–53
Upper airway, 134
Upper respiratory tract, 135f
Uvula, 136f

V

V_E. *See* Minute ventilation (V_E)
V_T. *See* Tidal volume (V_T)
Vacuum splint, 343f
Vagus nerve, 221f
Valium, 461
Valvular disruption, 190–191
Vapor, 459
Varicella, 466, 467f
Variola major, 466
Variola minor, 466
Vascular access, 203–204, 213–214,
   391–392
Vasogenic shock, 189

Vasovagal shock, 190
Vastus lateralis muscle, 336f
Vastus medialis muscle, 336f
Vecuronium, 150f
Vehicle incompatibility, 58–59
Vehicle positioning and warning devices,
   90–91
Venous bleeding, 114
Ventilation, 137, 293. *See also* Airway and
   ventilation; Breathing
Ventilatory devices, 152–154
Ventilatory rate
   airway management, 113f
   levels, 113–114
   pediatric patients, 384f
   shock, 196
Ventricular fibrillation/pulseless ventricu-
   lar tachycardia, 129
Vermiform appendix, 319f
Versed, 150f, 462
Vertebrae, 247
Vertebral column, 247–249
Vertebral foramen, 247
Vertical shear fractures, 344
Very high altitude, 550
Vesicant agents, 462–463
Vesicants, 372
Vestibular folds, 134
Vestibulocochlear nerve, 221f
Veterinary support, 581
Violent scene, 91–92
Viral hepatitis, 92–93
Visceral pleura, 293, 293f
Visualized orotracheal intubation, 172–173
Vital signs. *See also* individual component
   parts
   pediatric trauma, 388f
   secondary survey, 119–121
   shock, 195–196
Vocal cord, 136f
Volatility, 459
Volume resuscitation, 205–207, 208f
Voluntary dehydration, 482
Voluntary guarding, 324

W

Wadding, 77
Warm zone, 96, 97, 98f, 372, 449f, 450, 584
Warren, John Collins, 180
Water density, 48
Water intoxication, 484f, 487–489
Water moccasin (cottonmouth) snake, 574f
WBGT index. *See* Wet-bulb globe tempera-
   ture (WBGT) index
Weapon of mass destruction (WMD), 97,
   440–441. *See also* Explosion and
   weapons of mass destruction
Weather/light conditions, 89
Wet-bulb globe temperature (WBGT) index,
   492–493
White phosphorus (WP), 372, 458
Whole-body exposure, 470
Wilderness trauma care, 561–577
   backboard use, 568–569
   backcountry medical arrest, 572

Wilderness trauma care *(Continued)*
  bee sting, 572–573
  cervical spine, 565–566
  closing backcountry wounds, 571
  dislocation, 571
  elimination needs, 567
  food and water needs, 567–568
  hemostasis, 570
  improvised evacuations, 566–567
  injury patterns, 564
  prevention of injury, 570–571
  safety, 564–565

Wilderness trauma care *(Continued)*
  snakebite, 573–575
  sun protection, 569
  wound management, 569
Wind chill index, 513f
WMD. *See* Explosion and weapons of mass destruction; Weapon of mass destruction (WMD)
Work of breathing, 295f
Worker injury, 19, 29
Worker stress, 442–443
Worldwide injury-related statistics, 17

Wound botulism, 468
WP. *See* White phosphorus (WP)

Y
Years of potential life lost (YPLL), 18

Z
Zone of coagulation, 357, 357f
Zone of hyperemia, 357, 357f
Zone of stasis, 357, 357f
Zygomatic bone, 122f
Zygomaticus muscle, 336f